PRINCIPLES OF CLINICAL IMMUNOHEMATOLOGY

Principles of Clinical Immunohematology

Paul Weisz-Carrington, M.D.
Chief, Laboratory Services
Veterans Administration Medical Center
Shreveport, Louisiana

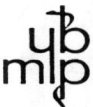

YEAR BOOK MEDICAL PUBLISHERS, INC.
Chicago • London

Copyright © 1986 by Year Book Medical Publishers, Inc. All rights reserved. No part of this publication may be reproduced, stored in a retrieval system, or transmitted, in any form or by any means, electronic, mechanical, photocopying, recording, or otherwise, without prior written permission from the publisher. Printed in the United States of America.

0 9 8 7 6 5 4 3 2 1

Library of Congress Cataloging-in-Publication Data

Weisz-Carrington, Paul.
  Principles of clinical immunohematology.

  Includes bibliographies and index.
  1. Immunohematology. 2. Compatibility testing
(Hematology) 3. Blood banks. I. Title. [DNLM:
1. Blood Banks. 2. Blood Groups—immunology.
3. Blood Transfusion. 4. Immunity. WB 356 W433p]
RB45.W4 1986   615'.65   85-20297
ISBN 0-8151-9199-5

Sponsoring Editor: Daniel J. Doody
Manager, Copyediting Services: Frances M. Perveiler
Production Project Manager: Etta Worthington
Proofroom Supervisor: Shirley E. Taylor

**To my wife Wendy,
and
my sons, Alexander and David**

A scientific concept should be explained as simply as possible, but no simpler.

Albert Einstein

Foreword

The vital role of blood in the maintenance of health has been recognized since antiquity. Goethe expressed this most eloquently in Faust, proclaiming "Blut ist ein ganz besonderer Saft." In addition to sustaining life it also carries out some kind of mysterious function in warding off disease and "evil." Individual variability to resist disease requires understanding and explanation. It was, therefore, not only blamed on the wish of the gods as a reward for good behavior but it was also directly ascribed to the vital vapors, such as blood. The great breakthrough came with Jenner's vaccination, employing the live virus of cowpox that all but eradicated the fear of the deadly smallpox by elimination of the disease. As these immunologic principles became better understood many other infections were prevented, not least of which is polyomyelitus. To this day there is great hope that a prevention of new and deadly diseases such as AIDS can yet be developed.

As host resistance became understood as the body's ability to distinguish "foreign" or "nonself" from "self," individual susceptibility to infection was no longer a mystery requiring metaphysical explanation. It was recognized that this process could break down because the body, like an old man who doesn't recognize his children, would confuse "self" with "nonself." This led Paul Ehrlich to also raise the spector of "horror autotoxicus," thereby laying the foundation for the understanding of autoimmune disease.

With the understanding of these basic principles transfusion of homologous blood components became a reality and not only saved lives in replacement of acute losses but opened new horizons to aggressive surgery and cytotoxic chemotherapy or radiation therapy. By application of essentially the same mechanism to tissue immunity, organ and bone marrow transplantation have now begun to find practical application.

Hemolytic disease of the newborn, dreaded by Rh negative mothers, can now be prevented by relatively simple application of immunohematologic principles.

Paternity and forensic identification are established with ever increasing certainty.

Principles of Clinical Immunohematology, by Dr. Paul Weisz-Carrington, represents a comprehensive text covering the clinical application of immunologic principles to hematology. It is neither a procedural or technical manual to manage a blood bank, nor is it a treatise on when or how to transfuse. Rather, immunologic concepts as they apply to the pathophysiology of blood and bone marrow diseases are portrayed as currently understood, leading to logical conclusions for appropriate therapy and case management. The experienced reader, the student, and the novice will not have to memorize endless facts; instead, the reader will find the learning process simplified by following Dr. Weisz-Carrington's logical reasoning.

Dr. Weisz-Carrington, an experienced hematologist and blood banker, has combined with skill the two related disciplines and provides a sound basis for the clinic. This well documented presentation constitutes a basic guide for further in-depth study or research.

Klaus Mayer, M.D.
Professor of Clinical Medicine
Memorial Sloan-Kettering Cancer Center
New York, New York

Preface

In today's practice of medicine, blood and blood component transfusions play a critical role in therapy. Without the availability of blood for transfusion, a variety of surgical procedures would not be feasible. Furthermore, blood and blood component transfusions are crucial for treating many nonsurgical patients.

The field of immunohematology has become increasingly complex as more information on the immunobiology and physiology of blood transfusion becomes available. The purpose of *Principles of Clinical Immunohematology* is to provide clinicians with a single up-to-date source of information, which encompasses the basic and clinical sciences comprising the field of immunohematology. The book first presents information dealing with basic sciences such as immunology and hematology, providing the foundations of immunohematology, and then presents more clinical chapters that are built on these foundations. The basic science chapters are intended to complement and perhaps explain some of the pathology described in the clinical chapters and to provide the scientific elements for rational transfusion therapy. Because of space limitations it was impossible to furnish an all-encompassing view of immunology or hematology. Therefore, the goal in preparing the basic science chapters was to present information relevant to the clinical practice of blood transfusion. An attempt has been made to present the basic science information as clearly as possible, but to preserve the necessary depth to retain the physician's interest. Since this work was written with a predominantly clinical audience in mind and its content geared to provide clinical information rather than detailed information on laboratory technique, readers are advised to consult the more technical blood banking texts if more detailed information is needed.

Following the basic science chapters are the clinically relevant chapters. These chapters include topics such as hepatitis and AIDS, two areas of high relevance to contemporary transfusion therapy. Much work in these areas is currently being conducted, making some of the data available at the time of writing this manuscript obsolete.

To conclude the book, information on quality assurance and transfusion practices is presented. This material is addressed mainly to physicians-in-training who are to become directors of blood banks.

It is my hope that nonphysicians will also find this book useful as a source of information on immunohematology. A concerted effort has been made to shy away from superfluous material, yet still provide a detailed, current bibliography to be used as a reference tool.

Nothing in my blood banking career has taught me as much about blood banking than preparing this text, and nothing would give me more pleasure than to know that the reader has learned from it as much as I did in writing it.

PAUL WEISZ-CARRINGTON, M.D.

Acknowledgments

When an exceptional genius such as Isaac Newton can attribute his discoveries to having climbed on the shoulders of giants, it behooves us, the less endowed, to acknowledge more so that we have also been inspired not only by the founders of the disciplines in which we have chosen to specialize, but also by those who were directly instrumental in encouraging and helping us to achieve some expertise in these fields. A page of acknowledgments places limitations on the number of individuals that can be directly named as having helped me complete this work, so I wish to apologize if I have failed to do so, but their names remain unmentioned due to the lack of space and not due to a lack of deep appreciation for their help.

I wish to thank Dr. Michael E. Lamm for introducing me to the field of immunology and for helping me acquire expertise in the experimental and theoretical aspects of this science. I also wish to thank Dr. Harold S. Kaplan for teaching me the foundations of blood banking and steering me into this very fascinating field that I have since adopted as a career. My debt to the staff of the N.Y.U. Blood Bank must also be mentioned here. Through their patience, I was able to learn practical blood banking. In addition, the staff of the Veterans Administration Laboratory at the Manhattan VA, and the laboratory and professional staff at the Shreveport VA have been a constant source of experience and help in my professional growth. I would like to acknowledge the help granted to me by many friends in the field of immunology, such as Dr. Vittorio Deffendi, Dr. Joel Oppenheim, Dr. Celso Bianco, Dr. Victor Nussensweig, Dr. Jeannette Thorbecke, Dr. Steven Emancipator, and Dr. Julia-Phillips Quagliata. I would also like to acknowledge those friends who have helped me in the field of blood banking: Dr. Klaus Mayer, Dr. Leonard Boral, Dr. Malcolm Levine, Dr. Robert Silbor, Dr. Edward Amorosi, Mr. Lawrie Marsh, Mr. Malcolm Beck, Ms. Kay Beattie, Ms. Katherine College, Mrs. Laura Wedeck, Mr. Peter Issit, Mr. George Garraty, Dr. Kris Murawski, Dr. Theodore Robertson, Dr. Shelley Brown, Dr. Johanna Pendyck, Dr. V. J. Malavade, Dr. Pablo Rubinstein, Dr. Ray Bryant, Dr. Parvis Lalezari, Dr. Fred Gorstein as well as many others too numerous to mention here. I would like to acknowledge my wife's patient and expert help in typing the first draft of this book. The final manuscript could not have been completed without the expert typing skills of my secretary, Ms. Elaine Botelho. I owe special thanks to the editorial staff at Year Book Medical Publishers: Mr. Daniel Doody for helping me prepare this book, Ms. Fran Perveiler, Manager of Copyediting Services, and Ms. Etta Worthington, Project Manager, all of whom, in addition to being very patient with me, have made excellent suggestions to improve the quality of the final product.

PAUL WEISZ-CARRINGTON, M.D.

Contents

Foreword vii
Preface ix

1 / A Historical Outline of Immunohematology 1

2 / Introduction to Hematology 5
    Blood as a Tissue: Normal Aspects 5
    Hematologic Values in Different Age Populations 6
    Red Blood Cells 6
    White Blood Cells. 17
    Neoplastic Disorders of Hematopoietic Cells: The Leukemias . . 29
    Pathology of Lymph Nodes 43

3 / Hemostasis and Thrombosis 71
    Structural Integrity of the Vessel Walls 71
    Role of Platelets in Hemostasis. 73
    Coagulation: The Soluble Phase of Hemostasis. 78

4 / Immunology 102
    Humoral Immunity 102
    The Complement System 113
    Cellular Immunity. 123
    Pathology of the Immune Response 129
    Autoimmunity 131
    Immediate and Delayed Hypersensitivity 132

5 / Blood Group Antigens 145
    Antigens That Usually Elicit Cold Antibodies 146
    The Warm-Reacting Antibodies 163
    High-Frequency Antigens 181
    Antigens of Low Incidence 182
    Polyagglutination 183

6 / Laboratory Aspects of Blood Banking 201
    Antigen-Antibody Testing in the Immunohematology Laboratory . 201
    The Coombs Test 202
    Antibody Detection and Identification 204
    The Crossmatch. 211
    RBC Antibodies 214
    Incompatibility In Vivo 215

7 / The HLA System **218**
Nomenclature of the HLA System 218
Biochemistry of the HLA Molecular Complex 219
Genetics of the HLA System 221
Immunobiology of the HLA System 223
Laboratory Identification of the HLA Antigens 224
HLA and Transplantation 225
HLA Typing in Platelet Transfusion Therapy 227
HLA Matching for Granulocyte Transfusions 228
HLA in Paternity Testing 228
HLA and Disease 228

8 / Components and Fractions **236**
Donor Selection 236
The Donation 238
Preparation, Storage and Use of Components 240
Fresh Frozen Plasma 245
Cryoprecipitate 246
Platelets 248
Granulocytes 253
Plasma Fractions 257
Bone Marrow Transplantation 264

9 / Apheresis Techniques and Autotransfusion **281**
Donor Apheresis 281
Therapeutic Apheresis 288
Management Techniques for an Apheresis Program 293
Autologous Transfusion 294

10 / Immune Hemolysis **303**
Autoimmune Hemolytic Anemia 303
Drug-Induced Immune Hemolysis 313

11 / Transfusion Reactions **325**
Hemolytic Transfusion Reactions 325
Immune Mediated Nonhemolytic Transfusion Reactions ... 333
Transfusion Reactions Caused by Plasma Protein Sensitivity ... 335
Non-Immune-Mediated, Nonhemolytic Transfusion Reactions to Blood ... 338
Infections Transmitted by Blood and Blood Component Transfusion ... 341
Incompatible IV Fluids 344
Other Complications of Transfusion 345
Reportable Cases in the United States 345

12 / Hepatitis ... 355
- Viral Hepatitis Type A ... 355
- Viral Hepatitis Type B ... 355
- NANB Hepatitis ... 367
- Concepts of Hepatitis Directly Related to Blood Banking ... 369

13 / Acquired Immunodeficiency Syndrome ... 377
- Epidemiology ... 377
- Analysis of Risk Factors ... 377
- Incidence and Etiology of AIDS ... 380
- Pathogenesis and Pathology ... 383
- Histopathology of Tissues From AIDS Patients ... 384
- Clinical Presentation of Patients With AIDS ... 385
- Other Complications Found in AIDS ... 386
- Laboratory Findings ... 386
- Treatment of Patients With AIDS ... 388
- Prevention ... 388
- AIDS in Reference to Blood Banking ... 389
- AIDS in Reference to Hepatitis B Vaccine ... 390
- Future Developments ... 391

14 / Concepts of Medical Genetics Useful in Immunohematology ... 397
- Basic Concepts of Genetics ... 397
- The Molecular Basis of Genetic Information ... 399
- Mendelian Genetics ... 403

15 / Paternity Testing and Forensic Immunohematology ... 409
- Identification, Testing, and Reporting ... 409
- Use of RBC Antigen Testing, RBC Enzymes, and Plasma Proteins in Criminology ... 417

16 / Perinatal Blood Banking ... 420
- Prenatal Immunohematology ... 420
- Management of Extrauterine Problems Caused by EF ... 430
- Special Aspects of Transfusion in Pediatric Practice ... 434
- Pediatric Diseases Needing Blood Banking Consultation ... 434
- Blood Transfusion in the Neonatal Period ... 435
- Other Diseases of the Newborn Requiring Components ... 436

17 / Quality Control and Legal Aspects of Immunohematology ... 444
- Quality Control in the Blood Bank ... 445
- Supplies ... 447
- Quality Control of Blood Component Preparation ... 449
- RPR and VDRL Testing of Donor Samples ... 451
- Quality Control of Forms and Record-Keeping ... 451

Inventory Control 452
Legal Aspects of Blood Banking 452
Legal Matters Affecting Blood Bank Management 454
Suggestions Regarding Legal Actions Against the Blood Bank 454
Blood Banking Organizations 455
Antitrust Laws Regarding Blood Banking 456

18 / Transfusion Practices **459**
External Regulatory Bodies 459
Internal Regulatory Bodies 459
Good Practices in the Use of Blood and Blood Components 460
The Transfusion of Blood 461
Special Problems in Transfusion Practice 466
Blood Bank Readiness Plan 469
Transfusion Practices in Open Heart Surgery Replacement Therapy 471
Blood Components in Patients With Cancer 474
Other Diseases in Which Special Transfusion Practices Are Recommended . . . 476
Plateletpheresis and Cytapheresis Practices 477

Index **697**

1

A Historical Outline of Immunohematology

THE THERAPEUTIC VALUE of blood was suspected for centuries before its specific biologic actions and effects were known. Transfusion technology as we know it today is the result of trials throughout the history of mankind to conquer disease.

The first transfusions were really blood drafts. Accounts of blood drafting can be found in ancient Roman chronicles. According to Celsus, Romans in the Coliseum drank the blood of dying gladiators in the belief that it had tonic effects. The first written account of the use of blood drafting as therapy describes the treatment of the ailing Pope Innocent VIII in 1492. The Pope's physicians had prescribed a draft of blood to the sick prelate, and three young healthy donors were sacrificed for their blood. Thus, the first recorded "transfusion" attempt resulted in the death of three donors, and, ironically, the death of the patient as well.[1]

Many religions have included the practice of drinking blood from animals or humans; similar rituals are followed even today by certain tribes and cults. The shedding of blood has always been a symbol of death, and from the beginning of recorded history, many have acknowledged the relationship between blood and the maintenance of life. However, it was not until 1616 that the circulation of blood through vessels was described by Sir William Harvey and blood circulation was approached scientifically.

We owe to Sir Christopher Wren the successful cannulation of veins. In experiments on dogs (around 1657) Wren introduced solutions into veins, using a primitive syringe. These experiments opened the door to intravenous transfusion therapy. However, the use of substances in solution injected intravenously was first attempted by Sir Robert Boyle in 1666, who used prisoners as subjects for his experiments.[2]

The actual transfusion of blood as a medication had to await the experiments of Richard Lower[3] and Jean Denys. Denys, a professor of philosophy and mathematics in France, successfully transfused blood from animals to some of his patients and in 1667 was the first to describe a transfusion reaction.[4] Many of these experiments were fatal to the patients. Consequently Denys was tried, his experiments were discontinued, and he was forced to leave the medical profession.

Nearly 150 years were to elapse before new experiments emerged in the field of transfusion. Although transfusion of blood from one human to another had been advocated as early as 1615 by Andreas Libavius,[5] it was not until 1818 that a British obstetrician, James Blundell, successfully performed the first human-to-human blood transfusion.[6] His experiments with animals led to the observations that animal blood was dangerous for transfusion to humans and that only human blood should be used for transfusion to patients. Only 4 of the 20 transfusions he performed were successful.

One of the main problems encountered in early transfusions was the tendency of blood to clot before it reached the recipient. This problem was not resolved until A. Hustin, L. Agote, and R. Lewishon discovered the use of sodium citrate as a blood anticoagulant. Each in a different country and approximately in the same year (1914–1915) reported results on safe anticoagulation with citrate for transfusion.[7]

Following the reports of Blundell, and throughout the Franco-German War, many transfusion reactions were reported, with a significant mortality. The cause of these reactions was unknown. It was Landsteiner (Fig 1–1) who, in 1901, discovered that donor blood could be agglutinated by serum from some patients but not from others. This led to the discovery of the ABO system. For this work, Landsteiner was granted the Nobel Prize in medicine and has since been considered the father of immunohematology.[8] The somewhat artificial separation of the fields of immunology and immunohematology was thus bridged by these kinds of scientific achievements.

It is appropriate to review here some of the historical developments in immunology. The term "immunization" was conceived under the general concept that the process was in essence a protective one. In 1796 Jenner observed that introduction of a relatively benign infection of cowpox could protect individuals against smallpox. This technique was inspired by the Chinese practice of using dermal scales from smallpox patients in remission for immunization. The term vaccination originates in the Latin word *vacca*, which means cow, recalling Jenner's discovery, and vaccination is used for most types of active immunization. In 1881 Pasteur (Fig 1–2) extended Jenner's work by active immunization against anthrax, and shortly thereafter Elie Metchnikoff proposed the founding ideas for what is now known as cellular immunity. These ideas were based on experiments conducted at the Pasteur Institute in 1887.[9] Equally important (although at that time, seemingly contradictory) concepts of humoral immunity were proposed by Pfeiffer and Bordet. Interestingly, Bordet did most of his research on the humoral theory of immunity in Metchnikoff's laboratory.[10]

The early chemical analysis of immunologic phenomena was set forth by Ehrlich (Fig 1–3).[11] Ehrlich proposed that antigens and antibodies react in a "key-lock" fashion, thus establishing the first model of antigen-antibody reactions. The term isoagglutinin, so frequently used in blood banking, was coined by Bordet, who observed that red blood cells (RBCs) from one species injected into another species agglutinated, whereas RBCs in same-species injections generally did not. These experiments afforded preliminary insight into the causes of some complications encountered by early transfusionists, namely, hemolytic reactions. These concepts were the basis for Landsteiner's blood group theories and

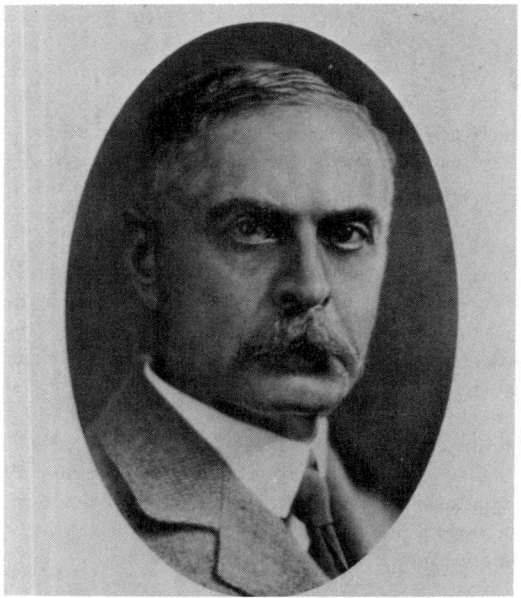

FIG 1–1.—Karl Landsteiner, discoverer of the ABO system.

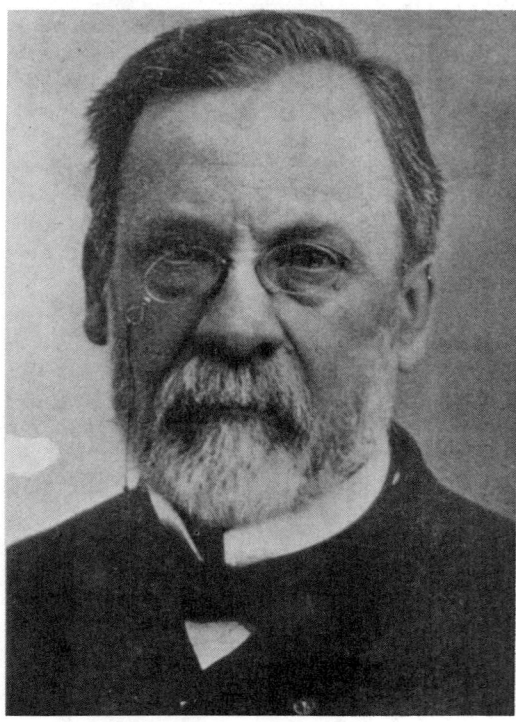

FIG 1–2.—Louis Pasteur: responsible for major developments in active immunization.

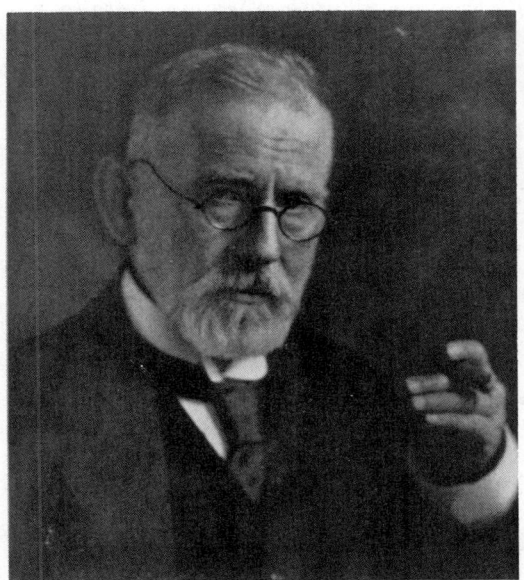

FIG 1–3.—Paul Erhlich: discovered the bivalence of antibodies.

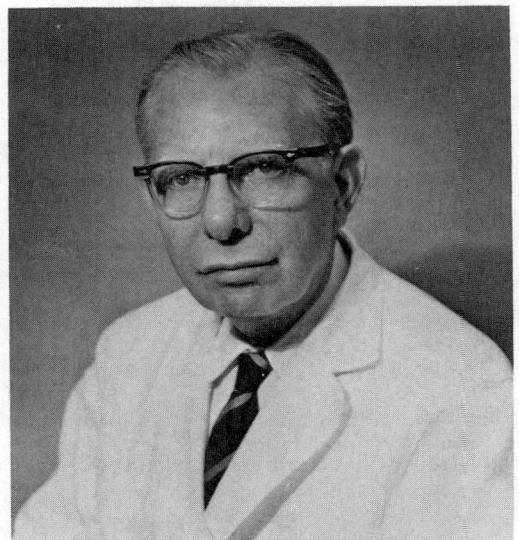

FIG 1–4.—Alexander Wiener, co-discoverer of the Rh system.

ultimately for the discovery of human RBC antigen groups. The next major breakthrough in the young science of immunohematology was the discovery of the Rh system and its relation to hemolytic disease of the newborn. In 1939 Levine and Stetson first reported hemolytic disease of the newborn and suggested it was caused by a serum factor capable of crossing the placenta and coating fetal cells.[12] In 1940 Landsteiner and his pupil Alexander Wiener (Fig 1–4) independently reported an agglutinin which reacted with most human RBCs but not all cells.[13] This agglutinin was obtained after immunizing guinea pigs with Rhesus monkey cells. The antibodies produced reacted with a common antigenic determinant, the Rh antigen.

Many RBC antigens and their respective antibodies have since been described and many phenomena explained. For example, the mathematician Bernstein discovered the co-dominant character of the ABO inheritance patterns.[14] The chemical analysis of the ABO substances has been developed principally on the basis of investigations undertaken by Kabat in 1948.[15] Initial research on the histocompatibility antigens and leukoagglutinins was performed by Dausset in 1952[16] and by Rapaport in 1958.[17] Among the more remarkable discoveries of modern immunology has been elucidation of the structure of the antibody molecule, reported by the Nobel laureates Porter and Edelman in 1959.[8, 19] Recent discoveries such as the finding of a correlation between the immune response and the major histocompatibility complex by Benacerraf in the early 1970s must also be mentioned here.[20]

The development of monoclonal antibodies by hybridoma technology has revolutionized the science of immunology and immunohematology. This technique was develped by Milstein in the early 1970s.[21]

Recently, through the development of gene splicing and DNA hybridization, Tonegawa[22] and Leder et al.[23] have defined how antibody diversity is produced.

It is now evident that the fields of immunology and immunohematology deal with extremely complex biologic phenomena, phenomena probably not suspected by investigators in the early years of these disciplines.

REFERENCES

1. Mathew A.H.: *The Life and Times of Rodrigo Borgia.* London, Stanley Paul and Co., Ltd., 1912.

2. Zmijewsky C.M.: *Immunohematology,* ed. 1. New York, Appleton-Century-Crofts, 1968, pp. 1–17.

3. Pepys S.: *Diary*. London, Wheatley, 1966.
4. Denys J.: *Philos. Trans.* 2:489, 1667.
5. Libavius A.: *Appendix Necessarius Syntagmatus Ancanorum Chymicorum Contra Henningum Sheunemannum.* Frankfort, 1615, vol. 4, p. 8.
6. Blundell J.: Successful case of transfusion. *Lancet* 1:431, 1829.
7. Agote L.: Nuevo procedimiento para la transfusión de sangre. *Ann. Inst. Clin. Med. (Buenos Aires),* 1915, p. 1.
8. Landsteiner K.: Über Agglutinationserscheinungen normalen menschlichen Blutes. *Klin. Wochenschr.* 14:1132, 1901.
9. Metchnikoff E.: *Traité de l'Immunité dans les Maladies Infectieuses,* ed. 2. Masson, Paris, 1937.
10. Bordet J.: *Traité de l'Immunité dans les Maladies Infectieuses,* ed. 2, 1937.
11. Ehrlich P.: *Gesammelte Arbeiten zur Immunitätsforschung.* Berlin, Hilshwald, 1904.
12. Levine P., Stetson R.E.: An unusual case of intragroup agglutination. *JAMA* 113:6, 1939.
13. Landsteiner K., Wiener A.S.: An agglutinable factor in human blood recognized by immune sera for rhesus blood. *Proc. Soc. Exp. Biol. NY* 43:223, 1940.
14. Bernstein F.: Ergebnisse einer biostatischen zusammenfassenden Betrachtungen über die erblichen Blutstrukturen des Menschen. *Klin. Wochenschr.* 3:1495, 1924.
15. Kabat E.A.: *Blood Group Substances: Their Chemistry and Immunochemistry.* New York, Academic Press, 1956.
16. Dausset J., Nenna A.: Présence d'une leuko-agglutine dans le sérum d'un cas d'aggranulocytose chronique. *Compt. Rend. Soc. Biol.* 146:1539, 1952.
17. Rapaport F.T., Dausset J. (ed.): *Human Transplantation.* New York, Grune & Stratton, 1968.
18. Porter R.R.: Structural studies of immunoglobulins. *Science* 180:713, 1973.
19. Edelman G.M., Galey J.A.: A model for the 7S antibody molecule. *Proc. Natl. Acad. Sci. USA* 51:846, 1964.
20. Benacerraf B., McDevitt H.O.: The histocompatibility-linked immune response genes. *Science* 175:273, 1972.
21. Köhler G., Milstein C.: Continuous cultures of fused cells secreting antibody of predefined specificity. *Nature* 256:495, 1975.
22. Tonegawa S.: Somatic recombination and mosaic structure of immunoglobulin genes. *Harvey Lect.* 75:61, 1981.
23. Leder P., et al.: The organization and diversity of immunoglobulin genes. *Proc. Natl. Acad. Sci. USA* 71:5109, 1974.

2

Introduction to Hematology

PHYSICIANS in charge of blood banks are often required to manage patients with hematologic diseases, because most hospital-based blood banks handle such cases in outpatient transfusion services. Patients with leukemia, lymphoma, and multiple myeloma, to mention a few of the hematologic diseases, are treated with blood and components in the outpatient transfusion service. It is necessary to have a general knowledge of hematology as well as of the laboratory evaluation of these hematologic diseases. Following is a review of the hematologic principles of interest in blood banking.

BLOOD AS A TISSUE: NORMAL ASPECTS

Blood is a fluid tissue composed of formed elements and a suspending medium, the plasma. The formed elements, mostly erythrocytes, constitute the packed cell volume, which can be expressed as the volume percent of red blood cells (RBCs) in a sample of whole blood. This in essence is the hematocrit. The hematocrit can be calculated in most donor rooms by filling a 7-cm heparinized capillary tube with venous blood and centrifuging at 5,000–10,000 rpm for 5–10 minutes. Males usually have values of 47% ± 7%, and females 42% ± 5%. A normal RBC count for men is 4.5–6.2 million/ml, and for women 4–5.5 million/ml.[1] Cell counts can be corroborated by electronic counting. In anemia, objective quantitative studies must be performed.

The several parameters introduced by Wintrobe are calculated as follows:[2]

1. MCV (mean corpuscular volume), the average volume of individual RBCs in cubic micra or microliters:

$$MCV = \frac{Hct (\%) \times 10}{RBC\ count/\mu l}$$

(Normal = 90 ± 8 cu μ)

2. MCH (mean corpuscular hemoglobin), the content in weight of hemoglobin of the average individual RBC, measured in micromicrograms or picograms:

$$MCH = \frac{Hb\ (gm/dl) \times 10}{RBC\ count/in\ millions/\mu l}$$

(Normal = 30 ± 3 pg)

3. MCHC (mean corpuscular hemoglobin concentration), the average hemoglobin concentration per 100 ml of packed RBC, given as a percentage:

$$MCHC = \frac{Hb\ (gm/dl) \times 100}{Hct\ (per\ unit)}$$

(Normal = 33 ± 2 gm/100 ml)

where Hb = hemoglobin and Hct = hematocrit. These values are very useful in assessing the type of anemia present. However, accurate determination is essential for them to be of any use in clinical practice.

HEMATOLOGIC VALUES IN DIFFERENT AGE POPULATIONS

Perinatal Hematology

Significant differences exist in the hematologic picture of the newborn as compared to children and adults. The mean hemoglobin level in cord blood is 16.8 gm/dl but values may vary between 14 and 20 gm/dl, depending on events such as intrauterine hypoxia.[3] A venous hemoglobin value less than 14 gm/dl is considered abnormal. Hemoglobin and hematocrit values can be expected to increase within the first several hours after birth, due to a shift of fluid from the intravascular space to the extravascular space.[4] Failure of these parameters to increase should be viewed as abnormal and warrants a hematologic evaluation.

Premature babies will have lower values than full-term babies,[5] but their reticulocyte counts are higher. Reticulocyte counts are high in the newborn, but can be expected to fall to below 1% after 6 days.[6] At birth the newborn's RBCs are macrocytic, but the size will decrease after the first week and reaches normal diameter by the ninth week.

The absolute number of white blood cells (WBCs) increases in the first 24 hours of life and progressively decreases[7] (Table 2-1).

The mean value for total blood volume in the first days of life is 86.3 ml/kg (89.4 ml/kg in prematures[8]) and decreases to a mean of 65 ml/kg at 3-4 months of age.

The oxygen affinity of cord blood is greater than that of maternal blood, because fetal hemoglobin has a lower affinity for 2,3-diphosphoglycerate (2,3-DPG) and adenosine triphosphate (ATP) than does adult hemoglobin.[9] The affinity curve in newborn infants is shifted to the left when compared to adult hemoglobin; this shift is more pronounced in prematures. Platelet counts in newborns are usually lower (223,000/μl) than in older children, and are not significantly different in premature from term infants.[10]

Prothrombin and factors V, VII, IX, X, XI, and XII are all lower in the newborn compared to maternal levels.[11]

Hematologic Values in the Elderly

Marrow stem cells have a limited proliferative capability, as has been shown in mice,[12] and the proliferative capacity progressively decreases with age. This concept becomes important as our elderly population increases. It is therefore relevant to review some hematologic values in the elderly.

Hemoglobin levels in men aged 60 years or older vary from 15 to 12.5 gm/dl[13] and may decrease further in the very old (96-106 years of age).[14] The WBC count may be normal in adults over 70, but increments during infection may be significantly lower than in young adults.[15] These changes can be correlated with a progressive decrease in bone marrow cellularity from 50% to 30% after age 65.[16]

The immune system becomes less effective with advancing age.[17, 18] Impaired functions are more noticeable in the T cell branch of the immune system, where T cells from aged individuals fail to undergo activation on exposure to antigens.[19] T cells from elderly individuals likewise fail to produce T cell growth factor after stimulation with phytohemagglutinin.[18] These and other changes make aging individuals increasingly susceptible to infections.[20]

RED BLOOD CELLS

Morphology and Physiology

RBCs are biconcave disks varying in diameter from 7.2 to 7.9 μ. The erythrocyte membrane is composed of a lipid bilayer formed by an orderly

TABLE 2-1.—Hematologic Values in Newborns and Infants*

AGE	HEMATOCRIT† (%)	HEMOGLOBIN† (gm/dl)	RETICULOCYTES† (%)	WBC‡ (per cu mm)
24 hr	61 ± 7	19 ± 2	3.2 ± 1	18,000
1 wk	54 ± 8	18 ± 2.5	0.5 ± 0.3	12,000
4 wk	36 ± 5	13 ± 1	1 ± 1	11,500

*Table modified from Schwartz and Gill.[6]
†Values are means ± 1 SD.
‡Values are means.

arrangement of phospholipids.[21] The polar ends of the molecules are oriented away from the middle layer and the nonpolar ends face each other toward the middle layer. Interspersed and embedded in the bilayer are proteins[22] and other complex molecules (Fig 2–1). Much of the exposed portion of these molecules is antigenic[23] and induces antibody formation if exposed to the appropriate host. The antigenic molecules are of major clinical and biologic interest to immunohematologists.

Erythrocytes are anucleate and do not contain mitochondria.[24] They are, however, capable of metabolic activity mediated by a variety of enzymes. The energy necessary for membrane integrity is obtained through glycolysis, mostly through the Embden-Meyerhof pathway, which provides ATP molecules for such needs.[25] Erythrocytes are mainly involved in the transport and delivery of oxygen to the tissues, but they also participate in maintaining the acid-base equilibrium of the blood. Hemoglobin is the key molecule in erythrocytes responsible for oxygen transport and delivery. It accounts for 90% of the erythrocyte dry mass.[26]

Hemoglobin is a 68,000-dalton protein composed of a heme portion and a globulin portion.[27] The heme portion is a prosthetic group composed of a porphyrin with four linked pyrrol groups and an iron molecule in the center.[27] The globin portion is a complex of two pairs of polypeptide chains, each pair termed α and β in adult hemoglobin. Each chain has an attached heme group. Deficiencies in sequence and structure of the globin portion result in various types of hemoglobins that can be characterized by their electrophoretic mobility. These characteristics may be inherited and constitute phenotypic markers. At times certain changes in hemoglobin structure result in disease (e.g., sickle cell anemia, thalassemia). In the developing human organism, fetal hemoglobin (Hb F) is found more abundantly in early stages. It contains two α chains and two δ chains. As soon as the fetus develops, the adult-type hemoglobulin increases in quantity and acquires an $\alpha_2\beta_2$ structure. The normal adult level is not reached until age 6 months. Hb F has a greater affinity for oxygen than does adult hemoglobin (Hb A).[28]

The laboratory method of choice for determining the hemoglobin value is the cyanomethemoglobin method read colorimetrically. However, most blood banks do not use this method for donor screening because instrumentation is usually lacking. A useful screening method is the specific gravity method. It measures the ratio of the weight of a volume of blood to the weight of the same volume of water at a temperature of 4° C in solutions of known specific gravity. Blood drops are observed to see if they sink within 15 seconds. Normal specific gravity values for men are 1.057, and for women, 1.053.[29, 30]

The molecular integrity of hemoglobin determines oxygen delivery to tissues. The hemoglobin molecule is capable of harboring 2,3-DPG. By an alosteric change in the β chains, 2,3-DPG establishes salt bridges. This phenomenon produces a decreased oxygen affinity in the heme groups of hemoglobin. In the presence of oxygen the phenomenon is reversed. Levels of 2,3-DPG in blood determine the shape of oxygen saturation curves of hemoglobin (Fig 2–2).[31] These saturation curves reflect the hemoglobin affinity for oxygen and ultimately its delivery to tissues. Changes in pH affect oxygen delivery as well, through the Bohr effect. These changes and the levels of 2,3-DPG are

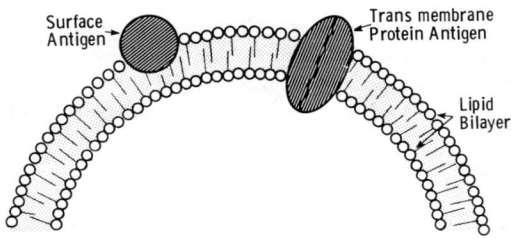

FIG 2–1.—Singer's bilayer model of biologic membranes. Surface antigens are shown exposed on the outer lipid layer. Transmembrane antigens, usually proteins, may have a stabilizing effect on the membrane.

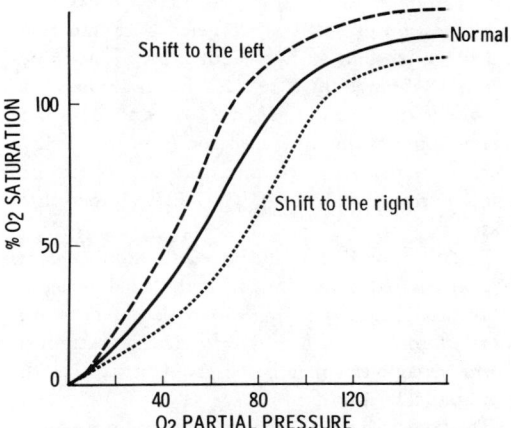

FIG 2–2.—Oxygen saturation curves. With a shift to the left, hemoglobin will bind oxygen more avidly; a shift to the right facilitates release of oxygen by the hemoglobin molecule.

responsible for oxygen binding and pH regulation by the erythrocyte.[32] Variations in 2,3-DPG levels in stored blood are discussed in chapter 8.

Development

Current concepts in RBC differentiation suggest that RBCs originate from a pluripotential stem cell which may give rise not only to RBCs but also to megakaryocytes and granulocytes.[33] A different stem cell is suggested as the origin of lymphocytes.[34] Theoretically, different compartments of stem cells respond to stimulation according to needs.[35] Self-replication of cells usually represents a loss of compartment stem cell numbers, and differentiation subsequently occurs after self-replication. Of these stem cells, a certain number are committed to differentiation in the direction of mature RBCs. Once the cell is committed, it undergoes changes according to the following stages: 1, early (pro and basophilic normoblasts); 2, intermediate; and 3, late development; after which the nucleus is ready for extrusion. A ratio of $1:4:4$ is noted in the general populations of cells in stages 1 to 3.

The morphological characteristics of these cells are fully described in standard hematology texts.[35] However, a short description of the development of the erythrocyte is in order. After the nucleus is lost, the cell becomes a reticulocyte (an RBC with remnants of Golgi apparatus, ribosomes, and mitochondria). A normal reticulocyte count ranges from 0.2% to 2%. The final stage of development is the mature RBC. Overall, these mature RBCs survive 110–120 days.

Maturation of RBCs is triggered by fluctuations in oxygen tension, such as occur in hypoxia. In hypoxia, erythropoietin is released by the kidney and its level returns to normal in 24 hours.[36] This hormone promotes the differentiation from stem cell to mature erythrocyte,[37] promoting the conversion of colony-forming unit cells (CFU-E) to proerythroblasts.[38]

In adults most erythroid precursor stem cells reside in the red bone marrow of the axial skeleton. In the context of bone marrow replacement by tumors, fibrosis, or failure due to aplasia, extramedullary hemopoiesis may be observed, usually in the liver and spleen.

The bone marrow is capable of maintaining a pool of stem cells or can divert cell production to differentiated cells. In the first case, the noncommitted cells are termed α cells. The more differentiated cells are called "n" cells.[39] Colony-forming stem cells (CFU) are cells capable of forming colonies by replication. This has been shown by growing stem cells in semisolid media to which a colony-stimulating factor has been added. The phenomenon is termed colony-stimulating activity (CSA). Colony-stimulating factors may be obtained from feeder cells (leukocytes are a good example). These products can be fractionated on columns which separate substances on the basis of molecular weight, and divided into CSA I, II, III, and IV, in order of decreasing molecular weight. Myeloid colonies in culture are termed CFU-C, whereas spleen colonies in extramedullary hematopoiesis are called CFU-S. CFU-E are colonies committed to RBC formation.[40] Once the cell is committed to differentiate into an erythroid line, the commitment is irreversible.[41] As outlined above, erythroid maturation is promoted by erythropoietin. This phenomenon can be demonstrated in vitro by culturing stem cells in semisolid medium with erythropoietin.[42]

Pathology

RBC pathology usually results in anemia of one sort or another. Anemia is reflected in a variety of symptoms, mainly dyspnea, fatigue, dizziness, and tachycardia. These symptoms are more pronounced according to the degree of anemia. In symptomatic anemia, the hemoglobin concentration usually falls below 10 mg/100 ml. Hypovolemic anemia is usually secondary to acute hemorrhage.

The main causes of anemia—decreased or abnormal RBC production, abnormal maturation, increased destruction or hemolysis, and hemorrhage—are discussed in detail below.

Anemias Due to Decreased or Abnormal Production of RBCs

Aplastic Anemias.—The etiology of aplastic anemia is poorly understood, and the disease generally has a poor prognosis. The diagnostic triad consists of cellular depletion, pancytopenia, and prolonged plasma iron clearance. It usually results from the effect of toxins on stem cells. It may be caused by any number of chemicals. However, certain chemicals are characteristically responsible for such types of anemia. Benzene and chloramphenicol are classic examples of this type of toxic effect on the bone marrow. Patients treated with chloramphenicol may exhibit thrombocytopenia, decreased reticulocyte counts, an increase in serum iron levels, and vacuolization of bone marrow cells.[43] Chloramphenicol given parenterally will also produce aplasia.[44] Other therapeutic agents such as tetracycline, penicillin, hydantoin, and phenylbutazone are frequently involved as etiologic agents of this type of anemia, as well.[45] Radiation has been found to cause aplastic anemia, probably by damage to the microenvironment (presumably due to fibrosis of capillaries).[46] Infection has also been found to be a causative agent, as in aplastic anemia secondary to miliary tuberculosis,[47] viral hepatitis,[48] and infectious mononucleosis.[49] However, most causes of aplastic anemia are idiopathic. The disease generally manifests with anemia, mild purpura, and fever secondary to infection.[50] Bone marrow biopsy reveals a very hypocellular marrow, with fatty replacement and a few lymphocytes.[51] The serum iron level is always elevated in these cases. Treatment is by avoiding the causative agent and preventing or treating opportunistic infections. Transfusions of RBCs are usually in the form of frozen-thawed cells to avoid graft-versus-host disease and to decrease platelet and WBC contaminants, which are potentially immunogenic. Androgens like bone marrow stimulants may be used.[52] Recently bone marrow transplantation has been used, with good results.[53] The better results have been obtained (as would be expected) using marrow from syngeneic donors. Pure RBC aplasia, otherwise known as Diamond-Blackfan syndrome, occurs as a constitutional defect.[54] However, it can occur in association with thymic tumors (usually thymomas),[55] and it appears to be associated with an immune defect.[56] There are idiopathic types of pure RBC aplasia as well. Occasionally the patient has a history of viral infections or drug intake (e.g., hydantoin).[57] Chronic forms of aplastic anemia have been described and include both congenital and acquired variants. Treatment is supportive, and if the etiology is diagnosed (e.g., thymoma), surgery is indicated.

Renal failure is a cause of aplastic anemia that may act both by bone marrow block and by destroying mature RBCs in the periphery. The anemia is usually normocytic. Peripheral smears exhibit schistocytes. Some patients respond to dialysis.

Endocrine diseases such as pituitary deficiency, hypothyroidism, hyperthyroidism, Addison's disease, and gonadal disease may also cause anemia with a normocytic-normochromic picture. Bone marrow replacement or myelophthisis is observed in patients with malignancies that infiltrate the bone marrow and in patients with diseases like myelofibrosis or granuloma. The anemia in these cases is normocytic-normochromic, and there may be a leukoerythroblastic phenomenon, in which marked anisocytosis and poikilocytosis are seen. Anemias due to decreased iron stores result in a "production deficiency" type of anemia. The anemia in chronic blood loss is compounded by the actual loss of blood and iron. Whatever the reason for hypochromic anemias, there is usually a decreased mean corpuscular hemoglobin concentration, and frequently there is an associated microcytosis due to increased cell division, with resulting smaller RBCs. The major causes of hypochromia are iron deficiency, pyridoxine-responsive anemia, lead poisoning, and impaired globulin synthesis. Impaired globulin synthesis gives rise to a distinct group of hypochromic anemias, examples of which are α- and β-thalassemias.

Iron Deficiency Anemias.—Iron is an essential component of the hemoglobin molecule and is responsible for the ability to bind oxygen. An average 70-kg adult has 3.5 gm of total body iron.[58] With a daily 15-mg iron intake, a normal adult accumulates about 5% of the total iron ingested.[59] Menstruation, pregnancy, and growth increase iron requirements. The regulation of iron assimilation depends on intestinal absorption through the ferritin-apoferritin cycle, as suggested by in vitro experiments.[60] Other factors include dietary iron, pancreatic secretions, and gastroferrin (which may depress iron absorption). Hydrochloric acid facilitates Fe^{+++} intestinal absorption. Iron is mostly transported in the plasma by a β-globulin called transferrin and is stored in the tissues as ferritin and hemosiderin. A molecular heterogeneity exists in transferrin. These molecules are called isotransferrins and have functional iron-binding differences.[61]

In iron deficiency anemia, the total body iron content is decreased. It is the most common nutritional deficiency in this country. Inadequate intake may be present in undernourished children or adults. Excessive losses of iron are usually secondary to bleeding from the gastrointestinal tract. Angular stomatitis, esophageal webbing, achlorhydria, and atrophic gastritis are common findings. A bone marrow study will show erythroid hyperplasia with "ragged normoblasts." An increased iron-binding capacity and a decreased serum iron level are the rule. Usually therapy is geared toward correcting the underlying disorders and supplying additional dietary iron. The usual daily dose for adults is 100–200 mg of elemental iron.[62]

Hypochromic Anemias Due to Faulty Heme and Porphyrin Portions of Hemoglobin.—Porphyrins and the heme group are composed of a ring of four pyrrole molecules.[63] Most heme is synthesized by the erythroid elements in the bone marrow. These are highly stable compounds that fluoresce in ultraviolet light. Normally they are not very abundant. However, when excess porphyrinogen is synthesized, they are eliminated in the urine as uroporphyrins. There are three forms of porphyrias: (1) true porphyrias with increased porphyrins, characterized by photosensitive dermatitis; (2) erythropoietic porphyria, a rare autosomal recessive disease; and (3) porphyria associated with anemia of lead poisoning.[64] Hypochromic anemia and basophilic stippling are characteristic of lead poisoning anemia. There is an increase in RBC protoporphyrins, and urinary coproporphyrin levels as well as urinary δ-amino levulenic acid levels are likewise elevated.[65] Lead interferes with the cation pump, possibly through membrane ATPase inhibition.[66]

Anemias Due to Faulty Maturation

Megaloblastic Anemias.—Megaloblastic anemias are usually secondary to folate or vitamin B12 deficiency. Folate deficiency may result from a variety of causes, including decreased intake (dietary malnutrition, alcoholism, or impaired absorption from intestinal disease), increased requirement (pregnancy, neoplasm), and blocked activation (folic acid antagonists).

Megaloblastic hematopoiesis, glossitis, cytologic abnormalities, and elevated serum lactic dehydrogenase (LDH) levels (especially isoenzymes 1 and 2)[67] are among the findings in patients with megaloblastic anemia secondary to folate deficiency.[68] Decreased serum folate levels, decreased RBC folate levels, and increased forminoglutamic acid (FIGLU) excretion after a loading dose of histamine suggest the diagnosis of folate deficiency. A response to folate therapy further suggests the cause of the megaloblastic anemia in these cases.[69]

Vitamin B12 Deficiency.—Vitamin B12 deficiency can be caused by decreased uptake. This may be due to diet, impaired absorption, intrinsic factor (IF) deficiency (e.g., pernicious anemia, gastrectomy, anti-IF antibodies, familial malabsorption, ileal resection, sprue, lymphomas, fish tapeworm, chronic pancreatic disease), and increased requirements (e.g., pregnancy, neoplasia, hyperthyroidism).[70]

The daily requirements of vitamin B12 are usually 5–30 μg, of which only 1–5 μg is absorbed. Cyanocobalamine resembles a porphyrin macroring with a central cobalt ring. This is the more frequent molecular form of the cobalamines forming the B12 complex. It is an important factor for the isomerization of methylmalonil coenzyme A (CoA) and therefore for the catabolism of propionate. Cyanocobalamine also affects the synthesis of methyl and thus regeneration of tetrahydrofolate, which impairs DNA synthesis.[71]

Intrinsic factor is deficient in pernicious anemia. It is secreted by the gastric mucosa and acts as a transport molecule, binding vitamin B12.[72, 73] There is a specific receptor for the IF B12 complex on intestinal cells. A good diagnostic test for absorption of vitamin B12 is the Schilling test. In this test a dose of radioactive vitamin B12 is given orally. Urine is collected after 24 hours and radioactivity is counted. Then a flushing dose of nonradioactive vitamin B12 is given. If excretion is low, the test is repeated with hog IF administered by mouth. If urinary excretion is still low, other causes for the deficiency are sought.[74]

Clinical features of vitamin B12 deficiency include (1) decreased vitamin B12 levels in plasma, (2) neurologic deficit (symmetric paresthesias, loss of vibratory sense), (3) methylmalonic aciduria, and (4) therapeutic response to vitamin B12. Other findings commonly associated with folate deficiency are megaloblastic anemia, neutrophilic hypersegmentation,[75] glossitis, elevated LDH levels, and weight loss. Other enzymes may be also increased, such as serum muramidase[76] and thymidine kinase.[77] Vitamin B12 therapy results in a prompt increase in the reticulocyte count and disappearance of most clinical manifestations, but a neurologic deficit may persist in spite of therapy. Pernicious anemia has long been identified as a risk factor for the development of gastric carcinoma.[78]

Megaloblastic Anemias Unresponsive to Vitamin B12.—Megaloblastic anemia may be present in the absence of vitamin B12 or folate deficiency. It is sometimes caused by therapy with antimetabolites (e.g., 6 MP, Immuran, and 6 TG). It is possible that the megaloblastic changes produced by these drugs are due to the drugs' inhibitory effect on DNA or RNA synthesis.[79] 6AzUR, Ara-C, and hydroxyurea, as well as other pyrimidine inhibitors, may also cause megaloblastic anemia.

Certain inborn errors of metabolism, such as hereditary orotic aciduria and deficiency,[80] are accompanied by megaloblastic changes. Pyridoxine-responsive anemias and erythremic myelosis, Di Guglielmo's syndrome, may be present also with megaloblastic anemia.

Anemias Due to Increased Destruction

Hemoglobinopathies.—Earlier in this chapter, some characteristics of the hemoglobin molecule were outlined. However, to understand the pathology that may occur in the synthesis of this molecule, it is advisable to study the structure in more detail.

Each molecule of hemoglobin is composed of four heme groups and one molecule of globin. The globin molecule consists of two pairs of polypeptide chains. The chains are either 141 α amino acids or 146 non-α amino acids joined in an α helical configuration alternating with short nonhelical regions.[81]

Synthesis of the Globin Molecule.—Synthesis of the globin portion of hemoglobin takes place in a similar fashion as the synthesis of other proteins: information from DNA is transmitted to RNA, and the globin molecule is synthesized at ribosomes. The structural genes for globin have been defined.[82,83] As with many proteins, the genes coding for amino acid sequences of hemoglobin have "introns" or intervening sequences which separate the coding sequences. When the DNA is transcribed into RNA, introns are included in the transcription. When the protein is decoded at the ribosomes, the intervening RNA sequences are eliminated and the coding sequences are joined; this process is termed splicing. Translation takes place from this mature mRNA. These intervening sequences appear to be necessary for adequate transcription at the DNA or RNA level, a fact which has not been completely clarified.[84] With the help of restriction endonuclease techniques and blotting on nitrocellulose filters, DNA fragments can be studied.[85]

Each globin gene of most species studied (mouse, rabbit, goat) contains two intervening sequences: a short (IVS-1) sequence which is located between codons 30 and 31 of all globin genes except α genes (i.e., ϵ, γ, δ, and β), and a long intervening sequence, IVS-2, which is located between codon 104 and 105.[86]

The 3' end of the structural gene contains 75 to 100 noncoding nucleotides which identify the polyadenylation site (poly-A addition).[87]

Polyadenylation is clearly a posttranscriptional event.[88] The 5' end of the globin-gene transcript where transcription begins is the "cap" region.[89] There are sequences which are essentially conserved during transcription. The δ and β genes, which are separated by 5.5 kilobases (Kb), are used in the synthesis of adult hemoglobin A ($\alpha_2\beta_2$) and hemoglobin A_2 ($\alpha_2\delta_2$).

The ϵ, γ, δ, and β genes are coded for on chromosome 11, whereas α_1 and α_2 genes are coded for on chromosome 16.[90]

Polyadenylation occurs at an extremely rapid rate in the nucleus. The 5'-methylation and the capping of globin mRNA occur in the nucleus.[88] Polyadenylated globin mRNA becomes linked to cytoplasmic proteins such as the eukaryotic initiating factor (eIF), elongation factor, and termination factor. The first event is linkage to eIF-2 and eIF-2-stimulating protein; eIF-3, -4A, and -4B are all needed for adequate linkage of mRNA to ribosomes. The mRNA there interacts with different tRNAs in the presence of elongation factor EF-1 to form the globin protein until a termination sequence is reached.[91,92]

Each molecule folds in such a way as to preserve a hydrophilic internal area. Each globin has a reversible bond to a prosthetic heme group. Fe^{++} atoms are fixed in the center of the porphyrin rings.

A single gene for each of the normal globin chains (α, β, γ, δ, ϵ) is inherited from each parent. However, there is some evidence suggesting that there may be more than one gene coding for the α-globulin chain.

Most pathologic genetic variants are the result of single amino acid substitutions.[93] For instance, sickle cell hemoglobins (Hb S) is a hemoglobin with an $\alpha_2\beta_2$ structure in which a glutamine β is substituted for a valine in the sixth amino acid from the N-terminal end of the β_2 chain.[93] The substituted amino acid is coded by an abnormal allelic gene. Affected persons may have heterozygous, doubly heterozygous (two chain pairs affected), or homozygous phenotypes. The amino acid substitution usually results in a net charge change, reflected in the electrophoretic migration patterns. This difference in mobility allows investigators to recognize such substitutions.[94]

The biochemical functions of hemoglobin variants may be affected in the following ways: (1) ability to transport oxygen, (2) change in solubility, and (3) instability of their quaternary configuration, making them more susceptible to drug-induced denaturation.[95]

Many of the abnormal hemoglobins are seen almost exclusively in the black population. Individuals carrying the heterozygous trait are usually asymptomatic. The heterozygous sickle cell trait occurs in 9% of the American black population. The next more frequent type of hemoglobinopathy is Hb C (3% of cases). Although anemia is not the rule in Hb C, target cells are frequently seen. American blacks show the following per 1,000 distribution of these traits: A/S, 90; S/S, 2; A/F, 10; S/C, 0.6; A/C, 30; C/C, 0.1.[96]

Sickle Cell Anemia.—Sickle cell anemia is a recessive hereditary disease mostly confined to the black population. The abnormal hemoglobin behaves differently from normal hemoglobin in that it has a tendency to precipitate at low oxygen tension, especially if the condition includes a drop in pH. The aggregation requires the substitution of valine for glutamic acid in the β-6 position, since only this type of substitution undergoes sickling.[97] The sickling of RBCs appears to be due to aggregation of hemoglobin molecules which form microtubular structures that are not due to membrane defects.[98] However, the repeated process of sickling and unsickling will eventually produce membrane damage. Membrane phosphorylation is deranged in sickle cells.[99] The result of RBC sickling is a tendency to stasis and obstruction of capillaries.

Many patients present in sickle cell crisis, consisting of pain in bones and joints and abdominal pain mimicking visceral diseases of various kinds. Sickle cell crisis has sometimes led to exploratory surgery. Scleral icterus is frequently found in these patients, and cerebral thrombosis may be a complication of the disease. Other complications include bone infarction, leg ulcers, cholelithiasis, and pulmonary thrombosis.[100]

Laboratory testing reveals a normochromic anemia, target cells, high LDH level, and decreased or absent haptoglobin. Screening tests are a positive metabisulfite test or a positive solubility test with sodium dithionite as a reducing agent and saponin as a precipitating agent. Sickle cell disease is confirmed by detecting the abnormal hemoglobin by electrophoresis.

The treatment of sickle cell anemia is mostly supportive. Alkalinization, oxygen therapy, and vasodilators have been used with some success during sickling crisis.[101] Transfusions are frequently necessary. Exchange transfusion has been used during severe sickle cell crisis, with some success.[102]

Sickle Cell Trait.—Sickle cell trait is infrequently symptomatic. Affected persons have the A/S hemoglobin genotype. They should not be exposed to high-altitude flying or other conditions that may cause a depression of oxygen tension or a low blood pH. Patients with sickle cell trait have a slightly higher incidence (1%) of hematuria and pulmonary embolism than the general population.[103]

S/C Hemoglobin Disease.—The symptoms and signs of S/C disease are similar to those of sickle cell anemia but are usually less severe. Patients with this hemoglobinopathy have positive results on tests for sickle cell anemia. Target cells are prominent and should be useful in establishing the differential diagnosis. On electrophoresis there are almost equal amounts of Hb S and Hb C.

Sickle Thalassemia.—Patients with sickle thalassemia have increased amounts of Hb A2 and Hb S hemoglobins. Symptoms, when present, are similar to those of sickle cell disease. The disease is usually less severe than S/C disease. Diagnosis is confirmed by electrophoresis (Fig 2–3).

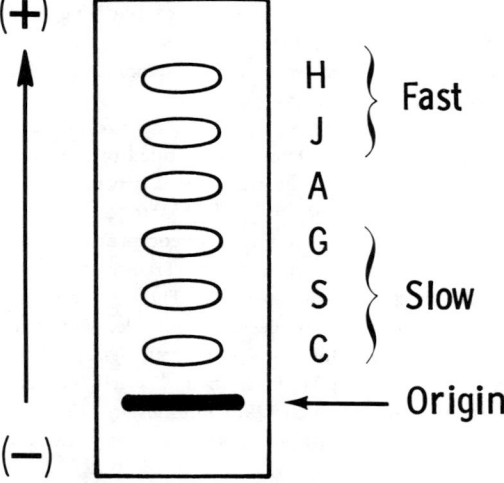

FIG 2–3.—Hemoglobin electrophoresis—fast, intermediate, and slow hemoglobins. The method is used to diagnose hemoglobinopathies.

TABLE 2–2.—Different Hemoglobins and the Composing Chains During Development

HEMOGLOBIN	CHAINS
Adult	
A	$\alpha_2\beta_2$
A2	$\alpha_2\delta_2$
Fetal	
F	$\alpha_2\gamma_2$
Embryonic	
Gower 1	$\zeta_2\epsilon_2$
Gower 2	$\alpha_2\epsilon_2$
Portland	$\zeta_2\gamma_2$

Hereditary Persistence of Fetal Hemoglobin.—Persons with persistent Hb F are rarely symptomatic. The condition is more frequent in blacks than in whites. Hb F may reach 20% of the total hemoglobin content.

The Thalassemias.—In thalassemia, there is a disequilibrium in the synthesis of the different chains composing the globin molecule. This results in insufficient production of hemoglobin to fill the RBCs, resulting in targeting of cells. It has been proposed that there is an mRNA deficiency which is expressed in the disequilibrium of hemoglobin synthesis. The defect may involve the α chains (α-thalassemia) or may result in decreased production of β chains (β-thalassemia).[104]

Adult hemoglobin consists mostly of hemoglobin A, with a minor component (2.5%) of hemoglobin A2. Fetal hemoglobin is mostly hemoglobin F. The chain composition of hemoglobin A1, A2, and F is given in Table 2–2.

Before the eighth week in utero, three embryonic hemoglobins are present, Gower 1, Gower 2, and Portland (see Table 2–2).[105] During fetal development an orderly switch from ζ to α, from ϵ to γ, and from β to δ occurs.[106]

In thalassemia the chains are synthesized at a reduced rate.[107] The syndromes are classified according to which chain is affected by the reduced rate of synthesis. The main forms of thalassemia are α, β, $\delta\beta$, δ, and $\gamma\delta\beta$ (Table 2–3).

β-Thalassemia is the form more frequently seen in the United States. it affects mostly populations of Mediterranean or Chinese descent; some blacks may also be affected. In β-thalassemia compensatory chains are found (e.g., γ and δ chains). This results in an increased Hb F if γ chains are present and an increased Hb A2 if δ chains are present.

Two types of thalassemia are recognized most frequently: thalassemia major, which is the homozygous trait, and thalassemia minor, which is the heterozygous trait.[107]

TABLE 2–3.—Main Forms of Thalassemia*

THALASSEMIA TYPE		GENETIC DEFECT	DISEASE
β°	Homozygous Hb F (97%–98%) Hb A2 (1%–3%)	Gene deletions; defective mRNA splicing	Thalassemia major
	Heterozygous Hb A2 (4%–7%) HbF (1%–3%)	Heterogeneous	Thalassemia trait
$\beta+$	Homozygous Hb F (60%–90%) Hb A2 (1%–5%) Hb A present	Defective mRNA transcription and splicing	Thalassemia intermedia
	Heterozygous		Thalassemia trait
$\delta\beta^\circ$	Homozygous Heterogeneous Hb F	Deletion of $\delta\beta$ genes; $\delta\beta$ fusion	δ,β-Thalassemia
α°	Homozygous Heterogeneous	Deletion of α gene from Chr. 16	α°-Thalassemia; hemoglobin H disease; Bart's hydrops fetalis
$\alpha^{3.7}$	Homozygous Heterogeneous	$\alpha^{3.7}$ deletion	Thalassemia trait normal
$\alpha+$	Heterozygous Homozygous Hb Bart (5%–15%)		Thalassemia similar to α°-thalassemia

*Adapted from Wetherall and Clegg.[107]

In thalassemia major there is usually anemia, which may be very severe. Onset is in infancy, when there may be a severe hepatosplenomegaly and jaundice. A microcytic-hypochromic anemia with severely deformed cells and targeting is seen. Serum bilirubin is usually elevated and there is decreased haptoglobin. Hb F may be very elevated. Skeletal x-rays show a hair on-end appearance of the skull and long bones with thinning of the cortex. Leg ulcers, hemosiderosis, and cardiac failure may complicate this disease. Treatment is symptomatic and supportive with transfusions.

The anemia of thalassemia minor is persistent but usually less severe than in thalassemia major. The spleen may be enlarged. Frequently the disease is asymptomatic. Usually Hb A2 is increased twofold to threefold. Iron therapy is usually not necessary and should be avoided. Transfusions may occasionally be necessary.[108]

Hemoglobin H disease is α-thalassemia. The homozygous trait is usually lethal. Heterozygotes present with similar clinical findings as in thalassemia minor. Silent carriers are usually asymptomatic but have decreased amounts of Hb A on electrophoresis. The RBC morphology is more striking than in thalassemia minor. This disorder is more frequently found in Chinese, Philippinos, and Thais. The brilliant cresyl blue test is usually positive in α-thalassemia. However, the diagnosis is achieved by electrophoresis.[109–111]

Anemias Due to Increased Destruction of RBCs

Anemias secondary to membrane and metabolic disorders may be divided into two groups: (1) defects of the RBC membrane, and (2) defects of glucose metabolism.

Defects of the RBC Membrane.—Most of these diseases exhibit a defect of the membrane components. Membranes are composed of a bilayer of lipids asymmetrically organized, endowing the membrane with the properties of a two-dimensional fluid.[22] Proteins are interspersed in the lipid bilayer, and some are firmly anchored to the cytoskeleton. Nevertheless, they are mobile in the membrane, and their mobility is affected by physical and biochemical phenomena. The proteins linked to the underlying cytoskeleton are attached to molecules composed of spectrin and actin. Certain membrane proteins are enzymes which are essential to the ion exchange across the membrane. Na^+-K^+-ATPase is one such enzyme and is responsible for the Na^+-K^+ pump.

Changes in the membrane may result in decreased deformability of the RBCs, increased fragility, or changes in shape, all of which can impair RBC functions. These changes affect the survival of those RBCs that are damaged or trapped by organs such as the spleen and the liver as they try to squeeze their way through the fenestrations of the sinuses in these organs.

Anemias Caused By Membrane Defects.—*Hereditary spherocytosis* is an inherited autosomal dominant disease. It occurs in about 20 per 100,000 population and frequently appears in the neonatal period as neonatal jaundice. The disease is characterized by mild to moderate anemia. Erythroid hyperplasia and reticulocytosis are observed as part of the ongoing hemolytic process. High bilirubin levels, low haptoglobin levels, and a tendency to gallstone formation are frequently found. Peripheral smears show characteristic spherocytes.[112] It is speculated that the pathogenesis involves a defect in the membrane Na^+ pump[113] and an altered binding of the cytoskeleton to the membrane.[114] The cells become spherical in shape due to a decreased surface-to-volume ratio. Affected persons have been treated by splenectomy, thus improving the survival of RBCs. The RBCs, however, retain their abnormal shape.

Hereditary elliptocytosis is also inherited as an autosomal dominant disease. Usually more than 60% of the cells are elliptical. Few patients present with severe hemolysis. In this disease as well as in hereditary spherocytosis there is increased osmotic fragility of the cells.[115] It appears that the abnormal RBC membrane in elliptocytes is linked to an abnormality in the structure of spectrin in these cells.[116]

In *disorders of cation permeability* there is leakage of sodium or potassium from the cells. The result is the formation of stomatocytes, and therefore the disease has been termed hereditary stomatocytosis.[117] Many target cells as well as spiculated cells are seen.[118] These disorders are improved by splenectomy.

Acanthocytes and target cells are the result of *abnormal lipid composition*. Biliary obstruction causes damage to the lipid component of the RBC membrane in certain diseases. Acanthocytes or "spur" cells are sometimes the result of these severe hepatocellular diseases. RBCs do not survive normally, and at times hemolytic anemia is seen in patients with advanced hepatocellular disease. Physical injury or chemical injury may affect the RBC membrane in a variety of ways. Acanthocytes are also seen in a β-lipoproteinemia[119] and familial neurologic disorders.[120] Of interest to blood bankers is the finding of membrane abnormalities leading to acanthocytosis in the McLeod syndrome. However, the abnormality in this syndrome is probably due to membrane proteins.[121, 122]

Paroxysmal Nocturnal Hemoglobinuria.—Paroxysmal nocturnal hemoglobinuria (PNH) appears to be an acquired stem cell disorder which makes the matured RBCs arising from these stem cells more susceptible to the lysis by complement.[123] Susceptibility varies from case to case. PNH cells can be divided into PNH I, II, and III, depending on the increasing susceptibility of the cells to complement lysis.[124] The proof of monoclonality of stem cells giving rise to PNH erythrocytes is based on the finding that PNH patients who are heterozygous for G6PD will only show a single G6PD phenotype in PNH erythrocytes.[123] Acetyl cholinesterase activity is markedly decreased in PNH erythrocytes.[125] However, this finding does not explain the increased susceptibility of these cells to lysis by complement. Paroxysmal nocturnal hemoglobinuria may arise as a complication of aplastic anemia,[126] and may be a prelude to both erythroleukemia[127] and myelomonocytic leukemia.[128]

Clinical Manifestations of PNH.—PNH usually appears insidiously in the third to fifth decades of life, but it may occur in children or the very old.[129] The cause for nocturnal exacerbation has been explained on the basis of decreased nocturnal plasma pH, or on the circadian rhythm of cortisol.[129] However, the course of hemolysis is most probably correlated with an increase in the number of abnormally susceptible RBCs. Characteristically the hemolysis appears at night; hence the name nocturnal hemoglobinuria.

In PNH, bouts of hemolysis may appear during stressful situations (surgery, infections). At the laboratory level there is usually severe anemia, usually microcytic-hypochromic.[130] The leukocyte alkaline phosphatase (LAP) level is very decreased or immeasurable. Some granulocytes may have the enzyme whereas others do not.[131]

Leukopenia is often present. Thrombocytopenia may give rise to a bleeding diathesis.[132] An erythroid hyperplasia is frequently seen in PNH, but the reticulocyte count may be normal. The diagnosis of PNH is arrived at by performing serologic tests which demonstrate the high susceptibility of PNH cells to complement. One such test is the Ham test, which uses an acidified solution to which fresh complement has been added.[133] The sugar water test enhances attachment of complement to RBCs. Thus PNH cells, which are more sensitive to complement lysis, often lyse in this solution.[134]

Complications of PNH.—Patients may develop severe bleeding or thrombosis, presenting with the Budd-Chiari syndrome.[135, 136] Renal failure may gradually develop.[137] Aplastic anemia and leukemia can be terminal complications of PNH.

Therapy of PNH.—Treatment of patients with PNH is usually supportive, although bone marrow grafting has occasionally been performed in patients who developed bone marrow failure.[138] Nevertheless, it appears necessary to pretreat these patients with cyclophosphamide to eliminate the abnormal stem cells.[139] Patients with PNH often need transfusions; these should be in the form of washed cells or frozen-thawed cells[140] to avoid adding plasma proteins consumed during activation of complement and to prevent the formation of antibodies capable of inducing future hemolysis. Dextran can be given with transfusions to avert possible hemolysis.[141] About 1,000 cc of Dextran is given immediately prior to transfusion.

Defects in RBC Metabolism.—Mature RBCs do not consume oxygen, due to their lack of mitochondria. Therefore, most of the RBC energy expenditure is by glycolysis, through either the Embden-Meyerhof glycolytic pathway or through the hexose monophosphate shunt pathway.[142] Glucose in the RBC thus is transformed into ATP, with lactate produced as a metabolite. Glycolysis also provides NADH, which is essential for several oxidative reactions as a cofactor. 2,3-DPG is another byproduct of the glycolytic process via the Rapoport-Luebering shunt. Not all the glucose entering the metabolic pathways results in the formation of high-energy phosphate ATP. After the formation of 1,3-DPG there is some flexibility as to the amount of ATP formed.[143] The 1,3-DPG formed can be converted to 2,3-DPG. Hydrogen ion concentrations regulate the DPG mutase reaction; thus 2,3-DPG levels are extremely sensitive to changes in pH.[144] This fact is of importance in the storage of RBCs in the blood bank. The 2,3-DPG formed is essential to the erythrocyte's capacity to release oxygen.[143] It acts as an oxygen transport modulator by interacting with hemoglobin. The hexose monophosphate shunt is the main source of NADPH in the RBC. NADPH is important in the synthesis of glutathione, which protects RBCs against intracellular and extracellular oxidants.

Anemias Caused by Metabolism Defects.—Among the disorders of hemolysis secondary to hexose monophosphate shunt deficiency, the most common is G6PD deficiency.[145] G6PD results in (1) oxydation of hemoglobin to methemoglobin, (2) production of sulfhemoglobin, and (3) intracellular precipitation of hemoglobin, forming Heinz bodies. All these changes result from an inability of RBCs to prevent noxious oxidative changes. The cells are pitted by the spleen in an attempt to rid them of Heinz bodies. As a result, patients have various degrees of cell damage.

The genes controlling G6PD synthesis are located on chromosome X and are juxtaposed to the genes for color blindness and hemophilia A.[146] Males are affected more often than females, who in turn are affected only in the homozygous state. The enzyme has predominantly two electrophoretically different allotypes, G6PDA and G6PDB. G6PDA is common in Africa, whereas G6PDB is common in caucasians. They differ by only a single amino acid substitution.[147] This difference in the electrophoretic migration of G6PD has been used to demonstrate clonality of tumors. Thus, in heterozygous individuals who develop tumors, the clonal expansion of the tumor cell will reflect only one of the two G6PD's.[148] The G6PD deficiency results from a variety of defects which affect the structural genes coding from G6PD enzymes. In the more common African (A) mutation, the enzyme may be normal in quantity but is of decreased stability.[145] The Mediterranean variety of G6PD deficiency, however, appears to result in enzymes with decreased activity.[149] It is assumed that most of the variants arise as point mutations, resulting in single amino acid substitutions, such as occurs in the Hektoen variant of G6PD.[150]

Just why G6PD-deficient RBCs are hemolyzed is not entirely clear. The G6PD-deficient cells have a limited ability to generate NADPH and reduced glutathione (GSH) which is necessary to reduce hydrogen peroxide and free radicals generated during RBC metabolism. These radicals may be produced in greater amounts when certain drugs such as primaquine are used.[151,152]

Most patients with a G6PD deficiency are asymptomatic. When symptoms do appear, these are in the form of episodic hemolytic anemia. The hemolysis may be triggered by a variety of factors (Table 2–4). Three main clinical presentations can be distinguished: (1) acquired hemolysis, (2) congenital nonspherocytic hemolytic anemia, and (3)

TABLE 2–4.—SOME FACTORS THAT TRIGGER HEMOLYSIS IN G6PD-DEFICIENT INDIVIDUALS

CAUSE	REMARKS
Drugs[145]	
Antimalarials (e.g., primaquine)	Varies in different individuals
Sulfonamides (e.g., sulfamethoxazole)	″ ″
Sulfones (e.g., diphenylsulfone)	″ ″
Nitrofurans (e.g., nitrofurantoin)	″ ″
Analgesic (e.g., acetanilid)	″ ″
Infection	
Bacterial infection (e.g. *Salmonella*,[153] *E. coli*,[154] *Rickettsia*,[155] viral (hepatitis)[156]	Bacterial infection more common cause than drugs; infection more severe if fever present, hemolysis more severe in viral hepatitis
Favism[145]	Caused by *Vicia fava* beans; often seen in people of Mediterranean origin
Diabetic acidosis[157]	
Neonatal icterus[158]	No evidence of immunologic incompatibility to cause kernicterus
Hereditary nonspherocytic hemolytic anemia[159,162]	Rare; usually chronic anemia; isoenzymes are markedly unstable

favism. Some of the features are outlined in Table 2–4. The diagnosis of this disease is best arrived at once reticulocytosis has decreased and the hemolytic process has been controlled. Enzyme testing should be performed on cells separated by density gradients. The older, more deficient cells can thus be selected by separating the cell bands with higher density.[160] The cells are then subjected to one of the better screening procedures to detect G6PD deficiency, such as the fluorescent spot test. The test measures G6PD activity by generation of NADPH in the presence of RBC membranes, G6P, and NADP.[161] Two main types are frequently seen, GdA and GdG, depending on different electrophoretic mobility of the enzymes.[145] Rare G6PD deficiencies can be very heterogenous.[149] The treatment is preventive, avoiding drugs or foods that trigger the hemolytic episode. Transfusion is usually unnecessary. Exchange transfusion may be considered if the possibility of kernicterus is present. Splenectomy is not indicated.[162] High-dose vitamin E therapy may be useful in some cases.[163]

Anemias Due to Other Enzyme Defects

Other RBC enzyme deficiencies are rare in comparison to G6PD deficiency. Defects of glutathione can be the result of either a lack of γ-glutamylcysteine synthetase or a defect in glutathione synthetase.[164] Lifelong hemolytic anemia, an isocytosis, poikilocytosis, and polychromatophilia are seen in these cases. Another inherited RBC enzyme abnormality is glutathione reductase deficiency, but it is rare.[165]

Other Causes of Hemolysis

The major cause for hemolysis that is of interest to the blood banker is immune-mediated hemolysis. This topic is addressed in detail in chapter 10. Hemolytic disease of the newborn is discussed in chapter 16.

WHITE BLOOD CELLS

Morphology, Physiology, and Pathology

WBCs are varied in morphology and constitute an important part of the cellular defense mechanisms of the body. The WBC forms include granulocytes, lymphocytes, and monocytes. Some of the characteristics of each of these cell types are described below. Other cells, especially lymphocytes, and their role in the immune response are discussed in more detail in chapter 4.

Granulocytes

Granulocytes are studied in peripheral smears or in bone marrow material from patients. Diagnostic conclusions can be derived on the basis of morphology alone. Many diseases are manifested by abnormal stages of maturation of the myeloid series. The more immature forms of granulocyte precursors should be seen only in the bone marrow. Their presence in peripheral smears should arouse great concern.

Immature WBC Forms

The various forms of the WBCs from the least to the most mature are described below.

The *myeloblast* is about 12–15 μ in diameter and contains a large purple nucleus with scant cytoplasm that stains blue with Wright's stain. Myeloblasts constitute about 1% of a normal bone marrow population. The nuclear chromatin is distributed in fine chromatin strands. One or more nucleoli are present, in contrast to lymphoblasts, which usually contain a single nucleolus. The myeloblasts are the more immature of the granulocyte precursors. By definition these cells do not contain cytoplasmic granules.[166] Myeloblasts show a basophilic (blue) cytoplasm due to the high cytoplasmic RNA content. These cells are difficult if not impossible to distinguish from lymphoblasts by routine microscopy. Stem cells committed to granulocytic development as myeloblasts may be of two types, CFU-NM, giving rise to neutrophils and macrophages, and CFU-EOS, giving rise to eosinophils.[167]

Promyelocytes are the next stage of development. Characteristically the cytoplasm reveals type A azurophilic, nonspecific granules.[168] Promyelocytes show a more clumped chromatin pattern than myeloblasts and contain nucleoli.

Myelocytes display large cytoplasmic purple granules containing myeloperoxidase and hydrolases.[168] These granules are type B or secondary granules and do not seem to derive from type A granules. The granule enzymes can be detected by staining with special enzyme stains.

Myelocytes derive from promyelocytes. A further increase in nuclear chromatin clumping is observed. Nucleoli are not present in these cells. It is possible at this stage to recognize subtypes of granulocytes by their staining characteristics: neutrophils have purple granules, eosinophils have reddish granules, and basophils have deep blue granules. Both myeloblasts and promyelocytes are immobile, which may explain why these forms are present mostly in the marrow. Primary granules are packaged and released from the inner, concave surface of the Golgi apparatus, whereas secondary (specific) granules are formed in the outer surface of the Golgi apparatus.[169] Primary granules are lysosomes which store hydrolases, myeloperoxidases, neutral proteases, and bactericidal cationic proteins.[170] Characteristically, secondary granules are peroxidase negative.[171] These findings have been obtained by separating the granules by isopyknic density gradient centrifugation.[170] With this method, primary granules separate into two bands, band A at 1.22 sg and band B at 1.20 sg.[172] The secondary granules separate as a single band at 1.18 sg. A comparison of primary and secondary granules is given in Table 2–5.

Metamyelocytes, which are the next stage of differentiation, are smaller in size; there is more pronounced clumping of chromatin, and prominent indentation of the nucleus is observed. Multiple primary but predominantly secondary granules are seen in the cytoplasm. A tertiary granule may also be present.[174]

Band forms are smaller than metamyelocytes. The nucleus shows evidence of elongation and indentation, suggesting areas where the mature granulocyte will show nuclear segmentation.

The *segmented polymorphonuclear cell* is the mature stage of granulocytes. Mature granulocytes normally exhibit two to four lobulations. In certain diseases, such as pernicious anemia, hypersegmentation of granulocyte nuclei is noted, where five or more lobules are seen. A clear separation of nuclear lobes is necessary to distinguish mature cells from band forms if the counts are to be of diagnostic significance.[175]

TABLE 2–5.—Characteristics of Human Neutrophil Granules*

PRIMARY (AZUROPHILIC)	SECONDARY (SPECIFIC)
Myeloperoxidase	Lactoferrin
Acid hydrolases	Cobalophilin
Glycosidases	Acidic proteins
Acid phosphatase	
Neutral proteases	Collagenase (specific)
Lysozyme	Lysozyme
Acid mucopolysaccharide	

*Data from Wright[171] and Olssen and Verge.[173]

Mature Granulocytes

Polymorphonuclear neutrophils represent fully mature granulocytes. Characteristically the cytoplasm contains azurophilic granules. These are the most numerous of the granulocytes, and their phagocytic functions are important to the primary cellular defense line. Each nucleus has three to five lobules. Glycogen stained by PAS and lipid stained by Sudan black B are conspicuous components of granulocytes.

Granulocyte Kinetics

Granulocytes are produced in the bone marrow from multipotential stem cells. To understand the replication of myelocytic stem cells it is necessary to understand some concepts regarding DNA synthesis.

Dividing cells enter a cell cycle that involves the S phase, or DNA synthesis phase, and the M phase, or mitotic phase. The G phase is defined as that part of the cycle just prior to DNA synthesis (which is the S phase). GS is the stage following S phase. Cells are defined as being in G_0 when they are in the resting state.[174]

Cells synthesizing DNA can be counted by allowing uptake of tritiated thymidine and assessing the cells undergoing S phase. Myeloblasts, granuloblasts, and myelocytes are precursors capable of division and can therefore be studied in this context. It is possible by these means to calculate a "labeling index," which gives one an idea of the rate at which cells are dividing. Generation time is the time required for cells to go through the full cycle. Counting labeled cells in mitosis permits the calculation of the generation times, which is the interval between two waves of labeled mitosis.[174]

Granulocytes derive from a totipotent hematopoietic stem cell (THSC) capable of giving rise to erythrocytes, megakaryocytes, mononuclear phagocytes, and granulocytes.[175] THSC cells give rise to committed stem cells in the form of colony-forming unit cells (CFU). This has been shown by injecting marrow cells into lethally irradiated mice. The grafted cells form colonies in the spleen (CFU-S).[176] Furthermore, a multipotent hemopoietic cell can be stimulated to produce colonies of erythroblasts, granulocytes, and megakaryocytes.[177] Additional evidence of the combined origin of granulocytes and megakaryocytes is the finding of defects in megakaryocytes and granulocytes in CFU-S-deficient W/W^v mice.[178] It has been possible to show that monocytes and granulocytes derive from the same stem cell by stimulating transformation in vitro of granulocyte-type cells into monocytes.[179]

The clonality of CFU-S is suggested by the linear relation of induced/CFU ratios.[175] Differentiation of CFU-S cells is driven by microenvironmental factors, as was demonstrated by abrogation of CFU-S differentiation into granulocytic cells after blockage of erythropoietin.[175] CFU-S cells have a prolonged generation time, remaining in G_0 phase, as shown by tritiated thymidine suicide experiments.[180] Many factors interact to form the hemopoietic microenvironment.[181] The thymus is crucial to the adequate formation of CFU-S. This can be shown in vitro with soluble T cell factors.[182] CFU-S presumably gives rise to CFU-NM, a cell capable of further differentiating into CFU-N (neutrophils) and CFU-M (monocytes/macrophages).[183] The stimulus to induce such differentiation is both the microenvironment, as mentioned above, and colony-stimulating factors (CSF). Colony-stimulating factors are 30,000-dalton glycoproteins,[184] mostly produced by monocytic phagocytes,[185] T cells,[186] and endothelial cells.[187]

Three kinetic compartments can be identified for neutrophils: bone marrow, blood, and tissues. Approximately five divisions occur from the myeloblast stage to the metamyelocyte. A myeloblast gives rise to 32 mature polymorphonuclear cells. The divisions, however, are not constant, as shown by ^{32}P labeling.[188] The marrow can be functionally divided into a proliferative compartment (myeloblasts to metamyelocyte) and a maturation compartment (metamyelocyte to mature polymorph). The maturation process lasts about 5–7 days and occurs in an orderly fashion, that is, the first cells leaving the proliferative compartment are also the first cells to mature and leave the marrow.[189]

Blood Neutrophil Kinetics.—Two populations of cells are identified: (1) the circulating pool and (2) the marginated pool, which consists of cells attached to the endothelial surface. The movement of neutrophils leaving the bone marrow, entering the circulation, and reaching the tissues is unidirectional. Certain substances will induce increments in the circulating neutrophil pool. Animals made neutropenic with endotoxin possess in their serum a substance capable of inducing leukocytosis, termed leukocytosis-inducing factor (LIF).[190] Of interest to blood banking, and granulocyte collection for transfusion, is that glucocorticoids are capable of increasing the granulocyte count. Increments of up to 4,000/μl can be achieved 5 hours after one dose of cortisol.[191] Paradoxically, dexamethasone promotes migration of WBCs to inflammatory sites.[192] Dexamethasone is used in granulocyte collections as a single IV dose of 4 mg/m.[2, 193] Exercise will likewise increase the granulocyte count.[193] Substances in serum termed chalones (4,000 daltons) have the opposite effect, inhibiting proliferation of neutrophils in the marrow.[194]

Granulocyte Functions

Endocytosis is the general process by which granulocytes internalize a portion of the membrane to which particles have attached.[195] The process of phagocytosis causes neutrophils to degranulate.[196] Primary granule degranulation is usually confined to internalized phagocytic vacuoles, whereas secondary degranulation is primarily directed to the outside of the cell.[197]

Concanavalin A[198] and phorbol esters[199] will cause selective secondary granule degranulation with exocystosis of granule contents. Using these substances it has been shown that secondary granule degranulation occurs before primary granule degranulation. More importantly for defense mechanism is the triggering of granulocyte degranulation by C5a.[200] Many of the degranulating stimuli decrease the negative surface charge, thereby increasing the adhesiveness of granulocyte outer membranes.[201] On stimulation by phagocytosis, neutrophils undergo a "burst" of respiratory activity,[202] probably by mediation of a membrane-bound oxidase.[203] This oxygen "burst" is necessary for the microbicidal activity of granulocytes. In addition to the oxygen formed in the respiratory burst, neutrophils have the capacity to produce superoxide ion ($O\dot{\div}$), a highly toxic byproduct of the respiratory burst.[204] The formation of the superoxide is mediated by myeloperoxidase (MPO) via the MPO-H_2O_2-halide antimicrobial system.[205]

Neutrophil Chemotaxis.—Chemoattractants are formed during bacterial invasion or tissue destruction of various sorts. A general mechanism of formation of chemoattractants is the independent or coordinated interaction of the complement, coagulation, and kinin-generating systems.[206] Other cells in the inflammatory infiltrate are likewise capable of producing chemoattractants. These may be in the form of lymphokines produced by lymphocytes or monocytes.[207] The most chemotactic complement factors are C5a, C4a, and C3a. Of these the most effective chemoattractant is C5a.[208] C5a is inactivated by a carboxypeptidase B, which converts

C5a to C5a-des-Arg; nevertheless, the chemotactic activity can be restored by a plasma cofactor which has not been characterized to this date.[209] When the clotting system is activated, activated factor XIIa catalyzes the conversion of prekallikrein to kallikrein, which is chemotactic.[210] Another byproduct of the coagulation system with chemotactic activity is fibrinopeptide B, which results from the cleavage of fibrin by plasmin.[211] Formyl peptide is a potent chemotactic factor. A receptor for formyl peptide has been identified on the membrane of neutrophils. This receptor is a protein of 60,000 daltons.[212] How neutrophils cross endothelial barriers to reach the chemoattractant has been the subject of recent research. In culture, neutrophils adhere preferentially to endothelial cells as opposed to other cells.[213] It appears that laminin, a basement membrane protein, has a critical role in the attachment of granulocytes to endothelial cells.[214] The process of transepithelial migration of neutrophils does not appear to alter the permeability of these epithelia.[214] The exact mechanism of ligand/receptor interaction during chemotaxis has not been fully elucidated. However, integrity of membrane glycoproteins appears to be needed.[215] Ready access to ATP and an integral cytoskeleton are likewise necessary to adequate motility, as has been shown in tritiated human neutrophils.[214] The cytoskeleton of the neutrophil is formed by filament networks of polymerized actin,[216] comprising 10% of the protein in a neutrophil, and myosin, which comprises about 1% of the protein in a neutrophil.[217]

Actin and myosin behave in a fashion similar to that found in muscle cells. Thus, the globular heads of the myosin heavy chains cross-link with actin monomers to form filaments. The cross-bridge formation requires ATP hydrolysis, and results in a sliding filament mechanism which results in contraction, as has been shown in platelets.[218] Another protein, termed actin-binding protein, concentrates at the periphery of the cell during phagocytosis. This protein cross-links with actin, forming a gel-like structure in the pseudopodia.[217] The actual gelation process, and contraction of the actin-myosin mechanism, appear to be controlled by variations in the concentration of calcium.[218] If the concentration of calcium is greater than $0.2\mu M$, the actin gel is dissolved by the protein gelsolin. If calcium concentrations decrease, gelsolin is inactivated and the gel structure is reconstituted.[219]

However, it appears that other transducer/excitation mechanisms apart from calcium concentration alone are at play in the neutrophil activation mechanism, as has been shown by chemotactic stimuli of neutrophils with formylmethionylleucylphenylalanine (FMLP).[220]

In addition to receptors for chemotactic factors, neutrophils have Fc receptors for immunoglobulin[221] as well as receptors for complement,[222] such as receptors for Clq[223] and C3b.[224]

Eosinophils

The granules of eosinophils stain red on Wright's stain, hence their name eosinophils. Eosinophils are both mobile and phagocytic. They increase in number in several clinical conditions, notably those associated with allergic reactions (bronchial asthma and allergic rhinitis). Eosinophils have surface receptors for IgE and are involved in phagocytosis of immune complexes. Their number decreases remarkably in patients treated with steroids.

Eosinophil Kinetics.—Eosinophil promyelocytes can be detected in the bone marrow. Together with myelocytes, they form the bone marrow mytotic pool. Morphologically mature eosinophils remain in the marrow several days before release.[225] An eosinophil-releasing factor has been described.[226] It has been shown, by culturing bone marrow on soft agar, that eosinophils arise from a different progenitor cell than do basophils, neutrophils, and monocytes, which appear to originate from a common stem cell precursor.[227] Presumably the above-mentioned eosinophilopoietin bears a function in both maturation and release of eosinophils from the bone marrow.[228] However, this maturation process must not be a simple one. For instance, it has been shown that the thymus is crucial to eosinophil development. Neonatal thymectomy in mice results in a poor eosinophilic response to infection by intestinal parasites. This abnormality can be corrected by reconstituting the thymus in these animals.[229] The exact kinetics of eosinophil circulation are not fully elucidated, but it is estimated that once eosinophils enter the circulation, cell survival is 24–35 hours.[230]

Eosinophil Functions.—Eosinophils do not appear to provide adequate cellular defense, even though these cells are known to share many of the characteristics which neutrophils possess (i.e., lysosomes, chemotactic responses, phagocytic ability, and oxidative metabolic responses).[231] This assumption is derived from the observation that patients with neutropenia and eosinophilia readily become infected.[232, 233] The reason may be that eosinophils are not as actively phagocytic as neutrophils,[234] have a decreased bactericidal ability,[235] and the actual eosinophil count, which is initially increased in infections, subsequently drops.[236] Although high levels of corticosteroids are sometimes seen in acute infection, and this increase in hormonal levels is accompanied by eosinopenia, other factors may be at play. This is suggested by the fact that most infections are not accompanied by significant elevations of circulatory adrenal steroids,[237] and certain stressful situations such as asthma and parasitic infections are accompanied by eosinophilia.[231] It appears that serum proteins such as eosinophil cationic proteins may be involved in the eosinopenia of infections.[238]

Role of Eosinophils in Host Defenses.— The precise role of the eosinophil in defending the host against metazoal parasites has not been fully elucidated. Initially (12–18 hours) a neutrophilic response is observed after invasion of a metazoal parasite such as trichinella. Then an infiltrate predominantly composed of eosinophils and macrophages appears.[239] The predominance of an eosinophilic infiltrate suggests that the cells are involved in actually controlling the progression of a parasitic infestation. The observation is further supported by the finding that antieosinophil antiserum blocks immunity to *Schistosoma mansoni* and *Trichinella spiralis* in mice.[240]

However, the possibility that such antisera may block neutrophils must be ruled out.[231] Eosinophils have been shown to be larvicidal to *S. mansoni* and *T. spiralis*;[241] however, neutrophils[242] and monocytes[243] are likewise capable of damaging these parasites. The damage of parasites by eosinophils appears to be more serious when these organisms are coated with antibody.[244] Actual attachment of eosinophils to parasites seems to be mediated by prior attachment of C3b to the parasite and subsequent attachment of the eosinophil to C3b via its C3b receptors.[245]

The direct damage to the parasite tegument may be via eosinophil peroxidase with production of toxic H_2O_2,[246] or via a toxic protein termed major basic protein (MBP).[247]

Eosinophil receptors for the Fc portion of IgE immunoglobulin are termed FcεR.[248] The FcεR receptors on eosinophils appear to be antigenically related to FcεR on lymphocytes,[249] as has been demonstrated with anti-FcεR antibodies. It appears that the affinity of IgE for FcεR is lower on lymphocytes and macrophages than it is on basophils and mast cells.[250] It is believed that eosinophils modulate anaphylactic reactions by ingesting IgE immune complexes.[251]

Furthermore, eosinophils release a variety of factors (arylsulfatase, phospholipase D, histaminase, prostaglandins, and MBP) capable of inhibiting mast cell mediators of hypersensitivity reactions.[241] Granules in eosinophils are very characteristic at the electron microscopic level. These granules have an electron-dense core and an electron-lucent matrix.[252] The granules are composed of a variety of proteins, among which are peroxidase[253] and MBP, an 11,000-dalton protein[254] that is highly toxic to schistosomules[247] and that enhances adherence of eosinophils to schistosomules.[255] MBP can also damage intestinal, splenic, and respiratory epithelium of mammalian origin,[256] which perhaps explains some of the tissue damage observed in hypersensitivity reactions where eosinophils are numerous.[256] Other proteins characteristic of eosinophils include the eosinophil cationic protein (ECP), which neutralizes heparin,[257] and the Charcot-Leyden crystal protein (CLC), which appears to be a lysophospholipase.[258]

Eosinopenia.— Acute infections, glucocorticoid therapy, epinephrine,[259] and prostaglandins[260] may all cause eosinopenia.

Eosinophilia.— Eosinophilia may be caused by a variety of diseases (Table 2–6).

In certain cases of eosinophilia arising from carcinomatosis, it has been possible to demonstrate a tumor-derived eosinophilopoietic factor.[262] At high dilutions, this factor was capable of stimulating the development of eosinophil colonies in vitro. Tu-

TABLE 2–6.—MAJOR CAUSES OF EOSINOPHILIA*

DISORDER	CAUSE
Parasitoses	Protozoans (e.g., amebiasis)
	Nematodes (e.g., trichinosis)
	Cestodes (e.g., cysticercosis)
	Arthropodes (e.g., scabies)
Allergy	Asthma, serum sickness (e.g.)
Dermatitis	Psoriasis, dermatitis herpetiformis (e.g.)
Gastrointestinal disease	Ulcerative colitis, regional enteritis (e.g.)
Malignancy	Hodgkin's disease, leukemia, melanoma (e.g.)
Other	Chronic renal disease, hypoadrenocorticism (e.g.)

*Modified from Zucker-Franklin.[261]

mor-associated eosinophilic factor has been characterized as a 45,000-dalton glycoprotein.[263]

It has been shown that the eosinophilic leukemoid reaction present in some tumors is associated with tumor necrosis, or wide dissemination of the tumor.[264]

Basophils and Mast Cells

Basophils are the least common of blood granulocytes (0.5% of the total leukocytes[265]). Ultrastructurally, basophils contain rounded to oval granules with characteristic dense particles and a less dense matrix.[266] Basophils originate from a common stem cell precursor which also gives rise to granulocytes and monocytes.[267] Most, if not all, mast cells originate in the bone marrow.[268] Basophils are mostly found in the circulation and, though similar in function, are distinct from mast cells.[269] The granules of basophils and mast cells contain sulfated glycosaminoglycans, one of which is heparin; however, the predominant glycosaminoglycan is chondroitin sulfate.[270] Basophils and mast cells have high affinity receptors for IgE (FcεR).[271] The binding of IgE to FcεR is greater to basophil and mast cell FcεR than to macrophage FcεR.[272] When basophils or mast cells sensitized with IgE or other antibodies bind specific antigen they rapidly degranulate, releasing histamine, serotonin, and other mediators of inflammation to the external milieu.[273]

It has been demonstrated by electron microscopy that the membrane coating the granules first binds to the plasma membrane, before exocytosis of granule content.[274]

Mediator release by basophils and mast cells may be antibody independent. In these circumstances, complement fragments, insect venoms, as well as certain drugs are capable of producing basophil degranulation.[275] Basophils possess about 170,000 receptors for IgE, but the number varies, depending on the serum IgE concentration.[276] This suggests that IgE levels may in some way determine the number of FcεR on these cells. Mast cells possess hormone receptors for hormones that modulate cyclic AMP (cAMP), such as β-adrenergic agonists,[277] prostaglandin (PGE$_2$), adenosine, and histamine.[278, 279]

One major difference between basophils and mast cells is that a 30-fold higher dose of anti-IgE is necessary to degranulate mast cells than to degranulate basophils.[280] The larger, more mature cells display a greater sensitivity to the stimulus produced by aggregated IgE and degranulate readily, whereas the smaller cells appear to be more immature.[277] IgE cross-linking on the surface of rat mast cells produces a rapid increase in cAMP[281] which is inversely related to histamine release; however, this phenomenon is not present in humans,[277] which suggests that the second signal following IgE aggregation to degranulation is not cAMP in human mast cells. Other mediators with a proinflammatory effect are lypoxygenase metabolites or arachidonic acid,[282] such as 5-hydroperoxyeicosatetraenoic acid (5-HPETE), which have a histamine release effect.[283]

Basophilopenia.—Basophilopenia occurs in situations similar to eosinopenia, such as infection and neoplasia,[284] and is often associated with an elevated level of circulatory steroids.

Basophilia.—Basophilia is associated with a number of disorders (Table 2–7).

Monocytes, Lymphocytes, and Plasma Cells

The more salient characteristics of monocytes, lymphocytes and plasma cells are reviewed in chapter 4. However, to complete this discussion of normal blood cells, a succinct discussion is given below.

Monocytes.—Monocytes may be considered precursors of macrophages. They are adherent to glass, similarly to macrophages, and if cultured may mature into cells indistinguishable from mac-

TABLE 2–7.—Diseases Associated With an Increase in Circulating Basophils*

DISEASE	EXAMPLES
Allergic	Drugs and foods
Inflammatory	
Digestive tract	Ulcerative colitis
Autoimmune	Rheumatoid arthritis
Endocrine disease	Diabetes, myxedema
Infections	
Viral	Influenza, chicken pox
Mycobacterial	Tuberculosis
Neoplasia	
Carcinoma	Various types
Leukemia	Myelogenous leukemia
Mastocytosis	

*Modified from Zucker-Franklin D.: Basophilopenia, basophilia and mastocytosis, in Williams W.J., et al. (eds.): *Hematology.* New York, McGraw-Hill Book Co., 1983, p. 828.

rophages obtained from other sites. As such, these cells exhibit immunoglobulin Fc receptors as well as complement receptors. Their function is mainly presenting antigen to immunocytes and phagocytosis. Monocytes are medium to large cells (12–15 μ). They stain positively with nonspecific esterases not inhibited by sodium fluoride, in contrast to esterases found in neutrophils, which are inhibited by these substances.[285]

Lymphocytes.—Lymphocytes are the main cells involved in the immune response both at the humoral level and at the cellular level.[286] They are mononuclear cells which may exhibit round or indented nuclei with condensed chromatin. Nucleoli are usually absent in these cells. The cytoplasm is characteristically scant and stains light blue with Wright's stain. Few azurophilic granules can be detected in them. Their diameter may vary, but is usually about 10 μ. There is evidence that lymphocytes originate from a different stem cell in the marrow than do myeloid elements. Lymphocytes can be segregated into at least two populations, T (thymus-derived) and B cells (derived from the bursa equivalent in humans). The functions of these cells are discussed in chapter 4.[286]

Plasma Cells.—Plasma cells are basophilic cells measuring 9–20 μ with an excentric nucleus and a perinuclear halo. The nuclear chromatin exhibits a characteristic cartwheel appearance. The perinuclear halo is the Golgi apparatus.[286] These cells have a very developed endoplasmic reticulum, adapted to the synthesis and secretion of immunoglobulins. They are thought to represent the end stage of development of B lymphocytes and exhibit abundant cytoplasmic immunoglobulin. Mature plasma cells do not have surface receptors for immunoglobulin but contain abundant immunoglobulin in their cytoplasm.[287]

WBC Pathology

Congenital and Acquired Abnormalities of Granulocytes

The more important granulocyte abnormalities include defects in mobility, granule structure, and the enzymes contained in them. These defects may result in an increased susceptibility to infection due to defective phagocytosis and killing by granulocytes.

Morphological Changes.—Döhle bodies are gray-blue cytoplasmic inclusions that have been shown by electron microscopy to be lamellar aggregates of rough endoplasmic reticulum containing RNA.[288] Döhle bodies are found in granulocytes of patients with severe infections,[289] severe burns,[290] and advanced neoplastic disease, and in patients treated with cyclophosphamide.[291] Structures similar to Döhle bodies are seen in the May-Hegglin anomaly, a rare autosomal dominant disease.[292] The endoplasmic structures in the May-Hegglin anomaly also seem to contain RNA.[293] Giant platelets with an abnormal survival time are another attribute of the syndrome.[294]

In the Alder-Reilly anomaly, granulocytes show large, coarse cytoplasmic granules. These result from disorders of polysaccharide metabolism, such as Hurler's disease and Morquio's syndrome.[295] The basic defect in these syndromes is the altered degradation of protein-carbohydrate complexes, resulting in accumulation of incompletely degraded mucopolysaccharides in lysosomes.[295]

Chédiak-Higashi Syndrome.—The Chédiak-Higashi syndrome is a rare familial disease characterized by partial albinism, photophobia, and severe recurrent infections.[296] Massive intracellular inclusions are present in granulocytes as well as other tissues such as epithelial cells of the gastric mucosa, small intestine, and pancreas. The leukocyte inclusions are 2–4 μ in diameter. In Chédiak-Higashi neutrophils, the granules are very much like those seen in normal cells and contain myeloperoxidase in nonspecific azurophilic granules,[297] lactoferrin and lysozyme in specific granules.[298] The neutrophils display abnormal chemotaxis[299] as well as bactericidal activities.[300]

A delayed fusion of phagocytic vacuoles into a phagosome is also observed in the neutrophils and other phagocytic cells of these patients.[301] A deficiency in the microtubular mechanism of the cell may be responsible for some of these defects.[302] The abnormal granules are formed during maturation of the cells by progressive aggregation and fusion of initially normally formed granules.[298] It was initially thought that the abnormal chemotaxis was due merely to a mechanical defect caused by the size of the granules, but it has been shown since that these cells are metabolically ineffective as well.[303]

In affected patients, IgE antibodies against *S. aureus* were described. In contrast, IgE-normal individuals infected with *S. aureus* do not usually possess IgE-anti-*S. aureus* antibodies.[304, 305] This was demonstrated showing IgE binding to *S. aureus* Wood, which does not have protein A and thus does not bind Fc from immunoglobulins nonspecifically. These antibodies were directed against the cell wall protein peptidoglycan.[306]

Patients with the hyperimmunoglobulin E syndrome are very susceptible to staphylococcal infections by *S. aureus* and *C. albicans*.[304] Furthermore, these patients have markedly abnormal hypersensitivity on skin testing,[307] and abnormal lymphocyte proliferative responses.[308] It must be noted, however, that some patients with increased IgE and atopic eczema with a significant skin colonization by *S. aureus* may not develop severe infections.[304]

Patients with the hyperimmunoglobulin E syndrome have neutrophils with a markedly altered chemotactic response.[307] This could explain to a certain degree their susceptibility to infections.

Chronic Granulomatous Disease of Childhood

Chronic granulomatous disease (CGD) of childhood is a lethal X-linked disease affecting mostly male infants.[309] Occasionally autosomal inheritance has been demonstrated.[310] Measurement of postphagocytic release of $^{14}CO_2$ from glucose-1-^{14}C or reduction of nitroblue tetrazolium can be used to detect the defect in neutrophils and to screen for female heterozygotes, who have a milder disease (Table 2-8).[310]

The disease is characterized by severe infections caused by otherwise low-grade pathogens such as *Serratia marcescens* or by pathogens such as staphylococci.[311] These patients develop eczematoid granulomatous skin lesions and purulent infections. These infections resolve slowly and many times incompletely. Most often the patient dies during childhood,[312] but survival into adolescence has been described,[313] and milder forms have been reported in adults.[314] Normally phagocytosis is accompanied by increased anaerobic glycolysis and consumption of ATP, a respiratory oxidative burst with production of H_2O_2 toxic to bacteria. In CGD, however, there is reduced oxygen uptake by phagocytes during phagocytosis and a reduced shift to the hexose monophosphate shunt, with a resulting low accumulation of H_2O_2 and hence a decreased bactericidal activity in the phagosome.[315, 316] Neutrophils and monocytes are both affected in this syndrome.[317] Interestingly, pneumococci and streptococci, which are catalase-negative bacteria, are capable of producing H_2O_2, which is autotoxic to bacteria in phagosomes.[318] Patients with CGD are especially susceptible to fungal infections. In one series of 245 patients, 20% had fungal infection, most often by *Aspergillus* pneumonia.[319]

CGD in Immunohematology

A remarkable association between CGD and the absence of Kell antigens on RBCs has been described.[320] Two types of CGD can be defined, based on the presence or absence of the Kx antigen: Type I CGD, in which RBCs and WBCs have normal Kx antigens,[321] and type II CGD, in which the Kx antigens are greatly weakened.[320] The finding led to the assumption that Kell antigens in some way were necessary for the adequate function of granulocytes.[322]

However, a Kx-negative individual with normal neutrophil function has been reported.[323] This finding suggests that the genes responsible for CGD are closely linked but distinct from Kell antigen genes and that the antigens are not essential to granulocyte function. Both genes are located on the X chromosome.[324] Patients with the McLeod syndrome (very weak Kx) have acanthocytic RBCs and may present with hemolytic anemia.[325] Although the exact membrane abnormality of RBCs has not been determined in the McLeod syndrome, the RBCs do show a defect in permeability to water.[326]

Abnormalities in cells other than RBCs are likewise present in the McLeod syndrome. In one series of 11 patients with the McLeod syndrome but without CGD, all had high CPK-MM isoenzymes.[327] In some of these patients microscopic evidence of muscle damage was found. Patients with the McLeod syndrome associated with CGD may or may not have elevated enzyme levels.[327]

The absence of Kell antigens on RBCs of some patients with CGD may cause severe problems in terms of providing compatible blood for transfusion.[328] Another disease associated with CGD is

TABLE 2-8.—NITROBLUE TETRAZOLIUM SCREEN FOR CHRONIC GRANULOMATOUS DISEASE*

POPULATION	% POSITIVE NBT CELLS
Normals	90
Nonaffected father, sister, brother	75
Carrier sister	50
Heterozygote	50
Hemizygote (CGD patient)	10

*Data modified from Windhorst et al.[310]

systemic lupus erythematosus in mothers of CGD patients.[329]

Treatment for CGD is basically supportive and symptomatic. Granulocyte transfusions provide only transient benefit and should be reserved exclusively for emergencies, where they can be life-saving.[330] Nevertheless, these transfusions may cause the development of hemolytic transfusion reactions due to sensitization to Kell antigens.[328] A hope for curing these patients is the use of bone marrow transplantation. A successful bone marrow transplant with an unrelated HLA-compatible bone marrow donor prior to ablation with cyclophosphamide has been reported.[331]

Other Diseases Associated With Neutrophil Function Abnormalities

Patients with mannosidosis,[332] ichtiosis,[333] and G6PD deficiency[334] may have chemotactic and microbicidal defects in their neutrophils.

Quantitative Disorders of Neutrophils.

—Normal adults have from 3,000–8,000 neutrophils/μl. Counts below 500/μl are considered to indicate agranulocytosis. Infection is an important clinical complication of granulocytopenia, but the susceptibility to infectious disease is variable: patients with 200 or fewer cells per microliter have survived years without serious infections.[335] A compensatory monocytosis is present in these patients, and the defense mechanisms are shifted to these cells.[335]

The etiology of agranulocytosis is obscure. However, it has been shown that different causative agents will affect granulocyte kinetics in various stages (Table 2–9). Furthermore, a causative classification can be combined with a kinetic classification (Table 2–10).

The salient etiologic agents or conditions will be discussed briefly.

Noncommitted Stem Cell Neutropenia.

—*Reticular dysgenesis* is a congenital immunologic defect with severe neutropenia and low serum immunoglobulins. The defect is at the level of the pluripotential stem cells.[338] The bone marrow is devoid of hemopoietic cells, and death is due to bacterial infection.[338]

Hereditary T and B cell disorders with neutropenia may be autosomal dominant[339] or X-linked[340] disease. There is severe persistent neutropenia, with lack of maturation beyond the myelocyte stage in

TABLE 2–9.—Classification of Neutropenia According to Etiology

TYPE	EXAMPLE	KINETICS
HEREDITARY		
Stem cell disorders	Reticular dysgenesis	I
T and B lymphocytic disorder	Disgammaglobulinemia	I
Progenitor cell disorder	Infantile genetic agranulocytosis	I, II
ACQUIRED		
Stem cell disorder	Preleukemia	I, II
T and B lymphocytic disorder	Chronic hypoplastic neutropenia	I, II
Progenitor cell disorder	Severe bacterial sepsis	I–IV
	Mycobacterial infections	
Autoimmune	Autoimmune neutropenia	III, IV
	SLE	III, IV
DRUG-INDUCED		
Analgesics	Aminopyrine	III
	Aspirin	?
Antibiotics	Ampicillin	I
	Cephalothin	I, III
Sulfonamides	Sulfisoxazole	I
Anticonvulsants	Diphenylhydantoin	I, III
Antihistamines	Cimetidine	I
Anti-inflammatories	Indomethacin	I
Antimalarials	Hydrochloroquine	I
Cardiovascular	Quinidine	I
Diuretics	Chlorothiazide	I

*Data from Howard et al.[336]

TABLE 2–10.—CLASSIFICATION OF NEUTROPENIAS
ACCORDING TO CELL KINETICS

Type I: Reduced neutrophil production (e.g., drug-induced: alkylating agents, antibiotics)
Type II: Intramedullary destruction of granulocytes (e.g., drug-induced: methotrexate, diphenylhydantoin)
Type III: Reduced neutrophil survival (e.g., sepsis, hypersplenism, autoimmune neutropenia)
Type IV: Combined (I, II, III)
Type V: Pseudoneutropenia (e.g., due to shifts of neutrophils to tissues)

*Modified from Finch.[337]

the bone marrow.[339] There may be an increase in circulating immunoglobulins, but it is usually at the expense of increased IgM or IgA.[341]

Cyclic neutropenia is an autosomal dominant inherited defect of bone marrow stem cells which usually appears in childhood.[342] Affected patients undergo cycles of infections occurring about every 21 days, with severe neutropenia, fever, adenitis, and skin infections. Mucosal infections are also present and can lead to severe complications such as intestinal perforation.[343] The use of steroids has been beneficial in selected cases.[344] Interestingly, the syndrome has a tendency to occur in gray collie dogs and has become the experimental model for this disease.[345]

Progenitor "Committed Stem Cell Neutropenias."—*Infantile genetic agranulocytosis (Kostmann's disease)* is an autosomal recessive disease, showing linkage with certain HLA phenotypes.[346] Stem cells mature to the myelocyte stage and produce normal numbers of colony-forming units, but normal maturation is impaired.[347] Death from this disorder is usually during childhood due to fatal infections, but prolonged survival has been described on occasion,[348] although leukemia has developed as a complication in these cases.[348] Antibiotic therapy improves survival. Bone marrow transplantation has corrected the agranulocytosis in certain cases.[349]

Acquired Stem Cell Disorders Leading to Neutropenia.—*Preleukemia* may give rise to neutropenia[350] as well as other malignant disorders involving replacement of bone marrow, such as lymphoma, myeloma, myelofibrosis, and carcinoma.

Acquired Committed Stem Cell (Progenitor Cell) Disorders.—Acquired chronic neutropenia, previously termed idiopathic neutropenia, may represent an incapacity of neutrophils to mobilize to sites of inflammation. A defective granulopoiesis[351] or altered marrow release mechanisms[352] may be the cause of these neutropenias.

Neutropenia of Infections.—Bacterial sepsis may induce a significant neutropenia,[353] as well as disseminated mycobacterial infections.[354] Viral infections have likewise induced severe neutropenia. Examples of these are hepatitis,[355] infectious mononucleosis,[356] and Kawasaki's disease.[357] Megaloblastic anemias may be accompanied by neutropenia, probably due to ineffective myelopoiesis.[358]

Immune-Mediated Neutropenias.—Antibodies against neutrophils produce neutropenia either by destroying cells in the periphery or by destroying intramedullary precursor cells.[359]

Isoimmune neonatal neutropenia is due to the passage of IgG antineutrophil maternal antibodies across the placenta.[360] These antibodies are produced by the mother prior to placental passage of granulocytes into the maternal circulation.[361] The mother then produces antineutrophil-specific antibodies against NA[362] and NB neutrophil antigens.[363] In one series, anti-NB1 was the most frequently found antibody, and anti-NA1 was the next most frequently found antibody.[364] In a prospective study of 200 pregnant women, 3% had antibodies against their husband's granulocytes.[365] The groups currently described are NA1, NA2, NB1, ND1, and NE1 as well as polymorphic HGA-3.[366]

Autoimmune Neutropenia.—Acquired autoimmune neutropenia caused by an anti-NA2 was first described in a 7-month-old child.[367] The bone marrow contained progenitor cells, but only 3% neutrophils were seen in the periphery. Anti-NB1 antibodies have also been shown to cause autoimmune neutropenia,[368, 369] and a new anti-ND1 auto-antibody has also been shown to produce neutropenia.[370] Treatment with steroids has been achieved[367] but steroids should be used with extreme caution because of possible enhancement of pre-existing infections due to the neutropenia. Plasmapheresis may be used in selected cases of neonatal isoimmune neutropenia[371] and in autoimmune neutropenias.

Acquired Pseudoneutropenia.—Pseudoneutropenia may be the result of hypersensitivity, severe endotoxemia, and other immune mediated mechanisms such as complement activation with release into the fluid phase of C5a, a potent chemoattractant, resulting in leukocyte margination and pseudoleukopenia.[372] It is believed that the development of transient neutropenia during filtration leukapheresis may be induced by liberation of C5a by neutrophils.[373] This phenomenon can be observed in hemodialysis[374] and cardiopulmonary bypass.[375] During cardiopulmonary bypass C3a increases but not C5a. Following recovery from bypass, C5-activated granulocytes may be trapped in the pulmonary capillaries, producing pseudoneutropenia.[375]

Drug-Induced Neutropenia.—Agranulocytosis is a severe disease with a mortality ranging from 5% to 20%, depending on the time of initiation of antibiotic therapy to combat infections.[376]

Agranulocytosis is probably the most common of severe drug reactions, accounting for about 40% of all severe drug reactions.[377] Two types of onset can be identified, an indolent slow onset, usually caused by direct injury to marrow cells, and a rapid onset, immune mediated type of neutropenia.

The direct injury to marrow cells is evident in many chemotherapeutic regimens for the treatment of neoplasia. Antimetabolite chemotherapy is currently the most important cause of neutropenia in these protocols. Chemotherapeutic drugs probably affect pluripotential stem cells directly in the marrow. Other drugs such as phenothiazines also affect granulocytes at the stem cell level. For instance, chlorpromazine inhibits nucleic acid synthesis in vitro in granulocytes of susceptible individuals.[378] The second mechanism is that affecting marrow and peripheral cells on an immune basis. This immune response is variable from individual to individual. This susceptibility has a genetic basis. For instance, individuals with HLA-B27 in their phenotype and who suffer from rheumatoid arthritis are at risk of developing agranulocytosis when treated with levamisole.[379]

The exact mechanism for destruction of granulocytes by antibody has not been completely elucidated due to technical problems in assessing these antibody-mediated effects in vitro. It is quite possible that cell destruction by antibodies is multifactorial, like drug-mediated autoimmune hemolytic anemia. Possibly drugs act as haptens, binding to the neutrophil membrane. Another mechanism may be formation of soluble immune complexes with activation of complement, and neutrophil injury as an "innocent bystander" effect.[380, 381]

With newer technology, the process of cell destruction by antibodies in immune mediated neutropenia can be elucidated.[382]

Bone marrow recovery usually occurs a few days after the drug is discontinued. Neutrophil counts increase with peripheralization of immature forms, a picture that may resemble leukemia.[383] Phenothiazines and chlorpromazine have been frequently involved in inducing neutropenia;[377] recently introduced semisynthetic antibiotics such as oxacillin, cloxacillin, nafcillin, and methicillin are also frequent inducers of neutropenia.[384] Chloramphenicol induces arrest of bone marrow colony growth when given in therapeutic doses.[385] The mortality from cloramphenicol-induced neutropenia may reach 50%.[386]

An extensive list of other therapeutic agents that cause neutropenia is available[337] and will not be reproduced here. However, the more common causes of neutropenia are listed in Table 2–9, and clinical findings are given in Table 2–11.

Management of Patients With Neutropenia.—Cross-contamination in a hospital environment should be prevented by careful adherence to infection control procedures such as wearing a mask when near the patient and hand-washing before physical examination of the patient. Fever in these patients usually announces the presence of infection.[387] The more frequent bacteria found in infections of granulocytopenic patients are S. aureus and gram-negative bacteria.[388]

Therapy may include empirical antibiotic therapy with intravenous ticarcillin disodium and gentamicin.[388] Granulocyte transfusion may be considered in cases where antibiotic response has been ineffective (see chapter 8).

Splenectomy and glucocorticoids have been used in chronic neutropenias, with little or no success.[389] Lithium carbonate stimulates stem cells and may be

TABLE 2–11.—COMMON FINDINGS IN NEUTROPENIA PATIENTS*

FREQUENT CLINICAL PRESENTATION
  Cutaneous abscesses
  Furunculosis
  Pneumonia
  Septicemia

COMMONLY ISOLATED ORGANISMS
  S. aureus
  P. aeruginosa
  E. coli
  Klebsiella sp.

*Data from Howard et al.[336]

of value in cases of agranulocytosis; however it is a toxic substance, and its long-term effects are unknown.[390]

Pancytopenia.—Many of the causes of neutropenia, such as aleukemic leukemia, bone marrow replacement by other neoplasms, and infectious diseases, also produce pancytopenia. The main causes are summarized in Table 2–12. Pancytopenia should be regarded as a complex syndrome resulting in the peripheral blood disease of RBCs, WBCs, and platelets. The possible pathogenesis is summarized in Table 2–13. Although many cases are irreversible, some patients do recover.[409] Fatal infections are a dreaded complication. Carbenicillin and cephalothin are used prophylactically to avert infection. When infections are present, they are treated with selected antibiotics after testing for organism sensitivities.

The bone marrow may be hypoplastic or hyperplastic, depending on the etiology and pathogenesis of the syndrome. Aplastic anemia and pure RBC aplasia were discussed at the beginning of this chapter.

Neutrophilia.—Neutrophilia is an increase in the peripheral WBC count above 7,500/µl. Leukocytosis is usually a response to inflammation.[410] An extreme benign granulocytic proliferation may result in a leukemoid reaction, which is difficult to differentiate from leukemia even with bone marrow aspiration.[411] The mechanisms of neutrophilia are summarized in Table 2–14. Neutrophilia may be stimulated by a variety of factors. A rapid neutrophilia occurs after exercise, stress, and other factors. Adrenalin may be a common triggering substance in these conditions,[414] but this assumption has not been conclusively proved.

Inflammation, infection, and steroids cause a more gradual increase in neutrophils, probably due to release of neutrophils from the marrow, possibly due to humoral releasing factors[415, 416] such as complement components. Glucocorticoids by themselves can stimulate neutrophilia.[417] This characteristic has been used to improve granulocyte yields during leukapheresis. Additional causes of neutrophilia are myocardial infarction and other diseases causing tissue necrosis. Extreme neutrophilia resulting in a leukemoid reaction can be seen in disseminated tuberculosis[418] and neoplasias, such as bronchogenic carcinoma[419] and renal carcinoma.[420] This type of tumor may produce a leukoerythroblastic type of leukemoid reaction, with an increase in nucleated RBCs. Neonatal leukocytosis has been described in Down's syndrome.[421] A rare type of hereditary neutrophilia has also been described.[422] The leukemoid reaction may be present after severe hemolysis. A good test to differentiate a leukemoid reaction from leukemia is the leukocyte alkaline phosphatase test, which is normal in leukemoid reactions.[423]

Lymphocytosis.—Lymphocytosis is considered to exist when the lymphocyte count is above 4,000/µl, although this value may vary with age.

TABLE 2–12.—MAIN CAUSES OF PANCYTOPENIA

BONE MARROW INFILTRATION
  Leukemia, lymphoma, myeloma[391]
  Carcinoma[392]
  Myelofibrosis[393]
  Osteopetrosis[394]

HYPERSPLENISM
  Congestive splenomegaly[395]
  Splenic lymphoma[396]
  Lipid storage diseases[397]
  Infectious: kala-azar, disseminated mycobacterial infection[398]

VITAMIN DEFICIENCIES
  Pernicious anemia[399]

OTHER
  Paroxysmal nocturnal hemoglobinuria[400]
  Systemic lupus erythematosus[401]
  Aplastic anemia[402]
  Toxic substances: benzene,[403] ionizing radiation,[404] hair dyes[405]

TABLE 2–13.—PATHOGENESIS OF PANCYTOPENIA

Ineffective hematopoiesis[406]
Defective cell formation with subsequent destruction[391] in the periphery
Immune-mediated destruction (e.g., aplastic anemia due to drugs)[407]
Trapping of normal cells by hypertrophied RES[408]

TABLE 2–14.—MECHANISMS OF NEUTROPHILIA

Mobilization from marrow or storage pools[412]
Increased neutrophil survival due to immaturity[410]
Increased granulopoiesis due to:[413]
  Increased stem cell differentiation
  Shortening of mytotic cell cycles
  Stimulation of resting neutrophilic cells

TABLE 2–15.—MAJOR CAUSES
OF LYMPHOCYTOSIS

VIRAL
  CMV[424]
  Infectious lymphocytosis[425]
  EBV (infectious mononucleosis)[426]

BACTERIAL
  Bordetella pertussis[427]
  Toxoplasma gondii[428]
  Brucellosis[429]
  Hypersensitivity reactions

NEOPLASTIC
  Lymphocytic leukemia

ENDOCRINE
  Thyrotoxicosis

Causes of absolute lymphocytosis are listed in Table 2–15. The lymphocytosis observed in whooping cough is caused by the production of a substance termed lymphocytosis-promoting factor, responsible for the redistribution of lymphocytes, which results in a peripheral lymphocytosis.[426]

Lymphocytopenia.—Lymphocyte counts below 1,500/µl are considered lymphocytopenic; in children a count below 3,000/µl is considered abnormal. The mechanisms producing lymphocytopenia can be secondary to decreased production, increased destruction, or increased loss (Table 2–16).

TABLE 2–16.—MAJOR CAUSES OF
LYMPHOCYTOPENIA

DECREASED PRODUCTION
  Immune deficiencies (e.g., DiGeorge syndrome, ataxia telangiectasia)
  Aplastic anemia
  Disseminated carcinoma
  Disseminated infection
  Hodgkin's disease

INCREASED DESTRUCTION
  Irradiation
  Chemotherapy
  Steroid therapy

INCREASED LOSS
  Thoracic duct drainage
  Whipple's disease

OTHER
  Sarcoid
  SLE

*Modified from Cassileth.[430]

NEOPLASTIC DISORDERS OF HEMATOPOIETIC CELLS: THE LEUKEMIAS

Preleukemia

Preleukemia is a preneoplastic condition that may result in acute leukemia in about 25% of cases[431] manifested as acute myelogenous leukemia (AML) or rarely as acute lymphocytic leukemia (ALL). It is currently thought that about 31% of AML cases have a preleukemic stage,[432] although in one series, up to 50% of cases of AML prospectively studied had a preleukemic stage.[433] The preleukemic syndrome can be manifested in a variety of manners (Table 2–17). It usually occurs in men in the sixth decade,[434] but it has been reported in children.[435] The etiology of preleukemia is unknown, but it is quite possible that there is a "promoter" phase wherein a virus is introduced in the genome, probably an RNA virus.[443] The tumor may subsequently be "initiated" by initiator factors such as radiation or carcinogens.[444] It is thought that the lesion occurs at the stem cell level, where a stem cell develops a clonal expansion, as demonstrated by single G6PD preleukemic cells from a heterozygous individual with G6PDA and B.[445] The preleukemic syndrome may be initially asymptomatic but may also appear as anemia, which is present in 85% of cases.[446] Predisposing diseases and factors are listed in Table 2–18. Abnormalities in RBC maturation are seen and include the appearance of nucleated RBCs in the periphery, increased Hb F,[458] and, rarely, acquired Hb H disease.[459] On occasion preleukemic states result in expression of "i" antigen on RBCs, or in loss of ABH antigens from RBCs.[460] Neutropenia occurs in about 50% of cases,[461] and neutrophils may exhibit abnormal chemotaxis and phagocytosis.[462] Thrombocytopenia is present in 25% of cases.[463]

TABLE 2–17.—PRELEUKEMIC SYNDROME

INEFFECTIVE HEMOPOIESIS
  Pancytopenia with marrow hyperplasia[436]
  Refractory sideroblastic[437] or nonsideroblastic anemia[438]

HYPOPLASTIC HEMOPOIESIS
  Hypoplastic neutropenia[439]
  Aplastic anemia[440]
  Paroxysmal nocturnal hemoglobinuria[441]

OLIGOBLASTIC LEUKEMIAS[442]

TABLE 2–18.—CONDITIONS LEADING TO PRELEUKEMIA OR LEUKEMIA

HEMATOLOGIC DISEASE THAT MAY CONVERT TO LEUKEMIA
    Polycythemia vera (especially after treatment with chlorambucil)[447]
    Myelofibrosis[448]
    Fanconi's anemia[449]
    Paroxysmal nocturnal hemoglobinuria[450]
    Hodgkin's disease[451]
    Aplastic anemia[452]

NONHEMATOLOGIC DISEASE THAT MAY CONVERT TO LEUKEMIA
    Down's syndrome,[449] Bloom's syndrome[449]
    Various congenital immunodeficiencies[453]

THERAPEUTIC REGIMENS THAT ARE OFTEN COMPLICATED BY LEUKEMIC TRANSFORMATION
    Chemotherapy for tumors or to induce immune suppression[454]
    Patients who are immunosuppressed for transplantation[455]

AGENTS PROVED TO BE LEUKEMOGENIC
    Ionizing radiation[456]
    Benzene[457]

Neutrophils may exhibit the Pelger-Huët anomaly,[464] present in 10%–20% of cases.[465] The neutrophils in these patients may have abnormal leukocyte alkaline phosphatase as well as poorly formed specific and nonspecific cytoplasmic granules.[466] Auer rods are not seen. A compensatory monocytosis is usually present. In the marrow, RBC precursors may appear as megaloblastoid; sideroblasts may be present. However, the presence of blasts in the marrow will determine the course to overt leukemia. Patients with 10%–40% blasts most frequently develop subsequent leukemia.[467]

Colony-forming units for neutrophils and monocytes may be increased on culturing marrow on soft agar.[468] The rate of transformation from a preleukemic state to overt leukemia is difficult to predict. However, about 10% of patients with sideroblastic anemias eventually develop overt AML.[469] About 50% of patients with pancytopenia develop AML. Chromosome alterations in patients with preleukemia have been reported. Up to 30% of patients in a series of 80 suspected preleukemics had abnormal chromosome morphology.[470] These studies have a prognostic significance; 81% of patients with preleukemia and chromosomal abnormalities eventually develop acute nonlymphocytic leukemia (ANLL), whereas only 37% of preleukemics with normal chromosomal studies develop ANLL.[470] The more frequent abnormal chromosomes in preleukemics are monosomy of chromosome 7, trisomy of chromosomes 8, 9, and 21 and the long arm of chromosome 1 (1q), deletions of chromosome 5 and 20 (5q−, 20q−)[471] or deletions of chromosome 21, and isochromosome 17 (iso 17q).[470] Chromosomal abnormalities are more frequent in sideroblastic anemias.[472] Deletions of chromosome 21 may be associated with primary thrombocythemia.[473]

Translocation of t(8;21) is frequent in M2 type of leukemias, whereas this abnormality is rarely seen in preleukemia.[470]

Patients with preleukemic syndromes are best managed conservatively, with RBC transfusions to control anemia. Chemotherapy may be used in certain cases[474] but its use is controversial because many patients with preleukemia never develop leukemia.[455] Recently a treatment consisting of a continuous infusion of low-dose cytarabine has been shown to improve peripheral blood counts of RBCs, WBCs, and platelets.[475] However, the group studied was small, and more evidence is needed to assess the validity of this treatment. Cytarabine appears to slow down DNA replication, allowing terminal differentiation to occur in the diseased cells.[476] In selected cases bone marrow transplantation may be considered in young patients with preleukemia.[477]

Chronic Myelogenous Leukemia

Chronic myelogenous leukemia (CML) is more common in men than women (57:43 ratio) and accounts for about 1 death per 100,000 population per year.[478] In the West, it accounts for about 20% of all cases of leukemia.[478] Its peak incidence is between the fourth and fifth decades.[479]

CML is a neoplastic disorder of hemopoietic stem cells[478] which, in about 90% of the cases, gives rise to cells that carry the group G, Philadelphia chromosome (Ph^1). This abnormality represents a deletion of about 50% of the long arm of chromosome 22[480] that is then translocated to chromosome 9.[481] Thus, in the new nomenclature, the translocation is written as t(9+, 22q−).[482] However, the 22q can be rarely translocated to other chromosomes.[483] The deletion in Ph^1 is distinct from the Down's syndrome 22− deletion[484] and is not usually present in other myeloproliferative disorders.[480] Ph^1 arises from a balanced translocation between the long arms of chromosome 9 and q11 in chromosome 22.[485] Immature and mature myeloid cells accumulate in the blood and bone marrow. Hepatosplenomegaly results from a compensatory extramedullary hemopoiesis due to a bone marrow "crowding" effect.

Etiologic Agents Associated With CML

Radiation exposure is a well-documented risk factor in the development of CML, (radiologists have about a ninefold higher risk of developing leukemia than physicians not routinely exposed to ionizing radiation[486]). Likewise, survivors of atomic bomb explosions have a high incidence of CML, but not their progeny.[487]

Patients irradiated therapeutically for several diseases such as ankylosing spondilitis have a higher incidence of CML than the general population.[488] The exact mechanism by which ionizing radiation induces leukemia is not known. A variety of factors have been shown to play a role in producing the disease, including modifying factors such as direct and indirect cell damage, hormonal factors, and activation of dormant viral agents.[478] A potentially good candidate is Epstein-Barr virus (EBV), which has been linked to Burkitt's lymphoma.[489] EBV transformation of B cells has been achieved in vitro.[489] T cells appear to block proliferation of B cells infected with EBV, and this block is HLA dependent.[490] Research conducted with molecular probes has suggested that a cellular gene, C-abl, similar to v-abl (a murine leukemia virus termed the Abelson virus), can be located in the fragment translocated from chromosome 9 to chromosome 22.[491] In spite of this evidence, not more than 0.5% of individuals exposed to high doses of ionizing radiation develop CML.[492] In animals, leukemia has been induced in CBA mice at fairly low doses of radiation.[493]

Benzene, as in preleukemia, has also been found to induce CML after heavy occupational exposure.[494] This is seen especially in patients who develope benzene-induced neutropenia prior to overt leukemia and who have WBC chromosomal abnormalities.[495]

The monoclonality of the CML neoplastic myeloid stem cells has been demonstrated by showing that the affected cells (granulocytes, erythrocytes, and monocytes as well as macrophages) had a single G6PD.[496] This monoclonality holds true for most cases, although new clones may appear late in the disease.[497]

It is very possible that the factors producing CML affect a primordial stem cell. Evidence for this idea is that some of the cells type positively for terminal deoxynucleotydil transferase (TdT), a T cell marker (see Chap. 4).[498]

Thus, transformation of CML, which is usually in the direction of granulocytic cells, or erythroid cells in erythroblastic transformation,[499] can, in certain cases, give rise to lymphoblastic leukemia.[500] This has been shown to occur in about 20% of cases of CML in transformation,[501] and can also give rise to lymphoblasts with Ph^1,[502] a change usually seen in myeloid cells. Furthermore, pre-B lymphocyte markers such as lymphoblastic leukemia antigen and Ia antigens are seen on cells bearing Ph^1.[503] In addition, about 25% of ALL patients exhibit Ph^1,[504] a sign of poor prognosis in some series.[505]

Using DNA probes, it has been shown that cells of chronic myelogenous leukemia undergoing lymphoid blast crises have heavy chain rearrangement expressing not only their B cell lineage, but different stages in B cell maturation.[506] The myeloid cell series, however, retain germ-like immunoglobulin genes which are not "turned on" at the time.

Neoplastic cells in CML, regardless of their lineage, may display better survival than normal cells in spite of their early stage of maturity.[507] It is quite possible that Ph^1-negative cells in CML are not leukemic and develop normally.[508] This concept is the basis for eradicating Ph^1-positive cells during treatment.[508] Occasionally chronic neutrophilic leukemia has been reported. This type of leukemia appears as a leukemoid reaction, with mostly mature granulocytes in the periphery.[509]

Clinical Presentation of CML

Malaise, weight loss, bone aches, and upper abdominal discomfort with hepatosplenomegaly are frequent presenting signs and symptoms. Bleeding, ecchymosis, and other signs of thrombocytopenia may also be initial or early signs and symptoms of CML. Hypercellularity of the bone marrow may cause demineralization of short bones, as well as other osteolytic lesions detectable by x-rays. Severe anorexia and weight loss are frequently seen in untreated patients or in relapses. The course with treatment runs approximately 1–4 years, depending on the number of relapses and the length of the remissions. By 5 years, blast crises have occurred in 70% of patients—about 50% of the peripheral cells may be blasts. Relapses are progressively more difficult to control.

Laboratory Findings

The WBC count is usually elevated over $50 \times 10^9/L$. The peripheral smear reveals a variety of myeloid cells at different stages of maturation. An absolute basophilia is usually present; however, the presence of markedly increased eosinophils and basophils is a poor prognostic sign.[492] Pronounced increases in the platelet count are found in 30%–40% of patients,[510] but the platelet count is decreased in 10% of patients.[511] The peripheral blood will show mostly neutrophilic cells, at all stages of development (i.e., myelocytes, promyelocytes, metamyelocytes, bands, and segmented cells). Myeloblasts and promyelocytes should not exceed 10% of the count.[511] The leukocyte alkaline phosphatase (LAP) score, normally 15%–70%, is markedly decreased or absent in 80%–90% of cases,[512] due to a net decrease in the quantity of LAP rather than to a qualitative defect.[513]

Myeloperoxidase detection identifies primary granules which appear in the promyelocyte stage.[514] Acute lymphocytic and "undifferentiated" leukemias are myeloperoxidase negative. Specific chloroacetate esterase is usually positive in granulocytes, whereas naphthylacetate esterase is predominantly a monocytic enzyme.[515] Lysozyme staining can be useful in detecting leukemic myeloblasts, for it is negative in normal myeloblasts. Simultaneous staining for peroxidase and lysozyme may be helpful in myelomonocytic leukemias.[516] As mentioned above, TdT staining is of use to define lymphoblastoid changes in CML.[517] For more details on enzyme stains and leukemia, see Table 2–19. The serum LDH level may be extremely high in CML.[518]

Some details on the peripheral smear are worthy of mention. An excess of 20% blasts should be considered a blast crisis. These immature myeloid cells are usually more prevalent in the higher WBC counts.[519] Cyclic variations in the WBC count are usually observed every 2–4 months.[520] These are true proliferative cycles rather than redistribution of cells in the different compartments. Leukostatic lesions (e.g., retinal hemorrhages) are due to very high WBC counts during blast crisis, but may be present in CML patients with high WBC counts not in crisis and may require intensive leukapheresis.[521]

Anemia is usually present in patients with CML but is initially mild.[522] At the morphologic level the WBCs reveal a nuclear cytoplasmic dysynchrony, with a more rapid development of the cytoplasm than the nucleus.[523] Auer rods are occasionally seen, but they are never as frequent as in acute myelogenous leukemia (AML).[524] Gaucher-like cells are identified in the bone marrow of patients with CML.[525] It is thought these are monocytoid cells that have undergone a hyperactive compensatory function storing cerebroside from neutrophil breakdown.

The bone marrow is markedly cellular with increased reticulum (65% of cases), and a high M:E ratio (10:1 to 30:1). As in the peripheral smear, all stages of myeloid cell maturation are seen. An increase in numbers of megakaryocytes is frequently present. This hypercellularity results in replacement of marrow fat by the proliferating cells. Mitoses are

TABLE 2–19.—Differentiated Morphological Classification of Acute Leukemias

FAB TYPE	CELL TYPE	ENZYMATIC STAINS						OTHER CHARACTERISTICS
		Peroxidase	Chloroacetate Esterase	Nonspecific Esterase	LDH	TdT*	Muramidase	
M1	Myeloblastic undifferentiated†	−	+	+	+	−/+	−	
M2	Myeloblastic†	−	+	+	+	−/+	+	
M3	Promyelocytic	+	+++	+	+	−	+	DIC +++ t(17–15)‡
M4	Myelomonocytic (Naegli)†	++	++	++	+	−	+++	
M5	Monocytic (Schilling)	++	+	+++	+	−	+	DIC +
M6	Erythroleukemia (Di Guglielmo)	++	++	+	+	−	−	PAS ++,§ megaloblasts
	Megakaryocytic	−	−	−	+++	−		Myelofibrosis, platelet peroxidase (+)
	Eosinophilic	+						
	Basophilic	−						Histamine +++

*Usually positive in lymphoid cells.
†Account for the majority of cases.
‡This translocation present in certain cases.
§Usually positive in lymphoid cells.

frequent. The proportion of immature to mature neutrophils tends to be higher in the marrow than in the blood,[526] suggesting that some control of immature cell release from the marrow is preserved. During the initial phases and during remission, CFU-C numbers appear normal (i.e., 10×10^6).[527]

CFU numbers, however, will increase to $10^3–10^6$ or more in blast crises, albeit the CFU-C units increase in a manner not directly related to the number of blasts.[528]

Granulocyte function in CML is abnormal during active disease but may be normal during remission. This abnormality is manifested by decreased efficiency in phagocytosis of bacteria, and chemotaxis.[529]

A difference in proliferative capabilities of marrow cells has been observed in CML patients with chronic anemia. Erythroblastic hyperplasia may be seen in these patients.[530] Serum vitamin B12 is very increased and may be 15-fold higher than normal.[531] This increase in vitamin B12 seems to be characteristic of leukemias with a predominantly myeloid cell population. The increased vitamin B12 appears to originate from granulocyte breakdown.[532]

Differential Diagnosis

CML must be differentiated from leukemoid reactions caused by disseminated infection (e.g., tuberculosis,[533] carcinomatosis, drug reactions, steroid therapy, Hodgkin's disease).

Leukoerythroblastic reactions constitute the appearance of few immature granulocytes and nucleated RBCs in the presence of a normal or slightly elevated WBC count. These reactions may occur in patients with metastatic tumors to the bone, multiple myeloma, and megaloblastic anemia.[534]

Other Variants of CML

Eosinophilic leukemia is a rare entity.[535] Extreme basophilia may also be noted (a basophilic leukemia)[536] and is of poor prognosis. Both these types may be Ph^1 positive. Erythroid involvement[537] as well as involvement of monocytoid cells[538] may also be observed in CML. Chronic myelomonocytic leukemia is occasionally seen.[539] It probably represents a single tumor cell with dual differentiation. CML is infrequently seen in children but is rapidly progressive in small children.[540]

Therapy of CML will be described only briefly here. A few more details are presented later in this chapter in relation to the effect of chemotherapeutic agents on the cell cycle.

Chemotherapy

Busulfan has proved to be an effective pharmacologic agent in the treatment of CML, causing few side effects when compared with radioactive phosphorus and ionizing radiotherapy.[541, 542] The median survival of patients treated with busulfan tends to be about 1 year longer than the median treated with radiation.[543] Other frequently used drugs are listed in Table 2–20. Some of the chemotherapeutic regimens result in a 50%–60% recovery of normal LAP scores,[544] considered to be an indication of a somewhat better prognosis. The main goal in the

TABLE 2–20.—Frequently Used Pharmacologic Agents in the Therapy of Chronic Myelogenous Leukemia*

GROUP	EXAMPLE	COMMENTS
Sulfonic acid esters	Busulfan†	Thrombocytopenia +++, Addison's disease Pulmonary fibrosis
Nitrogen mustards	Chlorambucil†	Thrombocytopenia +
	Cyclophosphamide†	Thrombocytopenia +
Antipurines	6-Mercaptopurine	Hepatotoxic
	Thioguanine	Veno-occlusive hepatic disease
Antipyrimidines	6-Azauridine	
Others	Vinblastine	Severe leukopenia, GI hemorrhage
	Dibromannitol	Addison's disease, dysplasia of uroepithelium, pulmonary fibrosis
	Hydroxyurea	Short remissions

*Data summarized from Rundles R.W.: Chronic myelogenous leukemia, in Williams W. (ed.): *Hematology*, ed. 3. New York, McGraw Hill Book Co., 1983, p. 196.
†More frequently used due to effective remissions and relatively lower toxicity.

treatment of CML is to achieve control of the neoplastic proliferation of leukemic cells. This goal is not successfully achieved permanently, as shown by the continued presence of Ph^1 in over 90% of the dividing bone marrow cells.[545] Curative attempts with chemotherapy have been made, combining busulfan, splenic radiotherapy, and induction of marrow hypoplasia with other chemotherapeutic agents. A decrease in Ph^1-positive cells is noted in these patients. However, the general median survival (50 months) of these patients is not statistically different from more conservative schedules to warrant this therapeutic protocol.[546] Recently the susceptibility of CML cells to different chemotherapeutic agents has been tested in vitro. This method may be routinely used in the future to assess the effectiveness of therapy.[547]

Leukapheresis has been used experimentally to treat CML; however, the repeated use of leukapheresis as sole therapy in the treatment of leukemia is not warranted. The main indication for leukapheresis in patients with CML is to reduce the WBC count drastically over a short period of time during leukostasis, until chemotherapy has acted on the marrow cell precursors.[548] Control of leukostasis and thrombocytosis is essential, for these complications of CML are often fatal. Intensive granulocyte removal usually results in rapid alleviation of leukostasis symptoms,[548] with neurologic and pulmonary improvement. It is customary to start cytotoxic therapy at the same time as leukapheresis, so that by 2 days chemotherapy will have achieved a reduction in the cell counts.[549] More than one leukapheresis procedure is usually necessary to reduce the WBC count.[549] The long-term use of leukapheresis as treatment for CML is not advisable for it is very expensive and does not significantly improve either the well-being of the patient or the final outcome of the disease, compared with chemotherapy.[550] Another indication for leukapheresis currently under study is to collect granulocyte progenitors during the chronic phase of CML, freeze-store these cells, and transfuse them during the nadir of chemotherapy as autologous granulocyte transfusions.[551]

Recently aggressive chemotherapy and radiation to eradicate Ph^1-positive stem cells, followed by HLA-identical bone marrow transplantation from a twin, has been successfully achieved[552] and holds promise as a therapeutic modality for CML in the future. Likewise, autologous bone marrow has been preserved in the frozen state and given to patients treated aggressively with chemotherapy during blast crisis. Revertion to chronic phase CML has been seen after successful re-engraftment of the patient's own bone marrow. Leukemia may recur after sibling marrow engraftment. Remission has occasionally occurred subsequent to the development of a graft-versus-host reaction to the engrafted marrow.[554]

Treatment of Other Neoplastic Disease States Resulting in Leukemia.—Acute leukemia may result from any of the causative agents discussed under chronic myeloid leukemia. Of great concern to hematologists and oncologists is the advent of leukemia as a consequence of therapy of certain neoplasms. For instance, of 2,067 patients given Semustine (methyl-CCNU) for gastrointestinal cancer, 14 developed leukemia. This number of patients was significantly greater than the number of patients who developed leukemia while on other chemotherapy protocols.[555] Leukemia has also developed as a late complication of other neoplasms,[556] especially as a result of treatment of Hodgkin's disease[557] and ovarian carcinoma.[558]

Prognosis of CML

CML has an average course of 1–5 years, terminating in acute phases lasting 2–6 months. Patients who were initially Ph^1 negative and who presented with CML have a poorer prognosis than those who were initially Ph^1 positive.[559] The presence of marked eosinophilia and basophilia is considered a bad prognostic sign, as is the presence of more than 10% blasts.

Lytic bone lesions with hypercalcemia are a sign that blast transformation may be present.[560] A return to normal of the LAP score is considered a good prognostic sign, but the LAP score may be markedly increased rather than decreased in blast crisis.[561]

Acute Myelogenous Leukemia

Like chronic myelogenous leukemia, acute myelogenous leukemia (AML) is a neoplastic disease of multipotential hemopoietic stem cells. AML is predominantly seen in the eighth and ninth decade, accounting for about 80% of acute leukemias in adults. However, it is also seen in children, in whom it accounts for 20% of the acute leukemias. AML is the most frequent acute leukemia in infants.[562] The incidence may be up to 2.5 per 100,000 population and appears to be increasing in urban areas.[563]

Morphologically, acute leukemia can affect almost any myeloid precursor; thus there are myelomonocytic, monocytic, erythroid, eosinophilic, and basophilic variants. Anemia, fatigue, malaise, and pallor are often seen and are the result of the replacement of normal marrow by neoplastic cells. The same mechanism is responsible for the thrombocytopenia, with resulting hematomas, epistaxis, and fatal hemorrhage. Infections are frequently seen due to immune system suppression. Hence, fever is often a presenting sign,[564] although febrile episodes can be due to causes other than infection. Hepatosplenomegaly is common in AML; lymphadenopathy is rare.

Laboratory Findings

Anemia and thrombocytopenia are almost universal, i.e., 70% of patients have hematocrits below 30%, and about 50% of patients have low platelet counts. Leukocytosis of up to 34,000 WBC/μl is found in 50% of patients and rises to over 100,000/μl in 11% of patients.[565] Normal or decreased counts are seen in the remaining patients. Some 15%–95% of the cells in the periphery may be blasts. A few to most of the cells in the marrow may be immature cells, depending on the individual case. Pelger-Huet cells can often be identified. Auer rods appear in 10% of cases, and myeloperoxidase granules identify myeloblasts.

Hyperuricemia and increased serum LDH are also seen in AML. Hypercalcemia is occasionally present.

AML Variants

In order to better classify the various subtypes of AML, an international group of French, American, and British researchers have proposed the FAB classification (Table 2–21).[566] M1 corresponds to undifferentiated cells without promyelocytes, in M2 there are a few promyelocytes, and M3 is predominantly promyelocytic.[567] M3 very frequently exhibits many Auer rods. Characteristically M3 leukemics have a tendency to develop disseminated intravascular coagulopathy (DIC). M6 has abundant PAS-positive granules, more often seen in lymphocytic leukemias; however, 30% of M1, M2, and M3, 60% of M4, and 80% of M5 patients also have abundant PAS-positive granules. The ASD acetate esterase stain is intense in monocytes, less intense in granulocytes, and negative in lymphoid cells. In monocytic leukemia, ASD esterase is markedly reduced by sodium fluoride.

PAS-positive granules do not appear on these cells and are considered more characteristic of lymphoblasts, but may be prominent in erythroleukemia.[568] Erythroleukemia M6 (Di Guglielmo's syndrome) accounts for about 3% of cases of childhood leukemias, and erythropoiesis is markedly abnormal in these cases.[569] The marrow picture may resemble that of megaloblastic anemia,[570] but B12 and folic acid levels are normal, and the changes are evidently refractory to vitamin B12 and folate therapy.

Chromosomal Abnormalities in AML

Loss of chromosomal material from chromosome 7 is consistently observed in many cases of AML. Gains of chromosomal material have also been seen in chromosome 8.

An 8;21 translocation between a group C and a group G chromosome has been observed.[571] The translocation can be summarized as [t(8;21) band (q22;q22)], and appears to occur mostly in M2 type leukemias, a few M4 cases, and in about 10% of all AML cases.[572] Interestingly, t(8;21) translocations are accompanied by a loss of X or Y chromosomes.[572] Acute promyelocytic leukemias are associated with a rearrangement of chromosomes 15 and 17.[573] The break in chromosome 15 is distal to band q21 and in chromosome 17 it is in q21. In one series,[572] 50 of 82 patients with acute promyelocytic leukemia had t(8;21). Other translocations involving t(9;22) have been described.[572] By means

TABLE 2–21.—Immunologic Markers in Acute Leukemia*

TYPE OF LEUKEMIA	TdT	Ia	cALL	E	HuTLA	SIg	CIg	HTA-1
AML (M1)	+	+/−	−	−	−	−	−	−
AML (M2)	+/−	+/−	−	−	−	−	−	−
B cell ALL	−	+	+/−	−	−	−	+/−	−
T cell ALL	+	−	−	+/−	+	−	−	+/−
Null cell ALL	+	+	+/−	−	−	−	−	−

*TdT, terminal deoxynucleotydil transferase; Ia, HLA-DR antigens; cALL, common leukemia antigens; E, erythrocyte receptor; HuTLA, human T cell leukemia antigen; SIg, surface immunoglobulin; CIg, cytoplasmic immunoglobulin; HTA-1, human T cell antigen.

of premature condensation analysis (PCC) it is possible to predict AML relapses. High PCC ratios may indicate a higher susceptibility to leukemia relapse.[574] By culturing bone marrow cells of a leukemia in relapse, it has been possible in certain cases to define points during maturation of the stem cell at which transformation occurs. For instance, in one case a t(1q−;11q+) translocation was found in all colonies of granulocyte/macrophage lineage, suggesting the translocation occurred at the granulocyte/macrophage progenitor stage.[575] This finding also suggests that AML, like CML, may be a stem cell disorder, thus explaining the presence of cells of different lineage yet with a common clonal origin in the same patient.

In general, patients in whom chromosomal abnormalities are detected tend to have a worse prognosis.[576] About 50% of AML patients have such chromosomal abnormalities.[576]

Other Laboratory Features

Leukemia-associated antigens can be tested for with the use of monoclonal antibodies (see Table 2-21). It is not known whether antibodies against leukemic cells are cell-associated antigens or virus-associated antigens. Most of the specificities currently available are against lymphoid cells;[577] however, an AML-associated antigen has been described.[578] The presence of leukemia-associated antigens may forecast imminent relapse, as detected by heterologous antisera.[579]

Differences have been observed between adult AML and childhood AML with respect to the expression of HLA-DR antigens. Older patients tend to produce cells which induce lower immune responses in vitro, as compared to cells from younger AML patients. Older patients also show increased HLA-DR antigen expression on cell surfaces, these cells tend to grow more rapidly in vitro.[580]

Correlation of Subclassification With Clinical Outcome of AML

In myeloblastic leukemia M1 and M2 the cells are very immature in appearance with three to five nucleoli. Lymphadenopathy is present in about 50% of cases. Leukemic infiltration of tissues is frequently seen (granulocytic sarcoma).[581] ASD staining of tissues should be performed to distinguish this form of leukemia from lymphoma.

In promyelocytic leukemia, the M3 variant, abnormal granules are present. This type of leukemia has a tendency to be complicated by DIC.[582] The granules appear to be responsible for the coagulopathy, owing to their thromboplastinic activity.[583] The granule release is particularly dangerous during therapy, when the neoplastic cells are lysed.

Myelomonocytic M4 and monocytic M5 variants are characterized by the presence of at least 20% of monocyte lineage cells in the bone marrow. FcR and CR markers are usually present in these cells, which characteristically adhere to glass and plastic surfaces in culture. These cells likewise stain positive with Sudan black B, PAS, and nonspecific esterase and are inhibited by sodium fluoride.[584] Urinary and serum lysozyme levels are usually increased in these patients. Tissue infiltration is common, and lymphadenopathy is seen in at least 76% of cases. M5 leukemias are frequently complicated by DIC,[585] and these patients tend to have a shorter life span than patients with the M4 type of AML.[586] Tn-polyagglutinability has been associated with the M4 type of leukemia.[587] Prognostically, M6 (erythroleukemia) does not appear to be very different from other common AML variants.[588]

Treatment of AML

The differential diagnosis between AML and ALL must be made, for the treatment of these two types of acute leukemia is very different. Once the diagnosis of AML has been made, the goal is to induce aplasia of the marrow by vigorous treatment. The treatment of choice is combination therapy to achieve remission induction. Six drugs are currently favored: 6-mercaptopurine (6-MP), thioguanine (TG), cytosine arabinoside (CA), daunomycin (D), adriamycin (AM), and 5-azacytidine (AZ). A combination of D, CA, and 6-MP or TG appears to be the treatment of choice,[589] producing up to 78% complete remission. Patients must be supported vigorously during the aplastic stage to prevent death from infections or thrombocytopenia with fatal hemorrhage.[590] Treatment of DIC with anticoagulants and components improves the survival of patients with this complication. Support during aplasia is critical; hence prior planning with the blood bank physician of the components to be used is of vital importance. Patients with leukemia tolerate relatively low platelet counts without major bleeding, but constant monitoring is essential to provide platelet support. HLA-typed platelets may be needed in patients who become refractory to random donor platelets. Maintenance therapy with chemotherapeutic agents is essential to maintain patients in remission.[591] The prevention of infection will also enhance survival. Oral gentamicin, vancomycin, and nystatin help to prevent infection, as does environmental isolation; however, infection control has no influence on the rate or duration of remission.[592] *S. aureus, E. coli, K. pneumoniae,* and *P. aeruginosa* account for about 58% of the isolates.[593]

Prognosis

Since cytarabine and the anthracyclines have been introduced in the therapy of AML, about 17% of patients treated with the newer protocols are complete responders to therapy. These patients are expected to remain in complete remission after 5 years.[594]

Recently complete marrow ablation followed by bone marrow transplantation has proved to be very successful, especially in patients under 40 years of age.[595] The prognosis is better if bone marrow transplants are given during the first remission. Autologous marrow transplantation, with the separation of neoplastic from normal cells on albumin gradients, has been attempted, with some success.[596]

Patients with circulating immune complexes appear to have fewer complete remissions than patients without them.[597]

AML has resulted as a complication of therapy for other neoplasms, such as therapy with alkylating agents for ovarian carcinoma,[598] and treatment for non-Hodgkin's lymphoma, although the diseases may appear simultaneously in the same patient, without prior antineoplastic treatment.[599] Treatment of myeloma with melphalan-cyclophosphamide-carmustine combinations has a 7% risk of inducing AML after 50 months.[600] Treatment of these patients with cytarabine has induced remissions.[601]

Chronic Lymphocytic Leukemia

Chronic lymphocytic leukemia (CLL) is a monoclonal neoplasm of small lymphocytes which type as B cells in about 95% of cases.[602] The cells bear IgM and IgD isotypes in most cases; occasionally IgG or IgA can also be seen.[602] About 2%–5% of cases type as T cells (Table 2–22). Age and genetic factors as well as some other leukemogenic factors seem to play a role in etiology. Ionizing radiation does not appear to be a causative agent. The disease incidence is about 2 per 100,000 population.[562] Two variants of the disease can be discerned, one in which there is prominent marrow infiltration with relatively few peripheral lymphocytes, and one in which cells are found mostly in the circulation. The first type tends to have a poorer prognosis,[603] and should probably be considered non-Hodgkin's lymphoma of the marrow.

A familial tendency has been found in certain clusters of CLL cases.[604] The 14q+ translocation found in other lymphoproliferative diseases has also been described in certain cases of CLL.[605] Trisomy of chromosome 12 has likewise been observed in this disease[606] and appears to be the most frequent chromosomal abnormality.[607] Abnormal karyotypes tend to reveal a poorer prognosis in CLL cases. An unusual translocation [t(2;14) (p13;q32)] has been described in a child with CLL, which in itself is a rare occurrence and has a poor prognosis.[608]

TABLE 2–22.—SUBTYPES OF CHRONIC LYMPHOCYTIC LEUKEMIA AND RELATED DISEASES*

DISEASE	SIg	CIg	EaC	BAg	Th	Ts	Ia	TdT	ADA	COMMENTS
B cell CLL	+	−	+	+	−	−	+/−	−	+/+++	NHL often in lymph node
T cell CLL	−	−	−	−	+/−	+/−	−	−	++/+++	Poor response to therapy
Sézary's syndrome	−	−	−	−	+	−	+/−	−	−	Poor response to therapy
LS-CLL (lymphosarcoma)	+	−	+/−	+/−	−	−	+/−	+/−	−	NHL (PD) often in lymph node
Hairy cell leukemia	+/−	−	−	−	+/−	+/−	+/−	−	−	Cytoplasmic acid phosphatase present
Waldenström's macroglobulinemia	+	+	−	+/−	−	−	+/−	−	−	Usually high serum IgM
Prolymphocytic leukemia	++	−	+	+/−	+/−	+/−	+	−	−	Poor response to therapy

*SIg, surface immunoglobulin; CIg, cytoplasmic immunoglobulin; EaC, complement-coated RBC rosettes; BAg, B cell antigen; Th, T helper cells; Ts, T suppressor cells; Ia, HLA-DR; TdT, terminal deoxynucleotidyl transferase; ADA, adenosine deaminase.

Clinical Features of CLL

Up to 30% of patients with CLL may be asymptomatic at presentation. It is the most benign of the leukemias, with a median survival of 10 years.[609] Lymphadenopathy and splenomegaly are the commonest presenting signs; later in the disease hepatomegaly is observed. Anemia (seen in 15% of cases) and thrombocytopenia (30% of cases) may be seen in advanced cases. Infections are also seen later in the disease. About 94% of patients have WBC counts greater than 10,000/µl, and about 18% have counts greater than 100,000/µl. The lymphocyte count may be as high as $1,000 \times 10^9$, but more frequently it does not exceed 100×10^9. Autoimmune hemolytic anemia with a positive direct Coombs test is occasionally present.

Hypogammaglobulinemia may occur in up to 50% of patients.[610] A decrement in serum IgA is particularly seen in these cases.[611] Serum acrylamide electrophoresis shows a decreased P band, and a prominent X band.[612]

A decreased concentration of i antigen is present on the lymphocytes[613] of some patients with CLL. Patients with CLL frequently fail to produce new RBC antibodies after transfusion, in contrast to patients with AML, who usually produce antibodies after immunization by transfusion.[614] Patients with CLL frequently present with harmful cold agglutinins, many of which may have anti-I specificity.[615]

Because T and B cells are morphologically indistinguishable, and because in most cases of CLL the cells are fairly well differentiated, the diagnosis is made by a combination of peripheral blood cell counts, bone marrow assessment, and surface marker and enzyme studies (see Table 2–22). In the prevalent B cell type of CLL, the surface immunoglobulin (SIg) is frequently of the IgM and/or IgD classes with either κ or λ but rarely both, denoting the monoclonality of this disease. Capping of SIg receptors is usually more sluggish than that of normal cells.[616]

TdT is usually absent in these cells.[617] LDH isoenzyme levels in T and B cells vary; LDH-1 is higher in T cells than in B cells, whereas LDH-3 and LDH-5 are lower in T cells than in B cells. Thus, this enzyme may be used to assess disease activity in CLL. Similarly, acid phosphatase isoenzyme 3 is lower in B cells than in T cells, which is reflected in patients with CLL bearing one of the two subtypes of CLL.[617]

When CLL affects lymph nodes, it does so in the pattern expected from the cell lineage of the CLL subtype. For instance B cell CLL produces a diffuse lymphomatous infiltrate, the "lymphosarcoma type"; CLL produces a nodular pattern; and the T cell type causes a paracortical infiltration.[618] For clinical staging see Table 2–23.

Therapy

The therapy of CLL will not be reviewed in detail here. In most cases treatment should be delayed until marrow malfunction is observed, but this rule is applied individually after evaluation of each case. Chlorambucil is useful in eliminating the expanding growth of well-differentiated small lymphocytes, whereas cyclophosphamide is superior in eliminating the less mature lymphocytes.[620] Prednisone can be used as a good therapeutic adjunct to chemotherapy, especially if autoimmune hemolytic anemia complicates the disease.[621] Local irradiation of enlarged nodes is useful as adjunctive therapy.

Prognosis

The prognosis of patients with CLL depends on the CLL subtype and the clinical stage (see Table 2–23). The prognosis is markedly dependent on the response of the neoplastic cells to chemotherapy.

Acute Lymphocytic Leukemia

Acute lymphocytic leukemia (ALL) is a neoplasm composed of immature-looking lymphocytes. It is the most frequent neoplasm of childhood and the most frequent of the childhood leukemias accounting for the majority of the 2,500 cases of childhood leukemia seen each year in the United States.[623]

It is usually seen between the ages of 2 years and 10 years, representing the most common malignancy in childhood.[624] However, a second peak is seen after middle age. Unlike CLL, impairment of the immune response is not routinely seen in ALL.

TABLE 2–23.—CLINICAL STAGING OF CLL*

STAGE	CHARACTERISTICS	SURVIVAL WITH THERAPY†
A	Lymphocytosis ($15,000 \times 10^9$/L); marrow involvement	Normal
B	As above, and 3 lymph node areas involved	7 yr
C	As above, and anemia and thrombocytopenia	2 yr

*Summarized from Binet et al.[619]
†T cell CLL has an expected survival of 6 months.[622]

Four types can be identified: common type ALL (cALL),[625] T cell ALL, B cell ALL, and acute undifferentiated leukemia (null cell ALL).

cALL cells display the common ALL antigen (cALLa), which is a glycoprotein.[626] This type of ALL is the most frequent. The second most frequent type is T cell ALL. These cells express T cell markers such as binding sheep RBCs and expressing T cell antigens (Table 2–24).[627] TdT is present both in cALL and T cell ALL, denoting their immature stage of development, for this enzyme is normally found only on immature T cells.[628] B cell leukemias are usually identified by their surface immunoglobulins (SIg). The fourth type, acute undifferentiated leukemia, is difficult to distinguish from undifferentiated acute AML unless lymphocyte markers can be detected on them.

The FAB classification may be used to distinguish among the acute lymphocytic leukemias (Table 2–25).[629] The L1 variant is a lymphoblastic leukemia with small cells and homogeneous nuclear chromatin. The nucleoli are not conspicuous, and the cytoplasm is slightly basophilic. L2 cells are large and heterogeneous. Irregularly distributed heterogeneous nuclear chromatin is seen, irregular clefting and indentation of the nucleus are moderately abundant, and the cells stain a deeper blue color than L1 cells. L3 cells are homogeneously large cells with nuclear chromatin which is finely stippled and homogeneous. Deeply basophilic cytoplasm and prominent vacuolation of the cytoplasm are seen. L1 is common in childhood, whereas L2 is not. L3 is characterized by the presence of B cell markers in 75% of cases and T cell markers in the remaining 25%. These cells should be differentiated with enzyme studies to define their lymphoid origin. TdT is present in high levels in ALL and is therefore diagnostically useful.[630] It is of paramount importance to differentiate AML from ALL cases; when this is not possible, the above-mentioned enzyme studies should be performed. Surface markers should also be tested for (see Table 2–24).

The great majority of cases of ALL (80%) are of the null cell type; that is, the cells cannot be identified as T or B cells.[631] There is reason to believe that most of these null cells are early B cells, because in 20% of patients intracytoplasmic μ chains are seen,[632] and most of these cells show gene rearrangement characteristic of immunoglobulin variable region development, even though detectable expression of immunoglobulins by these cells is lacking.[633]

Furthermore, using the forbol ester TPA test, it has been shown with DNA probes that gene rearrangement, with induction of differentiation of null ALL cells to B type cells, can be achieved.[634]

Rarely, ALL may be followed by AML. In these

TABLE 2–24.—IMMUNOLOGIC AND CYTOCHEMICAL CHARACTERIZATION OF ALL*

TYPE	FREQ. (%)	ANTIGENIC CHARACTERISTICS								ENZYMES		
		cALLa	E	Ia	SIg	CIg	B-Ag	HTA-1	HTLA	TdT	AP	PAS
cALL	70–80	+	−	+	−	−	−	−	−	+	−	Coarse
T cell ALL	20–25	−	+	−	−	−	−	+	+	+	Focal	Variable
B cell ALL	< 5	−	−	+/−	+	+/−	+	−	−	−	−	−
Null cell ALL	< 1	−	−	+/−	−	−	−	−	−	+/−	−	−

*cALLa, common acute leukemia antigen; E, spontaneous rosetting with sheep RBCs; Ia, HLA-DR; SIg, surface immunoglobulin; CIg, cytoplasmic immunoglobulin; B-Ag, B cell–specific antigen; HTA-1, human T cell antigen; HTLA, human T cell leukemia antigen; TdT, terminal deoxynucleotidyl transferase; AP, acid phosphatase; PAS, periodic acid schiff.

TABLE 2–25.—FAB MORPHOLOGICAL CHARACTERIZATION OF ALL*

TYPE	SIZE	NUCLEUS	CYTOPLASM	PROGNOSIS
L1 ALL	8–10 μm	Fine; homogenous cytoplasm	Scant, basophilic	Good
L2 ALL	10–14 μm	Variable nuclear shape; variable nuclear chromatin	Moderately abundant, basophilic	Moderate
L3 ALL	> 14 μm	Large round regular nuclei, prominent nucleoli	Vacuoles, lipid inclusions	Bad

*Summarized from Bennett et al.[629]

cases a stem cell disorder may be invoked, but the existence of a secondary neoplasm must be considered.[635] Most children present with the L1 variant of ALL (75% of cases), whereas most adults with ALL present with the L2 variant (68% of cases).[636] The distinction between the adult and the childhood variant is significant, for the adult variant has a poor prognosis and a lower remission rate (80%) than the childhood variant. Some T cell ALL cells have been shown to be suppressor T cells, causing hypogammaglobulinemia.[637]

Chromosomal Abnormalities

A t(9;22) translocation has been observed in both AML and ALL; however, two thirds of the patients in whom this translocation was seen had ALL.[638] Three nonrandom translocations are particularly found in ALL: t(4;11) (q21;q23); t(9;22) (q34;q11); and t(8;14) (q24;q32). All have a poor prognosis.[639] A deletion of the long arm of chromosome 6 is also seen but does not appear to carry the poor prognosis of the translocation mentioned above.[639] The t(8;14) translocation is frequently seen in the B cell type (Burkitt's-like) ALL.[640]

Etiology of ALL

Four main etiological factors—irradiation, viruses, chemicals, and genetic factors—have been mentioned as possible causes of ALL. Irradiation has been shown to be related in some way to the development of ALL as well as other forms of leukemia. This observation has been made in survivors of atomic bomb blast exposure,[641] as well as in patients exposed to therapeutic irradiation.[642]

Viral agents have long been suspected in the etiology of leukemias. Recently oncoviruses have been isolated from patients with ALL.[643] The human T cell leukemia virus is an example of a virus isolated from ALL[644] as well as from other lymphomas.

EBV has been suspected as an etiologic agent in Burkitt's lymphoma[645] and Burkitt's-type ALL[646] but this relationship has not been conclusively proved. It is not known at this time how a virus would induce the leukemic transformation, if this is indeed an etiologic agent in ALL. EBV has been shown to infect and transform hairy cell leukemia cells.[647] Other factors function as carcinogens or co-carcinogens. One such chemical is benzene, known to induce AML and ALL on prolonged exposure.[648] Genetic factors must also play a role in the pathogenesis of leukemia, as attested by the chromosomal translocation mentioned above, plus observations that HLA-A and Ia antigens seem to play a role in the susceptibility to develop ALL.[649]

Therapy for ALL

Current therapy for ALL is to attempt remission with vigorous chemotherapy using mainly vincristine and prednisone with or without the addition of other agents such as anthracycline or asparaginase. Remission is present when no leukemic cells are demonstrable in the bone marrow or other sites of the body.[650] Initial therapy is designed to decrease the WBC count from 10^{12}/L to 10^9/L, and consolidation therapy decreases the number to 10^6/L. Therapy is directed at various stages of cellular DNA synthesis. Vincristine arrests cells in M phase, prednisone lyses lymphoblasts in their resting or G_0 phase, mercaptopurine inhibits DNA synthesis, and methotrexate inhibits DNA and RNA synthesis. These drugs are used sequentially to affect all stages of the cycle and to prevent resistant clones from arising.[651]

The protocol is as follows: vincristine, 2 mg/m^2, is given IV once a week for 4 weeks, with prednisone, 1 mg/kg day, given orally for initial remission. Methotrexate is given orally, 15 mg/m^2, twice a week. To destroy CNS sanctuaries, radiation to the CNS axis is given at a dose of 2,400 rad. Intrathecal methotrexate is also given. However, a combination of CNS irradiation and intrathecal chemotherapy is currently under evaluation.[652]

In males, testicular irradiation should be considered to eliminate testicular leukemic cell sanctuaries. Testosterone insufficiency usually results from this type of treatment.[653]

Bone marrow transplantation with HLA-matched sibling donor marrow may be attempted after the first relapse, during the second remission.[654]

Prognosis

The best prognosis is in young patients, aged 2–10 years. Patients who present before and after this age range tend to have a worse prognosis. Patients with the Philadelphia chromosome, B cell markers, or high blast counts have a poor prognosis. Fifty percent of children with ALL succumb before 5 years. The remainder have a relatively better prognosis. Seventy-five percent of adults with ALL are dead before 5 years.

Tumor Cell Kinetics

In order to understand the rationale of therapy of the leukemias and lymphomas as well as other neoplasms, it is important to review some aspects of tumor cell kinetics.

Twenty-seven cell doublings usually occur before a tumor can be first detected clinically; at this stage, tumors are about 0.5 cm in diameter. A tumor 1 cm in diameter usually has undergone about 30 doublings. Neoplasms usually become lethal after 35–40 doublings.[655] These findings underscore the necessity to act promptly in the treatment of malignancies.

Neoplasms exhibit a gompertzian type of growth. This type of tumor growth is characterized by a sigmoid curve. During the first phase, the growth is rapid and linear, but upon reaching a certain size, the cells in the tumor tend to slow their mitotic rate, presumably because of limitations imposed by adjacent tissues. When chemotherapy is given, the tumor load is lowered, and therefore exponential growth can be expected. It is at this time, however, when cells are again in G_1, that chemotherapy becomes effective.[656]

Effect of Chemotherapeutic Agents on the Cell Cycle

Blood bankers are frequently involved at some stage in the treatment plan of leukemics as well as other cancer patients. These patients have a variety of hematologic complications requiring blood and blood components and, on occasion, require treatment by apheresis (see chapters 8 and 9). In order to better understand how these patients may require blood banking components, it is necessary to review the effects that many of these drugs have, first, in terms of their therapeutic effects, and second, in terms of their toxic effects on hemopoietic organs.

Each cell mitosis is sandwiched between two "resting" phase or interphase periods. DNA synthesis (S phase) occurs between gap 1 and gap 2 (G_1 and G_2) phases. During the G_1 postmitotic phase, enzymes necessary for DNA synthesis are manufactured. Corticosteroids and L-asparaginase appear to be most active in this phase of the cell cycle. During the S phase, when DNA replication occurs, cell cycle–specific agents are most active; examples of these drugs are cytarabine and methotrexate.[657] During G_2, the short premitotic phase, chemotherapeutic agents such as bleomycin seem to be most active. Alkaloids of the vinca and podophylotoxin type are most active at the M or mitotic phase. Cancer cells in the G_0 phase are usually not susceptible to most chemotherapeutic agents.

Concepts in Chemotherapy Useful to the Blood Banker

Quite often chemotherapeutic drugs are given in combination to cancer patients. These combinations are selected on the basis of different toxicities so as to avoid synergistic toxicity. For instance, vincristine is often used in the combinations, for it is mainly neurotoxic, as opposed to cytoxan, which is markedly myelosuppressive. Other nonmyelosuppressive agents are steroids, bleomycin, and asparaginase. The onset of myelosuppression can often be predicted; this onset is termed the nadir of the chemotherapy. In certain combinations, such as combinations of nitrosoureas with 5-FU, the nadir is at 7–14 days.

When nitrosoureas are used alone, maximum myelosuppression occurs between 21 and 35 days.[658] Perhaps one of the most dreaded toxic effects of chemotherapeutic agents, and the one of highest concern to the blood banker, is bone marrow suppression, due to the variety and number of blood components used by patients in marrow suppression. The kinetics of the particular agents in the chemotherapeutic combinations will, in the end, determine the severity of bone marrow suppression.

The rate of disappearance of the different peripheral blood cell elements depends on the half-life of the cell affected by the chemotherapeutic agent. Thus, the impact on the RBC population, whose cells have a viability of 120 days after cell division, will be often less noted than, for instance, the effect on granulocytes and platelets, with half-lives of 6 hours (granulocytes) and 5–7 days (platelets). Nevertheless, RBC suppression may be noted when the effect of these agents is prolonged. Alkylators such as mechlorethamine (nitrogen mustard) classically suppress bone marrow directly. Nitrosoureas such as lomustine (CCNU) and semustine (methyl-CCNU) will likewise suppress the marrow.

Bone marrow recovery usually originates from cells not affected by these agents—stem cells in the resting or G_0 phase. The rate of nadir and recovery depends on the phase of the cell cycle which the agent interferes with. Antimetabolites such as 5-FU and methotrexate produce nadirs very rapidly, with short duration, granulocytopenia, and rapid recovery. Cyclophosphamide and doxorubicin, which are cell cycle but not phase specific, produce relatively more prolonged nadirs and recoveries.

The more prolonged bone marrow depressions should be expected from the nitrosoureas.[659] It is a good idea for physicians in charge of blood banks to become familiar with the expected nadirs and recovery times of different agents. A close cooperation with the treating physician will usually avert panic episodes with last-minute arrangements for supportive therapy such as compatible blood, granulocytes, and platelets. A summary chart of the more frequent nadirs and recoveries is given in Table 2–26.

Other Types of Leukemias

Hairy Cell Leukemia

In this disorder, lymphoid cells with cytoplasmic projections have the appearance of a hairy surface on electron microscopy.[660] Hairy cells are characteristically tartrate-resistant, acid phosphatase-positive.[661] Many patients with hairy cell leukemia have antibodies against EBV, suggesting this virus may be an etiologic agent.[662] Most cases of hairy cell leukemia have been typed as B cells,[663] a lineage which has been corroborated with monoclonal antibodies to B cell markers.[664] The course is more benign than in other leukemias. Chemotherapy is not indicated. Splenectomy may be beneficial in certain cases. Infections are frequent in patients with hairy cell leukemia and may be the cause of death.[665] Alpha-interferon has been useful in inducing remission in patients with hairy cell leukemia.[666]

Sézary Syndrome

This is a T cell leukemia which characteristically infiltrates the skin. It resembles mycosis fungoides, another disease also produced by neoplastic T cells.[667] The T cells often type as T helper cells.[668] Chemotherapy with mechlorethamine is indicated for both diseases. Superficial irradiation of skin lesions may be beneficial.

Malignant Mastocytosis

Malignant mastocytosis is characterized by a neoplastic systemic increase in the mast cell count. Although mastocytosis may be present in leukemia

TABLE 2–26.—Effect of Chemotherapy on Bone Marrow*

DRUG	DEGREE OF MYELOSUPPRESSION†	NADIR (Days)	RECOVERY (Days)	BLOOD ELEMENT AFFECTED
Alkylating agents				
Mechlorethamine	I	7–15	28	Pancytopenia
Melphalan	I	10–12	40–50	WBCs, platelets
Busulfan	I	10–30	20–55	WBCs, platelets
Chlorambucil	I	15–30	30–40	WBCs, platelets
Cyclophosphamide	II	8–14	18–25	WBCs
Nitrosoureas				
Carmustine	I	25–30	35–40	WBCs, platelets, RBCs
Lomustine	I	40–50	60	WBCs, platelets, RBCs
Semustine	I	30–60	80–90	WBCs, platelets, RBCs
Antimetabolites				
Ara-C	I	10–15	20–25	WBCs, platelets
5-FU	I	7–14	15–25	WBCs, platelets
MTY	II	7–14	15–25	WBCs, platelets
GMP	II	7–14	20–35	WBCs, platelets
Vinca alkaloids				
Vincristine	III	4–5	7	WBCs
Velban	I	5–10	15–20	WBCs
Antibiotics				
Mitomycin	II	30–40	40–55	Pancytopenia
Mithramycin	III	14	20–30	Platelets
Anthracyclines				
Actinomycin	II	15–20	20–25	WBCs, platelets
Doxorubicin	II	10–15	20–25	WBCs
Others				
Procarbazine	II	25–35	35–50	WBCs, platelets
Dacarbazine	II	20–30	30–35	WBCs, platelets
Cisplatin	III	14	21	Pancytopenia

*Modified from Dorr and Fritz.[659]
†I, directly myelosuppressive; II, myelosuppressive plus serious dose-limiting toxicity; III, myelosuppression, not dose-limiting at usual dosage.

and myelofibrosis, an independent neoplastic proliferation of mast cells does exist. Urticaria pigmentosa of the adult type is the result of systemic mastocytosis of various kinds. Antihistamines and steroids may be beneficial in certain cases.[669] Leukemia may develop in the malignant form of mastocytosis. This occurs in about 15% of cases.[670]

Myeloproliferative Disorders

Myeloproliferative diseases are grouped together because they may convert or progress to (usually) a less differentiated form of neoplasm of the same myeloid series.

Polycythemia Vera.—Polycythemia vera is a myeloproliferative disorder that may affect several bone marrow cells (RBCs, WBCs, and platelets) in varying degrees.[671] Interestingly, erythropoietin is usually decreased,[672] and marrow from polycythemia vera patients responds abnormally to erythropoietin in vitro.[673] Clinically, patients display a dusky redness of the mucous membranes. Headache and malaise are present.[674] The RBC count is markedly increased (6–10 million/cu mm). Hemoglobin is above 18 gm/100 ml, and the hematocrit is usually above 55%. Platelets are usually above 1 million/cu mm. Increased megakaryocytes are seen in the bone marrow, and there is as well a general increase of cellularity. Polycythemia of other types should be ruled out.[675] Gastrointestinal bleeding and cerebral thrombosis are frequent complications. Development of myelofibrosis is reported in certain instances of polycythemia vera. Chromosomal abnormalities can be detected in up to 26% of cases of polycythemia vera before treatment.[676]

Radioactive phosphorus, 3–5 mCi given IV at 2-week intervals, is the treatment of choice. Remission is observed in most cases. Chlorambucil, cyclophosphamide, or melphalan may be used alternatively in the course of the disease.[677] There is, however, the risk of developing hematologic, as well as nonhematologic neoplasms after myelosuppressive treatment of polycythemia vera.[678]

Agnogenic Myeloid Metaplasia.—Agnogenic myeloid metaplasia is a monoclonal neoplasm of hematopoietic stem cells as proved by G6PD enzyme isotypes.[679] The disease is usually accompanied by varying degrees of mesenchymal tissue proliferation in the bone marrow (myelofibrosis) which is most probably reactive[680] and probably induced by megakaryocyte and platelet growth factors.[681]

The bone marrow fibrosis produces a secondary extramedullary hemopoiesis in the liver and spleen.[682] In 10% of cases the myelofibrosis is preceded by polycythemia vera. Fibrosis of the marrow may be associated with chronic infections, hairy cell leukemia, or metastatic neoplasms.

The spleen is usually markedly enlarged, and there may be hepatomegaly as well. The combination of anemia and a dry bone marrow tap is an indication that myelofibrosis may be present. Initially the WBC count as well as the platelet count may be increased. LAP levels are usually markedly increased. A bone marrow biopsy proves the diagnosis. A major complication of myelofibrosis is the development of acute myeloblastic leukemia. Other complications are thrombocytopenia and hemolytic anemia.

The use of androgenic steroids has been advocated if anemia is severe. Busulfan may be necessary if splenomegaly becomes painful. Blast crises are treated as in acute leukemia.

PATHOLOGY OF LYMPH NODES

First we will review a few nonneoplastic changes, then concentrate mostly on the primary neoplasms of lymph nodes.

Acute Reactive Hyperplasia.—Lymph nodes are the site of antigenic concentration for a variety of antigenic insults from the environment. As such, they are subject to reactive changes, of which acute reactive hyperplasia is the most common.

Histologically, acute reactive hyperplasia is characterized by enlarged germinal centers, within which reactive histiocytes reveal phagocytic activity. Lymph node enlargement may be due to edema and an acute inflammatory infiltrate mostly present within sinusoids. Abscess formation may be seen.

Chronic Nonspecific Reactive Hyperplasia.—When lymph nodes are chronically exposed to immunogenic challenges these patterns may be noted:

(1) B cell immunogenes will cause mainly a germinal center hypertrophy, whereas

(2) T cell immunogenes will cause a paracortical type of hypertrophy. In these reactions, germinal centers are almost obliterated. This obliteration may be worrisome for it resembles lymphoma and

may be cause of confusion. However, in these lesions, the cell populations are not monotonous and histiocytes will show evidence of phagocytosis.

(3) Sinus histiocytes, where lymphoid sinusoids are obliterated by reactive histiocytes, are the third pattern seen in chronic reactive hyperplasia.[683]

The Lymphomas: Hodgkin's Disease

The major primary neoplasms of lymph nodes are lymphomas. Lymphomas can be Hodgkin's type lymphomas or non-Hodgkin's type lymphomas. Hodgkin's disease accounts for about 1900 deaths a year in the United States.[684] The incidence of the disease is bimodal, with a peak in the second decade and another peak after age 45. A viral etiology for Hodgkin's disease has been suggested by epidemiologic studies.[685] Family studies in which siblings or parents of patients with Hodgkin's disease have developed the disease tend to support this assumption.[686] Patients with Hodgkin's disease tend to appear in areas epidemiologically related to those of EBV. Hodgkin's disease patients tend to have a higher titer of antibodies to EBV than controls.[687] However, no evidence of EBV genes has been detected in tissues of patients with Hodgkin's disease using sensitive DNA probes.[688] However, RNA sequence homology between Rauscher murine leukemia virus and DNA from certain tissues obtained from patients with Hodgkin's disease has been found.[689] Other risk factors such as hydantoin therapy[690] and immune system deficiencies[691] have also been linked to Hodgkin's disease.

Immunologic, Morphological, and Chromosomal Abnormalities

T cell–mediated immunity is significantly altered in patients with advanced Hodgkin's disease, as evidenced by a decreased responsiveness to *Candida* and other organisms[692] as well as a decreased response to PHA stimulation in vitro. These changes are infrequently seen in early stages of Hodgkin's disease.[693] B cell functions, such as humoral immunity, are essentially intact in these patients. Of special interest to the blood bank, some patients with Hodgkin's disease develop warm autoimmune hemolytic anemia.[694]

Chromosomal abnormalities found in cells from patients with Hodgkin's disease are limited to the neoplastic cells. The changes include hypotetraploid cells as well as added chromatin to the long arm of chromosome 14 (14q+). This abnormality can also be detected in non-Hodgkin's lymphomas.[695]

Hodgkin's lymphomas almost always arise in and remain confined to lymph nodes. They are morphologically distinct from non-Hodgkin's lymphomas in that they have a clear-cut morphological pattern under the microscope, especially a distinguishable type of giant cell, the Reed-Sternberg cell. Although some pathologists will not make the diagnosis of Hodgkin's disease without the finding of Reed-Sternberg cells, others will diagnose it when "Reed-Sternberg-like" cells, which do not fit the absolute criteria of Reed-Sternberg cells, are seen.

Reed-Sternberg cells are large bilobed nucleated histiocytoid cells with two reddish nucleoli resembling owl's eyes. Recent studies on cell markers have shown that these cells may be indeed histiocytes, but the final origin of Reed-Sternberg cells has not been conclusively determined. The marked derangement of T cell function in patients with Hodgkin's disease may be due in part to phagocytosis of lymphocytes by Reed-Sternberg cells.[696]

Classification

Hodgkin's disease was classified by a panel convened at Rye, New York; the Rye classification is currently the standard means of classifying this kind of lymphoma (Table 2–27).[697]

As is evident from Table 2–27, Hodgkin's lymphoma can be categorized quite clearly according to morphology. It is important to add a few facts to the information in the table. When obliteration of lymph node architecture suggests a lymphomatous process and a heterogeneous population of cells containing both eosinophils and plasma cells is seen, the diagnosis of Hodgkin's disease should be entertained and Reed-Sternberg cells should be sought. The more favorable prognosis is seen in those lesions with better-differentiated morphology.

A few points should be kept in mind:

1. In lymphocyte predominance, a lymphohistiocytic pattern is often seen with scattered Reed-Sternberg cells. This type has a better prognosis, and about 50% of these patients can be cured with current therapeutic modalities.[698]

2. In mixed cellularity eosinophils, plasma cells and many Reed-Sternberg cells are seen and pseudogranulomas may be observed.

3. In lymphocyte depletion and fibrosis, lymphocytes are lacking; a few Reed-Sternberg cells and occasional histiocytes are seen. This has a grave prognosis.

4. In nodular sclerosis, lymphoid islands are separated by broad fibrous bands. Histiocytes and

TABLE 2–27.—HISTOLOGIC CLASSIFICATION OF HODGKIN'S DISEASE (RYE CONFERENCE)*

TYPE	REED-STERNBERG CELLS	LYMPHOCYTES	COLLAGEN BANDS	DIFFUSE FIBROSIS	EOSINOPHILS	PLASMA CELLS	FREQUENCY (% of Total HD Patients)	5-YEAR SURVIVAL (% of Pts.)
1. Lymphocyte predominance	Rare	2–3	0	0	0	0	10	90
2. Mixed cellularity	3	1–3	0	2	2	1	35–60	70
3. Lymphocyte depletion a. Diffuse fibrosis	1–2	0	0	5	1	1	5–10	20
4. Nodular sclerosis	2	1–3	1–4	1	1	1	35–60	55–70

*Modified from Rosenthal D.S.: The malignant lymphomas, in Beck W.S. (ed.): *Hematology*, ed. 2. Cambridge, M.I.T. Press, 1977, p. 437. Values represent relative numbers except where specified. HD, Hodgkin's disease.

Reed-Sternberg cells appears as "lacunar" cells due to retraction of histiocytes secondary to a fixation artifact.

Extranodal Hodgkin's disease has been described but is not frequently seen. The clinical staging of Hodgkin's disease is given in Table 2–28.[699]

Symptoms

Hodgkin's disease usually manifests with lymphadenopathy (70% of cases), often localized to a single group of nodes (usually cervical) in early stages of the disease. Fever, excessive sweating, fatigue, and pruritus appear late in the course of the disease. A weight loss of more than 10% is not a good prognostic sign. Autoimmune hemolytic anemia, intractable itching, and compression of several anatomical structures by neoplastic tissue are frequent complications of advanced Hodgkin's disease.

The clinical staging of the disease is important for treatment and to assess prognosis.[699] Staging procedures include laparotomy, splenectomy, and lymphangiography. The final diagnosis, however, is based on histopathologic examination. Stage I is characterized by involvement of single node group. Stage IE represents disease localized to a single extranodular site. Stage II represents involvement of two lymph node regions on the same side of the diaphragm. Stage III represents lymphatic or extralymphatic involvement on the two sides of the diaphragm. Stage IV is equivalent to disseminated disease.

Intensive radiation therapy may be curative for patients with stage I or II disease. Up to 4,400 rad delivered per field may be necessary to achieve cure.[700] Radiation may be delivered in a mantle pattern to the neck and chest, in a paraortic field to the abdomen, or in an inverted Y pattern to the pelvic area, according to the areas of involvement. Stage III disease is treated by radiation and chemotherapy, and stage IV disease is treated by chemotherapy alone. Chemotherapy is usually given as a combination that includes nitrogen mustard, vincristine, procarbazine, and prednisone (MOPP).[701]

TABLE 2–28.—CLINICAL STAGES OF HODGKIN'S AND NON-HODGKIN'S LYMPHOMAS (ANN ARBOR CLASSIFICATION)*

STAGE†	DISTRIBUTION OF DISEASE
I	Involvement of a single lymph node region or involvement of a single extralymphatic organ or site (IE).
II	Involvement of two or more lymph node regions on the same side of the diaphragm alone (II) or with involvement of limited contiguous extralymphatic organ or tissue (IIE).
III	Involvement of lymph node regions on both sides of the diaphragm (III), which may include the spleen (IIIS) and/or limited contiguous extralymphatic organ or site (IIIE, IIIES).
IV	Multiple or disseminated foci of involvement of one or more extralymphatic organs or tissues with or without lymphatic involvement.

*Modified from Carbone P.T., et al.: Symposium (Ann Arbor): Staging in Hodgkin's Disease. *Cancer Res.* 31:1707, 1971.
†All stages are further divided on the basis of absence (A) or presence (B) of the following systemic symptoms: significant fever, night sweats, and/or unexplained weight loss of greater than 10% of normal body weight.

The Non-Hodgkin's Lymphomas

In order to better understand the current developments in typing lymphomas it is necessary to review some of the immunology dealt with in more detail in chapter 4.

The immune system is compartmentalized into basically T cells, B cells, and macrophages. T and B cell lymphocytes derive from a common progenitor cell, before they migrate to the bursa of Fabricius, in the case of avian B cells, or to the fetal liver in mammals, and to the thymus in the case of T cells. During ontogenic development, B and T cells display different surface markers as outlined in Tables 2–29 and 2–30.

Histopathologic Classification

Since histopathologic classifications are useful in assessing prognosis, an outline of each of three of the most popular classifications is given in Tables 2–31 to 2–33.

Rappaport's original classification (see Table 2–31) is useful but does not include immunologic markers.[704] In contrast, the Lukes-Collins classification does use immunologic markers[705] differentiating B and T cell lymphomas. The cells are classified morphologically into four categories:

1. Small cleaved: usually B cells at intermediate stages.
2. Large cleaved: stimulated B cells.
3. Small noncleaved: may be immature B cells or T cells.

TABLE 2–29.—B Cell Markers in Ontogeny*

FETAL TISSUE	AGE	CELL TYPE	Ia	cALL	MRBC	FcR	C3R	EBV	SIgM	SIgD	SIg(A,G,E)	CIg
YS, liver		Stem cell	±	+	–	–	–	–	–	–	–	–
SP, LN, BM	7 wk	Pre B	+	+	+/–	–	–	–	–	–	–	–
Liver	9 wk	Early B	+	–	+	±	–	–	+	–	–	–
SP, PB	12 wk	Maturing B	+	–	+	+	–	–	+	+	–	–
PB	Term	Circulating B	+	–	+	++	++	+	+	+	+	–
LN, BM	Term	Plasma cell	–	–	–	–	±	–	–	–	–	+

*YS, yolk sac; SP, spleen; LN, lymph node; BM, bone marrow; PB, peripheral blood; Ia, HLA-DR; cALL, common acute lymphocytic leukemia; MRBC, mouse RBC receptor; FcR, Fc receptor; C3R, C3b receptor; EBV, Epstein-Barr virus receptor; SIg, surface immunoglobulin; CIg, cytoplasmic Ig.

TABLE 2–30.—T Cell Receptors During Ontogeny*

						OKT SURFACE ANTIGENIC MARKERS†				
LOCATION	CELL TYPE	TdT	HTLA	PHA	PAR	10	9	8	4	3
YS, liver	Stem cell	–	–	–	+	+	–	–	–	–
BM, thymus	Pre-T cell	+	+	+/–	–	+	+	–	–	–
Thymus	Thymocyte	–	+	+	–	+	–	+/–	+/–	+/–
LN, PB	T cell	–	+	+	–	+	–	+/–	+/–	+

*Modified from Parker[702] and Reinherz and Schlossman.[703] YS, yolk sac; LN, lymph node; TdT, terminal deoxynucleotidyl transferase; HTLA, human T cell leukemia antigen; PAR, peanut agglutinin receptor; PHA, phytohemagglutinin.
†OKT, monoclonal antibodies: 10, all T cells; 9, immature T cells; 8, T suppressor cells; 4, T helper cells; 3, immature T cells.

TABLE 2–31.—Rappaport Classification of Non-Hodgkin's Lymphoma

HISTOLOGIC TYPE	SUBTYPE
Nodular (follicular) lymphomas	Poorly differentiated lymphocytic
	Mixed cell
	"Histiocytic"
Diffuse lymphomas	Well-differentiated lymphocytic
	Poorly differentiated lymphocytic
	Lymphoblastic
	Convoluted
	Nonconvoluted
	"Histiocytic"
	Burkitt's type
	Undifferentiated (non-Burkitt's type)

TABLE 2–32.—LUKES-COLLINS CLASSIFICATION OF NON-HODGKIN'S LYMPHOMA

CELL TYPE	SUBTYPE
B cell	Small lymphocyte (B cell)
	Plasmacytoid lymphocyte
	Follicular center cell (FCC)
	Small cleaved
	Large cleaved
	Small noncleaved
	Large noncleaved
	Immunoblastic sarcoma (B cell)
T cell	Sézary syndrome–mycosis fungoides
	Convoluted lymphocyte
	Immunoblastic sarcoma (T cell)
Histiocytes	
U (undefined) cell type	

4. Large noncleaved: mature B cells (immunoblasts), or may be stimulated T cells.

Since many pathologists have disagreed, using a variety of classifications, the National Cancer Institute convened an international workshop to classify non-Hodgkin's lymphoma (see Table 2–33).[706]

Etiology and Pathogenesis

The mechanisms by which lymphoid organs develop neoplasms are unknown. Although these seem to be complex, in certain cases a viral etiology is suspected. Among the viruses suspected to induce these neoplasms is the Epstein-Barr virus.[707] Diffuse polyclonal B cell lymphomas have arisen in clusters during EBV infections in individuals in the same community.[708] Using cloned probes and Southern blotting techniques, EBV DNA has been demonstrated in tissues of patients with Burkitt's lymphoma.[709] Furthermore, Bam H1 K fragments of EBV-FF41 were capable of hybridizing to DNA obtained from CNS lymphomas, suggesting an EBV etiology for certain CNS lymphomas.[710]

Type C RNA viruses have likewise been associated with Burkitt's lymphoma and lymphocytic leukemia.[711] Proto-oncogenes or c-oncogenes are sequences of DNA which bear sequence homology with v-oncogenes of acute transforming viruses. These oncogenes are highly conserved during evolution and are associated with cell growth control and differentiation.[712] However, following inducement of mutations and deletions at the sites of these oncogenes in mice, development of neoplasia is likely.[712] If mutations occur at the c-myb locus, for instance, unusual sizes of c-myb RNA as well as c-myb DNA rearrangements are likely to result in the development of lymphoid neoplasia. Burkitt's lymphoma cell lines show translocations between oncogene c-myc and immunoglobulin gene loci. Translocations [t(2;8) (p12;q24), t(8;14) (q24;q32), and t(8;22) (q24;q11)] indicate the potential importance of a gene locus in the long arm of chro-

TABLE 2–33.—CLASSIFICATION OF NHL ACCORDING TO NCI WORKING FORMULATION STUDY*

NOMENCLATURE	TYPE	COMMENTS
Small lymphocytic (low grade)	A	Well-differentiated, slow-growing, usually infiltrates nodes diffusely.
Follicular pattern:		
Small cleaved (low grade)	B	Slow-growing, favorable prognosis. Several follicular center cell types present. Consistently types as monoclonal B cell.
Mixed small cleaved and large cell (low grade)	C	Usually follicular, with diffuse areas. Types as B cell.
Predominantly large cell (intermediate)	D	Follicular and frequent diffuse areas determine poorer prognosis. Usually types as B cell.
Diffuse pattern:		
Small cleaved cell (intermediate)	E	Diffuse growth, may be B or T cell.
Mixed small and large cell (intermediate)	F	Diffuse growth, may be B or T cell.
Large cell (intermediate)	G	Diffuse growth, may be B or T cell.
Large cell, immunoblastic (high grade)	H	Unfavorable prognosis.
Lymphoblastic (high grade)	I	Unfavorable prognosis.
Small noncleaved (high grade)	J	Burkitt's type, unfavorable.

*Modified from reference 706.

mosome 8 at band q24 (8q24) in the development of lymphomas. The very interesting finding has been the mapping of c-myc oncogenes at precisely this q24 (8q24) location. Another oncogene that is a transforming gene is the Blym-1 gene, not physically associated with the c-myc gene located on chromosome 1. This gene has been found to be activated in Burkitt's lymphomas.[713]

Chromosomal Abnormalities of NHL

About 12%–50% of the cells in a lymph node affected by non-Hodgkin's lymphoma contain normal cells. In the abnormal cells, the most common anomaly is a 14q+ chromosome, found in about 80% of the cases. A translocation between chromosome 14 and 18 is the most frequent, usually to band 14q32.[714] In Burkitt's lymphoma the most common translocation is t(8;14), but t(2;8) and t(8;22) can also be seen in these cells. Of great significance in B cell lymphomas is that heavy chain immunoglobulin genes are located on chromosome 14,[715] and that κ and λ light chain genes are located on chromosome $2p^{716}$ and chromosome $22,^{717}$ respectively.

Clinical Aspects of Non-Hodgkin's Lymphoma

The first complaint or incidental finding during physical examination is a nonpainful cervical lymphadenopathy, found in over 60% of patients, although inguinal as well as other node groups are also enlarged in many cases. Extranodal lymphoma is seen in 20% of cases. Frequent sites are the GI tract, the basement membrane, and skin.[718]

Staging Procedures

A good clinical history is essential. A history of night sweats, weight loss, and GI symptoms is an important clue to the diagnosis of the disease and its extent. Careful physical examination to detect involved lymph node groups must be made. Abdominal examination to assess hepatosplenomegaly is important. A bone marrow biopsy of selected sites is mandatory in most cases. Radiologic studies must be performed to assess thoracic and abdominal lymph node involvement. A computed tomography scan is extremely useful to evaluate suspicious masses. Percutaneous liver biopsies are also useful. Staging is similar to that for Hodgkin's lymphomas.

About 15%–30% of both nodular and diffuse lymphomas are found to be in stages (I, IE, II, or IIE). The remaining patients usually present with widespread disease (stages III or IV).

Correlation of Histopathology with Stage and Prognosis

Low-grade non-Hodgkin's lymphoma accounts for about 10% of cases. Cases are histologically almost always of the diffuse type, have a blood component, and probably represent a tissue phase of CLL. They are usually of the B cell type and follow an indolent course.[719]

Follicular lymphomas (nodular) are mostly of B cell lineage. In certain cases, cells with SIgG or SIgM but lacking SIgD may have a worse prognosis,[720] but in general these neoplasms follow an indolent course. However, large cell follicular (nodular) lymphomas in more than 25% of the node have a guarded prognosis.[721]

Diffuse Lymphomas.—Peripheral T cell lymphomas composed of small cleaved cells may have a relatively worse outcome than other types of lymphoma.[722] Diffuse large cell non-Hodgkin's lymphoma, mostly composed of B cell non-Hodgkin's lymphoma, accounts for about 20% of cases and usually has a poor prognosis. However, 30% will present in stages I, IE, II, or IIE, and some will respond to aggressive chemotherapy, especially those with large, round cell diffuse non-Hodgkin's lymphoma.[723] High-grade non-Hodgkin's lymphomas are consistently diffuse in their lymph node infiltration pattern. The immunoblastic type usually presents as stage III or IV. Poor responses to aggressive chemotherapy are characteristic.[724] Most of these tumors are of B cell origin and contain intracytoplasmic immunoglobulin,[725] although some diffuse large cell lymphomas are of T cell origin.[726] These usually are of high-grade invasiveness and carry a poor prognosis. The lymphoblastic lymphoma type, or poorly differentiated lymphocytic lymphoma, is usually a T cell lymphoma of T suppressor cells[727] which, in contrast to other lymphomas, affects children and young adults. It often appears as an intrathoracic mass suggesting thymic origin.[728]

Burkitt's lymphoma is another high-grade non-Hodgkin's lymphoma. It usually appears in African children, invading the jaw tissues. Association with EBV has been documented in many cases of Burkitt's lymphoma.[729] The tumor is very aggressive but susceptible to various types of chemotherapy such as cyclophosphamide.[730]

Laboratory

The main diagnosis is made by histopathologic analysis of a lymph node biopsy. Anemia is present late in the disease. A positive Coombs test may be seen in a few patients and may be the result of an IgM cold agglutinin, sometimes with anti-I specificity.[731]

About 10% of patients have a frank blood involvement by non-Hodgkin's lymphoma cells, although most patients do show varying degrees of peripheral blood involvement by non-Hodgkin's lymphoma cells, detectable by monoclonal antibody cytofluorometry.

Analysis of Cell Markers

A battery of cell markers is used to type lymphomas. Most have been listed in the tables at the beginning of this section. Other markers are given in Table 2–34.[732]

Treatment

Only a very brief summary of treatment of NHL is given below. Curative radiation therapy, 2,000–2,500 rad delivered locally, may be attempted in proved stages I, IE, II, and IIE if the histopathology indicates low-grade non-Hodgkin's lymphoma. Cases with proved stages I, IE, II, and IIE with intermediate to high-grade non-Hodgkin's lymphoma should receive 5,000–5,500 rad.[733] Some cures can be obtained with these treatments (i.e., 5-year survival in 94% in low-grade non-Hodgkin's lymphoma and 75% 5-year survival in high-grade non-Hodgkin's lymphoma in stages I, IE, II, and IIE).

Patients with stage III or IV disease usually have relapses even with aggressive radiotherapy and chemotherapy. However, chemotherapy with chlorambucil or cyclophosphamide may be helpful in reducing tumor loads of patients with advanced disease.[734] Total body irradiation and systemic chemotherapy can be employed in the multicentric types.[735] Combination chemotherapy has also been useful.[736]

Immunoblastic Lymphadenopathy

Patients present with similar symptoms are those found in Hodgkin's disease. Polyclonal hypergammaglobulinemia and hemolytic anemia are often observed. There is a proliferation of blood vessels in an arborescent fashion in lymph nodes, as well as deposition of acidophilic material in the lymph node stroma.[737]

Plasma Cell Myelomas and Macroglobulinemia

In order to understand the pathobiology of myelomas, a review of B cell ontogeny is useful. B lymphocyte precursors originate in the blood islands of several embryonic tissues, including the yolk sac. They then home to lymphoid tissues where they differentiate into mature B cells. In humans the primary lymphoid tissues these primitive B cells home to are the placenta, the fetal liver, and the bone marrow.[738] These primitive B cells are called type I pre-B cells. They contain intracytoplasmic IgM but no surface immunoglobulin.

Type II pre-B cells show allelic exclusion of IgM allotypes.

Primary or immature B cells derive from pre-B cells and are the first B cells to exhibit SIgM. These cells cannot recover their SIgM once they have capped, and are easily made immunotolerant in vitro.[739]

SIgM-bearing B cells then acquire IgD and may have both SIgM and SIgD simultaneously. When SIgD is lost, B cells are considered to be committed

TABLE 2–34.—Non-Hodgkin's Lymphoma Cell Surface Monoclonal Markers*

NHL CELL TYPE	OKB				OKT				
	B1	B2	B4	B7	T4	T8	T9	T10	T11
Pre-B	−	+	−	−	−	−	−	−	−
SIg and B cell	+/−	+	+/−	+/−	−	−	−	−	−
Follicular B cell	−	−	+	−	−	−	−	−	−
Mantle zone	+	+	−	+	−	−	−	−	−
Plasma cells	−	−	−	−	−	−	−	−	−
Th	+/−	−	−	−	+	−	−	−	−
Ts	+/−	−	−	−	−	+	−	−	−

*Data from Knowles et al.[732]

to a memory cell stage. B cells at this stage synthesize a large molecular weight nuclear RNA transcript of the heavy chain genes, coding for various constant heavy chain genes but with a single V_H gene.[740] Once the B cell is committed to a single chain immunoglobulin, the drive to differentiation to a single chain is irreversible. Plasma cells represent the final stage of commitment and maturation to the synthesis of single chain class, single specificity plasma cells.

Plasma Cell Myeloma

Myelomas are composed of a monoclonal, neoplastic expansion of plasma cells which can present at different stages of maturation (e.g., plasmacytoid or mature plasma cell types). Very little SIg is found on these cells, most of the Ig being confined to the cytoplasm. However, when SIg is present on these cells, the specificity is the same as that of the cytoplasmic Ig, although the Ig class may be different.[741]

On occasion, only the heavy chain of the immunoglobulin is synthesized, producing what is called a heavy chain disease (Franklin's disease). These can be IgG, IgA, or of other classes.[742]

Etiology

Little is known about the etiologic mechanisms of plasmacytomas. However, it has been shown experimentally that the repeated injection of mineral oil intraperitoneally in mice will induce myelomas. The injection of pristane into the peritoneal cavity will likewise induce plasmacytomas.[743] A genetic predisposition to the development of myelomas has been shown both in BALB/c mice and in humans.[744]

Other possible etiologic factors are the Aleutian disease virus (ADV), which causes a myeloma-like disease in minks and may infect humans, inducing anti-ADV antibodies. Development of ADV-induced myelomas in humans, however, has not been documented.[745]

Laboratory Diagnosis

Immunoelectrophoresis of serum and urine reveals a monoclonal spike. The different patterns will not be reviewed here. Light chain immunofluorescence with class-specific antibodies, of renal basement membrane deposits reveals monoclonality when present. Class-specific monoclonal antibodies against IgG, IgM, IgA, IgD, and IgE are likewise helpful in the diagnosis. About 0.5% of patients have two monoclonal proteins (e.g., IgG and IgM). Most cases, however, share idiotypic determinants suggesting a common cell of origin.[746]

Treatment

The main therapeutic agents in the treatment of plasma cell myeloma are alkylating agents (cyclophosphamide, chlorambucil, melphalan,[747] or carmustine), radiotherapy (directed at specific bone lesions), and prednisone.[748] High intake of fluids to prevent some of the damage produced by the paraproteins on the kidney is encouraged.

Waldenström's Macroglobulinemia

Waldenström's macroglobulinemia bears a resemblance to both multiple myeloma and CLL. Characteristically, the paraprotein of this monoclonal gammopathy is IgM. Hypermetabolism, hyperviscosity, weakness, and easy fatigability are characteristic. Rouleaux formation is often present and presents difficulties in blood bank laboratory testing. The disease may develop over a period of 4–5 years. Treatment is usually with chlorambucil. Plasmapheresis may be helpful to reduce hyperviscosity, because unlike myeloma, Waldenström's macroglobulinemia has mostly an intravascular paraprotein component.[749]

REFERENCES

1. Nelson D.A., Henry B.J. (ed.): Hematology and coagulation, in *Clinical Diagnosis and Management by Laboratory Methods,* ed. 16. Philadelphia, W.B. Saunders Co., 1979, p. 858.
2. Wintrobe M.M.: *Clinical Hematology,* ed. 8. Philadelphia, Lea & Febiger, 1981, p. 18.
3. Linderkamp O., et al.: The effect of intrapartum and intrauterine asphyxia on placental transfusion in premature and full term infants. *Eur. J. Pediatr.* 127:91, 1978.
4. Matoth Y., Zaizor R., Varsano I.: Postnatal changes in some red cell parameters. *Acta Paediatr. Scand.* 60:317, 1971.
5. Meberg A.: Haemoglobin concentrations and eryth-

ropoietin levels in appropriate and small for gestational age infants. *Scand. J. Haematol.* 24:162, 1980.
6. Schwartz E., Gill F.M.: Hematology of the newborn, in Williams W.J., et al.: *Hematology,* ed. 3. New York, McGraw-Hill Book Co., 1983, pp. 37–44.
7. Saarinen U.M., Siimes M.A.: Developmental changes in red blood cell counts and indices of infants after exclusion of iron deficiency by laboratory criteria and continuous iron supplementation. *J. Pediatr.* 92:412, 1978.
8. Bratteby L.E.: Studies on erythro-kinetics in infancy: XI. The change in circulating red cell volume during the first five months of life. *Acta Paediatr. Scand.* 57:215, 1968.
9. Oski F.A., Delivoria-Papadopoulos M.: The red cell, 2,3-diphosphoglycerate, and tissue oxygen release. *J. Pediatr.* 77:941, 1970.
10. Aballi A., et al.: Platelet counts in thriving premature infants. *Pediatrics* 42:685, 1968.
11. Biland L., Duckert F.: Coagulation factors of the newborn and his mother. *Thromb. Diath. Haemorrh.* 29:644, 1973.
12. Relucke U., et al.: Hayflick's hypothesis: An approach to in vivo testing. *Fed. Proc.* 34:71, 1975.
13. Lipschitz D.A., et al.: The anemia of senescence. *Am. J. Hematol.* 11:47, 1981.
14. Zaino E.C.: Blood counts in the nonagenarian. *NY State J. Med.* 81:1199, 1981.
15. Thomas J.H., Powell D.E.B.: Blood disorders in the elderly. Bristol, John Wright & Sons, 1971, p. 18.
16. Hartsock R.J., et al.: Normal variations with aging on the amount of hematopoietic tissue in bone marrow from the anterior iliac crest. *Am. J. Clin. Pathol.* 43:326, 1965.
17. Makinodan T.: Immunobiology of aging. *J. Am. Geriatr. Soc.* 24:249, 1976.
18. Gilles S., et al.: Immunological studies of aging: Decreased production of and response to T-cell growth factor by lymphocytes from aged humans. *J. Clin. Invest.* 67:937, 1981.
19. Sohnle P., et al.: Failure of lymphokine-producing lymphocytes from aged humans to undergo activation by recall antigens. *J. Immunol.* 124:2169, 1980.
20. Gardner I.D.: The effect of aging on susceptibility to infection. *Rev. Infect. Dis.* 2:801, 1980.
21. Danielli J.F.: The bilayer hypothesis of membrane structure. *Hosp. Pract.* 8:63, 1973.
22. Singer S.J., Nicholson G.L.: The fluid mosaic model of the structure of cell membranes. *Science* 175:720, 1972.
23. Pardoe G.I.: Topochemistry of erythrocyte antigens. *Nouv. Rev. Fr. Hematol.* 11:863, 1971.
24. Williams W.J., Beutler E., et al. (eds.): *Hematology,* ed. 3. New York, McGraw-Hill Book Co., 1983, p. 280.
25. Murphy J.R.: Erythrocyte metabolism. *J. Lab. Clin. Med.* 55:281, 1960.
26. Wintrobe M.M.: *Clinical Hematology,* ed. 8. Philadelphia, Lea & Febiger, 1981, p. 117.
27. Merritt J.E., Leoning K., IUPAC-IUB Joint Commission on Biochemical Nomenclature: Nomenclature of tetrapyrroles. *Eur. J. Biochem.* 108:1, 1980.
28. Garlick R.L., et al.: Synthesis of acetylated human fetal hemoglobin. *J. Biol. Chem.* 256:1727, 1981.
29. Barnes M.G., Komarmy L., Novack A.H.: A comprehensive screening program for hemoglobinopathies. *JAMA* 219:701, 1972.
30. Allred S.: Quality control in the donor room, Appendix L, in Dawson R.B., Fletcher J.L. (eds.): *Donor Room Procedures: A Technical Workshop.* Washington, D.C., American Association of Blood Banks, 1977, p. 44.
31. Ranney H.M., Sharma V.S.: Structure and function of hemoglobin, in Williams W.J., et al (eds.) *Hematology,* ed. 3. New York, McGraw-Hill Book Co., 1983, p. 353.
32. McGivery R.W.: *Biochemistry: A Functional Approach.* Philadelphia, W.B. Saunders Co., 1979, p. 237.
33. Lajtha L.G.: The common ancestral cell, in Wintrobe M.M. (ed.): *Blood, Pure and Eloquent.* New York, McGraw-Hill Book Co., 1980, p. 81.
34. Chervenick P.A., Boggs D.R.: Patterns of proliferation and differentiation of hematopoietic stem cells after compartment depletion. *Blood* 37:568, 1971.
35. Kubane K.B.: Regulation of erythropoiesis: XXIII. Dissociation between stem cell and erythroid response to hypoxia. *Blood* 32:586, 1968.
36. Wintrobe M.M.: *Clinical Hematology,* ed. 8. Philadelphia, Lea & Febiger, 1981, pp. 89–94.
37. Reissman K.R., et al.: Effect of erythropoietin on proliferation of erythroid stem cells in the absence of transplantable colony forming units. *Blood* 36:287, 1970.
38. Udupa K.B., Reissman K.R.: In vivo erythropoietin requirements of generating erythroid progenitors (BFU-E and CFU-E) in bone marrow of mice. *Blood* 49:855, 1977.
39. Erslev A.J., Weiss L.: Structure and function of the marrow, in Williams W.J., et al. (eds.): *Hematology,* ed. 3. New York, McGraw-Hill Book Co., 1983, pp. 75–82.
40. Heath D.S., Axelrod A.A., et al.: Separation of the erythropoietin responsive progenitors BFU-E and CFU-E in mouse bone marrow by unit gravity sedimentation. *Blood* 47:777, 1976.
41. Izak G.: Erythroid cell differentiation and maturation. *Prog. Hematol.* 10:1, 1977.
42. Roodman G.D., et al.: Stimulation of erythroid colony formation in vitro by erythropoietin immobilized on agarose-bound lectins. *J. Lab. Clin. Med.* 98:684, 1981.
43. Best W.R.: Chloramphenicol-associated blood dyscrasias. *JAMA* 20:181, 1967.

44. Plant M.E., Best W.R.: Aplastic anemia after parenteral chloramphenicol: Warning reviewed. *N. Engl. J. Med.* 306:1486, 1982.
45. Wintrobe M.M.: The therapeutic minimum and its price: A view from the haematopoietic system. *J.R. Coll. Physicians Lond.* 3:99, 1969.
46. Sykes M.P., et al.: The effects of varying dosages of irradiation upon sternal-marrow regeneration. *Radiology* 83:1084, 1964.
47. Cooper W.: Pancytopenia associatiated with disseminated tuberculosis. *Ann. Intern. Med.* 50:1497, 1959.
48. Levy R.N., et al.: Fatal aplastic anemia after hepatitis. *N. Engl. J. Med.* 273:1113, 1965.
49. Shadduck R.K., et al.: Aplastic anemia following infectious mononucleosis: Possible immune etiology. *Exp. Hematol.* 7:264, 1979.
50. Levine A.S. (ed.): *Proceedings of the Conference on Aplastic Anemia: A Stem Cell Disease,* NIH Publication No. 81–1008. Washington, D.C., 1981.
51. Robbins S.L., Cotran R.S.: *Pathologic Basis of Disease,* ed. 2. Philadelphia, W.B. Saunders Co., 1979, p. 739.
52. Shahidi N.T., Diamond L.K.: Testosterone induced remission in aplastic anemia of both acquired and congenital types. *N. Engl. J. Med.* 264:953, 1961.
53. Storb R., et al.: Marrow transplantation in thirty "untransfused" patients with severe aplastic anemia. *Ann. Intern. Med.* 92:30, 1980.
54. Diamond L.K., et al.: Congenital (erythroid) hypoplastic anemia. *Am. J. Dis. Child.* 102:403, 1961.
55. Dameshek W., et al.: "Pure" red cell anemia and thymoma. *Semin. Hematol.* 4:222, 1967.
56. Geary C.G., et al.: Thymoma associated with pure red cell aplasia, immunoglobulin deficiency and an inhibitor of antigen-induced lymphocyte transformation. *Br. J. Haematol.* 29:479, 1975.
57. Brittingham T.E., et al.: Reversible erythroid aplasia induced by diphenyl-hydantoin. *Arch. Intern. Med.* 113:764, 1964.
58. Beck W.S.: *Hematology,* ed. 2. Cambridge, Mass., MIT Press, 1977, p. 128.
59. Green R., Charlton R., Seftel H., et al.: Body iron excretion in man: A collaborative study. *Am. J. Med.* 45:336, 1968.
60. Pape L., et al.: In vitro reconstitution of ferritin. *Biochemistry* 7:606, 1968.
61. Okada S., et al.: In vivo evidence for the functional heterogeneity of transferrin bound iron: V. Isotransferrins. An explanation of the Fletcher-Huehns phenomenon in the rat. *J. Lab. Clin. Med.* 93:189, 1979.
62. Dagg J.H., Golberg A.: Detection and treatment of iron deficiency. *Clin. Hematol.* 2:365, 1973.
63. Merritt J.E., Leoning K.L., IUPAC-IUB Joint Commission on Biochemical Nomenclature: Nomenclature of tetrapyrrols. *Eur. J. Biochem.* 108:1, 1980.
64. White J.M., Selhi H.S.: Lead and the red cell. *Br. J. Haematol.* 30:133, 1975.
65. Bradley M., et al.: Medical microscopy and examination of other body fluids, in Henry J.B. (ed.): *Clinical Diagnosis and Management by Laboratory Methods.* Philadelphia, W.B. Saunders Co., 1979, p. 601.
66. Hernberg W., Nikkanen J.: Enzyme inhibition by lead under normal urban conditions. *Lancet* 1:63, 1970.
67. Winston R.M., et al.: Enzymatic diagnosis of megaloblastic anaemia. *Br. J. Haematol.* 19:587, 1970.
68. Streiff R.R.: Folic acid deficiency anemia. *Semin. Hematol.* 7:23, 1970.
69. Carmel R.: The laboratory diagnosis of megaloblastic anemias. *West. J. Med.* 128:294, 1978.
70. Castle W.B.: Current concepts of pernicious anemias. *Am. J. Med.* 48:541, 1970.
71. Sullivan L.W.: Vitamin B12 metabolism and megaloblastic anemia. *Semin. Hematol.* 7:6, 1970.
72. Ardeman S., et al.: Studies on the secretion of gastric intrinsic factor in man. *Br. Med. J.* 2:600, 1964.
73. Ardeman S., et al.: Studies on the secretion of gastric intrinsic factor in man. *Gut* 7:99, 1966.
74. Thorn G.W., et al.: *Harrison's Principles of Internal Medicine,* ed. 8. New York, McGraw-Hill Book Co., 1977, p. 1524.
75. Lindenbaum J., Nath B.J.: Megaloblastic anemia and neutrophil hypersegmentation. *Br. J. Haematol.* 44:511, 1980.
76. Perillie P.E., et al.: Significance of changes in serum muramidase activity in megaloblastic anemia. *N. Engl. J. Med.* 277:10, 1970.
77. Ellims P.H., et al.: Plasma thymidine kinase in megaloblastic anemia. *Br. J. Haematol.* 44:167, 1980.
78. Elsborg L., Mosbech J.: Gastric cancer as a risk factor in pernicious anemia, in *Vitamin B12: Proceedings of the Third European Symposium on Vitamin B12 and Intrinsic Factor.* New York, Zagalak B. and Friedrich W. Walter deGruyter, 1979, p. 1119.
79. Rosenfelt F.: Methotrexate and the need for continued research. *Yale J. Biol. Med.* 48:97, 1975.
80. Fallon H.J.: A genetic study of hereditary orotic aciduria. *N. Engl. J. Med.* 270:878, 1964.
81. Lehman H., Cappel R.W.: Variations in the structure of human hemoglobins. *Br. Med. Bull.* 25:H, 1969.
82. Lawn R.M., et al.: The nucleotide sequence of the human β globin gene. *Cell* 21:647, 1980.
83. Spritz R.: Nucleotide sequence of the human δ-globin gene. *Cell* 21:639, 1980.
84. Bank A., et al.: Globin gene pathology, in Nienhuis A.W., Stamatoyannopoulos G. (eds.): *Clues to Gene Function and Hemoglobin Switching in Globin Gene Organization and Expression,* New York, Alan R. Liss, 1981.

85. Little P.F.R., et al.: Structure of the fetal globin gene locus. *Nature* 278:227, 1979.
86. Efstratiadis A., et al.: The structure and evolution of the human beta-globin gene family. *Cell* 21:653, 1980.
87. Marotta C.A., et al.: Human beta-globulin messenger RNA: III Nucleotide sequences derived from complementary DNA. *J. Biol. Chem.* 252:5040, 1977.
88. Curtis P.J., et al.: Characterization and kinetics of synthesis of 15s beta-globulin RNA, a putative precursor of beta-globin mRNA. *Cold Spring Harbor Symp. Quant. Biol.* 42:971, 1977.
89. Revel J., Groner Y.: Post-transcriptional and translational controls of gene expression in eukaryotes. *Annu. Rev. Biochem.* 47:1079, 1978.
90. Bunn H.F., et al.: The thalassemias and the molecular genetics of human hemoglobin synthesis, in Smith L.H. (ed.): *Hemoglobinopathies.* Philadelphia, W.B. Saunders Co., 1977, pp. 28–94.
91. Ochoa S., deHaro C.: Regulation of protein synthesis in eukaryotes. *Annu. Rev. Biochem.* 48:549, 1979.
92. Weintraub H., et al.: Alpha-globin gene switching during the development of chicken embryos: Expression and chromosome structure. *Cell* 24:333, 1981.
93. Pauling L., et al.: Sickle cell anemia, a molecular disease. *Science* 110:543, 1949.
94. Milner P.F., Gooden H.M., General R.T.: Citrate agar electrophoresis in routine screening for hemoglobinopathies using a simple hemolysate. *Am. J. Clin. Pathol.* 64:58, 1975.
95. Reider R.F.: Human hemoglobin stability and instability: Molecular mechanisms and some clinical correlations. *Semin. Hematol.* 11:423, 1974.
96. Wallerstein R.O.: Blood, in Krupp M.A., Chatton M.J. (eds.): *Current Medical Diagnosis and Treatment.* Los Altos, Calif., Lange Medical Publishers, 1982, p. 286.
97. Dean J., Schechter A.N.: Sickle-cell anemia: Molecular and cellular basis of therapeutic approaches. *N. Engl. J. Med.* 299:752, 1978.
98. Goldberg M.A., et al.: The effect of erythrocyte membrane preparations on the polymerization of sickle hemoglobin. *J. Biol. Chem.* 256:193, 1981.
99. Dzanda J.K., Johnson R.M.: Membrane protein phosphorylation in intact normal and sickle cell erythrocytes. *J. Biol. Chem.* 255:6382, 1980.
100. Finch C.A.: Pathophysiologic aspects of sickle cell anemia. *Am. J. Med.* 53:1, 1972.
101. Sheehy T.W., Plumb V.J.: Treatment of sickle cell disease. *Arch. Intern. Med.* 137:779, 1977.
102. Davey R.J., et al.: Partial exchange transfusion as treatment of hemoglobin SC disease in pregnancy. *Arch. Intern. Med.* 138:937, 1978.
103. Heller P., et al.: Clinical implications of sickle-cell trait and glucose-6-phosphate dehydrogenase deficiency in hospitalized black male patients. *N. Engl. J. Med.* 300:1001, 1979.
104. Nathan D.G., Gunn R.B.: Thalassemia: The consequences of unbalanced hemoglobin synthesis. *Am. J. Med.* 41:815, 1966.
105. Gale R.E., et al.: Human embryonic hemoglobins Gower 1 and Gower 2. *Nature* 280:162, 1979.
106. Wood W.C., et al.: Developmental biology of human hemoglobins. *Prog. Hematol.* 10:43, 1977.
107. Wetherall D.J., Clegg J.B.: *The Thalassemia Syndromes,* ed. 3. Oxford, England, Blackwell Scientific Publications, 1981.
108. Nathan D.G.: Thalassemia. *N. Engl. J. Med.* 286:586, 1972.
109. Rigas D.A., et al.: Hemoglobin H. *J. Lab. Clin. Med.* 47:51, 1956.
110. Wasi P. et al.: The α thalassemia. *Clin. Haematol.* 3:383, 1974.
111. Higgs D.R., et al.: α thalassemias in black populations. *Johns Hopkins Med. J.* 146:300, 1980.
112. Valentine W.N.: Hereditary spherocytosis revisited. *West. J. Med.* 128:35, 1978.
113. Johnsson R., Salminen S.: Effect of ouabain on osmotic resistance, and monovalent cation transport of red cells in hereditary spherocytosis. *Scand. J. Haematol.* 25:323, 1980.
114. Hill J.S., et al.: Hereditary spherocytosis: Altered binding of the cytoskeleton to the red cell membrane. *Blood* 58(suppl. 1):43A, 1981.
115. Greenberg L.H., Tanaka R.K.: Hereditary elliptocytosis with hemolytic anemia: A family study of five affected members. *Calif. Med.* 110:389, 1969.
116. Coetzer T., Zail S.S.: Tryptic digestion of spectrin in variants of hereditary elliptocytosis. *J. Clin. Invest.* 67:12, 1981.
117. Lock S.P., et al.: Stomatocytosis: A hereditary red cell anomaly associated with hemolytic anemia. *Br. J. Haematol.* 7:303, 1961.
118. Lande W., et al.: Congenital anemia with abnormal cation permeability and cold hemolysis in vitro. *Blood* 54:29a, 1979.
119. Cooper R.A., et al.: Decreased fluidity of red cell membrane lipids in a beta lipoproteinemia. *J. Clin. Invest.* 60:115, 1977.
120. Bird T.D., et al.: Familial degeneration of the basal ganglia with acanthocytosis: A clinical, neuropathological, and neurochemical study. *Ann. Neurol.* 3:253, 1978.
121. Taswell H.F., et al.: Erythrocyte morphology in genetic defects of the Rh and Kell blood group systems. *Mayo Clin. Proc.* 52:157, 1977.
122. Galey W.R., et al.: Morphology and physiology of the McLeod erythrocyte. *Vox Sang.* 34:152, 1978.
123. Oni S.B., et al.: Paroxysmal nocturnal hemoglobinuria: Evidence for monoclonal origin of abnormal red cells. *Blood* 36:145, 1970.
124. Rosse W.F.: Variations in the red cells in paroxysmal nocturnal haemoglobinuria. *Br. J. Haematol.* 24:327, 1973.
125. Siriwittayakorn J., Yuthavong Y.: Relation between low erythrocyte acetyl cholinesterase activity

and membrane lipids in paroxysmal nocturnal hemoglobinuria. *Br. J. Haematol.* 41:383, 1979.
126. Kruatrachue M., et al.: Paroxysmal nocturnal haemoglobinuria in Thailand with special reference to an association with aplastic anemia. *Br. J. Haematol.* 39:267, 1978.
127. Cowall D.E., et al.: Paroxysmal nocturnal hemoglobinuria terminating as erythroleukemia. *Cancer* 43:1914, 1979.
128. Zitoun R., et al.: Acute myelomonocytic leukemia: Terminal complication of paroxysmal nocturnal hemoglobinuria. *Acta Haematol.* 35:241, 1975.
129. Dacie J.V., Lewis S.M.: Paroxysmal nocturnal hemoglobinuria: Clinical manifestations, hematology and nature of the disease. *Ser. Haematol.* 5:3, 1972.
130. Rosse W.F., Gutterman L.A.: The effect of iron therapy in paroxysmal nocturnal hemoglobinuria. *Blood* 36:559, 1970.
131. Craddock P.R., et al.: Complement mediated granulocyte dysfunction in paroxysmal nocturnal hemoglobinuria. *Blood* 47:931, 1976.
132. Gardner F.H., Murphy S.: Granulocyte and platelet functions in PNH. *Ser. Haematol.* 5:78, 1972.
133. Jenkins D.E. Jr.: Diagnostic tests for PNH. *Ser. Haematol.* 5:24, 1972.
134. Hartman R.C., et al.: Diagnostic specificity of sucrose hemolysis test for paroxysmal nocturnal hemoglobinuria. *Blood* 35:462, 1970.
135. Rosse W.F.: Paroxysmal nocturnal hemoglobinuria: Present status and future prospects. *West. J. Med.* 132:219, 1980.
136. Leibowitz A.I., Hartmann R.C.: Annotation: The Budd-Chiari syndrome and paroxysmal nocturnal haemoglobinuria. *Br. J. Haematol.* 48:1, 1981.
137. Clark D.A., et al.: The kidneys in paroxysmal nocturnal hemoglobinuria. *Blood* 57:83, 1981.
138. Fefer A., et al.: Paroxysmal nocturnal hemoglobinuria and marrow failure treated by infusion of marrow from an identical twin. *Ann. Intern. Med.* 84:692, 1976.
139. Storb R., et al.: PNH and refractory marrow failure treated by marrow transplantation. *Br. J. Haematol.* 24:743, 1973.
140. Gockerman J.P., Brouillard R.P.: RBC transfusions in patients with paroxysmal nocturnal hemoglobinuria. *Arch. Intern. Med.* 137:536, 1977.
141. Gardner F.H., et al.: The use of clinical dextran in patients with paroxysmal nocturnal hemoglobinuria. *J. Lab. Clin. Med.* 55:946, 1960.
142. Beutler E.: Energy metabolism and maintenance of erythrocytes, in Williams W.J., et al. (ed.): *Hematology,* ed. 3. New York, McGraw-Hill Book Co., 1983, p. 331.
143. McGilvery R.W.: *Biochemistry: A Functional Approach,* ed. 2. Philadelphia, W.B. Saunders Co., 1979, p. 235.
144. Baldwin J., Chothia C.: Haemoglobin: The structural changes related to ligand binding and its allosteric mechanism. *J. Mol. Biol.* 129:175, 1979.
145. Beutler E.: *Hemolytic Anemia in Disorders of Red Cell Metabolism.* New York, Plenum Medical Book Co., 1978.
146. McKusick V.A., Ruddle F.H.: The status of the gene map of the human chromosomes. *Science* 196:390, 1977.
147. Yoshida A., Beutler E.: G-6-PD variants: Another update. *Ann. Hum. Genet.* 47:27, 1983.
148. Fialkow P.J.: Clonal origin of human tumors. *Biochim. Biophys. Acta* 458:286, 1976.
149. Testa U., et al.: Genetic heterogeneity of glucose-6-phosphate dehydrogenase deficiency in Sardinia. *Hum. Genet.* 56:99, 1980.
150. Yoshida A.: Amino acid substitution (histidine to tyrosine) in a glucose-6-phosphate dehydrogenase variant (G6PD Hektoen) associated with over production. *J. Mol. Biol.* 52:483, 1970.
151. Kosower N.S., et al.: The generation of reduced glutathione in normal and glucose-6-phosphate dehydrogenase deficient human red blood cells. *Blood* 29:313, 1967.
152. Chan T.K., et al.: Drug-induced haemolysis in G6PD deficiency. *Br. Med. J.* 2:1227, 1976.
153. Constantopoulos A., et al.: Fulminant diarrhea and acute hemolysis due to G-6-PD deficiency in salmonellosis. *Lancet* 1:1522.
154. Burka E.R., et al.: Clinical spectrum of hemolytic anemia associated with glucose-6-phosphate dehydrogenase deficiency. *Ann. Intern. Med.* 64:817, 1966.
155. Whelton A., et al.: Acute renal failure complicating Rickettsial infections in glucose-6-phosphate dehydrogenase-deficient individuals. *Ann. Intern. Med.* 69:323, 1968.
156. Clearfield H.R., et al.: Acute viral hepatitis, glucose-6-phosphate dehydrogenase deficiency, and hemolytic anemia. *Arch. Intern. Med.* 123:689, 1969.
157. Gelladay A.M., Greenwood R.D.: G-6-PD hemolytic anemia complicating diabetic ketoacidosis. *J. Pediatr.* 80:1037, 1972.
158. Carpentieri U., et al.: Kernicterus in a newborn female with G-6-PD deficiency. *J. Pediatr.* 89:854, 1976.
159. Feldman R., et al.: Congenital nonspherocytic hemolytic anemia due to glucose-6-phosphate dehydrogenase: East Harlem. A new deficient variant. *J. Pediatr.* 90:89, 1977.
160. Herz F., et al.: Diagnosis of erythrocyte glucose-6-phosphate dehydrogenase deficiency in the Negro male despite hemolytic crisis. *Blood* 35:90, 1970.
161. Beutler E., Mitchell M.: Special modifications of the fluorescent screening method for glucose-6-phosphate dehydrogenase deficiency. *Blood* 32:816, 1968.
162. Beutler E., et al.: Biochemical variants of glucose-6-phosphate dehydrogenase giving rise to congenital nonspherocytic hemolytic disease. *Blood* 31:131, 1968.
163. Corash L., et al.: Reduced chronic hemolysis during high-dose Vitamin E administration in Mediterra-

nean type glucose-6-phosphate dehydrogenase deficiency. *N. Engl. J. Med.* 303:416, 1980.
164. Konrad P.N., et al.: Glutamyl-cysteine synthetase deficiency. *N. Engl. J. Med.* 286:557, 1972.
165. Roos D., et al.: Protection of phagocytic leukocytes by endogenous glutathione: Studies in a family with glutathione reductase deficiency. *Blood* 53:851, 1979.
166. Wintrobe M.M., et al.: *Clinical Hematology,* ed. 8. Philadelphia, Lea & Febiger, 1981, p. 192.
167. Dao C., et al.: Eosinophil and neutrophil colony-forming cells in culture. *Blood* 50:833, 1977.
168. Bainton D.F., et al.: The development of neutrophilic polymorphonuclear leukocytes in human bone marrow: Origin and content of azurophil and specific granules. *J. Exp. Med.* 134:907, 1971.
169. Scott R.E., Horn R.G.: Ultrastructural aspects of neutrophil granulocyte development in humans. *Lab. Invest.* 23:202, 1970.
170. Baggiolini M.: The neutrophil, in Weissman C. (ed.): *The Cell Biology of Inflammation.* Amsterdam, Elsevier North-Holland, 1980, p. 163.
171. Wright D.G.: The neutrophil as a secretory organ of host defense, in Gallin J., Fauci A.S. (eds.): *Phagocytic Cells: Advances in Host Defense Mechanisms.* New York, Raven Press, 1982, p. 75.
172. West B.C., et al.: Separation and characterization of human neutrophil granules. *Am. J. Pathol.* 77:41, 1974.
173. Olssen I., Verge P.: The role of the human neutrophil in the inflammatory reaction. *Allergy* 35:1, 1980.
174. Smith J.A.: The cell cycle and related concepts in cell proliferation. *J. Pathol.* 136:149, 1982.
175. Quesenberry P., Levitt L.: Hematopoietic stem cells. *N. Engl. J. Med.* 301:755, 1979.
176. Abramson S., et al.: The identification in adult bone marrow of pluripotent and restricted stem cells of the myeloid and lymphoid systems. *J. Exp. Med.* 145:1567, 1977.
177. Fauser A.A., Messner H.A.: Identification of megakaryocytes, macrophages, and eosinophils in colonies of human bone marrow containing neutrophilic granulocytes and erythroblasts. *Blood* 53:1023, 1979.
178. Tyler W.S., et al.: Effect of a congenital defect in hemopoiesis on myeloid growth and stem cell (CFU) in an in vivo culture system. *Blood* 47:413, 1976.
179. Metcalf D.: Transformation of granulocytes to macrophages in bone marrow colonies in vitro. *J. Cell. Physiol.* 77:277, 1971.
180. Iscove N.N., et al.: The proliferative states of mouse granulopoietic progenitor cells. *Proc. Soc. Exp. Biol. Med.* 134:33, 1970.
181. Trentin T.J.: Determination of bone marrow stem cell differentiation by stromal hemopoietic inductive microenvironments (HIM). *Am. J. Pathol.* 65:621, 1971.
182. Lusis A.J., et al.: Purification and characterization of a human T-lymphocyte-derived granulocyte-macrophage colony-stimulating factor. *Blood* 57 13, 1981.
183. Cline M.J., Golde D.W.: Cellular interactions in haematopoiesis. *Nature* 277:177, 1979.
184. Burgess A.W., Metcalf D.: The nature and action of granulocyte-macrophage colony-stimulating factors. *Blood* 56:947, 1980.
185. Guilbert L.J., Stanley E.R.: Specific interaction of murine colony-stimulating factors with mononuclear phagocytic cells. *J. Cell Biol.* 85:153, 1980.
186. Cline M.J., Golde D.W.: Production of colony-stimulating activity by human lymphocytes. *Nature* 248:703, 1974.
187. Quesenberry P.J., Gimbrone M.A., Jr.: Vascular endothelium as a regulator of granulopoiesis: Production of colony stimulating activity by cultured human endothelial cells. *Blood* 56:1060, 1980
188. Warner H.R., Athens J.W.: An analysis of granulocyte kinetics in blood and bone marrow. *Ann. NY Acad. Sci.* 113:523, 1964.
189. Vincent P.C.: The measurement of granulocyte kinetics. *Br. J. Haematol.* 36:1, 1977.
190. Boogs D.R., et al.: Mechanisms controlling homeostasis of neutrophilic leukocytes. *Haematol. Lat.* 10:43, 1967.
191. Dale D.C., et al.: Comparison of agents producing a neutrophilic leukocytosis in man: Hydrocortisone, prednisone, endotoxin and etiocholanolone. *J. Clin. Invest.* 56:808, 1975.
192. Peters W.J., et al.: Corticosteroid administration and localized leukocyte mobilization in man. *N. Engl. J. Med.* 286:342, 1972.
193. Huestis D.W.: Granulocyte collection with the haemonetics system: Normal and leukemic donors, in *Leukapheresis and Granulocyte Transfusions.* Washington, D.C., American Association of Blood Banks, 1975, p. 33.
194. Rytomaa T., Kiviniemi K.: Control of granulocyte production: II. Mode of action of chalone and antichalone. *Cell Tissue Kinet.* 1:341, 1968.
195. Klebanoff S.J., Clark R.A.: *The Neutrophil: Function and Clinical Disorders.* New York, Elsevier North-Holland, 1978, p. 1.
196. Lefell M.S., Spitznagel J.K.: Intracellular and extracellular degranulation of human polymorphonuclear azurophil and specific granules induced by immune complexes. *Infect. Immun.* 10:1241, 1974.
197. Lefell M.S., Spitznagel J.K.: Fate of human lactoferrin and myeloperoxidase in phagocytizing human neutrophils: Effects of immunoglobulin G subclasses and immune complexes coated on latex beads. *Infect. Immun.* 12:813, 1975.
198. Hoffstein S., et al.: Concanavalin A induces microtubule assembly and specific granule discharge in human polymorphonuclear leukocytes. *J. Cell Biol.* 68:781, 1976.
199. Wright D.G., et al.: The differentiated mobilization of human neutrophil granules: Effects of phor-

bol myristrate acetate ionophore A23187. *Am. J. Pathol.* 87:273, 1977.
200. Wright D.G., Gallin J.I.: Secretory responses of human neutrophils: Exocytosis of specific (secondary) granules by human neutrophils during adherence in vitro and during exudation in vivo. *J. Immunol.* 123:285, 1979.
201. Gallin J.I.: Degranulating stimuli decrease the negative surface charge and increase the adhesiveness of human neutrophils. *J. Clin. Invest.* 65:298, 1980.
202. Badwey J.A., Karnovsky M.L.: Active oxygen species and the functions of phagocytic leukocytes. *Annu. Rev. Biochem.* 49:695, 1980.
203. Babior B.M.: Oxygen-dependent microbial killing by phagocytes. *N. Engl. J. Med.* 298:659, 1978.
204. Klebanoff S.J.: Oxygen-dependent cytotoxic mechanisms, in *Advances in Host Defense Mechanisms:* Vol. 1. *Phagocytic Cells.* New York, Raven Press, 1982, p. 111.
205. Klebanoff S.J.: Oxygen intermediates and the microbicidal event, in Van Furth R. (ed.): *Mononuclear Phagocytes: Functional Aspects.* Boston, Martinus Nijhoff Publishers, 1980, p. 1105.
206. O'Flaherty J.T., Ward P.A.: Chemotactic factors and the neutrophil. *Semin. Hematol.* 16:163, 1979.
207. Ward P.A., et al.: The production by antigen-stimulated lymphocytes of a leukotactic factor distinct from migration inhibitory factor. *Cell. Immunol.* 2:162, 1970.
208. Hugli T.E., Müller-Eberhard H.J.: Anaphylatoxins: C3a and C5a. *Adv. Immunol.* 26:1, 1978.
209. Fernandez H.N., et al.: Chemotactic response to human C3a and C5a anaphylatoxins: I. Evaluation of C3a and leukotaxis in vitro and when stimulated in vivo conditions. *J. Immunol.* 120:109, 1977.
210. Kaplan A.P., et al.: The prealbumin activator of prekallikrein: III. Appearance of chemotactic activity for human neutrophils by the conversion of human prekallikrein to kallikrein. *J. Exp. Med.* 135:81, 1972.
211. Stecher V.J., Sorkin E.: The chemotactic activity of fibrinolysis products. *Int. Arch. Allergy Appl. Immunol.* 43:879, 1972.
212. Niedel J., et al.: Covalent affinity labeling of the formyl-peptide chemotactic receptor. *J. Biol. Chem.* 255:7063, 1980.
213. Hoover R.L., et al.: The adhesive interaction between polymorphonuclear leukocytes and endothelial cells in vitro. *Cell* 14:423, 1978.
214. Gallin J.I., Snyderman R.: Leukocyte chemotaxis. *Fed. Proc.* 42:2852, 1983.
215. Arnaut M.A., et al.: Deficiency of a granulocyte membrane glycoprotein (gp150) in a boy with recurrent bacterial infections. *N. Engl. J. Med.* 306:693, 1982.
216. Boxer L.A., et al.: Neutrophil actin dysfunction and abnormal neutrophil motility. *N. Engl. J. Med.* 293:1093, 1974.
217. Boxer L.A., Stossel T.P.: Interactions of actin, myosin and an actin binding protein of chronic myelogenous leukemic leukocytes. *J. Clin. Invest.* 57:964, 1976.
218. Adelstein R.S., Pollard T.D.: Platelet contractile proteins. *Prog. Hemost. Thromb.* 4:37, 1978.
219. Yin H.L., et al.: Ca^{2+} control of actin gelation: Interaction of gelsolin with actin filaments and regulation of actin gelation. *J. Biol. Chem.* 255:9494, 1980.
220. Pozzan T., et al.: Is cytosolic ionized calcium regulating neutrophil activation? *Science* 221:1413, 1983.
221. Messner R.P., Yelinek J.: Receptors for human γ-globulin on human neutrophils. *J. Clin. Invest.* 49:2165, 1970.
222. Newman S.L., Johnston R.B. Jr.: Role of binding through C3b and IgG in polymorphonuclear neutrophil function: Studies with trypsin-generated IgG. *J. Immunol.* 123:1839, 1979.
223. Tenner A.J., Cooper N.R.: Identification of types of cells in human peripheral blood that bind C1q. *J. Immunol.* 126:1174, 1981.
224. Lay W.H., Nussenzweig V.: Receptors for complement on leukocytes. *J. Exp. Med.* 128:991, 1968.
225. Mahmoud A.A.F., Austin K.F. (eds.): *The Eosinophil in Health and Disease.* New York, Grune & Stratton, 1980, p. 1.
226. Mahmoud A.A.F., et al.: Eosinophilopoietin: A circulating low molecular weight peptide-like substance which stimulates the production of eosinophils in mice. *J. Clin. Invest.* 60:675, 1977.
227. Zucker-Franklin D., et al.: Granulocyte colonies derived from lymphocyte fractions of normal human blood. *Proc. Natl. Acad. Sci. USA* 71:2711, 1974.
228. Mahmoud A.A.F., et al.: Eosinophilopoietin: A low molecular weight peptide stimulating eosinophil production in mice. *Trans. Assoc. Am. Physicians* 90:127, 1977.
229. The mechanism of eosinophilia (editorial). *Lancet* 2:1187, 1971.
230. Anderson V., et al.: Autoradiographic studies of the kinetics of eosinophils. *Ser. Haematol.* 4:33, 1968.
231. Bass D.A.: Eosinophil behavior during host defense reactions, in Gallin J., Fauci A.S. (eds.): *Phagocytic Cells. Advances in Host Defense Mechanisms.* New York, Raven Press, 1982, p. 211.
232. Bjorksten B., Lundmark K.M.: Recurrent bacterial infections in four siblings with neutropenia, eosinophilia, hyperimmunoglobulinemia A, and defective neutrophil chemotaxis. *J. Infect. Dis.* 133:63, 1976.
233. Andrews J.P., et al.: Lethal congenital neutropenia with eosinophilia occurring in two siblings. *Am. J. Med.* 29:358, 1960.
234. Ishikawa T., et al.: *In vitro* and *in vivo* studies on uptake of antigen-antibody complexes by eosinophils. *Int. Arch. Allergy Appl. Immunol.* 46:230, 1974.
235. DeChatelet L.R., et al.: Comparison of intracellular bactericidal abilities of human neutrophils and eosinophils. *Blood* 52:609, 1978.

236. Beeson P.B., Bass D.A.: *The Eosinophil.* Philadelphia, W.B. Saunders, 1977, p. 1.
237. Beisel W.B., Rapoport M.I.: Inter-relations between adrenocortical functions and infectious illness. *N. Engl. J. Med.* 28:541, 1969.
238. Venge P., et al.: Neutrophil and eosinophil granulocytes in bacterial infection: Sequential studies of cellular and serum levels of granule proteins. *Br. J. Haematol.* 38:475, 1978.
239. Walls R.S., et al.: Macrophage-eosinophil interactions in the inflammatory response to *Trichinella spiralis. Blood* 44:131, 1974.
240. Mahmoud A.A.F., et al.: Production of monospecific rabbit anti-human eosinophil serums and demonstration of a blocking phenomenon. *N. Engl. J. Med.* 290:417, 1974.
241. Dessein A.J., David J.R.: The eosinophil in parasitic diseases, in Gallin J.I., Fauci A.S. (eds.): *Phagocytic Cells.* Volume 1 in *Advances in Host Defense Mechanisms.* New York, Raven Press, 1982, p. 243.
242. Askenase P.W.: Effector and regulatory functions of cells in the immune response to parasites: Summary. *Fed. Proc.* 42:1742, 1983.
243. Mahmoud A.A.F., et al.: In vitro killing of schistosomula of *Schistosoma mansoni* by BCG and *C. parvum*-activated macrophages. *J. Immunol.* 122:1655, 1979.
244. Vadas M.A., et al.: A new method for the purification of human eosinophils and neutrophils, and a comparison of the ability of these cells to damage schistosomata of *Schistosoma mansoni. J. Immunol.* 122:1228, 1979.
245. Anwar A.R.E., et al.: Killing schistosomula of *Schistosoma mansoni* coated with antibody and/or complement by human leukocytes in vitro: Requirement of complement in preferential killing by eosinophils. *J. Immunol.* 122:628, 1979.
246. Gleish G.J., et al.: The eosinophil: New aspects of structure and function. *J. Allergy Clin. Immunol.* 60:73, 1977.
247. Butterworth A.E., et al.: Interactions between human eosinophils and schistosomula of *Schistosoma mansoni* induced directly by eosinophil major basic protein. *J. Immunol.* 122:221, 1979.
248. Capron M., et al.: Fc receptors for IgE on human and rat eosinophils. *J. Immunol.* 126:2087, 1981.
249. Capron M., et al.: Role of IgE receptors in effector function of human eosinophils. *J. Immunol.* 132:462, 1984.
250. Melewicz F.M., et al.: Comparison of the Fc receptors for IgE on human lymphocytes and monocytes. *J. Immunol.* 129:563, 1982.
251. Ishikawa T., et al.: In vitro and in vivo studies on uptake of antigen antibody complexes by eosinophils. *Int. Arch. Allergy* 66:230, 1974.
252. Miller F., et al.: The structure of the leukocyte granules in rodents and man. *J. Cell Biol.* 31:349, 1962.
253. Archer G.T., Hirsch J.G.: Isolation of granules from eosinophil leukocytes and study of their enzyme content. *J. Exp. Med.* 118:277, 1963.
254. Gleich G.J., et al.: Physiochemical and biological properties of the major basic protein from guinea pig eosinophil granules. *J. Exp. Med.* 140:313, 1974.
255. Butterworth A.E., et al.: Interactions between human eosinophils and schistosomula of *Schistosoma mansoni*: II. The mechanisms of irreversible eosinophil adherence. *J. Exp. Med.* 150:1456, 1979.
256. Gleich G.J., et al.: Cytotoxic properties of eosinophil major basic protein. *J. Immunol.* 123:2925, 1979.
257. Venge P., et al.: Cationic proteins of human eosinophils and their role in the inflammatory reaction, in Mahmoud A.A.F., Austin K.F. (eds.): *The Eosinophil in Health and Disease.* New York, Grune & Stratton, 1980, p. 131.
258. Weller P.F., et al.: Identification of human eosinophil lysophospholipase as the constituent of Charcot-Leyden crystals. *Proc. Natl. Acad. Sci. USA* 77:7440, 1980.
259. Therathasan O.J., Gordon A.S.: Adrenocortical-medullary interactions on the blood eosinophils. *Acta Haematol.* 19:162, 1958.
260. Kurosawa M., et al.: Prostaglandin-induced eosinopenia in splenectomized rats. *J. Allergy Clin. Immunol.* 62:33, 1978.
261. Zucker-Franklin D.: Eosinopenia and eosinophilia, in Williams W., et al. (eds.): *Hematology,* ed. 3. New York, McGraw-Hill Book Co., 1983, p. 825.
262. Slungaard A., et al.: Pulmonary carcinoma with eosinophilia: Demonstration of tumor-derived eosinophilopoietic factor. *N. Engl. J. Med.* 309:779, 1983.
263. Slungaard A., et al.: Tumor induced eosinophilia and endocardial fibrosis: Evidence for ectopic eosinophilopoietin production and O_2-radical mediated endothelial damage. *Clin. Res.* 30:569A, 1982.
264. Viola M.V., et al.: Eosinophilia and metastatic carcinoma. *Med. Ann.* 41:1, 1972.
265. Juhlin L.: Basophil leukocyte differential in blood and bone marrow. *Acta Haematol.* 29:89, 1963.
266. Hastie R.L.: A study of the ultrastructure of human basophil leukocytes. *Lab. Invest.* 31:223, 1974.
267. Denburg J.A., et al.: Basophil production. *J. Clin. Invest.* 65:390, 1980.
268. Kitamura Y., et al.: Distribution of mast cell precursors in hematopoietic and lymphopoietic tissues of mice. *J. Exp. Med.* 150:482, 1979.
269. Galli S.J., Dvorak H.F.: Basophils and mast cells: Structure, function and role in hypersensitivity, in Gupta S., Good R.A. (eds.): *Cellular, Molecular and Clinical Aspects of Allergic Disorders.* New York, Plenum, 1979, p. 1.
270. Porter J.F., Mitchell R.G.L.: Distribution of histamine in human blood. *Physiol. Rev.* 52:361, 1972.
271. Ishizaka K., Ishizaka T.: Immunoglobulin E: Biosynthesis, and immunological mechanisms of IgE-mediated hypersensitivity, in Gupta S., Good R.A.

(eds.): *Cellular, Molecular, and Clinical Aspects of Allergic Disorders.* New York, Plenum, 1979, p. 153.
272. Finbloom D.S., Metzger H.: Binding of immunoglobulin E to the receptor of rat peritoneal macrophages. *J. Immunol.* 129:2004, 1982.
273. Metzger H., Ishizaka T.: Transmembrane signaling by receptor aggregation: The mast cell receptor for IgE as a case study. *Fed. Proc.* 41:7, 1982.
274. Dvorak A.M., et al.: Basophil and mast cell degranulation: Ultrastructural analysis of mechanisms of mediator release. *Fed. Proc.* 42:2512, 1983.
275. Ho P.C., et al.: Mediators of immediate hypersensitivity, in Gupta S., Good R.A. (eds.): *Cellular, Molecular, and Clinical Aspects of Allergic Disorders.* New York, Plenum, 1979, p. 179.
276. Malveaux F.J., et al.: IgE receptor on human basophils: Relationship to serum IgE concentration. *J. Clin. Invest.* 62:176, 1978.
277. MacGlashan D.W., et al.: Comparative studies of human basophils and mast cells. *Fed. Proc.* 42:2504, 1983.
278. Lichtenstein L.M., Margolis S.: Histamine release in vitro: Inhibition by catecholamines and methylxanthines. *Science* 161:902, 1968.
279. Tung R.S., Lichtenstein L.M.: cAMP agonist inhibition increases at low levels of histamine release from human basophils. *J. Pharmacol. Exp. Ther.* 218:642, 1981.
280. Peters S.P., et al.: The pharmacology of dispersed human lung mast cells. *Am. Rev. Respir. Dis.* 126:1034, 1982.
281. Halgate S.T., et al.: Role of adenylate cyclase in immunologic release of mediators from rat mast cells: Agonist and antagonist effects of purine- and ribose-modified adenosine analogs. *Proc. Natl. Acad. Sci. USA* 77:6800, 1980.
282. Dahlen S.E., et al.: Leukotrienes are potent constrictors of human bronchi. *Nature* 288:484, 1980.
283. Peters S.P., et al.: Lipoxygenase products modulate histamine release in human basophils. *Nature* 292:455, 1981.
284. Juhlin L.: Basophil and eosinophil leukocytes in various internal disorders. *Acta Med. Scand.* 174:249, 1963.
285. Ackerman S.K.: Morphology of lymphocytes, in Williams W., et al. (eds.): *Hematology,* ed 3. New York, McGraw-Hill Book Co., 1983, p. 837.
286. Douglas S.D.: Morphology of plasma cells, in Williams W., et al. (eds.): *Hematology,* ed 3. New York, McGraw-Hill Book Co., 1983, p. 883.
287. Uhr J.W., Finkelstein M.S.: The kinetics of antibody formation. *Prog. Allergy* 10:37, 1967.
288. McCall C.E., et al.: Lysosomal and ultrastructural changes in human "toxic" neutrophils during bacterial infection. *J. Infect. Dis.* 127:26, 1973.
289. Wiener W., Topley E.: Döhle bodies in leucocytes of patients with burns. *J. Clin. Pathol.* 8:324, 1955.
290. Laszlo J., Wayne Rundles R.: Morphology of neutrophils and neutrophil precursors, in Williams W., et al. (eds.): *Hematology,* ed 3. New York, McGraw-Hill Book Co., 1983, p. 719.
291. Itoga T., Laszlo J.: Döhle bodies and other granulocyte alterations with cyclophosphamide. *Blood* 20:668, 1962.
292. Cawley J.C., Hayhoe F.G.J.: The inclusions of the May-Hegglin anomaly and Döhle bodies of infection: An ultrastructural comparison. *Br. J. Haematol.* 22:491, 1972.
293. Jordan S.W., Larsen S.W.: Ultrastructural studies of the May-Hegglin anomaly. *Blood* 25:921, 1965.
294. Wintrobe M., et al. (eds.): *Clinical Hematology.* Philadelphia, Lea & Febiger, 1981, p. 1333.
295. Groover R.V., et al.: The genetic mucopolysaccharidosis. *Semin. Hematol.* 9:371, 1972.
296. Blume R.S., Wolff S.M.: The Chédiak-Higashi syndrome: Studies in four patients and a review of the literature. *Medicine* 51:247, 1972.
297. Higashi O.: Congenital gigantism of peroxidase granules: The first case ever reported of qualitative abnormality of peroxidase. *Tohoku J. Exp. Med.* 59:315, 1954.
298. Rausch P.G., et al.: Immunocytochemical identification of azurophilic and specific granule markers in the giant granules of Chédiak-Higashi neutrophils. *N. Engl. J. Med.* 298:693, 1978.
299. Clark K.A., Kimbell H.R.: Defective granulocyte chemotaxis in the Chédiak-Higashi syndrome. *J. Clin. Invest.* 50:2645, 1971.
300. Root R.K., et al.: Abnormal bactericidal metabolic and lysosomal functions in Chédiak-Higashi syndrome. *J. Clin. Invest.* 51:649, 1972.
301. Stossel T.P., et al.: Phagocytosis in chronic granulomatosis disease and the Chédiak-Higashi syndrome. *N. Engl. J. Med.* 286:120, 1972.
302. Oliver J.M.: Impaired microtubule function correctable by cyclic GMP and cholinergic agonists in the Chédiak-Higashi syndrome. *Am. J. Pathol.* 85:395, 1976.
303. Boxer L.A., et al.: Correction of leukocyte function in Chédiak-Higashi syndrome by ascorbate. *N. Engl. J. Med.* 295:1041, 1976.
304. Quie P.G.: Neutrophil dysfunction and recurrent infection, in Gallin J.I., Fauci A. (eds.): *Phagocytic Cells.* Volume 1 in *Advances in Host Defense Mechanisms.* New York, Raven Press, 1982, p. 163.
305. Schopfer K., et al.: Staphylococcal IgE antibodies, hyperimmunoglobulinemia E and *Staphylococcus aureus* infections. *N. Engl. J. Med.* 300:835, 1979.
306. Schopfer K., et al.: Immunoglobulin E antibodies against *Staphylococcus aureus* cell walls in the sera of patients with hyperimmunoglobulin E and recurrent staphylococcal infection. *Infect. Immun.* 27:563, 1980.
307. Gallin J.I., et al.: Disorders of chemotaxis. *Ann. Intern. Med.* 92:520, 1980.
308. Buckley R.H., Becker W.G.: Abnormalities in regulation of human IgE synthesis. *Immunol. Rev.* 41:288, 1978.
309. Johnston R.B., Baehner R.L.: Chronic granulomatous disease: Correlation between pathogenesis and clinical findings. *Pediatrics* 48:730, 1971.
310. Windhorst D.B., et al.: The pattern of genetic transmission of the leukocyte defect in fatal granu-

lomatous disease of childhood. *J. Clin. Invest.* 47:1026, 1968.
311. Klebanoff S.J., Clark R.A.: Chronic granulomatous disease, in *The Neutrophil: Function and Clinical Disorders*. New York, Elsevier North-Holland Publishing Co., 1978, p. 641.
312. Bridges R.A., et al.: A fatal granulomatous disease of childhood: The clinical, pathological, and laboratory features of a new syndrome. *Am. J. Dis. Child.* 97:387, 1959.
313. Mandell G.L., Hook E.W.: Leukocyte function in chronic granulomatous disease of childhood. *Am. J. Med.* 47:473, 1969.
314. Dilworth J.A., Mandell G.L.: Adults with chronic granulomatous disease of childhood. *Am. J. Med.* 63:233, 1977.
315. Holmes B., et al.: Studies of the metabolic activity of leukocytes from patients with a genetic abnormality of phagocytic function. *J. Clin. Invest.* 46:1422, 1967.
316. Klebanoff S.J.: Intraleukocytic microbicidal defects. *Annu. Rev. Med.* 22:39, 1971.
317. Rodey C.E., et al.: Defective bactericidal activity of monocytes in fatal granulomatous disease. *Blood* 33:813, 1969.
318. Kaplan E.L., et al.: Studies of polymorphonuclear leukocytes from patients with chronic granulomatous disease of childhood: Bactericidal capacity for streptococci. *Pediatrics* 41:591, 1968.
319. Cohen M.S., et al.: Fungal infection in chronic granulomatous disease: The importance of the phagocyte in defense against fungi. *Am. J. Med.* 71:59, 1981.
320. Giblett E.R., et al.: Kell phenotypes in chronic granulomatous disease: A potential transfusion hazard. *Lancet* 1:1235, 1971.
321. Marsh W.L., et al.: Chronic granulomatous disease and the Kell blood groups. *Br. J. Haematol.* 29:247, 1975.
322. Petz L.D., Swisher S.N.: *Clinical Practice of Blood Transfusion*. New York, Churchill Livingstone, 1981, p. 89.
323. Densen P., et al.: Kx: Its relationship to chronic granulomatous disease and genetic linkage with Xg. *Blood* 58:34, 1981.
324. Marsh W.L.: The Kell blood groups and their relationship to chronic granulomatous disease, in *Cellular Antigens and Disease*. Washington, D.C., American Association of Blood Banks, 1977, p. 52.
325. Symmans W.A., et al.: Hereditary acanthocytosis associated with the McLeod phenotype of the Kell blood group system. *Br. J. Haematol.* 42:575, 1979.
326. Galey W.R., et al.: Morphology and physiology of the McLeod erythrocyte. *Vox Sang.* 34:152, 1978.
327. Marsh W.L., et al.: Elevated serum creatinine phosphokinase in subjects with McLeod syndrome. *Vox Sang.* 40:403, 1981.
328. Brzica S.M., et al.: Chronic granulomatous disease and the McLeod phenotype: Successful treatment of infection with granulocyte transfusions resulting in subsequent transfusion reaction. *Mayo Clin. Proc.* 52:153, 1977.
329. McFarlane P.S., et al.: Fatal granulomatous disease of childhood and benign lymphocytic infiltration of the skin (congenital dysphagocytosis). *Lancet* 1:408, 1967.
330. Chusid M.J., Tomasulo P.A.: Survival of transfused normal granulocytes in a patient with chronic granulomatous disease. *Pediatrics* 61:556, 1978.
331. Foroozonfar N., et al.: Bone marrow transplant from an unrelated donor, for chronic granulomatous disease. *Lancet* 1:210, 1977.
332. Gallin J.I., et al.: Defective leukocyte chemotaxis in mannosidosis. *Clin. Res.* 24:344a, 1976.
333. Pincus S.H., et al.: Defective neutrophil chemotaxis with variant ichthyosis, hyperimmunoglobulinemia E and recurrent infections. *J. Pediatr.* 87:908, 1975.
334. Cooper M.R., et al.: Stimulation of leukocyte hexose monophosphate shunt activity by ascorbic acid. *Infect. Immun.* 3:851, 1971.
335. Dale D.C., et al.: Chronic neutropenia. *Medicine* 58:128, 1979.
336. Howard M.W., et al.: Infections in patients with neutropenia. *Am. J. Dis. Child.* 131:788, 1977.
337. Finch S.: Neutropenia, in Williams W.J., et al. (eds.): *Hematology*, ed. 3. New York, McGraw-Hill Book Co., 1983, p. 773.
338. Alonso K., et al.: Thymic alymphoplasia and congenital aleukocytosis (reticular dysgenesia). *Arch. Pathol.* 94:179, 1972.
339. Mentzer W.C., et al.: An unusual form of chronic neutropenia in a father and daughter with hypogammaglobulinemia. *Br. J. Haematol.* 36:313, 1977.
340. Lonsdale D., et al.: Familial granulocytopenia and associated immunoglobulin abnormality: Report of three cases in young brothers. *J. Pediatr.* 71:790, 1967.
341. Bjorksten B., Lundmark K.M.: Recurrent bacterial infections in four siblings with neutropenia, eosinophilia, hyperimmunoglobulinemia A and defective neutrophil chemotaxis. *J. Infect. Dis.* 133:63, 1976.
342. Evans D.I., Holzel A.: Cyclical neutropenia. *Proc. R. Soc. Med.* 61:302, 1968.
343. Gulhoed G.W., et al.: Colon ulceration and perforation in cyclic neutropenia. *J. Pediatr. Surg.* 8:379, 1973.
344. Wright D.C., et al.: Correction of human cyclic neutropenia with prednisolone. *N. Engl. J. Med.* 298:295, 1978.
345. Dale D.C., et al.: Studies of neutrophil production and turnover in grey collie dogs with cyclic neutropenia. *J. Clin. Invest.* 51:2190, 1972.
346. Chusid M.J., et al.: Congenital neutropenia: Studies of pathogenesis. *Am. J. Hematol.* 8:315, 1980.
347. Parmley R.T., et al.: Congenital dysgranulopoietic neutropenia: Clinical, serologic, ultrastructural, and in vitro proliferative characteristics. *Blood* 56:465, 1980.
348. Gilman P.A., et al.: Congenital agranulocytosis:

Prolonged survival and terminal acute leukemia. *Blood* 36:576, 1970.
349. Rappeport J.M., et al.: Correction of infantile agranulocytosis (Kostmann's syndrome) by allogeneic bone marrow transplantation. *Am. J. Med.* 68:605, 1980.
350. Kamada N., Uchino H.: Haematological abnormalities in six cases with the preleukemic stage for 5-13. *Acta Haematol. Jpn.* 37:32, 1974.
351. Dale D.C., et al.: Chronic neutropenia. *Medicine* 58:128, 1979.
352. Price T.H., et al.: Neutrophil kinetics in chronic neutropenia. *Blood* 54:581, 1979.
353. Murdoch J.M., Smith C.C.: Hematological aspects of systemic disease. *Infect. Clin. Haematol.* 1:619, 1972.
354. Bagby G.C., Gilberet D.N.: Suppression of granulopoiesis by T-lymphocytes in two patients with disseminated mycobacterial infection. *Ann. Intern. Med.* 94:478, 1981.
355. Nagaraju M., et al.: Viral hepatitis and agranulocytosis. *Am. J. Dig. Dis.* 18:247, 1973.
356. Stevens D.L., et al.: Infectious mononucleosis with severe neutropenia and opsonic neutrophil activity. *South. Med. J.* 72:519, 1979.
357. Calabro J.J., et al.: Kawasaki syndrome. *N. Engl. J. Med.* 306:287, 1982.
358. Perillie P.E., et al.: Significance of changes in serum muramidase activity in megaloblastic anemia. *N. Engl. J. Med.* 277:10, 1967.
359. Logue G.L., Shimm D.S.: Autoimmune granulocytopenia. *Annu. Rev. Med.* 31:191, 1980.
360. Lalezari P.: Neutrophil antigens: Immunology and clinical implications. *Prog. Clin. Biol. Res.* 13:209, 1977.
361. Boxer L.A.: Immune neutropenias: Clinical and biological implications. *Am. J. Pediatr. Hematol. Oncol.* 3:89, 1981.
362. Van Der Weerdt, Lalezari P.: Another example of isoimmune neonatal neutropenia due to anti-NA1. *Vox Sang.* 22:438, 1972.
363. Lalezari P., et al.: NB1, a new neutrophil-specific antigen involved in the pathogenesis of neonatal neutropenia. *J. Clin. Invest.* 50:1108, 1971.
364. Lalezari P., Radel E.: Neutrophil-specific antigens: Immunology and clinical significance. *Semin. Hematol.* 11:281, 1974.
365. Verheugt F.W.A., et al.: A family with allo-immune neonatal neutropenia: Group-specific pathogenicity of maternal antibodies. *Vox Sang.* 36:1, 1979.
366. Claas F.H.J., et al.: NE1: a new neutrophil-specific antigen. *Tissue Antigens* 13:129, 1979.
367. Lalezari P., et al.: Chronic autoimmune neutropenia due to anti-NA2 antibody. *N. Engl. J. Med.* 293:744, 1975.
368. Verheugt F.W., et al.: Serological, immunochemical, and immunocytological properties of granulocyte antibodies. *Vox Sang.* 35:294, 1978.
369. Verheugt F.W.A., et al.: Autoimmune granulocytopenia: The detection of granulocyte auto antibodies with the immunofluorescence test. *Br. J. Haematol.* 39:339, 1978.
370. Verheugt F.W.A., et al.: ND1, a new neutrophil granulocyte antigen. *Vox Sang.* 35:13, 1978.
371. Weetman R.M., Boxer L.A.: Childhood neutropenia. *Pediatr. Clin. North Am.* 27:361, 1980.
372. Craddock P.R.: Granulocyte aggregation as a manifestation of membrane interactions with complement: Possible role in leukocyte margination, microvascular occlusion, and endothelial damage. *Semin. Hematol.* 16:140, 1979.
373. Schiffer C.A., et al.: Transient neutropenia induced by transfusion of blood exposed to nylon fiber filters. *Blood* 45:141, 1975.
374. Craddock P.R., et al.: Hemodialysis leukopenia: Pulmonary vascular leukostasis resulting from complement activation by dialyzer cellophane membranes. *J. Clin. Invest.* 59:879, 1977.
375. Chenoweth D.E.: Complement activation during cardiopulmonary bypass (letter). *N. Engl. J. Med.* 305:51, 1981.
376. Arneborn D., Palmblad J.: Drug induced neutropenias in the Stockholm region 1976–77. *Acta Med. Scand.* 206:241, 1979.
377. Wintrobe M.M.: The therapeutic minimum and its price: A view of the haemopoietic system. The Lilly Lecture, 1968. *J. R. Coll. Physicians Lond.* 3:99, 1969.
378. Pisciotta A.V., et al.: Studies on agranulocytosis: IX. A biochemical defect in chlorpromazine-sensitive marrow cells. *J. Lab. Clin. Med.* 78:435, 1971.
379. Symoens J., et al.: Adverse reactions to levamisole. *Cancer Treatment Rep.* 62:1721, 1978.
380. Magis C.C., et al.: Serological study of an allergic agranulocytosis due to noramidopyrine. *Clin. Exp. Immunol.* 3:989, 1968.
381. Hartl W.: Drug allergic agranulocytosis (Schultz's disease). *Semin. Hematol.* 2:313, 1965.
382. Weitzman S.A., Stossel T.P.: Drug induced immunological neutropenia. *Lancet* 1:1068, 1978.
383. Levine P.H., Weintraub L.R.: Pseudoleukemia during recovery from Dapsone-induced agranulocytosis. *Ann. Intern. Med.* 68:1060, 1968.
384. Carpenter J.: Neutropenia induced by semisynthetic penicillin. *South. Med. J.* 73:745, 1980.
385. Yuvis A.A., Gross M.A.: Drug induced inhibition of myeloid colony growth: Modifying effect of colony stimulating factor. *Clin. Res.* 23:49A, 1975.
386. Polak B.C., et al.: Blood dyscrasias attributed to chloramphenicol: A review of 576 published cases and unpublished cases. *Acta Med. Scand.* 192:409, 1972.
387. Gurwith M.J., et al.: Granulocytopenia in hospitalized patients: I. Prognostic factors and etiology of fever. *Am. J. Med.* 64:121, 1978.
388. Schimpff S.C.: Therapy of infection in patients with granulocytopenia. *Med. Clin. North Am.* 61:1101, 1977.
389. Crosby W.H.: How many "polys" are enough? *Arch. Intern. Med.* 123:722, 1969.

390. Hall R.C., et al.: Lithium therapy and toxicity. *Am. Fam. Physician* 19:133, 1979.
391. Ketchel S.J., Rodriguez V.: Acute infections in cancer patients. *Semin. Oncol.* 5:167, 1978.
392. Contreras E., et al.: Value of the bone marrow biopsy in the diagnosis of metastatic carcinoma. *Cancer* 29:778, 1972.
393. Jacobson R.S., et al.: Agnogenic myeloid metaplasia: A clonal proliferation of hematopoietic stem cells with secondary myelofibrosis. *Blood* 51:189, 1978.
394. Besselman D.M.: Splenectomy in the management of the anemia and thrombocytopenia of osteopetrosis (marble bone disease). *J. Pediatr.* 69:455, 1966.
395. Wiseman B.K., Doan C.A.: A newly recognized granulocytopenic syndrome caused by excessive splenic leukolysis and successfully treated by splenectomy. *Ann. Intern. Med.* 16:1097, 1942.
396. Lester E.P., Ultmann J.E.: Non-Hodgkin's lymphoma, in Williams W.J., et al. (eds.): *Hematology*, ed. 3. New York, McGraw-Hill Book Co., 1983, p. 1035.
397. Amorosi E.L.: Hypersplenism. *Semin. Hematol.* 2:249, 1965.
398. Engstrom P.F., et al.: Disseminated *Mycobacteria kansasii* infection. *Am. J. Med.* 52:533, 1972.
399. Megaloblastic leukopenia (editorial). *N. Engl. J. Med.* 277:50, 1967.
400. Gardner F.H., Blum S.F.: Aplastic anemia in paroxysmal nocturnal hemoglobinuria: Mechanism and therapy. *Semin. Hematol.* 4:250, 1967.
401. Speck B., et al.: Immunologic aspects of aplasia. *Transplant. Proc.* 10:131, 1978.
402. Gale R.P., et al.: Aplastic anemia: Biology and treatment. *Ann. Intern. Med.* 95:477, 1981.
403. Snyder R., et al.: Bone marrow depressant and leukemogenic actions of benzene. *Life Sci.* 21:1709, 1977.
404. Kirshbaum J.D., et al.: A study of aplastic anemia in an autopsy series with special reference to atomic bomb survivors in Hiroshima and Nagasaki. *Blood* 38:17, 1971.
405. Toughill P.J., Wilcox R.G.: Aplastic anemia and hair dye. *Br. Med. J.* 1:502, 1976.
406. Bishop C.R., et al.: Leukokinetic studies: XIV. Blood neutrophil kinetics in chronic, steady state neutropenia. *J. Clin. Invest.* 50:1678, 1971.
407. Hoffman R., et al.: Antibody-mediated aplastic anemia and diffuse fasciitis. *N. Engl. J. Med.* 300:718, 1979.
408. Eichner E.R.: Splenic function: Normal, too much and too little. *Am. J. Med.* 66:311, 1979.
409. Pisciotta A.V.: Studies in agranulocytosis: Patterns of recovery. *J. Lab. Clin. Med.* 63:445, 1964.
410. Cartwright G.E., et al.: Blood granulocyte kinetics in conditions associated with granulocytosis. *Ann. NY Acad. Sci.* 113:963, 1964.
411. Welsh J.D., Denny W.F.: Diagnostic problems presented by the leukemoid reaction. *Med. Times* 88:16, 1960.
412. von Schulthess G.K., Mazer N.A.: Cyclic neutropenia (CN): A clue to the control of granulopoiesis. *Blood* 59:27, 1982.
413. Cronkite E.P.: Kinetics of granulopoiesis. *Clin. Haematol.* 8:351, 1979.
414. Mishler J.M., Sharp A.A.: Adrenaline: Further discussion of its role in the mobilization of neutrophils. *Scand. J. Haematol.* 17:78, 1976.
415. Ghebrehiwet B., Müller-Eberhard H.J.: C3e: An acidic fragment of human C3 with leukocytosis-inducing activity. *J. Immunol.* 123:616, 1979.
416. Chikkappa G., et al.: Kinetics and regulations of granulocyte precursors during a granulopoietic stress. *Blood* 50:1099, 1977.
417. Shoenfeld Y., et al.: Prednisone-induced leukocytosis: Influence of dosage, method, and duration of administration on the degree of leukocytosis *Am. J. Med.* 71:773, 1981.
418. Cameron S.J.: Tuberculosis and the blood: A special relationship? *Tubercle* 55:55, 1974.
419. Robinson W.A.: Granulocytosis in neoplasia. *Ann. NY Acad. Sci.* 230:212, 1974.
420. Rubins J., Wakem C.J.: Hypoglycemia and leukemoid reaction with hypernephroma. *NY State J. Med.* 77:406, 1977.
421. Weinstein H.J.: Congenital leukemia and the neonatal myeloproliferative disorders associated wtih Down's syndrome. *Clin. Haematol.* 7:147, 1978.
422. Herring W.B., et al.: Hereditary neutrophilia. *Am. J. Med.* 56:729, 1974.
423. Leonard B.J.: Alkaline phosphatase in the white cells in leukemia and the leukemoid reaction. *Lancet* 1:289, 1958.
424. Weller J.H.: The cytomegaloviruses: Ubiquitous agents with protean clinical manifestations. *N. Engl. J. Med.* 285:203, 1971.
425. Nrvumah F.K., Addy P.A.K.: Acute infectious lymphocytosis. *Lancet* 1:1257, 1973.
426. Andiman W.A.: The Epstein-Barr virus and EB virus infections in childhood. *J. Pediatr.* 95:171, 1979.
427. Adler A., Morse S.I.: Interaction of lymphoid and nonlymphoid cells in the lymphocytosis-promoting factor of *Bordetella pertussis*. *Infect. Immunol.* 7:461, 1973.
428. Remington J.S.: Toxoplasmosis in the adult. *Bull. NY Acad. Med.* 50:211, 1974.
429. Wintrobe M.M., et al. (eds.): *Clinical Hematology*, ed. 8. Philadelphia, Lea & Febiger, 1981, p. 1302.
430. Cassileth P.A.: Lymphocytopenia, in Williams W.J., et al. (eds.): *Hematology*, ed. 3. New York, McGraw-Hill Book Co., 1983, p. 955.
431. Biemer J.J.: The preleukemic syndrome. *Ann. Clin. Lab. Sci.* 13:156, 1983.
432. Saarhi M.I., Linman J.W.: Preleukemia: The hematologic syndrome preceding acute leukemia. *Am. J. Med.* 55:38, 1973.
433. Pierre R.V.: Preleukemic syndromes. *Virchows Arch. [Cell Pathol.]* 29:29, 1978.
434. Pierre R.V.: Preleukemic states. *Semin. Hematol.* 11:73, 1974.

435. Weber R.F., et al.: The preleukemic syndrome: I. Clinical and hematological findings. *Acta Med. Scand.* 207:391, 1980.
436. Blank J., Lange B.: Preleukemia in children. *J. Pediatr.* 98:565, 1981.
437. Cheng D.S., et al.: Idiopathic refractory sideroblastic anemia. *Cancer* 44:724, 1979.
438. Lindman J.W., Bagby G.C. Jr.: The preleukemic syndrome (hemopoietic dysplasia). *Cancer* 42:854, 1978.
439. Woods W.G., et al.: The occurrence of leukemia in patients with the Shwachman's syndrome. *J. Pediatr.* 99:425, 1981.
440. Cohen T., Creger W.P.: Acute myeloid leukemia following seven years of aplastic anemia induced by chloramphenicol. *Am. J. Med.* 43:762, 1967.
441. Zittoun R., et al.: Acute myelomonocytic leukemia: A terminal complication of paroxysmal nocturnal haemoglobinuria. *Acta Haematol.* 53:241, 1975.
442. Najean Y., Pecking A.: Refractory anemia with excess of myeloblasts in the bone marrow: A clinical trial of androgens in 90 cases. *Br. J. Haematol.* 37:23, 1977.
443. Bishop J.M.: The molecular biology of RNA tumor viruses. *N. Engl. J. Med.* 303:675, 1980.
444. Ashley D.B.: The two "hit" and multiple "hit" theories of carcinogenesis. *Br. J. Cancer* 23:313, 1969.
445. Prchal J.T., et al.: A common progenitor for human myeloid and lymphoid cells. *Nature* 274:590, 1978.
446. Linman J.W., Bagby G.C. Jr.: The preleukemic syndrome: Clinical and laboratory features, natural course, and management. *Blood Cells* 2:11, 1976.
447. Berk P., et al.: Increased incidence of acute leukemia in polycythemia vera associated with chlorambucil therapy. *N. Engl. J. Med.* 304:441, 1981.
448. Polliack A., et al.: Lymphoblastic leukemic transformation (lymphoblastic crisis) in myelofibrosis and myeloid metaplasia. *Am. J. Hematol.* 9:211, 1980.
449. Miller R.W.: Relation between cancer and congenital defects: An epidemiological evaluation. *JNCI* 40:1079, 1968.
450. Kaufmann R.W., et al.: Paroxysmal nocturnal hemoglobinuria terminating in acute granulocytic leukemia. *Blood* 33:287, 1969.
451. Rosner F., Grunwald H.: Hodgkin's disease terminating in acute leukemia: Report of eight cases and review of the literature. *Am. J. Med.* 58:339, 1975.
452. Brauer M.J., Dameshek W.: Hypoplastic anemia and myeloblastic leukemia following chloramphenicol therapy. *N. Engl. J. Med.* 277:1003, 1967.
453. Spector B.D., et al.: Genetically determined immunodeficiency disease and malignancy: Report from the immunodeficiency-cancer registry. *Clin. Immunol. Immunopathol.* 11:12, 1978.
454. Sieber S.M., Adamson R.H.: Toxicity of antineoplastic agents in man: Chromosomal aberrations, antifertility effects, congenital abnormalities, and carcinogenic potential, in Klein G., et al. (eds.): *Advances in Cancer Research.* New York, Academic Press, 1975, vol. 22, p. 57.
455. Biemer J.J.: The preleukemic syndrome. *Ann. Clin. Lab. Sci.* 13:156, 1983.
456. Bross I.D., Natarajan N.: Leukemia from low-level irradiation: Identification of susceptible children. *N. Engl. J. Med.* 257:107, 1972.
457. Aksoy M., et al.: Leukemia in shoeworkers exposed chronically to benzene. *Blood* 44:837, 1974.
458. Rochant H., et al.: Hypothesis: Refractory anemias, preleukemic conditions and fetal erythropoiesis. *Blood* 39:721, 1972.
459. Streichman S., et al.: Red cell inclusion bodies in a case of preleukemia. *Scand. J. Haematol.* 22:263, 1979.
460. Worlledge S.M.: Red cell antigens in dyserythropoiesis, in Lewis S.M., Verwilghen R.A.L. (eds.): *Dyserythropoiesis.* New York, Academic Press, 1977.
461. Economopoulos T., et al.: Myelodysplastic syndrome. *Acta Haematol.* 65:97, 1981.
462. Runtu P., et al.: Function of neutrophils in preleukaemia. *Scand. J. Haematol.* 18:317, 1977.
463. Maldonado J.E.: Platelet granulopathy: A new morphologic feature in preleukemia and myelomonocytic leukemia. *Mayo Clin. Proc.* 51:452, 1976.
464. Dreyfus B.: Preleukemic states. *Blood Cells* 2:33, 1976.
465. Panani A., et al.: Cytogenetic studies in preleukaemia using the G-banding staining technique. *Scand. J. Haematol.* 18:301, 1977.
466. Breton-Gorius J.: Abnormalities of granulocytes and megakaryocytes in preleukemic syndromes, in Schmalzl F., Helbriegel K.P. (eds.): *Preleukemia.* New York, Springer-Verlag, 1979. p. 24.
467. Najean Y., Pecking A.: Refractory anemia with excess of blast cells: Prognostic factors and effects of treatment with androgens or cytosine arabinoside. Results of a prospective trial in 58 patients. Cooperative Group for the Study of Aplastic and Refractory Anemias. *Cancer* 44:1976–1982, 1979.
468. Lidbeck J.: In vitro colony and cluster growth in haemopoietic dysplasia (the preleukemic syndrome): II. identification of a maturation defect in agar cultures. *Scand. J. Haematol.* 25:113, 1980.
469. Lewy R.I., et al.: Leukemia in patients with acquired idiopathic sideroblastic anemia. *Am. J. Hematol.* 6:323, 1979.
470. Nowell P.C.: Preleukemias. *Hum. Pathol.* 12:522, 1981.
471. Van den Berghe H., et al.: Simultaneous occurrence of 5q− and 21q− in refractory anemia with thrombocytosis. *Cancer Genet. Cytogenet.* 1:63, 1979.
472. Sandberg A.A.: *The Chromosomes in Human Cancer and Leukemia.* New York, Elsevier, 1980.
473. Petit P., Van den Berghe H.: A chromosomal abnormality (21q−) in primary thrombocytosis. *Hum. Genet.* 50:105, 1979.
474. Armitage J.O., et al.: Effect of chemotherapy for the dysmyelopoietic syndrome. *Cancer Treat. Rep.* 65:601, 1981.

475. Wisch J., et al.: Response of preleukemic syndromes to continuous infusion of low-dose cytarabine. *N. Engl. J. Med.* 309:1599, 1983.
476. Griffen J., et al.: Induction of differentiation of human myeloid leukemia cells by inhibitors of DNA synthesis. *Exp. Hematol.* 10:774, 1982.
477. Bhaduri S., et al.: A case of preleukemia: Reconstitution of normal marrow function after bone marrow transplantation (BMT) from identical twins. *Blut* 38:145, 1979.
478. Dameshek W., Gunz F.: *Leukemia,* ed. 2. New York, Grune & Stratton, 1964.
479. Cutler S.J., et al.: Ten thousand cases of leukemia: 1940–62. *JNCI* 39:993, 1967.
480. Gahrton G., et al.: Origin of the Philadelphia chromosome: Tracing the chromosome 22 to patients with chronic myelocytic leukemia. *Exp. Cell Res.* 79:246, 1973.
481. Rowley J.D.: A new consistent chromosomal abnormality in chronic myelogenous leukemia identified by quinacrine fluorescence and Giemsa staining. *Nature* 243:290, 1973.
482. Sandberg A.A.: Chromosomes and causation of human cancer and leukemia: XL. The Ph^1 and other translocations in CML. *Cancer* 46:2221, 1980.
483. Oshimura M., et al.: Variant Ph^1 translocation in CML and their incidence, including two cases with sequential lymphoid and myeloid crises. *Cancer Genet. Cytogenet.* 5:187, 1982.
484. O'Riordan M.L., et al.: Distinguishing between the chromosomes involved in Down's syndrome (trisomy 21) and chronic myelogenous leukemia (Ph^1) by fluorescence. *Nature* 230:167, 1971.
485. Rowley J.D.: Ph^1-positive leukaemia, including chronic myelogenous leukaemia. *Clin. Haematol.* 9:55, 1980.
486. March H.C.: Leukemia in radiologists, ten years later. *Am. J. Med. Sci.* 242:137, 1961.
487. Neel J.V., et al.: Search for mutations affecting protein structure in children of atomic bomb survivors: Preliminary report. *Proc. Natl. Acad. Sci. USA* 77:4221, 1980.
488. Graham D.C.: Leukemia following x-ray therapy for ankylosing spondylitis. *Arch. Intern. Med.* 105:51, 1960.
489. De-Thé G., et al.: Epidemiological evidence for causal relationship between Epstein-Barr virus and Burkitt's lymphoma from Ugandan prospective study. *Nature* 274:756, 1978.
490. Rickinson A.B., et al.: HLA-restricted T-cell recognition of Epstein-Barr virus-infected B cells. *Nature* 283:865, 1980.
491. deKlein A., et al.: A cellular oncogene is translocated to the Philadelphia chromosomes in chronic myelocytic leukaemia. *Nature* 300:765, 1982.
492. Rundles W.: Chronic myelogenous leukemia, in Williams W.J., et al. (eds.): *Hematology,* ed. 3. New York, McGraw-Hill Book Co., 1983, p. 197.
493. Major I.R., Mole R.H.: Myeloid leukemia in x-ray irradiated CBA mice. *Nature* 272:455, 1978.
494. Infante P.I., et al.: Leukemia in benzene workers. *Lancet* 2:76, 1977.
495. Tough I.M., Brown W.M.: Chromosome aberrations and exposure to ambient benzene. *Lancet* 1:684, 1965.
496. Fialkow P.J., et al.: Chronic myelomonocytic leukemia: Clonal origin in a stem cell common to the granulocytic, erythrocyte, platelet and monocyte/macrophage. *Am. J. Med.* 63:125, 1977.
497. Kohno S., Sandberg A.A.: Chromosomes and causation of human cancer and leukemia: Usual and unusual findings in Ph^1-positive CML. *Cancer* 46:2227, 1980.
498. Marks S.M., et al.: Terminal transferase as a predictor of initial responsiveness to vincristine and prednisone in blastic chronic myelogenous leukemia. *N. Engl. J. Med.* 298:812, 1978.
499. Rosenthal S., et al.: Erythroblastic transformation of chronic granulocytic leukemia. *Am. J. Med.* 63:116, 1977.
500. Fialkow P.J., et al.: Chronic myelocytic leukemia: Origin of some lymphocytes from leukemia stem cells. *J. Clin. Invest.* 62:815, 1978.
501. Philadelphia chromosome positive leukemias (editorial). *Lancet* 1:857, 1979.
502. Philip P., et al.: Philadelphia chromosome in acute lymphocytic leukemia. *Hereditas* 84:231, 1976.
503. LeBieu T.W., et al.: Origin of chronic myelocytic leukemia in a precursor of pre-B lymphocytes. *N. Engl. J. Med.* 301:144, 1979.
504. Alimena G.: Meeting report: Second International Workshop on Chromosomes in Leukemia. *Cancer Res.* 40:4826, 1980.
505. Bloomfield C.D.: The Philadelphia chromosome in acute leukemia. *Virchows Arch. [Cell Pathol.]* 29:81, 1978.
506. Bakhshi A., et al.: Lymphoid blast crises of chronic myelogenous leukemia represent stages in the development of B-cell precursors. *N. Engl. J. Med.* 309:826, 1983.
507. Chervenick P.A., Boggs D.R.: Granulocyte kinetics in chronic myelocytic leukemias. *Ser. Haematol.* 1:24, 1968.
508. Fefer A., et al.: Disappearance of Ph^1-positive cells in four patients with chronic granulocytic leukemia after chemotherapy, irradiation and marrow transplantation from an identical twin. *N. Engl. J. Med.* 300:333, 1979.
509. You W., Weisbrut M.: Chronic neutrophilic leukemia: Report of two cases and review of the literature. *Am. J. Clin. Pathol.* 72:235, 1979.
510. Mason J.E., et al.: Thrombocytosis in chronic granulocytic leukemia: Incidence and clinical significance. *Blood* 44:483, 1974.
511. Hyur B.H., Gulati G.: Myeloproliferative disorders: Blood and bone marrow changes. *Lab. Med.* 12:341, 1981.
512. Moloney W.C.: Chronic myelogenous leukemia. *Cancer* 43:865, 1978.
513. Rosenblum D., Petzald S.: Neutrophil alkaline phosphatase: Comparison of enzymes from normal

subjects and patients with P. vera and CML. *Blood* 45:335, 1975.
514. Bainton D.F., et al.: Development of neutrophilic polymorphonuclear leukocytes in human bone marrow. *J. Exp. Med.* 134:907, 1971.
515. Strauchen J.: Enzymatic markers in hematologic malignancy. *Laboratory Management*, July 1980, p. 33.
516. Kageoka T., et al.: Simultaneous demonstration of peroxidase and lysozyme activities in leukemic cells. *Am. J. Clin. Pathol.* 67:483, 1977.
517. Morse E., et al.: Use of terminal deoxynucleotidyl transferase in the diagnosis of leukemia. *Ann. Clin. Lab. Sci.* 13:128, 1983.
518. Magill G.B., et al.: Serum lactic dehydrogenase and serum transaminase in human leukemia. *Blood* 14:870, 1959.
519. Wintrobe M.M., et al. (eds.): *Clinical Hematology*, ed. 8. Philadelphia, Lea & Febiger, 1981, p. 1568.
520. Rodriguez A.R., Lutcher C.L.: Marked cyclic leukocytosis-leukopenia in chronic myelogenous leukemia. *Am. J. Med.* 60:1041, 1976.
521. Stirling M.L., et al.: Leukapheresis for papilloedema in chronic granulocytic leukemia. *Br. Med. J.* 2:676, 1977.
522. Witts L.J., et al.: Chronic granulocytic leukemia: Comparison of radiotherapy and busulphan therapy. Report of the Medical Research Council's Working Party for Therapeutic Trials in Leukemia. *Br. Med. J.* 1:201, 1968.
523. Asano M., Kawahara I.: Ultramicroscopic characteristics of bone marrow cells in human chronic myeloid leukemia. *Shinsu Univ. Med. J.* 13:109, 1968.
524. Wilkinson J.F., Turner R.L.: Chemotherapy of chronic myeloid leukemia with special reference to myleran, in Tocantis C.M. (ed.): *Prog. Hematol.* New York, Grune and Stratton, 1959, p. 225.
525. Lee R.E., Ellis L.D.: The storage cells of chronic myelogenous leukemia. *Lab. Invest.* 24:261, 1971.
526. Boggs D.R.: The kinetics of neutrophilic leukocytes in health and disease. *Semin. Hematol.* 4:359, 1967.
527. Goldman J.M., et al.: Chronic granulocytic leukemia: Selective removal of immature granulocytic cells by leukapheresis. *Ser. Haematol.* 8:28, 1975.
528. Leong S.S., et al.: Circulating colony forming cells in different stages of chronic myelocytic leukemia. *Cancer Res.* 39:2704, 1979.
529. Odelberg H., et al.: Granulocyte function in chronic granulocytic leukaemia: I. Bactericidal and metabolic capabilities during phagocytosis in isolated granulocytes. *Br. J. Haematol.* 29:427, 1975.
530. Goodman S.B., Block M.H.: Increased red blood cell production in chronic myelocytic leukemia. *JAMA* 200:141, 1968.
531. Beard M.F., et al.: Serum concentrations of vitamin B12 in patients from leukemia. *Blood* 9:789, 1954.
532. Zittoun J., et al.: The three transcobalamines in myeloproliferative disorders and acute leukemia. *Br. J. Haematol.* 31:287, 1975.
533. Twomey J.J., Leavell B.W.: Leukemoid reactions to tuberculosis. *Arch. Intern. Med.* 116:21, 1965.
534. Levine P.H., Hanstra R.D.: Megaloblastic anemia of pregnancy simulating acute leukemia. *Ann. Intern. Med.* 71:1141, 1969.
535. Chusid M.J., et al.: The hypereosinophilic syndrome: Analysis of fourteen cases with review of the literature. *Medicine* 54:1, 1975.
536. Youman J.D., et al.: Histamine excess symptoms in basophilic chronic granulocytic leukemia. *Arch. Intern. Med.* 131:560, 1973.
537. Sheridan B.L., et al.: The patterns of fetal haemoglobin production in leukemia. *Br. J. Haematol.* 32:487, 1976.
538. Altman A.J., et al.: Juvenile chronic granulocytic leukemia: A panmyelopathy with prominent monocytic involvement and circulating monocytes colony-forming cells. *Blood* 43:341, 1974.
539. Skinnider L.F., et al.: Chronic myelomonocytic leukemia: An ultrastructural study by transmission and scanning electron microscopy. *Am. J. Clin. Pathol.* 67:339, 1977.
540. Hays T., et al.: Cytogenetic studies of chronic myelocytic leukemia in children and adolescents. *Cancer* 44:210, 1979.
541. Gollerkeri M.P., Shah G.B.: Management of chronic myeloid leukemia: A five-year survey with a comparison of oral busulfan and splenic irradiation. *Cancer* 27:596, 1971.
542. Hauch T., et al.: Treatment of chronic granulocytic leukemia with melphalan. *Blood* 51:571, 1978.
543. Conrad F.G.: Survival in chronic granulocytic leukemia: Splenic irradiation, busulfan. *Arch. Intern. Med.* 131:684, 1973.
544. Carbone P.P., et al.: The effect of treatment in patients with chronic myelogenous leukemia: Hematologic and cytogenetic studies. *Ann. Intern. Med.* 59:622, 1963.
545. Tough I.M.: Cytogenetic studies in cases of chronic myeloid leukemia with a previous history of radiation, in Hayhoe F.G.J. (ed.): *Current Research in Leukemia*. London, Cambridge University Press, 1965, p. 47.
546. Cunningham I., et al.: Result of treatment of Ph^1 positive chronic myelogenous leukemia with an intensive treatment regimen (L-5 protocol). *Blood* 53:375, 1979.
547. Goldberg J., et al.: The in vitro effects of vincristine on peripheral blood leukocyte progenitor cells (CFU-C) in patients in blast crisis of chronic granulocytic leukemia: Correlation with clinical response. *Am. J. Hematol.* 14:149, 1983.
548. Lowenthal R.M., et al.: Intensive leukapheresis as initial therapy for chronic granulocytic leukemia. *Blood* 46:835, 1975.
549. Goldfinger D.: Clinical applications of therapeutic cytapheresis, in Berkman E.M., Umlas J. (eds.): *Therapeutic Hemapheresis: A Technical Workshop*. Washington, D.C., American Association of Blood Banks, 1980, p. 65.
550. Huestis D.W., et al.: Leukapheresis of patients with chronic myelogenous leukemia (CGL), using the Haemonetics blood processor. *Transfusion* 16:225, 1976.

551. Goldman J.M.: Modern approaches to the management of chronic granulocytic leukemia. *Semin. Hematol.* 15:420, 1978.
552. Fefer A., et al.: Disappearance of Ph^1-positive cells in four patients with chronic granulocytic leukemia after chemotherapy, irradiation and marrow transplantation from an identical twin. *N. Engl. J. Med.* 300:333, 1979.
553. Thomas M.R., et al.: Autologous marrow transplantation for patients with chronic myelogenous leukemia (CML) in blast crisis. *Am. J. Hematol.* 16:105, 1984.
554. Odom L.F., et al.: Remission of relapsed leukemia during a graft versus host reaction: A graft-versus-leukemia reaction in man? *Lancet* 2:537, 1978.
555. Boice J.D., et al.: Leukemia and preleukemia after adjuvant treatment of gastrointestinal cancer with semustine (methyl-CCNU). *N. Engl. J. Med.* 309:1079, 1983.
556. Harris C.C.: A delayed complication of cancer therapy—cancer. *JNCI* 63:275, 1979.
557. Petersen-Bjergaard J., Larsen S.O.: Incidence of acute nonlymphocytic leukemia, preleukemia and acute myeloproliferative syndrome up to 10 years after treatment of Hodgkin's disease. *N. Engl. J. Med.* 307:965, 1982.
558. Greene M.H., et al.: Acute nonlymphocytic leukemia after therapy with alkylating agents for ovarian cancer: A study of five randomized trials. *N. Engl. J. Med.* 307:1416, 1982.
559. Kardinal C.G., et al.: Chronic granulocytic leukemia: Review of 536 cases. *Arch. Intern. Med.* 136:305, 1976.
560. Walter R.M., Greenberg B.R.: Hypercalcemia in the accelerated phase of chronic myelogenous leukemia. *Cancer* 46:1174, 1980.
561. Boggs D.R.: The pathogenesis and clinical patterns of blastic crisis of chronic myeloid leukemia. *Semin. Oncol.* 3:289, 1976.
562. Cutler S.J., Young J.L. (eds.): *Third Cancer Survey*, monograph 41. Washington, D.C., National Cancer Institute, 1975.
563. Fraumeni J.A. Jr., Miller R.W.: Epidemiology of human leukemia: Recent observations. *JNCI* 38:593, 1967.
564. Goodall P.T., Vosti K.L.: Fever in acute myelogenous leukemia. *Arch. Intern. Med.* 135:1197, 1975.
565. Rowe J.M.: Clinical and laboratory features of myeloid and lymphocytic leukemias: Focus. *Am. J. Med. Technol.* 43:103, 1983.
566. Bennett J.M., et al.: Proposals for the classifications of the acute leukemias. *Br. J. Haematol.* 27:7, 1974.
567. Galton D.A.G., et al.: Classification of acute leukemia. *Ann. Intern. Med.* 87:740, 1977.
568. Quaglino D., Hayhoe F.G.J.: Periodic-acid-Schiff positivity in erythroblasts with especial reference to DiGuglielmo syndrome. *Br. J. Haematol.* 6:26, 1960.
569. Crossen P.E., et al.: Chromosomal abnormality, megaloblastosis, and arrested DNA synthesis in erythroleukemia. *J. Med. Genet.* 6:95, 1969.
570. Baldini M., et al.: The anemia of the DiGuglielmo syndrome. *Blood* 14:334, 1959.
571. Rowley J.D.: Identification of a translocation with quinacrine fluorescence in a patient with acute leukemia. *Ann. Genet.* 16:109, 1973.
572. Rowley J.D.: Chromosome abnormalities in leukemia and lymphoma. *Ann. Clin. Lab. Sci.* 13:87, 1983.
573. Rowley J.D., et al.: Further evidence of a non-random chromosomal abnormality in acute promyelocytic leukemia. *Int. J. Cancer* 20:869, 1977.
574. Hittelman W.N., et al.: Predicting relapse of human leukemia by means of premature chromosome condensation. *N. Engl. J. Med.* 303:479, 1980.
575. Reid M.M., et al.: Detection of leukemia-related karyotypes in granulocyte/macrophage colonies from a patient with acute myelomonocytic leukemia. *N. Engl. J. Med.* 308:1324, 1983.
576. Kobrinsky N.L., et al.: Acute nonlymphocytic leukemia. *Pediatr. Clin. North Am.* 27:345, 1980.
577. Metzger R.S., Mohanaklumar R.: Tumor associated antigens of leukemia cells. *Semin. Hematol.* 15:138, 1978.
578. Henderson E.S.: Acute leukemia—general considerations, in Williams W., et al. (eds.): *Hematology*, ed. 3. New York, McGraw-Hill Book Co., 1983, p. 221.
579. Baker M.A., et al.: Early diagnosis of relapse in acute myeloblastic leukemia: Serologic detection of leukemia-associated antigens in human marrow. *N. Engl. J. Med.* 301:1353, 1979.
580. Giannoulis N., et al.: Difference between young and old patients in characteristics of leukemic cells: Older patients have cells growing excessively in vitro, with low antigenicity despite high HLA-DR antigens. *Am. J. Hematol.* 16:113, 1984.
581. Ersboll J., et al.: Granulocytic sarcoma preceding acute myeloid leukemia. *Scand. J. Haematol.* 24:435, 1980.
582. Galton D.A.G., et al.: The relation between morphology and other features of acute myeloid leukemia, and their prognostic significance. *Br. J. Haematol.* 31:165, 1975.
583. Groopman J., et al.: Acute promyelocytic leukemia. *Am. J. Hematol.* 7:395, 1979.
584. Shaw M.T.: Monocytic leukemias. *Hum. Pathol.* 11:215, 1980.
585. Tobelem G.: Acute monoblastic leukemia: A clinical and biologic study of 74 cases. *Blood* 55:71, 1980.
586. Wiernik P.H., et al.: Randomized clinical comparison of daunorubicin, cytosine arabinoside (NSC-63878), 6-thioguanine (NSC-752), and pyrimethamine (NSC-3061) for the treatment of acute nonlymphocytic leukemia. *Cancer Treat. Rep* 60:41, 1976.
587. Baldwin M.L., et al.: Tn-polyagglutinability associated with acute myelomonocytic leukemia. *Am. J. Clin. Pathol.* 72:1024, 1979.
588. Wintrobe M.M., et al. (eds.): *Clinical Hematology*, ed. 8. Philadelphia, Lea & Febiger, 1981, p. 1542.
589. Gale R.R., Cline M.J.: High remission induction

rate in acute myeloid leukemia. *Lancet* 1:497, 1977.
590. Wiernik P.H.: Advances in management of acute nonlymphocytic leukemia. *Arch. Intern. Med.* 136:1399, 1976.
591. Armitage J.O., Burns C.P.: Maintenance of remission in adult acute non-lymphoblastic leukemia using intermittent courses of cytosine arabinoside and 6-thioguanine. *Cancer Treat. Rep.* 60:585, 1976.
592. Infection prevention in acute leukemia (editorial). *Lancet* 2:769, 1978.
593. Balducci L., et al.: Acute leukemia and infections: Perspectives from a general hospital. *Am. J. Hematol.* 15:57, 1983.
594. Keating M.J., et al.: Improved prospects for long-term survival in adults with acute myelogenous leukemia. *JAMA* 248:2481, 1982.
595. Thomas E.D., et al.: Marrow transplantation for acute nonlymphoblastic leukemia in first remission. *N. Engl. J. Med.* 301:597, 1979.
596. Dicke K.A., et al.: Autologous bone-marrow transplantation in relapsed acute leukaemia. *Lancet* 1:514, 1979.
597. Carpentier N.A., et al.: Circulating immune complexes and the prognosis of acute myeloid leukemia. *N. Engl. J. Med.* 307:1174, 1982.
598. Green M.H., et al.: Acute nonlymphocytic leukemia after therapy with alkylating agents for ovarian cancer: A study of five randomized clinical trials. *N. Engl. J. Med.* 307:1416, 1982.
599. Kapadia S.B., Kaplan S.S.: Simultaneous occurrence of non-Hodgkin's lymphoma and acute myelomonocytic leukemia. *Cancer* 38:2557, 1976.
600. Bergsagel D.E., et al.: The chemotherapy of plasma-cell myeloma and the incidence of acute leukemia. *N. Engl. J. Med.* 301:743, 1979.
601. Preisler H.D.: Therapy of secondary acute nonlymphocytic leukemia with cytarabine. *N. Engl. J. Med.* 308:21, 1983.
602. Kosiner B., et al.: Characterization of B-cell leukemias: A tentative immunomorphological scheme. *Blood* 56:815, 1980.
603. Zippin C., et al.: Survival in chronic lymphocytic leukemia. *Blood* 42:367, 1973.
604. Gunz F.W., Veale A.M.O.: Leukemia in close relatives: Accident or predisposition? *JNCI* 42:517, 1969.
605. Mitelman F.: Marker chromosome 14q+ in human cancer and leukemia. *Adv. Cancer Res.* 34:141, 1981.
606. Gahrton G., et al.: Nonrandom chromosomal aberrations in chronic lymphocytic leukemia revealed by polyclonal B-cell stimulation. *Blood* 56:640, 1980.
607. Han T., et al.: Prognostic importance of cytogenetic abnormalities in patients with chronic lymphocytic leukemia. *N. Engl. J. Med.* 310:288, 1984.
608. Sonnier J., et al.: Chromosomal translocation involving the immunoglobulin kappa-chain and heavy-chain loci in a child with chronic lymphocytic leukemia. *N. Engl. J. Med.* 309:590, 1983.
609. Boggs D.R., et al.: Factors influencing the duration and survival of patients with chronic lymphocytic leukemia. *Am. J. Med.* 40:243, 1966.
610. Slungaard A., Smith M.J.: Serum immunoglobulin levels in chronic lymphatic leukemia. *Scand. J. Haematol.* 12:112, 1974.
611. Fidder P., et al.: Clinical correlations with immunoglobulin levels in chronic lymphatic leukaemia. *Aust. NZ J. Med.* 2:346, 1972.
612. Werthamer S., Avaral L.: Electrophoretic abnormalities in chronic lymphocytic leukemia and cancer sera. *Am. J. Clin. Pathol.* 65:40, 1976.
613. Shumak K.H., et al.: Diagnosis of haematological disease using anti-i: I. Disorders with lymphocytosis. *Br. J. Haematol.* 41:399, 1979.
614. Blumberg N., et al.: The immune response to chronic red blood cell transfusion. *Vox Sang.* 42:212, 1983.
615. Pruzanski W., Shumak K.H.: Biologic activity of cold-reacting autoantibodies. *N. Engl. J. Med.* 297:583, 1977.
616. Cohen H.J.: Human lymphocyte surface immunoglobulin capping: Normal characteristics and anomalous behavior of chronic lymphocytic leukemic lymphocytes. *J. Clin. Invest.* 55:84, 1975.
617. LaFuente R., et al.: Isoenzymatic study of leucoacid phosphatase in haematologic diagnosis. *Scand. J. Haematol.* 23:146, 1979.
618. Berard C.W., et al.: Immunologic aspects and pathology of the malignant lymphomas. *Cancer* 42:911, 1978.
619. Binet J.L., et al.: A new prognostic classification of chronic lymphocytic leukemia derived from multivariate survival analysis. *Cancer* 48:198, 1981.
620. Huguley C.M.: Long-term study of chronic lymphocytic leukemia: Interim report after 45 months. *Cancer Chemother. Rep.* 16:241, 1962.
621. Galton D.A.G., et al.: The use of chlorambucil and steroids in the treatment of chronic lymphocytic leukemia. *Br. J. Haematol.* 7:73, 1961.
622. Matsumoto M., et al.: Adult T-cell leukemia-lymphoma in Fagoshima District, Southwestern Japan: Clinical and hematological characteristics. *Jpn. J. Clin. Oncol. Suppl.* 9:325, 1979.
623. Miller D.R.: Acute lymphoblastic leukemia. *Pediatr. Clin. North Am.* 27:269, 1980.
624. Zippin C., et al.: Variations in survival among patients with acute lymphocytic leukemia. *Blood* 37:59, 1971.
625. Thiel E., et al.: Multimarker classification of acute lymphoblastic leukemia: Evidence for further T subgroups and evaluation of their clinical significance. *Blood* 56:759, 1980.
626. Ritz J., et al.: A monoclonal antibody to human acute lymphoblastic leukemia antigen. *Blood* 54(suppl.):204a, 1979.
627. Tsukimoto I., et al.: Surface markers and prognostic factors in acute lymphoblastic leukemia. *N. Engl. J. Med.* 294:245, 1976.

628. McCaffrey R., et al.: Terminal deoxynucleotidyl transferase in human leukemic cells and in human thymocytes. *N. Engl. J. Med.* 292:775, 1975.
629. Bennett J.M., et al.: Proposals for the classification of acute leukemias. French-American-British cooperative group. *Br. J. Haematol.* 33:451, 1976.
630. Coleman M.S., et al.: Serial observation on terminal deoxynucleotidyl transferase activity and lymphoblast surface markers in acute lymphoblastic leukemia. *Cancer Res.* 36:120, 1976.
631. Greaves M.F., et al.: Antisera to acute lymphoblastic leukemia cells. *Clin. Immunol. Immunopathol.* 4:67, 1975.
632. Vogler L.B., et al.: Pre-B-cell leukemia: A new phenotype of childhood lymphoblastic leukemia. *N. Engl. J. Med.* 298:872, 1978.
633. Korsmeyer S.J., et al.: Developmental hierarchy of immunoglobulin gene rearrangements in human leukemic pre-B-cells. *Proc. Natl. Acad. Sci. USA* 78:7096, 1981.
634. Cossman J., et al.: Induction of differentiation in a case of common acute lymphoblastic leukemia. *N. Engl. J. Med.* 307:1251, 1982.
635. Spector G., et al.: Acute lymphoblastic leukemia followed by acute granulocytic leukemia in a pediatric patient. *Am. J. Clin. Pathol.* 72:242, 1979.
636. Brouet J.C., et al.: Immunological classification of acute lymphoblastic leukemias; evaluation of its clinical significance in a hundred cases. *Br. J. Haematol.* 33:319, 1976.
637. Broder S., et al.: Characterization of a suppressor-cell leukemia: Evidence for the requirement of an interaction of two T cells in the development of human suppressor effector cells. *N. Engl. J. Med.* 298:66, 1978.
638. Trujillo J.M.: Cytogenetics in hematology. *Curr. Hematol.* 1:276, 1981.
639. Lawler S.D.: Significance of chromosome abnormalities in leukemia. *Semin. Hematol.* 19:257, 1982.
640. Mitelman F., et al.: Reciprocal 8;14 translocation in EBV-negative B-cell acute lymphocytic leukemia with Burkitt-type cells. *Int. J. Cancer* 24:27, 1979.
641. Kamada N.: The effects of radiation on chromosomes of bone marrow cells: III. Cytogenetic studies on leukemia in atom bomb survivors. *Acta Haematol. Jpn.* 32:249, 1969.
642. Hutchinson G.B.: Leukemia in patients with cancer of the cervix uteri treated with radiation: A report covering the first five years of an international study. *JNCI* 40:951, 1968.
643. Gallo R.C., Meyskens F.L.: Advances in viral etiology of leukemia and lymphoma. *Semin. Hematol.* 15:379, 1978.
644. Popovic M., et al.: Isolation and transmission of human retrovirus (human T-cell leukemia virus). *Science* 219:856, 1983.
645. O'Conner G.T.: Persistent immunologic stimulation as a factor in oncogenesis with special reference to Burkitt's tumor. *Am. J. Med.* 48:279, 1970.
646. Levine P.H., et al.: Infectious mononucleosis prior to acute leukemia: A possible role for the Epstein-Barr virus. *Cancer* 30:875, 1972.
647. Sairenji T., et al.: Analysis of transformation with Epstein-Barr virus and phenotypic characteristics of lymphoblastoid cell lives established from patients with hairy-cell leukemia. *Am. J. Hematol.* 15:361, 1983.
648. Vigliali E.L., Sarta G.: Benzene and leukemia. *N. Engl. J. Med.* 271:872, 1964.
649. Svejgaard A., et al.: HL-A and disease associations: A survey. *Transplant. Rev.* 22:3, 1975.
650. Cline M.J.: Acute leukemia: Biology and treatment. *Ann. Intern. Med.* 91:758, 1979.
651. Mauer A.M.: Review: Therapy of acute lymphoblastic leukemia in childhood. *Blood* 56:1, 1980.
652. Steinhorn S.C., Myers M.H.: Progress in the treatment of childhood acute leukemia: A review. *Med. Pediatr. Oncol.* 9:333, 1981.
653. Brauner R., et al.: Leydig-cell function in children after direct testicular irradiation for acute lymphoblastic leukemia. *N. Engl. J. Med.* 309:25, 1983.
654. Johnson F.L., et al.: A comparison of marrow transplantation with chemotherapy for children with acute lymphoblastic leukemia in second or subsequent remission. *N. Engl. J. Med.* 305:846, 1981.
655. Collins V.P., Loeffler R.K., Tivey H.: Observations on growth rates of human tumors. *AJR* 76:988, 1956.
656. Silvergleid A.J.: Acute leukemia, in Silvergleid A.J. (ed.): *Clinical Hematology for Blood Bankers*. Washington, D.C., American Association of Blood Banks, 1979, pp. 18, 19.
657. Dorr R.J., Fritz W.L.: *Cancer Chemotherapy Handbook*. New York, Elsevier, 1980, pp. 3–4.
658. Schein P.S., et al.: Bleomycin, adriamycin, cyclophosphamide, vincristines and prednisone (BACOP) combination chemotherapy in the treatment of advanced diffuse histiocytic lymphoma. *Ann. Intern. Med.* 85:417, 1976.
659. Dorr R.T., Fritz W.L.: *Cancer Chemotherapy Handbook*. New York, Elsevier, 1980, pp. 102, 104–106.
660. Burke J.S., Byrne G.E. Jr., Rappaport H.: Hairy cell leukemia. *Cancer* 33:1399, 1974.
661. Katayama I., Yang I.P.: Reassessment of a cytochemical test for differential diagnoses of leukemic reticuloendothelioses. *Am. J. Clin. Pathol.* 68:268, 1977.
662. Casareale D., et al.: Sera of patients with hairy cell leukemia immunoprecipitate EBV-related antigens. *Leukemia Res.* 5:107, 1981.
663. Turner A., Kjeldsberg C.R.: Hairy cell leukemia: A review. *Medicine* 57:477, 1978.
664. Jansen J., et al.: The phenotype of the neoplastic cells of hairy cell leukemia studied with monoclonal antibodies. *Blood* 59:609, 1982.
665. Golomb H.M., Hanauer S.B.: Infectious complications in HCL. *J. Infect. Dis.* 143:639, 1981.
666. Quezada J.R., et al.: Alpha interferon for induction of remission in hairy-cell leukemia. *N. Engl. J. Med.* 310:15, 1984.

667. Lutgner M., et al.: Cutaneous "T" cell lymphomas: The Sézary syndrome, mycosis fungoides, and related disorders. *Ann. Intern. Med.* 83:534, 1975.
668. Broder S., et al.: The Sézary syndrome: A malignant proliferation of helper T-cells. *J. Clin. Invest.* 58:1297, 1976.
669. Clinicopathologic Conference: Systemic mastocytosis. *Am. J. Med.* 61:671, 1976.
670. Lennert K., Parwaresch M.R.: Mast cells and mast cell neoplasia: A review. *Histopathology* 3:349, 1979.
671. Ellis J.T., Peterson P.: The bone marrow in polycythemia vera. *Pathol. Ann.* 14:383, 1979.
672. Ersley A.J., et al.: Plasma erythropoietin in polycythemia. *Am. J. Med.* 66:243, 1979.
673. Prchal J.F., et al.: Polycythemia vera: The in vitro response of normal and abnormal stem cell lives to erythropoietin. *J. Clin. Invest.* 61:1044, 1978.
674. Willison J.R., et al.: Effect of high hematocrit on alertness. *Lancet* 1:846, 1980.
675. Berlin N.I., et al.: Symposium on polycythemia. *Semin. Hematol.* 12:355, 13:1, 1976.
676. Wurster-Hill D., et al.: Cytogenetic studies in polycythemia vera. *Semin. Hematol.* 13:13, 1976.
677. Wasserman L.R.: The management of polycythemia vera. *Br. J. Haematol.* 21:371, 1971.
678. Berk P.D., et al.: Non-hematologic malignancies in patients receiving myelosuppressive treatment for polycythemia vera. *Clin. Res.* 30:558A, 1982.
679. Kahn A., et al.: A deficient G-6-PD variant with hemizygous expression in blood cells of a woman with primary myelofibrosis. *Hum. Genet.* 30:41, 1975.
680. Van Slyck E.J., et al.: Chromosomal evidence for the secondary role of fibroblastic proliferation in acute myelofibrosis. *Blood* 36:729, 1970.
681. Ross R., Vogel R.: The platelet-derived growth factor. *Cell* 14:203, 1980.
682. Laszlo J.: Myeloproliferative disorders (MPD): Myelofibrosis, myelosclerosis, extramedullary hemopoiesis, undifferentiated MPD, and hemorrhagic thrombocythemia. *Semin. Hematol.* 12:409, 1975.
683. Robbins S.L., Cotran R.S.: *Pathologic Basis of Disease*, ed. 2. Philadelphia, W.B. Saunders, 1979, p. 758.
684. Gutensohn N., Cole P.: Childhood social environment and Hodgkin's disease. *N. Engl. J. Med.* 304:135, 1981.
685. Newell G.R.: Etiology of multiple sclerosis and Hodgkin's disease. *Am. J. Epidemiol.* 91:119, 1970.
686. Graza K., et al.: Hodgkin's disease in monozygotic twins: A case report. *J. Surg. Oncol.* 12:221, 1979.
687. Langerhuysen M.M.A.C., et al.: Antibodies to Epstein-Barr virus, cytomegalovirus, and Australia antigen in Hodgkin's disease. *Cancer* 34:262, 1974.
688. Lindahl T., et al.: Relationship between Epstein-Barr virus (EBV) DNA and the EBV-determined nuclear antigen (EBNA) in Burkitt-lymphoma biopsies and other lymphoproliferative malignancies. *Int. J. Cancer.* 13:764, 1974.
689. Aulakh G.S., Gallo R.C.: Rauscher-leukemia-virus-related sequences in human DNA: Presence in some tissues of some patients with hematopoietic neoplasias and absence in DNA from other tissues. *Proc. Natl. Acad. Sci. USA* 74:353, 1977.
690. Li F.P., et al.: Malignant lymphomas after diphenylhydantoin (Dilantin) therapy. *Cancer* 36:1359, 1975.
691. Waldemann T.P., et al.: Immunodeficiency disease and malignancy. *Ann. Intern. Med.* 77:605, 1972.
692. Ziegler J.B., et al.: Intrinsic lymphocyte defect in Hodgkin's disease: Analysis of the phytohemagglutinin dose-response. *Cell. Immunol. Immunopathol.* 3:451, 1975.
693. Shulof R.S., et al.: Multivariate analysis of T-cell functional defects and circulating serum factors in Hodgkin's disease. *Cancer* 48:964, 1981.
694. Levine A.M., et al.: Positive coombs test in Hodgkin's disease: Significance and implications. *Blood* 55:607, 1980.
695. Fukakara S., Rowley J.D.: Chromosome 14 translocations in non-Burkitt lymphomas. *Int. J. Cancer* 22:14, 1978.
696. Poppema S.: Sternberg-Reed cells with intracytoplasmic lymphocytes: Phagocytosis or emperipolesis? *Virchows Arch. [Pathol. Anat.]* 380:355, 1978.
697. Lukes R.J., et al.: Report of the nomenclature committee. *Cancer Res.* 26:1311, 1966.
698. Wright C.J.E.: Prospects of cure in lymphocyte-predominant Hodgkin's disease. *Am. J. Clin. Pathol.* 67:507, 1977.
699. Carbone P.T., et al.: Staging in Hodgkin's disease: Symposium. *Cancer Res.* 31:1707, 1971.
700. Kaplan H.S.: *Hodgkin's Disease.* Cambridge, Mass., Harvard University Press, 1980, p. 371.
701. Kaplan H.S., Rosenberg S.A.: The management of Hodgkin's disease. *Cancer* 36(suppl.):796, 1975.
702. Parker J.W.: A new look at malignant lymphomas. *Diagn. Med.* June 1981, p. 79.
703. Reinherz E., Schlossman S.F.: The differentiation and function of human T lymphocytes. *Cell* 19:821, 1980.
704. Rappaport H.: Tumors of the hematopoietic system, in *Atlas of Tumor Pathology.* Washington, D.C., Armed Forces Institute of Pathology, 1966, Sec. III, fasc. 8.
705. Lukes R.J.: The immunologic approach to the pathology of malignant lymphomas. *Am. J. Clin. Pathol.* 72:657, 1979.
706. The Non-Hodgkin's Lymphoma Pathologic Classification Group: NCI sponsored study of classifications of Non-Hodgkin's lymphomas: Summary and description of a working formulation for clinical usage. *Cancer* 49:2112, 1982.
707. Andiman W.A.: The Epstein-Barr virus: EB virus infections in childhood. *J. Pediatr.* 95:171, 1979.
708. Robinson J.E., et al.: Diffuse polyclonal B-cell lymphoma during primary infection with Epstein-Barr virus. *N. Engl. J. Med.* 302:1293, 1980.

709. Andiman W., et al.: Use of cloned probes to detect Epstein-Barr viral DNA in tissues of patients with neoplastic and lymphoproliferative diseases. *J. Infect. Dis.* 148:967, 1983.
710. Hochberg F.H., et al.: Central-nervous-system lymphoma related to Epstein-Barr virus. *N. Engl. J. Med.* 309:745, 1983.
711. Robert-Guraff M., et al.: Natural antibodies to human retrovirus HTLV in a cluster of Japanese patients T-cell leukemia. *Science* 215:975, 1982.
712. Mushinski F.J., et al.: DNA rearrangement and altered RNA expression of the c-myb oncogene in mouse plasmacytoid lymphosarcoma. *Science* 220:795, 1983.
713. Morton C.C., et al.: Mapping of the human blym-1 transforming gene activated in Burkitt lymphomas to chromosome 1. *Science* 223:175, 1983.
714. Rowley J.D., Fukuhara S.: Chromosome studies in non-Hodgkin's lymphomas. *Semin. Oncol.* 7:255, 1980.
715. Croce C.M., et al.: Chromosomal location of the genes for human immunoglobulin heavy chains. *Proc. Natl. Acad. Sci. USA* 76:3416, 1979.
716. McBride O.W., et al.: Chromosomal localization of human immunoglobulin light chain constant region genes, in *Human Gene Mapping Conference VI*. New York, National Foundation, 1981.
717. Erickson J., et al.: Assignment of human genes for lambda immunoglobulin chain to chromosome 22. *Nature* 294:173, 1981.
718. Patchefsky A.S., et al.: Non-Hodgkin's lymphomas: A clinicopathologic study of 293 cases. *Cancer* 34:1173, 1974.
719. Jones S.E., et al.: Non-Hodgkin's lymphomas: IV. Clinicopathologic correlation in 405 cases. *Cancer* 31:806, 1973.
720. Rudders R.A., et al.: Surface marker identification of small cleaved follicular center cell lymphomas with a highly favorable prognosis. *Cancer Res.* 42:349, 1982.
721. Warnke R.A., et al.: The coexistence of nodular and diffuse patterns in nodular non-Hodgkin's lymphomas: Significance and clinicopathologic correlation. *Cancer* 40:1229, 1977.
722. Waldron J.A., et al.: Malignant lymphoma of peripheral T-lymphocyte origin. *Cancer* 40:1604, 1977.
723. Armitage J.O., et al.: Clinical usefulness and reproducibility of histologic subclassification of advanced diffuse histiocytic lymphoma. *Am. J. Med.* 67:929, 1979.
724. Rudders R.A., et al.: Surface marker and histopathologic correlation with long-term survival in advanced large-cell non-Hodgkin's lymphoma. *Cancer* 47:1329, 1981.
725. Nathwani B.N.: A critical analysis of the classifications of non-Hodgkin's lymphomas. *Cancer* 44:349, 1979.
726. Palutke M., et al.: T-cell lymphomas of large cell type. *Cancer* 46:87, 1980.
727. Nadler L.M., et al.: Heterogeneity of T-cell lymphoblastic malignancies. *Blood* 55:806, 1980.
728. Boucheix C., et al.: Lymphoblastic lymphoma/leukemia with convoluted nuclei. *Cancer* 45:1569, 1980.
729. Lindahl T., et al.: Relationship between Epstein-Barr virus (EBV) DNA and the EBV-determined nuclear antigen (EBNA) in Burkitt lymphoma biopsies and other lymphoproliferative malignancies. *Int. J. Cancer* 13:764, 1974.
730. Ziegler J.L.: Management of Burkitt's lymphoma: An update. *Cancer Treat. Rev.* 6:95, 1979.
731. Mollison P.L.: *Blood Transfusion in Clinical Medicine*, ed. 7. Oxford, England, Blackwell Scientific Publications, 1983, p. 445.
732. Knowles D.M. II, et al.: The application of monoclonal antibodies to the characterization and diagnosis of lymphoid neoplasms: A review of recent studies. *Diagn. Immunol.* 1:142, 1983.
733. Sweet D.L., et al.: Survival of patients with localized diffuse histiocytic lymphoma. *Blood* 58:1218, 1981.
734. Portlock C.S., Rosenberg S.A.: Chemotherapy of the non-Hodgkin's lymphomas: The Stanford experience. *Cancer Treat. Rep.* 61:1049, 1977.
735. Hellman S., et al.: The place of radiation therapy in the treatment of non-Hodgkin's lymphomas. *Cancer* 39(suppl.):843, 1977.
736. Voakes J.B., et al.: The chemotherapy of lymphoblastic lymphoma. *Blood* 57:186, 1981.
737. Lukes R.J., Tinelle B.J.: Immunoblastic lymphadenopathy: A hyperimmune entity resembling Hodgkin's disease. *N. Engl. J. Med.* 292:1, 1975.
738. Owen J.J.T., et al.: In vitro generation of B-lymphocytes in mouse fetal liver, a mammalian 'bursa' equivalent. *Nature* 249:361, 1974.
739. Metcalf E.S., Klinman N.R.: In vitro tolerance induction in neonatal murine B cells. *J. Exp. Med.* 143:1327, 1976.
740. Liu C.P., et al.: Mapping of the heavy chain genes for mouse immunoglobulin M and D. *Science* 209:1348, 1980.
741. Heller P., et al.: Surface immunoglobulins of circulating lymphocytes in mouse and human plasmacytoma. *Trans. Assoc. Am. Physicians* 85:192, 1972.
742. Seligman M.: Immunochemical, clinical, and pathological features of α-chain disease. *Arch. Intern. Med.* 135:78, 1975.
743. Potter M., et al.: Brief communication: Growth of primary plasmacytosis in the mineral oil conditioned peritoneal environment. *JNCI* 49:305, 1972.
744. Warner N.L., et al.: *Multiple myeloma and related immunoglobulin-producing neoplasms*. UICC Technical Report Series, vol. 13. Geneva, International Union Against Cancer, 1974.
745. Henry L.W.: Multiple myeloma in a mink handler following exposure to Aleutian disease. *Cancer* 44:273, 1979.
746. Hopper J.E.: Immunofluorescent evidence for a

common clonal origin of IgM-λ and IgG-κ paraproteins. *Clin. Res.* 21:557, 1973.
747. McArthur J.R., et al.: Melphalan and myeloma: Experience with a low-dose continuous regimen. *Ann. Intern. Med.* 72:665, 1970.
748. McIntire O.R.: Multiple myeloma. *N. Engl. J. Med.* 301:193, 1979.
749. Blumberg N., Katz A.J.: Partial plasma exchange: Diseases in which it is of reported efficacy, in Berkman E.M., Umlas J. (eds.).: *Therapeutic Hemapheresis.* Washington, D.C., American Association of Blood Banks, 1980, p. 79.

3

Hemostasis and Thrombosis

BLOOD BANK PHYSICIANS are often called on to treat patients with hemostatic disorders. Patients needing blood components or factors may have a variety of hemostatic disorders. These disorders can often be complex, involving the formed elements of hemostasis (platelets), endothelium, or the soluble factors of coagulation. In order to treat these patients with the appropriate therapy, one must have some understanding of the process of hemostasis. For instance, in modern blood banking, treatment of hemophiliacs with severe factor deficiencies may require the use of concentrates; the potential complications of such therapy include hepatitis and AIDS. Leukemics treated with aggressive chemotherapy will present at the nadir, with severe neutropenia and thrombocytopenia, and a variety of components will be needed to improve hemostasis. Open heart surgery patients frequently need massive replacement with a variety of components such as fresh frozen plasma (FFP) and platelets. In many surgical patients and oncology patients disseminated intravascular coagulation (DIC) is a dreaded complication, both of the disease and, occasionally, of the therapy. Thus, a knowledge of hemostatic and thrombotic processes is of great value in providing the appropriate treatment.

This chapter discusses the biochemistry, physiology, and pathology of hemostasis. The specific use of blood components and fractions for the treatment of hemostatic disorders is discussed in Chapter 8.

Hemostatic mechanisms interact to prevent the loss of blood from the circulatory system. When these mechanisms break down, bleeding occurs and preservation of blood within the vessels is compromised. Several factors interact to prevent bleeding and to repair certain types of damage to the circulatory system.

Vascular integrity and good platelet function as well as integrity of the biochemical components of the plasma clotting factors are necessary for hemostasis. So, in essence, hemostasis depends on the structural integrity of the vessel walls, platelets, and clotting factors. The function of each is described below.

STRUCTURAL INTEGRITY OF THE VESSEL WALLS

Although blood vessel contraction is one of the first mechanisms of hemostasis to be activated after injury, it is also one of the least known mechanisms in the hemostatic process.

Endothelial cells form a monolayer of cells, joined to each other through tight cell-cell junctions varying in width from 0 to 1 nm.[1] Fluids traverse the endothelial barrier via endothelial cell pinocytosis or in the spaces between cells. The endothelial cells rest on an amorphous matrix, the subendothelium secreted by the endothelial cells. It contains both type IV and type V (AB_2) collagen fibers.[2]

In addition to collagen, fibronectin, elastin, mucopolysaccharides, and laminin form part of the subendothelial matrix.[3] Certain blood cells such as granulocytes[4] and lymphocytes are capable of adhering to and crossing the endothelium, although lymphocytes appear to interact with specialized types of endothelium more readily.[5] Although endothelial integrity is crucial to adequate hemostasis, it is now known that the vasculature and its endothelium have a much more dynamic role in hemostasis than was previously thought. Endothelial cells synthesize a variety of substances active during hemostasis. Prostaglandins such as PGI_2 (prostacyclin) are examples of substances synthesized by the endothelium. Prostacyclin is a potent vasodilator[6] and inhibitor of platelet function; it binds to a specific receptor on platelets,[7] with a resulting increase in intraplatelet adenosine monophosphate (AMP) and platelet shape modifications. Prostacyclin synthesis is stimulated by thrombin,[8] angiotensin II,[9] hypoxia,[10] and other factors. Aspirin inhibits the effects of prostacyclin.[11] Furthermore, endothelial cells regulate platelet adhesion by enzymes capable of inactivating adenosine diphosphate (ADP) and ATP, which are strong inhibitors of platelet function.[12] These cells are also involved in anti-thrombin III inactivation.[13] When the endothelium is denuded, as occurs in a variety of pathologic circumstances, subendothelial collagen types IV and V (AB_2) are exposed to platelets. Platelets aggregate and release thromboxane A_2 on exposure to these collagen fibers.[14]

Clotting Factors Produced by Endothelial Cells

It is now clear that the vW (von Willebrand) portion of factor VIII is synthesized in endothelial cells.[15]

Although disruption of endothelial cells will induce formation of tissue factor clotting activity, the effect is minor when compared with the tissue factor activity of disrupted smooth muscle cells and fibroblasts.[16] This suggests that relatively superficial damage to the endothelium will cause less activation of platelets and coagulation factors than deeper damage involving smooth muscle cells and fibroblasts.

Endothelial cell microsomes are capable of activating factor XII, which in turn is capable of activating prekallikrein.[17] It is clear from this finding, that endothelial cells make an important contribution to the hemostatic process; however, these cells also contribute to fibrinolysis and anticoagulation. Endothelial cells contain plasminogen activator[18] and are capable of inactivating thrombin-antithrombin III complexes.[19] These cells have the capacity of activating protein C,[20] which cleaves factors V and VIII enzymatically.

Platelets are significantly involved in the maintenance of endothelial integrity, as evidenced by leakage of RBCs[21] and dyes from the intravascular space[22] in thrombocytopenic patients.

Abnormal Hemostasis Due to Derangement of the Endothelium

Disorders of endothelial integrity as well as other vascular disorders resulting in bleeding can be divided into four groups: degenerative changes of collagen and supporting structures; infections which damage the vessels and their endothelium; a variety of noninfectious inflammatory diseases, usually autoimmune or having a direct toxic effect on endothelial cells; and purpura of other causes. A short discussion of each follows.

1. Examples of bleeding susceptibility due to degenerative changes of collagen are:

  a. Senile purpura, in which hematomas occur in sun-exposed areas. Actinic radiation destroys collagenous supporting structures, creating a fragile vascular bed.[23] Decreased procoagulants in elderly individuals may add to the bleeding tendency.

  b. Vitamin C deficiency. Ascorbic acid is an essential constituent of collagen biosynthesis. When vitamin C is lacking in the diet, a structurally abnormal collagen results;[24] consequently the vascular bed becomes more fragile and the bleeding tendency increases.

  c. Ehlers-Danlos syndrome. The abnormally extensible collagen produced by this syndrome likewise results in an increased bleeding tendency due to fragility of small and intermediate-sized vessels.[25]

  d. Purpuras caused by chronic stasis, such as the Majocchi-Schamberg progressive pigmentary purpura, are also due to vascular fragility.[26]

  e. Other diseases such as the Rendu-Osler-Weber syndrome, pseudoxanthoma elasticum, and Marfan's syndrome present with purpuras due to increased vascular fragility.

2. Nonthrombocytopenic purpura secondary to infection probably results from toxic damage to the endothelium or to microemboli. Bacterial, rickettsial,[27] and viral infections will result in purpuric bleeding manifestations.

3. Noninfectious inflammatory diseases such as

the Henoch-Schönlein syndrome also result in purpura. The purpura in these instances affects mostly children and is secondary to immune-mediated lesions. Anaphylactoid purpura may be secondary to insect bites, toxic agents, food allergy, or infections. A β-hemolytic streptococcal infection may precede the development of anaphylactoid purpura.[28] Patients with Henoch-Schönlein purpura often have circulating immune complexes, mainly composed of IgA complexes,[29] C3c, C3d, and C5;[30] the purpura may be associated with gastrointestinal lesions and renal disease. Histologically the lesions consist of microvascular plugging with fibrinoid necrosis.

4. Other causes of purpuric lesions are neoplastic diseases, such as Kaposi's sarcoma. Recently this tumor has been found in younger individuals with AIDS.[31]

ROLE OF PLATELETS IN HEMOSTASIS

Apart from their role in the formation of a clot plug when a small vessel is severed, platelets also maintain the integrity of the endothelium, with which they interact constantly. When platelets are reduced in number or when their function is impaired, vessels tend to become more permeable, and escape of blood ensues. Platelets are anucleate disks that derive from the "pinching off" of polypoid projections of megakaryocyte membranes.[32] Megakaryocytes arise from marrow stem cell precursors capable of differentiating into granulocyte/macrophage precursors, megakaryocyte precursors, and erythroid precursors. The colony-forming unit which differentiates into megakaryocytes is the CFU-M.[33] CFU-M cells can be subdivided into an earlier CFU-M1 stage and a later CFU-M2 stage. CFU-M1 cells can give rise to promegakaryoblasts directly or proceed to CFU-M2.[34] Promegakaryoblasts are cells that have entered polyploidization (2N polyploidy). When these cells appear blastic they are termed megakaryoblasts, and their polyploidy ranges from 4N to 64N.[35] Megakaryoblasts give rise to non-DNA-synthesizing promegakaryocytes and subsequently to megakaryocytes that are capable of liberating platelets; however, platelets can be liberated from 8N polyploidy on. Platelets are produced from cytoplasmic processes that contain an array of longitudinally oriented microtubules. These processes gradually undergo attentuation and develop constrictions which "pinch off" as platelets.[36]

Kinetics of Platelet Production

A normal platelet count varies between 150,000 and 300,000/cu mm of blood. Several thousand platelets are released by each megakaryocyte during its life span, and over 44,000 platelets are produced daily.[37] The adequate growth of CFU-M requires erythropoietin and other growth factors.[38] Thus, at least two factors are necessary for megakaryocyte production; however, erythropoietin appears to be capable of overriding the deficit of the second factor if supplied in large doses.[39] Another hormone, thrombopoietin, has been shown to be synthesized in the kidney.[40] It stimulates platelet production directly.[41] Other factors such as acetylcholinesterase also affect platelet production. Neostigmine, a cholinesterase inhibitor, induces an increase in CFU-M.[42]

In the circulation, platelets have an overall survival time of approximately 10 days.[43] It appears that the bone marrow, rather than the liver or spleen,[44] plays a significant role in removal of senescent platelets.

Platelet Structure

Platelets are diskoid structures measuring about 2 μ in diameter. They can be functionally divided into three structures: the outer or peripheral zone, primarily involved in adhesion; the sol-gel zone, involved in the contractile phases of these disks; and the organelle zone, involved in the secretory functions of platelets.

The peripheral zone is composed of at least three parts: an *amorphous coat*, which is about 100–200 Å thick[45] and recently has been shown to have some structural organization;[46] a *membrane;* and a *submembrane*. The peripheral zone interacts with the immediate environment and is responsible for first-phase aggregation, consisting of a cycle of adhesion → release → aggregation.[47] The membrane is a trilaminar structure and is responsible for maintaining the integrity of the internal milieu of platelets and supplying phospholipids necessary for thrombus formation.[48] Furthermore, the membrane exhibits a thrombin receptor.[49] The innermost submembrane area of the peripheral zone is closely associated with the cytosol of platelets. Fine filaments form part of this submembrane.[50]

The sol-gel zone is responsible for maintaining the platelets' diskoid shape. Arrays of fibers attached to the submembrane and microtubules which form a complex microcanalicular system as the cytoskeleton of these cells. This microcanalicular system is instrumental in transporting substances extruded from organelles to the cell exterior.[51] The cytoskeleton is also responsible for platelet contraction.[52] The tubular system that connects with the exterior is termed the open canalicular system (OCS). A second membrane tubular system that originates from the parent megakaryocyte cell is termed the dense tubular system (DTS).[53] The two tubular systems appear to be connected, as demonstrated by peroxidase activity which delineates the two systems.[54] This dual tubular system appears to operate as the sarcoplasmic reticulum in the muscle, channeling calcium ions to the closely associated contractile structures containing actomyosin capable of reversible depolymerization.[55] These proteins are platelet actin, a 55,000-dalton globular protein, which polymerizes with an axial periodicity of 3.5 nm, and myosin, a large 460,000-dalton, asymmetric protein.[56]

The organelle zone contains platelet granules. Granules can be alpha granules, lysosomes, or dense bodies. The alpha granules contain platelet factor 4, fibrinogen, β-thromboglobulin, thrombin-sensitive protein, and growth-promoting factor.[57,58] Dense bodies are 0.05–0.15 μ in diameter and play an important role in thrombus formation, storing serotonin, nucleotides, calcium ions, and catecholamines.[59] ADP has likewise been found in these granules.[60] During aggregation, these dense bodies are shifted to the cell center.[61]

In addition to granules, platelets contain a few mitochondria, which contribute significant amounts of ATP, and other small organelles such as glycogen and ferritin granules.

The platelet has an energy metabolism very similar to that of skeletal muscle and is capable of active carbohydrate glycolysis and synthesis of glycogen.[62]

Platelet Turnover

Platelets have an approximate turnover rate of about 35,000 ± 4,300/μl/day.[63] Senescent and damaged platelets are preferentially trapped by the spleen[64] and bone marrow.

There is a morphological as well as a physiologic heterogeneity in the platelet population. This is probably due to a difference in size and age of these corpuscles.[65] Survival of different platelet subpopulations varies. Determination of platelet survival is possible by platelet cohort label studies with ^{75}Se-selenomethionine.[66] It is by these means that an 8- to 11-day mean survival for normal platelets has been determined.

Platelet Physiology During Hemostasis

When the endothelial surface is broken and blood comes in contact with the components of the disrupted surface, platelets adhere to collagen fibers, microfibers, and other endothelial and subendothelial structures.[67] Under these conditions platelets have a tendency to adhere, thus initiating a cycle of activation. Adhesion triggers a secretory process in the platelet. This process as stated before, involves adhesion → release reaction → ADP-induced platelet aggregation and accounts for the primary arrest of bleeding.

Adhesion

Upon denudation of endothelium with exposure of subendothelial structures, platelets adhere especially to collagen.[67] The quaternary structure of collagen appears to be necessary for adherence to occur. Other elements important in platelet adhesion are galactosyl residues,[68] free sulfhydryl groups,[69] and ε-amino groups of lysine.[70] Recent evidence supports the view that fibronectin on the platelet membrane constitutes the molecular receptor for exposed collagen during adhesion, in which factor XIII is also involved.[71]

Platelet Aggregation

This is a phenomenon that involves attachment of platelets to one another. Aggregation can be primary or secondary. Primary aggregation is induced by certain substances directly, while secondary aggregation occurs after an indirect stimulus that triggers endogenous aggregating-factor release by platelets per se. ADP, thrombin, epinephrine, and vasopressin are the primary aggregating factors. ADP is considered to be a key factor in primary aggregation and is calcium and fibrinogen dependent.[72] Epinephrine produces a biphasic wave on the aggregometer. The first wave is not accompanied by platelet shape changes, but the second wave is accompanied by shape changes and a release reaction.[73] Secondary aggregation can be induced by collagen,[74] ristocetin,[75] and factor VIII.[76]

The exact mechanism of ADP-induced aggregation is not fully understood. It is thought that platelets possess an ADP receptor on the membrane

tion is not fully understood. It is thought that platelets possess an ADP receptor on the membrane similar to receptors found in drug interactions, and that activation of actomyocin is probably involved.[77] Thromboxane A_2 is capable of both causing aggregation and release.[78]

The Release Reaction

When platelets become activated through various stimuli, these corpuscles degranulate, releasing bioactive substances. These substances not only activate clotting but result in aggregation of platelets to the endothelium.

There are two types of platelet granule release from platelets.[79] In release type 1, ADP and serotonin are liberated from dense granules. ADP and epinephrine stimulate release type 1; aspirin usually inhibits it. Type 2 release originates in alpha granules. It is stimulated by catepsins and hydrolases. Thrombin stimulates both release type 1 and release type 2 from platelets.

Platelets, which are normally disk shaped, become deformed and "spiny shaped," as well as adherent to damaged endothelium upon contact. The deformability and contraction of platelets are due to the actin content of platelets. Platelets adhere to the ϵ-amino group of lysine in native collagen, and this radical becomes accessible when the vascular endothelium is damaged.[80]

It has been suggested that a prostaglandin precursor may also mediate aggregation, whereas prostaglandins such as $PGF_{2\alpha}$ and PGE_2 may inhibit platelet aggregation and release of the corpuscles.[81]

Additional Concepts on Release Type 1. —The release reaction of platelets is considered to be an energy-dependent reaction resulting in the gathering of various platelet organelles to the center of the platelet due to microtubule contraction. Secretion with the release of ADP, ATP, serotonin, and calcium from electron-dense platelet cytoplasmic organelles, or dense bodies, is seen during type 1 release.[82] The activity of these organelles can be monitored via release and uptake of labeled serotonin.[83] The release reaction is accompanied by disappearance of granules from platelets, as assessed by electron microscopy. A variety of substances, most of which act at the membrane of the platelet, are capable of inducing the release reaction. Of these substances, calcium, magnesium, ADP, ATP, fibrinogen, factor VIII, and prostaglandins are the most important.

Platelet Pathology

Due to the scope of this book, only a brief description of selected platelet disorders which are representative of the listed categories will be given here. A classification is outlined in Table 3–1.

Congenital Defects of Platelets

Congenital defects of platelet function can be intrinsic, caused by abnormalities of platelets per se,

TABLE 3–1.—MAJOR PLATELET DISORDERS

Congenital	
QUALITATIVE	QUANTITATIVE
Intrinsic	*Decreased production*
Defects of adhesion (e.g., Bernard-Soulier syndrome)	(e.g., hereditary thrombocytopenia)
Defects of aggregation (e.g., Glanzmann's disease)	*Increased destruction*
	(e.g., erythroblastosis faetalis)
Extrinsic	
(e.g., von Willebrand's disease)	

Acquired	
QUALITATIVE	QUANTITATIVE
Uremia	*Decreased production*
Liver disease	(e.g., aplastic anemia, thiazides, alcoholism)
Disproteinemia	
Drug-induced	*Increased destruction*
	Nonimmune (e.g., infection, DIC, TTP)
	Immune (e.g., ITP, drug-induced, posttransfusional)

Thrombocytosis	
PRIMARY	SECONDARY
Examples: essential thrombocythemia, myeloproliferative disorders	Examples: infections, neoplasia, postoperative

or extrinsic, caused by lack of external factors necessary for adequate platelet function. Platelets may be congenitally defective in the adhesion phase or may display abnormalities during aggregation.

Defects of Adhesion and Aggregation.—
An example of a defect of adhesion is the Bernard-Soulier syndrome, although defective aggregation is also seen in this disease. The Bernard-Soulier syndrome is a rare autosomal recessive disease of platelets. Giant platelets which display a dilated canalicular system[84] are observed on the peripheral blood smear. Platelet adhesion to glass beads is decreased. A defect in a membrane receptor for factor VIII has been suggested as the etiology of this syndrome.

A lack of membrane type Ib and Is glycoproteins has likewise been described in this syndrome.[85] Autoantibodies seen in quinine-induced thrombocytopenia fail to react with Bernard-Soulier platelets lacking Ib and Is proteins.[86] Platelet aggregation is normal in the presence of ADP and collagen but abnormal in the presence of ristocetin and thrombin;[87] the abnormality is not corrected by factor VIII vW. Treatment for the Bernard-Soulier syndrome is supportive. Platelets do not respond to ristocetin. Patients can be managed with transfusion of platelets if bleeding is anticipated or if major trauma has caused bleeding.

Glanzmann's thrombasthenia, an autosomal recessive disease of platelets, is characterized by spheroidal platelets that do not respond to ADP aggregation.[88] A deficit in clot retraction is also noted. The defect is in the primary aggregation curve and is partially due to a membrane glycoprotein abnormality, such as aberrations of platelet membrane glycoproteins types IIb, III, and IIIa.[89] These proteins appear to be molecular anchors to actin.

Abnormal Platelet Aggregation Due to Clotting Factor Abnormalities.—An example of poor platelet function associated with abnormalities extrinsic to the platelet is von Willebrand's disease. This disease is an autosomal dominant or recessive disorder in which a portion of the factor VIII molecular complex, factor VIII vW, is deficient quantitatively or qualitatively. Factor VIII vW, which exists in plasma as multimers weighing about 20×10^6 daltons, is composed of smaller subunits (0.22×10^6 daltons).[90] The multimeric quaternary structure is necessary for adequate function of this portion of factor VIII.[91] Some patients with von Willebrand's disease lack such multimers,[92] but others do not. In addition, certain patients with von Willebrand's disease have factor VIII vW molecules with an abnormal carbohydrate moiety[93] whereas others do not.[94] Evidently, the disease is in reality a syndrome that may be caused by qualitative as well as quantitative abnormalities of factor VIII vW. It is not clear, however, why, when factor VIII vW is restored, levels of factor VIII C simultaneously are almost immediately restored in these patients. This suggests that factor VIII vW functions as a stabilizer of factor VIII C or that it regulates its synthesis; the answer to this question is currently not known. At the clinical laboratory level, the bleeding time is prolonged, reflecting the activity of factor VIII vW on platelet aggregation. Most patients with von Willebrand's disease exhibit an abnormal ristocetin aggregation test.[95] Two main patterns of autosomal dominant von Willebrand's disease are recognized, type I and type II. In type I there are decreased levels of factor VIII R:Ag, factor VIII R:R CO, and factor VIII:C, but the multimeric quaternary structure is usually normal.[96] In type II von Willebrand's disease these factors are not decreased—in fact the VIII portion is usually increased[96]—but the multimeric quaternary structure is abnormal.[96]

In the treatment of von Willebrand's disease, cryoprecipitate is preferred, because this preparation contains more intact factor VIII vW in its quaternary structure than do concentrates of factor VIII in the lyophilized form.[91] Factor VIII levels usually rise shortly after infusion of cryoprecipitate.

Acquired Qualitative Disorders

Drug-Induced Platelet Abnormalities.—
A variety of drugs are capable of disrupting normal platelet function. A good example is aspirin, a potent inhibitor of the platelet release reaction due to irreversible acetylation by the drug of active sites on platelet cyclo-oxygenase.[97] The inhibition of this enzyme blocks the synthesis of PGE_2, $PGF_{2\alpha}$, and thromboxane A_2. Collagen-induced aggregation and epinephrine-induced aggregation are deficient in aggregometric studies of aspirin-treated platelets.[98] Aspirin-induced defects are considered to be primary release defects with normal levels of platelet ADP. In contrast, ADP-storage pool defects where the release mechanism is normal are termed "storage pool defect."[99] By blocking release mechanisms, aspirin produces a deficient release of ADP, ATP, and serotonin (Fig 3–1).[100]

It is critical that platelets from aspirin-treated donors not be used because aspirin produces a dras-

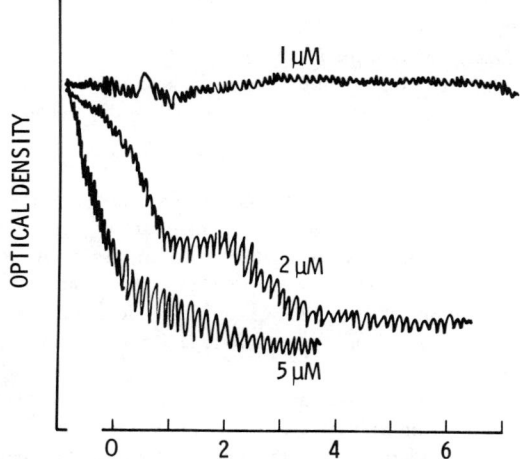

FIG 3–1.—Platelet aggregometer curves; no aggregation *(top curve)* and aggregation *(middle and lower curves)*, as indicated by the decrement in optical density.

tic and irreversible defect in platelet release for the life span of the affected platelet. In contrast, indomethacin, which also inhibits prostaglandins, does so in a reversible manner.[101]

Other substances such as carbenicillin,[102] antihistaminics,[103] infusion of Dextran, melphalan, and ethanol ingestion produce abnormal platelet function via different mechanisms. Uremia causes a variety of platelet defects. In severe cases of uremia, ADP-induced aggregation may be grossly abnormal.[104–105] Likewise, severe liver disease will produce qualitative defects in platelet aggregation.[106] Platelet defects in uremia are improved by deamino-8-D-arginine vasopressin by restoring factor VIII vW.[107] This type of therapy has also been used in mild cases of hemophilia, and in von Willebrand's disease.[108] Of great interest to blood bankers, because of its prevalence in centers where open heart surgery is performed, is the damage to platelets by the cardiopulmonary pump, which produces an "acquired" platelet storage pool defect.[109]

Thrombocytopenia

Thrombocytopenia may be congenital or acquired.

Congenital Thrombocytopenias.—Some thrombocytopenias may be associated with other malformations such as bilateral bone malformations (absent radius syndrome). Rubella has been implicated as the cause in certain cases.[110] The prognosis is poor, and therapy is supportive.

In the Wiskott-Aldrich syndrome, congenital cellular and humoral immune deficiency and thrombocytopenia are present. Platelets exhibit abnormal ultrastructure on electron microscopy. Splenectomy may be useful in selected cases.[111]

The May-Hegglin anomaly is an autosomal dominant disease with giant platelets and Döhle body-bearing granulocytes.

Acquired Thrombocytopenias.—The acquired thrombocytopenias are generally divided into thrombocytopenias due to lack of production of platelets or increased destruction.

Acquired Thrombocytopenia Due to Lack of Platelet Production.—Thrombocytopenia is frequently seen in bone marrow aplasia. During recovery, platelet normalization lags several months behind erythrocyte and granulocyte recovery and remains as a permanent complication of aplasia.[112] Isolated megakaryocytic aplasia may be seen.[113] Many of these cases develop into leukemias after a few months or years. Marrow infiltration by tumor can often result in thrombocytopenia. Gaucher's disease and miliary tuberculosis[114] can likewise obliterate the marrow, causing thrombocytopenia.

In today's cancer therapy, bone marrow transplantation has become more feasible, and patients are therefore more frequently exposed to whole body irradiation, which produces an immediate drop in the lymphocyte and granulocyte count. Platelet counts, however, drop after 7 days, exposing these patients to bleeding diathesis.[115] Although all myelosuppressive drugs cause thrombocytopenia, such drugs vary in their capacity to reduce the platelet count. Cytosine arabinoside has a very toxic effect on megakaryocytes.[116] Vinca alkaloids have a relatively low thrombocytopenic effect.[117]

Drugs Capable of Inhibiting Platelet Production.—Many substances are capable of inhibiting platelet production. Thiazides, however, have very often caused thrombocytopenia. The effect may be a direct pharmacologic toxicity or secondary to the formation of platelet antibodies.[118] Estrogens[119] and ethanol[120] can also be directly toxic to megakaryocytes. Conditions such as viral infections,[121] renal failure,[122] and malnutrition[123] can also cause thrombocytopenia.

Thrombocytopenia Due to Increased Platelet Destruction.

Thrombocytopenia due to increased destruction of platelets can be caused by immune or nonimmune mechanisms.

Immune-Mediated Thrombocytopenias.—Idiopathic thrombocytopenic purpura (ITP) is now known to be caused, for the most part, by an autoimmune process, caused by binding in the majority of cases of IgG1 to platelets,[123] hence the term *immune thrombocytopenic pupura* is now more appropriate. Although the etiology to date is not fully clarified, a decreased T cell suppression function is present in many cases.[124] A major site of destruction of IgG-coated platelets is the spleen,[125] which is also a major site of platelet autoantibody synthesis.[126] The preponderance of ITP in females may be due to an estrogen effect[127] or to increased Fc receptor expression on platelets in females.[128] ITP is frequently associated with other autoimmune diseases (e.g., SLE,[129] scleroderma[130]).

At the laboratory level, the platelet count is usually reduced, although bleeding may occur at relatively high platelet counts due to the fact that attached antibodies inhibit adequate platelet function.[131] Steroids are useful, due to inhibition of platelet phagocytosis by RES macrophages[132] and inhibition of autoantibody synthesis. Platelet therapy is reserved for life-threatening hemorrhage.[133] Splenectomy is beneficial in the majority of cases, for it removes both the site of autoantibody synthesis as well as the site of platelet destruction.[134] In refractory patients, immunosuppressive therapy has resulted in improvement of the thrombocytopenia. Azathioprine in combination with prednisone has been used in these cases.[134] Vinblastin-loaded platelets have also been used in an attempt to kill macrophages that ingest platelets; the method has been useful in cases of short platelet survival.[135]

At least two mechanisms exist regarding *drug-induced, immune-mediated* thrombocytopenia. In the one case, drugs bind to platelets and act as haptens, stimulating the production of an autoantibody.[136] In the second case, drug-antibody complexes may bind secondarily to platelets,[137] possibly via platelet surface Fc receptors.[138] Sedormid,[139] quinidine,[140] and quinine[141] are among the more common causes of drug-induced thrombocytopenia. Cimetidine has been reported to cause immune-mediated thrombocytopenia.[142] Sensitive techniques such as platelet factor 3 release can be used to detect IgG binding to platelets.[143] The direct detection of IgG has been elusive but may be resolved in the future.[144]

Treatment includes withdrawal of all medications potentially responsible for the thrombocytopenia. Treatment is similar to that of ITP.

A rarer form of immune-mediated thrombocytopenia is seen in cases of Tn activation and polyagglutination.[145]

Non-immune-Mediated Platelet Destruction.—Several diseases cause destruction of platelets by non-immune-mediated mechanisms. Examples include thrombocytopenia accompanying a cavernous hemangioma, DIC, TTP, and hypersplenism. Hypoxia, snake bites, and graft rejection can likewise be complicated by thrombocytopenia. Of great interest to the blood banker is the thrombocytopenia seen during and after cardiopulmonary bypass surgery.[146] Platelets are probably damaged in the cardiopulmonary pump; therefore aggregates form that are trapped in the filter system and lungs,[147] with a subsequent decrease in circulatory platelets. Massive hemorrhage may produce a "washout" effect and result in thrombocytopenia if platelets are not included in the replacement therapy.[148]

Thrombocytosis

Thrombocytosis may be caused by a variety of disorders (Table 3-2). Thrombocytosis may cause thrombosis. Overproduction of platelets in reactive thrombocytosis is probably related to a thrombopoietic substance. The fact that thrombocytosis appears after acute hemorrhage has suggested that erythropoiesis and thrombopoiesis are in some way related, although erythropoietin and thrombopoietin are chemically and physiologically distinct.[158] With few exceptions, reactive thrombocytosis is not treated by lowering the platelet count unless there is a true risk of thrombosis.

Coagulation: The Soluble Phase of Hemostasis

Plasma has the capacity to clot. This has been shown to be due to enzymatic reactions that convert fibrinogen, a solute, to fibrin, an insoluble polymer. Two major enzymes are involved in this process. The first enzyme is thrombin, a derivative of prothrombin which cleaves arginine-glycine bonds in each fibrinogen molecule.[159] Four fibrinopeptides are the cleavage products of this enzymatic breakdown of fibrinogen. The free fibrinogen monomers then polymerize to form fibrin. Thrombin cleaves a

TABLE 3–2.—MAJOR CAUSES OF THROMBOCYTOSIS

CATEGORY	EXAMPLE
Myeloproliferative disease	Polycythemia vera (50% of cases on diagnosis)[149]
Chronic inflammation	Rheumatoid arthritis[150]
Malignancy	Carcinoma[151]
	Hodgkin's disease[152]
Drug-induced	Vincristine[153]
Other	Prematurity[154]
	Acute hemorrhage[155]
	Postsplenectomy[156]
	Infection[157]

second enzyme (factor XIII, a transamidinase which acts as a fibrin-stabilizing factor), converting it into its active form, which generates stabilizing bonds within fibrin strands. This in essence constitutes the basic process of clot formation. However, several factors termed procoagulants must participate in a chain reaction in order to activate the above-mentioned enzymatic process.

In order to understand the process, a review of the biochemistry of clotting factors is relevant.

Biochemistry of Clotting Factors

Clotting factors are numbered with Roman numerals (Table 3–3). No factor VI exists.

Fibrinogen (Factor I)

Fibrinogen is a 340,000-dalton glycoprotein synthesized by hepatocytes and composed of three pairs of peptidic chains linked by disulfide bonds, which tend to be biochemically heterogeneous, probably due to their sialic acid content.[160] These chains are designated Aα, Bβ, and γ. Upon cleavage by thrombin, chain Aα yields fibrinopeptide A from

TABLE 3–3.—SOME CHARACTERISTICS OF CLOTTING FACTORS*

FACTOR	NAME	MOLECULAR WEIGHT (Daltons)	SITE OF SYNTHESIS	ACTIVE HALF-LIFE (hr)	FUNCTION
I	Fibrinogen	340,000	Liver	72–170	Precursor to fibrin
II	Prothrombin†	69,000	Liver	48–96	Precursor to thrombin, a serine protease
III	Tissue thromboplastin	Variable	Tissues		Lipoproteins, cholesterol, and phosphatides with procoagulant activity
IV	Calcium				Involved in several phases of clotting
V	Labile factor or proaccelerin	300,000–1,000,000	Liver	15–24	Cofactor
VII	Proconvertin†	50,000	Liver	4–6	Activated form has esterase activity
VIII	Antihemophilia A factor (AHF), VIII:C	50,000	Liver	12	Cofactor
VIII	von Willebrand's factor, multimers; FVIII:vWF	200,000	Endothelium	12	Anchors platelets to subendothelium
IX	Christmas factor,† antihemophilia B factor	55,000	Liver	18–30	Activated form has peptidase activity
X	Stuart-Prower factor†	59,000	Liver	40–60	Activated form has prothrombin activity
XI	Plasma thromboplastin antecedent, CPTA	180,000	Liver	45–54	Activated form has serine protease activity
XII	Hageman factor	80,000	Liver?	48–96	Serine protease
XIII	Fibrin-stabilizing factor	300,000	Liver and megakaryocytes	96	Stabilizes fibrin polymers as a transamidase
Prekallikrein (Fletcher factor)		85,000	Liver?		Serine protease
Kininogen (Fitzgerald factor)		110,000	Liver?		Cofactor for factor XII

*Data compiled from multiple sources. Factor VI is not currently assigned.
†Vitamin K dependent.

the N-terminal portion of the chain, Bβ yields fibrinopeptide B, and the γ chain is not attacked by thrombin.[161] Thrombin cleavage of fibrinogen yields more fibrinopeptide A than B, and although many potentially susceptible arginil groups exist in the molecule, only four are attacked by this enzyme.[162] In addition to thrombin, viper venoms are capable of removing fibrinopeptide A, but copperhead venom will preferentially remove fibrinopeptide B.[163]

The removal of fibrinopeptide A is essential for coagulation, whereas the removal of fibrinopeptide B is not. Nevertheless, further exposure to thrombin results in more active release of fibrinopeptide B with further polymerization.[164] The tertiary structure of fibrinogen reveals a dimeric configuration and three nodular structures in the polar central aspect of the molecule.[165] Integrity of the N-terminal disulfide nodule appears crucial to binding during fibrin polymerization.[166] The remaining clotting factors are discussed in terms of their vitamin K dependency.

Vitamin K–Dependent Factors

Prothrombin Factor II.—Prothrombin is a single-chain 69,000-dalton polypeptide with an N-terminal alanine.[167] γ-Carboxyglutamic acid (Gla) is an integral component of this peptide and is added by carboxylation in an enzymatic reaction which requires vitamin K.[168] The polypeptide chain is folded on itself and attached by a disulfide bond. Thrombin is generated when peptide bonds of prothrombin are hydrolyzed by factor Ia and by newly generated thrombin,[169] a reaction that is calcium-dependent. This hydrolysis results in the formation of two fragments, a 35,000-dalton fragment that is a reaction peptide and thrombin that is the remaining 34,000-dalton two-chain fragment (α, β), which preserves the disulfide bond. The larger β-chain contains the enzymatic active site.[170]

Factor VII.—Factor VII is a 50,000-dalton safety pin-shaped single polypeptide chain proenzyme,[171] connected by disulfide bonds, that, when acted on by factor Xa in the presence of phospholipid, produces a two-chain structure with enhanced procoagulant activity.[172] Both the single- and the double-chain forms of factor VII have a significant esterase activity.[173] It is possible that factor VII is either synthesized or stored in the kidney.[174]

Factor IX.—Factor IX is a 55,000-dalton procoagulant with the capability of becoming enzymatically active[175] after cleavage by factor XIa, which hydrolizes two peptide bonds. As with other factors, the activated form of factor IX (IXa) is a 46,000-dalton double-chain structure linked by disulfide bonds.[176] The heavier chain contains the factor IXa enzyme active site.

Factor X.—Like prothrombin and factors VII and IX, the synthesis of factor X is vitamin K dependent. Factor X is essential to the formation of prothrombinase, which is the crossroad of both the intrinsic and extrinsic pathways of the clotting system. Factor X is a 59,000-dalton α-globulin.[177] Although factor X is usually isolated as a two-chain structure with a disulfide bond, it is apparent that this is due to degradation. It seems logical to consider that the factor X structure is initially a single-chain structure, similar to other procoagulants, and that it then becomes a two-chain structure on cleavage.[178] As with other enzymatic vitamin K–dependent procoagulants, the active site is located on the heavy chain. On activation, factor Xa exhibits a serine protease activity.[179] Protein S, a plasma procoagulant, seems to be homologous to the factor X heavy chain.[180]

Protein C.—Protein C, a single chain polypeptide with a molecular weight of 62,000 daltons, is also a vitamin K–dependent coagulation factor.[180] It has serine protease activity and appears to be involved in factor V activation.[181]

Non-Vitamin K–Dependent Factors

Factor V.—Factor V participates in the common pathway of blood coagulation, although its biochemical role is not clear at present. Due to its lability, the precise chemical structure of factor V has been elusive, with molecular weights ranging from 300,000 to 1,000,000 daltons.[182] Although it may be a large molecular weight complex with subunits, there is evidence that the major portion of the molecule is a single-chain glycoprotein[183] containing galactose, a sugar that is essential to its activity.[184] Activation of factor V involves hydrolysis of three peptide bonds.[183] Factor V appears to be synthesized in the liver.

Factor VIII.—Factor VIII is a 162 million–dalton protein complex composed of two subunits which participates in the intrinsic pathway. A low molecular weight component has the coagulant activity (FVIII:C), whereas the high molecular weight component is a carrier protein that is termed factor VIII–related protein (FVIII R:Ag). This heavier molecular weight protein contains the von Willebrand factor VIII portion (FVIII:vWF).[185] Another component of this heavier protein is the FVIII R:RCo, or ristocetin cofactor, which participates in the aggregation of platelets by ristocetin. On activation by thrombin, the low molecular weight component of factor VIII possesses the same activity as the full factor VIII molecule.[186] The two components are bound by relatively weak bonds. The synthesis of each of these molecules is regulated by genes located in different chromosomes; the gene coding for the low molecular weight FVIII:C is located in chromosome X, whereas control for FVIII R is controlled by an autosome.

The high molecular weight F VIII R:Ag is synthesized by endothelial cells,[187] whereas no FVIII:C has been identified in endothelial cell cultures. It appears that the low molecular weight portion of the complex is synthesized by the liver.[188] Factor VIII:C appears to function as a cofactor in the enzymatic activation of factor X by factor IXa.[189] The activation of factor VIII as cofactor appears to be mediated by thrombin.[189]

Factor VIII R exists in a multimeric arrangement and has different properties. It appears to function as an anchor during platelet aggregation stimulated by ristocetin. This anchorage requires a platelet counterpart that is deficient in the Bernard-Soulier syndrome.[190] The ristocetin cofactor activity and the FVIII R:Ag are different. Thus, only larger polymers will act as ristocetin cofactor.[191]

Factor XI.—This proenzyme is part of the intrinsic pathway and its synthesis does not depend on vitamin K. This glycoprotein has been purified and constitutes a 180,000-dalton protein composed of two 80,000- to 90,000-dalton subunits connected by disulfide bonds.[192] Activated factor XII (XIIa) or trypsin are capable of cleaving these 80,000-dalton subunits into smaller 35,000- and 50,000-dalton units.[193] The active site is in the lower molecular weight component. On activation factor XIa appears to be a serine protease.

Factor XII.—Factor XII is an 80,000-dalton single-chain polypeptide.[194] Factor XII has the capacity of becoming activated on exposure to glass and collagen, upon which it undergoes physico-chemical changes.[195] Contact activation of factor XII yields a 52,000-dalton fragment and a 28,000-dalton fragment.[196] Serine esterases present in the body, such as trypsin, kallikrein, and plasmin, can likewise activate factor XII.[197] These enzymes cleave factor XII at two sites, yielding fragments of 52,000 daltons, 40,000 daltons, 28,000 daltons, and 12,000 daltons.

In both cases, the contact activation and the enzymatic activation result in the binding of the heavier fragment (52,000 daltons) to the surface. On further activation this fragment splits into smaller fragments capable of activating prekallikrein to kallikrein.[198]

Prekallikrein.—Prekallikrein is an 85,000- to 88,000-dalton polypeptide which is converted into a two-chain enzyme on activation by factor XIIa.[199] Kallikrein is then capable of activating plasminogen and high molecular weight kininogen. Its activity on high molecular weight kininogen results in the formation of bradykinin. Further digestion of kallikrein on kininogen results in a two-chain structure. The lighter chain has procoagulant activity.[200] Prekallikrein is a factor XII cofactor.

Factor XIII.—Factor XIII is a four-unit α-globulin weighing 300,000 daltons. The subunits are composed of two α chains weighing about 75,000 daltons each and two β chains weighing 80,000 daltons each.[201] On activation by thrombin, factor XIII is converted to factor XIIIa.[202] Factor XIII is involved in the common coagulation pathway, where it acts as a stabilizing molecule, forming covalent bonds between fibrin strands.

Tissue Factor.—Thromboplastin is termed tissue factor or factor III. It is a particulate agglomerate of lipoproteins, cholesterol, and phosphatides. None of these component molecules is active on its own. However, significant procoagulant activity will be present if these substances are combined.

Physiology of Blood Coagulation

Some of the reactions leading to the formation of a clot were reviewed at the beginning of this section. An integrated view will now be given. A waterfall mechanism has been suggested whereby a sequence of previously inactive plasma proteins become enzymatically activated. Subsequently these proteins act on the next precursor that becomes enzymatically active.[203] Evidently certain steps do not result in activated enzymes, such as the final step of the conversion of fibrinogen to fibrin and its subsequent polymerization. For practical purposes, the activation of the clotting cascade can be divided into two main forms: (1) the intrinsic system initiated by activation of factor XII, and (2) the extrinsic system, initiated by activation of factor VII (Fig 3–2).

The Intrinsic System

Activation of the intrinsic system is initiated, in vitro by the activation of factor XII on exposure to a foreign surface, such as glass, collagen, or fatty acids. Activation probably results from a non-calcium-dependent change in the stereochemical configuration of factor XII.[204] This activation results in factor XIIa and can be self-perpetuating, for XIIa acts on surface-bound factor XII to generate more XIIa.[205] Factor XIIa is now capable of activating the next step of clotting, and that is the activation of factor XI to XIa, a reaction which occurs in the presence of high molecular weight kininogen.[206] At this stage factor XIIa is likewise involved in the conversion of prekallikrein to kallikrein, also requiring high molecular weight kininogen.[207] Kininogen seems to bind the factor XI, or prekallikrein (Fletcher factor) to form kallikrein, orienting these molecules in the proper activation stereochemical configuration.[208] Kallikrein also has the capability of activating factor XII, markedly amplifying the generation of XIIa. The enzymatically active site of factor XII is present in a small 28,000-dalton fragment liberated during the reaction. The larger inactive fragment remains in the bound phase. Factor XIIa is enzymatically active on factor VII of the extrinsic system and thus is capable of activating this pathway.[209] Activation of factor XI to XIa by factor XIIa seems to be the main pathway of factor XI activation; however, factor XII–independent activation of factor XI is possible via platelets.[210] Activated factor XI (XIa) functions, similarly to other enzymatically active clotting factors, as a serine esterase, inhibitable by heparin-antithrombin III.[211] Factor XIa acts on factor IX enzymatically, and this reaction is calcium dependent.[212] Next comes the activation of a critical factor, factor X, which represents the crossroads of the intrinsic and extrinsic pathways, beyond which it becomes a common pathway between the two systems.

Activation of factor X involves a complex interaction between IXa, phospholipid or platelet surfaces, and calcium. This reaction is accelerated by thrombin[212] and is perpetuated by factor Xa.[213]

Factor Xa, like factor XIa, is a serine protease inhibited by heparin-antithrombin III complex.[214] This enzymatic property of factor Xa is capable of one of the more critical steps in clotting, namely the conversion of prothrombin to thrombin. Factor Va (resulting from cleavage of factor V by thrombin), phospholipid or platelets, and calcium supply positive catalysis to this reaction.[215] Thrombin is strongly proteolytic and hydrolyzes fibrinogen at four peptide bonds, releasing fibrinopeptides A and B. The end result is fibrin monomers capable of polymerizing to form an insoluble mesh of fibrin. The enzymatic activity of thrombin can be neutralized by complexes of heparin-antithrombin III.[216] Thrombin also acts enzymatically on factor XIII, yielding factor XIIIa, a transamidase responsible for the formation of peptidic bonds linking glutamine and lysine groups of adjacent fibrin monomer molecules.[217]

The Extrinsic System

The extrinsic system comprises the calcium-dependent activation of factor VII by tissue factor, forming a procoagulant complex which is particulate and enzymatically active.[218] Factor VII, like other procoagulants, exists in the form of a single-chain structure. Factor Xa acts enzymatically on factor VII to yield an enzymatically active two-chain structure capable of cleaving factor X to yield more factor Xa.[219] Plasma, which is contact activated, enhances the activity of factor VII due to the presence of XIIa, Xa, thrombin, plasmin, and kallikrein.[220] Phospholipid appears to be necessary in

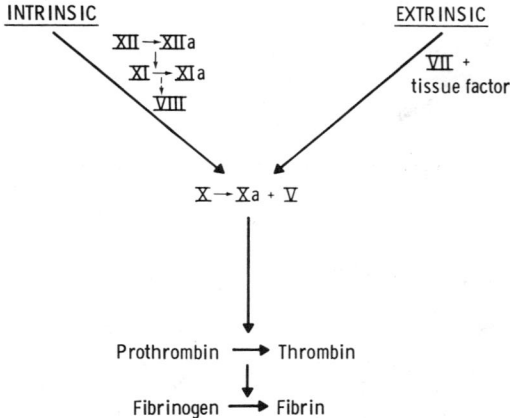

FIG 3–2.—Coagulation cascade. Intrinsic pathway is initiated by the activation of factor XII; extrinsic pathway is initiated by the activation of tissue factor and factor VII. Both pathways activate factor X.

both the intrinsic and the extrinsic systems; in the intrinsic pathway, phospholipid is supplied by platelets, whereas in the extrinsic system, the phospholipid is supplied by tissue factor.

The role of the extrinsic system is viewed today as a pathway for the rapid formation of small thrombin supplies responsible for the immediate initiation of clotting.

With the intrinsic system, the extrinsic system shares the common pathway of activation, from Xa to the formation of fibrin polymers. It is unlikely that either of the two pathways acts independently in vivo; rather, it is thought that the extrinsic system rapidly supplies a small amount of thrombin which then allows the intrinsic system to be activated.[221]

Control Mechanisms of Coagulation

The formation of a clot requires regulatory mechanisms to prevent this repair process from becoming a threat to the host. Thus, mechanisms to regulate the amplitude of the clotting process exist at three levels: regulation at the clot site, humoral processes involving inactivators; cellular processes at the RES which clear the circulation from activated procoagulants; and the fibrinolytic system.

Local Controls

Blood flow acts as a control by preventing the local accumulation of procoagulants. Fibrin also acts locally by adsorbing thrombin and blocking its activity. However, this block is only physical, for active thrombin can be obtained from fibrin mesh; this effect of fibrin adsorption is termed antithrombin I. This thrombin adsorption by fibrin is significant, and must have an important coagulation inhibitory function.[222]

Humoral Inhibitors.—Antithrombins have been designated with Roman numerals; in certain cases (e.g., antithrombin I) there is a physical effect of fibrin adsorption. Antithrombin II (heparin cofactor I) and antithrombin III are located on the same molecule but appear to be on different moieties.

Antithrombin III is a 67,000-dalton α_2-glycoprotein.[223] It appears that antithrombin III attaches to a serine residue located in the thrombin active site, forming an irreversible bimolecular complex.[224] Heparin functions as a catalytic factor which accelerates the formation of the complex, involving lysine residues on the inhibitor.[225] After inhibitor–clotting factor complexes are formed, heparin is released, renewing the process.

Antithrombin III also inhibits factor Xa.[226] Other heparin cofactors exist. Heparin cofactor II forms an inactive complex with thrombin, a process accelerated by heparin.[227] Unlike antithrombin III, heparin cofactor II does not appear to inhibit factor Xa.

α_2-**Macroglobulin Inhibitor.**—The α_2-macroglobulin forms an irreversible complex with thrombin which results in its inhibition.[228] Plasmin and thrombin compete for binding sites on the α_2-macroglobulin inhibitor. This inhibitor appears to act by engulfment of the enzymatic binding site, preventing interaction with the substrate.[229] It is likewise capable of inhibiting other proteolytic enzymes.[230]

Other Inhibitors.—Many other inhibitors exist at various stages of coagulation. However, only the more important ones will be summarized here.

A specific 65,000-dalton α-globulin inhibitor exists for factor XIa.[231] α_1-Antitrypsin is another factor XIa and plasmin inhibitor. It also acts as a slow thrombin inhibitor.[232] Cl-inactivator of the complement system is also inhibitory to XIa.[233] The inactivator of factor VIII:C and Va is thrombin.

Cellular Clearance of Procoagulants

Activated procoagulants are actively removed by macrophages in the RES, especially the liver.[234] However, removal of thrombin appears to be mediated by endothelial cells.[235]

Macrophages have likewise been shown to "pick up" and catabolize fibrin and fibrin split products (FSP), as has been demonstrated in vitro with alveolar macrophages. Catepsin in macrophage lysosomes degrades fibrin and FSP.[236]

Fibrinolysis

Aside from natural inhibitors, control of clotting is achieved by a counteracting proteolytic system termed the fibrinolytic system. This system, when activated, has anticoagulant properties. The fibrinolytic system is primarily regulated by activated plasminogen, which then becomes plasmin. Plasminogen is an 88,000-dalton single-chain protein composed of 790 amino acid residues.[237] Activation of plasmin occurs when plasminogen monomer is cleaved at the Arg_{560}-Val peptide bond to form a double-chain enzyme with two disulfide bonds.[238] The light chain contains the serine active site, a site which can be blocked by α_2-antiplasmin.[239]

Plasmin has five loops or "kringles," most of which are capable of binding to lysin binding sites on the fibrin molecule.[240] These binding sites are also occupied by antiplasmin during inactivation. Plasmin, like trypsin, acts on a variety of protein and nonprotein substrates by cleaving arginyl-lysine bonds.[241] In addition to fibrin, plasmin degrades factors V, VIII, and complement components. Plasminogen is converted to plasmin by a number of proteolytic enzymes present in lysosomes of most cells.[242] These activators are usually named according to their tissue of origin and are immunologically distinct.[243]

Degradation Steps of Fibrin.—The end product of plasmin degradation of fibrin is the formation of fragments generally termed fibrin split products (FSP). The larger fragments are antigenically similar to fibrin.[244]

In the first plasmin-digestion phase, an α chain C-terminus fragment is cleaved from fibrinogen. This fragment (fragment X) constitutes about 20% of the fibrinogen molecule.[245] Fragment X is a 250,000-dalton fibrinogen fragment that retains thrombin-binding sites.[246]

The next cleavage products of fibrin degradation are two fragments, a larger 150,000-dalton fragment Y and a smaller 90,000-dalton fragment D.[247] Further degradation of fragment Y will result in an additional fragment D and a 30,000- to 50,000-dalton fragment E.[248] Antigenically fragment E is very distinct and can be considered neoantigenic. Its epitopic determinants are located within the fibrin γ-chain residues 36–53.[249]

Inhibition of Plasmin.—The main inhibitor of plasmin is α_2-antiplasmin, which binds irreversibly to the lysine binding sites of the active center of plasmin.[250] Lysine analogs such as EACA block this reaction, retarding the effect of the inhibitor.[251]

Detection of plasmin is today possible with labeled synthetic plasmin substrates such as S-2251, substrate which contains the H-D-Val-Leu-Lys-pNA sequence which reacts with the plasmin cleavage site.[252] In essence, this method can be adapted to the study of any of the serine proteases of the coagulation cascade for which a substrate is known.[253]

Fibrin Degradation Product Detection.—Due to its importance in the diagnosis of DIC and fibrinolysis, the detection of FSP is crucial. The more sensitive tests are immunologic tests that detect neoantigens; these include the tanned RBC hemagglutination inhibition immunoassay (TRCHII) and a latex agglutination test.[254]

Abnormalities of Coagulation

Only a brief review of clotting abnormalities will be given, summarizing the more frequent congenital and acquired abnormalities. A thorough clinical workup that includes a complete clinical history and physical examination is necessary to evaluate bleeding disorders. These elements of the workup may reveal a history of bleeding, joint deformity due to hemarthrosis, and other useful data. A laboratory evaluation is usually performed on samples carefully collected in plastic tubes using 3.2% sodium citrate in a 1:9 ratio with blood; this amount is adjusted to changes in plasma volume due to concomitant changes in the hematocrit. Care must be taken not to draw samples from heparinized lines.

Initially a coagulation screen is performed. The more general screen will outline derangements of the intrinsic or the extrinsic pathways. The prothrombin time (PT) screens for derangements of the extrinsic pathway and measures both factor VII activity as well as the common pathway. The normal reaction is 10–12 seconds, depending on the laboratory. The activated partial thromboplastin time (PTT) screens for alterations in the intrinsic system and therefore does not detect factor VII deficiencies. A normal reaction time ranges between 32 and 52 seconds. The thrombin time essentially measures the conversion of fibrinogen to fibrin and is useful in detecting abnormalities at that level. A normal thrombin time is 3–4 seconds. Contemporary instrumentation using photometry is employed to measure these parameters. Fibrinogen is measured by immunologic or chemical methods. Serum measurement of FSP is available by immunoassay, as outlined above.

Congenital Disorders of Coagulation

Most patients with a congenital coagulopathy have either hemophilia A (factor VIII deficiency), von Willebrand's disease (factor VIII:vW deficiency) or hemophilia B (factor IX deficiency).

Hemophilia A.—Hemophilia A is an X-linked recessive clotting disorder which affects the adequate synthesis of the C portion of factor VIII. Its incidence is about 1 in 10,000. Usually levels of factor VIII:C in carriers range from 25% to 75% of normal, a finding which can help to screen carriers. The mutation in hemophilia A is at a locus found about 50 centimorgans from the Xg blood group locus.[255] Most patients with hemophilia A have negligible amounts of factor VIII:C activity, but some have the antigenic FVIII:CAg moiety.[256] Monoclonal antibodies against different moieties of factor VIII have been produced.[257] These antibodies have helped characterize the FVIII:C molecule and can now be used to quantitate FVIII:C in hemophiliacs. At the laboratory level, hemophiliacs characteristically have a prolonged PTT if the FVIII:C is below 35% of normal. Activated PTT with Kaolin or celite enhances the sensitivity of the PTT test. A distinction from von Willebrand's disease should be made by assessing the bleeding time and performing a ristocetin platelet aggregation test, for about 5% of patients with hemophilia may also have von Willebrand's disease. Usually FVIII:C is below 40%, and FVIII Ag and FVIII R:RCo are normal in cases of hemophilia A.

In general, blood samples from persons with suspected hemophilia and a prolonged PTT will correct with normal plasma. A specific factor assay which is a modified PTT test is then performed. In this test, serial dilutions of a control plasma are made and combined with a mixture of (1) a plasma known to be deficient in the putative factor, (2) kaolin-lipid mixture, and (3) calcium, to construct a standard curve. A linear curve plotting percentage dilution against PTT in seconds should result. The patient's plasma is then diluted two or more dilutions and plotted against the standard curve.

Management.—Preventive management is very important in severe hemophilia. The presurgical prophylaxis for hemophilia is described in the chapter on components. Recently, great concern has arisen from the finding that factor VIII concentrates not only carry a high risk of hepatitis but may also transmit AIDS.[258] Cryoprecipitate has therefore become more popular to treat mild to moderate cases of hemophilia A preoperatively. A classification of hemophilia A and its complications is given in Tables 3–4 and 3–5.

Hemophilia B.—Hemophilia B, also known as Christmas disease, is a deficiency of factor IX and, like hemophilia A, carried as a sex-linked recessive trait with an incidence of 1 in 100,000 population. Some affected individuals have excess factor IX (hemophilia B Leyden). In other cases the molecule is defective, of higher molecular weight and deficient in its capacity to bind calcium, probably due to the additional peptide residues.[259] The PTT is usually prolonged when factor IX levels are below 30%. Specific factor IX antigen testing can now be performed with monoclonal antibodies to factor IX. The diagnosis of both hemophilia A and hemophilia B can be made by radioimmunoassay of clotting factors obtained by fetoscopy.[260] The diagnosis is arrived at by specific factor IX activity assays. Therapy is discussed in detail in the chapter on components. Patients are treated with plasma in mild cases, and with prothrombin complex concentrates which contain prothrombin, factors VII, IX, and X. These concentrates carry the risk of transmitting hepatitis[261] and AIDS, although the risk of transmission of AIDS from factor IX concentrates is slightly less than with factor VIII concentrates.[262]

Von Willebrand's Disease.—Von Willebrand's disease is caused by a FVIII:vW defect. The FVIII:vW protein is synthesized by endothelial cells.[263] This factor is involved in platelet aggregation and apparently also is involved in either stimulating synthesis of FVIII:C, or chemically stabilizing the molecule, the procoagulant portion of FVIII

TABLE 3–4.—CLASSIFICATION OF HEMOPHILIA A

DEGREE OF SEVERITY	% FVIII:C	COMPLICATIONS
Severe	<1	Frequent hemarthroses and arthropathy; severe bleeding
Moderate	1–5	Occasional hemarthroses; often bleeding during minor surgery
Mild	6–40	Rare hemarthroses; increased bleeding during surgery

TABLE 3–5.—COMPLICATIONS OF HEMOPHILIA

PROCEDURE/CONDITION	SECONDARY COMPLICATION
Dental extractions	Hemorrhage, asphyxia
Intramuscular hematomas	Organ compression, gangrene
Neurologic	Intracranial hemorrhage (frequently fatal); nerve compression
Hemarthroses	Knee, ankle, hip, elbow

which is not synthesized by endothelial cells. The FVIII:vW protein is capable of binding both to platelets and to the subendothelium.[264] The disease may be inherited as a dominant or recessive autosomal trait.[265] Different varieties of von Willebrand's disease are found; thus the disease is really a syndrome (Table 3-6).[266]

Symptoms in von Willebrand's disease appear in childhood and in some cases disappear in adulthood, an observation difficult to explain. Excessive bleeding during minor surgery and mucosal or cutaneous hemorrhage are the more frequent symptoms. At the laboratory level, the bleeding time and aggregation tests are very useful in the diagnosis. Platelets of patients with von Willebrand's disease have a tendency not to adhere to glass beads. Ristocetin-induced aggregation is consistently decreased in most patients with 25% or less FVIII:vW, although certain variants of von Willebrand's disease may have a normal ristocetin aggregation test.

The multimeric structure of FVIII:vW can be determined by SDS-agarose electrophoresis or by crossed immunoelectrophoresis.[266] Therapy for von Willebrand's disease is supportive. Prevention of bleeding preoperatively is achieved with cryoprecipitate. Factor VIII concentrates contain unpredictable levels of FVIII:vW in the high molecular weight form.

Recently DDAVP (1-deamino-8-D-arginine vasopressin) has been used to increase factor VIII levels in patients with von Willebrand's disease as well as patients with hemophilia A.[267]

Other inherited coagulopathies.—A deficiency of factor XI is an autosomal recessive trait affecting mostly persons of European Jewish ancestry. The bleeding abnormality is mild.[268] The APTT is abnormal, revealing the intrinsic pathway abnormality. Two-stage fluorogenic assays using the synthetic substrate Boc-Leu-Thr-Arg-4-methylcoumarin amide are available to define the factor XI deficiency.[269] These patients may bleed only at surgery. Infusions of FFP at a dosage of 10–20 ml/kg are employed to treat the deficiency prophylactically.[270]

A deficiency of factor XII (Hageman factor) is inherited as an autosomal recessive trait. The disease is not characterized by hemorrhagic episodes but may instead be associated with thromboembolic phenomena. There is marked heterogeneity in factor XII deficiencies.[271]

Factor XIII deficiency occurs in populations where consanguinity is prevalent. Umbilical vein bleeding is characteristic in infants born with a deficiency of this transamidase.[272] The PT, APTT, and bleeding time are usually normal. The disease is diagnosed by thromboelastographic patterns.[273] Therapy is usually prophylactic, with FFP.[274]

Factor V deficiency is usually inherited as an autosomal recessive trait. Some patients have an increased bleeding time, probably due to low factor Xa binding sites on platelets.[275] A combined deficiency of factors V and VIII is occasionally seen in Sephardic Jews. This deficiency is most probably due to a deficiency of protein C, not to a gene deletion of factor V[276] or to factor VIII.

Factor VII deficiency is rare and is usually inherited as an autosomal recessive trait. A prolonged PT is characteristic. Severe bleeding may be present in homozygotes. Paradoxically, thromboembolism may be a complication in certain cases. The defect may be qualitative or quantitative.[277] Treatment is with FFP or lyophilized prothrombin complex. Congenital deficiencies of fibrinogen are autosomal and usually found in consanguineous populations. Prolonged PT, PTT, and thrombin time are characteristic. Deficiencies in fibrinogen may be quantitative or qualitative. Qualitative defects may

TABLE 3-6.—CLASSIFICATION OF VON WILLEBRAND'S DISEASE*

| TYPE | RESPONSE TO RISTOCETIN | MULTIMERS | FACTOR COMPONENT LEVELS | | | INHERITANCE |
			VIII:C	VIIIR:Ag	VIIIR:RCo	
I	Low	Nl.	Low	Low	Low	AD
IIA	Very low	Abnl.	Nl.	Low	Very low	AD
IIB	High	Abnl.	Nl. or low	Nl. or low	Nl.	AD
IIC	Low	Abnl.	Nl.	Nl. or low	Low	AR
III	Very low	Variable	Very low	Very low	Very low	AR

*From Zimmerman and Ruggieri.[266]
Abbreviations: Nl., normal; AD, autosomal dominant; AR, autosomal recessive.

be at the fibrinopeptide release on cleavage by thrombin[278] or during cross-linking.[279] Patients are treated prophylactically with cryoprecipitate.

Acquired Coagulopathies

Acquired coagulopathies encompass the majority of diseases associated with abnormal coagulation and bleeding diathesis. The more frequent acquired coagulopathies are summarized in Table 3–7 according to laboratory abnormalities.

Liver Disease Coagulopathy.—The vitamin K–prothrombin complex (factors II, VII, IX, and X) is synthesized in the liver[280] and is generally decreased in severe liver disease, although single factor deficiencies (e.g., factor IX deficiency) have rarely been documented.[281] This decrement is not corrected by vitamin K therapy. Most of the non-vitamin K–dependent factors, including the procoagulant portion C of factor VIII, are synthesized in the liver.[282] However, FVIII:C levels in fact are increased in most cases of liver disease.[283] Thus multiple derangements of the clotting system can be expected in patients with liver disease, to the extent that about 15% of patients with severe liver disease have severe bleeding episodes.[284]

Moderate to severe liver disease is associated with a slow but progressive drop in factor V.[285] Severe liver disease is usually associated with depletion of fibrinogen.[286] FSP can be expected to be increased due to lack of hepatic inactivation of fibrinogenolysis activators.[287] Thromboembolic phenomena may also occur in liver disease, due to the development of an antithrombin III deficiency in liver disease. This finding is a reason not to use prothrombin lyophilized concentrates in severe liver disease.[288] If necessary the coagulopathy of liver disease can be corrected temporarily with infusions of FFP.[289]

Coagulopathy of Vitamin K Deficiency.—Vitamin K is essential as a cofactor in the conversion of glutamic acid residues on coagulation proteins in the prothrombin complex by a vitamin K–dependent hepatic carboxylase.[290] When a deficiency of vitamin K is present, the amounts of γ-carboxyglutamic acid in these proteins decreases, rendering them biologically inactive.[291]

Humans do not have a storing mechanism for vitamin K and therefore rely on dietary intake as well as bacterial synthesis in the gut for adequate supplies of vitamins K1 and K2. In the vitamin K–deficient patient the procoagulants disappear in the following order: first factor VII, followed by factors IX and X, and finally prothrombin.[292] Bleeding in the newborn is frequently due to a vitamin K deficiency, although other causes must be ruled out (DIC, hereditary disorders, etc.). In the adult, the more frequent cause of vitamin K deficiency is the intestinal sterilization syndrome[293] caused by the decimating effect of antibiotics on the vitamin K–synthetizing flora of the gut.

Acquired Clotting Factor Inhibitors.—Acquired inhibitors or anticoagulants are usually antibodies that bind to an active site of the procoagulant inhibiting them. They can be assumed to be present when a prolonged PTT does not correct when the sample is mixed in a 1:1 ratio with normal plasma. Neutralization studies with isolated clotting factors may reveal the specificity of the factor inhibited by the antibody. Theoretically, inhibitors may develop against any procoagulant, for any of these proteins may act as an antigen. The more relevant ones are described below.

Factor VIII inhibitors usually arise in patients with hemophilia A who have been transfused. Some 6%–8% of hemophiliacs with severe hemophilia A will develop anti-FVIII:C antibodies.[294] Most of the classified inhibitors have proved to be of the IgG4

TABLE 3–7.—LABORATORY FINDINGS IN MAJOR ACQUIRED CLOTTING DISORDERS*

CONDITION	PT	PTT	TT	FI	FV	FX	FSP	BT	PLTS
Liver disease	↑	↑	Var.	Nl. or ↓	↓	↓	Nl. or ↑	Nl. or ↓	Nl. or ↓
Vitamin K deficiency	↑	↑	Var.	Nl.	Nl.	↓	Nl.	Nl.	Nl.
DIC	↑	↑	Var.	↓	↓	↓	↑	↑	↓
Fibrinolysis	↑	↑	Var.	Nl. or ↓	Nl. or ↓	Nl. or ↓	↑	↑	Nl. or ↓
Cardiac bypass	↑	↑	↑	Nl. or ↓	Nl. or ↓	Nl. or ↓	Nl. or ↑	↑	Nl. or ↓
Inhibitors	Var.	Var.	Var.	Nl.	Var.	Var.	Nl.	Nl.	Nl.

*Abbreviations: Var., variable; Nl., normal; PT, prothrombin time; PTT, partial thromboplastin time; TT, thromboplastin time; F, factor (i.e., I, II, III); FSP, fibrin split products; BT, bleeding time; Plts, platelets.

(κ light chain) subclass,[295] although concomitant IgG1 and IgG3 have also been identified in these cases.[296] The finding of single κ chains in most IgG4 anti-FVIII:C samples suggests oligoclonality.

Single λ chains have been described in a few cases, also suggesting oligoclonality.[297] Inhibitors to FVIII:C only rarely affect FVIII:vWF.[298] At the laboratory level, Bethesda units can be used to measure acquired inhibitors. A Bethesda unit is the amount of inhibitor required to reduce to 50% the factor VIII activity of 1 ml of normal plasma after a 2-hour incubation period at 37° C.[299]

Inhibitors to factor VIII may arise in nonhemophilic patients. Usually an underlying autoimmune disease such as SLE[300] or a myeloid dyscrasia[301] may be present, but multiparous as well as other healthy individuals may develop these inhibitors. IgG inhibitors of factor VIII have developed as a result of penicillin[302] as well as phenytoin therapy.[303] The incidence of factor IX inhibitors in hemophilia B is 2.8%, much lower than the incidence of FVIII:C inhibitors found in hemophilia A.[304] Non-hemophilia B patients with factor IX inhibitors may have an underlying autoimmune disease such as SLE.[305] These antibodies, like factor VIII antibodies, also tend to be of the IgG4 subclass.[306] Factor XI inhibitors usually occur in patients with congenital factor XI deficiency, although factor XI inhibitors appear spontaneously in patients with autoimmune disease[307] and do not usually cause a major bleeding diathesis.

Factor V inhibitors are rare, may occur in factor V–deficient patients, and have been found in non-congenitally factor V–deficient patients who received streptomycin.[308] Bleeding in these cases may be very severe.

Inhibitors of fibrinogen have likewise been described in congenital afibrinogenemic patients[309] and in previously normal individuals.

Treatment of patients with acquired inhibitors will depend on the factor inhibited and on the severity of the disease. When factor VIII inhibitors appear, giving large doses of factor VIII may stop the bleeding episode.[310] Bovine and porcine factor VIII have been used successfully in the treatment of these patients,[311] as have activated factor IX concentrates.[312]

Disseminated Intravascular Coagulation.—Disseminated intravascular coagulation (DIC) is of interest to the blood banker for a variety of reasons. Patients who have not been transfused and who present with DIC almost invariably require varying amounts of blood and blood components, and patients who have been transfused with an incompatible unit may develop DIC and usually require components, blood bank testing, and consultation by the blood bank physician. DIC may be present as an acute medical emergency or as a smoldering process accompanying chronic disease.

Acute DIC.—Acute DIC may be caused by a variety of mechanisms. For example, introduction of thromboplastinic substances such as RBC stroma into the circulation will activate the extrinsic system. This type of mechanism may play a significant part in the physiopathology of DIC in ABO-incompatible transfusion reactions.[313]

The major causes of DIC are outlined in Table 3–8. Apart from the introduction of thromboplastins into the circulation, other mechanisms such as destruction of the endothelium and exposure of subendothelial surfaces to plasma may trigger DIC. This mechanism is seen in the Shwartzman reaction, such as is seen after IV injection of endotoxins.[315] The clotting cascade activation may occur at various stages, such as activation at the factor X level (e.g., tumor extracts).[316] Some substances such as certain snake poisons act directly on fibrinogen, cleaving it to release fibrin monomers.[317]

Activation of the clotting cascade in DIC may occur at the intrinsic pathway level as well. It is very possible that triggering of the intrinsic pathway by endotoxins (lipid A fraction of bacterial lipopolysaccharides) is caused by direct activation by the endotoxin of factor XII,[318] although the role of factor XII activation in DIC is controversial.[319] For example, preventing activation of factor XII with lysozyme does not abrogate DIC.[320] However, other intrinsic pathway factors such as factor XI can be activated by collagen and may be a triggering mechanism of DIC.[321] Of interest in ABO-incompatible reactions is the finding that the release of thromboplastin from RBC membranes may not be the only factor triggering DIC in these reactions;[322] the activation of complement may itself trigger DIC.[323] However, depletion of C3 by cobra venom factor in the Shwartzman phenomenon does not prevent DIC.[324] Platelets on aggregation may also induce clotting by making platelet factor 3 available.[325] This platelet release probably tends to accelerate DIC, as has been demonstrated experimentally by the fact that endotoxin induces platelet release of serotonin and platelet factor 3.[326]

The DIC phenomenon is usually composed of two main processes—activation of clotting, with

TABLE 3–8.—MAJOR CAUSES OF DIFFUSE
INTRAVASCULAR COAGULATION*

CONDITION	CAUSES
Intravascular hemolysis	ABO incompatibility
	Other incompatible transfusions
	Hemolysis due to infection
	Other
Obstetric complications	Placenta abruptio
	Amniotic fluid embolism
Tissue trauma	Multiple fractures
	Major trauma
	Burns
	Cardiopulmonary bypass
Malignancies	Rapidly growing tumors with extensive necrosis (e.g., prostatic, pancreatic, and other carcinoma)
	Leukemias
Vascular tumors	Giant hemangiomas
Snake bites	
Shock	Cardiogenic
	Other
Infections	Bacterial (gram-negative bacteria, meningococcal septicemia, etc.)
	Viral (hemorrhagic fever)
	Mycoses: histoplasmosis, aspergillosis
	Protozoal: malaria, kalaazar
	Rickettsial: Rocky Mountain spotted fever
Autoimmune disease	SLE, polyarteritis

*Modified from Wintrobe.[314]

consumption of clotting factors and platelets, and activation of the fibrinolytic system by plasmin, with subsequent degradation of fibrin to FSP.

The acute DIC clotting activation consumes factors inactivated by thrombin, namely, fibrinogen and factors V, VIII, and XIII, although these factors may be increased in the chronic type of DIC. Triggering of the clotting mechanism results in the activation of thrombin which cleaves two N-terminal peptides from the α and β chains of fibrinogen. These are fibrinopeptide A and fibrinopeptide B. The residual fibrin monomers form soluble fibrin complexes which are subsequently stabilized by factor XIII. A concomitant activation of plasmin in DIC results in degradation of fibrin and the formation of FSP. Fibrin split products (X, Y, D, and E) may form complexes with soluble fibrin monomers, resulting in defective fibrin structures.[327] This complex formation has been demonstrated chromatographically by showing that fragment D binds to immobilized fibrin monomers,[328] although controversy still exists regarding complexing of fibrin monomers and fragments Y, D, and E.[329] It appears that high molecular weight plasmin degradation products of fibrin (e.g., fragment X) are likewise capable of forming complexes with fibrin,[330] but not the lower molecular weight fragments Y, D, and E.

There is evidence that for a classic Shwartzman reaction to occur in DIC, the RES must first be saturated with soluble complexes before the microangiopathic findings are seen.[331] Leukocytes play a significant role in amplifying the DIC phenomenon. Leukopenia seems to interfere with DIC induced by endotoxin.[332]

A factor that plays a significant part in the physiopathology of DIC is tissue necrosis due to ischemia. Not all types of DIC are accompanied by fibrin thrombi in small vessels. For example, experimental endotoxemia may not reveal microvessel thrombosis,[333] and DIC secondary to abruptio may not be accompanied by cortical necrosis due to fibrin microthrombosis. Based on experiments in which the RES was blocked with Thorotrast, it appears that the development of microthrombosis depends on the capacity of the RES to clear activated procoagulants from the circulation.[334]

Laboratory Diagnosis of DIC.—A quick estimate of the platelet count and of the presence of schistocytes can be made by observing the peripheral smear. A prolonged bleeding time is usually present due to consumption of platelets.[335]

Evidence of Factor Consumption.
Fibrinogen and factors VIII, V, and XIII are usually decreased due to cleavage by thrombin and consumption during clotting. Other factors only minimally reduced in DIC are factors VII, IX, X, and XI.[336] The factor decrements result in a prolonged PT, PTT, and a low fibrinogen.

In certain cases of DIC, however, an increase in individual clotting factors may be seen.

Evidence of Fibrinolysis.
Gelation tests are designed to demonstrate soluble fibrin complexes resulting from fibrinolysis. The protamine sulfate gelation test is one such test, but false negative and false positive results have been reported.[337]

Fibrinogen as well as fragments Y, D, and E inhibit the formation of fibrin polymers, a phenomenon which can be detected in the thrombin time test, which is sensitive to plasma levels of fibrinogen.[338] The test is of use if mixing thrombin tests with normal plasma are performed. To study patients in DIC who have received heparin, reptilase, which polymerases fibrin but is not inhibited by heparin and is blocked by FSP and fibrinogen, is added to the sample.[339]

The more widely used tests today to detect FSP are immunoassays which utilize antibodies to neoantigens D and E, a latex agglutination test for X and Y antigens,[340] and a tanned RBC agglutination inhibition test.[341] With immunoassays, as little as 2–4 μg/ml of fibrinogen on FSP can be detected.

A *Staphylococcus* clumping test is also available but is based on a different principle. Fibrinogen Aα and Bβ chains bind specifically to staphylococci membrane proteins. Fragment E does not bind. The test is very sensitive, detecting 2–600 ng/ml of fibrinogen or FSP.[342]

Other Tests.
Plasma levels of antithrombin III may be useful in detecting early cases of DIC. Neoantigens of antithrombin III can be demonstrated immunochemically.[343] Antithrombin III can be assayed through its inhibitory effect on proteases such as factors IXa, Xa, and XIa as well as on other proteases, using synthetic chromogenic substrates.[344]

Therapy for DIC.
Blood bankers may be called in to consult on the management of DIC cases. The management of this disorder must be tailored to the individual case. Removing the cause of intravascular clotting is the primary target. Supportive therapy with components is almost always warranted in severe cases of DIC. Fresh frozen plasma, cryoprecipitate, and blood may be necessary to correct hemostasis and oxygen-carrying capacity. Some authors recommend 3–4 units of cryoprecipitate per 10 kg of body weight and 10–15 ml/kg of FFP.[345] Heparin may be indicated in selected cases to control indiscriminate clotting during the clotting phase of this disorder. If heparin is given, it must be given at a therapeutic dose (e.g., 70–140 units/kg/4 hours) IV in patients with relatively normal platelet counts, and 50 units/kg/4 hours in thrombocytopenic patients.[346, 347] Heparin should not be used in patients with massive surface bleeding hemorrhage, as is seen in obstetric catastrophic DIC.[348] Antithrombin III has been used experimentally in DIC, with encouraging results.[349] It should be noted here that heparin has not been very effective in certain cases of acute DIC, and its routine use is controversial.[350] The use of ε aminocaproic acid has no place in the treatment of DIC.[351] Platelet transfusions may be indicated in DIC patients with thrombocytopenia; 2 units/10 kg is recommended.[352]

Hemostasis in Cardiac Surgery

The alterations of hemostasis in cardiopulmonary bypass surgery are complex. The use of heparin alters many coagulation parameters. Circulation of blood through the bypass pump will induce severe changes in hemostasis, and replacement therapy as well as hemodilution will alter clotting test results. Patients undergoing bypass surgery are premedicated with heparin.[353] Protamine sulfate, used to reverse the heparin effect in these patients, may be rapidly metabolized, allowing anticoagulation by circulating excess heparin. This effect is termed "heparin rebound phenomenon." It may likewise be caused by reentry of heparin from the tissues to the circulation.

Thrombocytopenia may be present in open heart surgery patients as a consequence of DIC or hemodilution. Abnormal platelet function in cardiopulmonary bypass surgery is probably due to depletion of alpha granules.[354] Often, therefore, these patients are treated with units of platelets postoperatively. Up to 50% of patients with intrathoracic bleeding secondary to bypass have an unchecked bleeding vessel responsible for the hemorrhage.[355]

Bleeding Associated With Massive Transfusion

A "washout" phenomenon can be observed in the massively transfused patient. The major hemostatic deficit that develops in these patients is thrombocytopenia,[356] but this only occurs after 15–20 units of platelet-pools have been given. No significant clotting factor deficiencies are likely to be present. Furthermore, units of platelets given to these patients usually contain significant amounts of clotting factors.[357]

REFERENCES

1. Simionescu M., et al.: Segmental differentiation of cell junctions in the vascular endothelium: The microvasculature. *J. Cell Biol.* 67:863, 1975.
2. Madri J.A., et al.: The collagenous components of the subendothelium: Correlation of structure and function. *Lab. Invest.* 43:303, 1980.
3. Sage H., Pritzl P., Bornstein P.: Characterization of cell matrix associated collagens synthesized by aortic endothelial cells in culture. *Biochemistry* 20:436, 1981.
4. Biesley J.E., Pearson J.D., Hutchings A., et al.: Granulocyte migration through endothelium in culture. *J. Cell Sci.* 38:237, 1979.
5. Butcher E.C., Scollay R.G., Weissman I.L.: Organ specificity of lymphocyte migration: Mediation by highly selective lymphocyte interaction with organ specific determinants on high endothelial venules. *Eur. J. Immunol.* 10:556, 1980.
6. Weeks J.R., Compton G.D.: The cardiovascular pharmacology of prostacyclin. *Prostaglandins* 17:501, 1979.
7. Schafer A.I., et al.: Identification of platelet receptors for prostaglandin I_2 and D_2. *J. Biol. Chem.* 254:2914, 1979.
8. Weksler B.B., Ley C.W., Jaffe E.A.: Stimulation of endothelial cell prostacyclin production by thrombin, trypsin, and the ionophore A23187. *J. Clin. Invest.* 62:923, 1978.
9. Louchaupt M., et al.: The effect of angiotensin II on PGI_2 production by endothelial cells in culture. *Thromb. Haemost.* 46:39, 1981.
10. Roberts A.M., Messina E.J., Kaley G.: Prostacyclin (PGI_2) mediates hypoxic relaxation of bovine coronary strips. *Prostaglandins* 21:555, 1981.
11. Preston F.E., et al.: Inhibition of prostacyclin and platelet thromboxane A_2 after low-dose aspirin. *N. Engl. J. Med.* 304:76, 1981.
12. Crutchley D.J., Ryan U.S., Ryan J.W.: Effects of aspirin and dipyridamole on the degradation of adenosine diphosphate by cultured cells derived from bovine pulmonary artery. *J. Clin. Invest.* 66:29, 1980.
13. Busch P.C., Owen W.G.: Identification in vitro of an endothelial cell surface cofactor for anti-thrombin III. *J. Clin. Invest.* 69:726, 1982.
14. Barnes M.J., et al.: Platelet aggregation by basement-associated collagens. *Thromb. Res.* 18:375, 1980.
15. Piovella F., et al.: The ultrastructural localization of factor VIII antigen in human platelets, megakaryocytes and endothelial cells utilizing a ferritin labeled antibody. *Br. J. Haematol.* 39:209, 1978.
16. Maynard J.R., et al.: Tissue factor activity of cultured human endothelial and smooth muscle cells and fibroblasts. *Blood* 50:387, 1977.
17. Wiggins R.C., et al.: Activation of rabbit Hageman factor by homogenates of cultured endothelial cells. *J. Clin. Invest.* 65:197, 1980.
18. Lang W.E.: Secretion of plasminogen activators by cultured bovine endothelial cells: Partial purification, characterization and evidence for multiple forms. *Thromb. Haemost.* 45:219, 1981.
19. Wasteson A., et al.: Effect of a platelet endoglycosidase on cell surface associated heparin sulphate of human cultured endothelial and glial cells. *Thromb. Res.* 11:309, 1977.
20. Owen W.G., Esmon C.T.: Functional properties of an endothelial cell cofactor for thrombin-catalyzed activation of protein C. *J. Biol. Chem.* 256:5532, 1981.
21. Roy A.J., Djerassi I.: Effects of platelet transfusions: Plug formation and maintenance of vascular integrity. *Proc. Soc. Exp. Biol. Med.* 139:137, 1972.
22. Weiss H.J.: Platelet physiology and abnormalities of function. *N. Engl. J. Med.* 293:531, 580, 1975.
23. Shuster A., Scarborough H.: Senile purpura. *Q. J. Med.* 30:33, 1961.
24. Grant M.E., Prockop D.J.: Biosynthesis of collagen. *N. Engl. J. Med.* 286:194, 242, 291, 1972.
25. Kivirkko K.I., Risteli L.: Biosynthesis of collagen and its alterations in pathologic states. *Mea. Biol.* 53:159, 1976.
26. Nichamin S.J., Brough A.J.: Chronic progressive pigmentary purpura: Purpura anularis telangiectoides of Majocchi-Schamberg. *Am. J. Dis. Child.* 116:429, 1968.
27. Mengel C.E., Trystad C.: Thrombocytopenia in Rocky Mountain spotted fever. *JAMA* 113:886, 1963.
28. Ayoub E.M., Hoyer J.: Anaphylactoid purpura: Streptococcal antibody titers and B_{1c}-globulin levels. *J. Pediatr.* 75:193, 1969.

29. Kauffman R.H., Herrmann W.A., Meyer C.J.L.M., et al.: Circulating IgA-immune complexes in Henoch-Schoenlein purpura: A longitudinal study of their relationship to disease activity and vascular deposition of IgA. *Am. J. Med.* 69:859, 1980.
30. Nakamoto Y., et al.: Primary IgA glomerulonephritis and Schoenlein-Henoch purpura nephritis: Clinicopathological and immunohistochemical characteristics. *Q. J. Med.* 178:495, 1978.
31. Durack D.T.: Opportunistic infections and Kaposi's sarcoma in homosexual men. *N. Engl. J. Med.* 305:1465, 1981.
32. Tavassoli M.: Megakaryocyte-platelet axis and the process of platelet formation and release. *Blood* 55:537, 1980.
33. Williams N.: Megakaryocyte progenitor cells in vitro, in Evatt B.L., et al. (eds.): *Megakaryocytes in vitro*. Amsterdam, Elsevier-North Holland, 1981, pp. 101–108.
34. Mazur M.E., Hoffman R., Bruno E., et al.: Identification of two classes of human megakaryocyte progenitor cells, in Evatt B.L., et al. (eds.): *Megakaryocytes in vitro*. Amsterdam, Elsevier-North Holland, 1981, pp. 283–287.
35. Levine R.F., Bunn P.A. Jr., Hazzard K.C., et al.: Flow cytometric analysis of megakaryocyte ploidy: Comparison with Feulgen microdensitometry and discovery that 8N is the predominant ploidy class in guinea pig and monkey marrow. *Blood* 56:210, 1980.
36. Radley J.M., Scurfield G.: The mechanism of platelet release. *Blood* 56:996, 1980.
37. Paulus J.M., Deschamps J.F., Prenant M., et al.: Kinetics of platelets, megakaryocytes and their precursors: What is measure? *Blood Cells* 6:215, 1980.
38. Williams N., Eger R.R., Jackson H.M., et al.: Two factor requirement for murine megakaryocyte colony formation. *J. Cell. Physiol.* 110:101, 1982.
39. Evatt B.L., Spivak J.L., Levin J.: Relationships between thrombopoiesis and erythropoiesis: With studies of the effects of preparations of thrombopoietin and erythropoietin. *Blood* 46:547, 1976.
40. McDonald T.P., Clift R., Lange R.D., et al.: Thrombopoietin production by human embryonic culture. *J. Lab. Clin. Med.* 85:59, 1975.
41. Ebbe S.: Thrombopoietin. *Blood* 44:605, 1974.
42. Burnstein S.A., Adamson J.W., Harker L.A.: Megakaryocytopoiesis in culture: Modulation by cholinergic mechanisms. *J. Cell. Physiol.* 103:201, 1980.
43. Corush L., Shafer B., Porlow M.: Heterogeneity of human blood platelet subpopulations: II. Use of a subhuman primate model to analyze the relationship between density and platelet age. *Blood* 52:726, 1978.
44. Klonizakis I., Peters A.M., Fitzpatrick M.L., et al.: Radionuclide distribution following injection of 111 indium-labeled platelets. *Br. J. Haematol.* 46:595, 1980.
45. White, J.G.: Platelet morphology, in Johnson S.A. (ed.): *The Circulating Platelet*. New York, Academic Press, 1971, pp. 46–122.
46. Cooper H.A., Mason R.G., Brinkhous K.M.: The platelet surface membrane: Membrane and surface reactions. *Annu. Rev. Physiol.* 38:501, 1976.
47. Weiss, H.J.: Platelet physiology and abnormalities of platelet function. *N. Engl. J. Med.* 293:531, 1975.
48. Schick P.K.: The role of platelet membrane lipids in platelet hemostatic activities. *Semin. Hematol.* 16:221, 1979.
49. Davney M.G., Luscher E.F.: Actions of thrombin and other coagulant and proteolytic enzymes on blood platelets. *Nature* 216:857, 1967.
50. Nachmias V.T.: Cytoskeleton of human platelets at rest and after spreading. *J. Cell Biol.* 86:795, 1980.
51. Fukami M.H., Salganikoff L.: Human platelet storage organelles. *Thromb. Haemost.* 38:963, 1977.
52. Cohen I., Gerrard J.M., Bergman R.N., et al.: The role of contractile filaments in platelet activation, in *Protides of the Biological Fluids*. Oxford, Pergamon, 1979, p. 55.
53. White J.G.: Interaction of membrane systems in blood platelets. *Am. J. Pathol.* 66:295, 1972.
54. Breton-Gorius J., Guichard J.: Ultrastructural location of peroxidase activity in human platelets and megakaryocytes. *Am. J. Pathol.* 66:277, 1972.
55. White J.G., Gerrard J.M.: Platelet ultrastructure in relation to platelet function, in Jamieson G.A., Greenwalt T.J. (eds.): *The Blood Platelet in Transfusion Therapy*. New York, Allan R. Liss, 1978, p. 5.
56. Pollard T.D., et al.: Contractile proteins in platelet activation and contraction. *Ann. NY Acad. Sci.* 283:218, 1977.
57. Kaplan K.L., Broekman M.J., Chernoff A., et al.: Platelet α-granule proteins: Studies on release and subcellular organization. *Blood* 53:604, 1979.
58. Bentfeld M.E., Bainto D.F.: Cytochemical localization of lysosomal enzymes in rat megakaryocytes and platelets. *J. Clin. Invest.* 56:1635, 1975.
59. Day H.J., Holmsen H.: Concepts of the blood platelet release reaction. *Ser. Haematol.* 4:3, 1971.
60. Holmsen H., Day J., Stormorken H.: The blood platelet release reaction. *Scand. J. Haematol. Suppl.* 8:3, 1969.
61. White J.G.: Fine structural alterations induced in platelets by adenosine diphosphate. *Blood* 31:604, 1968.
62. Karpatkin S., et al.: Glycogenesis and glyconeogenesis in human platelets: Incorporation of glucose, pyruvate, and citrate into platelet glycogen, glycogen synthetase and fructose-1,6 diphosphate activity. *J. Clin. Invest.* 49:140, 1970.
63. Harker L.A., Finch C.A.: Thrombokinetics in man. *J. Clin. Invest.* 48:963, 1969.
64. Aster R.H.: Studies of the fate of platelets in rats and man. *Blood* 34:117, 1969.
65. Paulus J.M., Bury J., Grosdent J.C.: Control of platelet territory development in megakaryocytes. *Blood Cells* 5:51, 1979.
66. Brodsky I., Ross E.M., Petkov G., et al.: Platelet and fibrinogen kinetics and ^{75}Se-selenomethionine

in patients with myeloproliferative disorders. *Br. J. Haematol.* 22:179, 1972.
67. Baumgartner H.R.: Morphometric quantitation of adherence of platelets to an artificial surface and components of connective tissue. *Thromb. Diath. Hemorrh. Suppl.* 60:39, 1974.
68. McChesney C., et al.: Critical role of carbohydrate side-chain of collagen in platelet aggregation. *J. Clin. Invest.* 51:2693, 1972.
69. Al-Moudhiry H., Spaet T.H.: Inhibition of platelet adhesion to collagen by sulfhydryl inhibitors. *Proc. Soc. Exp. Biol. Med.* 135:878, 1978.
70. Wilner G.D., et al.: Aggregation of platelets by collagen. *J. Clin. Invest.* 47:2616, 1968.
71. Zucker M.B., et al.: Release of platelet fibronectin (cold insoluble globulin) from alpha granules induced by thrombin and collagen: Lack of requirement for plasma fibronectin in ADP-induced platelet aggregation. *Blood* 54:8, 1979.
72. Marguerie G.A., Plow E.F., Edgington T.S.: Human platelets possess an inducible and saturable receptor specific for fibrinogen. *J. Biol. Chem.* 254:5357, 1979.
73. O'Brien J.R.: A comparison of platelet aggregation produced by seven compounds and a comparison of their inhibitors. *J. Clin. Pathol.* 17:275, 1964.
74. Santoro S.A., Cunningham L.W.: Collagen mediated platelet aggregation. *J. Clin. Invest.* 60:1054, 1977.
75. Zucker M.B., et al.: Binding of factor VIII to platelets in the presence of ristocetin. *Br. J. Haematol.* 35:535, 1977.
76. Solum N.O., et al.: Platelet membrane glycoproteins and the interaction between bovine factor VIII related protein and human platelets. *Thromb. Haemost.* 38:914, 1977.
77. Booyse F.M., Rafelson M.E. Jr.: Human platelet contractile proteins: location, properties and function. *Ser. Haematol.* 4:152, 1971.
78. Meyers K.M., Seachord C.L., Holmsen H., et al.: A dominant role of thromboxane formation in secondary aggregation of platelets. *Nature* 282:331, 1979.
79. Day H.J., Holmsen H.: Concepts of the blood platelet release reaction. *Semin. Hematol.* 41:3, 1971.
80. Wilner G.D., Nossel H.L., Procupez J.L.: Aggregation of platelets by collagen: Polar active sites of insoluble human collagen. *Am. J. Physiol.* 22:1074, 1971.
81. Marquis N.R., et al.: Platelet aggregation: III. An epinephrine-induced decrease in cyclic AMP synthesis. *Biochem. Biophys. Res. Commun.* 39:783, 1970.
82. Holmsen A., Day J., Stormorken H.: The blood platelet release reaction. *Scand. J. Haematol. Suppl.* 8:3, 1969.
83. Holmsen H., Ostvold A.C., Day H.J.: Behavior of endogenous and newly absorbed serotonin in the platelet release reaction. *Biochem. Pharmacol.* 22:2599, 1973.
84. Maldonado J.E., et al.: Ultrastructure of platelets in Bernard-Soulier syndrome. *Mayo Clin. Proc.* 50:402, 1975.
85. Solum N.O., et al.: Platelet membrane glycoproteins and the interaction between bovine factor VIII related protein and human platelets. *Thromb. Haemost.* 38:914, 1977.
86. Caen J.P., et al.: Bernard-Soulier syndrome: A new platelet glycoprotein abnormality. *J. Lab. Clin. Med.* 87:586, 1976.
87. Jamison G.A., Kumura T.: Reduced thrombin binding and aggregation in Bernard-Soulier platelets. *J. Clin. Invest.* 61:861, 1978.
88. Cohen I., et al.: Effects of ADP and ATP on bovine fibrinogen and ristocetin-induced platelet aggregation in Glanzmann's thrombasthenia. *Br. J. Haematol.* 31:343, 1975.
89. Jamieson G.A., et al.: Platelet membrane glycoproteins in thrombasthenia, Bernard-Soulier syndrome and storage pool disease. *J. Lab. Clin. Med.* 93:652, 1979.
90. Zimmerman T.S., Meyer D.: Factor VIII/von Willebrand's factor and the molecular basis of von Willebrand's disease, in Colman R., Hirsh, J., Marder V.J., et al. (eds.): *Hemostasis and Thrombosis.* Philadelphia, J.B. Lippincott Co., 1982, p. 54.
91. Weinstein M., Deykin D.: Comparison of factor VIII related von Willebrand factor proteins prepared from human cryoprecipitate and factor VIII concentrate. *Blood* 53:1095, 1979.
92. Ruggieri Z.M., Zimmerman T.S.: Variant von Willebrand's disease: Characterization of two subtypes by analysis of multimeric composition of factor VIII/von Willebrand's factor in plasma and platelets. *J. Clin. Invest.* 65:1318, 1980.
93. Gralnick H.R.: Factor VIII/von Willebrand factor protein galactose, a cryptic determinant of von Willebrand factor activity. *J. Clin. Invest.* 62:496, 1978.
94. Zimmerman T.S., Wilson R., Edgington T.S.: Carbohydrate of factor VIII von Willebrand factor in von Willebrand's disease. *J. Clin. Invest.* 64:1298, 1979.
95. Weiss H.J.: Defects of factor VIII and platelet aggregation: Use of ristocetin in diagnosing the von Willebrand's syndrome. *Blood* 45:403, 1975.
96. Meyer D., Obert B., Pietu G., et al.: Multimeric structure of factor VIII/von Willebrand factor in von Willebrand's disease. *J. Lab. Clin. Med.* 95:590, 1980.
97. Majerus P.W., Stanford N.: Comparative effects of aspirin and diflurisal on prostaglandin synthetase from human platelets and sheep seminal vesicles. *Br. J. Clin. Pharmacol.* 4:155, 1977.
98. Pareti F.I., Day H.J., Mills D.C.B.: Nucleotide and serotonin metabolism in platelets with defective secondary aggregation. *Blood* 44:789, 1974.
99. Homsen H., Weiss H.J.: Further evidence for a deficient storage pool of adenine nucleotides in platelets of some patients with thrombocytopathia—"storage pool disease." *Blood* 39:197, 1972.
100. Baele G., et al.: Inhibitory effect of acetylsalicylic

acid on human platelet function in normal volunteers and in women using a combined oral contraceptive regimen. *Thromb. Haemost.* 36:623, 1976.
101. Rane A., et al.: Relation between plasma concentration of indomethacin and its effect on prostaglandin synthesis and platelet aggregation in man. *Clin. Pharmacol. Ther.* 23:658, 1978.
102. Harburchak D.R., et al.: Postoperative hemorrhage associated with carbenicillin administration. *Am. J. Surg.* 134:630, 1977.
103. Mills D.O.B., Roberts G.C.K.: Membrane active drugs and the aggregation of human platelets. *Nature* 213:35, 1967.
104. Davis J.W., et al.: Effects of exogenous urea, creatinine, and guanidinosuccinic acid on human platelet aggregation in vitro. *Blood* 39:388, 1972.
105. Remuzzi G., et al.: Prostacyclin-like activity and bleeding in renal failure. *Clin. Nephrol.* 12:127, 1979.
106. Ballard H.S., Marcus A.J.: Platelet aggregation in portal cirrhosis. *Arch. Intern. Med.* 136:316, 1976.
107. Mannucci P.M., Remuzzi G., Pusineri F., et al.: Deamino-8-D-arginine vasopressin shortens the bleeding time in uremia. *N. Engl. J. Med.* 308:8, 1983.
108. Ruggeri Z.M., Mannucci P.M., Lombardi R., et al.: Multimeric composition of factor VIII von Willebrand's factor following administration of DDAVP: Implications for pathophysiology and therapy of von Willebrand's disease subtypes. *Blood* 59:1272, 1982.
109. Harker L.A., et al.: Mechanism of abnormal bleeding in patients undergoing cardiopulmonary bypass: Acquired transient dysfunction association with selective α-granule release. *Blood* 56:824, 1980.
110. Luthy D.A., Hall J.G., Graham C.B.: Prenatal diagnosis of thrombocytopenia with absent radii. *Clin. Genet.* 15:495, 1979.
111. Lum L.G., Tubergen D.G., Corash L., et al.: Splenectomy in the management of the thrombocytopenia of the Wiskott-Aldrich syndrome. *N. Engl. J. Med.* 302:892, 1980.
112. Shahidi N.T., Diamond L.K.: Testosterone-induced remission in aplastic anemia in both acquired and congenital types. *N. Engl. J. Med.* 264:953, 1961.
113. Hirsch E.H., Vogler W.R., McDonald T.P., et al.: Acquired hypomegakaryocytic thrombocytopenic purpura: Occurrence in a patient with absent thrombopoietic stimulating factor. *Arch. Intern. Med.* 140:721, 1980.
114. Cameron S.J.: Tuberculosis and the blood: A special relationship? *Tubercle* 55:55, 1974.
115. Storb R., Weiden P.L.: Transfusion problems associated with transplantation. *Semin. Hematol.* 18:163, 1981.
116. Karnofsky D.A.: Cancer chemotherapeutic agents. *Cancer* 18:80, 1968.
117. Morse B.S., Stohlmum F. Jr.: Regulation of erythropoiesis: XVIII. The effect of vincristine and erythropoietin on bone marrow. *J. Clin. Invest.* 45:1241, 1966.
118. Eisner E.V., Crowell E.R.: Hydrochlorothiazide dependent thrombocytopenia due to IgM antibody. *JAMA* 215:480, 1971.
119. Cooper B.A., Bigelow F.S.: Thrombocytopenia associated with the administration of diethylstilbestrol in man. *Ann. Intern. Med.* 52:907, 1960.
120. Cowan D.H., Graham R.C. Jr.: Studies on the platelet defect in alcoholism. *Thromb. Diath. Haemorrh.* 33:310, 1975.
121. Mitrakul C., Poshiachinda M., Sagawibha N., et al.: Hemostatic and platelet kinetic studies in dengue hemorrhagic fever. *Am. J. Trop. Med.* 26:975, 1977.
122. Ingeberg S., Stoffersen E.: Platelet dysfunction in patients with vitamin B12 deficiency. *Acta Haematol.* 61:75, 1979.
123. Rosse W.F., Adams J.P., Yount W.J.: Subclasses of IgG antibodies in immune thrombocytopenic purpura (ITP). *Br. J. Haematol.* 46:109, 1980.
124. Trent R., Adams E., Ehrhardt C., Basten A.: Alterations in T-gamma-cells in patients with chronic idiopathic thrombocytopenic purpura. *J. Immunol.* 127:621, 1981.
125. Ries C.A., Price D.C.: Platelet kinetics in thrombocytopenia: Correlation between splenic sequestration of platelets and response to splenectomy. *Ann. Intern. Med.* 80:702, 1974.
126. Karpatkin S., Stuck N., Siskind G.W.: Detection of splenic antiplatelet antibody synthesis in idiopathic autoimmune thrombocytopenic purpura (ATP). *Br. J. Haematol.* 23:167, 1972.
127. Laros R.K., Sweet R.L.: Management of idiopathic thrombocytopenic purpura during pregnancy. *Am. J. Obstet. Gynecol.* 122:182, 1975.
128. Moore A., Weksler B.B., Nachman R.L.: Platelet Fc IgG receptor: Increased expression in female patients. *Thromb. Res.* 21:469, 1981.
129. Budman D.R., Steinberg A.D.: Hematologic aspects of systemic lupus erythematosus: Current concepts. *Ann. Intern. Med.* 86:220, 1977.
130. Neuks S.H., Moore T.L., Lichtenstein J.R., et al.: Localized scleroderma and idiopathic thrombocytopenia. *J. Rheumatol.* 7:741, 1980.
131. Karpatkin S.: Autoimmune thrombocytopenic purpura. *Blood* 56:329, 1980.
132. Handin R.I., Stossel T.P.: Effect of corticosteroid therapy on the phagocytosis of antibody-coated platelets by human leukocytes. *Blood* 51:771, 1978.
133. Abraham J., Ellman L.: Platelet transfusion in immune thrombocytopenic purpura. *JAMA* 236:1847, 1976.
134. McMillan A.: Chronic idiopathic thrombocytopenic purpura. *N. Engl. J. Med.* 304:1135, 1981.
135. Nenci G.G., Agnelli G., Decunto M., et al.: Infusion of vincristine-loaded platelets in acute ITP refractory to steroids: An alternative to splenectomy. *Acta Haematol.* 66:117, 1981.
136. Ackroyd J.F.: The immunological basis of purpura due to drug hypersensitivity. *Proc. R. Soc. Med.* 55:30, 1962.
137. Shulman N.R.: A mechanism of cell destruction in individuals sensitized to foreign antigens and its

138. Moore A., Ross G.D., Nachman R.L.: Interaction of platelet membrane receptors with von Willebrand factor, ristocetin and the Fc region of immunoglobulin G. *J. Clin. Invest.* 62:1053, 1978.
139. Ackroyd J.F.: Allergic purpura, including purpura due to food, drugs and infections. *Am. J. Med.* 14:605, 1953.
140. Kekomaki R., Rajamaki A., Myllyla G.: Detection of quinidine-specific antibodies with platelet ^{125}I-labeled staphylococcal protein A test. *Vox Sang.* 38:12, 1980.
141. Helmly R.B., et al.: Quinine-induced purpura. *Arch. Intern. Med.* 120:59, 1967.
142. Isaacs A.J.: Cimetidine and thrombocytopenia. *Br. Med. J.* 280:294, 1980.
143. Karpatkin M., Siskind G.W., Karpatkin S.: The platelet factor 3 immunoinjury technique re-evaluated: Development of a rapid test for antiplatelet antibody. Detection of various clinical disorders, including immunologic drug-induced and neonatal thrombocytopenias. *J. Lab. Clin. Med.* 82:400, 1977.
144. Kelton J.G., et al.: Drug-induced thrombocytopenia is associated with increased binding of IgG to platelets both in vivo and in vitro. *Blood* 58:524, 1981.
145. Cartron J.P., Nurden A.T.: Galactosyl transferase and membrane glycoprotein abnormality in human platelets from Tn-syndrome donors. *Nature* 282:621, 1979.
146. Bick R.L.: Alterations of hemostasis associated with cardiopulmonary bypass: Pathophysiology, prevention, diagnosis, and management. *Semin. Thromb. Hemostas.* 3:59, 1976.
147. Solis R.T., Kennedy P.S., Beall A.C. Jr., et al.: Cardiopulmonary bypass: Microembolization and platelet aggregation. *Circulation* 52:163, 1975.
148. Counts R.B., et al.: Hemostasis in massively transfused trauma patients. *Ann. Surg.* 190:91, 1979.
149. Berlin N.J.: Diagnosis and classification of the polycythemias. *Semin. Hematol.* 12:339, 1976.
150. Bean R.H.D.: Thrombocytosis in auto-immune disease. *Bibl. Haematol.* 23:43, 1965.
151. Tranum B.L., Haut A.: Thrombocytosis: Platelet kinetics in neoplasia. *J. Lab. Clin. Med.* 84:615, 1974.
152. Davis R.B., Theologides A., Kennedy B.J.: Comparative studies of blood coagulation and platelet aggregation in patients with cancer and nonmalignant diseases. *Ann. Intern. Med.* 71:67, 1969.
153. Robertson J.H., Crozier E.H., Woodard B.E.: The effect of vincristine on the platelet count in rats. *Br. J. Haematol.* 19:331, 1970.
154. Lundstrom U.: Thrombocytosis in low birth weight infants: A physiologic phenomenon in infancy. *Arch. Dis. Child.* 54:715, 1979.
155. Ingram M., Coppersmith A.: Reticulated platelets following acute blood loss. *Br. J. Haematol.* 17:222, 1969.
156. Boxer M.A., et al.: Thromboembolic risk of post-splenectomy thrombocytosis. *Arch. Surg.* 113:808, 1978.
157. Marchasin S., Wallerstein R.D., Aggeler P.M.: Variation of the platelet count in disease. *Calif. Med.* 101:95, 1964.
158. Kruytman M.: Influence of repeated acute thrombocytopenias on the reappearance of circulatory blood platelets. *Blood* 37:323, 1971.
159. Mann K.G., Downing M.R.: Thrombin generation, in Lundblod R.L., Fenton J.W., Mann K.G. (eds.): *Chemistry and Biology of Thrombin.* Ann Arbor, Mich., Ann Arbor Science Publisher, Inc., 1977, pp. 11–19.
160. Wolfenstein-Todel C., Mosesson M.W.: Human plasma fibrinogen heterogeneity: Evidence for an extended carboxyl terminal sequence in a normal γ chain variant (γ^1). *Proc. Natl. Acad. Sci. USA* 77:5069, 1980.
161. Blombäck B., Johnson A.J.: Joint Report of the Subcommittee on Nomenclature and on Fibrinolysis, Thrombolysis, and Intravascular Coagulation. *Thromb. Diath. Haemorrh.* 51(suppl):251, 1972.
162. Mihalyi E., Godfrey J.E.: Digestion of fibrinogen by trypsin: I. Kinetic studies of the reaction. *Biochim. Biophys. Acta* 67:73, 1963.
163. Herzig R.H., et al.: Studies on a procoagulant fraction of southern copperhead snake venom: The preferential release of fibrinopeptide β. *J. Lab. Clin. Med.* 76:451, 1970.
164. Blombäck B., Hessel B., Hogg D., et al.: A two step fibrinogen-fibrin transition in blood coagulation. *Nature* 275:501, 1978.
165. Doolittle R.F., et al.: Fibrinogen: A highly evolved regulatory agent for maintaining the integrity of the vertebrate circulatory system, in Lo C.H. (ed.): *Versatility of Proteins.* New York, Academic Press, 1978, p. 393.
166. Blombäck B., Hessel B., Okada M., et al.: Mechanism of fibrin formation and its regulation. *Ann. NY Acad. Sci.* 370:536, 1981.
167. Mann K.G., Elion J., Butkowsky R.J. et al.: Prothrombin. *Methods Enzymol.* 80:286, 1981.
168. Esmon C.T., Suttie J.W.: Vitamin K-dependent carboxylase: Solubilization and properties. *J. Biol. Chem.* 251:6283, 1976.
169. Seegers W.H., Walz D.A., Renterby J., et al.: Isolation and some properties of thrombin-E and other prothrombin derivatives. *Thromb. Res.* 4:829, 1974.
170. Doolittle R.F.: Structural aspects of the fibrinogen to fibrin conversion. *Adv. Protein Chem.* 27:1, 1973.
171. Jesty J., Nemerson Y.: Purification of factor VII from bovine plasma: Reaction with tissue factor and activation of factor X. *J. Biol. Chem.* 249:509, 1974.
172. Broze G.J. Jr., Majerus P.W.: Purification and properties of human coagulation factor VII. *J. Biol. Chem.* 255:1242, 1980.
173. Zur M., Nemerson Y.: The esterase activity of coagulation factor VII: Evidence for intrinsic activity of zymogen. *J. Biol. Chem.* 253:2203, 1978.
174. Dodds W.J., et al.: Storage, release, and synthesis

of coagulation factors in isolated perfused organs. *Am. J. Physiol.* 217:879, 1969.
175. Lindquist P.A., et al.: Activation of bovine factor IX (Christmas factor) by factor XIa (activated thromboplastin antecedent) and a protease from Russell's viper venom. *J. Biol. Chem.* 253:1902, 1978.
176. DiScipio R.G., Kurachi K., Davie E.W.: Activation of human factor IX (Christmas factor). *J. Clin. Invest.* 61:1528, 1978.
177. DiScipio R.G., et al.: Activation of human factor X (Stuart factor) by a protease from Russell's viper venom. *Biochemistry* 16:5253, 1977.
178. Mattok P., Esnouf M.P.: A form of bovine factor X with a single polypeptide chain. *Nature* 242:90, 1973.
179. Chuang T.F., et al.: The intrinsic activation of factor X in blood coagulation. *Biochim. Biophys. Acta* 273:287, 1972.
180. DiScipio R.G., et al.: A comparison of human prothrombin, factor IX (Christmas factor), factor X (Stuart factor), and protein S. *Biochemistry* 16:698, 1977.
181. Kisiel W., et al.: Anticoagulant properties of bovine protein C following activation by thrombin. *Biochemistry* 16:5824, 1977.
182. Bartlett S., et al.: High molecular weight factor V of bovine and human plasma. *Biochemistry* 19:273, 1980.
183. Kane W.H., Majerus P.W.: Purification and characterization of human coagulation factor V. *J. Biol. Chem.* 256:1002, 1981.
184. Saraswathi S., et al.: Role of galactose in bovine factor V. *J. Biol. Chem.* 250:811, 1975.
185. Baugh R., Brown J., Sargeant R., et al.: Separation of human factor VIII activity from the von Willebrand's antigen and ristocetin platelet aggregating activity. *Biochim. Biophys. Acta* 371:360, 1974.
186. Rick M.E., Hoyer L.W.: Activation of low molecular weight fragments of antihemophilic factor (factor VIII) by thrombin. *Nature* 252:404, 1974.
187. Jaffe E.A.: Endothelial cells and the biology of factor VIII. *N. Engl. J. Med.* 296:377, 1977.
188. Webster W.P., et al.: Plasma factor VIII synthesis and control as revealed by canine organ transplantation. *Am. J. Physiol.* 220:1147, 1971.
189. Hoyer L.W.: The factor VIII complex: Structure and function. *Blood* 58:1, 1981.
190. Howard M.A., Hutton R.A., Hardisty R.M.: Hereditary giant platelet syndrome: A disorder of a new aspect of platelet function. *Br. Med. J.* 2:586, 1973.
191. Doucet-de Bruine M.H.M., Sixma J.J., Over J., et al.: Heterogeneity of human factor VIII: II. Characterization of forms of factor VIII binding to platelets in the presence of ristocetin. *J. Lab. Clin. Med.* 92:96, 1978.
192. Bouma B.N., Griffin J.H.: Human blood coagulation factor XI: Purification properties, and mechanism of activation by activated factor XII. *J. Biol. Chem.* 252:6432, 1977.
193. Mannhalter C., Schiffman S., Jacobs A.: Trypsin activation of human factor XI. *J. Biol. Chem.* 255:2667, 1980.
194. Revak S.D., Cochrane C.G., Johnston A.R., et al.: Structural changes accompanying enzymatic activation of human Hageman factor. *J. Clin. Invest.* 54:619, 1974.
195. Donaldson V.H., Ratnoff O.D.: Hageman factor: Alterations in physical properties during activation. *Science* 150:754, 1964.
196. Revak S.D., Cochrane C.D., Griffin J.H.: The binding and cleavage characteristics of human Hageman factor during contact activation: A comparison of normal plasma with plasma deficient in factor XI, prekallikrein, or high molecular weight kininogen. *J. Clin. Invest.* 59:1167, 1977.
197. Cochrane C.G., Revak S.D., Wuepper K.D.: Activation of Hageman factor in solid and fluid phases: A critical role of kallikrein. *J. Exp. Med.* 138:1564, 1973.
198. Revak S.D., Cochrane C.G.: The relationship of structure and function in human Hageman factor. The association of enzymatic and binding activities with separate regions of the molecule. *J. Clin. Invest.* 57:852, 1976.
199. van der Graaf F., Tans G., Bouma B.N., et al.: Isolation and functional properties of the heavy and light chains of human plasma kallikrein. *J. Biol. Chem.* 257:14300, 1982.
200. Kerbirou D.M., Griffin J.H.: Human high molecular weight kininogen: Studies of structure-function relationships and proteolysis of the molecules occurring during contact activation of plasma. *J. Biol. Chem.* 254:12020, 1979.
201. Chung S.I., Lewis M.S., Folk J.E.: Relationships of the catalytic properties of human plasma and platelet transglutaminase (activated blood coagulation factor XIII) to their subunit structures. *J. Biol. Chem.* 249:940, 1974.
202. Schwartz M.L., Pizzo S.V., Hill R.L., et al.: Human factor XIII from plasma and platelets: Molecular weights, subunit structures, proteolytic activation and cross-linking of fibrinogen and fibrin. *J. Biol. Chem.* 248:1395, 1973.
203. Davie E.W., Ratnoff O.D.: Waterfall sequence for intrinsic blood clotting. *Science* 145:1310, 1964.
204. Fair B.D., Saito H., Ratnoff O.D., Rippon W.B.: Detection of fluorescence of structural changes accompanying the activation of Hageman factor (factor XII). *Proc. Soc. Exp. Biol. Med.* 155:199, 1977.
205. Silverberg M., Thompson R., Miller G., et al.: Initiation of the intrinsic coagulation pathway: Autoactivability of human Hageman factor and mechanisms by which the light chain derived from HMW-kininogen functions as a co-factor in the activation of prekallikrein, factor XI and Hageman factor, in Mann K.G., Taylor F.B. Jr. (eds.): *The Regulation of Coagulation.* New York, Elsevier-North Holland, 1980, p. 531.
206. Kington H.S., Lundblad R.L.: Factors affecting the evolution of factor XIa during coagulation. *J. Lab. Clin. Med.* 85:826, 1975.
207. Cochrane C.G., Wuepper K.D.: The first compo-

nent of the kinin-forming system in human and rabbit plasma: Its relationship to clotting factor XII (Hageman factor). *J. Exp. Med.* 134:986, 1971.
208. Meier H.L., Pierce J.V., Colman R.W., et al.: Activation and function of human Hageman factor: The role of high molecular weight kininogen and prekallikrein. *J. Clin. Invest.* 60:18, 1977.
209. Kisiel W., Fujikawa K., Davie E.W.: Activation of bovine factor VII (proconvertin) by factor XIIa (activated Hageman factor). *Biochemistry* 16:4189, 1979.
210. Walsh P.N., Griffin J.H.: Contribution of human platelets to the proteolytic activation of blood coagulation factors XII and XI. *Blood* 57:106, 1981.
211. Rosenberg R.D.: The effects of heparin on factor XIa and plasmin. *Thromb. Diath. Haemorrh.* 33:51, 1974.
212. Switzer M.E.P., McKee P.A.: Reactions of thrombin with human factor VIII/von Willebrand factor protein. *J. Biol. Chem.* 255:10606, 1980.
213. Hultin M.B.: Role of human factor VIII in factor X activation. *J. Clin. Invest.* 69:950, 1982.
214. Yiu E.T., Wessles S., Stall P.J.: Biological properties of the naturally occurring plasma inhibitor of activated factor X. *J. Biol. Chem.* 246:3703, 1971.
215. Walsh P.N.: Platelets and coagulation proteins. *Fed. Proc.* 40:2086, 1981.
216. Rosenberg R.D., Damus P.S.: The purification and mechanism of action of human antithrombin-heparin cofactor. *J. Biol. Chem.* 248:6490, 1973.
217. Greenberg C.S., Shuman M.A.: The zymogen forms of blood coagulation factor XIII bind specifically to fibrinogen. *J. Biol. Chem.* 257:6096, 1982.
218. Pitlik F.A., et al.: Peptidase activity associated with the tissue factor of blood coagulation. *Biochemistry* 10:2650, 1971.
219. Bajaj S.P., Rapaport S.I., Brown S.F.: Isolation and characterization of human factor VIII: Activation of factor VII by factor Xa. *J. Biol. Chem.* 256:253, 1981.
220. Laaki K., Østerud B.: Activation of purified plasma factor VII by human plasmin, plasma kallikrein, and activated components of the human intrinsic blood coagulation system. *Thromb. Res.* 5:759, 1974.
221. Williams W.J.: The tissue factor system and its possible role in thrombosis, in Sherry S., Brinkhous K.M., Genton E., et al. (eds.): *Thrombosis.* Washington, D.C., National Academy of Sciences, 1969, p. 345.
222. Ogston D., Bennett B.: Naturally occurring inhibitors of coagulation, in Ogston D., Bennett B. (eds.): *Hemostasis: Biochemistry, Physiology and Pathology.* New York, John Wiley & Sons, Inc., 1977, p. 202.
223. Miller-Andersson M., et al.: Purification of antithrombin III by affinity chromatography. *Thromb. Res.* 5:439, 1974.
224. Matheson N.R., Travis J.: Inactivation of human thrombin in the presence of human α-1-proteinase inhibitor. *Biochem. J.* 159:495, 1976.
225. Rosenberg R.D., Damus P.S.: The purification and mechanism of action of human antithrombin-heparin cofactor. *J. Biol. Chem.* 248:6490, 1973.
226. Yin E.T.: Effect of heparin on the neutralization of factor Xa and thrombin by the plasma alpha-2-globulin inhibitor. *Thromb. Diath. Haemorrh.* 33:43, 1974.
227. Tollefsen D.M., Majerus D.W., Blank M.K.: Heparin cofactor II. Purification and properties of a heparin dependent inhibitor of thrombin in human plasma. *J. Biol. Chem.* 257:2162, 1982.
228. Abildgaard U.: Inhibitor of the thrombin-fibrinogen reaction by α-2-macroglobulin, studied by N-terminal analysis. *Thromb. Diath. Haemorrh.* 21:173, 1969.
229. Harrel P.C.: Studies on human plasma alpha-2-macroglobulin-enzyme interactions. *J. Exp. Med.* 138:508, 1973.
230. Ogston D., Bennett B.: Biochemistry of naturally occurring inhibitors of the fibrinolytic enzyme system, in Ogston D., Bennett B. (eds.): *Hemostasis: Biochemistry, Physiology and Pathology.* New York, John Wiley & Sons, Inc., 1977, p. 230.
231. Niemetz J., Nossel H.L.: Method of purification and properties of anti-XIa (inhibitor of the contact product). *Thromb. Diath. Haemorrh.* 17:335, 1967.
232. Burrows C.E., Movat H.Z.: Isolation of antithrombin-III from human plasma. *Biochem. Biophys. Res. Commun.* 74:140, 1977.
233. Forbes C.D., et al.: Inhibition of activated Hageman factor and activated plasma thromboplastin antecedent by purified serum C1 inactivator *J. Lab. Clin. Med.* 76:809, 1970.
234. Deykin D., Lochios F., DeCamp G., et al.: Hepatic removal of activated factor X by the perfused rabbit liver. *Am. J. Physiol.* 214:414, 1968.
235. Lollar P., Hoak J.C., Owen W.G.: Binding of thrombin to cultured human endothelial cells: Non-equilibrium aspects. *J. Biol. Chem.* 255:10279, 1980.
236. Bang N.U., Chang M.L., Mattler L.E, et al.: Monocyte/macrophage-mediated catabolism of fibrinogen and fibrin. *Ann. NY Acad. Sci.* 370:568, 1981.
237. Sottrup-Jensen L., Peterson T.E., Magnusson S.: Plasminogen, in M.O. Dayhoff (ed.): *Atlas of Protein Sequence and Structure,* vol. 5, suppl. 3, 1978, p. 91.
238. Wohl R.C., Summaria L., Robbins K.C.: Kinetics of activation of human plasminogen by different activator species at pH 7.4 and 37° C. *J. Biol. Chem.* 255:2005, 1980.
239. Collen D.: On the regulation and control of fibrinolysis. *Thromb. Haemost.* 43:77, 1980.
240. Rakoczi I., et al.: On the biological significance of the specific interaction between fibrin, plasminogen and antiplasmin. *Biochim. Biophys. Acta* 540:295, 1978.
241. Reagan C.R., et al.: Isolation and biological characterization of fragments of human growth hormone produced by digestion with plasmin. *Endocrinology* 96:625, 1975.
242. Soszka T.: Partial purification and some properties

of the tissue plasminogen activator from the human myometrium. *Thromb. Res.* 10:823, 1977.
243. Bernik M.B., Rijken D.C., Wijngaards G.: Production of two immunologically distinct Plasminogen activators by human tissue culture (abstract). *Thromb. Haemost.* 42:414, 1979.
244. Chang M.L., Bang N.U.: Biological behavior of higher molecular weight products of fibrinolysis. *J. Lab. Clin. Med.* 90:216, 1977.
245. Gaffney P.J.: The biochemistry of fibrinogen and fibrin degradation products, in Ogston D., Bennett B. (eds.): *Hemostasis: Biochemistry, Physiology and Pathology.* New York, John Wiley & Sons, Inc., 1977, p. 106.
246. Mills D., Karpatkin S.: The initial macromolecular derivatives of human fibrinogen produced by plasmin. *Biochim. Biophys. Acta* 271:163, 1972.
247. Marder V.J., et al.: High molecular weight derivatives of human fibrinogen produced by plasmin. *J. Biol. Chem.* 247:4775, 1972.
248. Marder V.J., Budzinski A.Z.: Data for defining fibrinogen and its plasmic degradation products. *Thromb. Diath. Haemorrh.* 33:199, 1975.
249. Wilner G.D., Thomas D.W., Nossel H.L., et al.: Immunochemical analysis of rabbit antihuman fibrinopeptide B antibodies. *Biochemistry* 18:5078, 1979.
250. Wiman B., Collen D.: On the mechanisms of the reaction between human α-2-antiplasmin and plasmin. *J. Biol. Chem.* 254:9291, 1979.
251. Wiman B., Collen D.: On the kinetics of the reaction between human antiplasmin and plasmin. *Eur. J. Biochem.* 84:573, 1978.
252. Friberger P., Knos M., Gustavsson S., et al.: Methods for determination of plasmin, antiplasmin and plasminogen by means of substrate (S-2251). *Haemostasis* 7:138, 1978.
253. Fareed J., Messmore H.L., Walenga J.M., et al.: Diagnostic efficacy of newer synthetic-substrates methods for assessing coagulation variables: A critical overview. *Clin. Chem.* 29:225, 1983.
254. Wilner G.D.: Molecular basis for measurement of circulating fibrinogen derivatives. *Prog. Hemost. Thromb.* 4:211, 1978.
255. Davies S.H., et al.: The linkage relations of hemophilia A and hemophilia B (Christmas disease) to the Xg blood group system. *Am. J. Hum. Genet.* 15:481, 1963.
256. Reisner H.M., Price W.A., Blatt P.M., et al.: Factor VIII coagulant antigen in hemophilic plasma: A comparison of five alloantibodies. *Blood* 56:615, 1980.
257. Sultan Y., Sola B., Avner P.H., et al.: Monoclonal antibodies against factor VIII procoagulant activity. *Thromb. Haemost.* 46:166, 1981.
258. Menitove J.E., Aster R.H., Casper J.T., et al.: T-lymphocyte subpopulations in patients with classic hemophilia treated with cryoprecipitate and lyophilized concentrates. *N. Engl. J. Med.* 308:83, 1983.
259. Bertina R.M., vander Linden I.K.: A genetic variant of factor IX with an abnormal high molecular weight. *Thromb. Haemost.* 46:125, 1981.
260. Firshein S.I., Hoyer L.W., Lazarchick J., et al.: Prenatal diagnosis of classic hemophilia. *N. Engl. J. Med.* 300:937, 1979.
261. Hoffnagle J.H., et al.: Serologic evidence for hepatitis B virus infection in patients with hemophilia B. *Thromb. Diath. Haemorrh.* 33:606, 1975.
262. Cable R.G., et al.: Influence of plasma source on T-lymphocyte subpopulations in hemophiliacs using factor VIII concentrate. *N. Engl. J. Med.* 309:1057, 1983.
263. Wall R.T., Counts R.V., Harker L.A., et al.: Binding and release of factor VIII/von Willebrand's factor by human endothelial cells. *Br. J. Haematol.* 46:287, 1980.
264. Sakariassen K.S., Bolhius P.A., Sixma J.J.: Human blood platelet adhesion to artery subendothelium is mediated by factor VIII-von Willebrand factor bound to the subendothelium. *Nature* 279:636, 1979.
265. Sultan Y., Simeon J., Caen J.P.: Detection of heterozygotes in both parents of homozygous patients with von Willebrand's disease. *J. Clin. Pathol.* 28:309, 1975.
266. Zimmerman T.S., Ruggieri Z.M.: Von Willebrand's disease. *Clin. Hematol.* 12:175, 1983.
267. Marwick C.: New ways to boost factor VIII in hemophilia: DDAVP for mild hemophilia A, von Willebrand's [news]. *JAMA* 249:3278, 1983.
268. Seligsohn U.: High gene frequency of factor XI (PTA) deficiency in Ashkenazi Jews. *Blood* 51:1, 1978.
269. Iwanaga S., Kato H., et al.: Fluorogenic peptide substrate for proteases in blood coagulation, kallikrein-kinin, and fibrinolysis systems: Substrate for plasmin and factor XIa. *Thromb. Haemost.* 42:49, 1979.
270. Triplett D.A.: Congenital coagulation factor deficiencies (excluding abnormalities of factor VIII, in Triplett D.A. (eds.): *Laboratory Evaluation of Coagulation.* Chicago, American Society of Clinical Pathologists Press, 1982, pp. 53–114.
271. Saito H., Scott J.G., Movat H.Z., et al.: Molecular heterogeneity of Hageman trait (factor XII deficiency): Evidence that two of 49 subjects are cross-reacting material positive (CRM+). *J. Lab. Clin. Med.* 94:256, 1974.
272. Kitchens C.S., Newcomb T.F.: Factor XIII. *Medicine* 58:413, 1979.
273. Duckert F.: Fibrin stabilizing factor (factor XIII): Consequence of its deficiency. *Thromb. Diath. Haemorrh.* 13(suppl.):115, 1964.
274. Steinberg P., Henriksson P., Nilsson I.M.: Factor XIII deficiency. *Lancet* 1:136, 1980.
275. Miletich J.P., Majerus D.W., Majerus P.W.: Patients with congenital factor V deficiency have decreased factor Xa binding sites on their platelets. *J. Clin. Invest.* 62:824, 1978.
276. Seligsohn U., Zinelin A., Zwang E.: Combined factor V and factor VIII deficiency among non-Ashkenazi Jews. *N. Engl. J. Med.* 307:1191, 1982.
277. Fair D.S., Plow E.F., Edington T.S.: Combined functional and immunochemical analysis of normal

and abnormal factor X. *J. Clin. Invest.* 64:884, 1979.
278. Soria J., Soria C., Samama M., et al.: Fibrinogen Troyes-Metz: Two new cases of congenital dysfibrinogenemia. *Thromb. Diath. Haemorrh.* 27:619, 1972.
279. Samori T., Yatabe M., Ukita M., et al.: A new congenital dysfibrinogenemia (fibrinogen Tokyo) with defective stabilization of fibrin polymer. Abstract, *V International Congress of the International Society for Thrombosis and Haemostasis*, 1975, p. 64.
280. Shah D.V., Suttie J.W.: The vitamin K dependent in vitro production of prothrombin. *Biochem. Biophys. Res. Commun.* 60:1397, 1974.
281. Lee S., et al.: Factor IX deficiency in liver disease. *JAMA* 221:410, 1972.
282. Shaw E., Giddings J.C., Peake I.R., et al.: Synthesis of procoagulant factor VIII, factor VIII-related antigen, and other coagulation factors by the isolated, perfused rat liver. *Br. J. Haematol.* 41:585, 1979.
283. Baele G., et al.: Antihaemophilic factor A activity, FVIII-related antigen and von Willebrand factor in hepatic cirrhosis. *Acta Haematol.* 57:290, 1977.
284. Deutsch E.: Blood coagulation changes in liver disease, in Poper H., Schaffner H. (eds.): *Progress in Liver Diseases*. New York, Grune & Stratton, Inc., 1965, vol. 2.
285. Rapaport S.I.: Plasma clotting factors in chronic hepatocellular disease. *N. Engl. J. Med.* 263:278, 1960.
286. Clark R., et al.: Coagulation abnormalities in acute liver failure: pathogenic and therapeutic implications. *Scand. J. Gastroenterol.* 19(suppl.):63, 1973.
287. Merskey C., et al.: Quantitative estimation of split products of fibrinogen in human serum: Relation to diagnosis and treatment. *Blood* 28:1, 1966.
288. Blatt P.M., Lundblad R.L., Kingdon H.S., et al.: Thrombogenic materials in prothrombin complex concentrates. *Ann. Intern. Med.* 81:766, 1974.
289. Spector I., Corn M., Ticktin H.E.: Effect of plasma transfusions on the prothrombin time and clotting factors in liver disease. *N. Engl. J. Med.* 275:1032, 1966.
290. Suttie J.W.: Vitamin-K-dependent carboxylation. *CRC Crit. Rev. Biochem.* 8:191, 1980.
291. Blanchard R.A., Furie B.C., Jorgensen M., et al.: Acquired vitamin-K-dependent carboxylation deficiency in liver disease. *N. Engl. J. Med.* 305:242, 1981.
292. Kazmier F.J., et al.: Effect of oral anticoagulants on factors VII, IX, X, II. *Arch. Intern. Med.* 115:667, 1965.
293. Klippel A.P., Pitsinger B.: Hypoprothrombinemia secondary to antibiotic therapy and manifested by massive gastrointestinal hemorrhage. *Arch. Surg.* 96:266, 1968.
294. Biggs R.: Jaundice and antibodies directed against factor VIII and IX in patients treated for hemophilia or Christmas disease in the United Kingdom. *Br. J. Haematol.* 26:313, 1974.
295. Hultin M.B., London F.S., Shapiro S.S., et al.: Heterogeneity of factor VIII antibodies: Further immunochemical and biological studies. *Blood* 49:807, 1977.
296. Lavergne J.M., Meyer D., Reisner H.: Characterization of human anti-factor VIII antibodies purified by immune complex formation. *Blood* 48:931, 1976.
297. Poon M.C., et al.: Heterogeneity of human circulating anticoagulants against antihemophilic factor (factor VIII). *Blood* 46:409, 1975.
298. Koutts J., Meyer D., Richard K., et al.: Heterogeneity of biological activity of human factor VIII antibodies. *Br. J. Haematol.* 29:99, 1975.
299. Kasper C.K., et al.: A more uniform measurement of factor VIII inhibitor. *Thromb. Diath. Haemorrh.* 34:869, 1975.
300. Shapiro S.: The immunologic character of acquired inhibitors of antihemophilic globulin (factor VIII) and the kinetics of their interaction with factor VIII. *J. Clin. Invest.* 46:147, 1967.
301. Brody J.F., Haider M.E., Rossman R.E.: A hemorrhagic syndrome in Waldenström's macroglobulinemia secondary to immunoadsorption of factor VIII. *N. Engl. J. Med.* 300:408, 1979.
302. Vera J.C., Herzig E.B., Sise H.S., et al.: Acquired circulating anticoagulant to factor VIII. *JAMA* 232:1038, 1975.
303. Ratnoff O.D., Rabaa M.S.: Autologous antibodies to AHF and phenytoin. *Blood* 51:768, 1978.
304. Roberts H.R.: Acquired inhibitors in hemophilia B. *Thromb. Diath. Haemorrh.* 45(suppl.):217, 1971.
305. Largo R., et al.: Acquired factor IX inhibitor in a nonhaemophilic patient with autoimmune disease. *Br. J. Haematol.* 26:129, 1974.
306. Pike I.M., Yount W.J., Puritz E.M., et al.: Immunochemical characterization of a monoclonal γG4λ human antibody to factor IX. *Blood* 40:1, 1972.
307. Reece E.A., Clyne L.P., Romero R., et al.: Spontaneous factor XI inhibitors: Seven additional cases and a review of the literature. *Arch. Intern. Med.* 144:525, 1984.
308. Frantantoni J.C., Hilgartener M., Nachman R.L.: Nature of the defect in congenital factor V deficiency: Study in a patient with an acquired circulating anticoagulant. *Blood* 39:751, 1972.
309. Menache D.: Abnormal fibrinogens. *Thromb. Diath. Haemorrh.* 29:525, 1973.
310. Edson J.R., et al.: Successful management of a subdural hematoma in a hemophiliac with an anti-factor VIII antibody. *Blood* 41:113, 1973.
311. Strauss H.S.: Acquired circulating anticoagulants in hemophilia A. *N. Engl. J. Med.* 281:866, 1969.
312. Kasper C.K., et al.: Effect of prothrombin complex concentrates on factor VIII inhibitor levels. *Blood* 54:1358, 1979.
313. Goldfinger D.: Complications of hemolytic transfusion reactions: Pathogenesis and therapy, in Dawson R.B. (ed.): *New Approaches to Transfusion Reactions*. Washington, D.C., American Association of Blood Banks, 1974, p. 15.

314. Wintrobe M.M.: *Clinical Hematology*. Philadelphia, Lea & Febiger, 1981, p. 1214.
315. Josey W.E., Hoch W., Moon E.C., et al.: Analysis of 21 septic abortion deaths with special reference to the Shwartzman phenomenon. *Obstet. Gynecol.* 28:335, 1966.
316. Gordon S.G., Franks J.J., Lewis B.: Cancer procoagulant A: A factor X activating procoagulant from malignant tissue. *Thromb. Res.* 6;127, 1975.
317. Weiss H.J., Allan S., Davidson E., et al.: A fibrinogenemia in man following the bite of a rattle snake (*Crotalus adamanteus*). *Am. J. Med.* 47:625, 1969.
318. Morrison D.C., Cochrane C.G.: Direct evidence for Hageman factor (factor XII) activation by bacterial lipopolysaccharides (endotoxins). *J. Exp. Med.* 140:787, 1974.
319. Muller-Berghaus G.: Pathophysiology of generalized intravascular coagulation. *Ser. Thromb. Haemost.* 3:209, 1977.
320. Muller-Berghaus G., Schneberger R.: Hageman factor activation in the generalized Shwartzman reaction induced by endotoxin. *Br. J. Haematol.* 21:513, 1971.
321. Walsh P.N., Griffin J.H.: The role of human platelets in the contact phase of blood coagulation. *Clin. Res.* 26:509A, 1978.
322. Rock R.C., et al.: Heparin treatment of intravascular coagulation accompanying hemolytic transfusion reactions. *Transfusion* 9:57, 1969.
323. Bang Nu: Disseminated intravascular coagulation, in Triplett D.A. (ed.): *Laboratory Evaluation of Coagulation*. Chicago, American Association of Clinical Pathologists Press, 1982, p. 158.
324. Bergstein J.M., Michael A.F. Jr.: Failure of cobra venom to prevent the generalized Shwartzman reaction and loss of renal cortical fibrinolytic activity. *Am. J. Pathol.* 75:195, 1974.
325. Spaet T.H., Cintron J.: Studies on platelet factor 3 availability. *Br. J. Haematol.* 11:269, 1965.
326. Horowitz H.I., Des Prez R.M., Hook E.W.: Effects of bacterial endotoxin on rabbit platelets: II. Enhancement of platelet factor 3 activity in vitro and in vivo. *J. Exp. Med.* 116:619, 1962.
327. Bang Nu: Normal and abnormal fibrin polymerization. *Thromb. Diath. Haemorrh. Suppl.* 13:131, 1964.
328. Kudryk B., Reuterby J., Blomback B.: Adsorption of plasmic fragment D to thrombin modified fibrinogen-sepharose. *Thromb. Res.* 2:297, 1973.
329. Latallo Z.S., et al.: Analysis of soluble fibrin complexes (agarose gel chromatography and protamine sulfate gelation). *Biochim. Biophys. Acta* 420:69, 1976.
330. Chang M.L., et al.: Evidence for aggregation of fibrin fragments D and E in soluble fibrin complex formation. *Thromb. Res.* 5:719, 1974.
331. Lee L., McCluskey R.T.: Immunohistochemical demonstration of the reticuloendothelial clearance of circulating fibrin aggregates. *J. Exp. Med.* 116:611, 1962.
332. Forman E.N., Abildgaard C.F., Bolger J.F., et al.: Generalized Shwartzman reaction: Role of the granulocytes. *Lab. Invest.* 18:101, 1968.
333. Lee L.: Reticuloendothelial clearance of circulating fibrin in the pathogenesis of the generalized Shwartzman reaction. *J. Exp. Med.* 115:1065, 1962.
334. Gans H., Lowman J.T.: The uptake of fibrin and fibrin degradation products by the isolated perfused rat liver. *Blood* 29:526, 1967.
335. Hamilton P.J., Stalker A.L., Douglas A.S.: Disseminated intravascular coagulation: A review. *J. Clin. Pathol.* 31:609, 1978.
336. Spero J.A., Lewis J.H., Hasiba U.: Disseminated intravascular coagulation: Findings in 346 patients. *Thromb. Haemost.* 43:28, 1980.
337. Hedner U., Nilsson I.M.: Parallel determinations of fibrin degradation products and fibrin monomers with various methods. *Thromb. Diath. Haemorrh.* 28:268, 1972.
338. Latallo Z.: Critical evaluation of the thrombin time test, in *Proceedings of the 8th Congress of the European Society of Hematologists*. Basel, Switzerland, S. Karger, 1961, p. 423.
339. Arnesen H., Kierult P., Godal H.C.: The influence of fibrinogen degradation products on the reptilasetime of plasma. *Scand. J. Haematol.* 11:360, 1973.
340. Allington M.J.: Detection of fibrin(ogen) degradation products by a latex clumping method. *Scand. J. Haematol. Suppl.* 13:115, 1971.
341. Merskey C., Lalezari P., Johnson A.J.: A rapid, simple, sensitive method for measuring fibrinolytic split products in human serum. *Proc. Soc. Exp. Biol. Med.* 131:871, 1969.
342. Hawiger J., Hamond D.K., Timmons S.: Human fibrinogen possesses binding site for staphylococci on Aα and Bβ polypeptide chains. *Nature* 258:643, 1975.
343. Collen D.: Emergence in plasma during activation of the coagulation and fibrinolytic systems of neoantigens, associated with the complexes of thrombin or plasmin with their inhibitors. *Thromb. Res.* 5:777, 1974.
344. Fareed J., Messmore H.L., Walenga J.M., et al.: Synthetic peptide substrates in hemostatic testing. *CRC Crit. Rev. Clin. Lab. Sci.* 19:71, 1983.
345. Hehne H.J., et al.: Management of bleeding disorders in traumatic-haemorrhagic shock state with deep frozen fresh plasma. *Eur. J. Intensive Care Med.* 2:157, 1976.
346. Colman R.W., Robboy S.J., Minna J.D.: Disseminated intravascular coagulation: An approach. *Am. J. Med.* 52:679, 1972.
347. Hardisty R.M., Ingram G.I.C.: *Bleeding Disorders*. Oxford, Blackwell Scientific Publications, 1965.
348. Beller F.F., Uszynski M.: Disseminated intravascular coagulation in pregnancy. *Clin. Obstet. Gynecol.* 17:250, 1974.
349. Schipper H.G., et al.: Antithrombin III transfusion in disseminated intravascular coagulation. *Lancet* 1:854, 1978.

350. Bang Nu: Disseminated intravascular coagulation, in Triplett D.A. (ed.): *Laboratory Evaluation of Coagulation.* Chicago, American Society of Clinical Pathologists Press, 1982, p. 192.
351. Minna J.D., et al.: *Disseminated Intravascular Coagulation in Man.* Springfield, Ill., Charles C Thomas, 1974.
352. Wintrobe M.W., Lee G.R., Boggs D.R., et al.: *Clinical Hematology,* ed. 8. Philadelphia, Lea & Febiger, 1981, p. 1224.
353. Marengo-Rowe A.J., et al.: The evaluation of hemorrhage in cardiac patients who have undergone extracorporeal circulation. *Transfusion* 19:426, 1979.
354. Harker L.A., et al.: Mechanism of abnormal bleeding in patients undergoing cardiopulmonary bypass: Acquired transient platelet dysfunction associated with select α-granule release. *Blood* 56:824, 1980.
355. Wintrobe M.M., Lee G.R., Boggs D.R., et al.: *Clinical Hematology,* ed. 8. Philadelphia, Lea & Febiger, 1981, p. 1234.
356. Sherman L.A.: Alterations of hemostasis during massive transfusion, in Nusbacher J. (ed.): *Massive Transfusion.* Washington, D.C., American Association of Blood Banks, 1978, p. 53.
357. Simon T.L., Henderson R.: Coagulation factor activity in platelet concentrates. *Transfusion* 19:186–189, 1979.

Immunology

HEMAGGLUTINATION REACTIONS often used in the blood bank as diagnostic procedures are antigen-antibody reactions. These reactions as well as many other types of reactions are interpreted in the blood bank during typing, screening, and antibody identification. This chapter provides a brief review of immunology with an emphasis on the biochemical and physiologic bases of these phenomena.

Functions of the immune system are of two kinds, humoral immunity and cellular immunity. These two major divisions of function stem from the organizational division, in most mammalians, of two cell populations. Humoral immunity is mainly associated with the activity of B cells and their immunoglobulin products. Cellular immunity is mainly associated with a population of T cell lymphocytes. However, most immune factors require the interaction of both B and T cells.

HUMORAL IMMUNITY

Immunoglobulins

Immunoglobulins are the major component of humoral immunity.[1] Immunoglobulins are glycoproteins composed, in most cases, of 82% polypeptide and 18% carbohydrate. Their main function is binding to antigen. Each immunoglobulin contains at least one basic unit or monomer (Fig 4–1). The monomer unit is subdivided into four chains, two heavy chains and two light chains. As in any protein, the chains have a carboxyl terminal and an amino terminal determined by the end-to-end linkage of the amino acids forming the sequence. The carboxyl terminal is called C, or *constant region,* whereas the amino terminal is called V, or *variable region.* Each chain is folded, forming loops, linked by disulfide bonds, in specific areas of each chain. The loops are called *domains* (see Fig 4–1).[2]

Light Chains.—Light chains have a molecular weight of approximately 23,000 daltons and possess a C and V region. They may be present in two forms, κ or λ. These forms are determined by a difference in the amino acid sequence. Light chains have two domains, V_L and C_L.

Heavy Chains.—These proteins have molecular weights of 50,000–70,000 daltons and are grouped into immunoglobulin classes on the basis of weight. Heavy chains have one V_H domain and three C_H domains (C_H1, C_H2, C_H3). Some heavy chains have a fourth C_H domain, called C_H4. Some of the functions of these domains are known. The C_H1 domain participates in the three-dimensional orientation of the combining site. The C_H2 domain is involved in binding C1q as demonstrated by the fact that C_H3 cleaved molecules can still bind complement, but Fab fragments cannot. C_H3 is involved in effector functions such as binding to FcR on macrophages.[3]

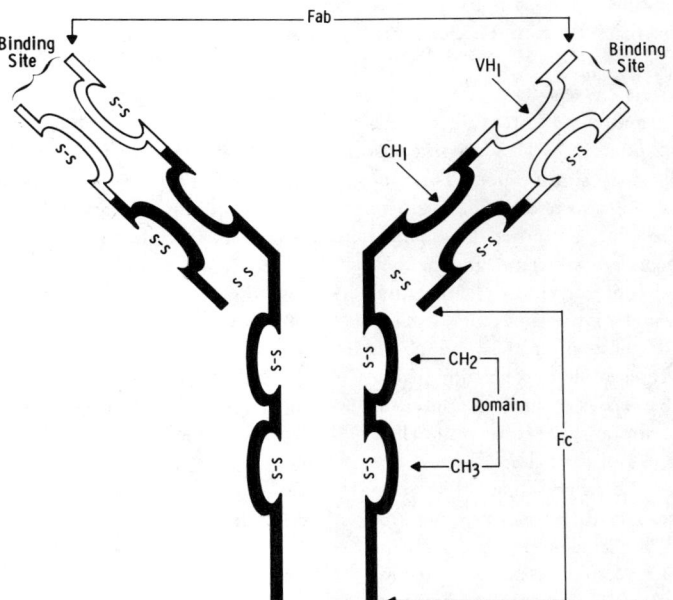

FIG 4–1.—Structure of immunoglobulin monomer Fab fragment with two binding sites. Fc fragment is bottom portion of the monomer.

It has been shown recently that both $C1q^4$ as well as *Staphylococcus* protein A^5 are capable of binding to the C_H2 domain, but these molecules must bind to different areas of the C_H2 domain, since binding of protein A does not inhibit binding of $C1q.^6$

Hinge Region.—The hinge region where the Fab fragment and the Fc fragment meet is coded by a separate minigene;[7] this region appears to have a double-stranded helical configuration on crystalography studies.[6]

Determinant of Specific Binding (Antibody Combining Site).—The antibody binding site has recently been clarified by experiments with labeled haptens and by measuring binding ability to amino acid sequences. These specific binding sites have been traced to the variable region. Radiolabel tracing experiments have helped define binding sites in much more detail. These experiments show that the V regions of H chains have more binding capability than the light chains alone.

Once the hapten is attached to the binding site of an immunoglobulin Fab fragment, the chains resist denaturation. The inference to be drawn from these denaturation experiments is that antibody hypervariable regions are spaced along the variable region of the binding site.[8]

Several new experiments suggest that the combining site does not change significantly in chemical conformation after combining with antigen; however, this phenomenon needs further study before we can assume that a conformational change can be made.[6]

The sizes of combining sites are similar to those found on enzymes.[6] Depending on the shape of the antigen, the combining site may be groove-like or pocket-like.[9] Although the "pocket" or "groove" arrangement of the binding site may have a role in specificity, linkage is more probably by means of a surface-to-surface hydrophobic bond between the antigen and the combining site.

For the combining site to operate properly, both the hypervariable regions of the heavy chain and the light chain must interact to produce a relatively strong association yielding a stable three-dimensional structure.[1] This association of heavy and light chains also provides a wider combinational diversity. Researchers using artificial monoclonal cell hybrids have proved that most heavy chains and light chains can combine randomly to produce new combining possibilities on immunoglobulins.

Immunoglobulin Classes

Immunoglobulins are divided into five classes, IgG, IgM, IgA, IgE, and IgD.[10] This division has a structural and functional significance. The immunoglobulin classes are characterized both by their primary structure (i.e., amino acid sequence) as well as by their secondary, tertiary, and quaternary structures (spatial configurations).[11] Structural differences are manifested in the different physicochemical properties of these molecules, which in turn are reflected in their biologic behavior in the immune reactions. The classes of immunoglobulins vary principally in the amino acid sequences of their heavy chains. Thus, the amino acid sequence of the Fc portion determines the heavy chain class category. The characteristics of different immunoglobulin classes are listed in Table 4–1. Heavy chains are further subdivided into subclasses. Each immunoglobulin has particular biologic characteristics, as described below.

IgG.—IgG is the main immunoglobulin of the secondary immune response. It is usually a monomer with sedimentation rate of 7S and a molecular weight of 150,000 daltons. IgG constitutes about 75% of the total plasma immunoglobulin content.

The various IgG subclasses (Fig 4–2) differ in concentration, ability to bind complement, ability to cross the placenta, and ability to bind to macrophages.[12] These characteristics are determined by the Fc fragment. Interestingly, the amount of antibody may vary from individual to individual. It has been shown that the ability to produce certain amounts of IgG subclasses may be under genetic regulation.[13]

IgM.—IgM is usually composed of five monomers linked by S-S bonds and a J chain. It is found mainly in the primary antibody response when an animal is stimulated with an antigen for the first time. As a pentamer (see Fig 4–1) it has ten binding sites (two for each monomer), weighs about 900,000 daltons, and has a sedimentation rate of 19S.[14] The heavy chain of IgM possesses one extra domain, C_H4.[15] IgM is the main immunoglobulin in the so-called natural antibodies (e.g., anti-A, anti-B in the ABO system) and the major immunoglobulin of cold-reacting antibodies. Along with IgD, IgM is found on the surface of immature B cells. It does *not* cross the placenta, and in its pentameric form it is an efficient complement-binding immunoglobulin.

IgA.—IgA is the main immunoglobulin in secretions and thus protects mucosal surfaces from infection. It is usually found in secretions as a dimer, and the two monomers are linked by a J chain. When secreted, IgA acquires a secretory piece (see Fig 4–2) provided by the epithelial cells, which secrete the immunoglobulin into the lumina of the exocrine glands.[16] IgA may be found in the serum as a monomer, with a molecular weight of 160,000, and in secretions as a dimer, with a molecular weight of about 400,000. IgA constitutes about 15% of serum immunoglobulin. IgA pos-

TABLE 4–1.—Chemical And Biologic Properties Of Immunoglobulins*

PROPERTY	CLASS				
	IgG	IgA	IgM	IgD	IgE
Subclasses	1, 2, 3, 4	1, 2	—	—	—
Domains	4	4	5	4	5
Sedimentation coefficient	6–7	7	19	7–8	8
MW (daltons)	150,000	160,000–400,000	900,000	180,000	190,000
Serum concentration (mg/dl)	1,000	200	120	3	0.05
Biologic activity	Main serum Ig; CF+, PT+++	Main Ig, in secretions	Main Ig in primary response, and in isoantibodies (i.e., ABH); CF+++	Ig switch for B cell differentiation	Main reagin

*M, monomer; D, dimer; CF, complement fixation test; PT, placental transfer.

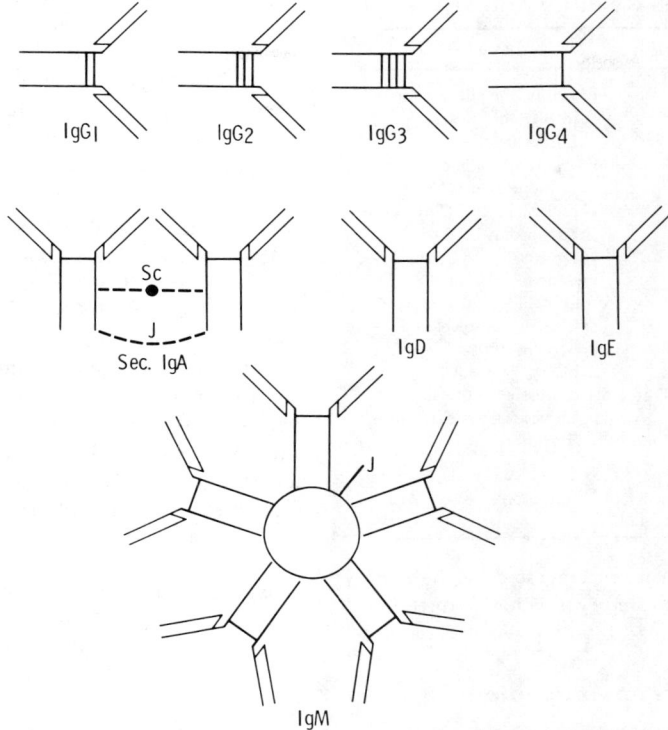

FIG 4–2.—*Top,* subclasses of IgG. The vertical lines joining the heavy chains are S-S bonds. *Middle,* secretory IgA. The monomers are bound by a J chain and secretory component *(Sc)*. *Bottom,* IgM pentamer. IgM monomers are joined by a J chain.

sesses two subclasses, A1 and A2. A2 is usually a monomer with a molecular weight of about 190,000. It is found in trace amounts in serum, constituting 0.004% of the immunoglobulin content of serum.[17] It is important in blood banking because anti-IgA antibodies may cause severe transfusion reactions (see Chap. 11).

IgE.—IgE is the main reaginic immunoglobulin and is responsible for allergic reactions. Mast cells and basophils have specific receptors for the Fc portion of the IgE molecule. These cells may degranulate on binding IgE on their surface and exposure to antigen, with release of leukotrienes and histamine.[18] IgE is not known to have any subclasses.

IgD.—IgD is a monomer with a molecular weight of approximately 180,000 and with a sedimentation coefficient of 7S to 8S. It constitutes about 0.2% of the total immunoglobulin content. It may play a role in the differentiation of B lymphocytes to plasma cells. It is envisioned as a cell "switch" on the surface of B cells which triggers maturation of B cells and plays a role in immune tolerance.[19]

Genetic Markers on Antibodies: Allotypes

IgG has determinant amino acid sequences on its heavy chains which are called Gm markers.[20] These allotypes, as they are called, are inherited sequences that make one individual different from another and are therefore phenotypic manifestations of genetically determined sequences. Such markers can be used in genetic studies as well as in paternity testing. Over 20 Gm allotypes have been described. Each IgG subclass has its own allotypes (Table 4–2). IgA also has genetic markers, termed Am 1 and Am 2 allotypes. In contrast to Gm allotype antibodies, Am allotype antibodies can cause very dangerous transfusion reactions.[21]

Allotype markers for light chains are termed Inv allotypes. At least three Inv allotypes are known,

TABLE 4–2—HEAVY CHAIN ALLOTYPES*

IG SUBCLASS	ALLOTYPE	FREQUENCY
IgG1	1, 2, 17	Probably one allele present in 60% of West Europeans
	3, 4, 22	Probably one allele present in more than 90% of caucasians and Chinese but in only 13% of Japanese
IgG2	23	Present in 50% of caucasians, 90% of Chinese, no blacks
IgG3	5, 6, 10, 11, 13, 14, 21	Present in 100% of blacks, 90% of caucasians, 90% of Chinese, no Australian aborigines
IgG4	4a, 4b	

*Modified from Eisen H.N.: *Immunology.* New York, Harper & Row, 1974, p. 421.

but there may be others, as suggested by the finding of individuals who are negative for all three Inv allotypes.[21]

Genetic Markers on Antibodies: Idiotypes

The term idiotype was originally coined by Oudin in 1966[22] to describe a unique antigenic determinant found on the variable regions of antibody molecules from a single clone of antibody-secreting cells. Idiotypic determinants are recognized by anti-idiotypic antibodies. These determinants are composed of varying amino acid sequences on V_H or V_L regions of the immunoglobulin molecule. There are two types of idiotypes: individual idiotypes, which arise from somatic mutation (IdIs) and are recognized by anti-IdIs antibodies, and inherited idiotypes (IdXs), which are recognized by anti-IdXs antibodies.[23]

The Network Theory of Jerne.—According to Niels Jerne, the immune system interacts via idiotypic determinants in the V-region domains.[24] It is assumed that there are about 10^7 different combining sites per individual; thus there are 10^7 idiotypic determinants. Combining sites recognize through the same molecular compatibility both antigen and a specific idiotypic determinant. In this way, the organism possesses an "internal image" of external antigens (Fig 4–3). At the same time, cells in the immune system recognize idiotypic specificities through anti-idiotype antibodies. This creates a closed network. By the same token, idiotype-anti-idiotype interactions lead to clonal selection by the expansion or elimination of specific lymphocyte clones. The system remains in equilibrium until antigen enters the system, inducing clonal expansion of selected idiotypic clones by cells bearing anti-idiotypic specificities.[25]

Generation of Antibody Diversity.—V regions contain a single domain with an intrachain disulfide bridge. The N-terminus defines a V region as κ or λ. The first 100 amino acids of the V region have an area that varies independently; this region is called the J segment,[26] which is not to be confused with the J chain of IgA and IgM. There are two ways of increasing the number of combining sites in V regions. The first is intrachain rearrangements uniting V regions and J segment genes. The second is interchain combinational amplification between V_H and V_L gene products.[27]

Somatic Mutation

Mutations occur at the rate of one mutation per gene per 10^6 cell dimension. Mutations are very likely to occur in lymphocytes, which divide rapidly during ontogeny. This phenomenon was shown experimentally in A-J mice immunized to arsonate: the genetic framework of the mice was the same, yet the antibody diversity against arsonate was different.[28]

The combining site diversity is achieved through changes in single amino acids during clone amplification.[29] Network interactions inducing clonal expansion aid in the development of antibody diver-

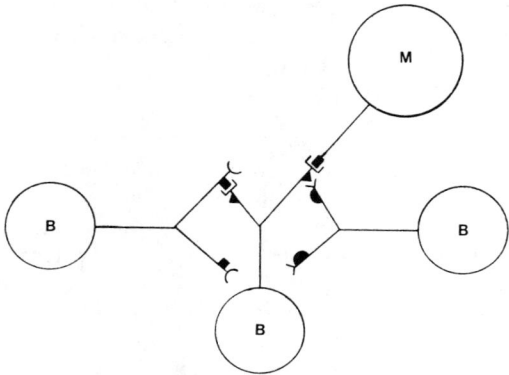

FIG 4–3.—Jerne's network model. Macrophage *(M)* presents antigen to B cells *(B)*. Idiotypes are the determinants in the hypervariable region. B cells and T cells recognize these idiotypic determinants, providing the network recognition system.

sity.[30] Jerne has proposed that germ line genes code for receptors of the major histocompatibility system (MHS). During lymphocyte ontogeny, lymphocytes recognizing the MHS via these receptors are driven to proliferation and may be considered autoreactive clones.[31]

Genetics of Antibody Diversity

Antibodies are proteins and, as such, their amino acid sequence is determined by DNA coding. The puzzle of how, with a limited number of genes, antibody diversity is achieved has been partially resolved, and we now have information that may explain this antibody diversity. The total complement of genes in the genome is about 1 million.[32] Rather than possessing a complete set for all antibody genes, the germ line cells have a "kit" of essential component genes to provide the necessary permutation information to lymphocytes. These genes are then shuffled during maturation of B cells. The end result is the production of a unique antibody combining site.

Antibody genes coded for in the DNA in the form of codons do not exist as a continuous codon array but are separated by noncoding intervening sequences. The information at the DNA level is transmitted to the RNA along with the noncoding sequences. At the RNA level the codons are joined by splicing, which consists of the joining of codons into a sequence of meaningful information.

Dreyer-Bennet Hypothesis.—According to the Dreyer-Bennet hypothesis, genes coding for antibodies are not arranged as for other proteins in a continuous array of codons. Rather, Dreyer and Bennet propose that a single gene exists for the constant region, whereas variable region genes are multiple (hundreds or thousands). In order for this mechanism to work, split genes and joining mechanisms must exist to encode a coherent message that would result in an antibody molecule.[33] Through reverse transcriptase experiments, the Dreyer-Bennet hypothesis has proved to be essentially correct. The method studies the rate of hybridization kinetics with a radioactive probe. If a gene sequence coding for the constant region is hybridized, the rate of hybridization is low and can be equated with low or no shuffling of C region genes. This is not so for V regions, where many separately encoded regions exist. The most economical way to achieve a coherent sequence would be by somatic recombination or gene shuffling. This has been shown by Tonegawa et al.[34] to be correct.

Embryonic somatic cells, on their way to becoming mature B cells, shuffle the variable genes through endonucleases which cleave DNA at specific sites. Nonsignificant sequences are eliminated during division, thus bringing V region genes closer together as well as closer to C region genes.[35]

Antibody diversity is achieved by the alternative joining of one of about 150 V gene sequences to one of five different J region sequences, accounting for the hypervariable region of the combining site. Joining of V genes to another gene sequence termed D (for diversity) genes also provides diversity. The D genes account for the major portion of the third hypervariable region of the combining site. Thus, the different permutations possible between V, D, and J genes provide a potential for about 18 billion antibodies with different specificities.

Active light chain genes are assembled by somatic recombination and splicing of RNA.[35] Each V region gene is separated by a leader (L) sequence recognized during recombination and splicing. The leader sequences are cleaved off as they pass through the membrane. The entire gene is transcribed from DNA to RNA, including intervening sequences, which are spliced off as the formation of coherent sequences takes place. The end product achieves adjoining sequences of L/V-J-C sequences.

Immunoglobulin Class Switching

B lymphocyte immunoglobulin class switching depends on two mechanisms: differential RNA transcription and splicing, and DNA recombination. Active heavy chain genes are assembled from four sets of genes in the germ line L/V, D, J, and C. L/V, D, and J are brought together by somatic recombination. Constant (C) regions are coded downstream—that is, from the 5' end of the DNA sequence to the 3' end of the sequence. RNA transcription and splicing are responsible for the successive appearance of μ and δ constant heavy chains with the same V regions. Switching signals (S) and long noncoding segments separate γ-3, 1, 2b, 2a, ϵ, and α genes. The switch is accomplished by DNA recombination. Switching signals apparently mediates recombination that joins V/D/J sequences to one of the downstream C region sequences.[32]

Binding of Immunoglobulins to Membranes

The sequence of amino acids of Fc portions of membrane-bound immunoglobulin differs from free immunoglobulin. The intramembrane portion is coded by two exons, M_1 and M_2.[6] Interestingly, this intramembrane portion of the molecule is similar in amino acid sequence to other intramembrane proteins.[36] It contains 26 amino acids, which are characteristically hydrophobic. The hydrophobic intracellular portion of the immunoglobulin varies between immunoglobulin classes. For instance, membrane-associated IgM (mIgM) has three amino acid residues, whereas mIgG has 28 residues.[37]

Effect of Surface-Bound Immunoglobulin on Cells

The precise mechanism by which surface-bound immunoglobulin affects the cells bearing immunoglobulin is not known, but some data are available. For instance, clustered immunoglobulin mobilizes bound Ca^{2+}.[38] There is evidence of association between the clustered immunoglobulin with underlying cytoskeleton.[39] Furthermore, methylation of phospholipids, activation of serine esterase, and generation of cytoplasmic factors have all been associated with immunoglobulin clustering on the membrane of cells,[6] but these effects require mediation by cellular factors such as interleukins.[6]

The size and persistence of immunoglobulin clusters are dependent on the affinity of antibody to antigen, and may be of significance in the immunoglobulin effect on the immunoglobulin receptor-bearing cell.[40]

Binding of Fc receptors has also been investigated. A decapeptide from domain C_H3 of IgG has affinity for the receptor, but this decapeptide is hidden in the molecule.[41] Another point of interest is that β-microglobulin, the light chain of the MHS, has affinity for the Fc receptor of macrophages,[42] which may have some bearing on immunoglobulin receptor interactions with effector cells.

The integrity of certain areas of the Fc appears to be necessary for Fc binding. For instance, cleavage of the hinge region distorts the binding capacity of Fc from IgG1 to granulocytes,[43] and binding of *S. aureus* to Fc interferes with binding of IgG1 to granulocytes but not to monocytes.[44] It is currently believed that in synthesis, the penultimate carboxy terminal C_H domain is critical to the binding of Fc to receptors.

Fc Receptors on Mononuclear Cells.—It

has recently been shown that receptors on mononuclear phagocytes for Fc (FcR) vary: some receptors bind IgG2a in monomeric or aggregated form (these are called FcRI), whereas other receptors bind only immune aggregates of IgG1 and IgG2b subclasses (these are termed FcRII). Evidently these two kinds of receptors are of different chemical composition, for they vary in their trypsin sensitivity.[45–47] Other Fc receptors have also been described. For instance, IgE receptors have been observed on human monocytes in up to 20% of peripheral blood monocytes.[48, 49] Some authors report tissue macrophages from spleen which bear IgM receptors.[50]

The Fc receptor in mice accounts for about 0.01% of the total cell protein.[51] Its chemical structure has been partially characterized. This has been possible, using monoclonal antibodies against FcR to enable separation.[52, 53] Furthermore, monoclonal antibodies are available against FcRI and FcRII.[52] The receptor is thought to weigh approximately 60,000 daltons, according to some authors.[51] However, these authors find that the molecular weights of peptides vary in FcR of different mouse macrophage tumor cell lines (J774 and P388D). Using a monoclonal antibody termed 2.4g2 IgG to bind the FcR molecule, it has been shown that two poorly resolved peptides, one weighing 47,000 daltons and the second weighing 60,000 daltons, can be defined.[51]

Antigens

The capacity of a substance to induce an antibody response by the immune system is known as antigenicity or immunogenicity. Antigens are usually multivalent, macromolecular compounds such as proteins, mucopolysaccharides, and other high molecular weight complexes. Under normal conditions, antibodies are formed against chemicals "foreign" to the organism. This capacity to induce a response depends on how "foreign" the substance is to the host. However, immunogenicity in reality entails a complex interaction between the antigen and the immune system of the host. High molecular weight and increased structural complexity of the compound make an antigen more immunogenic, but these are not the only factors creating immunogenicity. It is known, however, that highly immunogenic molecules have molecular weights in the range of 100,000 daltons. Molecules low in immunogenicity have a significantly lower molecular weight (e.g., 20,000 daltons).

Recent research emphasizes the variability of responsiveness determined by genetic factors. Individuals of the same species may have different ability to respond to a certain antigen. The ability to respond may be inherited as an autosomal dominant trait.

The dose of antigen and the route of administration have long been known to be determining factors in immune induction.

Certain portions of the antigen molecule are more antigenic than others. These areas elicit specific antibody formation for such areas. Such regions in the antigen are called *antigenic determinants*.

Small molecules may become antigenic if they are coupled to a carrier protein. These molecules linked to a "carrier" molecule are referred to as *haptens*.

Karl Landsteiner pioneered the research of haptenic determinants on carrier molecules. His experiments demonstrated that haptens such as arsenate and its isomers in the ortho, meta, or para position varied in ability to induce antibody formation. This is due to differences in "closeness of fit" in their keylock arrangement.[54] Some determinants may resemble the steric arrangement of other determinants; this similarity is responsible for cross-reactivity.

Synthetic antigens have helped remarkably in the study of antigenic determinants. Synthetic antigens are produced by chemically attaching haptens to side chains of carrier proteins. The more exposed a portion of an antigenic determinant is, the more likely it will become antigenic.

Also, the branching character of certain antigenic determinants will elicit more vigorous immune reactions than nonbranching determinants. Here again, steric configuration plays a role in the final outcome of antibody formation.

Antigens with only one antigenic determinant will elicit T cell–mediated responses. When more than one antigen determinant is present, B cells are predominantly involved.

In complex antigens, B cells respond to the haptenic portion of the antigen, while T cells respond to the carrier portion of the antigen.[55]

Certain types of molecules induce purely B cell responses. These antigens characteristically have repeating units (e.g., polysaccharides).[56]

Antigen-Antibody Reaction Kinetics

Antibodies bind to ligands (i.e., antigens) by noncovalent forces, and therefore these bonds, though firm, are reversible. Assuming the two binding sites of an antibody molecule bind independently, the stoichiometry of intrinsic association constants can be calculated by the following formula:

$$K = \frac{k}{K1} = \frac{[SL]}{[S][L]}$$

where S is the binding site, L is the ligand, k is the association constant, and K1 is the dissociation constant.

Antibody valence for each antibody can be calculated on the basis of the above formula.[57] Since antibody specificities are heterogeneous, the equilibrium of any given antibody-ligand binding reaction is given by the sum of the bound specificities of the antibody to the ligand. Changes in pH affect ionic ligands. Nonionic ligands are minimally affected by changes in pH. Binding is affected by temperature, depending on the antibody class. Most reactions are speeded up by increases in temperature. Those which are not are termed exothermal.

The entropy of these reactions can be derived from the following formula:[58]

$$\Delta F° = \Delta H° - T\Delta S°$$

where $\Delta F°$ is the change in free energy, $\Delta H°$ is the change in enthalpy in calories, T is the absolute temperature, and $\Delta S°$ is the entropy change.

Hydrophilic ligands tend to form less stable antigen-antibody complexes. These bonds may be ionic, hydrophobic (hydrogen) bonds or charge transfer bonds. Steric hindrance may appear when bulky substituents inhibit the approach of antibody to antigen.

The antigen-antibody reactions with soluble molecules were first quantitatively studied by Michael Heidelberger. Heidelberger was also the first investigator to demonstrate that macromolecular antigens other than proteins are antigenic.[57] He showed that in antigen-antibody reactions, an optimum zone of equivalence is attained for each antibody-antigen reaction, where the antibody concentration and the antigen concentration reach a state of binding equilibrium (Fig 4–4).

Precipitin Reaction

Usually many antibody (Ab) molecules combine simultaneously with one molecule of antigen (Ag). Since antibodies are bivalent and antigens are multivalent, a lattice formation results. This changes the physicochemical behavior of the reactants (the antibody and the ligand).

Upon the formation of Ab/Ag lattice complexes, the previously soluble reactants tend to come out of solution and precipitate. However, less complex structures, called soluble complexes, tend to form during this reaction as well. The multivalency of antigens depends on a variety of antigenic determinants rather than on repeated units of the same determinant (Fig 4–5).

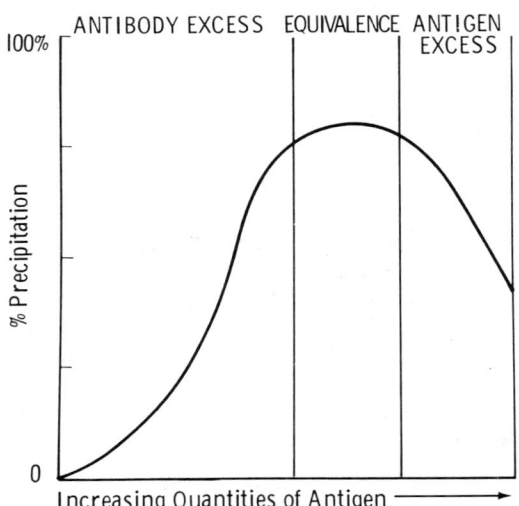

FIG 4–4.—Heidelberger's curve of antibody-antigen reactions. Maximum precipitation occurs at equivalence, where the number of antigen sites are saturated by equal numbers of antibody-binding sites.

The shape of an antigen-antibody precipitation curve can be described by using Langmuir plots. Relatively homogeneous antibodies (e.g., monoclonal antibodies from myelomas with known specificity) produce linear Langmuir curves. Less homogeneous antibodies (more frequently found in normal immune responses) give compounded Langmuir curves due to varying specificities and avidities of antibodies composing these sera.[59]

Interaction of Antibodies With Antigens

Usually molecular interactions between antibody and antigen are both concentration dependent and time dependent. This is clearly appreciable in blood banking tests, where serum and RBCs react to cause agglutination. When the serum to cell ratios are increased, the sensitivity of reactions is usually increased. When percentage agglutination is plotted against the logarithm of the antiserum concentration, a sigmoid curve is produced (Fig 4–6). This occurs both because of saturation of binding sites and because of a decreasing chance of molecular interactions. When antibody concentrations are such that all antigen sites are blocked, "prozoning" occurs. This usually occurs with avid antibodies (e.g., anti-D). When antibodies and antigens combine, the avidity is determined by the "best fit" or compatibility between the interacting structures. The actual fit will depend on the number of points

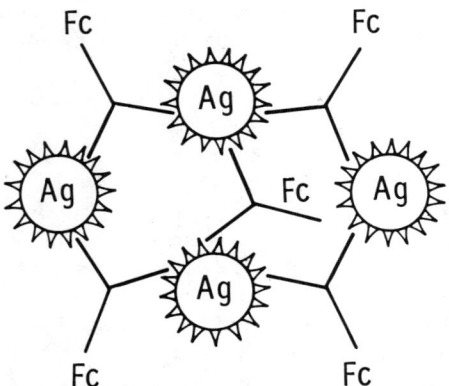

FIG 4–5.—Antigen-antibody lattice formation. Antibody-binding sites are attached to antigenic sites. Free terminals of the monomers are Fc fragments with no antibody-binding site activity.

of contact between the combining site and the antigen. Thus, the affinity of antibody for antigen will be greater if the number of points of contact is large (Fig 4–7). These points of contact are the hypervariable regions (three found in the light chain[60] and four on the heavy chain[61] of the immunoglobulin molecule). The amino acids actually involved in bonding to antigen are quite limited.[62] Arginine, histidine, tyrosine, and tryptophan are often involved in hypervariable regions. In contrast, proline, cysteine, and cystine are more often involved in the three-dimensional folding of the antibody molecule.

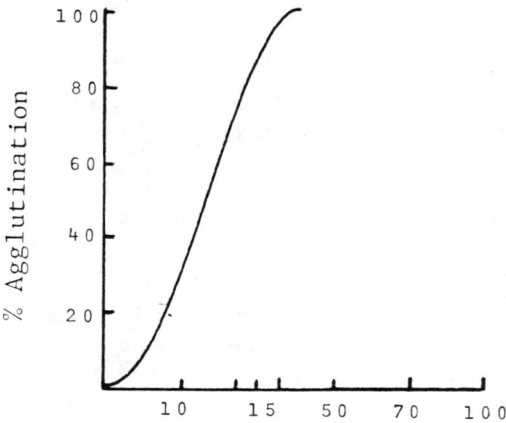

FIG 4–6.—Concentration of antibody plotted against percent agglutination is not linear. After a certain concentration is reached, no further agglutination occurs.

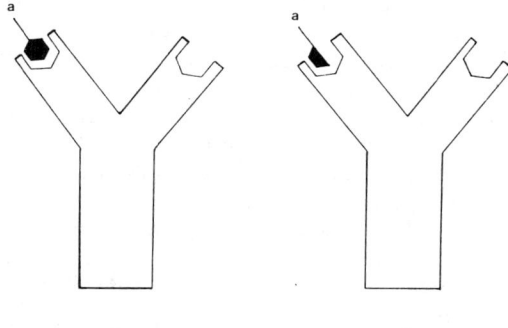

FIG 4–7.—Complementarity of antibody and antigen. **A,** antibody and antigen (a) are fully complementary. Several points of contact ensure greater strength in bonding. **B,** antibody and antigen (a) are partially complementary. The bond is less strong than in **A**.

The actual forces involved in the bond are electrostatic, hydrogen bonding, dipolar, hydrophobic, and van der Waals forces. Of these, the hydrogen bond appears to be the most significant.[58] Evidently these molecular bonds are affected by pH and ionic strength (see Chap. 6).

Different amino acids in the combining site have different functions (Table 4–3). Why RBCs agglutinate on addition of antibody is a complex phenomenon. It is quite possible that RBCs remain separate due to zeta potential (see Chap. 6) and also due to a hydration envelope provided by the RBC's membrane sialic acid affinity for water.[63] Along with other factors, such as actual binding, antibodies very probably affect this water envelope, thus promoting agglutination.[63]

Monoclonal Antibodies

Polyclonal antibodies are the primary tool for the detection and study of antigens in the immunology and immunohematology laboratory. Furthermore, antibodies have become part of the clinical armory of medicine in the form of passive immunization, examples of which are prevention of Rh immunization of Rh-negative mothers, passive immunization against hepatitis, and enhancing survival of a transplanted organ.

Nevertheless, cross-reactivity and multispecificity present in polyclonal antibodies have haunted researchers and clinical laboratory scientists in both testing and therapeutic applications of antibodies. These unwanted characteristics of polyclonal antibodies are absent in monoclonal antibodies. Monoclonal antibodies are produced by tumoral clones of B cells in their end stage of differentiation, namely plasma cells. Since these antibodies are secreted by cells originating from a single clone, the spectrum of specificity and cross-reactivity is narrowed to the point where specificity will be unique, and cross-reactivity will be limited by one type of combining site alone.[64]

The problem that remained to be solved was how to control or induce the specificity of antibody formation by a cell which had already been committed to monoclonal neoplastic proliferation, the specificity of which was likewise predetermined and selected at random by the tumoral process. This seemingly insurmountable problem was solved by a technique developed by Kohler and Milstein:[65] the artificial fusion of lymphocytes from deliberately immunized animals, with a clone of plasma cells capable of antibody secretion. This technique has caused a veritable revolution in immunology and its related sciences. It has provided scientists with an extraordinarily powerful tool, that of a homogeneous, monospecific antibody of selected specificity.

The technique[66] is summarized as follows: Mice or rats are immunized to a specific antigen. Good antibody responders are selected and sacrificed for their spleens. Lymphocyte single cell suspensions from these spleens are mixed with a line of drug-marked, cultured, secreting mouse myeloma cells. The mixture of cells is fused by adding polyethylene glycol, an agent that acts on cell membranes, allowing two different cells to become one fused cell. The cell mixture contains single lymphocytes, single myeloma cells, and fused cells of the same

TABLE 4–3.—Bonds Produced by Different Amino Acid Groups*

BOND	AMINO ACID
van der Waals, hydrophobic	Alanine
	Valine
	Leucine
	Isoleucine
	Phenylalanine
	Methionine
	Tryptophan
Electrostatic	Aspartic acid
	Glutamic acid
	Lysine
	Arginine
Hydrogen bond	Serine
	Threonine
	Tyrosine
	Asparagine
	Glutamine

*Modified from Stean.[58]

type, but, most important, it also contains hybrids of antigen-specific primed lymphocytes and myeloma cells. The lymphocyte-myeloma hybrids can now be selectively grown in medium containing hypoxanthine, aminopterin, and thymidine (HAT medium). This culture medium does not encourage the growth of the other cells. Lymphocytes do not thrive in culture unless special conditions are met. Drug-marked myeloma cells and myeloma-myeloma hybrids will not thrive because of the genetic deletion of hypoxanthine-guanine phosphoril transferase and the absence of HPRT, which in HAT medium is toxic to these cells. However, lymphocyte-myeloma cells will survive because the lymphocyte genome provides the hybrid with enzymes capable of metabolizing adequately in HAT culture medium.

In order to select a single hybrid per culture well, the cells are diluted to the point where one cell alone will be expected per defined cell suspension volume. This volume is then placed in each of 96 wells of culture microplates. It can be expected that 100–1,000 different hybrids result from this procedure. Of these, very few produce the antibody specific to the priming antigen. About 0.5 mg/ml of antibody is produced in culture medium. In order to select the clone of interest, a screening method is necessary to determine which wells contain the antibody of selected specificity. This is achieved by radioimmunoassay[56] or by enzyme-linked immunoassays.[66] Both methods are highly sensitive and involve binding of antigen to polystyrene wells and the addition of supernates to assess binding to antigen linked to well walls. The amount of antibody bound after washing is determined by adding labeled antimouse κ antibodies to determine monoclonality.

Counting is performed by placing the cut wells in a gamma counter, in the case of a radiolabeled assay, or testing the supernatants fluids for color reaction, in the case of chromogenic enzyme-linked assays.[66] The selected clones are then propagated in larger culture flasks. In order to obtain significant amounts of antibody, the clones are injected intraperitoneally into mice, which develop tumors and ascites containing large amounts of monoclonal antibodies. The ascites fluid will contain up to 5 mg/ml of antibody, 90% of which is monoclonal antibody.[67, 68]

It is quite possible that in vitro immunization prior to fusion will allow the development of monoclonal antibodies in a less cumbersome manner.[69] The multitude of different actual and potential uses of monoclonal antibodies is beyond the scope of this review. However, it must be stressed that monoclonal antibodies are today a reality; they will become increasingly available as different clones to specific antigens are developed and may eventually replace many of the reagents currently used as polyclonal reagents, such as Coombs reagents and blood typing reagents. We will, however, outline some of the uses of monoclonal antibodies of most interest to immunohematology.

In most laboratories specializing in immunology workups, lymphocyte enumeration by subtyping using monoclonal antibodies is a routine test. This is possible due to the development of monoclonal antibodies which react with stable glycoproteins present on the surface of the different lymphocyte subpopulations.[70] T cells can be subdivided into their different subpopulations using monoclonal antibodies and enumerating cells by immunofluorescence. Monoclonal antibodies against helper/inducer T cells bind to the T4 antigen, whereas anti-T8 antibodies bind to cytotoxic/suppressor T cells. The trade designations for these reagents are OKT4 (Leu-3) and OKT8 (Leu-2), respectively. OK reagents are produced by Ortho Diagnostics (Raritan, N.J.) and Leu reagents are produced by Becton-Dickinson (Mountain View, CA). Other monoclonal antibodies against T cells are likewise available. Anti-T1 will detect all thymocytes. T9 and T10 detect early thymocytes,[71] but these antigens may be present on malignant non-T cells and in mitogen-stimulated T cells.[72] Mature postthymic resting T cells lack T10 antigens.[73] The studies with these reagents is critical in the diagnosis of various congenital and acquired immune deficiencies (see Chap. 13).

At the blood banking level, monoclonal antibodies have been obtained against several antigens. Some examples are monoclonal antibodies against all the products of the HLA-A, B, and C loci, and HLA-DRw1, 2 and 6.[74] Monoclonal antibodies against group A substance[75] and against group B substance[76] have also been obtained. Likewise, hybridomas have been raised which produce anti-M and anti-N antibodies.[77, 78] Monoclonal antibodies against IgG have not been very satisfactory;[79] however, anticomplement hybridoma antibodies have been raised against C3 and C4.[80] These reagents are commercially available from Ortho Diagnostics (Raritan, N.J.).

Even though monoclonal antibodies appear to have great promise as reagents in the blood bank, there are some difficulties involving the use of these reagents. (1) It is difficult to produce monoclonal antibodies against weak immunogens. (2) Monoclonal antibodies are quite sensitive to changes in pH and temperature.[81] (3) Hybridoma lines may become unstable and lose their ability to synthesize the required antibody structure.[82] (4) Monoclonal antibodies do not form the complex lattice structures necessary for agglutination. This could be bypassed by combining antibodies with distinct antigenic determinants on the same antigen.[83] (5) Paradoxically, monoclonal antibodies may be cross-reactive if they have high affinity to antigen, and this may pose problems in those monoclonal antibodies of high affinity.[84] (6) Finally, monoclonal antibodies are very expensive to manufacture.

Monoclonal Antibodies in the Analysis of Clotting Factors.—Monoclonal antibodies have been raised against factor VIII (von Willebrand factor),[85] against factor VIII coagulant protein (VIII:C),[86] and against factor IX,[87] factor V,[88] and fibrinogen.[89] Platelet surface glycoprotein gpIb, which is a likely receptor for FVIII/vWF, has been characterized with the help of monoclonal antibodies.[90] Likewise, glycoprotein gpIIb/IIIa which is the likely receptor for fibrinogen, has also been characterized with the help of monoclonal antibodies.[91] The relative proximity of the different molecular components of factor VIII has been determined by calculating a logarithmic index of radiolabeled monoclonal antibody binding.[92]

Laboratory Methods for Detecting Antigen-Antibody Reactions

Immunodiffusion.—Immunodiffusion entails the detection of antigen-antibody reactions by visible precipitation on a gel matrix. The precipitation patterns depend to a great extent on the concentration of both the antigen and the antibodies in the system. A prozone in such system is the incomplete or suboptimal precipitation due to antibody excess. Dilutions of antisera usually correct this deficiency. The immunodiffusion method was discovered by Oudin and standardized for use in laboratory by Ouchterlony. Since then it has been called the double immunodiffusion or Ouchterlony technique (Fig 4–8).

If the antibody is blended with the gel and a well is cut to permit diffusion of antigen into the matrix, antigen concentration can be measured by

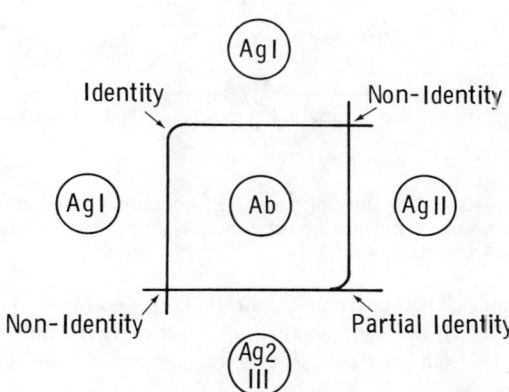

FIG 4–8.—Ouchterlony plate. Identity *(upper left)* is shown by fusion of precipitin lines. Nonidentity *(upper left and lower left)* is depicted by crossing precipitin lines. Partial identity *(lower left)* is depicted by fused precipitin lines and a spur.

plotting diameters of diffusion rings against controls (Fig 4–9). This type of plate is called a Mancini plate.

Electrophoresis.—The separation of proteins on a gel matrix subjected to an electrical field was first demonstrated by Tiselius; the technique is called *zone electrophoresis*.[93] Proteins are separated on the basis of their electrical charge. If the matrix is then stained and washed, protein bands can be identified (Fig 4–10). *Immunoelectrophoresis* is an extremely informative method in laboratory immunology.[93] The method combines zone electrophoresis with immunodiffusion. The method is outlined in Figure 4–11. Many variations of methods have been used to study proteins of various sorts.

In *affinity chromatography,* antigens or antibodies are coupled with gel beads and their respective antibodies or antigens are passed through chromatographic columns.[94] The substance of interest can then be eluted with specified solutions.

Other methods that may help define antigen-antibody reactions are differential centrifugation, radioimmunoassays, nephelometry, and immunofluorescence. Details of these methods are found in general references.[95, 96]

THE COMPLEMENT SYSTEM

Characteristics and Nomenclature

The complement system can be regarded as the principal effector arm of antibody-mediated reac-

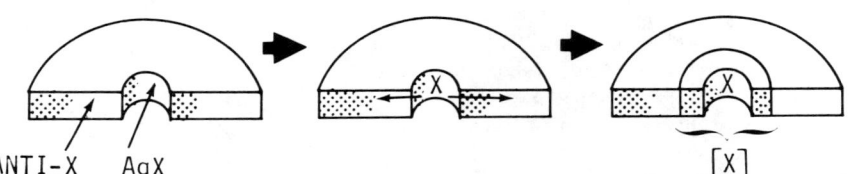

FIG 4–9.—Mancini plate. *Left gel* contains anti-*x* antibody in gel matrix, antigen *x* in well. *Middle gel* shows diffusion of antigen into the gel. *Right gel* shows a precipitin circle, the diameter of which is equivalent to the concentration of *x* [x].

tions. That is, complement is often necessary for antibody to bring about lysis of cells (e.g., hemolysis) and therefore is of great interest to blood bankers. However, lysis is not the only function of complement. The major functions of the system can be summarized as follows: (1) lytic functions, (2) production of anaphylatoxins, and (3) sensitization of cells during opsonization.

The complement system, like the coagulation cascade, is activated as a chain of enzymatic reactions which convert previously inert plasma proteins into enzymes capable of limited proteolytic cleaving of the proteins involved in subsequent steps in the chain of activation; this constitutes the initial stage of activation and encompasses the first components of complement, C1–C5, and factor B. The second part of the activation involves the formation of protein-protein complexes (C5b–C9) capable of membrane lysis.[97]

The complement system consists of a group of at least 20 plasma proteins designated C1 to C9 and by trivial names such as properdin, factor B, and factor D.

The system comprises about 15% of the plasma protein,[98] adding to a total of about 300 mg/dl.[99]

The third component (C3) exists in plasma in a concentration of over 1 mg/dl, making it the fourth more abundant protein, after immunoglobulin, albumin, and transferrin. Some physicochemical characteristics of complement components are given in Table 4–4.

On activation, the components are designated with an overlying bar, e.g., $\overline{C1s}$ or $\overline{C42}$. If a component is enzymatically cleaved during activation, the split products are designated with a lower case letter. For example, the split products of C3 are C3a and C3b. When a component is labile, it is followed by an asterisk e.g., C3b.*

Complement Activation

There are two pathways for the activation of complement, the classical pathway[100] and the alternative pathway.[101, 102]

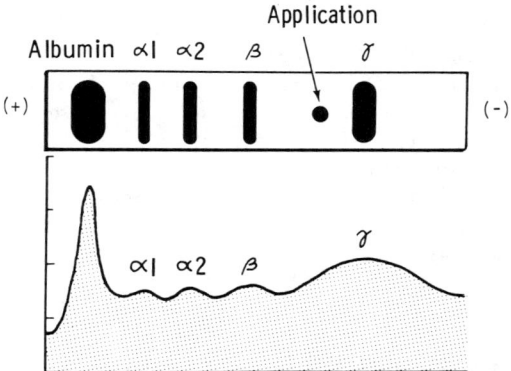

FIG 4–10.—Zone electrophoresis. γ-Globulins migrate to the negative pole from the application site, whereas β-, α_1-, and α_2-globulins as well as albumin migrate to the positive pole.

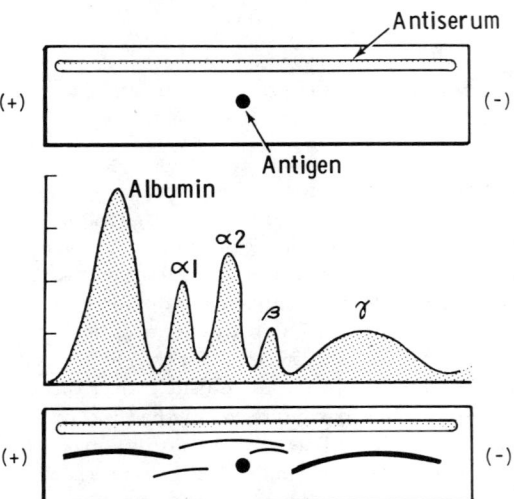

FIG 4–11.—Immunoelectrophoresis. Heavy precipitin arc on the right is produced by γ-globulin. Heavy arc on the left is produced by albumin.

TABLE 4–4.—Characteristics of Complement Components, by Pathway

COMPONENT	CONCENTRATION (mg/ml)	MW (daltons)	ELECTROPHORESIS AT pH 8.6	NUMBER OF CHAINS	SITE OF SYNTHESIS*	COMPONENT USED AS ENZYMATIC SUBSTRATE	ACTIVATION PRODUCTS
			Classical Pathway				
Recognition unit							
C1q	0.15	400,000	γ_2	6 × 3	IE		
C1r	0.05	166,000	β	2	IE	C1s	$\overline{C1r}$
C1s	0.05	83,000	α	1	IE	C4,C2	$\overline{C1s}$
Activation unit							
C4	0.45	200,000	β	3	M		C4a,C4b
C2	0.03	100,000	β	1	M	C3,C5	C2a,C2b
C3	1.20	200,000	β	2	Lv, M		C3a,C3b
Membrane attack unit							
C5	0.07	200,000	β	2	Sp, M		C5a,C5b
C6	0.06	130,000	β_2	1			
C7	0.05	120,000	β_2	1	Lv		
C8	0.08	154,000	γ	3	Sp		
C9	0.15	77,000	α	1	Lv		
			Alternative Pathway				
Factor B	0.20	90,000	β_2	1	Lv, M, L	C3,C5	Ba,Bb
Factor D	0.001	23,000	α_2	1		B	
			Control Proteins				
C1-INH	0.19	100,000		1			
Factor I (C3b inactivator)	0.035	100,000	β	2			C3b,C4b,C5b
Factor H	0.475	150,000	β	1			
C4-binding protein	0.250	590,000		8			
Anaphylatoxin inactivator	Trace	310,000		1			C3a,C4a,C5a
Properdin	0.025	185,000	γ_2	4			
S protein	0.500	84,000		2			

*IE, intestinal epithelium, Lv, liver; Sp, spleen; M, macrophages; L, lymphocytes.

Classical Pathway

The components involved in the classical pathway are C1 to C3. From the formation of C3b on, this pathway shares the lytic components with the alternative pathway. In order to understand some of the mechanisms involved in the complement system it is necessary to briefly review some of the biochemistry of the components.

Most of the components C1–C9 are glycoproteins found as single-chain or multichain units.[99] They constitute families of proteins with enough similarities to suggest that they resulted from gene duplication from common ancestors.[101, 103]

The first component of complement is composed of three major proteins: C1q, C1r, C1s. The C1q molecule is a γ_2-globulin whose appearance on electron microscopy has been likened to a bunch of six tulips.[104] The heads are globular proteins, and the stalks are 18-polypeptide chains with collagen-like amino acid sequences.[105] The six globular heads can each attach to the Fc portion of a molecule of IgG or IgM which in turn has bound to antigen. It is necessary for two Fc portions of the antibody molecules to be close together in order to bind C1q. Therefore, IgM can bind C1q on its own account.[106]

If IgG is involved, two molecules must be attached in a proximity of between 250 and 400 Å before C1q can be bound.[106] The attachment of these structures is probably to the C_H2 domain of the Fc portion of immunoglobulins capable of binding complement.[107]

Not all immunoglobulins have the same capacity to bind complement, and some are not known to bind complement (Table 4–5).

C1r is a β-globulin composed of two 83,000-dalton chains linked by disulfide bonds. C1s is a single-chain α-globulin.

C2 is a single-chain β_1-globulin and is structurally very similar to factor B of the alternative pathway.[108] C4 is composed of three chains and runs as a β_1-globulin on electrophoresis.

C3 and C5 only have two chains and run as β_2- and β_1-globulins, respectively. C3 and C4 are initially synthesized as a single chain, and the multichain structure is most probably formed by postsynthetic cleavage.[103] It is thought that ancestrally, C3, C4, and C5 have a common origin.[99]

C6 and C7 have a similar molecular weight and some homology, likewise suggesting a common gene ancestry.[109] They are both single-chain β_2-globulins (see Table 4–4).

C8 is a γ-globulin composed of three chains. C9 is a single-chain α-globulin.

Biosynthesis of Complement Components

Little is known about the detailed biosynthesis of complement components. Some of the known data are shown in Table 4–4. Other data are discussed below.

By in vitro studies it has been shown that macrophages synthesize C2, C3, C4, C5, FD, FB, I, and H in vitro.[103, 110] Hepatocyte in vitro studies, hepatoma cell studies, and liver transplantation studies showing allotype conversion of complement components in the recipient[111] demonstrate that the hepatocyte can synthesize C1, C3, C6, C8, and C9 as well as factor B.

The intestinal epithelium and the urothelium are likewise capable of synthesizing C1q, C1r, and C1s.[103] Under special conditions, tumor cells in culture, such as HeLa cells, will synthesize C4.[112]

Activation of the Classical Pathway.—Activation of the classical pathway is initiated by the

TABLE 4–5.—DIFFERING FC-DEPENDENT CHARACTERISTICS OF IMMUNOGLOBULINS

CLASS	BINDING OF COMPLEMENT		PLACENTAL TRANSPORT	BINDING TO MONOCYTES	BINDING TO SECRETORY CELLS	BINDING TO MAST CELLS
	Classical	Alternative				
IgG1	+ +	+	+ + +	+ +	+	+
IgG2	+	0	+	0	0	0
IgG3	+ + +	+	+ +	+ + +	+	+
IgG4	0	0	+	0	0	0
IgA	0	+ +	0	0	+ + +	0
IgM	+ + +	+	0	±	+	0
IgD	0	0	0	0	0	0
IgE	0	?	0	0	0	+ + +

binding of C1q, primarily to immunoglobulins and, less importantly from a biologic viewpoint, to other molecules. This activation of C1 produces a molecular structure that is termed recognition unit. C1 is a calcium-dependent trimolecular complex that in its native form exists as a single molecule of C1q plus two polypeptide chains each of C1r and C1s. Thus the molecule is designated C1q C1r2 C1s2.[113] This molecular composition has been determined with equimolar concentrations of purified C1r and C1s in the presence of calcium, and shown to sediment as dimers, at rates of 8.5–8.7 with the structure C1r2 C1s2.[114] In the presence of C1q a 16S complex is formed, C1q C1r2 C1s2.[115]

There are several conditions for the activation of C1: (1) The complex C1q C1r2 C1s must be present. (2) Immunoglobulins or other activating substances must exist in aggregates. (3) Several globular heads of C1q must be "occupied."[116]

Knowledge that it is the globular heads that are involved in binding to immunoglobulins has come from studies where collagenase-digested C1q inhibited binding of C1q to immunoglobulins.[117] Earlier in this section we reviewed the capacity of different immunoglobulins to bind C1q (see Table 4–5).

Nevertheless, the aggregated Fc portions of, for instance, IgA and IgG4 immunoglobulins are indeed capable of binding C1q, which suggests that the native molecules are incapable of exposing binding sites to the globular heads of C1q.[118] For instance, one molecule of IgM, bent in the "staple" configuration on binding to one molecule of the D antigen of Rh is sufficient for exposure of the Fc areas capable of binding C1q.[118] The area of the Fc fragment capable of binding C1q has been shown to be the $C_H 2$ domain of the constant region.[107]

Apart from aggregated immunoglobulin, other diverse chemicals can activate C1q. Some examples are mitochondrial and other cellular membranes,[119] monosodium urate crystals, lipid A lipopolysaccharides, gram-negative bacteria, parasites, and heparin.[113]

The binding of C1q C1r2 C1s2 to activating surfaces results in the conversion of C1r to an active enzyme, $\overline{C1r}$. $\overline{C1r}$ hydrolyzes C1s zymogen to $\overline{C1s}$, which cleaves C4 to C4b and C4a, thereby initiating activation of the classical pathway. $\overline{C1r}$ has as its sole substrate C1s, which it splits to form $\overline{C1s}$; however, $\overline{C1s}$ can split a variety of amino acid esters (e.g., arginine and tyrosine esters), and it cleaves its natural substrates, C4 and C2.

$\overline{C1s}$ splits an 8,000-dalton fragment from the N-terminus of the α chain of C4; this fragment is C4a. The remaining larger fragment is C4b. C4b is capable of binding hydrophobically to cell surfaces within its vicinity. Only 10%–15% of C4b binds to cell membranes. The remainder stays in solution.

C4b reacts reversibly with C2 in the presence of magnesium ions. $\overline{C1q}$ can now split C2 in two fragments: a larger C2b fragment (MW = 74,000), formerly called C2a, and a smaller C2a fragment (MW = 34,000), formerly called C2b. The larger fragment remains attached to C4b, forming a C4b2b complex,[120] also termed $\overline{C42}$ or C3b convertase. $\overline{C42}$ is enzymatically active and capable of cleaving C3 into a small fragment, C3a, and a larger fragment, C3b (Fig 4–12).

C3a has anaphylatoxin activity and goes to the fluid phase.[121] It is at the C3b stage of activation that the classical and alternative pathways meet. However, for the sake of clarity we will continue with the analysis of the classical pathway and discuss the alternative pathway later (Fig 4–13).

The Membrane Attack Unit.—Unlike the activation unit (C1–C5), the membrane attack unit (C5–C9) is not a sequential enzymatic process. Instead, the attack unit involves the close association

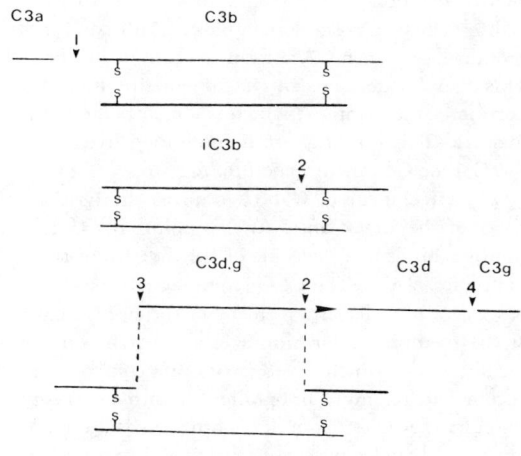

FIG 4–12.—C3 cleavage products: Formation of C3a and C3b *(1)*, iC3b *(2)*, C3d,g *(3)*, and C3d,C3g *(4)*.

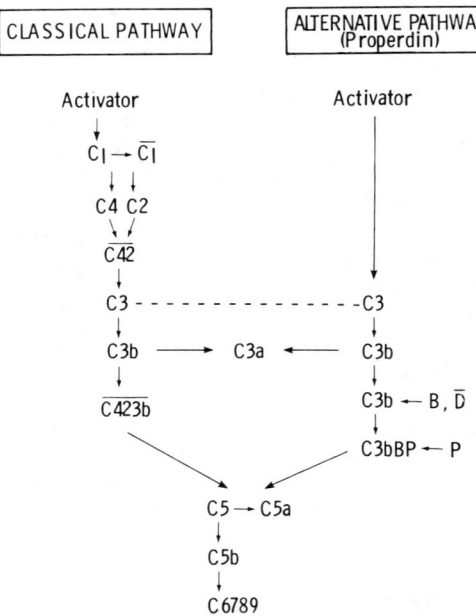

FIG 4–13.—Activation of complement via the classical and alternative or properdin pathways. Both pathways share activation of complement from C5 to C9.

of protein molecules in a protein-protein interaction.

C$\overline{42}$ also splits C5 into two fragments, C5a and C5b. C5a is a potent anaphylatoxin that acts directly on the contractility of smooth muscle cells in vitro.[122]

C3b binds loosely to C5b, but it does so sufficiently to allow C5b to bind to C6 and to form C5b6, which is a stable complex. C5b6 combines spontaneously with C7 to form the complex C5b67. This complex develops an attachment site in the C5 portion of the complex, which is a membrane binding site. This binding site is more long-lived than the C3b or C4b membrane binding sites.

The attachment of C5b67 localizes the lytic activity of the attack unit. At this point, the C5b67 complex binds one molecule of C8 and two or three molecules of C9. The C5–9 complex is thought to produce a micellar arrangement of the lipid bilayer of the membrane, forming a "leaky patch" on the membrane,[123] which, as it recruits its components, becomes increasingly lipophilic.[124] An older theory suggests that C5–9 complexes function as a doughnut-shaped molecule that is inserted in the membrane.[125]

Regardless of which model is correct, there is evidence that C5b–9 complexes and to a lesser degree C5b–8 complexes will produce transmembrane channels of varying diameter (1–4 mm).[126]

The difference in speed of lysis between cells exposed to C5b–8 and C5b–9 is probably due to the fact that C5b–8 lesions are smaller than those produced by C5b–9.[127]

Lysis of anucleated cells is much more effective than lysis of nucleated cells because nucleated cells are capable of membrane repair. Nucleated cells treated with a metabolic inhibitor such as Puromycin become more susceptible to C567-initiated cytolysis.[128]

The Alternative Pathway of Complement

Activation of complement via the alternative pathway is biologically important because it can occur in the absence of antibody and therefore is an important defense mechanism.[129] The alternative pathway is similar to the classical pathway in that it will produce an attack unit by enzymatic cleavage of C3 and subsequent recruitment of C5b–9. It is different from the classical pathway in that it has a positive feedback amplification mechanism, resulting in membrane attachment of several units of C3b.

The alternative pathway is composed of six serum proteins, one of which (C3) is shared with the classical pathway. For details on the chemistry and properties of the components of the alternative pathway, see Tables 4–5 and 4–6.

Activation of the Alternative Pathway.—
Activation of the alternative pathway can be considered in two parts: initiation and amplification.[129]

Initiation of the Alternative Pathway.—
The alternative pathway can be initiated by a variety of substances in the absence of antibody. It preferentially consumes C3–C9 without utilization of C1, C2, or C4. Endotoxin from gram-negative organisms,[130] viruses, virus-infected cells, tumor cells, parasites, agarose, and inulin can trigger the alternative pathway.[131,132] Furthermore, aggregated immunoglobulin (especially IgA and certain subclasses of IgG) can also activate the alternative pathway, bypassing C1, C4, and C2 activation.[102] Aggregated immunoglobulin may also be involved in enhancing the alternative pathway.[133] There is some question as to whether the alternative pathway can be activated by immunoglobulin aggregates, due to possible contamination of these prep-

TABLE 4–6.—CHARACTERISTICS OF PROTEINS INVOLVED
IN THE ALTERNATIVE PATHWAY

COMPONENT	MW (daltons)	CHAINS	SERUM CONCENTRATION (mg/ml)	ELECTROPHORETIC MOBILITY
C3	200,000	2	1.200	β
Factor B	90,000	1	0.200	β_2
Factor D	23,000	1	0.001	α_2
H (β_1-H)	150,000	1	0.475	β
I (C3b inactivator)	100,000	2	0.035	β
P (properdin)	185,000	4	0.025	γ_2

arations with endotoxin, which in itself may activate the alternative pathway.[99] IgG antibodies may be involved in the activation of the alternative pathway by measles virus–infected cells.[134]

Initiation occurs by one of the above-mentioned substances, which act on C3 to produce metastable C3b.[135] Metastable C3b is probably produced constantly in the fluid phase at a slow rate,[136] attaching randomly to nearby surfaces. A cleaving of the internal thiol ester of C3 produces a C3b-like molecule, which is C3(H_2O) or hydrolyzed C3. C3(H_2O) interacts with factor B in the presence of magnesium to form C3bB complexes only when bound to C3b. Factor B is susceptible to proteolysis by factor D, which is a serine protease.[137] Cleavage of factor B releases a 33,000-dalton fragment, Ba, which forms C3bBb. C3bBb is the central enzyme of the alternative pathway[138] and essentially is a C3 convertase. The Bb portion of the molecule is a serine protease.[139] This molecule splits C3 into C3a and C3b. In addition C3b can be generated by tissue enzymes and enzymes from the fibrinolytic or coagulation cascade, which can combine with factors B and D to form C3bBb. Thus, C3b generated can bind to cell membranes and initiate lysis. C3b bound to membranes is protected from the usual inactivators of the alternative pathway,[140] namely factors H and I (Fig 4–14) (see Table 4–6 for details on the alternative pathway components).

C3bBb is converted to C3bPBb when it binds to properdin. Properdin, though not essential to the activation of the alternative pathway, does provide a 10-fold increase in stability and protects the complex from the destabilized activity of factor Bb.

Amplification of the Alternative Pathway.—Amplification of the alternative pathway is a C3b-dependent positive feedback process.[138] It works as follows. On formation of C3bBb, which is a C3 convertase, generation of many molecules of C3b by splitting of C3 takes place. In the presence of excess factor B, more C3bBb is formed, which in turn cleaves more available C3, resulting in a significant positive feedback system capable of activating the system geometrically. When the C3b so generated attaches to cell membranes, the control proteins H and I inactivate many of the C3b molecules. However, when C3b attaches to activators, such as polysaccharides, viruses, and parasites,[129] these structures in themselves restrict the effective control by factors H and I.[132] At the same time,

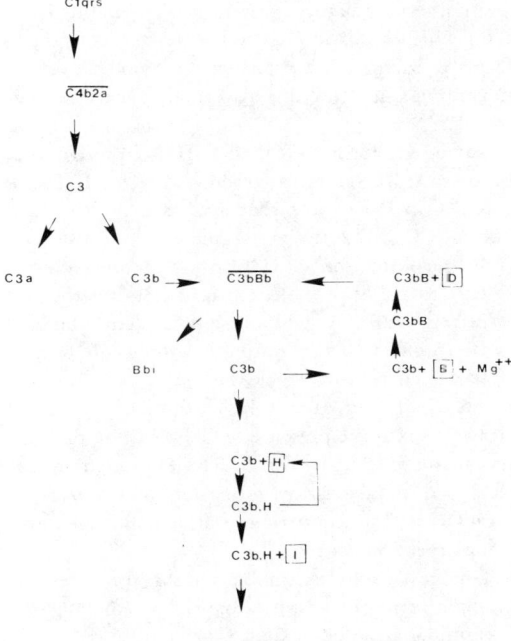

FIG 4–14.—Classical (C1qrs) activation interacting with alternative (C3bBb) activation. The C3b formed acts as a feedback cycle. On combination with factor B, a self-amplifying loop is formed (center). Factor H and factor I are regulatory proteins.

the great quantity of C3b that is generated interacts in close proximity to activator-bound $\overline{\text{C3bPBb}}$ and $\overline{\text{C3bBb}}$, resulting in the formation of modified enzymes $\overline{\text{C3b}_n\text{Bb}}$ and $\overline{\text{C3b}_n\text{PBb}}$ ($n > 1$), which have the ability to cleave C5 and initiate the membrane attack mechanism, just as described earlier for the classical pathway.

Control Mechanisms of the Complement System

It is not surprising that higher organisms possess the ability to control a mechanism of cell lysis as potent as the complement system. The control mechanisms involve various regulatory proteins.

In the classical pathway, a C1 inhibitor exists,[141] a glycoprotein containing 40% carbohydrate, that acts stoichiometrically on $\overline{\text{C1r}}$ and $\overline{\text{C1s}}$. This inhibitor is a protease inhibitor and therefore also capable of inhibiting plasmin, kallikrein, activated factor XII, and activated factor XI. The molecule is responsible for preventing the nonrestricted action of $\overline{\text{C1}}$ on C4. Its genetic deficiency causes hereditary angioedema due to the formation of C4, C2, C3, and C5 cleavage units, which are vasoactive.

Another regulatory protein is C4-binding protein, which binds to C4b and serves as a cofactor to factor I. Factor I is a proteolytic enzyme capable of degrading C4b, cleaving it to smaller inactive fragments.[142]

Factor H, formerly called β-1H, a protein that binds to C3b, serves as cofactor to factor I. Factor I is a C3b inactivator that acts as a protease and degrades C3b to inactive fragments.[143] It also controls the formation of C3bBb.[144] Factor I cleaves C3b at two sites of the α chain of C3b but the two resulting small fragments remain covalently bonded to the β chain;[145] this results in a molecule termed iC3b which on further cleavage gives rise to fragments C3c, C3d, and C3e.[146] Similarly, factor I cleaves C4b in the presence of C4b-binding protein, producing C4c and C4d.[147] The S protein modulates and regulates the formation of C5–9 complexes and thus controls the attack unit phase of complement activation.[148]

Finally, anaphylatoxin inactivator abrogates the biologic action of anaphylatoxins by removing the C-terminal arginine of C3a, C4a, and C5a.[149]

Complement Receptors on Cells

There is evidence from experiments of radioactively labeled C1q that a receptor for C1q exists on granulocytes, monocytes, B lymphocytes, and a small percentage of T cells and null cells.[97] Granulocytes, for instance, are thought to possess from 150,000 to 600,000 C1q receptors.[150]

The C1q receptor is sensitive to trypsin, but no other knowledge is available as to the physicochemical properties of the receptor. The C1q receptor-ligand interaction mediates a respiratory burst and activation of the cell bearing the receptor.[150]

The C3b receptor, also termed CR1, exists on RBCs, neutrophils, eosinophils, monocytes, macrophages, B and T cells, mast cells, and glomerular podocytes.[151]

With the help of polyclonal and monoclonal antibodies, this receptor has been further characterized.[152,153] The C3b receptor has thus been shown to be a 250,000-dalton membrane glycoprotein.[152] The structure of the receptor is an inherited polymorphic trait, as evidenced by the interindividual differences in CR1 electrophoretic mobility.[151]

There is an average of 500–600 C3b receptors per RBC. Receptors on cells from patients with SLE are decreased. This is an inherited rather than acquired condition and may be related to the physiopathology of SLE.[153] Neutrophils have about 140,000 receptors per cell.[153] Temperature increases in the live culture incubation of these cells produce a dramatic increase in the number of CR1 receptors. Chemotactic factors also produce increments in the number of C3b receptors on cells.[154] C3b receptors on RBCs are thought to serve as carriers of immune complexes, which are then transferred to cells in the reticuloendothelial system.[155] CR1 on macrophages and neutrophils has long been known to be associated with phagocytosis.[151] C3 receptor type 2 (CR2) is present on B cells but not on T cells, monocytes, or neutrophils.[156]

CR2 is a 72,000-dalton glycoprotein and may likewise be the receptor of C3d.[157] The number of CR2 receptors on cells is not presently known. CR2 probably plays a role in B cell/T cell communication and cell-cell interactions, as shown by the inhibitory effect of F(ab')$_2$ antibody to CR2 on lymphocyte proliferative responses.[158]

The CR3 receptor is present on monocytes, neutrophils, lymphocytes, and glomerular podocytes.[152] It is thought that CR3 and the Mac-1 antigen of macrophages are the same molecule, but evidence in support of this suggestion is not conclusive.[151]

It is possible that C3d,g is the ligand of CR3.[159] About 60,000 receptors per cell have been calculated for CR3.[151] Cells bearing CR3 receptors degranulate on incubation with C3d,g.[151]

Factor H receptors exist on leukocytes in a density of about 157,000 receptors per cell. This has been determined using Raji B lymphoblastoid cells.[160] Protein polypeptides of 100,000 daltons and 50,000 daltons have been immunoprecipitated with H ligand, which suggests that the receptor is within this molecular weight range.[160] Receptors for diffusible factors also exist on effector cells. Strong evidence for the existence of C3a receptors on mast cells has been available for a long time.[161]

C3a and C4a both share a functional homology,[162] as evidenced by abolition of the contractile response of ileum by C3a or C4a if the tissue is preincubated with either C3a or C4a.[162] Mast cells, basophils, neutrophils, eosinophils, monocytes, and macrophages respond to the stimulus of C5a[151] by degranulation or a respiratory burst, as shown by chemiluminescence.[163]

Role of Complement in Phagocytosis

C3b is involved in the attachment of the target particle to be engulfed and the phagocyte, which, as discussed above, has receptors of various types for the different components of complement. If immunoglobulin coats the target, it is mainly IgG that is actually involved in the process of phagocytosis by nonactivated macrophages.[164] Thus, complement and IgG potentiate each other during phagocytosis.[165] It should be noted, however, that activated macrophages may exhibit C3b receptor-dependent phagocytosis in the absence of IgG.[166] Complement-independent lysis of IgG-coated particles such as anti-D coated RBCs can be lysed by killer lymphocytes in the absence of complement.[167] There is evidence that when cells are incubated with Ig and complement at low ionic strength, it is complement (probably C4) that helps binding of antibody to target cells.[168]

Complement-sensitized RBCs that are not taken to the lytic phase of complement activation (C5–9), are usually trapped by the liver, later released, and survive normally.[169] Presumably such trapping is via Kupffer cells[169] and the subsequent release into the circulation is due to C3b inactivator. This enzyme would cleave C3b, C3c would remain attached to the macrophage, and C3d would remain attached to the coated particle, in this case the RBC.[169] Some of the cells are converted into spherocytes in this process and exhibit a shortened survival in cases of immune hemolysis mediated by complement coating.

The relationship between complement coating and receptors for complement on phagocytic cells has been further elucidated by recent studies.

It is necessary to discuss this information regarding IgM antibody-mediated complement coating of target particle versus coating mediated by IgG because IgG-mediated binding involves Fc receptor binding in addition to complement binding, and phagocytic cells often have both Fc receptors as well as complement receptors.

As far as is known today, the role of IgM in the extravascular destruction of RBCs lies in the attachment of complement,[170] although some evidence exists that IgM is capable of inducing cell injury in the absence of complement.[171]

Binding of C4b3b (which has not been cleaved by β_1-H) to RBCs will bind to CR1 via the C3c cleavage portion of C4b3b. The binding occurs on the membrane of monocytes, macrophages, granulocytes, or other cells bearing the CR1 receptor.[170] Once C4b3b has been cleaved by β_1-H, this complement complex will also adhere to CR2 and CR3 receptors. Cells coated with C4d3d attach to CR2, which serves as a ligand for this complex. Since CR2 is present only on lymphocytes and not on monocytes, macrophages, or granulocytes, C4d3d-coated cells can be expected to bind only to lymphocytes. C3b attaches to CR3 via a portion of C3 lying between C3d and C3c, the C3e portion of the molecule.[172] This portion of C3b is exposed after cleavage by β_1-H, making it available to the CR3 receptor.[173]

CR2 attachment of coated RBCs to lymphocytes does not appear to damage the cells.

The presence of C3d and C4d on the surface of RBCs is further indication of attachment of C3b on these cells. This explains why cells initially trapped by the liver then circulate with remaining C3d and C4d, which prevents further antibody binding to them.[174]

Role of Soluble Components of Complement

An important role of complement is the vasoactive and chemotactic effect of some of the byproducts of complement activation. Some of the byproducts are characteristically low molecular weight substances such as C3a and C5a. C3a, also called anaphylatoxin 1, has a 9,000-dalton molecular weight and results from the cleavage of one of the ends of the α chain of C3.[151] As has been mentioned, C3a and C5a are capable of inducing contraction of smooth muscle fibers, a reaction that may be mediated not by histamine[175] but by leukotrienes.[176] Another small peptide product of C3 cleavage is C3e, a 12,000-dalton molecular weight peptide which is the cleavage product from the α-chain of C3c. It has the capacity of inducing leukocytosis in rabbits.[177] Anaphylatoxin 2, also termed C5a, is a 12,000-dalton molecule that results from the cleavage of C5 by $\overline{C42}$. It is capable of binding to basophils, producing degranulation and release of histamine,[151] but the biologic effects can likewise be produced by the stimulation of C5a on cells that release leukotrienes.[176]

The cleavage of the C-terminal arginine (C5a-des-Arg) increases the anaphylactic activity of C5a 1,000-fold.[178] These anaphylatoxins may well be responsible for many of the symptoms found in ABO hemolytic transfusion reactions, such as flushing, wheezing, and vascular collapse.[98] C3a,[161] C5a[179] and the trimolecular complex of $\overline{C567}$ are chemotactic factors for monocytes and neutrophils.[180]

Evolutionary Genetics of the Complement System

Complement appears relatively early in evolution and is found in elasmobranch fish, the most primitive animal to possess such a system. Complement has survived in evolution by a mechanism of gene duplication. This occurs by either tandem duplication, which provides copies of the gene in close proximity in the same chromosome, or by chromosomal duplication, which results in chromosomal rearrangement, and the genes appear on different chromosomes.

Tandem duplication permits mutation without compromising the function of the gene. The complement proteins are polymorphic and run differently on electrophoresis.[181] A good example is factor B: the less common alleles are found on the Bb fragment, while the more common ones are found on the Ba fragment.[181] Two alleles of C4 are known, C4F and C4S. C4F is the Chido antigen on RBCs and C4S is the Rogers antigen on RBCs, both having been adsorbed from plasma.[182] C2, C4, and factor B are coded for near the HLA-B genes of the HLA system.[181]

It is quite possible that the primitive ancestor genes of the complement system coded for molecules that were very similar or identical to C3 and factor B. This would provide a primitive organism with the capability of producing C3b as a result of the splitting of C3 by leukocyte enzymes.

The classical pathway present in the more evolved species has probably evolved by gene duplication from the primitive type of complement system. C3, C4, and C5 are all proteins derived from a 200,000-dalton precursor and result from splits at the N-terminus of the α heavy chain, yielding a small, 9,000-dalton polypeptide.

There is evidence of genetic linkage among C3, C4, and C5. C6 and C7 may be closely linked, and so are C2 and factor B. C1r, C1s, and factor D are probably linked.[183]

Inborn abnormalities are rare in humans.[184] Most are inherited in an autosomal recessive fashion. Complement components may be very decreased in concentration. This abnormality has been described for C1r, C1s, C4, C2, C3, C5, C6, and C7. Most patients with these deficiencies have not been sick. However, individuals who are C3 defective do develop pyogenic infections more frequently than normal individuals, and develop a lupus erythematosus-like syndrome.[185] The most frequent hereditary defect of complement, however, is hereditary angioedema, resulting from a defective C1 esterase inhibitor. The inhibitor level may be very low (10% of normal), normal, or increased; if it is increased, the molecule is nonfunctional.[186, 187]

Complement in Disease

Complement deposits causing tissue injury are found in a variety of diseases. Patients with IgA nephritis and Henoch-Schönlein purpura have been shown to develop complement deposits, via the alternative pathway of complement activation, in the glomerulus.[188] In SLE, however, complement deposition is via both the classical and alternative pathways.[103] Clinically, complement utilization in vivo can be assessed by measuring byproducts such as C4d. Rheumatoid arthritis complicated by vasculitis is usually accompanied by hypocomplementemia.[189] Patients with membranoproliferative glomerulonephritis (MPGN) have normal levels of C1, C4, and C2, whereas the level of C3 is very reduced. Nephritic factor (NeF), an IgG capable of activating the alternative pathway, is usually present in MPGN. C3 deficiencies are accompanied by failure of opsonization, hemolytic activity, and a decreased WBC response to infection.[103] These patients are characteristically susceptible to *Neisseria* infections. Persons with C4 and C2 deficiencies have a higher incidence of SLE than the general population, probably because the susceptibility gene for SLE codes near the C4, C2 complement genes. Susceptibility for SLE may correlate with a higher incidence of the disease in patients who type for HLA-A10, Bw18, and DRw2. The same HLA phenotypes have a higher incidence of C1 inhibitor deficiency patients with hereditary angioedema.[187]

The activity of NeF resides in the $F(ab')_2$.[190] Another cause of complement consumption of interest to blood bankers is that found in patients undergoing extracorporeal circulation. Plasma complement can be activated when exposed to dialysis membranes, with generation of C5a from activation of the alternative pathway. The liberation of C5a under these conditions may cause adult respiratory distress syndrome.[191] The same activation of complement can be seen during cardiopulmonary bypass surgery.[192]

Significance of Complement in the Blood Bank

IgM antibodies against ABO blood group substances are involved in most of the fatal hemolytic transfusion reactions. These antibodies produce hemolysis through their ability to bind complement (see Chap. 5). Other IgM antibodies likewise are capable of binding complement, such as anti-I antibodies (see Chap. 5). IgM antibodies do not remain attached to the RBC but produce binding of complement and then elute off the RBC, leaving bound complement attached to the RBC membrane. C3b, C4b, and C5b remain on the membrane and are detectable by the routine antiglobulin test[99] or by the use of monoclonal antibodies directed against C3b or C4b. The cells remaining in circulation with complement attached to them are acted on by circulating complement enzymes which cleave C3b, releasing C3c and C4c and leaving C3d and C4d attached to cells. These components of complement can be detected only with antiglobulin antisera capable of detecting C3d and C4d specific-

TABLE 4–7.—COMPLEMENT BINDING BY DIFFERENT RBC ANTIBODIES*

ANTIBODY TO:	IgM	IgG	BINDING TO COMPLEMENT (%)	HEMOLYTIC IN VITRO (%)
ABH	Yes	Yes	Most	>20
Ii	Yes	Rare	Most	>20
Lewis	Yes	Rare	Most	>10
P	Yes	Rare	Most	<5
Fy^a	Rare	Yes	19	0
Fy^b	Rare	Yes	50	0
K	Rare	Yes	15	0
k	Rare	Yes	17	0
Jk^a	Rare	Yes	71	<5
Jk^b	Rare	Yes	57	<5
S	Rare	Yes	33	0

*Data from Garraty[99] and Mollison.[196]

TABLE 4–8.—AUTOIMMUNE HEMOLYTIC ANEMIA AND BINDING OF COMPLEMENT OR IMMUNOGLOBULIN* ON RBCs

GLOBULIN ON RBC	% OF CASES
Complement alone	30
Immunoglobulin and complement	34
Immunoglobulin alone	36

*Data from Garraty.[99]

ities, and by monoclonal antibodies specific for C3d and C4d. IgG antibodies can likewise bind complement to RBCs. These are usually of the IgG1 or IgG3 subclass. Interestingly, Rh antibodies, which are usually of the IgG1 subclass,[193] do not bind complement unless the cells are very heavily coated with anti-D.[194] This is probably due to the relatively low numbers of Rh sites on RBC membranes.[195]

Details on the binding of complement by specific antibodies to blood group antigens are given in Table 4–7.

In laboratory studies of autoimmune hemolytic anemia and drug-induced hemolytic anemia, combinations of complement and immunoglobulin can be found (Table 4–8).

CELLULAR IMMUNITY

The two main lymphoid cell subtypes are B cells and T cells. In mammals, T cells originate in the bone marrow as pre-T cells which then migrate to the thymus gland. The thymus evolved from the third and fourth branchial pouches. It is composed of lobules which possess a cortex and a medulla. The lymphocytes mature within the cortex, then migrate to the medulla. From there they gain access to the circulation.[197] In humans, the thymus regresses abruptly in late adolescence. B cells in chickens derive from the bursa of Fabricius. In mammals several organs have been considered candidates, including bone marrow, fetal liver, and gut-associated lymphoid tissue. None of these organs has been conclusively identified as the B cell precursor organ of origin.

The Lymphatic System

The lymphatic system is composed of lymphatic vessels and lymphatic organs. The smaller vessels, the lymphatic capillaries, constitute a wide network throughout the body and end as blind tubes. The network forms larger trunks as vessels join into their larger tributaries.

Lymphatic Organs

Lymph nodes are large accumulations of lymphatic tissue organized as a definite lymphatic organ. They are usually kidney-shaped and have a slight indentation, the hilus, where blood vessels enter and leave the organ. Lymphatic vessels enter the node at many places but leave only from the hilus. Lymph nodes are covered by a capsule. Trabeculae of dense connective tissue arise from the capsule and penetrate the lymph node. These septae divide the lymph node into roughly rounded alveoli. Suspended from this framework is the reticular framework. Loose areas in this framework constitute the lymph sinuses, through which the lymph percolates.

The cellular stroma of lymph nodes is made up of reticular cells and fixed macrophages. Free cells in the mesh are mostly various types of lymphocytes.

Functional Anatomy of Lymph Nodes

Antigens are transported to lymph nodes via the lymphatic system into the subcapsular sinus, but antigen retention is only transitory in this area. The flow continues to the trabecular and medullary sinuses, where fixed macrophages are located. It has been shown that antigen is phagocytized and retained intracellularly by macrophages at this location for prolonged periods of time. It appears probable that antigens are then transported to germinal centers, where dendritic cells and fixed macrophages bind antigen superficially and present it to lymphocytes.[197-199]

The lymphatic flow in a lymph node is centripetal. Access to the lymph node is through multiple afferent lymphatics which drain into the subcapsular sinus. The lymph moves through the cortex, the lymph node medulla, and leaves it via the main efferent lymphatic vessels. Primary lymphoid follicles are located mostly within the cortex at the periphery. Between the core or medulla of the lymph node and the cortex is the paracortical area. This area has a functional significance in the maturation of lymphoid cells in lymph nodes.[200]

The primary follicles exhibit germinal centers on stimulation (e.g., infection). Germinal centers are mostly composed of rapidly dividing B cells. B cells from the follicles mature and migrate toward the medullary portion of the node, where they are often found as the end stage of B cells (e.g., plasma cells), which actively secrete antibody.[200] The paracortical area usually contains most of the T cell population of the lymph node (Fig 4–15).

Lymphocyte Subpopulations

B cells are essentially committed to the production of specific antibodies when they reach the plasma cell stage of maturation. They are therefore responsible for humoral immunity. T cells are mostly responsible for cellular immunity. However, the two populations of cells cooperate in many immune responses for adequate production of antibody.

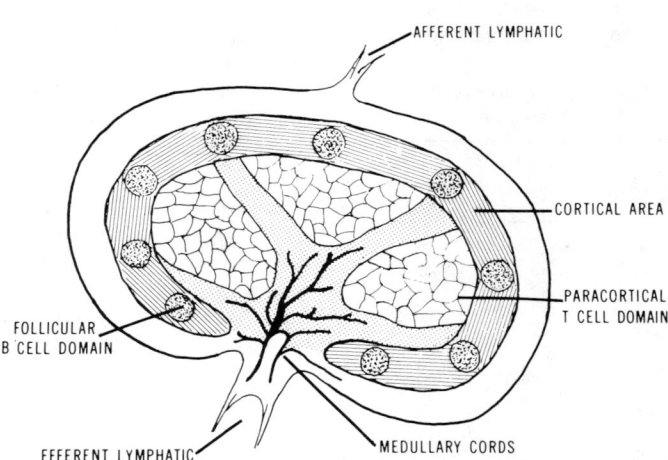

FIG 4–15.—Functional anatomy of a peripheral lymph node. B cells are mainly found in follicular areas of the cortex. T cells are mainly found in the paracortical areas of the lymph node.

B Cells.—Evidence for a difference between B cells and T cells was first discovered in the chicken. The avian bursa of Fabricius is epithelial in origin and is secondarily seeded by lymphoid cells that arise in other organs.

Membrane IgM is the first immunoglobulin to be found on B cells in the bursa. Days after maturation, however, IgG-bearing B cells can be detected. This suggests that B cell precursors bearing IgM later differentiate into B cells bearing other immunoglobulins—IgG, IgM, or IgA. In humans, the precursor cells have been identified at various stages of development in the bone marrow, the fetal liver, and the spleen.

It has been shown experimentally that B cells bear IgM in early stages, may bear IgM and IgD simultaneously, and are then committed to specific immunoglobulins (IgG, IgM, IgA, or IgE). IgD has been proposed as a "switch" for differentiation. Committed B cells subsequently lose their surface immunoglobulins and become plasma cells with full ability to synthesize and secrete immunoglobulins.[201, 202]

It has recently been shown that genes responsible for immunoglobulin class isotype expression are closely linked in the following order: $C\mu$, $C\delta$, $C\gamma$ 3, 1, 2b, and 2a, $C\epsilon$, and $C\alpha$. The expression of the isotypes is achieved by the activation of genes through translocation of the V-D-J complex.[201]

B cells can be identified by readily detectable surface immunoglobulin. The ability to retain immunoglobulin on the surface apparently is due to the existence of receptors for the Fc portion of the immunoglobulins. Complement receptors in addition to the Fc receptors have also been described on lymphocytes. Fc receptors are mobile and float on the lipid bilayer membranes of the lymphocytes. There is subcellular organelle control of the movement of these molecules, which explains the tendency of Fc receptors to cap under certain physicochemical changes.

B cells can be quantified by exposing them to sheep RBCs coated with immunoglobulin. This is another method of showing that B cells bind the Fc fragments of the immunoglobulin coating sheep RBCs.[203] However, surface immunoglobulin studies by fluorescence are also useful,[203] and the recent introduction of monoclonal antibodies against specific B cell markers has become the method of choice for enumerating B cells.[204]

T Cells.—T cells derive from the bone marrow and migrate to the thymus gland, where they mature. The thymus, which arises in the third and fourth branchial pouches, is the first lymphoid organ to develop. The organ is epithelial in origin but later is populated by cells arising in other organs, such as fetal liver and bone marrow. These cells arrive via the cortical sinus of the thymus gland. The thymus regulates the transformation of these prethymic cells arising from other sites and during development converts them to mature thymocytes. Human T cells have the capacity to spontaneously form rosettes with uncoated sheep RBCs. They also react with antibrain antiserum and with antisera produced by injecting human thymocytes into rabbits. Another characteristic of T cells is that they react with soluble phytohemagglutinin and are stimulated by other lymphocytes in mixed lymphocyte cultures (MLC). This can be measured in the laboratory by measuring uptake of radioactively labeled thymidine from cells in mitosis.

In the mouse, a main experimental animal in the study of these cells, several different antigens have been described: (1) Thy-1, previously called theta, (2) TL (thymus leukemia) present on precursor cells, and (3) Ly+, or lymphocyte cell antigen, present on Lyt-1, Lyt-2, and Lyt-3. Lyt-1 cells are helper/inducer cells in T and B cell cooperation, whereas Lyt-2 and Lyt-3 cells are suppressor/cytotoxic cells in mice.[205]

Ortho Diagnostics Laboratories (Raritan, New Jersey) have produced monoclonal antibodies against human T cell markers. OKT4 antibodies recognize helper T cells, OKT8 antibodies recognize suppressor T cells,[206] OKT3 define T cells in the peripheral circulation,[207] and OKM1 binds to natural killer (NK) cells[208] and monocytes.[209]

T killer cells are the third category of T cells that have been identified.[210] These cells are involved in cytolytic activity. It appears, however, that cytolytic cells may be subsets of T cells. The cytotoxicity is caused by HLA- or non-HLA-dependent large granular lymphocytes (LGL). LGL non-HLA-dependent cytotoxic cells can be killer cells (K cells), which are seen in primed recipients and require coating of target cells with antibody, or NK cells, which are seen in nonprimed recipients.[211]

Macrophages.—Macrophages are an important cellular element of the immune response. Initially recognized as phagocytic cells, they are now known to be involved in more complex interactions with B and T cells in the process of antibody formation as well as in cellular immunity. Macrophages are cells bearing Fc membrane receptors as well as complement receptors. These membrane structures help cells in ingesting antibody-coated or complement-coated particles on cells. Macrophages are involved in processing as well as presenting antigen to B and T cells, and they also store antigen for various periods of time. The presentation of antigens to B or T cells is specific in that different subpopulations of macrophages are involved in presenting antigen to either T or B cells.[212]

Cooperation of Cells in the Immune Response

The cellular basis of the immune response comprises both the interaction of antigens to elicit the production of specific immunoglobulins against them, and the purely cellular responses, usually directed against more complex antigens. Just how antigens elicit the production of specific antibody responses has been the subject of intensive research. In the last hundred years, selective theories on stimulation by the immunogen of precommitted antibody-producing cells have been proposed. "Instructive" theories propose that cells synthesize antibodies de novo, adapting antibody molecules in a "template" manner to the specific production of a particular immunoglobulin with specificity for that antigen. It now seems clear that the clonal theory of Burnett is more probable in terms of explaining antibody production.[213] This theory suggests that precommitted antibody-producing cells can reproduce by clonal division, which explains physiologic antibody levels to a specific antigen. In this theory it is assumed that cells are precommitted to a specific antibody. When these cells are stimulated by a particular antigen, the clones of cells expand to produce antibody.

Antibody Production

The development of the antibody response can be better understood by following the sojourn of antigen, its fate, and the subsequent development of specific antibodies against it.

When antigens penetrate the body and come in contact with the immune defense systems, they are usually ingested and/or trapped by macrophages. Macrophages are phagocytic cells which are capable of trapping antigen and either ingesting and destroying it or presenting it on their membrane to the two main cells of the immune system, the B and T cells.[214] Antigens ingested by phagocytes such as monocytes are at times degraded and converted into nonantigenic particles. However, antigens exposed on the membrane of macrophages usually become more antigenic. This is probably due to the availability and configuration in which these antigens are exposed to T and B cells. Macrophages can be mobile or fixed in tissues. Circulating phagocytes, such as monocytes, are capable of traveling to sites where antigenic substances may be present. Fixed tissue macrophages are usually found attached to the endothelium of several organs and trap antigens that circulate by them. The surface of macrophages is usually sticky, a characteristic which enhances their trapping ability. It has also been shown that macrophages possess receptors for the Fc portions of IgG and in certain cases IgM, as well as complement.[215] These receptors allow macrophages to bind antibodies with specificities for certain antigens, thus making the process of antigen presentation to B or T cells a more selective one. This function also allows macrophages to make their phagocytic function more specific.

The molecular structure of antigens can elicit either a predominantly B cell stimulation or a response requiring both B and T cells to elicit adequate antibody formation.

In predominantly B cell stimulation, responses are elicited by rather large molecules with repetitive units, such as large polysaccharides. These are referred to as T cell–independent antigens. Often these antigens produce an IgM response.[216] Conversely, there are antigens, usually of a complex structure (e.g., hapten plus carrier), which require the interaction of both B and T cells. Macrophages are crucial for the adequate interaction of these cells. In T cell–dependent antibody formation, helper T cells are responsible for mediating production of antibody against the carrier portion of the protein, whereas B cells are responsible for production of antibody against the haptenic portion of the molecule. IgG antibodies and IgE antibodies are usually T cell–dependent responses. Both T and B cells synthesize surface recognition molecules for antigen. T cell surface receptors for antigen have been studied recently, and found to be a two chain structure. Ia gene products and other components of the histocompatibility complex have been proposed as possible candidates for antigen receptor molecules on T cells. This aspect, however, is not entirely defined to date.[217] However, it appears that a cDNA probe obtained from copies of ribosome-bound mRNA codes for proteins which are rearranged in all T cells tested for. This seems to point to the fact that the T cell receptor gene has been isolated with the aid of these DNA hybridization techniques.[218] Furthermore, a monoclonal antibody against the receptor for antigen and the MHC on human helper/inducer T cells has been obtained. This antibody identifies a 20,000-dalton monomorphic T3 molecule and a clonotypic heterodimer Ti with a molecular weight of 90,000 daltons. The antibody is capable of activating clonal proliferation of helper/inducer T cells in the absence of antigen and MHS complex.[219]

Surface Stimulation of B and T Cells

B cells synthesize membrane-bound immunoglobulin, which makes them easily recognizable. However, it has been shown that helper T cells are capable of producing immunoglobulin that is structurally similar to IgM and is called IgT. The IgT is present in much smaller quantity on T cells than on B cells. There is evidence that IgT may be the membrane antigen receptor for T cells. Although the stimulation of B and T cells is mediated by antigen, there are mitogenic substances that function as inductive substances and stimulate these cells to divide.

Concanavalin A (ConA) binds to both B or T cells but stimulates only T cells to divide. *Escherichia coli* lipopolysaccharide stimulates B cells only. Anti-immunoglobulin antiserum will stimulate both T and B cells to divide, provided there are no specific helper substances in the incubation medium.

In mice and humans, antisera to surface glycoproteins exist to define helper T cells.[210] B cells may produce IgM antibodies to certain antigens unaided.[214, 216] To produce IgG, IgA, and IgE, T cell help is necessary. Macrophages act nonspecifically by presenting antigen to B and T cells. It is now evident that Ia and other histocompatibility antigens are necessary for adequate T and B cell immune responses.[217]

Development of B Cells into Plasma Cells

B cells may have IgM and IgD on their surface in immature stages. With further differentiation (through T cell mediation) they develop into committed B cells to produce IgM, IgG, IgA, or IgE. On commitment, only one immunoglobulin is produced by each plasma cell, which is the final stage of development of B cells. IgD on immature B cells may function as a "switch" membrane molecule which triggers commitment to single immunoglobulin synthesis.[219, 220]

Ontogeny of T Cells

Stem pre-T cells derived from the marrow migrate to the thymus, where they develop their specificity repertoire.[221] Pre-T cells are stem cells from the bone marrow which are committed to T cell differentiation and are identified by their ability to express terminal deoxynucleotidyl transferase (TdT), an enzyme present in cortical thymocytes. These cells can be shown to express T cell markers after incubation with thymopoietin.[222] These markers have been defined with the help of monoclonal antisera.[223] In humans, T surface markers are defined numerically (T1, T2, T3 . . . T11).[224] Prethymic cells are characterized by the expression of T9 and T10 markers. Helper T cells are characterized by T4 antisera, whereas T suppressor cells are characterized by T8 antisera.

T Cell Idiotypes

It has been shown in rats that T cells have receptors for idiotypes with the same specificity as serum antibody specificities.[225] Genetic analysis reveals that T cell idiotype expression is linked to expression of heavy chain allotype of the MHS. Thus it appears that MHS genes code for part of the T cell receptor or influence T cell specificity repertoires.[226]

Most of the available data point to the fact that T cell repertoires are coded for on V_H-type sequences, termed V_T. We now know that the T-cell antigen receptor has an alpha and a beta chain. This receptor, much like Ig molecules, has VDJ and constant regions.[227]

Cell-Cell Interactions in the Immune Response

T and B cells cooperate to produce adequate immune responses. This cooperation is through cell interactions of essentially two sorts: lymphocyte activation or lymphocyte suppression. Soluble factors also mediate cell interactions between T and B cells. The fact that T and B cells are both needed for an adequate response became evident after thymus and bone marrow reconstitution of lethally irradiated mice.[228]

Two types of responses occur in animals challenged with complex antigens, a hapten-specific response mediated by B cells and a carrier-specific response mediated by T cells.[229] Apparently both responses are necessary for adequate immune function. Cell-cell interactions are necessary[230] and probably the most significant, for no soluble factors to date have been shown to be antigen specific in lymphocyte cooperation during immune responses.

In mice, Ly1+ cells function as T helper cells, and Ly2+ and Ly3+ cells function as suppressor cells in cell-mediated lympholysis (CML) reactions.[231] In humans, helper cells are characterized with monoclonal anti-T4 antibodies. Helper cells are also essential for adequate IgG responses in vitro, where the addition to B cells will enhance lysis in plaque-forming cell assays. Other T cells mediate suppression of the immune response; these are termed T suppressor cells. Evidence for T cell suppression was first obtained by Gershon.[232] Neoplastic T cells may be of the helper-type lineage, as in Sézary syndrome, or of the suppressor-type lineage, as in Japanese T cell leukemia.[233]

The two-receptor theory of Benacerraf proposes that T cells, in order to recognize antigenic and/or idiotopic specificities, must also recognize the products of the histocompatibility complex.[234] The balance of T helper and T suppressor functions depends on the expression of certain antigenic molecular determinants when T cells encounter the antigen. For instance, if the globulin hen eggwhite lysozyme (HEL) is cleaved with cyanogen bromide, a large LII fragment is obtained. T cells from responder strains of mice recognize this fragment as a T helper determinant during an antibody response against a smaller N-C peptide portion of the HEL molecule. This response is mediated by histocompatibility antigens, for $H-2^b$ and $H-2^s$ nonresponder strains fail to produce a response due to high numbers of N-C peptide-specific suppressor T cells.[235]

Macrophage-Lymphocyte Interactions

Immunogenicity of antigen depends on antigen modification by macrophages.[236] It has been suggested that such immunogenicity of high molecular weight protein or peptide antigens depends on primary amino acid sequence association with products of the MHS on macrophage surfaces.[237] The enzymatic cleavage of this highly immunogenic macrophage membrane-bound antigen renders macrophages unable to reconstitute this antigenicity. This suggests that there is no antigen reservoir in these cells.[236]

The Major Histocompatibility Complex and the Immune Response

The MHC is so important to blood banking and tissue transplantation that it will be discussed separately in a later chapter. The present discussion is limited to the MHC as it relates to immune system function.

T cells do not recognize antigen alone but in the context of the MHC. The MHC genes are close to other genes important to the immune system and may even reflect homology, such as the Ig genes.[238] This homology does not mean that they are the same genes. The structure of the MHC and its function are distinct and independent from other factors important to cell communication in the immune system. Nevertheless, the concept of a supergene, in which several genes such as complement, Ig, and MHC genes are clustered together as a result of genetic selection pressures, may well be correct.[239]

The MHC codes for two major classes of molecules, class I and class II.[240] Class I glycoproteins are usually 44,000-dalton chains, possess three extra membrane domains,[241] and have a functional role in T cell cytolytic functions. Class II glycoproteins are composed of an α chain (34,000 MW) and a β chain (28,000 MW). Their function has been linked to the recognition of T helper cells and T suppressor cells.[242] Class I molecules in humans are HLA-A, -B, and -C, whereas class II molecules are HLA-D and HLA-DR antigens.

It appears that lymphocytes, in order to recognize antigen, must do so by the proper "diplomatic channels"—namely, in relation to the MHC.

This association of antibody-presenting function and the MHC has been shown in research where cytotoxic T cells from mice infected with lymphocyte choriomeningitis virus could only kill infected target cells that expressed the same MHC H-2 haplotype,[243] and was an example of MHC restriction. This implies that T cells have a dual recognition system or function under "the altered self" mechanism. The dual recognition mechanism appears to be the more likely mechanism through which the MHC and T cells communicate. In the mouse, the K and D serologically defined regions are critical gene products for proper cytotoxic T cell function[244] as well as for intrathymic T cells development. The MHC "environment" in which intrathymic T cells develop is important to subsequent H-2 haplotype restriction.[245]

The process of MHC restriction can be summarized as three stages: (1) antigen-independent phase, mediated by prethymic stem cells; (2) stem cells reach the thymus, where they are exposed to MHC restriction, termed thymic phase; and (3) T cells go to the circulation, and only those T cells with the appropriate MHC products undergo clonal expansion on exposure to antigen, clonal expansion phase.

Two major types of genes control the immune response, the immunoglobulin V region Ir genes that code for immunoglobulins and the Ir genes that do not code for Ig sequences but for MHC products, responsible for T cell interactions. The Ir MHC genes influence the level of T cell responses and only rarely[246] influence the specificity of the antibody response. Antigen-specific T suppressor cells may also be under MHC control.[247]

The lack of a specific MHC product can result in inappropriate presentation of antigen or in lack of appropriate T cells for a given antigenic specificity.[248] The first case may be associated with MHC expression on macrophages, whereas the second may be related to specific expression of receptors on T cells. These two mechanisms may or may not be mutually exclusive, and more evidence is needed to clarify this phenomenon.

Interleukin

T and B cell activation occurs, not only on the basis of cell-cell interactions but through the mediation of a variety of soluble factors. The more important of these factors are termed interleukins. Interleukin 1 (Il-1) is a 15,000-dalton protein produced by mononuclear phagocytes which stimulates T cell proliferation in vitro in the absence of mitogens.[249] Interleukin 2 (Il-2) is a 15,000-dalton protein produced by human T cells which induces the proliferation of antigen/mitogen-stimulated T cells.[249] Il-1 cannot induce proliferation of stimulated T cells but can induce Il-2–producing T cells to proliferate.[250] It is possible that Il-2 may also be involved in B cell proliferation, but the data on this phenomenon are not conclusive.[251]

Tolerance

Immunologic tolerance is an acquired lack of response to a particular immunogenic stimulus. Two mechanisms may be operating: (1) Specific clonal deletion, or (2) specific suppression by suppressor T cells. In effect, both mechanisms may be responsible for the phenomenon of tolerance. Neonatal inbred mice injected with partially histocompatible hemopoietic stem cells develop tolerance to skin grafts from the partially histocompatible strain.[252,253]

Tolerance to T cell–dependent antigens affects both B and T cells, as has been shown by adoptive transfer to irradiated mice. In these studies, T cell tolerance persisted for 150 days and B cell tolerance for 50 days.[254] Evidently, tolerance by development of T suppressor clones allows recovery once the store of antigen has been exhausted. This type of tolerance may occur at stages not critical to ontogeny of T cells.[255] Recently, such T suppressor cells in rats made tolerant to polyvinyl alcohol (PVA) have been demonstrated.[256] However, tolerance induction in organisms that have been primed to an antigen after T cell ontogeny is much more difficult to demonstrate. Nevertheless, this type of tolerance is much more relevant clinically, for it would be therapeutically significant to hypersensitive patients. Two ways to achieve this have been shown: tolerance induction to non-T cell antigens, and suppression control manipulation.

In the first case, high doses of polymeric flagellin, POL, have been shown to bypass T cell regulation by inactivating B cells.[257] In the second case, anti-idiotypic T cells delivering suppressor signals cause unresponsiveness. Thus, manipulating the auto-anti-idiotypic response suppression to transplantation antigens can be achieved.[258]

Closely related antigens can block tolerance, as has been shown by injection of heterologous thyroglobulin into rabbits; the injection induced T cell help and induced antithyroglobulin antibodies to "self" thyroglobulin antigenic determinants.[259]

PATHOLOGY OF THE IMMUNE RESPONSE

Congenital Immunodeficiencies

Thymic Hypoplasia.—Thymic hypoplasia, also known as DiGeorge's syndrome, results from an embryologic developmental failure of the third and fourth pharyngeal pouches with consequent loss of parathyroids and thymus.[260] This results in poor immune responses—the serum immunoglobulin is mainly IgM, with deficient IgG. The thymus-dependent paracortical areas of lymph nodes are hypoplastic.[261] The severity of the syndrome is variable.[262] Patients with thymic hypoplasia often succumb to fatal viral infections. Thymus transplantation has been successful in certain cases, with an increase in lymphocyte counts and phytohemagglutinin responses.[263] Spontaneous improvement does occur without treatment.

Infantile X-Linked Agammaglobulinemia (Bruton Type).—Infantile X-linked agammaglobulinemia is mainly a B cell defect. The block is in B cell development, for these patients have normal numbers of pre-B cells.[264] Very low immunoglobulin levels are found in the serum. Cellular immune responses such as reactivity to *Candida* antigens are normal, but no mature plasma cell formation is present in this disease. Fatal pyogenic infections develop once affected infants are no longer protected by maternal IgG. Gram-positive organisms and *Hemophilus influenzae* are frequently the causative agents of these infections. Patients are given immunoglobulin intramuscularly (IM), 300 mg as a loading dose followed by 0.6 ml/kg/month to maintain IgG levels at 200 mg/dl.[265] Immunoglobulin preparations for IV use are likewise available.

Severe Combined Immunodeficiency.—Severe combined immunodeficiency (SCID) may be inherited as an autosomal recessive trait or as an X-linked trait. Dysostosis and adenosine deaminase deficiency may also be present. Affected infants have severe infections beginning in the second or third month of life. *Escherichia coli*, *Salmonella*, and *Pseudomonas* infections kill patients within the first 2 years of life.[266] Bone marrow transplantation, the only available treatment, is often complicated by graft-versus-host disease.[267] Inducing tolerance before transplantation is currently being explored in mice.[268]

Wiskott-Aldrich Syndrome.—The Wiskott-Aldrich syndrome is also a combined B and T cell deficit that is associated with eczema and thrombocytopenia.[269] Abnormal platelet aggregation studies may help identify carriers.[270] These patients can be treated with a bone marrow transplant after the recipient has been prepared with antithymocyte antiserum.[271] Ataxia and telangiectasia may also be associated with immunodeficiency, especially of T cells. About 80% of patients with ataxia and telangiectasia have very low levels of IgE and 70% have low IgA levels.[272] About 5%–10% have low levels of IgG, and most have normal or high levels of IgM.[272] One case of transient improvement after marrow transplantation has been reported.[273]

Acquired Immunodeficiencies

Primary Acquired Agammaglobulinemia.—Primary acquired agammaglobulinemia has its onset in adulthood. Patients present with an increased susceptibility or a variety of pyogenic infections which may be manifested as respiratory pyogenic infections with severe bronchopneumonia or intestinal infections with diarrhea and malabsorption simulating a sprue syndrome. Autoimmune diseases are frequent in these patients.[274]

There is evidence that primary acquired agammaglobulinemia is produced by an abnormal suppressor T cell population which inhibits B cells from producing immunoglobulins. Treatment includes globulin replacement and, in the future, possible suppressor T cell reduction from the peripheral circulation by selective column cytapheresis.

Selective Immunoglobulin Deficiency.—The synthesis of any of the immunoglobulins may be inhibited, resulting in absence of serum IgA,[275] IgM,[176] or IgG.[277] Treatment with plasma or any other component containing the missing immunoglobulin may be hazardous if the patient has antibodies against the deficient immunoglobulin (Chapter 11).

Secondary Immunodeficiencies.—These diseases have as a secondary complication the development of cellular immunodeficiency. Sarcoidosis, for example, appears to be complicated by a deficiency of T cells that does not affect B cells.[277] This results in decreased reactivity to intradermal antigen challenge by various antigens, including *Candida* antigens. Serum immunoglobulins may be normal or increased.

The deficit in Hodgkin's disease appears to be a T cell defect, but B cells are not always intact. This may explain patients' increased susceptibility to herpes virus and cryptococcal infections.[278]

Acquired Immunodeficiency Syndrome (AIDS).—AIDS is the most important of the secondary immune deficiencies.[279] Because the epidemiology of AIDS is similar to that of transfusional hepatitis and therefore of great concern for transfusionists, AIDS is discussed at length in Chapter 13. Nevertheless, we will give a brief description of the disease here and outline some of its immunologic characteristics.

AIDS affects mostly young men, with most cases seen in homosexuals, IV drug abusers, and hemophiliacs.[280] However, it is by no means limited to these groups, having been reported in neonates and the very elderly, in heterosexual as well as homosexual men, and in the female consorts of male carriers.

The disease is characterized by a virtual loss of T cell help, reflected in inverted T4/T8 cell ratios.[281] Mitogen T cell stimulation studies show a markedly decreased responsiveness in these patients, with values of 10%–50% of normal.[281] B cell function abnormalities have also been described.[282] However, immunoglobulin levels are either normal or increased.[280] Cutaneous anergy to mumps, *Candida albicans*, and trycophyton has also been described.[279] α_1-Thymosin[283] as well as acid-labile α-interferon[284] levels are frequently elevated in patients with AIDS.

The immune deficiency observed in patients with AIDS results in severe life-threatening infections by opportunistic bacteria[279] and the development of a variety of tumors, commonly Kaposi's sarcoma.[279]

The Gammopathies

A neoplastic expansion of a clone of antibody-producing plasma cells may produce single heavy chains, light chains, or whole antibody molecules. Since these tumor cells originate from a single clone, only one antigenic specificity is expressed in the antibody produced. One type of heavy chain and one type of light chain (κ or λ) are present. This is the pathologic basis of multiple myeloma, which is characterized by widespread invasion of the bone marrow by neoplastic plasma cells. Anemia from bone marrow replacement, hypercalcemia, and susceptibility to infection are most often present in patients with myeloma. A single type of light chain may be present in the urine as Bence Jones protein (40% of myeloma cases). The increase in homogeneous immunoglobulin in serum is detected as a spike on the electrophoretic pattern. If only heavy chains (e.g., A, M, or G) are present, the disease is termed heavy chain disease and histologically resembles a lymphoma rather than a myeloma.[285,286] Amyloidosis may complicate this disease and is usually of late onset. This pathologic phenomenon constitutes the deposit of polymerized variable regions forming chain complexes.

Hyperviscosity, anemia, and thrombocytopenia are common complications. Analgesia, diuresis, and exercise can be used as supportive measures. Melphalan, 0.25 mg/kg orally for 4 days, and prednisone, 1 mg/kg orally for 4 days, are given together every 4 weeks.[287] The prognosis is approximately 2 years' survival after diagnosis in most cases.

Waldenström's Macroglobulinemia.—Waldenström's macroglobulinemia represents a malignant neoplastic expansion of B cells that do not fully mature into plasma cells, forming so-called plasmacytoid cells. These cells produce a monoclonal IgM, which is mostly intravascular in distribution and may thus cause a hyperviscosity syndrome. The disease responds symptomatically to plasmapheresis in certain cases. Cryoglobulinemia with Raynaud's syndrome may complicate these cases. Retinal hemorrhages, thrombocytopenia, and hemorrhage are frequently seen. Hemolytic anemia may be present.[288] Average survival is about 4 years. Treatment is with chlorambucil, 0.2 mg/kg day, or with melphalan.[289,290] Until these drugs act, suppressing the neoplastic cells, plasmapheresis is used to reduce the plasma viscosity (see Chap. 9).

Benign Monoclonal Gammopathy.—A benign monoclonal expansion of plasma cells is recognized. This disease is frequently found in Swedish populations. Prognostically good signs are low levels of γ-globulin when compared to myeloma levels, a normal serum albumin, absence of Bence Jones protein, and a normal hematocrit.[291]

AUTOIMMUNITY

Autoimmunity may be a transient disease or may represent a life-threatening malady. Several diseases are now known to be in some way associated with autoimmune phenomena. Hashimoto's thyroiditis, autoimmune-mediated hemolytic anemia, and rheumatoid arthritis are a few examples of these diseases. Autoimmunity is characterized by the production of antibodies by immunocompetent cells which react against antigens present on tissues of the host, resulting in destruction or impairment of the normal function of target cells. The exact mechanism by which this happens has not been fully elucidated. However, several parts of the puzzle are known, and these point to the fact that several types of cells are involved in the process, usually including B cells, subsets of T cells, and macrophages. Autoimmunity probably develops out of a complex interaction of genetic, immunologic, and environmental factors.

HLA-B8 antigen and its high frequency of association with chronic hepatitis and autoimmune thyroiditis is a good example of genetically determined factors in autoimmunity (see Chap. 7). Autoimmunity in many instances may represent a loss of immunologic tolerance. One should regard tolerance as a complex interaction of immunocytes and not just as a loss of immune response. It is now apparent that autoimmunity arises from cells capable of producing antibodies against self, by escaping a suppressor mechanism that is present in normal individuals. Tolerance may be produced by inhibition of T or B cells and can suppress antibodies to T- or non-T-cell-dependent antigens.[292]

There is evidence of soluble blocking agents which act by inhibiting effector cells. Some of these factors may block immunocytes, forming antigen-antibody complexes. Immunoparalysis due to antigen excess can result in the production of suppressor T cells to that antigen and the subsequent development of tolerance. Administration of antigen and antibody together to a host may abrogate the host's humoral or cellular immune response. Results from recent research in the field suggest that the injection of immunoglobulin may in effect produce a negative feedback inhibition of B memory and B effector cells. Just how this inhibition takes place is not fully elucidated, but there is evidence that it may be multifactorial. The coating of antigen sites, masking their immunogenicity, is one of the proposed mechanisms, but more complicated factors seem to be at work, at least for certain antigens. It is possible that the antigen-antibody complexes present the antigen in a configuration that stimulates suppressor cells, or perhaps anti-idiotypic antibodies coat B cells and T cells can become tolerant. This tolerance seems to be mediated by suppressor T cells. Suppressor T cells seem to be short-lived compared to helper T cells, and this may explain remissions. The most probable model at this time is a direct T cell recognition of antigens on the surface of B cells; these cells are then detected and suppressed by T cells.[293] Autoimmunity may thus be produced when the mechanisms of tolerance are overcome or bypassed. Viral infections or repeated innoculations of viruses induce autoimmune diseases in these hosts. This is probably due in part to the production of cross-reacting antigens on the viral envelope. Haptens and drugs may also produce autoimmunity by binding to host antigens. Interestingly, some animal models have been described for autoimmunity. One such animal is the New Zealand black mouse, which develops a lupus erythematosus-like syndrome.[294]

IMMEDIATE AND DELAYED HYPERSENSITIVITY

Tissue damage can be caused by the immune response in basically two ways: immediate and delayed hypersensitivity immune reactions. Many causes of these phenomena are understood today. The division of hypersensitivity diseases into two categories is useful, even though these terms do not accurately reflect the nature or even the time of onset of the disease. For practical purposes, immediate hypersensitivity is mediated by antibodies and may therefore be considered as caused by humoral factors rather than cellular factors. Delayed hypersensitivity, by contrast, is usually mediated by the cellular response or, more accurately, by a T-cell response.

Coombs and Gell have divided these mechanisms of tissue damage into 4 types:[295] type I, anaphylactic; type II, cytotoxic; type III, Arthus's disease and immune complex disease; and type IV, delayed hypersensitivity.

Type I Reactions

Anaphylactic reactions are of the immediate type. They occur on exposure of an immunized recipient to the antigen. The reaction is produced by the release of vasoactive amines from mast cells, which happens when mast cells bind to specific antibodies which have reacted with antigen and trigger the intracellular activation of a proesterase.[296] This enzyme acts on the microfilaments of the cells, producing amine release from mast cell granules.[297] The subsequent vasodilation and escape of plasma produce the pathologic changes. The homocytotropic antibodies or reagins are usually of the IgE class in humans. Binding of antibody by mast cells is specific for the Fc portion of IgE. The reaction may be local or systemic, depending on the route of administration of the antigen. It has been shown that IgE response may be genetically predetermined and under control of the MHS system.[298]

Reactions which are life-threatening are those of a systemic nature and are termed anaphylactic. Shock, laryngeal edema, and vascular collapse are frequent components of anaphylaxis. A dreaded anaphylactic reaction in immunohematology practice is seen after administration of blood products containing IgA to an individual who has IgA antibodies. This reaction is described in more detail in Chapter 11.

Anaphylactic reactions are frequently fatal and occur minutes after administration of the causative agent. Management is by the IM administration of 0.5–1 ml of a 1:1000 solution of epinephrine containing 1 mg in 1 ml. If necessary it can be followed by 0.1 ml of a 1:1000 epinephrine solution in 10 ml of saline given slowly IV. The patient should be recumbent with the legs elevated. An adequate airway is maintained by an endotracheal tube or by tracheostomy if laryngeal edema is suspected. Oxygen and IV fluids are given as needed to restore volume. Hydrocortisone sodium succinate, 100 mg in saline, may be added to the therapy to prevent prolonged reactions.[299]

Type II and Type III Reactions

Type II and III reactions are caused by antigen-antibody interaction binding of complement with subsequent tissue damage. The distinction of type II and type III reactions is based on the assumption that antigen-antibody reactions occurring directly on tissues (type II reactions) can be distinguished from damage occurring from the complexing of antibody to soluble antigen and subsequent attachment of the complex to tissues, thus causing cell injury (type III reactions). This distinction is sometimes difficult to demonstrate;[300] nevertheless, many cases of type II and III reactions share a common tissue injury mechanism, that of complement activation.

Direct tissue injury by antigen-antibody reactions can be produced by three general mechanisms: (1) conformational change of antigens after interaction with antibody, (2) blocking by antibody of an active site (e.g., a receptor) acting as antigen, and (3) cross-linking of antigen and antibody, forming complexes with or without activation of complement. Thus, in the first case, cells modified by antibody can be eliminated from the circulation via Fc or C receptors on reticuloendothelial cells. This occurs in a variety of immune injuries to RBCs and is discussed in the chapter on immune hemolysis (Chapter 10). These reactions are considered type II reactions. The second type of injury, that caused by blocking antibodies, can also be considered the result of a type II reaction. Several disease states can be explained on this basis. Anti-factor VIII antibodies inhibit the adequate function of factor VIII and thus function as factor VIII inhibitors. This is a serious complication in the treatment of hemophiliacs. Recently factor IX concentrates have been used to bypass the effect of these inhibitors.[301] Antibodies to factor IX have likewise been described in patients with hemophilia B.[302]

Antireceptor antibodies such as those found in myasthenia gravis are also type II reactions. In this case the antibody interferes with the modulation of acetylcholine receptors, with reduced activity at the synaptic junction, due to a decrease in the available receptors for acetylcholine.[303]

In Graves' disease, antibodies of the long acting thyroid stimulator (LATS) type compete for receptor sites, binding to thyrotropin receptors and stimulating adenylate cyclase activity and production of cyclic AMP by thyroid cells.[304] Receptor block could occur via three mechanisms:[300] (1) A direct block of the receptor by antibody. (2) Upon binding of antibody, receptors become internalized, becoming unavailable. (3) After binding to the receptor, the antibody-receptor complex is shed; the cell loses the receptor from the membrane. The humoral antibody response to incompatible tissue transplantation, as well as Goodpasture's syndrome,[305] are both type II reactions.

Type III reactions result in immune complex diseases, a group that includes systemic lupus erythematosus, rheumatoid arthritis, certain drug-induced hemolytic anemias (e.g., acetaminophen-induced), and thrombocytopenias. In these reactions, tissues are injured as "innocent bystanders" when antigen-antibody complexes attach to tissues (e.g., glomerular basement membrane) secondarily, promoting activation of complement and injury to the tissue. Deposition of fibrin, accumulation of neutrophils, and complement activation interact to produce such diseases. Vasculitis and vascular obliteration by fibrin are common findings in these diseases; IgG and IgM are the immunoglobulins more commonly involved in these reactions.

Immune complex disease can be acute or chronic. Acute immune complex disease (serum sickness) is produced when a sensitized patient is exposed, usually parenterally, to a foreign protein or a drug, resulting in the formation of circulating soluble immune complexes which can produce complement-dependent vasculitis.[306] The disease is characterized by malaise, arthralgia, neuropathy, and dermatitis.

Chronic immune complex disease is seen in conditions such as SLE and rheumatoid arthritis. Hepatitis B antigen may cause immune complex formation and polyarteritis in posttransfusional hepatitis. IgA may occasionally be involved in immune complex formation (e.g., IgA nephropathy).[307]

Type IV Reactions

Type IV reactions are known to immunologists as delayed hypersensitivity or cell-mediated hypersensitivity. There are two main pathways by which cell-mediated damage occurs:[308] (1) lysis is produced directly by T cells, which destroy cells bearing an antigen for which these T cells are specific, and (2) antigen induces secretion of lymphokines, which can be directly cytotoxic or cause the appearance of other inflammatory cells (e.g., neutrophils and macrophages). The ability of cytotoxic T cells to produce cellular damage is MHC dependent; therefore both antigen and autologous MHC molecules must be recognized before this type of cell lysis is produced.[309]

Live T cells are necessary for effective lysis; however, the target cell need not be alive, as has been shown in vitro, where T cells are capable of lysing glutaraldehyde-fixed cells or anucleated cells.[310] Cell contact is necessary for this type of lysis to take place. Immunized animals yield specific T cells that bind avidly to cells bearing antigen to which the host has been immunized. This adherence can be inhibited with cytochalasin B, which suggests that the mechanism of attachment is mediated by membrane movement modulation.[308] The cytolysis is probably energy independent.[308] The actual lesions are membrane defects that allow intracellular contents to escape. These lesions are calculated to be about 90 angstroms in diameter.[311] The lesion is most probably produced by interacting cell membranes, where an enzymatic system such as phospholipase intervenes to damage the lipid bylayer.[308] This lesion may be produced by enzyme activation associated with specific coupling of target cell membrane-bound antigen and specific T cell receptor for the antigen, or the target for the lytic attack may be the bilayer lecithin moiety.

Graft Versus Host Disease

Graft versus host disease (GVHD), once a rare disorder, has now become a frequent and serious complication of bone marrow transplantation and of the grafting of transfused cells in an immunocompromised (by chemotherapy) host. Indeed, the major threat to patients recovering from bone marrow transplantation is GVHD.[312]

GVHD is usually seen when the MHC systems of the host and donor are incompatible; however, up to 20% of MHC-compatible hosts who have undergone transplantation may develop this complication. The greater the degree of incompatibility, the more severe the GVHD.

GVHD is a type IV reaction mediated by immunocompetent T cells present in the graft that attack host tissues, which the T cells recognize as foreign. If the host's cells are capable of recognizing idiotypes on grafted T cells, the disease is limited. Experimentally, eliminating T cells from the graft effectively eliminates GVHD.[313] The main target tissues of acute GVHD are skin, GI tract mucosal epithelium, and liver. Chronic GVHD affects lymphoid tissues and bone marrow as well. The bronchial epithelium may be compromised, resulting in a lymphocytic bronchitis.[314]

The actual mechanism of injury is not clear. A remarkable paucity of graft immunocytes and of specific antibodies to the involved tissues has been observed. In contrast, most of the lymphoid cells in these lesions are of host origin. This finding suggests that the grafted T cells induce host immunocytes to produce the damage.[313] A decrease in suppressor T cells of the host is often noted in acute GVHD, whereas an increase in suppressor T cells is seen in chronic GVHD.[315]

The pathologic findings in GVHD can be graded from 1 to 4.[313] In grade 1 the skin and mucosa of the GI tract show focal vacuolization and necrosis. The liver shows atypia in less than 25% of the cells.

The degree of cell destruction may increase to grade 4 GVHD, with complete epidermolysis, diffuse mucosal necrosis, and 75% atypia of hepatocytes. Clinically a macular urticarial reaction and a focal acneiform eruption on the skin appear about 6 weeks after transplantation.[316] Deposition of IgM, IgG, IgA, and complement may be observed at the dermoepidermal junction.[317] In severe cases the GI tract mucosa shows a diffuse necrosis; less severe cases are marked by nonspecific degenerative changes, manifested clinically as diarrhea of varying severity.

The liver damage correlates with varying degrees of jaundice and elevation of liver enzymes (e.g., alkaline phosphatase and alanine amino transferase). Veno-occlusive disease with a Budd-Chiari type of syndrome is sometimes seen as a hepatic complication of GVHD.[318]

In chronic GVHD, the skin and appendages may show changes indistinguishable from those of scleroderma and Sjörgen's disease.[319]

To prevent GVHD, a regimen with methotrexate at spaced intervals during the first 102 days after the graft is recommended.[320] When methotrexate has not been tolerated, cyclosporin has been used with success to avert GVHD.[321]

Complement Deficiencies

The more severe complement deficiencies may be associated with severe infections and autoimmune diseases such as SLE. C1q deficiency and X-linked hypogammaglobulinemia have been frequently associated. Deficiencies of C1r and C1s have similarly been associated with hypogammaglobulinemia.[322]

C2 deficiency has also been associated with autoimmune deficiencies such as SLE, dermatomyositis, and anaphylactoid purpura.[323] Haplotypes A10, B18 in the HLA system are in linkage disequilibrium for C2 deficiency. Treatment with plasma may produce immune complexes. C3 deficiency may be present in type I and II reactions. The former is more severe. A type II reaction is milder and associated with lipodystrophy.[324]

C4 may be associated with SLE or may be asymptomatic. HLA-A2, B12, and D2 have been associated with C4 deficiency. C5 deficiency is usually associated with infection. Ineffective chemotaxis is observed in these cases.

C6 deficiency may be associated with meningococcal infections. C7 deficiency may be complicated by Raynaud's phenomenon. C8 deficiency has been associated with *Neisseria* infections. Secondary immunodeficiencies may be associated with multiple diseases such as chronic infections, malignancies, and malnutrition.[324]

Hereditary angioedema is present when there is a genetic absence of C1 inhibitor.[324]

REFERENCES

1. Silverton W.W., Navia M.A., Davies D.R.: Three-dimensional structure of an intact human immunoglobulin. *Proc. Natl. Acad. Sci. USA* 74:5140, 1977.
2. Merler E., Rosen F.S.: The gammaglobulins: I. The structure and synthesis of the immuno-globulin. *N. Engl. J. Med.* 275:480, 536, 1964.
3. Issitt P.D.: The structure and function of antigens and antibodies, in Dawson B.R. (ed.): *Blood Bank Immunology*. Washington D.C., American Association of Blood Banks, 1977, p. 24.
4. Yasmeen D., et al.: The structure and function of immunoglobulin domains: IV. The distribution of some effector functions among the C-gamma-2 and C-gamma-3 homology regions of human immunoglobulin G1. *J. Immunol.* 116:518, 1976.
5. Deisenhofer J.: Crystallographic refinement and atomic models of human Fc fragment and its complex with fragment B of protein A from *Staphylococcus aureus* at 2.9 and 2.8-A resolution. *Biochemistry* 20:2361, 1981.
6. Davies D.R., Metzger H.: Structural basis of antibody function. *Annu. Rev. Immunol.* 1:87, 1983.
7. Sakano H., et al.: Domains and the hinge region of an immunoglobulin heavy chain are encoded in separate DNA segments. *Nature* 277:627, 1979.
8. Capra J.D., Kehoe J.M.: Hypervariable regions idiotypy and the antigen-combining site. *Adv. Immunol.* 20:1, 1975.
9. Kabat E.A.: The structural basis of antibody complementarity. *Adv. Protein Chem.* 32:1, 1978.
10. Metzger H.: The chemistry of the immunoglobulins. *JAMA* 202:129, 1967.
11. Natvig J.B., Kunkel H.G.: Human immunoglobulins: Classes, subclasses, genetic variants and idiotypes. *Adv. Immunol.* 16:1, 1973.
12. Kochwa S., Kunkel H.G. (eds.): *Immunoglobulins*. Ann. NY Acad. Sci. 19:5, 1971.
13. Katz D.H., Benacerraf B.: The function and interrelationships of T-cell receptors, Ir genes and other histocompatibility gene products. *Transplant. Rev.* 22:173, 1975.
14. Metzger H.: Structure and function of gamma-M macroglobulins. *Adv. Immunol.* 12:57, 1970.
15. McConnell I., et al.: *The Immune System: A Course on the Molecular and Cellular Basis of Immunity*, ed. 2. Oxford, England, Blackwell Scientific Publications, 1981, pp. 3–21.
16. Bienenstock J., Befus A.D.: Some thoughts on the biologic role of immunoglobulin A. *Gastroenterology* 84:178, 1983.
17. Tomasi T.B., et al.: Mucosal immunity: The origin and migration patterns of cells in the secretory system. *J. Allergy Clin. Immunol.* 65:12, 1980.
18. Dahlen S.E., et al.: Leukotriens promote plasma leakage and leukocyte adhesion in postcapillary venules: In vivo effects with relevance to the acute inflammatory response. *Proc. Natl. Acad. Sci. USA* 78:3887, 1981.
19. Uhr J., Vitetta E.S.: Receptor-mediated triggering and tolerance in murine B cells, in Pernis B., Vogel H.J. (eds.): *Cells of Immunoglobulin Synthesis*. New York, Academic Press, 1979, p. 155.
20. Natvig J.B., Kunkel H.G.: Genetic markers of human immunoglobulins: The Gen and the InV systems. *Semin. Hematol.* 1:66, 1968.
21. Eisen H.N.: *Immunology*, ed. 2. New York, Harper & Row, 1974, pp. 419–425.
22. Oudin J.: The genetic control of immunoglobulin synthesis. *Proc. R. Soc. Lond.* [B] 166:207, 1966.
23. McConnell I., Munro A. Waldmann H.: *The Immune System: A Course on the Molecular and Cellular Basis of Immunity*, ed. 2. Oxford, England, Blackwell Scientific Publications, 1981, pp. 15,16.
24. Jerne N.K.: The immune system: A web of V-domains. *Harvey Lecture Series* 70:93, 1975, Academic Press, N.Y.
25. McConnell I., Munro A., Waldman H.: *The Immune System: A Course on the Molecular and Cellular Basis of Immunity*, ed. 2. Oxford, England, Blackwell Scientific Publications, 1981, p. 117.
26. Weigert M., et al.: Rearrangement of genetic information may produce immunoglobulin diversity. *Nature* 276:785, 1978.
27. Du Pasquier L., Wabl M.R.: Antibody diversity in amphibians: Inheritance of isoelectric focusing antibody patterns in isogenic frogs. *Eur. J. Immunol.* 8:428.

28. Capra J.D., Nisonoff A.: The complete amino acid sequence of the heavy-chain variable region of anti-p-azophenylarsonate antibodies from A/J mice bearing a cross-reactive idiotype. *J. Immunol.* 123:279, 1979.
29. Estess P., Nisonoff A., Capra J.D.: NH_2-terminal amino acid sequence analysis of the heavy- and light-chain variable regions of monoclonal anti-p-azophenylarsonate antibodies. *Mol. Immunol.* 16:1111, 1979.
30. Jerne N.K.: Towards a network theory of the immune system. *Ann. Inst. Pasteur* 125C:373, 1974.
31. Jerne N.K.: The somatic generation of immune recognition. *Eur. J. Immunol.* 1:1, 1971.
32. Leder P.: The genetics of antibody diversity. *Sci. Am.* 246:102, 1982.
33. Dreyer W.J., Bennet U.: The molecular basis of antibody formation: A paradox. *Proc. Natl. Acad. Sci. USA* 54:864, 1965.
34. Tonegawa S., et al.: Sequence of a mouse germ-line gene for a variable region of an immunoglobulin light chain. *Proc. Natl. Acad. Sci. USA* 75:1485, 1978.
35. Gorski J., Rollini P., Mach B.: Somatic mutations of immunoglobulin variable genes are restricted to the rearranged V gene. *Science* 220:1179, 1983.
36. Tyler B.M., et al.: mRNA for surface immunoglobulin gamma chains encodes a highly conserved transmembrane sequence and a 28-residue intracellular domain. *Proc. Natl. Acad. Sci. USA* 79:2008, 1982.
37. Rogers J., et al.: Two mRNAs with different 3' ends encode membrane-bound and secreted forms of immunoglobulin mu chain. *Cell* 20:303, 1980.
38. Braun J., et al.: Crosslinking by ligands to surface immunoglobulin triggers mobilization of intracellular 45Ca2+ in B-lymphocytes. *J. Cell Biol.* 82:755, 1979.
39. Braun, J., et al.: Ligand-induced association of surface-immunoglobulin with the detergent-insoluble cytoskeletal matrix of the B-lymphocyte. *J. Immunol.* 128:1198, 1982.
40. Metzger H.: A comment on the "speculation" of Jarvis and Voss. *Mol. Immunol.* 19:1071, 1982.
41. Ciccimmara F., et al.: Localization of the IgG effector site for monocyte receptors. *Proc. Natl. Acad. Sci. USA* 72:2081, 1975.
42. Painter R.H., et al.: Complement fixing and macrophage opsonizing activities associated with beta-2-microglobulin. *Immunol. Commun.* 3:19, 1974.
43. Foster D.E.B., et al.: Structure and function of immunoglobulin domains: VIII. An analysis of the structural requirements in human IgG1 for binding to the Fc receptor of human monocytes. *J. Immunol.* 124:2186, 1980.
44. Foster D.E.B., et al.: The effect of fragment B of staphylococcal protein A on the binding of rabbit IgG to human granulocytes and monocytes. *Mol. Immunol.* 19:407, 1982.
45. Unkeless J.C., Eisen H.N.: Binding of monomeric immunoglobulins to Fc receptors of mouse macrophages. *J. Exp. Med.* 142:1520, 1975.
46. Unkeless J.C.: The presence of two Fc receptors on mouse macrophages: Evidence from a variant cell line and differential trypsin sensitivity. *J. Exp. Med.* 145:931, 1977.
47. Walker W.S.: Separate Fc receptors for immunoglobulins IgG2a and IgG2b on an established cell-line of mouse macrophages. *J. Immunol.* 116:911, 1976.
48. Melewicz F.M., Spielberg H.L.: Fc receptors for IgE on a subpopulation of human peripheral blood monocytes. *J. Immunol.* 125:1026, 1980.
49. Capron A., et al.: Specific IgE antibodies in immune adherence of normal macrophages to *Schistosoma mansoni* schistosomules. *Nature* 253:474, 1975.
50. Roubin R., Zolla-Pazner S.: Markers of macrophage heterogeneity: I. Studies of macrophages from various organs of normal mice. *Eur. J. Immunol.* 9:972, 1979.
51. Unkeless J.C., et al.: Purifications and characterization of a mouse macrophage Fc receptor, in Forster O., Landy M. (eds.): *Heterogeneity of Mononuclear Phagocytes.* New York, Academic Press, Inc., 1981, pp. 91–96.
52. Yagawa K., Onoue K., Aida Y.: Structural studies of Fc receptors: I. Binding properties, solubilization, and partial characterization of Fc receptors of macrophages. *J. Immunol.* 122:366, 1979.
53. Kulczycki A. Jr., et al.: Purification of Fc gamma receptor from rabbit alveolar macrophages that retains ligand-binding activity. *J. Immunol.* 124:2772, 1980.
54. Kabat E.A.: The nature of an antigenic determinant. *J. Immunol.* 97:1, 1966.
55. Watson J., Trenkner E., Cohn M.: The use of bacterial lipopolysaccharides to show that two signals are required for the induction of antibody synthesis. *J. Exp. Med.* 138:699, 1973.
56. McConnell I., et al.: *The Immune System,* ed. 2. Oxford, England, Blackwell Scientific Publications, 1981, p. 131.
57. Heidelberger M.: *Lectures in Immunochemistry.* New York, Academic Press, 1956.
58. Stean E.A.: The interaction of antibodies with red cell surface antigens: Kinetics, noncovalent bonding, and hemagglutination, in Dawson R.B. (ed.): *Blood Bank Immunology: A Technical Workshop.* Washington, D.C., American Association of Blood Banks, 1977, p. 61.
59. Froese A.: Kinetic and equilibrium studies on 2,4-dinitrophenyl hapten-antibody systems. *Immunochemistry* 5:253, 1968.
60. Wu T.T., Kabat E.A.: An analysis of sequences of the variable regions of Bence-Jones proteins and myeloma light chains and their implications for antibody complementarity. *J. Exp. Med.* 132:211, 1970.
61. Givol D., et al.: Combining site and antigenic determinants of the V regions. *Haematologia* 12:15, 1979.
62. Givol D.: Affinity labeling and topology of the antibody combining site. *Essays Biochem.* 10:73, 1974.
63. Stean E.A.: The physical chemistry of hemaggluti-

nation, in Walker R.H. (ed.): *A Seminar on Polymorphisms in Human Blood.* Washington, D.C., American Association of Blood Banks, 1975, p. 105.
64. Potter M.: Immunoglobulin-producing tumors and myeloma proteins of mice. *Physiol. Rev.* 52:631, 1972.
65. Kohler G., Milstein C.: Continuous cultures of fused cells secreting antibody of predefined specificity. *Nature* 256:495, 1975.
66. Kennett R.H., McKearn T.J., Bechtol K.B. (eds.): *Monoclonal antibodies: Hybridomas. A New Dimension in Biological Analyses.* New York, Plenum Press, 1980.
67. Milstein C.: Monoclonal antibodies. *Sci. Am.* 243:56, 1980.
68. Diamond B., et al.: Monoclonal antibodies. *N. Engl. J. Med.* 304:1344, 1981.
69. Olsson L., Kaplan H.S.: Human-human hybridomas producing monoclonal antibodies of predefined antigenic specificity. *Proc. Natl. Acad. Sci. USA* 77:5429, 1980.
70. Reinherz E.L., Schlossman S.F.: The characterization and function of human immunoregulatory T-lymphocyte subsets. *Immunol. Today* 2:69, 1981.
71. Reinherz E.L., et al.: Discrete stages of human intrathymic differentiation: Analysis of normal thymocytes and leukemic lymphoblasts of T-cell lineage. *Proc. Natl. Acad. Sci. USA* 77:1588, 1980.
72. Terhorst C., et al.: Biochemical analysis of human T lymphocyte differentiation antigens T4 and T5. *Science* 209:520, 1980.
73. Reinherz E.L., et al.: A monoclonal antibody reactive with the human cytotoxic/suppressor T cell subset previously defined by a heteroantiserum termed TH2. *J. Immunol.* 124:1301, 1980.
74. Brodsky F., et al.: Monoclonal antibodies for analysis of the HLA system. *Immunol. Rev.* 47:3, 1979.
75. Voak D., et al.: Monoclonal anti-A from a hybrid myeloma: Evaluation as a blood grouping reagent. *Vox Sang.* 39:134, 1980.
76. Sacks S.H., Lennox E.S.: Monoclonal anti-B as a new blood-typing reagent. *Vox Sang.* 40:99, 1981.
77. Rubinstein P., quoted by Mollison P.L., in *Blood Transfusion in Clinical Medicine,* ed. 7. Oxford, England, Blackwell Scientific Publications, 1983, p. 416.
78. Fraser R.H., et al., quoted by Mollison P.L., in *Blood Transfusion in Clinical Medicine,* ed. 7. Oxford, England, Blackwell Scientific Publications, 1983, p. 419.
79. Mollison P.L.: *Blood Transfusion in Clinical Medicine,* ed. 7. Oxford, England, Blackwell Scientific Publications, 1983, p. 506.
80. Barker J., quoted by Mollison P.L., in *Blood Transfusion in Clinical Medicine,* ed. 7. Oxford, England, Blackwell Scientific Publications, 1983, p. 507.
81. Mossman T.R., et al.: Alterations of apparent specificity of monoclonal (hybridoma) antibodies recognizing polymorphic histocompatibility and blood group determinants. *J. Immunol.* 125:1152, 1980.
82. Yarmush M.L., et al.: Identification and characterization of rabbit-mouse hybridomas secreting rabbit immunoglobulin chains. *Proc. Natl. Acad. Sci. USA* 77:2899, 1980.
83. Steensgaard J., et al.: Preliminary communication: The development of difference turbidimetric analysis for monoclonal antibodies to human IgG. *Mol. Immunol.* 17:1315, 1980.
84. Mollison P.L.: *Blood Transfusion in Clinical Medicine,* ed. 7. Oxford, England, Blackwell Scientific Publications, 1983, p. 230.
85. Katzmann J.: Reactivity of mouse monoclonal antibodies with porcine and human Willebrand antigen. *Fed. Proc.* 40:834, 1981.
86. Fass D.N., et al.: Murine monoclonal antibody to porcine factor VIII:C. *Thromb. Haemost.* 46:155, 1981.
87. Goodall A.H., et al.: A monoclonal antibody to factor IX. *Thromb. Haemost.* 46:165, 1981.
88. Katzmann J.A., et al.: Isolation of functional human coagulation factor V using a hybridoma antibody. *Proc. Natl. Acad. Sci. USA* 78:162, 1981.
89. Sobel J.H., et al.: Characterization of a crosslink-containing fragment derived from the alpha-polymer of human fibrin and its application in immunologic studies using monoclonal antibodies. *Thromb. Haemost.* 46:240, 1981.
90. Ruan C., et al.: Effects of a monoclonal antibody to human platelet glycoprotein I on platelet-von Willebrand factor subendothelium interactions. *Thromb. Haemost.* 46:98, 1981.
91. McEver R.P., et al.: Isolation and quantitation of the platelet membrane glycoprotein deficient in thrombasthenia using a monoclonal hybridoma antibody. *J. Clin. Invest.* 66:1311, 1980.
92. Edington T.S., Meyer D.: Hybridoma antibody analysis of the molecular biology of coagulation proteins, in Masouredis S. (ed.): *Hybridomas and Monoclonal Antibodies.* Washington, D.C., American Association of Blood Banks, 1981, pp. 25–56.
93. Ouchterlony O., Nilsson L.A.: Immunodiffusion and immunoelectrophoresis, in Weir D.M. (ed.): *Handbook of Experimental Immunology,* ed. 3. Oxford, England, Blackwell Scientific Publications, 1978, p. 19.1.
94. Weir D.M.: (ed.): *Handbook of Experimental Immunology,* ed. 3. Oxford, England, Blackwell Scientific Publications, 1978, p. 5A.2.
95. Weir D.M. (ed.): *Handbook of Experimental Immunology,* ed. 3. Oxford, England, Blackwell Scientific Publications, 1978, pp. 1–47, 115.
96. Williams C.A., Chase M.W.: *Methods in Immunology and Immunochemistry.* New York, Academic Press, 1976, vol. 2, pp. 1–409.
97. Reid K.B.M., Porter R.R.: The proteolytic activation systems of complement. *Annu. Rev. Biochem.* 50:433, 1981.
98. Cooper N.R., Cochrane C.G.: The biochemistry and biologic activities of the complement and contact systems, in Williams W.J., et al. (eds.): *Hematology,* ed. 3. New York, McGraw-Hill Book Co., 1983, pp. 98–110.
99. Garraty G.: Immunobiology of complement, in Dawson B.R. (ed.): *Blood Bank Immunology.* Wash-

ington, D.C., American Association of Blood Banks, 1977, pp. 113–142.
100. McConnell I., Munro A., Waldmann H.: The Immune System, ed. 2. Oxford, England, Blackwell Scientific Publications, 1981, pp. 40–54.
101. Müller-Eberhard H.J.: Complement. *Annu. Rev. Biochem.* 44:697, 1975.
102. Götze O., Müller-Eberhard H.J.: The alternative pathway of complement activation. *Adv. Immunol.* 24:1, 1976.
103. Lachmann P.J., Peters D.K.: Complement, in *Clinical Aspects of Immunology*, ed. 4. Oxford, England, Blackwell Scientific Publications, 1982, p. 18.
104. Knobel H.R., et al.: Chemical analysis and electron microscopy studies of human $C1_q$ prepared by different methods. *Eur. J. Immunol.* 5:78, 1975.
105. Porter R.R.: Complement. *Int. Rev. Biochem.* 23:177, 1979.
106. Humphrey T.K., Dourmashkin R.R.: The lesions in red cell membranes caused by complement. *Adv. Immunol.* 11:75, 1969.
107. Klein M., et al.: Expression of biological effector functions by immunoglobulin G molecules lacking the hinge region. *Proc. Natl. Acad. Sci. USA* 78:524, 1981.
108. Kerr M.A.: Limited proteolysis of complement components C2 and factor B: Structural analogy and limited sequence homology. *Biochem. J.* 183:615, 1979.
109. Podack E.R., et al.: Structural similarities between C6 and C7 of human complement. *J. Immunol.* 123:1071, 1979.
110. Newell S.L., Atkinson J.P.: Biosynthesis of C4 by mouse peritoneal macrophages: II. Comparison of C4 synthesis by resident and elicited populations. *J. Immunol.* 130:834, 1983.
111. Alper C.A., et al.: Studies of hepatic synthesis in vivo of plasma proteins orosomucoid, transferrin, alpha-antitripsin, C8 and factor B. *Clin. Immunol. Immunopathol.* 16:84, 1980.
112. Colten H.R., Einstein L.P.: Complement metabolism: Cellular and humoral regulation. *Transplant. Rev.* 32:3, 1976.
113. Cooper N.R.: Activation and regulation of the first component of complement. *Fed. Proc.* 42:136, 1983.
114. Tschopp J., et al.: Assembly of subcomponents of $C1_r$ and $C1_s$ of first component of complement: Electron microscopic and ultracentrifugal studies. *Proc. Natl. Acad. Sci. USA* 77:7014, 1980.
115. Siegel R.C., et al.: Stoichiometry and sedimentation properties of the complex formed between the $C1_q$ and $C1_{r2}C1_{s2}$ subcomponents of the first component of complement. *J. Immunol.* 127:2447, 1981.
116. Hughes-Jones N.C., Gardner B.: Reaction between isolated globular subunits and the complement component $C1_q$ and IgG complexes. *Mol. Immunol.* 16:697, 1979.
117. Knobel H.R., et al.: Enzymatic digestion of the first component of human complement ($C1_q$). *J. Immunol.* 112:2094, 1974.
118. Feinstein A., Richardson N.E.: Tertiary structure of the constant regions of immunoglobulins in relation to their function, in Edebo L., Stendahl O. (eds.): *Endocytosis and Exocytosis in Host Defense.* Volume 17, *Monographs in Allergy.* Basel, S. Karger, 1981.
119. Storrs B.S., et al.: $C1_q$ binding and C1 activation by various isolated cellular membranes. *J. Immunol.* 131:416, 1983.
120. McConnell I., et al.: *The Immune System*, ed. 2. Oxford, England, Blackwell Scientific Publications, 1981, p. 44.
121. Bokisch V.A., et al.: Isolation of a fragment (C3a) of the third component of human complement containing anaphylatoxin and chemotactic activity and a description of an anaphylatoxin inactivator of human serum. *J. Exp. Med.* 129:1109, 1969.
122. Scheid C.R., et al.: Direct effect of complement factor C5a on the contractile state of isolated smooth muscle cells. *J. Immunol.* 130:1997, 1983.
123. Esser A.F.: Interaction between complement proteins and biological and model membrane, in Chapman D. (ed.): *Biological Membranes.* New York, Academic Press, vol. 4, 1981.
124. Podack E.R., et al.: Membrane attack complex of complement. *J. Exp. Med.* 151:301, 1980.
125. Mayer M.M.: Mechanism of cytolysis by complement. *Proc. Natl. Acad. Sci. USA* 69:2954, 1972.
126. Michaels D.W., et al.: Characterization of the complement lesion: The formation of transmembrane channels and their mechanism of assembly. *J. Immunol.* 120:1785, 1978.
127. Ramm L., et al.: Size of the transmembrane channels produced by complement proteins C5b-8. *J. Immunol.* 129:1143, 1982.
128. Baker P.J. et al.: C567-initiated cytolysis of lymphoid cells: Description of the phenomenon and studies on its control by C567-inhibitors. *J. Immunol.* 118:198, 1977.
129. Müller-Eberhard H.J., Schreiber R.D.: Molecular biology and chemistry of the alternative pathway of complement. *Adv. Immunol.* 29:1, 1980.
130. Gewurz H. et al.: Interactions of the complement system with endotoxin lipopolysaccharides: Consumption of each of the six terminal complement components. *J. Exp. Med.* 128:1048, 1968.
131. Reid K.B., Porter R.R.: The proteolytic activation systems of complement. *Annu. Rev. Biochem.* 50:433, 1981.
132. Pangburn M.K.: Activation of complement via the alternative pathway. *Fed. Proc.* 42:139, 1983.
133. Nelson B., Ruddy, S.: Enhancing role of IgG in lysis of rabbit erythrocytes by the alternative pathway of human complement. *J. Immunol.* 122:1994, 1979.
134. Joseph B.S., et al.: Immunologic injury of cultured cells infected with measles virus: I. Role of IgG antibody and the alternative complement pathway. *J. Exp. Med.* 141:761, 1975.

135. Pangburn M.K., Müller-Eberhard H.J.: Activation of the alternative complement pathway: Recognition of surface structures on activators by bound C3b. *J. Immunol.* 124:977, 1980.
136. Pangburn M.K., et al.: Formation of the initial C3 convertase of the alternative complement pathway: Acquisition of C3b-like activities by spontaneous hydrolysis of the putative thiol ester in native C3. *J. Exp. Med.* 154:856, 1981.
137. Johnson M.S., et al.: Factor D of the alternative pathway of human complement: Purification, alignment and N-terminal amino acid sequences of the major cyanogen bromide fragments, and localization of the serine residue at the active site. *Biochem. J.* 187:863, 1980.
138. Müller-Eberhard H.J., Götze O.: C3 proactivator convertase and its mode of action. *J. Exp. Med.* 135:1003, 1972.
139. Medicus R.G., et al.: The serine protease nature of the C3 and C5 convertases of the classical and alternative complement pathways. *Scand. J. Immunol.* 5:1049, 1976.
140. Fearon D.T., Austen K.F.: Activation of the alternative complement pathway with rabbit erythrocytes by circumvention of the regulatory action of endogenous control proteins. *J. Exp. Med.* 146:22, 1977.
141. Cooper N.R., Ziccardi R.J.: The nature and reaction of complement enzymes, in Ribbons D.W., Brew K. (eds.): *Proteolysis and Physiological Regulation.* New York, Academic Press, 1976, vol. 11, pp. 167–187.
142. Fujita T. et al.: Human C4 binding protein: I. Role in proteolysis of C4b and C3b inactivator. *J. Exp. Med.* 148:1044, 1978.
143. Pangburn M.K., Schreiber R.D., Müller-Eberhard H.J.: Human complement C3b inactivator: Isolation, characterization and demonstration of an absolute requirement for the serum protein B1H for cleavage of C3b and C4b in solution. *J. Exp. Med.* 146:257, 1977.
144. Whaley K., Ruddy S.: Modulation of the alternative pathway by beta-H globulin. *J. Exp. Med.* 144:1147, 1976.
145. Sim E., et al.: Pattern of degradation of human complement fragment, C3b. *FEBS Lett.* 132:55, 1981.
146. Lachman P.J., Pangburn M.K.: The breakdown of C3bi to C3c, C3d and C3e. Read before the 19th International Conference on Complement, Key Biscaine, Florida; quoted by Mollison P.L.: *Blood Transfusion in Clinical Medicine,* ed. 7. Oxford, England, Blackwell Scientific Publications, 1983, p. 261.
147. Nagasawa S., et al.: Cleavage of C4b by C3b inactivator: Production of a nicked form of C4b, C4b', as an intermediate cleavage product of C4b by C3b inactivator. *J. Immunol.* 125:578, 1980.
148. Podak E.F., Müller-Eberhard H.J.: Isolation of human S-protein, an inhibitor of the membrane attack complex of complement. *J. Biol. Chem.* 254:9908, 1979.
149. Bokisch V.A., Müller-Eberhard H.J.: Anaphylatoxin inactivator of human plasma: Its isolation and characteristics as a carboxypeptidase. *J. Clin. Invest.* 49:2427, 1970.
150. Tenner A.J., Cooper N.R.: Identification of types of cells in human peripheral blood that bind C1q. *J. Immunol.* 126:1174.
151. Fearon D.T., Wong W.W.: Complement ligand-receptor interactions that mediate biological responses. *Annu. Rev. Immunol.* 1:243, 1983.
152. Fearon D.T.: Identification of the membrane glycoprotein which is the C3b receptor of the human erythrocyte, polymorphonuclear leukocyte, B lymphocyte and monocyte. *J. Exp. Med.* 152:20, 1980.
153. Iida K., Mornaghi R., Nussenzweig V.: Complement receptor (CR1) deficiency in erythrocytes from patients with systemic lupus erythematosus. *J. Exp. Med.* 153:1427, 1982.
154. Fearon D.T., Collins L.A.: Increased expression of C3b receptors on polymorphonuclear leukocytes induced by chemotactic factors and purification procedures. *J. Immunol.* 130:370, 1983.
155. Herbert L.A., et al.: In vivo kinetics of the private erythrocyte-immune complex clearing mechanism (abstract). *Clin. Reg.* 30:350A, 1981.
156. Lambris J.D., Ross G.D.: Assay of membrane complement receptors (CR1 and CR2) with C3b- and C3d-coated fluorescent microspheres. *J. Immunol.* 128:186, 1982.
157. Lambris J.D., Dobson N.J., Ross G.D.: Isolation of lymphocyte membrane complement receptor type two (the C3d receptor) and preparation of receptor-specific antibody. *Proc. Natl. Acad. Sci. USA* 78:1828, 1981.
158. Schenkein H.A., Genco R.J.: Inhibition of lymphocyte blastogenesis by C3c and C3d. *J. Immunol.* 122:1126, 1979.
159. Ross G.D., Lambris J.D.: Identification of a C3bi-specific membrane complement receptor that is expressed on lymphocytes, monocytes, neutrophils and erythrocytes. *J. Exp. Med.* 155:96, 1982.
160. Lambris J.D., Ross G.D.: Characterization of the lymphocyte membrane receptor for factor H (beta 1H-globulin) with an antibody to anti-factor H idiotype. *J. Exp. Med.* 155:1400, 1982.
161. Johnson A.R., et al.: Release of histamine from rat mast cells by the complement peptides C3a and C5a. *Immunology* 28:1067, 1975.
162. Gorski T.P., et al.: C4a: The third anaphylatoxin of the human complement system. *Proc. Natl. Acad. Sci. USA* 76:5299, 1979.
163. Gerhard C., et al.: Response of human neutrophils to C5a: A role for the oligosaccharide moiety of human C5a-des-ARg-74 but not of C5a in biologic activity. *J. Immunol.* 127:1978, 1981.
164. Mantovani B., et al.: Phagocytosis of immune complexes by macrophages: Different roles of the macrophage receptor sites for complement (C3) and for immunoglobuin (IgG). *J. Exp. Med.* 135:780, 1972.
165. Ehlenberger A.G., Nussenzweig V.: The role of

165. membrane receptors for C3b and C3d in phagocytosis. *J. Exp. Med.* 145:357, 1977.
166. Griffin F.M., Mullinax P.J.: Augmentation of macrophage complement receptor function in vitro: III. C3b receptors that promote phagocytosis migrate within the plane of the macrophage plasma membrane. *J. Exp. Med.* 154:291, 1981.
167. Urbaniak S.J.: ADCC (K-cell) lysis of human erythrocytes sensitized with rhesus alloantibodies: Investigation into the mechanism of lysis. *Br. J. Haematol.* 42:315, 1979.
168. Szymanski I.O., et al.: Complement and Ig uptake by erythrocytes in low ionic strength solutions. *Vox Sang.* 41:151, 1981.
169. Schreiber A.D., Frank M.M.: Role of antibody and complement in the immune clearance and destruction of erythrocytes: I. In vivo effects of IgG and IgM complement-fixing sites. *J. Clin. Invest.* 51:575, 1972.
170. Engelfriet C.P., et al.: Immune destruction of red cells, in Bell C.A. (ed.): *A Seminar on Immune-Mediated Cell Destruction.* Washington, D.C., American Association of Blood Banks, 1981, p. 97.
171. Halburn A.M., et al.: Some biological effects of IgM anti-Rh(0). *Immunology* 20:681, 1971.
172. Ghebrehiwet B., Müller-Eberhard H.J.: Description of an acidic fragment (C3e) on Human C3 having leukocyte-producing activity. *J. Immunol.* 120:1774, 1978.
173. Ross G.D., Tack B.F., Robetino E.M.: Effects of beta-1H, C3b inactivator (C3bINA) and serum protease in the interactions of C3b with membrane receptors. *Fed. Proc.* 37:1270, 1978.
174. Engelfriet C.P., et al.: Autoimmune hemolytic anemias: V. Studies on the resistance against complement haemolysis of red cells of patients with chronic cold agglutinin disease. *Clin. Exp. Immunol.* 11:255, 1972.
175. Stimler N.P., et al.: Anaphylatoxin mediated contraction of guinea pig lung strips: A non-histamine tissue response. *J. Immunol.* 126:2258, 1981.
176. Stimler N.P., et al.: Release of leukotrienes from guinea pig lung stimulated by C5a-des-Arg anaphylatoxin. *J. Immunol.* 128:2247, 1982.
177. Ghebrehiwet B., Müller-Eberhard H.J.: C3e: An acidic fragment of human C3 with leukocytosis inducing activity. *J. Immunol.* 123:616, 1979.
178. Gerhard C., Hugli T.E.: Identification of classical anaphylatoxin as the des-Arg form of the C5a molecule: Evidence of a modulator role for the oligosaccharide unit in human des-Arg-^{74} C5a. *Proc. Natl. Acad. Sci. USA* 78:1833, 1981.
179. Shin H.S., et al.: Chemotactic and anaphylatoxic fragment cleaved from the fifth component of guinea pig complement. *Science* 162:361, 1968.
180. Snyderman R., et al.: Biological activity of complement in vivo: Role of C5 in the accumulation of polymorphonuclear leukocytes in inflammatory exudates. *J. Exp. Med.* 134:1131, 1971.
181. Lachman P.J., Hobart M.J.: The genetics of the complement system. *CIBA Symp.* 66:231, 1979.
182. O'Neill G.J., et al.: Chido and Rogers blood groups are distinct antigenic components of human complement C4. *Nature* 273:668, 1978.
183. McConnell I., et al.: *The Immune System,* ed. 2. Oxford, England, Blackwell Scientific Publications, 1981, pp. 69–82.
184. Frank M.M., Atkinson J.P.: Complement in clinical medicine. *DM,* January 1975.
185. Kohler P.F.: Inherited complement deficiencies and systemic lupus erythematosus: An immunogenetic puzzle. *Ann. Intern. Med.* 82:420, 1975.
186. Frank M.M., et al.: Hereditary angioedema: The clinical syndrome and its management. *Ann. Intern. Med.* 84:580, 1976.
187. Donaldson V.H., et al.: Role of the second component of complement (C2) and plasma in kinin release in hereditary angioneurotic edema (HANE) plasma. *Trans. Am. Assoc. Physicians* 40:174, 1977.
188. Uff J.S., et al.: In vitro fixation of guinea-pig complement by renal biopsies. *J. Clin. Lab. Immunol.* 1:299, 1979.
189. Nydegger U.E., et al.: Circulatory complement breakdown products in patients with rheumatoid arthritis: Correlation between plasma C3d, circulating immune complexes, and clinical activity. *J. Clin. Invest.* 59:682, 1977.
190. Scott D.M., et al.: The role of carbohydrate in the structure and function of nephritic factor. *Clin. Exp. Immunol.* 46:120, 1981.
191. Hammerschmidt D.E., et al.: Association of complement activation and elevated plasma-C5a with adult respiratory distress syndrome: Pathophysiological relevance and possible prognostic value. *Lancet* 1:947, 1980.
192. Chenoweth D.E., et al.: Complement activation during cardiopulmonary bypass: Evidence for generation of C3a and C5a anaphylatoxins. *N. Engl. J. Med.* 304:497, 1981.
193. Natvig J.B., et al.: Idiotypic specificities of anti-Rh antibodies. *J. Immunol.* 116:1536, 1976.
194. Hughes-Jones N.C., Ghosh S.: Anti-D-coated Rh positive red cells will bind the first component of the complement pathway, C1q. *FEBS Lett.* 128:318, 1981.
195. Mollison P.L.: *Blood Transfusion in Clinical Medicine,* ed. 7. Oxford, England, Blackwell Scientific Publications, 1983, p. 352.
196. Mollison P.L.: *Blood Transfusion in Clinical Medicine,* ed. 7. Oxford, England, Blackwell Scientific Publications, 1983, p. 267.
197. Moller G.: *T and B Lymphocytes in Humans. Transplant. Rev.*, vol. 16, 1975.
198. Gutman G.A., Weissman I.L.: Lymphoid tissue architecture: Experimental analysis of the origin and distribution of T-cells and B-cells. *Immunology* 23:465, 1972.
199. Nelson D.S.: *Immunobiology of the Macrophage.* New York, Academic Press, 1976, p. 45.
200. Weissman I.L., et al.: The lymphoid system: Its normal architecture and the potential for its under-

standing by the study of lymphoproliferative diseases. *Hum. Pathol.* 9:25, 1978.
201. Lawton A.R.: B lymphocyte development, heterogeneity and activation. *Fed. Proc.* 41:2492, 1982.
202. Warner J.L.: Membrane immunoglobulins and antigen receptors on B and T lymphocytes. *Adv. Immunol.* 19:153, 1974.
203. Winchester R.J., Ross G.: Methods for enumerating lymphocyte populations, in Rose N.R., Friedman H. (eds.): *Manual of Clinical Immunology.* American Society of Microbiologists, Washington D.C., 1976, p. 64.
204. Nadler L.M., et al.: Diagnosis and treatment of human leukemia and lymphomas utilizing monoclonal antibodies. *Prog. Hematol.* 12:187–225, 1981.
205. Canton H., Boyse E.A.: Functional subclasses of T lymphocytes bearing different Ly antigens: 1. The generation of functionally distinct T cell subclasses as a differentiative process independent of antigen. *J. Exp. Med.* 141:1376, 1975.
206. Aiuti F., et al.: Monoclonal antibodies in the characterization of human T and LGL cells. *Clin. Immunol. Newslett.* 4:23, 1983.
207. Chang T.W., et al.: Does OKT3 monoclonal antibody react with an antigen-recognition structure on human T-cells? *Proc. Natl. Acad. Sci. USA* 78:1805, 1980.
208. Zarling J.M., Kung P.C.: Distinction between human NK cells and cytotoxic T lymphocytes by monoclonal antibodies. *Nature* 288:394, 1980.
209. Breard J., et al.: A monoclonal antibody reactive with human peripheral blood monocytes. *J. Immunol.* 124:1943, 1980.
210. Cantor H., Boyse E.A.: Functional subclasses of T lymphocytes bearing different Ly antigens: 2. Cooperation between subclasses of Ly+ cells in the generation of killer activity. *J. Exp. Med.* 141:1390, 1975.
211. Herberman R.B., et al.: Natural cytotoxic reactivity of mouse lymphoid cells against syngeneic and allogeneic tumors. *Int. J. Cancer* 16:216, 1975.
212. Unanue E.R., Cerottini J.C.: The immunogenicity of antigen bound to the plasma membrane of macrophages. *J. Exp. Med.* 131:711, 1970.
213. Burnet F.M.: *The Clonal Selection Theory of Acquired Immunity.* Nashville, Tenn., Vanderbilt University Press, 1959.
214. Basten A., Mitchell J.: Role of macrophages in T cell-B cell collaboration in antibody production, in Nelson D.S. (ed.): *Immunobiology of the Macrophage.* New York, Academic Press, 1976, p. 45.
215. Lay W.H., Nussenzweig V.: Receptors for complement of leukocytes. *J. Exp. Med.* 128:991, 1968.
216. Gilliland B.C.: Clinical Immunology, in Isselbacher K., et al. (eds.): *Harrison's Principles of Internal Medicine,* ed. 9. New York, McGraw-Hill Book Co., 1980, p. 3.
217. Benacerraf B., McDevitt H.D.: The histocompatibility-linked immune response genes. *Science* 175:273, 1972.

218. Marx J.L.: Likely T cell receptor gene cloned. *Science* 221:1278, 1983.
219. Meuer S.C., et al.: Identification of the receptor for antigen and major histocompatibility complex on human-inducer T-lymphocytes. *Science* 222:1240, 1983.
220. Grey H.M.: Phylogeny of immunoglobulins. *Adv. Immunol.* 10:51, 1969.
221. Wallis V.J., et al.: On the sparse seeding of bone marrow and thymus in radiation chimeras. *Transplantation* 19:1, 1975.
222. Silverstone A.L., et al.: Terminal deoxynucleotidyl transferase is found in prothymocyte. *J. Exp. Med.* 144:543, 1976.
223. Milstein C., et al.: Monoclonal antibodies and cell surface antigens, in *Human Genetics: Possibilities and Realities. CIBA Symp.* 66:251, 1979.
224. Reinhertz E.L., Schlossman S.F.: The differentiation and function of human T lymphocytes. *Cell* 19:821, 1980.
225. Binz H., Wigzell H.: Antigen binding, idiotypic T-lymphocyte receptors, in Stutman, O. (ed.): *Contemp. Topics Immunol.* 7:113, 1977.
226. Krammer P.H., Eichmann K.: T cell receptor idiotypes are controlled by genes in the heavy-chain linkage group and the major histocompatibility complex. *Nature* 270:733, 1977.
227. Desforges J.F.: T cell receptors. *N. Engl. J. Med.* 313:376, 1985.
228. Claman H.N., et al.: Immunocompetence of transferred thymus-marrow combinations. *J. Immunol.* 97:928, 1966.
229. Mitchison N.A.: Carrier effects in secondary response to protein conjugates: I. Measurement of the effect of transferred cells and objection to the local environment hypothesis. *Eur. J. Immunol.* 1:10, 1971.
230. Phillips J., Waldmann H.: Monogamous T helper cell. *Nature* 268:641, 1977.
231. Cantor H., Boyse E.A.: Functional subclasses of T lymphocytes bearing different Ly antigens: I. The generation of functionally distinct T cell subclasses in a differentiative process independent of antigen. *J. Exp. Med.* 141:1376, 1975.
232. Gershon R.K.: T-cell control of antibody production. *Contemp. Top. Immunobiol.* 3:1, 1974.
233. Waldman T., et al.: Regulation of the humoral immune response: From immunoglobulin genes to regulatory T-cell networks. *Fed. Proc.* 42:2498, 1983.
234. Benacerraf B.: Overview of the major histocompatibility complex. *Science* 212:1229, 1981.
235. Adorini L., et al.: Fine specificity of regulatory T cells: II. Suppressor and helper cells are inducing different regions of hen egg white lysozyme in a genetically non-responder mouse strain. *J. Exp. Med.* 150:293, 1979.
236. McConnell I., et al. (eds.): *The Immune System,* ed. 2. Oxford, England, Blackwell Scientific Publications, 1981, pp. 204–215.
237. Benacerraf B.: An hypothesis to relate the specific-

ity of T lymphocytes and the activity of I-region-specific Ir genes in macrophages and B lymphocytes. *J. Immunol.* 120:1809, 1978.
238. Orr H.T., et al.: The heavy chain of the human histocompatibility antigen HLA-B7 contains an immunoglobulin-like region. *Nature* 282:266, 1979.
239. Bodmer W.F.: HLA: A super supergene. *Harvey Lect.* 72:91, 1976.
240. Klein J.: The major histocompatibility complex of the mouse. *Science* 203:516, 1979.
241. Nathenson S.G., et al.: Primary structural analysis of the transplantation antigen of the murine H-2 major histocompatibility complex. *Annu. Rev. Biochem.* 50:1025, 1981.
242. Klein J., Nagy Z.A.: MHC restriction and Ir genes. *Adv. Cancer Reg.* 37:233, 1982.
243. Zinkernagel R.M., Doherty P.C.: Activity of sensitized thymus-derived lymphocytes in lymphocytic choriomeningitis reflects immunological surveillance against altered self components. *Nature* 257:547, 1974.
244. Blanden R.V., et al.: Cytotoxic T-cell response to *Ectromelia* virus-infected cells: Different H-2 requirements for triggering precursor T cell induction or lysis by the effector T-cells defined by the Balb 1_c-H-2^{db} mutation. *J. Exp. Med.* 146:869, 1977.
245. Bevan M.J.: In a radiation chimera host H-2 antigens determine the immune responsiveness of donor cytotoxic cells. *Nature* 269:417, 1977.
246. Bluestein H.G., et al.: Specific immune response genes of the guinea pig. *J. Exp. Med.* 135:98, 1972.
247. Deline P., et al.: Genetic control of specific immune suppression. *J. Exp. Med.* 142:1447, 1975.
248. McConnell I., et al.: *The Immune System*, ed. 2. Oxford, England, Blackwell Scientific Publications, 1981, p. 197.
249. Aarden L.A., et al.: Revised nomenclature for antigen non-specific T cell proliferation and helper factors (letter). *J. Immunol.* 123:2928, 1979.
250. Maizel A.L., et al.: Effect of interleukin-1 on human thymocytes and purified human T cells. *J. Exp. Med.* 153:470, 1981.
251. Gillis S.: Interleukin biochemistry and biology: Summary and introduction. *Fed. Proc.* 42:2635, 1983.
252. Billingham R.E., et al.: Actively allergized tolerance of foreign cells. *Nature* 172:603, 1953.
253. von Boehmer, et al.: Tolerance to histocompatibility determinants in tetraparental bone-marrow chimeras. *J. Exp. Med.* 411:322, 1975.
254. Weigle W.O.: Recent observations and concepts in immunological unresponsiveness and autoimmunity. *Clin. Exp. Immunol.* 9:537, 1971.
255. Brent L., et al.: Transplantation tolerance. *Br. Med. Bull.* 32:101, 1976.
256. Rosen B., Dorsch S.: The cellular basis of transplantation tolerance in the rat. *Immunol. Rev.* 46:55, 1979.
257. Diener E., Feldmann M.: Relationship between antigen- and antibody-induced suppression of immunity. *Transplant. Rev.* 8:76, 1972.
258. Binz H., Wigzell H.: Specific transplantation tolerance induced by auto-immunization against the individual's own naturally occupying idiotypic, antigen-binding receptors. *J. Exp. Med.* 144:1438, 1976.
259. McConnell I., et al.: *The Immune System: A Course on the Molecular and Cellular Basis of Immunity*, ed. 2. Oxford, England, Blackwell Scientific Publications, 1981, p. 213.
260. Kretschmer R., et al.: Congenital aplasia of the thymus gland (DiGeorge's syndrome). *N. Engl. J. Med.* 279:1295, 1969.
261. Lischner H.W., Huff D.S.: T-cell deficiency in DiGeorge's syndrome. *Birth Defects* 11:16, 1975.
262. Conley M.E., et al.: The spectrum of DiGeorge syndrome. *J. Pediatr.* 94:883, 1979.
263. Thong Y.H., et al.: Successful restoration of immunity in the DiGeorge syndrome with fetal thymic epithelial transplant. *Arch. Dis. Child.* 53:580, 1978.
264. Pearl E.R., et al.: B lymphocyte precursors in human bone marrow: An analysis of normal individuals and patients with antibody deficiency states. *J. Immunol.* 120:1169, 1978.
265. Gelfand E.W., Biggar W.D., Orange R.P.: Immune deficiency: Evaluation, diagnosis and therapy. *Pediatr. Clin. North Am.* 21:745, 1974.
266. Rosen F.S.: The lymphocyte and the thymus gland: Congenital and hereditary abnormalities. *N. Engl. J. Med.* 279:643, 1968.
267. Bortin M.M., Rimm A.A.: Severe combined immunodeficiency disease: Characterization of the disease and results of transplantation. *JAMA* 237:591, 1977.
268. Anderson L.C., et al.: Induction of specific immune unresponsiveness using primed mixed leucocyte culture activated T lymphoblasts as autoimmunogen. *J. Exp. Med.* 146:1124, 1977.
269. Blaese R.M., et al.: The Wiskott-Aldrich syndrome: A disorder with a possible defect in antigen processing or recognition. *Lancet* 1:1056, 1968.
270. Shapiro R.S., et al.: Wiskott-Aldrich syndrome: Detection of carrier state by metabolic stress of platelets. *Lancet* 1:121, 1978.
271. Parkman R., et al.: Complete correction of the Wiskott-Aldrich syndrome by allogeneic bone marrow transplantation. *N. Engl. J. Med.* 298:921, 1978.
272. Hayward A.: Immunodeficiency, in Lachman P.J., Peters D.K. (eds.): *Clinical Aspects of Immunology*. Oxford, England, Blackwell Scientific Publications, 1982, p. 1658–1711.
273. Buckley R.H.: Bone marrow and thymus transplantation in ataxia telangiectasia, in Bergsma D., et al. (eds.): *Immunodeficiency in Man and Animals*. Sunderland, Mass., Sinauer Press, 1975.
274. Geha R.S., et al.: Heterogeneity of "acquired" or common variable agammaglobulinemia. *N. Engl. J. Med.* 291:1, 1974.
275. Ammann A.J., Houg R.: Selective IgA deficiency: Presentation of 30 cases and review of the literature. *Medicine* 50:223, 1971.

276. Hobbs J.R., Milner R.D., Watt P.J.: Gamma-M deficiency predisposing to meningococcal septicaemia. Br. Med. J. 2:583, 1967.
277. Schur P.H., et al.: Selective gamma-G globulin deficiencies in patients with recurrent pyogenic infections. N. Engl. J. Med. 283:631, 1970.
278. Shuster J., Eisen A.H.: Immunologic deficiency diseases, in Freedman S.O., Gold P. (eds.): Clinical Immunology, ed. 2. New York, Harper & Row, 1976, p. 410.
279. Kaposi's sarcoma and Pneumocystis pneumonia among homosexual men—New York City and California. MMWR 30:305, 1981.
280. Peter J.B.: Acquired immune deficiency syndrome: A new medical mystery. Diagn. Med. 6:25, 1983.
281. Pitchemik A.E.: Acquired immune deficiency syndrome in low risk patients. JAMA 250:1310, 1983.
282. Lane H.C., et al.: Abnormalities of B-cell activation and immunoregulation in patients with the acquired immunodeficiency syndrome. N. Engl. J. Med. 309:453, 1983.
283. Hersh E.M., et al.: Elevated thymosin alpha-1 levels associated with evidence of immune dysregulation in male homosexuals with a history of infectious diseases or Kaposi's sarcoma. N. Engl. J. Med. 308:45, 1983.
284. Eyster M.E., et al.: Acid labile alpha interpheron: A possible preclinical marker for the acquired immunodeficiency syndrome in hemophilia. N. Engl. J. Med. 309:584, 1983.
285. Hobbs J.R.: Paraproteins: Benign or malignant? Br. Med. J. 3:699, 1967.
286. Isaacson P.: Middle East lymphoma and α-chain disease: An immunohystochemical study. Am. J. Surg. Pathol. 3:431, 1979.
287. Bergsagel D.E.: The treatment of plasma cell myeloma. Br. J. Haematol. 33:443, 1976.
288. MacKenzie M.R., Fudenberg H.H.: Macroglobulinemia: An analysis of forty patients. Blood 39:874, 1972.
289. McCallister B.D., et al.: Primary macroglobulinemia: Review with a report on thirty-one cases and notes of value of continuous chlorambucil therapy. Am. J. Med. 43:394, 1967.
290. Deuel T.F. et al.: Waldenström's macroglobulinemia. Arch. Intern. Med. 143:986, 1983.
291. Zawadzki Z.A., Edwards G.A.: Nonmyelomatous monoclonal immunoglobulinemia. Prog. Clin. Immunol. 1:105, 1972.
292. Cohen I.R., Wekerle H.: Regulation of autosensitization: The immune activation and specific inhibition of self-recognizing thymus-derived lymphocytes. J. Exp. Med. 137:224, 1973.
293. Weigle W.O.: Recent observations and concepts in immunological unresponsiveness and autoimmunity. Clin. Exp. Immunol. 9:437, 1971.
294. Howie J.B., Heluer B.J.: The immunology and pathology of NZB mice. Adv. Immunol. 9:215, 1968.
295. Coombs R.R.A., Gell P.G.H.: Classification of allergic reactions responsible for clinical hypersensitivity and disease, in Gell P.G.H., et al. (eds.): Clinical Aspects of Immunology. Oxford, England, Blackwell Scientific Publications, 1975, p. 761.
296. Ishizaka T., et al.: Transmission and regulation of triggering signals induced by bridging of IgE receptors on rat mast cells, in Becker E.L., et al. (eds.): Biochemistry of the Acute Allergic Reactions. New York, Alan R. Liss, 1981, p. 213.
297. Morrison D.C., et al.: Two distinct mechanisms for the initiation of mast cell degranulation. Int. Arch. Allergy Appl. Immunol. 49:172, 1975.
298. Marsch D.G., et al.: Basal serum IgE levels and HLA antigen frequencies in allergic subjects: I. Studies with ragweed allergen Ra3. Immunogenetics 5:217, 1975.
299. Kelly J.F., Patterson R.: Anaphylaxis: Course, mechanisms and treatment. JAMA 227:1431, 1974.
300. Henson P.M.: Antibody and immune-complex-mediated allergic and inflammatory reactions, in Lachman P.J., Peters D.K. (eds.): Clinical Aspects of Immunology. ed. 4. Oxford, England, Blackwell Scientific Publications, 1982, p. 687.
301. Lusher J.M., et al.: Efficacy of prothrombin-complex concentrate in hemophiliacs with antibodies to factor VIII. N. Engl. J. Med. 303:421, 1981.
302. Reisner H.M., et al.: Immunochemical characterization of a polyclonal human antibody to factor IX. Blood 50:11, 1977.
303. Drachman D.B.: Myasthenia gravis. N. Engl. J. Med. 298:136, 1978.
304. van Herle A.J., et al.: Control of thyroglobulin synthesis and secretion. N. Engl. J. Med. 301:239, 1979.
305. Briggs W.A., et al.: Antiglomerular basement membrane: Antibody mediated glomerulonephritis and Goodpasture's syndrome. Medicine 58:348, 1979.
306. Cochrane C.G., Koffler D.: Immune complex disease in experimental animals and man. Adv. Immunol. 16:186, 1973.
307. Emancipator S., et al.: IgA-immune complex renal disease induced by mucosal immunization, in McGhee J.R., Mestecky J. (eds.): The Secretory Immune System. Ann. NY Acad. Sci. 409:171, 1983.
308. Henny C.S., Newman W.: T-cell-mediated tissue damage, in Lachman P.J., Peters D.K. (eds.): Clinical Aspects of Immunology, ed. 4. Oxford, England, Blackwell Scientific Publications, 1982, p. 710.
309. Simpson E., Matsunaga T.: Physiological function of major histocompatibility complex macromolecules. Transplantation 27:295, 1979.
310. Siciliano R.F., Henney C.S.: Enucleated cells as targets for cytotoxic attack. J. Immunol. 121:186, 1978.
311. Henney C.S.: Estimation of the size of a T-cell induced lytic lesion. Nature 249:456, 1974.
312. Reinherz E.L., et al.: Aberrations of suppressor T-cells in human graft-versus-host disease. N. Engl. J. Med. 19:1061, 1979.
313. Kay H.E.M.: Bone marrow transplantation, in Lachman P.J., Peters D.K. (eds.): Clinical Aspects of

Immunology, ed. 4. Oxford, England, Blackwell Scientific Publications, 1982, p. 1347.
314. Beschorner W.E., et al.: Lymphocytic bronchitis associated with graft-versus-host disease in recipients of bone-marrow transplants. *N. Engl. J. Med.* 299:1030, 1978.
315. Bacigalupo A., et al.: Suppressor T-cells after allogeneic bone marrow transplantation, in Thierfelder S., et al. (eds.): *Immunology of Bone Marrow Transplantation*. Berlin, Springer Verlag, 1980.
316. Sale G.E., et al.: The skin biopsy in the diagnosis of acute graft-versus-host disease in man. *Am. J. Pathol.* 89:621, 1977.
317. Tsoi M., et al.: Deposition of IgM and complement at the dermoepidermal junction in acute and chronic graft-vs-host disease in man. *J. Immunol.* 120:1485, 1978.
318. Berk P.D., et al.: Veno-occlusive disease of the liver after allogeneic bone marrow. *Ann. Intern. Med.* 90:158, 1979.
319. Graze P.R., Gale R.P.: Chronic graft-versus-host disease: A syndrome of disordered immunity. *Am. J. Med.* 66:611, 1979.
320. Thomas E.D., et al.: Bone marrow transplantation. *N. Engl. J. Med.* 292:832, 1975.
321. Kay H.E.M., et al.: Cyclosporin A in human marrow grafts, in Thierfelder S., et al. (eds.): *Immunology of Bone Marrow Transplantation*. Berlin, Springer Verlag, 1980, p. 255.
322. Gabrielson A.E., et al.: Reduced haemolytic C1 activity in serum of hypogammaglobulinemic chickens. *Immunology* 27:463, 1974.
323. Alper C.A., Rosen F.S.: Clinical applications of complement assays. *Adv. Intern. Med.* 20:61, 1975.
324. Lachman P.J., Rosen F.S.: Genetic defects of complement in man. *Springer Semin. Immunopathol.* 1:339, 1978.

5

Blood Group Antigens

THE STUDY OF blood group antigens is of paramount importance in immunohematology. An understanding of their chemistry as well as of the immunoglobulin characteristics of the antibodies elicited against them is necessary for making the ultimate decision on blood compatibility.

Red blood cell (RBC) antigens elicit hemagglutination reactions which vary at different thermal ranges[1] as well as at different pH[2,3] and ionic strengths.[3] To understand the kinetics of these reactions it is necessary to review some concepts of antigenicity as well as the localization of antigens on membranes. The chemical study of antigenic determinants was begun by Landsteiner and van der Scheer.[4] From these early studies came the classic concepts of specificity of antigen-antibody reactions. This specificity, as detailed in the previous chapter, is so high as to be able to discriminate between ortho, meta, or para orientations on amino benzene rings.[5]

Antigens usually involved in the induction of antibody responses lie on the external surface of the lipid bilayer of RBC membranes or on the external surface of other cells of formed elements exposed to the immune system via transfusion (granulocytes, platelets, etc.). Knowledge of the basic structure of a cell membrane stems from early studies conducted by Danielli and Davson[6] and allows some speculation as to where and how antigens are located in the lipid bilayer. Macromolecules are thought to be embedded in the lipid bilayer and are free-floating or anchored to underlying cytoplasmic proteins. They may be either superficial or transmembrane molecules (see Fig 2–1).[7] Transmembrane molecules are usually proteins, and many are glycoproteins.[8] Localization of membrane antigens on the RBC membrane has been made possible by the freeze-etching electron microscopy technique.[9] With this method it is possible to determine whether a particular protein is inside or outside the cell membrane. Specific proteins can be detected by ferritin-labeled antibodies against specific glycoproteins and localized by freeze-etching electron microscopy. Characteristically spectrin is considered an extrinsic protein, whereas glycophorin A is considered an integral protein of the RBC membrane.[10]

The mobility of the antigens on the fluid bilayer may determine the agglutination patterns of RBCs, as has been demonstrated by antigens in the Rh system.[11] Furthermore, it has been postulated that transmembrane proteins are crucial to the equilibrium of the membrane. This has been inferred from the osmotic fragility and abnormal deformability of RBCs bearing the Rh null phenotype, which lack this membrane antigen.[12] In contrast, certain antigens of the ABH system probably are extrinsic molecules. This is supported by the fact that Bombay group RBCs, which lack ABH substances, are normal in shape and have a normal life span.[13] Other antigens such as Lu, P, and i appear to be linked to ganglioside molecules.[14]

Antigen mobility on the membrane has been shown to be necessary for adequate hemagglutination. This has been demonstrated via cross-linking experiments with glutaraldehyde, which "freezes"

145

antigenic sites, preventing movement on the membrane. These cells show adequate coating by antibodies but poor agglutinability.[15]

Antigens vary in their representation on the RBC membrane. Rh antigens number approximately 30,000 per RBC,[16] whereas ABH molecules are far more numerous, approximately 1 million per RBC.[17] These figures have been derived using immunoferritin electron microscopy and radiolabeling experiments.

Antigenic representation is also thought to be significant in the kinetics of antigen-antibody binding on the RBC as well as in hemagglutination.

The following sections review the chemistry, agglutination reactivity of antibodies elicited, and the clinical significance of different antigens.

ANTIGENS THAT USUALLY ELICIT COLD ANTIBODIES

The ABO System

Agglutination across species was first described by Landois in 1875.[18] However, credit for the discovery of blood groups in man must be given to Landsteiner, who described his experiments in a 1901 publication, "The Cross-Agglutination Phenomenon of Normal Human Blood."[19] In this publication Landsteiner reported that sera from six normal individuals agglutinated or did not agglutinate saline suspensions of each of the other individual cells, thus discovering the three main blood types in the ABO system, namely, group A, B, and O cells. Two of his students discovered the fourth, rarer AB type in 1902.

Landsteiner also described the reciprocity of serum reactivity with RBC antigens (Landsteiner's rule). Briefly, group A individuals have anti-B antigens in their plasma, group B individuals have anti-A antibodies in their plasma, serum from group O individuals agglutinates both A and B cells, and serum from group AB individuals agglutinates neither A nor B cells (Fig 5–1). This phenomenon holds true in the vast majority of A and B individuals, with a few notable exceptions that will be described later.

The pattern of codominant inheritance in the ABO system was not fully understood until 1924, when F. Bernstein, a mathematician, proposed codominant alleles for blood groups, based on statis-

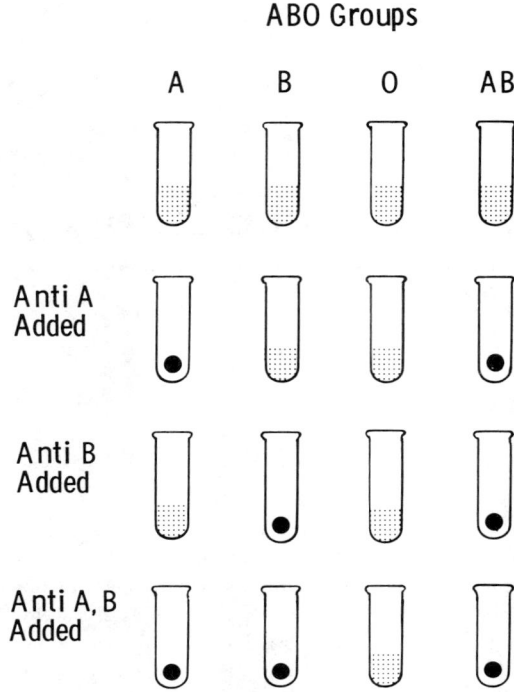

FIG 5–1.—Laboratory determination of ABO groups. Test tube reactions define A, B, O, and AB blood groups according to reaction. *Solid dot* identifies 4+ agglutination of RBCs incubated at room temperature.

tical analysis of blood groups in the population.[20]

Based on these findings the permutations given in Table 5–1 were shown to be possible.

Biochemistry of the ABH Substances

A, B, and H substances have a different chemical nature on membranes than when they exist in the soluble state in secretions. On membranes, they constitute part of band 3 proteins (70%) or glycosphingolipids (10%) which float on the bilipid membrane, with the antigenic terminal sugars exposed to the surface.[21, 22] However, in the soluble state (e.g., in secretions), these sugars form part of glycoproteins rather than glycosphingolipids.[23] On band 3, the major intrinsic protein on RBC membranes, they most likely represent type II chains.

Different terminal sugars are added to a common polysaccharide backbone or H substance present in all groups but forming all of the group substance in group O individuals. The H substance has a terminal fucose on the polysaccharide chain. However,

TABLE 5–1.—POSSIBLE PERMUTATIONS IN THE ABO SYSTEM

GENOTYPES	AA	AO	BB	BO	OO	AB
AA	AA	AA AO	AB	AB AO	AO	AA AB
AO	AA AO	AA AO OO	AB BO	AB OO	AO OO	AA AB BO
BB	AB AB	AB BO	BB	BB BO	BO	AB BB
BO	AB AO	AB OO AO BO	BB BO	BB OO BO	BO OO	AB BB AO BO
OO	AO	AO OO	BO	BO OO	OO	AO BO
AB	AA AB	AA AO AB BO	AB BB	AB AO BO BB	AO BO	AA AB BB

if one additional sugar is added, the specificity of the group substance is changed.[24] The backbone chains of the H substance can be type I or type II chains. The difference between type I or type II chains depends on β-1,3 or β-1,4 linkages of terminal sugars.[24]

Group A substance is composed of an H substance backbone to which N-acetyl-galactosamine has been added as a terminal sugar. Group B substance is formed when instead of N-acetylgalactosamine, D-galactose is added to the H substance backbone.[25] In the absence of H substance as backbone to these terminal sugars, A, B, and AB substances cannot be formed (Fig 5–2).

Both the formation of the backbone and the addition of terminal sugars depend on sugar transferases, which are proteins and as such are coded for by genes in nuclear DNA. The phenotypic expression of A, B, or H substances depends on the synthesis of transferases by ribosomes.[26] The H substance has been shown to be a precursor to antigens other than ABO which have a similar sugar backbone sequence. (e.g., group Ii).

Persons with the Bombay phenotype lack the capacity to produce and secrete H substance[27] because they lack fucosyltransferase.[28] In addition, they cannot produce A or B substances, though they may possess the N-acetylgalactosamine transferase (group A determinant) and/or the D-galactose transferase (group B determinant). These individuals can genetically transmit the transferase coding to their progeny, but their own cells will type as group O cells. Bombay-type transfusion recipients should be transfused with (h) phenotype blood.

Blood Group Substances on Cell Membranes

Many cells of various origins, such as epithelial cells (goblet cells)[29] and endothelial cells, appear to synthesize or bear ABH substances.[30] However, ABH antigens on platelets are secondarily absorbed from plasma glycolipid ABH substances.[31]

On RBC membranes, ABH substances may also be acquired from the plasma as part of a regular glycolipid exchange, but the bulk of the antigen is linked to band 3 protein as a type II carbohydrate chain,[32] in contrast to ABH substances in plasma, which are mostly type I chains.[33] *Ulex europaeus* detects only type II chains of H substance and therefore is useful in typing H-bearing cells.

ABH Blood Group Substances in Secretions

ABH blood group substances in secretions derive from epithelial cells which contain enzymes capable of synthesizing these antigens as glycoproteins. These substances are $3 \times 10^{5-6}$-dalton glycoproteins composed of 80%–90% carbohydrate and 10%–20% amino acids.[34] In secretory cells, type I chain acceptors will form H substances in the presence of α-L-fucosyltransferase by adding fucose to the terminal galactose. Once H substance is formed, Le^b substance can then be synthesized in the secretory cell if Le^b-transferase is present, which adds a second L-fucose to the chain. These individuals secrete ABH and Le^b substances. The fucose on the terminal galactose of the H substance is required for Le^b enzyme to act. Le^a individuals have an enzyme that converts type I acceptor molecules to Le^a substance by adding L-fucose to the subter-

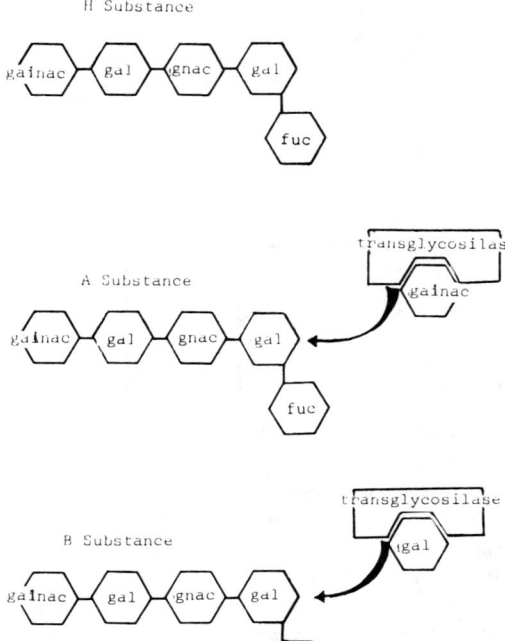

FIG 5–2.—Synthesis of group A and group B substances from each substance, mediated by a specific transglycosilase. Group A substance is synthesized by N-acetylgalactosamine transglycosilase. Group B substance is synthesized by D-galactose transglycosilase.

minal N-acetylglucosamine of the type I chain. This enzyme does not require H substance to add the subterminal fucose; instead, it acts as an enzyme stopper to prevent the addition of the second fucose.[35] Le^a individuals do not secrete ABH substances but do secrete Le^a substance. Clinically these substances are important because they are expressed on RBCs. Newborns have weaker ABH antigens than adults.[36] In infants, ABH antigens are not fully developed until age 6–18 months.[37]

ABH antigens are present on the membrane but are not crucial to the RBC membrane stability. This is evident in persons of the Bombay phenotype who lack ABH substances yet whose RBCs have a normal shape and survive as do cells with ABH substances.[38]

The expression of A, B, or H molecules on RBC membranes is abundant, reaching close to 1 million antigenic units per RBC.[39]

Groups in the ABO System

Group A.—Group A individuals constitute approximately 40% of the caucasian population in the United States. Group A substance can be manifested in different molecular forms, termed subgroups. It appears that the weaker expression of A antigens on A subgroup cells may be due to a difference in enzyme kinetics of the inherited glycosyltransferase.[40] At least four sets of A and H glycolipid variants in human group A and O erythrocytes, respectively, have been defined. These are A^{a-d} and H_{1-4} in order of carbohydrate complexity. There is a difference in steric hindrance to GalNAc transfer by the A_2 glycosyltransferase to H_3 and H_4 substrates, explaining to some extent phenotypic differences between group A_1 and A_2 individuals.[41]

The discovery of subgroups of A is attributed to Von Dungern and Hirszfeld (1911).[42] Differences in subgroups of A are usually quantitative, i.e., the relative amounts of A and H substances vary (Fig 5–3), but the differences may also be qualitative. Differences in expression of these substances on RBCs or in saliva are given in Table 5–2. Just how this variability results in antibody formation against one group or another is not completely known. A qualitative immunochemical difference has been reported.[43]

Subgroup A_1.—Subgroup A_1 is by far the most frequent, constituting 80% of the group A population.[44] A_1 individuals have the least amount of H substance[45] and may produce anti-H antibodies.[46]

A_1 cells react specifically with *Dolichos biflorus* lectin.[47] This plant glycoprotein can be used for resolving certain group A subgroup problems. The reactivity of this lectin with group A_1 cells must be adjusted by dilution to be of diagnostic value. Since group A_1 cells have the least amount of H substance, reactivity with *Ulex europaeus* lectin, which specifically detects H substance, is least with these cells. Anti-H antibodies also react weakly with A_1 cells.[45] Conversely, group A_1 individuals are the most likely of the A subgroups to produce anti-H antibodies, probably because the steric configuration between H substance and A substance is recognized as non-self, or due to a qualitative change.

Subgroup A_2.—The second most frequent

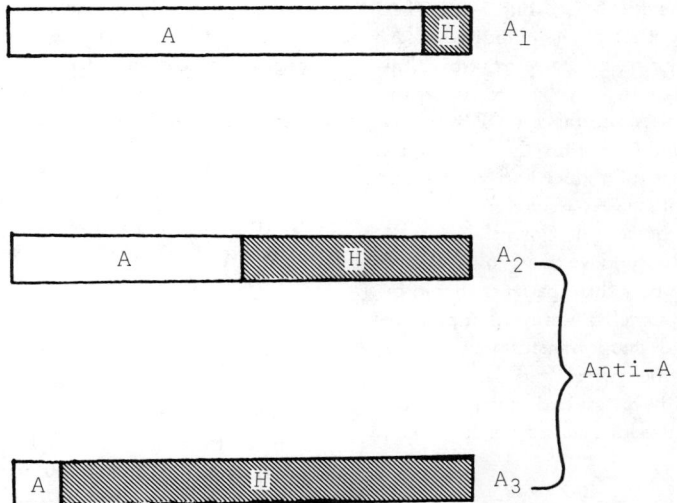

FIG 5–3.—Relative proportion of H substance in subgroups of A. Group A_1 individuals have small amounts of H and hence small likelihood of producing anti-A_1 antibodies. However, anti-H antibodies may be found *(tcp)*. *Middle* and *bottom*, represent relative amounts of A substance and H substance in subgroups A_2 and A_3. These two groups are more likely to produce anti-A antibodies and less likely to produce anti-H antibodies.

subgroup of A is subgroup A_2, seen in 20% of group A individuals and 1% of AB individuals typing A_2B.[48] About 17% of A_2 individuals and 25% of A_2B individuals produce anti-A_1 antibodies.[49] If A_2 and A_2B individuals have a greater amount of H substance than A_1 individuals, it is possible that these individuals see A_1 individuals as "foreign" and produce anti-A_1 antibodies (see Fig 5–3), although qualitative differences may also be responsible for the antigenic stimulus to produce anti-A_1.

Evidence for a qualitative difference is the finding in rabbits which have A-like RBCs of anti-A_1 but not anti-A_2 antibodies on challenge with human group A RBCs.[50] Biochemical studies on the two subgroups have yielded controversial results. Some results show qualitative differences based on differences in linkage of N-acetylgalactosamine to type I or type II precursor chains;[51] others have not been able to reproduce these findings and contend that the differences are purely quantitative.[52]

Subgroup A_3.—This subgroup was first described by Friedenreich.[53] When group A or A,B typing antisera are reacted with subgroup A_3 cells, a mixed field pattern is observed. This pattern is characterized by agglutinated cells against a background of nonagglutinated cells, similar to the pattern seen in incompatible transfusions. Patients with the secretor gene (to be described later) do not secrete A substance or H substance, as do secretor group A individuals.

Subgroup A_3 individuals have more group H

TABLE 5–2.—SEROLOGIC CHARACTERIZATION OF SUBGROUPS OF A

	REACTIONS OF CELLS WITH					
SUBGROUP	Anti-A	Anti-A,B	*Dolichos biflorus*	Anti-H	Anti-A in Eluates	Antigens in Saliva
A_1	+++	+++	+++	++	++	A + H
A_2	+	+	O	+++	+	A + H
A_3	Mixed field	Mixed field	O	+++	+	A + H
A_{int}	+	+	±	++	+	A + H
A_x	O	+	O	+++	+	H
A_m	W	W	O	+++	+	A + H

substance than A_2 individuals (see Fig 5–2). They represent about 0.1% of all group A individuals.[54] The variability in agglutination patterns responsible for the mixed field pattern may be due to a variability in expression of A substance on RBCs, but this hypothesis has not been proved conclusively. Group A_3 individuals may produce anti-A antibodies, for their cells recognize A_1 as foreign.

Because of the theoretical potential for A subgroup recipients to produce dangerous anti-A antibodies, it would appear these patients should be transfused with group O cells; however, in practice these patients rarely develop transfusion reactions unless an anti-A antibody reactivity at 37°C is found.[55] Some deaths have resulted when A_2 individuals with anti-A antibodies have been transfused with A_1 RBCs.[56]

Other Subgroups of A.—These are much less frequent than the subgroups described above. The A_x subgroup frequency is about 1 in 40,000.[57] A_x is always agglutinated by anti-A,B antisera.[58] These individuals exhibit H substance in the saliva but lack A substance in secretions.[58]

Group A_m individuals have cells that either are not agglutinated or are agglutinated very weakly by anti-A and anti-A,B. A_m secretors have A and H substances in saliva.[59] A_{int} denotes a subgroup of A with intermediate A substance content, the first example of which was reported by Landsteiner and Levine in 1930.[60] Other subgroups of A exist but are rare, and their description is available in general references.[61,62] For different reactivities to identify subgroups of A, see Table 5–2.

Most subgroups of A can be detected by the use of anti-A,B antiserum. Eluates of cells incubated with these antisera may resolve questionable cases. Secretions are usually investigated for A substances by agglutination inhibition techniques as well as by using specific lectins.

The main clinical significance of the subgroups of A is that they may be mistyped as group O cells and transfused to O individuals with high anti-A titers. Such a transfusion may cause hemolysis. The weaker expression of the A antigen appears to be due to a difference in the enzyme kinetics of the inherited glycosyltransferases.[40] A minimum of 2.5 $\times$ 10^5 A antigen sites are needed for anti-A_1 to produce agglutination.[63]

Group B.—Subgroups of B are considerably rarer than subgroups of A and will not be discussed in detail here. For their reactivity, see Table 5–3.[64,65]

Serologic Aspects of the ABO System

Antibodies to A, B, and H substances are usually of the IgM type, bind complement, and react at room temperature.[66] Nevertheless, a portion of saline-reacting immunoglobulin may be of the IgG class.[67]

These antibodies are formed, most probably, against colonic bacterial membrane polysaccharides (e.g., *Escherichia coli* group O 86 has a B-like antigen on its surface) and cross-react with antibodies to ABH substances.[68] Antibodies in the newborn are mostly maternal IgG antibodies.[69] However, on exposure to bacterial antigens, the host produces antibodies against these bacterial specificities. These antibodies reach adult levels at age 1–5 years.[70] An IgM response to ABH antigens is not surprising, because the molecules have repetitive sugar units, which characteristically induce IgM antibody formation.[71] The ABH pentameric antibody response is most likely T cell independent (see Chap. 4). Anti-A or anti-B antibodies can be neutralized with Witebsky substances, which have either group A specificity (hog stomach mucosa) or group AB specificity (horse stomach mucosa).[72] These substances can be used in the deliberate immunization of individuals to A or B antigens for the production of laboratory reagents.

Group O individuals have the capacity to make antibodies that react with group A and group B cells, the so-called anti-A,B antibodies. These antibodies may have a binding site capable of detecting steric configurations provided by the different

TABLE 5–3.—SUBGROUPS OF B

	REACTIVITY WITH		SALIVA IN SECRETORS		ANTIBODIES IN SERUM
GROUP	Anti-B	Anti-A,B	B Substance	H Substance	
I	Weak	Weak	+	+	Anti-B, anti-A
II	Weak	Weak	+	+	No anti-B in serum
III	Weak	Weak	−	+	No anti-B in serum

orientation or sugars on group A and group B substances. Anti-A,B antibodies are very often of the IgG type and can bind complement, but they may also be of the IgM class.[73] Eluates from A RBCs coated with anti-A,B have both anti-A and anti-B reactivity.[74] A separate C antigen, proposed by some early investigators,[75] probably doesn't exist as a separate entity; rather, the immune system of group O individuals "sees" the steric configuration of H substance plus the N-acetylgalactosamine of group A and the configuration of H substance with D-galactose of group B as foreign in a different way from, for instance, the group A individual's immune system would "see" group B, D-galactose. These specificities may cross-react due to similarity of fit at the antibody binding site (Fig 5–4).[76]

IgM anti-A or anti-B antibodies are not capable of crossing the placenta; however, IgG anti-A,B antibody is capable of crossing the placenta and may produce ABO hemolytic disease of the newborn (see Chap. 16). This transport is selective and is mediated by the Fc receptor in the placenta specific for the Fc portion of the IgG molecule.[77]

The major concern in clinical transfusion is that the IgM of anti-A or anti-B individuals avidly binds complement and is responsible for major hemolytic transfusion reactions. The capacity of anti-A or anti-B antibodies to hemolyze can be tested for in vitro to detect dangerous group A, B, or O plasmas, but is not routinely used in daily blood banking.

ABO IgG antibodies in group A or B individuals very frequently are secondary to immunization via routes other than the oral route (i.e., intramuscular injections of A or B substance). Anti-ABH IgG responses usually imply T cell dependency and may indicate that antigens presented to the immune system parenterally rather than orally stimulate such responses (see Chap. 4). Furthermore, group O individuals who "see" A and B antigens in a different way from group A or group B individuals respond to group A or group B substances with a T cell–mediated response with a significant IgG component without prior parenteral challenge. Rarely, IgM autoantibodies against ABH antigens are observed. These antibodies may not react with A_2B cells and may not be associated with hemolysis.[78]

Genetics of the ABO System

The ABO system is coded for on chromosome 9.[79] Linkage has been found with the "nail-patella" syndrome.[80] This disease is inherited as an autosomal dominant trait and characterized by onycho-osteodysplasia, webbed elbows, and mild chronic glomerulonephritis. ABO linkage to adenylate kinase coding has also been documented.[81] Genes coding for the A and B substances are on a different gene and may even be on a different chromosome from genes coding for the H substance, as manifested in the Bombay-group individual who may have the genes for the N-acetyl transglycosidase or the D-galactose transglycosidase but cannot produce these substances due to a lack of H substance.

ABO genes are inherited in a codominant pattern, as are most blood group antigens. That is, if a group A gene is present, it will be manifested on the RBC. If both the A and B genes are present the person will type as AB. Possible permutations in the ABO system are given in Table 5–1; possible genes involved are shown in Figure 5–5.

The Bombay Group.—Bombay group individuals lack H substance because of a defect in a fucosyltransferase necessary to add a terminal fucose to the group substance polysaccharide backbone. This phenotype is extremely rare in Europeans and occurs in about 1 in 13,000 Asian Indians, in whom it is most frequent.[82] The first case described in Bombay gave origin to the phenotype's name.

Since persons with the Bombay phenotype cannot produce the complete H substance backbone, their

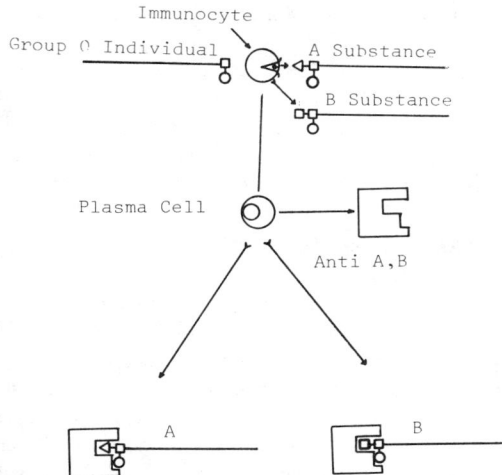

FIG 5–4.—Suggested mode of action of anti-A,B. *Top,* immunocytes from group O individuals assessing group A and group B substance antigenic differences. *Middle,* development of plasma cells producing anti-A,B. Bottom, cross-reactivity of antibodies agglutinating group A and group B substances.

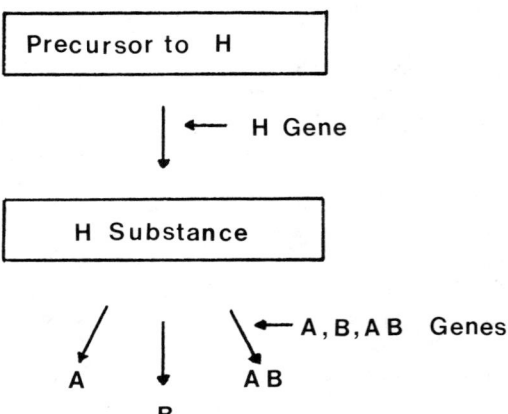

FIG 5–5.—Suggested genes involved in the synthesis of ABH substances.

enzymes, when these individuals are genetically group A or group B, cannot synthesize group A or B substances. The plasma of Bombay group A individuals contains N-acetylgalactosamine transferase and the plasma of Bombay group B individuals contains D-galactosamine transferase.[83]

ABH substances are also found in secretions[84] as well as in other tissues. The capacity to secrete is inherited and coded for by dominant genes different from ABH genes.[85] Therefore, these genes do not affect the expression of ABH antigens on RBCs or the capacity of cells to secrete H substance. This observation strongly suggests that genes for group A and B substances are separate from those of H substance. Individuals with the Bombay phenotype must be homozygous for the h gene (hh) in order to manifest the phenotype. Their cells front type as group O but their serum contains anti-A, anti-B, and anti-H antibodies because their immune system detects ABH antigens as foreign, or non-self.

The ABO System in the Laboratory

ABO antibodies of the IgM class (most isoantibodies in this system) produce agglutination at room temperature, are not enhanced by albumin, and may be weakened when incubated at higher temperatures (e.g., 37° C), though incubation at 37° C in LISS has been recently suggested by some authors.[86] Tube testing for these antigens is more accurate than slide testing. Conventionally, anti-A antiserum is colored blue with either 1:5,000 dilution of stock trypan blue dye or with methylene blue. Anti-B antiserum is colored yellow with natural acriflavin.[87] This substance may cause immunization. Occasional cases of ABO typing discrepancies have been described with this reagent, if the patient has antiacriflavin antibodies.[88] Anti-A,B reagents are usually colorless. ABH reagent antisera are obtained commercially. Plasma from immunized donors is usually employed in the preparation of these reagents. The antibodies are of high titer and obtained from individuals who have been immunized, in most cases with Witebsky substances. Detailed descriptions of laboratory techniques are beyond the scope of this work, and readers are referred to pertinent references.[89]

As in all other laboratory tests, it is essential that persons follow the manufacturer's directions when using these reagents. It is dangerous to change or abbreviate steps in most types of blood bank tests. Most commercial reagents are carefully tested in the blood bank beforehand, and the reactivity is evaluated based on the instructions given in reagent package inserts.

When subtypes of A are suspected, the RBCs can be tested with plant lectins to determine the nature of the subtype. Plant lectins used in the blood bank are glycoproteins of high molecular weight that react with specific blood group carbohydrates.[90] These reactions are so specific that they are routinely used to type certain RBCs.[91]

One of the more useful lectins is *Dolichos biflorus*,[92] which reacts specifically with A_1 cells and weakly with A_2 cells. This lectin will not react with group B or group O cells, even after enzyme treatment.

Aged seeds of *Bandeiraea simplicifolia* contain a lectin which has specificity for the group B antigen,[93] whereas *Ulex europaeus* has specificity for H antigens.[94] Many of these lectins are available commercially and useful in defining ABO discrepancies.

Monoclonal Antibodies to ABH Substances

Monoclonal antibodies from mouse/mouse hybridoma against group A cells[95] and group B cells[96] have recently been produced and may be added to the laboratory testing armory. It has been shown that these monoclonal reagents perform as well as or better than polyclonal reagents both in manual and automated testing, and have the added advantages of a constant immunochemical composition and an unlimited supply of reagent.[97]

Discrepancies in ABO typing.—Most discrepancies are due to clerical errors, and proper identification of specimens should be confirmed in any ABO discrepancy. Laboratory and technical errors can be the cause of discrepancies. Tests are repeated to detect possible mistakes. Dirty glassware and improper suspensions of cells after centrifugation may cause false positive results. Hemolysis may be overlooked if it is not searched for. Overcentrifugation and undercentrifugation of specimens may cause discrepancies in reading; proper centrifuge calibration prevents this problem. Warming test tubes is a frequent cause of ABO discrepancy, giving false negative results. Cell carryover from other specimens may contaminate reagents.

One must also suspect the less usual causes of ABO discrepancy, such as weakened A or B substances in infants[98] and in patients with advanced age, leukemia, or extensive carcinomatosis,[99] and acquired B substance in patients with intestinal infection, gangrene, or carcinoma of the colon.[100]

Transfused cells (e.g., group O blood transfused to a group A individual) may be responsible for discrepancies. Large fetomaternal bleeds, polyagglutinability, chimeras (which may have two different ABO populations of cells),[101] and cis-AB genes may also be the source of confusion in ABO typing.[102]

Other causes for laboratory discrepancy may be found in the patient's serum. A frequent problem is rouleaux formation due to increased plasma proteins (e.g., myeloma).[103] Saline replacement techniques and properly washed cells help prevent this problem.[104] An improperly clotted sample (e.g., due to heparin therapy) can cause confusion. Adding protamine or thrombin helps solve this problem. Increased fibrinogen,[103] dextran infusions, and some intravenous medications are other causes of rouleaux formation.[104,105]

Unexpected cold-reacting agglutinins such as anti-I antibodies, anti-A_1 in an A_2 individual, and anti-H may cause laboratory discrepancies in ABO typing. Testing against a panel will reveal whether unexpected antibodies are present. Autoabsorption with the patient's own cells if the patient has not been transfused helps solve this problem. Newborns and young infants may have decreased isoagglutinin levels as well as decreased expression of antigens. Debilitated, malnourished individuals may have decreased isoagglutinins. Hypogammaglobulinemia is a rare cause for discrepancy but should be kept in mind as a possible reason for mistyping. In these cases, a plasma protein profile as well as serum immunoelectrophoresis will reveal the source of the typing problem (e.g., myeloma or hypogammaglobulinemia).

Aspects of Clinical Significance.—Clinically the ABO system is most significant in incompatible transfusion. There is no doubt that hemolytic transfusion reactions due to ABO incompatibility are the most dangerous and the most frequently fatal.[106] The most frequent cause of ABO-incompatible transfusion reactions is clerical error.[107]

Many ABO antibodies avidly bind complement, activating it to lytic molecular units and causing rapid destruction of RBCs with liberation of thromboplastin from membrane debris, which can lead to disseminated intravascular coagulation, the most dreaded complication of transfusion errors (see discussion of DIC in Chap. 3).

Blood of the patient's own group should be transfused whenever possible. If blood of another group is given (Table 5–4), one can switch back to the patient's blood group when the patient's serum is nonreactive with test cells of his own blood group. Otherwise, the patient's transfusion therapy is continued with packed cells of the selected alternate blood group. Group O patients can be transfused only with group O blood. In emergencies, A plasma or B plasma can be given to group O individuals if group O plasma is not available.

In patients with other ABO groups, group-specific or group AB plasma is given. Platelets can be given out of group if the number of units does not exceed 5. Current methods for storage of platelets at room temperature require a minimum of 50 cc plasma volume per unit of platelets;[108] therefore, incompatible plasma may reach dangerous levels if numerous units are given.

Another aspect of clinical importance in the ABO system is hemolytic disease of the newborn. It results from anti-AB immune agglutinins of the IgG class, which can cross the placenta. In ABH-incompatible pregnancies, group O Rh-negative mothers with group A fetuses appear to be pro-

TABLE 5–4.—ABO GROUPS WHICH ARE COMPATIBLE

PATIENT'S GROUP	1ST ALTERNATIVE*	2ND ALTERNATIVE*
A	Group O	None
B	Group O	None
AB	A or B	Group O
A_2B	A_2 or B	Group O
A_2 with anti-A_1	A_2	Group O
A_1B	A_1 or B	Group O
A with anti-H	A_1	None

*All alternative groups should be given as packed cells.

tected in 90% of cases against Rh immunization, whereas group O Rh-negative mothers with group B fetuses become immunized in 45% of cases.[109] Other aspects of the ABH system and hemolytic disease of the newborn are discussed in chapter 15.

Weakening of ABO antigens should arouse concern, for it can be the manifestation of a malignant process (e.g., acute leukemia) or lymphoma with sideroblastic anemia. These patients may have normal ABH substances in secretions.[110] Congenital rubella may likewise be associated with weak ABH antigens.[111]

Of interest to oncogenesis is the association of elevated carcinoembryonic antigen (CEA) levels in plasma of patients with colorectal carcinoma. CEA is an incomplete antigen which can be converted to group A or group B substance with the appropriate transferases. It has been shown that in certain areas of colonic carcinomas, H substance and CEA are identified in the same area of the tumor.[112] It has likewise been shown that a loss of ABH antigenic representation in epithelium, seemingly normal, may be a sensitive marker for malignant transformation.[113] Similar claims have been made for evaluation of urothelial tumors,[114] but others report no statistical significance in their evaluations.[115]

ABH Antigens and Transplantation.—ABH compatibility must be respected during tissue transplantation. This fact is highlighted by the finding that a bone marrow transplant may be rejected by a recipient despite vigorous pretransplant plasmapheresis.[116] Furthermore, engrafted group O kidneys in group A individuals may give rise to "passenger" immunocompetent lymphocytes capable of inducing hemolysis due to anti-A or anti-B antibody production.[117]

The Anti-H Antibody in the Bombay Phenotype.—Bombay individuals of the Ah phenotype who are transfused with A cells destroy 65% of the transfused cells in a few hours. It appears that these patients must be transfused with Ah or Oh cells.[118]

ABH Antigens and Disease

Interesting correlations in clinical practice have been noted in disease incidence in different ABO groups. For instance, carcinoma of the stomach is more frequent in group A individuals,[119] as is pernicious anemia,[120,121] which has been found to co-occur with carcinoma of the stomach. Group O individuals have a higher incidence of benign peptic ulcer than other groups.[122] Groups, A, B, and AB individuals have a higher incidence of thromboembolism than group O individuals.[123] Acquired group antigens in gastrointestinal infections were discussed earlier and should be considered in clinical immunohematology workups.

It has recently been shown that group B cells can be converted into group O cells by cleaving the terminal D-galactose with an α-galactosidase.[124] This procedure, if feasible on a wide scale, could have important and far-reaching positive effects on blood bank inventories. Furthermore, group A cells could be transformed into group O cells by the use of an N-acetylgalactosidase in a similar fashion.[124]

The Lewis System

The Lewis system was first described by Mourant in 1946, who discovered the Le^a antigen.[125] These antigens are not synthesized by RBCs but instead are acquired from plasma glycolipids.[126] About 30% of circulating Lewis antigens are found on RBCs; the remainder are found in the plasma.[127] Two frequent phenotypes of the Lewis system are the Le^a antigen and the Le^b antigen, which are determined phenotypically by the presence or absence of Lewis genes (Le or le) and by the presence or absence of the secretor gene, Se or se.

Another important aspect of the Lewis System is that genes for the Lewis system and secretor genes (Se, se) interact to be expressed phenotypically in the secretion of both ABH and Lewis antigens in external secretions.[128] This interaction can be better understood after reviewing the Lewis system biochemistry.

Biochemistry

The Le gene codes for a fucosyltransferase capable of adding a fucose residue to type I chains. In the absence of H substance, most of the type I chains will be converted to Le^a substance by the addition of a fucose to the preterminal GNAc residue of the chain in the α-1,4 position (Fig 5–6).

In the presence of H substance, the Le-transferase can add a fucose at the α-1,4 position to the subterminal GNAc, in which case the resulting antigen will be Le^b.[129] It is possible the H fucosyltransferase has two isoenzymes, one that is responsible for plasma and RBC H substance and another that is produced in salivary and other epithelial cells and

day, for they are identical to type I-H molecules.[132] These types of molecules are found in Le$^{(a-b-)}$ individuals who are secretors.[132] These glycolipids (Le^c and type I-H) can also be adsorbed onto RBCs in vitro.[133]

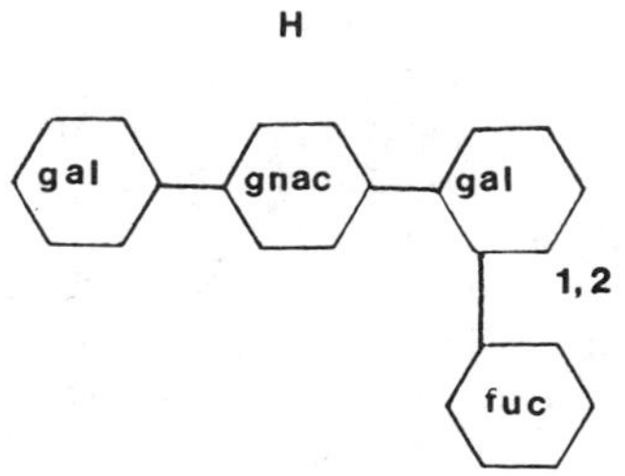

Serologic Aspects of the Lewis System

Antibodies against Lewis substances are mostly of the IgM class, with exceptional cases of IgG anti-Lewis antibodies.[134] Therefore, they do not cross the placenta. Hemolytic disease of the newborn caused by anti-Lewis antibodies has not been reported, possibly because of weak expression of Lewis antigens in the fetus as well as the IgM character of anti-Lewis antibodies in the mother.[134] However a weak positive antiglobulin in a newborn of a mother with IgG anti-Le^b has been reported[135] and in another case a strong anti-Le^a of the IgG class was seen in the cord blood of a newborn infant.[136]

The antigens are not well expressed on the cells of newborns.[137] This may also be why the antibodies are not responsible for hemolytic disease of the newborn. RBCs express Lewis antigens at about age 6 months. Lewis antigens may disappear from the RBCs of pregnant women[138] probably due to an increment in the ratio of glycolipids to RBC mass.[139] This may be in some way associated with the higher incidence of anti-Lewis antibodies in pregnant women.[140]

Since these antibodies bind complement they are capable of producing lysis in vitro, especially anti-Le^a. Hemolytic transfusion reactions in patients with anti-Lewis antibodies transfused with Lewis (+) cells has been described.[141]

An interesting phenomenon observed in the

FIG 5–6.—Comparison of the sugar sequence of H, Le^a, and Le^b substances. Notice the similarity of the backbone structure in these three blood group substances.

is regulated by a different gene, the Se gene (Fig 5–7). Thus, if Se is not present, as occurs in Le^a individuals, the H transferase might not be present in epithelium. Therefore, neither Le^b nor ABH substances, which need H substance as a substrate, would be secreted. Le^a substance will appear in the secretion of these individuals. Individuals who lack the Le gene (le, le), lack the Le-transferase and, therefore do not have Le (a or b) in their RBCs or secretions (Le$^{(a-b-)}$).

However, these Le$^{(a-b-)}$ individuals may or may not be secretors. If they are secretors they will secrete ABH substances but not Lewis substances, whereas if they are not secretors they will secrete neither ABH nor Lewis substances. Nonsecretors have the Le^c phenotype, whose biochemical structure has not been fully clarified[130] but may be type I chains. Le^c is also present on molecules of RBCs and secretions of individuals of the Bombay phenotype.[131] Le^d antigens are not accepted separately to-

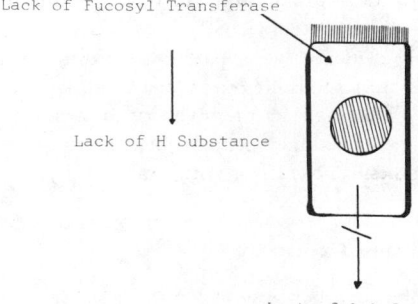

FIG 5–7.—Possible significance of the presence or absence of fucosyltransferase in the epithelium and the resulting expression of Lewis substances in secretions.

Lewis system and corroborated in vitro[127] is that Le^a RBCs can be converted to Le^b cells after transfusion into an Le^b recipient, and vice versa—Le^b cells can be converted to Le^a cells on transfusion into an Le^a recipient. This phenomenon is probably due to a continuous exchange of glycosphingolipid between the plasma and RBCs.[142] Anti-Lewis antibodies have been found in individuals who were never transfused. In one such case, the individual had a potent anti-Le^b of the IgG class.[143] Monoclonal antibodies against Lewis substances have been produced.[144] Some of these monoclonal antibodies bear the Le^{bH} specificity.[145]

Clinical Aspects of Lewis Antigens

Anti-Lewis antibodies are frequently found in multiparous women, especially during pregnancy (without a previous history of transfusion).[140] However, these antibodies are of the IgM class in the vast majority of cases and do not cross the placenta. IgG anti-Le^a has been reported in the literature but does not bind complement significantly.[146] In transfusion, anti-Le^a antibodies are to be respected since they have been known to occasionally produce hemolytic transfusion reactions, generally in $Le^{(a-b-)}$ individuals.[141] The clear clinical significance of screening for these antigens in future transfusions for patients with anti-Lewis antibodies, however, is the object of current analysis.[147] Anti-Le^b antibodies are less dangerous. In transfusion practice, Le^b antibodies can be neutralized by giving a unit of Le^b plasma prior to transfusion of RBCs to individuals with anti-Le^b antibodies. Anti-Le^a antibodies, though hemolytic, are partially neutralized in Le^b individuals, owing to partial expression of Le^a on cells of Le^b individuals.[148] In general, Lewis antibodies are slowly hemolytic, due to rapid clearance of the antibody from the RBCs by the reticuloendothelial system (RES).[149]

Recently evidence has appeared that anti-Lewis antibodies are responsible for kidney transplant rejection.[150] This suggests the necessity to screen for these antigens in kidney donors when the recipient has antibodies against Lewis antigens.

The Ii Blood Group

The Ii blood group was first defined by Wiener et al. in 1956.[151] The I antigen system is similar to the ABO antigen system in many ways and probably shares some of the biochemical pathways which produce the ABO antigens.[152] The agglutinin, as described originally, was capable of reacting with most adult cells but did not react with cord cells. It was therefore suggested that I be used to designate the adult antigen and i the cord cell antigen. I antigens can be found in WBCs[153, 154] and secretions (milk, urine, saliva).[155] Adult RBCs exhibit i antigens in the immature marrow stages, and then progressively lose these antigens as the RBC matures and becomes senescent (Fig 5–8).[156]

Biochemistry of the I System

The finding that combined reactivities of the I system and the ABH system (i.e., IH, IB, and IA),[157] as well as the finding that the digestion or breakdown of Lewis and ABO substances result in I antigenic reactivity, suggest that the I molecule may be a precursor to these antigens (Fig 5–9).[152] Further evidence that this might be the case is the enhancement of I antigens in individuals with the Bombay phenotype.[158] A precursor gene, probably a very primitive one, codes for this molecule, serving as a backbone molecule to other antigens. It has also been shown that the I antigen exists in many other species.[159]

The I molecule is probably a glycolipid on RBC membranes but it is a glycoprotein in secretions. Its antigenic determinant is a sequence of carbohydrates at the terminal end of a lipid, similar to that described for the ABO system. Furthermore, I antigen is obtained after mild hydrolysis of B substance.[152] In plasma, i is present as a 150,000-dalton glycoprotein.[160] The I antigen is more difficult to assess due to the heterogeneity of antibodies against it.[152] It is not known if the precursor molecule for I is the i antigen. The i antigen is present as the only antigen in the rare i adult phenotype.

Fetal Cells

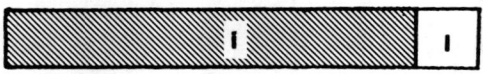

Adult Cells

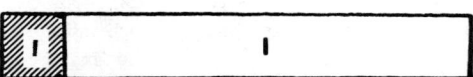

FIG 5–8.—Relative content of I and i substances in adult and fetal cells.

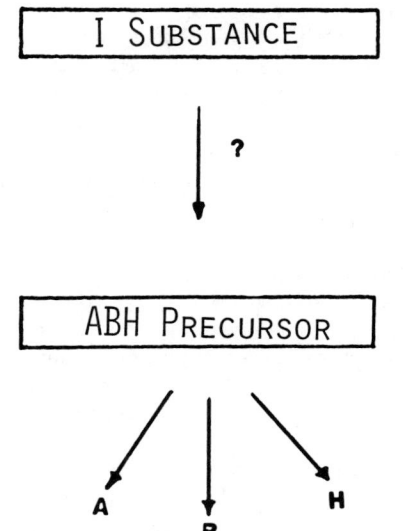

FIG 5–9.—Possible synthesis of ABO groups from group I substance.

The phenotypic product is antigenic and recognized by the presence of i antibodies in certain patients. It is thought that i antigens represent mostly non-branched polysaccharides, whereas I represents a branched variant of the chain.[161] Both type I and type II chains have been associated with OG, and F1 precursor-like substances thought to be very similar to I antigens.[162]

Genetics of the Ii System

The genetics of the Ii system are not fully understood. The very frequent gene Z putatively controls expression of I on RBCs. Thus the zz genotype would result in phenotypical i RBCs that do not preclude the expression of the I antigen in secretions such as saliva and milk.[163] The adult i variant may thus be similar to the A_m variant of the ABO system where RBCs lack the antigen but A substance is present in secretions.[164]

Subtypes of I

The I antigen has two components, I^F (fetal) and I^D (developed), as shown by Marsh et al.[165] Very rarely, an absence or decrement of I is present in adults. These are i_1 and i_2 adult types.[166] These i subtypes are found more frequently in the black population. The i_1 phenotype is more frequent than the i_2.[167] The i_1 and i_2 antigens are distinct from i found on cord cells. A transitional I^T has been described and is detected by antibodies to cells that react more strongly with cord cells than with adult cells and fail to agglutinate i adult;[168] however, anti-I^T reacts more strongly with fetal cells than with cord cells, and does not react with adult i.

Serology of the I System

Anti-I and anti-i antibodies usually present as cold-reacting agglutinins of the IgM class capable of binding complement, although in a few cases they may be of the IgG class.[169] Anti-I antibodies characteristically agglutinate all adult cells except the rare i adult and can be detected because of failure to agglutinate cord cells.

Most normal individuals have circulating anti-I of varying strengths of reactivity, reacting best at 4° C. However, this antibody may appear as a result of cold agglutinin disease at higher thermal ranges, becoming clinically significant. Anti-I antibodies can usually be ignored because of their low temperature reactivity. Nevertheless, a reason for concern would exist if the patient's temperature were to be lowered, as is customary in open heart surgery. This danger has been overestimated as, in practice, during bypass a significant hemodilution from the transfused electrolytes as well as the transfusion of plasma and blood diminish the concentration of antibody and hence the likelihood of hemolysis.[170] However, flushing the coronary circulation with crystalloid solution may be warranted,[171] and in selected cases plasmapheresis may be indicated before the procedure.[172]

Anti-I antibodies can be bothersome, clouding other clinically significant antibodies. In order to study samples from patients with strongly reactive IgM anti-I, its pentameric structure can be dissociated with mercaptoethanol or other disulfide bond–cleaving substances. Some anti-I antibodies may be reactive only in low ionic strength solutions.[173]

Clinical Aspects of the I/i Antigens

The I antigen becomes fully developed at age 18 months.[174] Before this, RBCs express i (see Fig 5–8). In adults, lymphocytes bear i throughout their life span.[175] In certain diseases (e.g., leukemia), the expression of the I antigen is weakened,[176] a fact that can be used in differentiating chronic lymphocytic leukemia from lymphocytosis.[177] Interestingly, during bone marrow stress (e.g., thalassemia), the circulating cells revert to expression of the i antigen.[178].

It is possible that this phenomenon is related to the finding of anti-i antibodies in patients with infectious mononucleosis. However, cross-reactivity with viral particles and the i antigen cannot be ruled out. Patients with hereditary erythroblastic multinuclearity have increased i antigen on their RBCs and are very susceptible to anti-i antibodies.[179] Strong anti-I antibodies can be found as polyclonal antibodies in patients with cold agglutinins secondary to respiratory bacterial infections[180] and viral pneumonias.[181] Cross-reactivity of specificity between mycoplasmal antigens and I antigens has been demonstrated.[182] *Listeria* antigens also cross-react with I antigens.[183] Monoclonal or oligoclonal antibodies with anti-I specificity are very frequent in cold agglutinin disease and in monoclonal antibodies secondary to lymphoma.[184] Most autoimmune hemolytic anemias of the cold-reacting type are caused by anti-I reactivity.[184] Many examples of anti-i antibodies in patients with infectious mononucleosis have been reported;[185] however, the presence of the anti-i antibody and the development of the i antigen are not necessarily causally related to the anemia.[186] In some cases, oligoclonal cold-reacting agglutinins have anti-I and anti-F1 specificities.[187]

Hemolytic anti-i antibodies secondary to infectious mononucleosis are usually of the IgM class and may exhibit anti-IgG specificity.[188]

In Japan, the association of the adult i phenotype and congenital cataract has been reported; however, recent reports of i adult not associated with cataract suggest that the genes for cataract are separate, though probably placed close to each other.[189]

The P System

The P system was initially described by Landsteiner and Levine in 1927, after immunizing rabbits with human RBCs.[190]

The P system represents a family of molecules with carbohydrate antigenic determinants. The main phenotypes are P1 (found in 80% of caucasians), P2 (found in most of the remaining population), and the very rare "p" phenotype. These variants are not allelic and are most probably coded for in different genes.

Biochemistry of the P System

The P antigens on RBCs bear a certain similarity to the ABO, Lewis, and I systems in that the antigenic determinant is a glycosphingolipid with repeating carbohydrate units.[191] It has been shown that α-D-galactose is crucial to the antigenic specificity of P1 substance obtained from hydatid cyst fluid, where P1 appears as a glycoprotein.[192] The specificity of other P group antigens or precursors to the P1 substance is determined by variation of terminal sugars, just as in other systems (ABO, Lewis, and I).[193] It has recently been shown that anti-Gd antibodies will react with "p" RBCs, but anti-F1 will not, which suggests that anti-Gd recognizes specificities present on "p" RBCs.[194]

Biosynthesis of the P System Substances

The P system substances are synthesized by two separate pathways departing from a common precursor, lactosyl ceramide. In the first pathway, the lactosyl ceramide backbone is converted to P^K substance (trihexosyl ceramide) by a glycosyltransferase coded by the P^K gene, which is then converted into P substance (globoside) by the addition of N-acetylgalactosamine to the trihexosyl ceramide molecule.[195]

The second pathway involves the conversion of lactosyl ceramide to paragloboside, which is then converted into P1 substance by an α-galactosyltransferase which can only interact with paragloboside. These, P1 individuals, in whom the two pathways are active will have P^K, P and P1 substances; conversely, in P2 individuals only the first pathway is active, and only P^K and P substances are produced (Fig 5-10).

P substance in humans can be found both as glycosphingolipids or as glycoproteins.[195]

It has recently been shown that the P system may be coded for on chromosome 6.[196]

Serology of the P System

As mentioned above, anti-P1 antibodies occur in P2 or the rare P individuals;[197] these antibodies are usually of the IgM class, are enhanced by enzyme treatment of RBCs, react at room temperature and in cold, and usually occur in P2 individuals. However, exceptions are seen in clinical practice, such as the anti-P antibodies responsible for the Donath-Landsteiner phenomenon found in luetic patients and patients with viral respiratory syndromes with paroxysmal cold hemoglobinuria.[198] This biphasic antibody is usually an IgG3[199] with anti-P but no anti-P^K specificity; it is capable of binding complement in the cold and lysing cells upon warming.[200] The antigen responsible for the Donath-Landsteiner reaction may be a Forssman-like antigen, which is present in several organisms usually responsible for inducing the syndrome.[201]

Anti-P, P1, and P^K antibodies, previously called

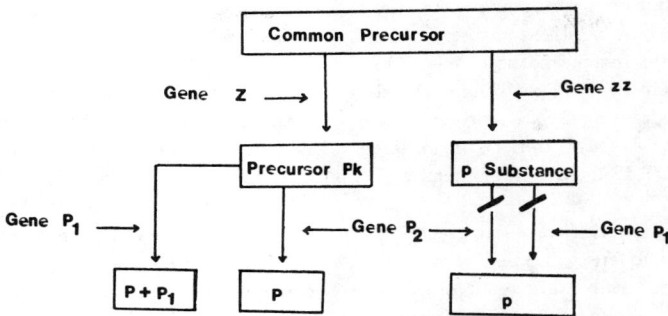

FIG 5–10.—Possible gene action for the synthesis of P substances.

anti-Tj^2, were initially described by Levine et al. in 1951 as a rare antibody.[202] These antibodies are frequently of the IgM class but may be of the IgG class, in which case they are capable of crossing the placenta and may produce hemolytic disease of the newborn.[203] Anti-P antibodies must be respected in transfusion practice, for they may be hemolytic, especially if the thermal reactivity reaches room temperature or above. Occasionally anti-P1 antibodies have been responsible for delayed transfusion reactions, in which case the evidence for the causative antibody may be delayed several days.[204]

Some parasites exhibit a P-like substance that will neutralize anti-P and anti-P^K antibodies (e.g., *Ascaris lumbricoides*,[205] but other worms such as *Faciola hepatica* will likewise produce P-like substances.[206] P2 patients may develop anti-P antibodies if infested by these parasites. Inosine present in test cell diluents may occasionally inhibit P1 antibodies, making an anti-P1 antibody difficult to identify.[207]

Clinical Aspects of the P System

Antibodies with P specificity may be hemolytic, occasionally producing fatal reactions when reactive at room temperature or above,[208] and should therefore be screened for. This is especially significant in patients who are to experience surgery under hypothermia and therefore are at greater risk, due to the increased thermal reactivity at low temperatures. However, only about 20% (those who are on the P2 phenotype) of patients are at risk of producing antibodies.

One out of 5 units screened may be negative for the antigen P1; but only 0.0024 unit will be compatible for p patients with anti-Tj^a antibodies (P, P1, P^K).[209] Almost 50% of patients with anti-Tj^a antibodies have spontaneous abortions;[210] these abortions have been associated with the presence of IgG anti-Tj^a antibodies.[211]

Hemolytic disease of the newborn, which may be very severe, is also a complication secondary to the development of IgG anti-P, P1, P^K (Tj^a) antibodies.[202]

Another complication outlined above is hemolysis due to anti-P antibodies in the Donath-Landsteiner phenomenon in paroxysmal cold hemoglobinuria. It should be suspected in patients who have biphasic hemolytic antibodies with anti-p reactivity. Auto-anti-P antibodies have also been reported. Some of these may be reactive only in low ionic strength solutions.[212]

It has been reported that pigeon-breeders of the P2 phenotype often develop anti-P1 antibodies because of a P1-like antigen present on pigeon erythrocytes.[213] Recently it has been shown that the P system antigens are involved in some way in the resistance of urothelial cells to infection by gram-negative bacteria such as *Escherichia coli*. This system may be a receptor site on urothelial cells for these bacteria.[214] The receptor site appears to reside in the P^K (ceramide) moiety and the P (globoside) moiety.[215]

The MNSs System

The MNSs system was discovered by Landsteiner and Levine in 1927 by deliberately immunizing rabbits.[216] The main antigens in the system are the pairs of allelic genes M,N and S,s, and a single high-frequency U gene with an amorphic allele closely placed to each other, showing very low crossover.[217] The Miltenberger complex, which will not be defined here in detail, is also associated with the MNSs gene complex.[218]

Biochemistry of the MNSs System

The M and N molecules are glycoproteins; therefore, to understand their biochemistry, one must understand the glycoprotein components of the RBC membrane that contain MNSs antigens. The major glycoproteins are listed in Table 5–5. On electrophoresis followed by PAS staining, several glycoprotein bands containing MNSs antigens can be demonstrated: PAS-1 (MN dimer), PAS-4,B (MNSs), C (Ss dimer), PAS-2 (MN monomer), and PAS-3 (Ss monomer).[219]

The M and N antigens reside in α-sialoglycoprotein (glycophorin A) and are composed of a 131-amino acid polypeptide chain and 16 oligosaccharides, 15 of which are linked to serine or threonine.[220]

It appears that the difference between M antigens and N antigens is basically the amino acid sequence of the terminal portion of the polypeptide chain most exposed to the surface. The N antigen has the sequence Glu-Thr-Thr-Ser-Leu whereas the M antigen has the sequence Gly-Thr-Thr-Ser-Ser.[220] To each of the three preterminal amino acids is attached a tetrasaccharide chain thought to be essentially identical in both M and N antigens (Fig 5–11).[221]

However, the NANA carbohydrate moiety may be important for anti-M or anti-N antigenic reactivity.[222] This idea is further supported by the finding that cells depleted of NANA by neuraminidase and exposed to different sialyltransferases and NANA can recuperate their MN antigenicity.[223] However, antibodies against desialized RBCs can be induced in rabbits. These antibodies will recognize polypeptide specificity differences between M and N but will not recognize intact antigens containing NANA.[224]

Unlike MN antigens, which are carried on glycophorin A, Ss antigens are carried on glycophorin B. These glycoproteins are shorter, containing about 100 amino acid residues Table 5–6; see also Table 5–5. The only difference between S and s is that the 29 methionine in S is substituted in s by a threonine.[225] There appears to be full homology between N and Ss antigens, in the first 26 amino acid residues,[226] as well as the anchoring positions of the oligosaccharides attached to the serine and threonine residues of both N and Ss antigens.[227]

This homology between N and Ss antigens may explain why M-positive, N-negative, S-positive individuals with anti-N will also agglutinate M cells, but will not agglutinate S-negative, s-negative cells.[226] Unlike MN, the Ss reactivity is not affected by neuraminidase or trypsin. It is possible that the U antigen is located on the same polypeptide chain as the Ss antigens, but closer to the lipid bilayer. This concept is supported by the fact that chymotrypsin and pronase, which cleave off Ss reactivity, do not affect U antigenicity.[228] Furthermore, cells negative for Ss may be positive for U, but U-negative cells (uu) can have normal MN antigens. U-negative cells lack PAS-3, PAS-4, and component C (δ2) glycoproteins, which carry Ss antigenicity.[229]

Certain specificities react with Ss glycoprotein that lack "N." Removal of NANA from M or N antigens uncovers the T cryptantigen responsible for polyagglutination, making the cells reactive to *Arachis hypogea* lectin.[230-232] Anti-M antibodies may have different specificities, as shown by the reactivity of anti-M antigen, which is dependent on the serine 1/glycine 5 amino acid sequence, and anti-Me, which is dependent only on glycine 5.[233] En^a antigens are polymorphic, as shown by Mi^v individuals who lack a normal MN sialoglycoprotein (SGP)

TABLE 5–5.—SDS-PAGE BANDS FOR RED CELL MEMBRANE GLYCOPROTEINS IN REFERENCE TO MNSs ANTIGENS*

ORIGIN	NOMENCLATURE	MNSs ANTIGENICITY	OTHER CHARACTERISTICS
1	Band 3	None	MW 83,000; 131 amino acid residues
2	PAS-1, α2, glycophorin A	MN	
3	PAS-4, B or αδ	MN, Ss	
4	Component C or δ2, glycophorin B	Ss	
5	PAS-2, or α	MN	MW 45,000
6	PAS-2′, D or β	None	
7	ε or γ	None	
8	PAS-3, δ, glycophorin B	Ss	MW 25,000; 100 amino acid residues

*Data from Mueller et al.,[219] Anstee et al.,[231] and Marquesi.[232]

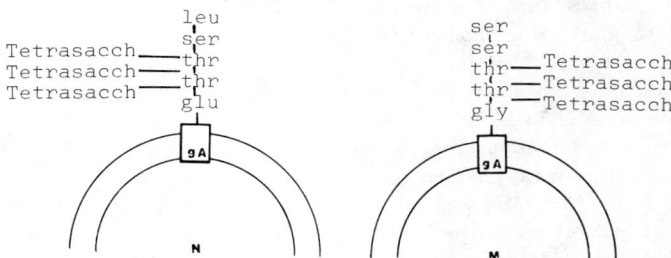

FIG 5–11.—M and N substances on RBC membranes. Note linkage of tetrasaccharides to terminal amino acid chain (*gA*, glycophorin A).

and have a normal Ss SGP.[234] Certain antibody specificities react with Ss glycoprotein which lacks "N" antigenicity.[235] Hybrid MNSs sialoglycoproteins have been described but are rare, and form part of En[a] heterogeneity.[236] Autoantibodies against Ss sialoglycoproteins may occasionally be detected.[237] A heterogeneity of antibodies to U has likewise been identified.[238]

Genetics of the MNSs System

The MNSs system is coded for on the q arm of chromosome 4, segment 2-9.[239] The two genes (M and N) are codominant and allelic (both are expressed if present). A dosage effect exists in heterozygous M/N individuals.[240] A dosage effect in the Ss antigens could be detected with an ELISA method.[241] The system is useful in paternity testing because they are codominant. Nevertheless, subtypes of M (e.g., Mg antigens) can cause misinterpretations and must therefore be considered in paternity exclusion cases.[242] This is a reason why the MNSs system is never used alone in paternity exclusion cases.[242]

Approximately 22% of the American population are negative for the M antigen and 28% are negative for the N antigen. About half the population are negative for S and 11% are negative for s.[243] Most people are U positive. These frequencies are useful in finding compatible units when antibodies against these antigens are present.

Serology of the MNSs System

Most antibody responses against the MN antigens are of the IgM class, react in the cold or at room temperature, and bind complement.[244] These antibodies do not appear to be dangerous under hypothermia.[245] In contrast to other cold antibody-generating antigens (I, P, H, etc.), the MN antigens are destroyed by enzymes, which reveals the protein nature of the antigen backbone. The fact that mostly IgM antibodies are produced against the MN antigens could be due to the exposed tetrasaccharides linked to the protein backbone. Another characteristic of certain anti-M antibodies is their improved reactivity in acid pH.[240] Some anti-N antibodies are likewise enhanced in acid pH.[246] Some

TABLE 5–6.—TERMINAL AMINO ACIDS OF MNSs ANTIGENS

		ANTIGENIC REACTIVITY		
	TERMINAL SEQUENCE	a-M	a-'N'	a-S or s
ANTIGEN				
M	Ser-Ser-Thr-Thr-Gly*	+	−	−
N	Leu-Ser-Thr-Thr-Glu*	−	+	+
S	Leu-Ser-Thr-Thr-Glu†	−	+	+
s	Leu-Ser-Thr-Thr-Glu‡	−	+	+
SUBGROUPS				
Mc	Ser-Ser-Thr-Thr-Glu*	−	−	−
Mg	Leu-Ser-Thr-Asn-Glu	−	−	−
En (a-)		−	−	+
En[MK]		wk	−	+

*Glycosilated in terminal amino acids 2, 3, and 4.
†Methionine in position 29.
‡Threonine in position 29.

MN antisera react better on RBCs stored in glucose solutions.[247] About 75% of anti-M antibodies have an IgG component. Rarely, anti-MN antibodies are purely of the IgG class,[248] can cross the placenta, and are therefore involved in hemolytic disease of the newborn.[249] In contrast to anti-MN antibodies, anti-S antibodies are usually of the IgG class and react at 37° C.[244] Anti-MN antibodies used as reagents in the laboratory are currently produced in rabbits.[250]

Anti-U antibodies are very rare and occur mostly in u blacks,[251] who are negative for U antigens. These individuals usually lack Ss antigens and make very strong anti-MNSs antibodies (the frequency of U-negative individuals is about 1.3%). Most U-negative caucasians are Rh null individuals.[252] This was thought to be related to a change in the sialic acid content of the RBC membrane, with a transformed steric configuration of the RBC membrane antigens, but now is thought to be due to a genetic absence of the membrane proteins carrying the MNSs and Rh antigens. Antibodies with anti-U specificity are usually of the IgG class, although they may react better at low temperatures, and may be involved in hemolytic disease of the newborn.[253]

In addition to antisera specific for MNSs, the M and N antigens can be detected by their reactions with *Vicia graminea* lectin.[254] M antigens alone react with lectins from *Iberis amara* seeds.[255] Monoclonal antibodies to N antigens have been developed.[256]

Clinical Aspects of the MNSs System

Anti-MN antibodies may occur as natural antibodies.[248] They may also cause rapid cell destruction by binding complement, and they produce hemolysis in the severe cases. As mentioned above, hemolytic disease of the newborn caused by anti-MN antibodies is rare and occurs only when antibodies are of the IgG class.[257] Delayed transfusion reactions due to anti-M have been described.[258]

The occurrence of anti-N antibodies in patients undergoing dialysis is well known.[259] The antibody may be responsible for rejection of a grafted kidney in a patient with anti-N antibodies when the kidney donor is N positive.[260] It is possible that the anti-N present in dialysis patients is secondary to changes on the RBC membrane that result from Formalin treatment of the dialysis tubing.[261] It is interesting that blood group M–specific hemagglutinins have been encountered in pyelonephritogenic strains of *Escherichia coli*,[262] *Proteus mirabilis,* as well as other bacteria[263] which may cause the so-called naturally occurring anti-M.

Cleavage of MN antigens reveals cryptantigens termed T, Tk, and Th antigens. Normal sera readily agglutinate these antigens, causing the polyagglutination syndrome. The exposure of T antigens is thought to occur due to cleavage by bacterial neuramidase of MN NANA residues, especially but not exclusively alkali-labile tetrasaccharides termed Thomas-Winzler tetrasaccharides,[264] although peptide proteolytic activity on MN backbone cannot be ruled out at present. Patients with inflammatory bowel disease may also reveal T and Tk activation. The finding of cryptantigen activation may be associated with proliferation of T-antigen-activating bacteria, with neuramidase release into the circulation.[265] Anti-Tm, for instance, has been shown to be reactive to the "N" polypeptide backbone.[266] Many anti-U antibodies cause hemolytic disease of the newborn; some others, however, do not, in spite of being of the IgG1 or IgG3 type and causing coating of fetal RBCs.[267]

The Lutheran System

The Lutheran system was discovered by Callender et al. in a multiply transfused patient with systemic lupus erythematosus.[268] The known phenotypes and frequencies are L^u (a+b−), 1%; L^u (a+b+), 7%; L^u (a−b+), 92%; and L^u (a−b−), rare. The L^u (a−b−) phenotype was first discovered by Crawford, who was also the propositus for the study.[269]

In contrast to other blood groups, L^u (a−b−) can be inherited in either recessive or dominant form.[270] The dominant type seems to be negative, owing to the action of an inhibitor gene (Jn), as shown by Crawford et al.[271] This inhibitor gene affects the expression of I, Au, and P antigens as well, and may be located on a different chromosome. The Lu system has proved to be very complex, with 20 known alleles.

Biochemistry and Genetics

Little is known about the biochemical structure of the Lu antigen. It may be a glycoprotein or a glycolipid with several repeating carbohydrate units, for it elicits an IgM response. There is evidence the Lu antigen shares the carbohydrate backbone structure of P and Ii,[14] although the antigenic moiety may be anchored to a protein, as suggested by the destruction of Lu activity by proteolytic enzymes.[272]

The antigen is inherited in a codominant pattern, but, as mentioned above, several modifier genes may be involved in the regulation of the Lutheran antigen expression. The secretor gene and the Lutheran genes are linked, as shown by crossover studies.[273] The antigens are present in RBCs of newborn infants but are less strong than in adults.[274] Lutheran antigens are not present on platelets.[275]

Serology of the Lu System

Lutheran antibodies are usually of the complete IgM type, although exceptions have been reported.[276] They are generally detected at room temperature and 12° C incubations, although a few 37° C antibodies to Lu have been described. A mixed field reaction may be seen in several cases. A monoclonal antibody reacting with Lu-positive cells but not with Lu-negative cells has been described.[277]

Clinical Aspects

Lutheran antibodies are usually of the IgM type and therefore rarely produce hemolytic disease of the newborn. Those that have been implicated in hemolytic disease of the newborn have been of the IgG type.[278] Anti-Lu antibodies are infrequently found in routine blood banking. They may be "natural"[279] or immune[280] in origin. It has been shown experimentally that antibodies directed against Lu can be inhibited by RNA derivatives.[281]

Anti-Lutheran antibodies very rarely, if ever, cause hemolytic reactions.

THE WARM-REACTING ANTIBODIES

Most of the antigenic systems that have been reviewed so far produce a cold antibody type of immune response (e.g., ABH, Lewis, Ii, P), although notable exceptions have been referred to in the description of each system. We will review here those antigenic systems responsible mainly for IgG reactions occurring at 37° C, and which therefore are called warm antibodies. Complex, branched antigens such as proteins often produce T cell–dependent, IgG-mediated antibody responses (see Chap. 4). It is believed, therefore, that many of the antigens inducing a warm antibody response are of a complex, branched nature. In the introduction to this chapter a general review of the membrane structure was given. More details are given here to better understand the role of these antigens on RBC membranes.

Some antigens are thought to be peripheral components of the RBC membrane, interacting electrostatically with the lipid bilayer, whereas other antigens are thought to be integral proteins that interact via hydrophobic associations with membrane lipids.[10] Some physicochemical properties of membrane proteins are given in Table 5–5. Singer has studied these molecules and advanced the hypothesis that loosely bound proteins that can be removed by gentle pH or low ionic strength changes are extrinsic proteins (e.g., spectrin), whereas those that require more aggressive mechanisms such as detergents, for extraction are intrinsic (e.g., glycophorin A).[7] These intrinsic membrane proteins have a transmembrane configuration spanning the full thickness of the lipid bilayer, as has been shown with glycophorin A using radioactive labeling. In these experiments glycophorin A is cleaved externally from nonpermeable RBCs. In these cells glycophorin A can no longer be labeled. If these RBCs are then made permeable, the internal aspect of the molecule can be labeled, proving that it spans the thickness of the membrane.[282] Furthermore, by analyzing the amino acid sequence of glycophorin A, it has been shown that the segment between amino acid 71 and amino acid 90 is the hydrophobic transmembrane segment of the molecule.[220]

Current data indicate that antigens of the MNs system[283] and probably the Rh system (Fig 5–12)[284] are integral proteins, whereas the Duffy Fy^a and Fy^b antigens are peripheral proteins.[285]

Warm antibodies are of clinical importance because they react at body temperature and are responsible for extravascular immune-mediated hemolysis. This type of hemolysis occurs because warm antibodies, which for the most part are of the IgG class, coat RBCs, which are then "picked up" and destroyed or damaged by macrophages bearing IgG-Fc receptors.[286] This type of hemolysis is slower by comparison to hemolytic cold antibodies of the IgM class, capable of inducing complement-mediated intravascular hemolysis. More details on immune system–mediated intravascular hemolysis are given in chapter 10.

A description of the more frequent antigenic systems producing warm antibody responses follows.

The Rh System

Levine and Stetson described an antibody causing intragroup hemagglutination which was shown to have caused hemolytic disease of the newborn and was capable of agglutinating RBCs of 80% of the population.[287] It was later shown by Landsteiner

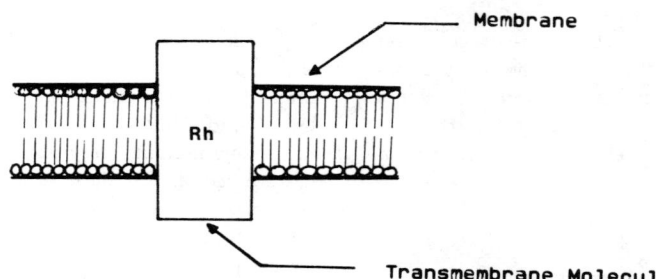

FIG 5–12.—Model of the Rh molecule as a transmembrane protein. This protein purportedly functions as a stabilizing protein.

and Wiener that an antibody obtained in rabbits and guinea pigs by immunization with human RBCs was capable of agglutinating most but not all human RBCs. This antibody, which proved to have a similar reactivity to that described by Levine and Stetson, was termed the Rh antigen.[288] Anti-Rh antibodies are responsible for most cases of severe hemolytic disease of the newborn and for many transfusion reactions of the warm antibody type.

Nomenclature of the Rh System

Various proposals for nomenclature of the Rh system have been set forth. The more useful ones are those described independently by Wiener, Fisher-Race, and Rosenfield. All three have useful characteristics and are used in today's blood banking. The terminology of each nomenclature is based on different theories which at the time the nomenclatures were established probably underestimated the complexity of the Rh system. A brief description of each of these systems follows (Fig 5–13).

Fisher-Race Nomenclature.—According to these workers the Rh system is coded by six frequently found genes, D (which codes for the most immunogenic antigen), d (an amorph), C, c, E, and e.[289] These genes are grouped in groups of three antithetical genes (D, C, E vs. d, c, e), which means that DD cannot occur on the same side of the genome (Figs 5–14 and 5–15). Thus, genotypes can be DCe/DCe if the individual is homozygous for the three genes D, C, e, or heterozygous if an individual has the genotype DCe/dcE, but the genotype DDE/CCE is never possible, for these genes are antithetical. On this basis, all possible permutations have been described. The more frequent genotypes are given in Table 5–7. The Rh genes are purported to be so closely placed to each other that virtually no crossing over takes place. Very rarely, however, crossing over in the Rh system has been documented.[290]

Due to its ease of use, the Fisher-Race nomenclature has been officially adopted by the World Health Organization (WHO).[291] More on the Fisher-Race nomenclature will be given in other sections.

Wiener Nomenclature.—Wiener did not believe the Rh antigen complex to be coded by three different genes (D, C, e), but by a single gene that coded for an agglutinogen.[292] This reasoning came from the lack of evidence of crossing over of the Rh genes (see Fig 5–13). Thus, DCe would be written as Rh1, which contains several factors or phenotypic determinants, namely Rh_o (D), rh' (C), hr'' (e), and rhi (Ce). The Wiener nomenclature is useful as a shorthand. For instance, DCe can be written as Rh1 or simply as R1, and DCe/DCe can be written as R1/R1. The Wiener nomenclature for the Rh genes and their possible permutations is given in Table 5–8 (see Fig 5–14).

Nevertheless, the Fisher-Race method is simpler to handle when defining the genotype and phenotype of the Rh complex; e.g., it is simpler to write DCe than Rh_o, rh', hr''.

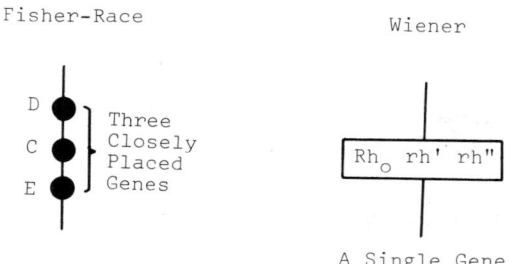

FIG 5–13.—*Left,* arrangement of genes according to the Fisher-Race theory. The theory assumes the existence of three closely placed genes in tandem. Such an arrangement would explain the lack or very rare existence of crossing over. *Right,* Wiener's theory of a single gene for a single agglutinogen.

Blood Group Antigens

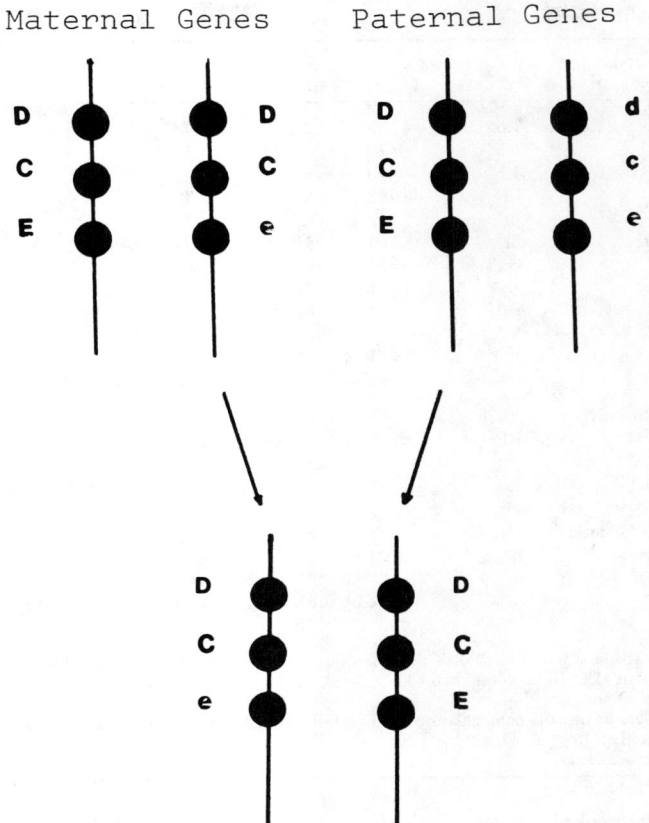

Progeny's Phenotype: DCCEe

FIG 5–14.—Rh gene inheritance. Notice expression of homozygous (CC) and heterozygous (E,e) phenotypes.

Rosenfield Nomenclature.—Rosenfield thought it better to designate the different Rh determinants by numbering them rather than by speculating on their order or display in the genome until more is known regarding the biochemistry of the Rh system.[293] He numbered each Rh antigenic specificity as Rh1, Rh2, etc. If one designates a specific phenotype, a positive sign indicates antigens present and a negative sign indicates antigens not present. For example, DCE is designated as Rh:1,2,3,−4,−5, whereas DCe is designated as Rh:1,2,−3,−4,5. This system lends itself to automated data processing, whereas neither the Fisher-Race nor the Wiener system has this advantage.

Chemistry of the Rh System Antigens

Due to the small amount of antigen present on each RBC and the complex antigenic polymorphisms of the Rh system, the precise structure of the antigens remains unknown at this time. However, some facts regarding the structure of the Rh system are known and are reviewed briefly here.

An absence of Rh antigens, as in Rh null individuals(—/—), causes membrane deformity, which suggests that Rh antigens are a part of a transmembrane protein.[294] Interestingly, recent studies using reversed RBC ghosts show that D-negative RBCs possess D antigens in the inner aspect of the RBC.[295] However, these data are now considered controversial. Furthermore, D antigenicity can be

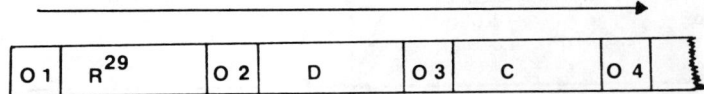

FIG 5–15.—Rosenfield's model for Rh genes. *O,* operon gene. R[29], D, and C are structural genes.

TABLE 5-7.—Frequently Used Nomenclature for the Rh System*

ROSENFIELD	FISHER-RACE OR OTHER	WIENER	% OF§	ROSENFIELD	FISHER-RACE OR OTHER	WIENER	% OF§
Rh 1	D	Rh_o	85	Rh 21	C^G	...	70
Rh 2	C	Rh'	70	Rh 22	CE	...	< 1
Rh 3	E	Rh''	30	Rh 23	D^w, Wiel	...	< 1
Rh 4	c	hr'	80	Rh 24	ET	...	30
Rh 5	e	hr''	98	Rh 25	LW 1–4	...	> 99
Rh 6	ce(f)	hr	64	Rh 26	C-like, Deal	hr^A	80
Rh 7	Ce	rhi	70	Rh 27	cE	...	30
Rh 8	C^w	rh^{w1}	1	Rh 28	...	hr^H	2
Rh 9	C^x	rh^x	< 1	Rh 29	"Total Rh"	...	> 99
Rh 10	Ce^s, V	hr^v	1	Rh 30†	Go^a, D^{cor}	...	< 1
Rh 11	E^w	rh^{w2}	< 1	Rh 31	e mosaic	hr^B	98
Rh 12	G	rh^G	85	Rh 32†	D (C) (e) Troll.	$\bar{\bar{R}}^N$ prod.	< 1
‡Rh 13	D^u mosaic	Rh^A	85	Rh 33	Har.	R^o Har. prod.	< 1
‡Rh 14	D^u IV	Rh^B	85	Rh 34	Bas.	Hr^B	100
‡Rh 15	D^u V	Rh^C	85	Rh 35	D (C) (e), 1114	...	< 1
‡Rh 16	D^uIII	Rh^D	85	Rh 36	Ber.	...	< 1
†Rh 17	D—Hr^o prod.	Hr_o	> 99	Rh 37	Evans	...	< 1
†Rh 18	D—Hr prod.	Hr, Hr^S	> 99	Rh 38	Duclos	...	> 99
Rh 19	e mosaic	hr^S	98	Rh 39	C-like	...	> 99
Rh 20	VS,e^S	...	1	Rh 40	Tar.	...	< 1
				Rh 41	Ce-like	Rhi-like	< 1
				Rh 42	Ce^S, Thor.	Rhi^S	< 1

*From references 406, 407, 408. Note: ·D·$^{(a)}$ is like –D–$^{(a)}$, but Evans positive, –D– is Evans negative. Both have enhanced D, but ·D· slightly less than –D–.
†Have enhanced D antigens.
‡Tippett's low-grade mosaic nomenclature do not fully correlate with Wiener's nomenclature; they are listed from I to VI rather than from A–D.
§Frequency in caucasians.

preserved in purified proteolipid micels.[296] Current studies suggest that Rh antigens are located in band 3 glycoprotein, represented in a 28,500-dalton polypeptide structure,[297] although different studies using radiation Rh-antigen destruction suggest a 140,000-dalton structure.[298] The presence of both phospholipids and sulfhydryl bonds appears to be important to preserve Rh antigenicity,[299] although the requirement for sulfhydryl bonds has not been fully proved.[300] It is currently believed that there are about 30,000–56,000 Rh_o (D) antigenic sites on each (·D·/·D·) homozygous Rh-positive RBC,[301] compared to 1 million sites for ABH antigenic sites.[302] At least 100–150 antigenic sites on immature RBCs are required for a positive Coombs test.[303] The number of these antigenic sites is about two times greater in homozygous D individuals than in heterozygous individuals.[304]

Other antigens in the Rh system reveal about 70,000–85,000 sites in homozygous cc and about

TABLE 5-8.—Rh Combinations of Genes and Frequency of Combinations

PHENOTYPE	MOST LIKELY GENOTYPE			2ND MOST LIKELY GENOTYPE		
	Wiener	Fisher-Race	% Freq.	Wiener	Fisher-Race	% Freq.
DCcee	R_1r	DCe/dce	33	R_1R_o	DCe/Dce	2
DCCee	R_1R_1	DCe/DCe	18	R_1r'	DCe/dCe	1
DCeEe	R_1R_2	DCe/DcE	12	R_1r''	DCe/dcE	1
DccEe	R_2r	DcE/dce	11	R_2R_o	DcE/Dce	1
DccEE	R_2R_2	DcE/DcE	2	R_2r''	DcE/dcE	<1
Dccee	R_or	Dce/dce	2	R_oR_o	Dce/Dce	<1
ccee	rr	dce/dce	15			
Ccee	$r'r$	dCe/dce	1			
ccEe	$r''r$	dcE/dce	1			

half as many in heterozygous Cc, whereas there are about 18,000–24,000 e sites in homozygous ee individuals and 13,500–14,500 e sites in heterozygous Ee individuals.[305]

Rh antigens are thought to be found exclusively on RBCs and their precursors. Their previous allocation to platelets is not supported by current studies.[275]

Genetics of the Rh System

The Rh molecular complex is likely part of a transmembrane protein. Therefore, the antigenic determinants are thought to be amino acid sequences, unlike antigenic determinants on antigens such as the ABH system, which are carbohydrate sequences. In view of these concepts, Rosenfield et al.[306] envision operating genes (operons) and structural genes, just as has been shown by Jacob and Monod for bacterial proteins (Figs 5–15 and 5–16).[307] The R^{29} gene of the Rh system, in the Rosenfield nomenclature, would function as an "on" switch; "off" switch genes would be located at other sites. This operon is designated OP1. The structural gene R^{29} coding for a precursor protein would then be activated and the phenotypic product R^{29} synthesized. This would activate OP2, which would turn on the structural gene for D. OP3 would turn on structural genes for C,c, and OP4 for E,e. OP1 to OP4 would be on line. Thus, if D and C are in the *cis* position, the products would be decoded as sequential amino acids; if the genes D and C were in the *trans* position, D amino acid sequences present as well as C amino acid sequences would be close to each other but not contiguous, though probably on the same protein. In the Jacob-Monod model, the products of structural genes act as a feedback mechanism to control the "off" switch of the operon gene sequences. Operons that are composed of an initiator, a promoter, and an operator are acted on respectively by a "turn-on" protein, RNA polymerase, and an inhibitory protein. In this way, RBC precursors would contain a set of operon and structural genes which would be decoded irreversibly, transcribed into RNA, and eventually translated in ribosomes to produce the Rh molecule on RBCs.

The genetic code for the Rh system is much more complicated than the simple gene action of six

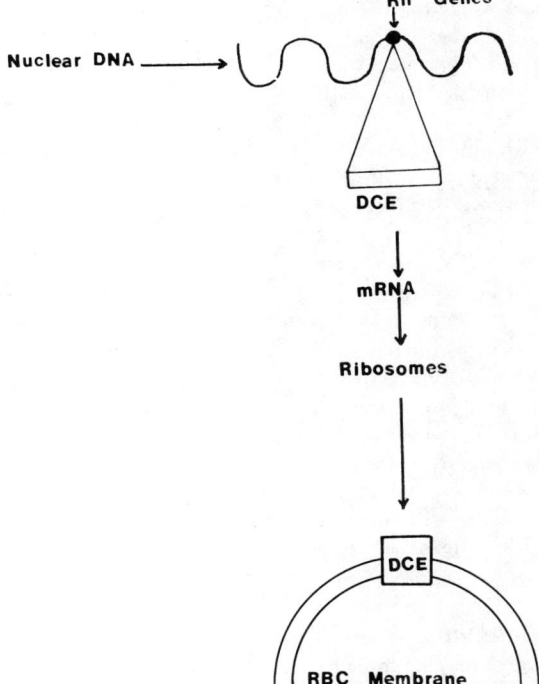

FIG 5–16.—Suggested mechanism of inheritance of Rh genes. Rh genes coded for by the nuclear DNA are translated to the messenger RNA. The information is decoded in ribosomes in a protein and a protein is synthesized. Subsequently it is affixed to the RBC membrane.

allelic genes (D, C, E, d, c, e). This is inferred in part from the finding of a mosaic structure of the D and e antigen as well as Rh antigen variants. If the antigens have various subunits (D has at least four subunits), then several genes must interact to produce a completed major antigenic determinant such as D. This probably occurs by interaction of several structural genes regulated by D+ or D− operon.[308] Weakened forms of the D antigen are reviewed in more detail below.

There is now conclusive evidence that the Rh antigens are coded for by chromosome 1,[309] although evidence of linkage between the Rh system and chromosome 1 was suspected much earlier.[310]

Altered Expression of Rh Antigens

Deletion, Suppression, and Amorphic Rh Genes

Rh Null Phenotype.—The Rh null phenotype was originally described by Vos et al., who showed that these cells completely lack Rh antigens.[311] Two types of Rh null phenotypes have been described. One is thought to be caused by amorphic genes at the Rh locus where the parental Rh phenotypes are normal.[312] Another is thought to be caused by a homozygous suppressor gene. Heterozygous parental Rh phenotypes are usually weakened in these cases.[313]

The antibody produced by Rh null individuals is termed anti-Rh29 and is directed to an antigen present on all other Rh-positive and Rh-negative cells.[314]

The lack of Rh molecules on RBCs makes these cells more permeable to potassium (Fig 5–17). However, it has been shown that the molecule for the potassium pump is located at a different site from the Rh molecule, for Rh null cells have an increased number of potassium pump sites.[315] These abnormal cells cause what is known as the Rh null syndrome, where RBCs appear as stomatocytes. Patients with the Rh null syndrome frequently develop hemolytic anemia.[315] Rh mod is another phenotype in which Rh antigens are very weak.[316]

Other Rh Antigen Deletions.—Certain parts of the Rh antigenic complex may be missing because of gene deletions. Examples of these are D-- or DC-. These may be represented schematically on the cell membrane, as shown in Figure 5–18. D-- was first reported by Race et al.[317]

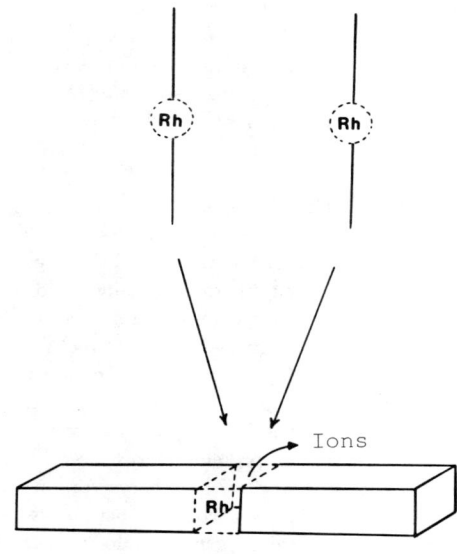

FIG 5–17.—Figure showing homozygous Rh null genes located in an allelic position and the resulting absence of the RBC membrane Rh molecular complex. The absence of Rh results in deformity of the membrane and escape of intracellular ions.

Almost any type of deletion combination is possible and is reflected antigenically by the lack of these structures on RBCs (Fig 5–19). Many deletions result in changes in the steric configuration of the Rh antigen, producing rare antibodies that otherwise would not be present. A D-- deletion, for instance, results in a greater antigenicity for the D antigen.[318] This enhancement has been explained on the basis that the D antigen may be much more accessible on the RBC surface, though such an explanation may turn out to be simplistic.

The Rh D^u Antigens.—Rh D^u antigens are weakened forms of the D antigen complex. They were first reported by Stratton and Renton.[319] These antigens do not react normally with Rh typing reagents and therefore may cause Rh mistypings. For this reason Rh-negative samples are routinely tested in some laboratories with Coombs reagent to assess the presence of D^u after they have been reacted with the anti-D reagent.

Traditionally, D^u antigens have been grouped into high-grade and low-grade D^u types. The high-grade D^u types are usually caused by a C antigen in

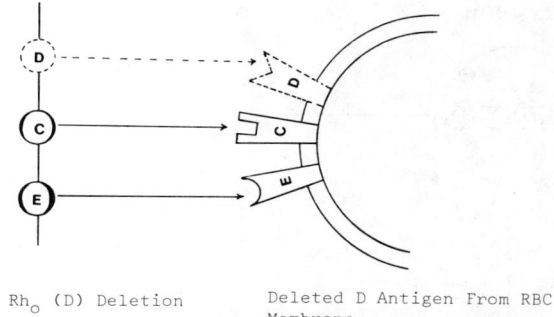

Chromosome Rh_o (D) Deletion   Deleted D Antigen From RBC Membrane

FIG 5–18.—Rh_o (D) deletion resulting in the absence of a portion of the Rh molecular complex at the RBC membrane.

the *trans* position, for instance Dce/dCe. Possibly steric hindrance causes a decrease in reactivity of the D antigen in this type of Rh D^u cell. Persons with high-grade D^u antigens very rarely produce anti-D. The low-grade D^u is caused by the deleted portions of the D molecule (D mosaic), first described by Shapiro (Fig 5–20,A).[320] Presumably, lack of some portions of the mosaic (Fig 5–20,B) causes cells to react weakly with anti-D reagents.

The reaction against mosaic D^u cells will depend on the specificity of antibodies directed against the various portions of the mosaic antigen (i.e., A, B, C, D, not to be confused with the Fisher-Race terminology for major Rh determinants). Persons with low-grade D^u antigens often produce anti-D antibodies and should be transfused with Rh_o (D) negative blood.[321]

A variant of the C antigen called C^w is sometimes found as an antigenic specificity in R_1R_1 individuals who form anti-c.[322] C^w can be considered a weak variant of C and gives different dosage effects in homozygous and heterozygous individuals.

In certain cases, RBC antigenic expression of C or e may be decreased, possibly because of a suppressor gene variant. These individuals' phenotype is written as D(c)(e) and was described for the first time by Rosenfield and co-workers.[323] A similar antigen is Rh33, written symbolically as (D)c(e).[324]

Enhanced Forms of the D Antigen.—Certain Rh gene products produce more "exposed" D antigen than other D antigens. One such case, already mentioned, is the D--/D-- genotype. However, other cases of enhanced D reactivity are found. Notably, D-positive cells lacking En^a antigens show increased reactivity with anti-D.[325] Another theory proposed to explain enhanced expressivity of D assumes that greater amounts of D substance are produced. However, this theory has not been proved experimentally.

Cells with M^g or M^r variants in the MNSs system have increased Rh_o (D) reactivity.[326] This increment may be due to the decreased sialic acid content in the membrane of these cells, but more evidence is needed to support this idea.

Interestingly, GO^a cells, which lack a portion of

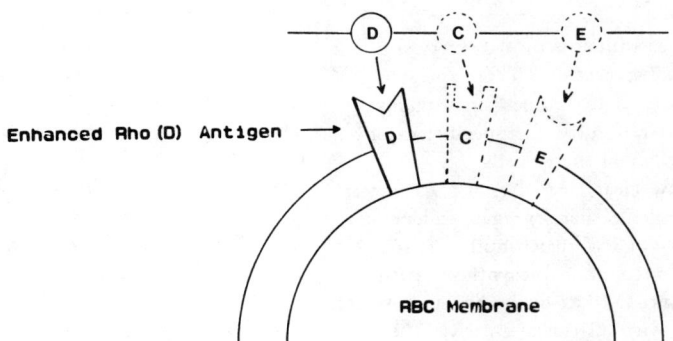

Enhanced Rho (D) Antigen

RBC Membrane

FIG 5–19.—CE deletion with enhancement of the D antigen. Such enhancement may result from the fact that the Rh_o (D) antigen in these deletions makes the Rh_o (D) antigen more accessible to the immune system.

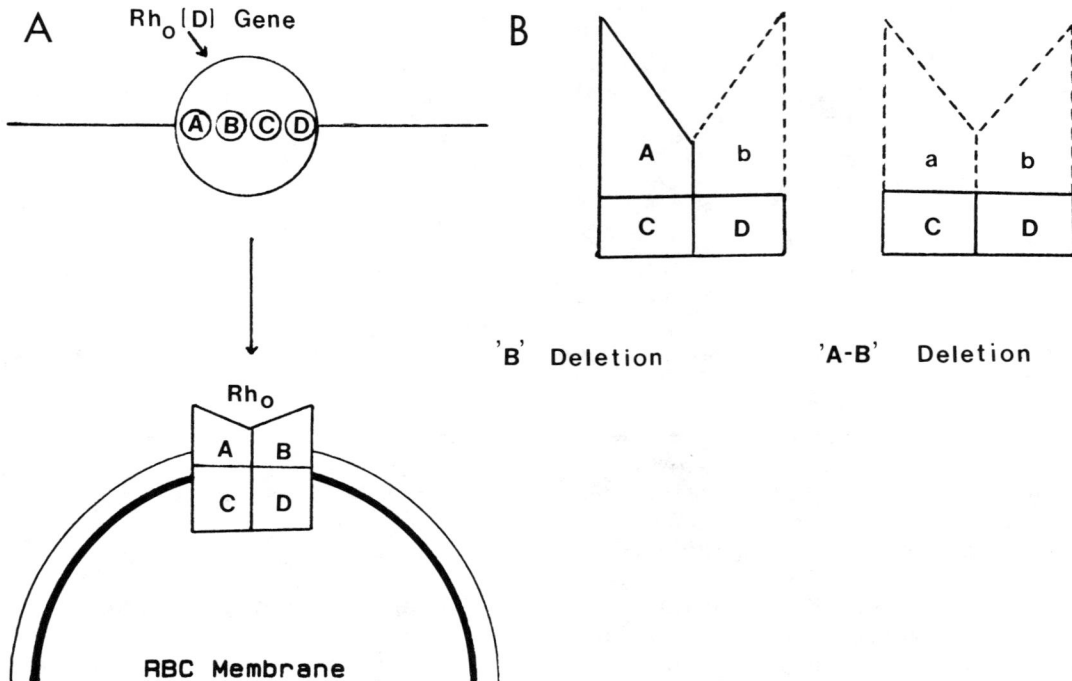

FIG 5–20.—**A,** inheritance of the mosaic structure of the Rh_o (D) molecule. The D gene is represented as containing four subset genes (a, b, c, d). These subset genes are decoded as proteins that form the D Rh molecule complex, which is subsequently anchored to the RBC membrane. The Wiener nomenclature for the mosaic subset genes must not be confused with the Fisher-Race nomenclature for non-D antigens. **B,** low-grade D^u resulting from mosaic deletions of the Rh_o (D) antigen.

the D mosaic, react more avidly with anti-D than other Rh-positive cells.[327] This reactivity may be secondary to steric hindrance.

The Landsteiner-Wiener Antigen

The LW (Landsteiner-Wiener) antigen is the antigen most likely described as the Rh antigen in the initial publication on Rh system. In those early experiments guinea pigs were immunized with rhesus monkey RBCs.[328]

The LW antigen determinants must be very similar to Rh precursor substances or Rh core antigens, since antibodies produced by guinea pigs against rhesus monkey RBCs recognize the specificity for both human Rh+ cells and rhesus cells.[329]

However, it is now clear that LW and Rh are coded for by separate genes that segregate independently.[330] The absence of LW in Rh null cells suggests they may share a common biosynthetic pathway.[331] However, anti-D-like antibodies can be elicited in rabbits with Rh-negative RBC extracts,[328] showing that Rh and LW are indeed distinct. Furthermore, the fact that certain immunosuppressed Rh-negative individuals develop anti-LW antibodies in the absence of anti-D antibodies[332] supports this concept.

There are at least four allelic variants of the LW gene, 1, 2, 3, and 4, against which antibodies have been found, revealing the heterogeneity of the LW system.[333]

New Rh Antigenic Specificities Resulting From Probable Antigen Proximity

The phenotypic product of Ce can induce, if transfused into an individual, an antibody that will react with cells where Ce are close to each other. This antigenic determinant is termed rhi.[334] This antibody reacts with dCe/dcE but not with dCE/dce. Another example of an antibody induced by antigenic proximity is ce, otherwise known as anti-f.[335] The ce antibody reacts with dce/DCE but not with dcE/DCe (Fig 5–21).

Other Specificities in the Rh System

Even though antibodies against the G determinant react with cells containing D and C, very rare RBC examples are Rh_o (D)-positive G-negative,[336]

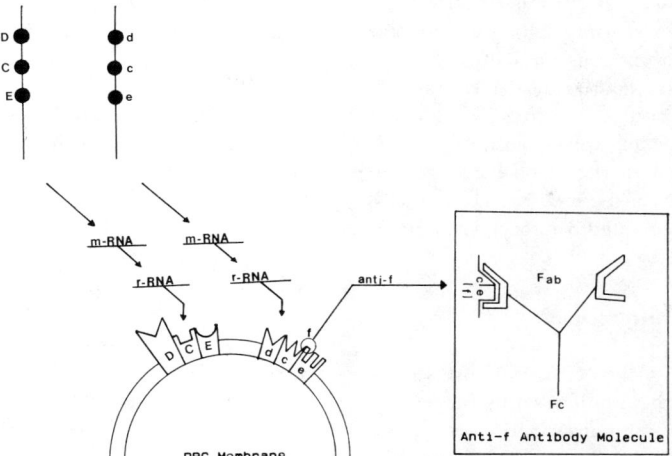

FIG 5–21.—Suggested mechanisms whereby maternal and paternal genes code for separate Rh molecule complexes. The message in the nuclear DNA is decoded by the ribosomes. Though amino acid sequences defining the maternal and paternal gene products are separate, they probably form part of the same protein on the membrane. Note that it is possible to detect molecular proximity of c and e antigens on one of the Rh molecular complexes provided by the parental Rh gene complex dce. Such proximity is detected by a specific antibody (f). The hypervariable region of the Fab fragment of the anti-f antibody molecule recognizes the ce complex.

or Rh_o (D)-negative G-positive,[337] which suggests the existence of an independent antigenic moiety, although this determinant may prove to be a shared amino acid sequence, common in both D and C determinants, which may be present even though the major determinant for D or C may be absent. Anti-G antibodies are best test-controlled by r^G cells.[338] C^w, also reviewed under weakened form of C, is present both in C and c-positive individuals.[339] The gene probably codes for amino acids in close proximity to Cc. It is not a frequent antigen in caucasians (2%). Many other Rh antigenic determinants have been described. In the Rosenfield nomenclature at least 42 antigenic specificities have been listed. Rh41, which has recently been described, may be associated with abnormalities in chromosome 1 genetic markers (see Table 5–7).[340]

Laboratory Aspects of Rh Antigen-Antibody Testing

A tube Rh typing test is the preferred method of antigen-antibody testing in immunohematology laboratories. Antiserum against the D antigen is added. Albumin is used to enhance the reaction. The test can produce false positive results in the following instances:

1. If the patient's cells are coated with antibody in vivo.
2. If the patient has hyperproteinemia. In this case the reaction is repeated with saline replacement after the cells are washed several times (see Chapter 6).
3. If the sample is improperly clotted. This may be seen in patients on anticoagulant therapy. The addition of protamine for full clotting may be necessary.
4. If other specificities are present in the antiserum.[341]
5. If a passively immunized individual with RhIG immunoglobulin has a transient serum anti-D.[342] Antilymphocyte globulin may have a similar effect.[343]

False negative results may be seen in the following situations:

1. Weak suspensions.
2. Weak reactions after saline replacement.
3. Weakly reactive cells (i.e., cells that have a weak dosage of antigens on their surface).[344]

More details on techniques are available in technical manuals and will not be discussed further here.

Rh antisera can be modified to increase the span of the IgG molecule. The modifications involve breaking an interchain disulfide bond distal to the Fc fragment. This allows testing for antigens without the need for anti-human globulin serum. The reagent is commercially available.[345] An interesting and very sensitive method for detecting antibodies of the Rh type coating Rh-positive cells is that described by Lalezari[346] using an autoanalyzer. This method allows detection of very small amounts of antibody coating RBCs that are missed on the direct Coombs test. Experimentally, a sensitive method to detect Rh antigens on RBCs, the fluoresceinated anti-D method, is available; this test detects Rh-positive cells in titers as low as 1:100,000.[347] Dosage of $Rh_o(D)$ antigens cannot routinely be tested for in the blood bank, but an enzyme immunoassay can be used to detect dosage of $Rh_o(D)$ in homozygous and heterozygous individuals.[348]

Clinical Significance of Rh Immunization

Rh immunization usually occurs in transfused individuals and in patients immunized by pregnancy. Very rarely, however, immunization is present in a person without a history of pregnancy or transfusion,[349] and immunization without transfusion may likewise occur in Rh null individuals.[350] Transient anti-D antibodies may occur in Rh_o (D)-positive individuals with dyserythropoietic anemia.[351]

In general, 80% of Rh individuals are capable of producing anti-D antibody, while 20% are nonresponsive.[352]

Rh Antigens and the Immune Response

Unlike other primary immune responses, it appears that a primary immune response to Rh antigens is always composed of an IgG and IgA component,[353] and rarely of an IgM component. Secondary responses to Rh antigens are usually of the IgG class; of this class, a predominance of IgG1 and IgG3 is observed,[354] although IgG2 and IgG4 responses have likewise been observed. Occasionally the main response is a nonagglutinating IgA antibody.[355] Most anti-D sera do not bind complement, probably due to the distance between $Rh_o(D)$ sites. Infrequently, complement-binding anti-D antibodies have been observed.[356] These probably represent antisera with more than one specificity, which allows two Fc portions to lie close to each other.

Recent evidence suggests that the immune response genes to Rh_o (D) are located in the extended 6P haplotype, which also contains BF*8F1, C2*C, C2*A*3C4B*QO complotypes.[357] The immunizing dose of Rh D-positive cells can be as small as 0.01 ml.[358] Therefore, care must be exercised when transfusing Rh-negative individuals with components (such as platelets) contaminated with RBCs, as there may be 1 ml or more of RBC contamination when the components are pooled. These patients must receive anti-D passive protection (with RhIG) as described for Rh-negative mothers delivering Rh-positive infants, discussed later in this chapter.

Of all Rh antigenic determinants, Rh_o (D) appears to be the most immunogenic. Individuals producing anti-D can produce antibodies to other determinants which they lack (e.g., C, G), but less frequently. Antibodies to C or E independently from a concomitant anti-D are infrequent.[359] D^u is substantially less antigenic than D or other Rh antigens.

The relative immunogenicity of Rh antigens is given in Table 5–9.[360] Immunization to Rh_o (D) may occur after extensive plasma exchange with Rh_o (D)-positive plasma replacement.[361]

Rh Antibodies in Pregnancy

Although hemolytic disease of the newborn is discussed in detail in chapter 16, a few aspects of the disease are pertinent here. It is not surprising that the Rh antigen system was described after the discovery of the causative antibody of Rh hemolytic disease of the newborn. It is now known that the antibody is an IgG antibody, usually of the IgG1 or IgG3 class, that is capable of crossing the placenta. The mother is usually an Rh-negative individual carrying an Rh-positive conceptus. A fetomaternal bleed may occur during pregnancy or, more frequently, at delivery (there is usually a 1-ml fetomaternal bleed in normal deliveries), thus causing immunization (Fig 5–22). Actual determination of the extent of a fetomaternal bleed with the Kleihauer-Betke test[362] is discussed in more detail in chapter 16. Another method using an erythrocyte rosetting technique has also been devised.[363] A

TABLE 5–9.—IMMUNOGENICITY OF RH ANTIGENS OTHER THAN Rh_o (D)*

ANTIGEN	% LIKELIHOOD OF IMMUNIZATION†
hr' (c)	2.05
rh" (E)	1.69
hr" (e)	0.5
rh' (C)	0.11
(C^w)	<.1

*The likelihood of immunization with Rh_o (D) is greater than 80% after the second transfusion on Rh_o (D)-positive blood to an Rh_o (D)-negative recipient.
†Dependent on the frequency of the phenotype in the population.

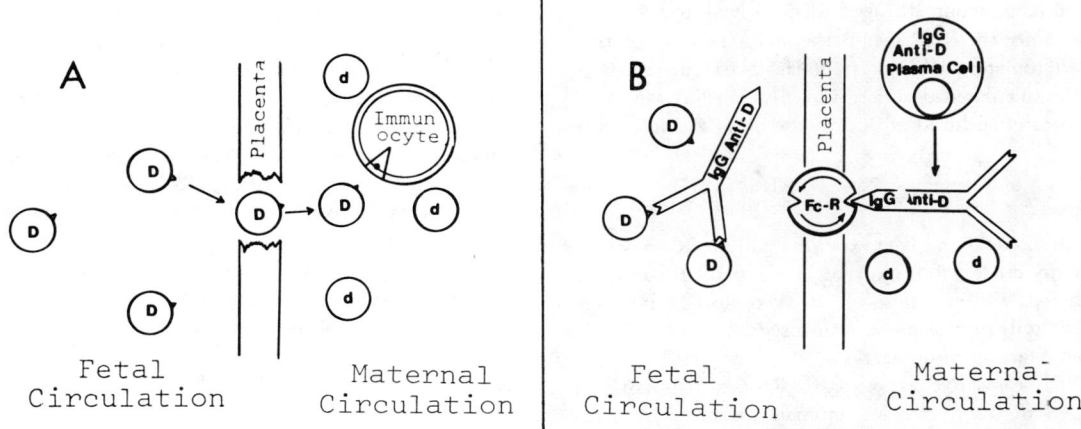

FIG 5–22.—Development of anti-Rh$_o$ (D) antibodies as a result of fetomaternal hemorrhage. **A,** penetration of fetal Rh$_o$ (D) RBCs into the maternal circulation. Immunocytes in the Rh-negative maternal circulation recognize Rh$_o$ (D) cells as non-self. **B,** IgG anti-Rh$_o$ (D) committed plasma cells in the maternal circulation produce IgG anti-Rh$_o$ (D) monomers. The Fc portion of these antibodies is compatible with a placental Fc receptor *(Fc-R)*, which transports IgG into the fetal circulation. Such antibodies will coat Rh$_o$ (D) fetal RBCs.

recent study on Rh immunization after induced abortion showed that Rh$_o$ (D)-positive RBCs of the conceptus entering the maternal blood during abortion were responsible for at least 3% of the immunizations of Rh-negative females of child-bearing age.[364] Whether an Rh$_o$ (D)-negative fetus can become immunized by a transplacental bleed from an Rh-positive mother is controversial.[365]

Rh Immunization and Fetomaternal Bleeding.—Transplacental hemorrhage was first documented by Chown in 1954.[366] However, in most cases fetomaternal bleeding is much less severe than in the case described by this author. The greatest amount of bleeding usually occurs in the third trimester[367] and during delivery.[368] About 50% of women have detectable fetal cells in their circulation in the postpartum period.[369] The average fetomaternal bleed is usually less than 1 ml at delivery.[370] However, less than 0.1 ml of Rh-positive cells is sufficient to immunize the mother against the D antigen.[367] Approximately 8% of Rh-negative women with ABO-compatible pregnancies will develop anti-D antibodies within 6 months of delivery[367] if unprotected by anti-D globulin (RhIG), and an additional 8% will develop antibodies with their second Rh-positive pregnancy,[371] or 47% of all Rh-negative women in their second Rh-positive pregnancy.[372] However, immunization to Rh in ABO-incompatible pregnancies is much less frequent[371, 373] because of the rapid destruction of ABO-incompatible cells in the circulation and because of transportation of Rh antigens to areas unfavorable to anti-Rh antibody synthesis.[374, 375] About 93% of cases of isoimmunization to the Rh complex are to the D antigen, and about 6% are of anti-c, anti-E, or anti-Ce specificity.[376] From this it can be inferred that the D antigen is about 30 times more immunogenic.[377] Rh$_o$ (D)-positive plasma has been shown to be occasionally capable of immunizing Rh$_o$ (D)-negative recipients.[378]

Prevention of Rh Immunization

The first experiments showing that antibodies against Rh antigens might prevent Rh immunization were performed by Stern et al.,[374] who found that RBCs coated with anti-D in vitro and transfused did not immunize Rh-negative individuals. Finn et al.[379] first attempted to passively immunize Rh-negative mothers with IgM anti-Rh antibodies. Further experiments were performed by Freda et al. using IgG fractions of anti-D human sera to avoid possible enhancement by the use of Rh antisera of the IgM class.[380] This enhancement is now thought not to occur when IgM anti-D is used.[381] Nevertheless, the use of IgG fraction is now universal and most effective in producing suppression of Rh immunization.[382] Rh$_o$ (D) immunoglobulin (RhIG) is the preparation used to prevent immunization of Rh-negative individuals who have been exposed to Rh$_o$ (D) antigenic material. Each unit of RhIG contains about 300 μg of immune globulin. It is administered intramuscularly and is capable of neutralizing about 30 ml of Rh-positive blood.[383]

Since the Kleihauer-Betke method for calculating a fetomaternal bleed is about 50% accurate, twice the calculated dose is given.[384] Therefore, for a fetomaternal bleed of 90 ml, the dose is as follows:

$$\frac{90 \text{ ml}}{30} \times 2 = 6 \text{ vials of RhIG}$$

RhIG has been given experimentally to Rh-negative individuals who received 1 unit of Rh-positive blood, and at a dose of 20 μg of anti-D antibody per milliliter of blood transfused, it was capable of abrogating immunization.[385]

If a massive exposure to Rh-positive RBCs is present (e.g., massive fetomaternal bleed or inadvertent transfusion of Rh-positive blood to a young female of child-bearing age), then the dosage of RhIG may be very high. If the decision has been made to attempt abrogating immunization, the dose may have to be divided to avoid severe pain at the injection site as well as hematomas.[386]

RhIG is given intramuscularly in this country because of the potential of inducing DIC with impure RhIG preparations. An intravenous preparation is available in Europe and may be more effective in controlling RhIG dosages.[386, 387] However, intravenous anti-D infusions may cause severe hemolytic reactions in certain cases,[388] as well as hypotensive episodes.[389]

RhIG may have to be given after cesarean sections,[390] manual removal of the placenta, and abortions.[391] It is advocated that Rh-negative women who have abortions receive RhIG preventatively at a smaller dosage (100 μg), for it abrogates immunization by cells from the conceptus that bear Rh antigens.[392] Other authors suggest Rh typing of blood from fetuses of second-trimester abortions to determine RhIG use, but this practice is by no means universal.[393] It has also been advocated that RhIG be given to Rh-negative mothers during pregnancy when an Rh-positive fetus may be present. Passage of RhIG through the placenta at the usual dosage seems not to affect the fetus.[394] A unit of RhIG is given at 28 weeks' gestation in selected cases and the dose is repeated post partum.[394]

RhIG is recommended in Rh_o-negative mothers undergoing amniocentesis as part of antenatal workups.[392] D^u-negative women of the mosaic type, although rare, are now considered as potentially capable of becoming immunized[395] and may require RhIG at the usual dosage. Although RhIG should be given as soon as possible after delivery of an Rh-positive baby by an Rh-negative mother, the 72-hour "grace" period[396] was established empirically in experiments on volunteers at Sing Sing.[397] This should not be a prevention to attempt abrogating immunization in individuals who missed receiving preventative therapy in the first 72 hours after exposure to Rh-positive cells.[397] RhIG is also given to Rh-negative recipients of Rh-positive units of platelets, for these units are usually contaminated with up to 0.5 ml of RBCs.[398] Desensitization to Rh immunization has been attempted by oral administration of Rh-positive stroma from RBCs, with initially promising results.[399] Reversal of Rh alloimmunization with RhIG has not proved successful.[400]

RhIG Failures.—Anti-D titers in passively immunized recipients may be positive up to 5 months after RhIG is given prophylactically. If the levels do not drop after 5 months, it is assumed that abrogation of sensitization has failed. This occurs in approximately 0.1% of women immunized after delivery.[401] Some failures can be explained on the basis of previous immunization not detected because the very small amounts of antibody present escaped laboratory notice.[397] Another cause of failure is intrapregnancy sensitization.[397]

Rh Immunization of Rh-Negative Mothers.—Rh-negative mothers not protected by RhIG show immunization to the D antigen in approximately 3.3% of women that have had abortions,[391] 1.8% of women after a first full-term pregnancy with an Rh-positive conceptus,[394] 4.3% of ABO-compatible Rh-positive women 6 months after delivery,[402] and about 17% of Rh-negative women in a second Rh-positive pregnancy.[403] Antibody levels may remain elevated for several years[404] or may decrease to practically undetectable levels and be boosted by transfusion even several years after the initial stimulus.[404]

Role of Plasmapheresis in Rh Immunization.—A topic of current interest because of the availability of automated plasmapheresis[405] is the attempt to reduce anti-D antibody levels in pregnant mothers and thus decrease the severity of Rh hemolytic disease of the newborn. The few studies reported in the literature have not had encouraging results with this therapeutic modality.[405]

The Duffy Blood Group System

The Duffy system was first described by Cutbush et al. in 1950.[409] Initially three phenotypes, Fy (a+b−), Fy (a+b+), and Fy (a−b+), were described and demonstrated on the basis of an antigen dosage effect. However, 68% of American blacks typed as Fy (a−b−), which suggested the existence of other phenotypes. These were revealed later, as was shown in an immunized Fy (a−b−) female patient, whose serum was able to agglutinate all cells carrying Fy^a or Fy^b but none of the cells showing the Fy (a−b−) phenotypes. Her cells were described as Fy3 cells.[410] Two other antigens have been added since to the Duffy system: Fy4[411] and Fy5.[412]

Biochemistry of the Duffy System

Knowledge of the biochemistry of the Duffy system is quite sparse. Nevertheless, some inferences can be made regarding its nature. Most IgG responses to antigens are secondary to antigenic stimulation by antigens of a fairly complex structure, such as proteins. Duffy antigens elicit IgG responses in the great majority of cases and are destroyed by proteolytic enzymes. Therefore, the structure of the antigen is probably partly protein. It has been calculated, from membrane eluates with an inhibitory effect on anti-Duffy antibodies, that the Duffy antigens weigh about 35,000–55,000 daltons.[413] In addition, Masouredis et al.[414] have demonstrated that there are about 12,000 Fy^a sites on Fy^{a}Fy^a RBCs.[414] Dosage studies using an enzyme immunoassay have revealed that homozygotes have about twice as many sites as heterozygotes.[348]

The Duffy system has become of critical importance in the understanding of host parasite interactions. Recent studies have revealed that RBCs negative for Duffy antigens possess a higher resistance to parasites of the *Plasmodium* genus than erythrocytes bearing Duffy antigens.[415] Though at first Duffy antigens were thought to be directly involved in the attachment invasion process, this notion was contested when En^a-negative and Wr^b-negative RBCs were shown to be also resistant to plasmodia.[416] These RBC phenotypes are known to be defective in glycophorins, and have an absence of MN sialoglycoprotein.[417] This finding suggests that the main receptor for plasmodia on erythrocytes is glycophorin, a possible common thread on the above-mentioned observations. Recently, a definitive affinity of a 155-kilodalton and a 130-kilodalton protein purified from membranes of plasmodial merozoites and both glycophorin A and B have been demonstrated in vitro.[418] These findings are strong evidence that the receptor for plasmodia on RBCs is indeed glycophorin (Fig 5–23).

Genetics of the Duffy System

If Duffy antigens are part of a protein, then coding takes place in the DNA in a similar manner as

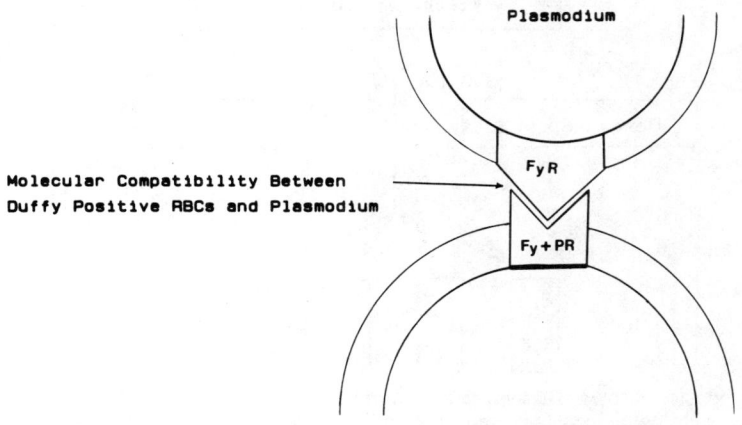

FIG 5–23.—Proposed mechanism by which *Plasmodium* parasites infect RBCs bearing Duffy antigens. Lack of such antigens supposedly results in resistance of RBCs to malarial infection. The *Plasmodium* receptor *(PR)* is glycophorin A and B.

in the now-prevalent model for Rh antigens. Thus, the Duffy complex may be initiated by an operon gene which lies in sequence with Fy^a, Fy^b, Fy^x, Fy3, Fy4, or Fy5.

Fy3 is always synthesized when Fy^a, Fy^b, and Fy^x (weak subgroup of Fy^b) are present, but not when Fy4 is present (Fig 5–24).[419] The Duffy system antigens along with the Rh antigens are coded for on chromosome 1.[420] The synthesis of some Duffy antigens (Fy5) appears to be linked in some way to the coding for the Rh system, as suggested by Colledge et al.[412] and as summarized graphically by Issitt and Issitt.[419] This is suggested by the fact that Rh null individuals are incapable of producing Fy5 and D-- deletions have reduced amounts of Fy5 antigen. This phenomenon is illustrated graphically in Figure 5–25.

The Duffy system may be used in paternity exclusion tests as an accessory genetic system as well as for anthropological studies because it is inherited in a codominant pattern, and individuals who are negative for one antigen can be phenotyped on the basis of a dosage effect.

Gene Frequencies

Extensive population studies show that about 66% of the caucasian population is Fy (a+), belonging to phenotypes of the Fy^aFy^a type or Fy^aFy^b; the remainder are Fy^bFy^b.[409] Fy (a−b−) people are usually black, although whites and Sephardic Jews have exhibited this phenotype in rare cases.

Laboratory Studies

Most cases of anti-Duffy antibodies against Fy^a or Fy^b are of the IgG_1 subclass and are well detected in the antiglobulin phase. It has been shown recently that Fy^a is restricted to V_HI or V_HII allotypes, whereas Fy^b are restricted to V_HII allotypes.[421] Certain saline-reactive IgM anti-Duffy antibodies have been described. About 50% of anti-Duffy antibodies bind complement.[422]

The Fy^a and Fy^b antigens are very susceptible to proteolytic enzymes such as papain and trypsin, which further suggests the protein nature of these substances. However, Fy3, Fy4, and Fy5 are not cleaved by these enzymes. This proteolytic enzyme

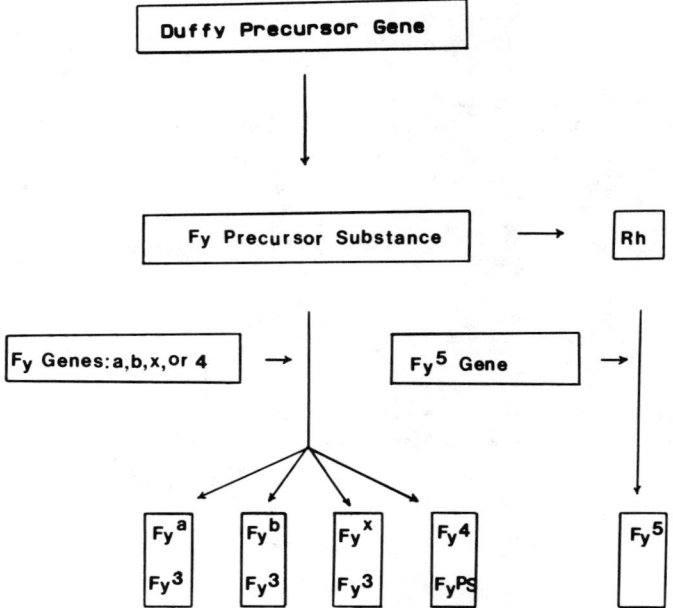

FIG 5–24.—Suggested pathway for the production of Duffy antigens. The production of Duffy a, b, and x antigens is associated with the concomitant production of Duffy 3 antigens. The production of Duffy 4 results in the expression of Duffy 4 antigens and Duffy precursor substance *(FyPS)*. The production of Duffy 5 antigens is not associated with the expression of FyPS; however, the expression of Duffy 5 is linked to the biosynthesis of Rh antigens. The phenotypic product is most probably a protein; thus an operon/structural gene mechanism is involved in the biosynthesis of these products.

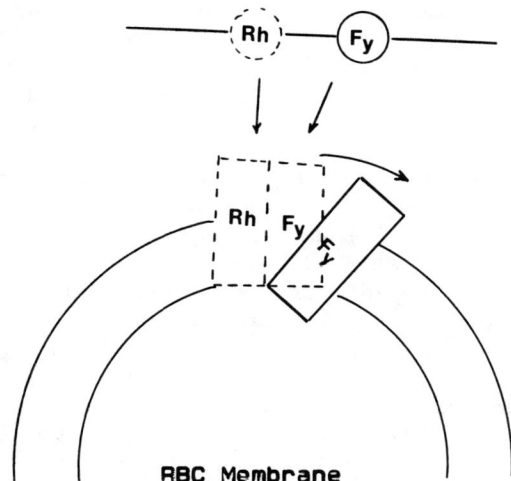

FIG 5–25.—A possible change of orientation of Fy antigens in Rh null cells resulting in the change of antigenic expression of Duffy antigens in Rh null individuals.

susceptibility is used in the laboratory as a diagnostic aid to single out anti-Duffy antibodies when multiple antibodies are present. Duffy antigens are likewise susceptible to prolonged storage at 12° C in saline, where Duffy-positive cells leach substances that inhibit anti-Duffy antibodies.[423] Duffy antigens do not appear to be present on platelets.[275]

Clinical Aspects

Anti-Duffy antibodies are usually produced after immunization by transfusion, with the subsequent production of an IgG antibody response. However, occasional cases of "natural" antibodies to the Duffy system have been reported.[424] These antibodies may be responsible for some hemolytic transfusion reactions, although very few terminate fatally.[425] Duffy antigens are well developed in fetuses as early as 40 days[426] and therefore capable of maternal immunization and occasionally responsible for hemolytic disease of the newborn, as they readily cross the placental barrier.[427]

Anti-Fy^b is rarer than anti-Fy^a on testing in immunohematology panels. Anti-Duffy autoantibodies can occur, albeit very rarely.[428]

The Kidd System

Antibodies against the Kidd system were first reported in 1951 by Allen et al., who described anti-Jk^a.[429] The rarer Jk^b antigen was discovered soon thereafter.[430] Since antibodies directed against Jk antigens are frequently evanescent and not very potent, it is often difficult to study their antigenic specificity. In addition, anti-Jk antibodies are very labile in vitro, further complicating their detection.

Jk (a−b−) individuals are usually of Oriental or Polynesian origin.[431] Rarely, if ever, is the phenotype present in caucasians (Table 5–10).[432]

Biochemistry

Little is known about the biochemistry of the Jk^a system. It is known, however, that the antigen is present on fetal cells[433] and that Kidd antigens are present on neutrophils.[434]

Antibodies to Jk antigens are usually of the IgG type,[435] which suggests that Kidd antigens may be partly protein. Nevertheless, IgM antibodies in this system have been described.[435]

It has been shown by radioimmunoassay that there are approximately 14,000 Jk^a sites per homozygous Jk^a cell.[414] A dosage effect in Jk (a+b+) is significant.

Genetics

The system behaves in an autosomal dominant fashion. The phenotypes and frequencies in cauca-

TABLE 5–10.—Statistical Frequencies of Routine Duffy, Kidd, and Kell Antigens*

GENE PRODUCT	FREQUENCIES		COMMENT
	Caucasians	Blacks	
Fy^a	0.425		
Fy^b	0.557		
Fy^x	0.016		
Fy (a+b+)	0.4735	0.0268	
Gy (a+b−)	0.1823	0.0982	
Fy (a−b+)	0.3302	0.1987	
Fy (a−b−)	>.0001	0.6763	Plasmodium resistant
Jk^a	0.5142		
Jk^b	.4858		
Jk3	>.9999		
Jk (a+b+)	0.6539	.3400	
Jk (a+b−)	0.3461	.5700	
Jk (a−b+)	0.2360	.0900	
Jk (a−b−)	<0.0001	<.0001	Frequent in Polynesians
K	0.0457		
k	0.9543		
KK	0.00235	<.001	
Kk	0.0872	.350	
kk	0.9107	.965	
Kp^a	0.0228	…	
Kp^b	0.9800	…	
Js^a	0.001	0.2000	Frequent in blacks
Js^b	.999	0.9051	

*Data from Race R.R., Sanger R.: *Blood Groups in Man*, ed. 6. Oxford, England, Blackwell Scientific Publications, 1975.

sians are Jk (a+b−), 35%; Jk (a+b+), 65%; and Jk (a−b+), 24%.[436] A dosage effect is present in heterozygotes.[437] The Jk (a−b−) phenotype may be the result of an amorphic gene or possibly a suppressor gene Jk. These individuals may produce an anti-Jk3 antibody reactive with a determinant present on both Jk^a-positive and Jk^b-positive cells.[431] The fact that anti-Jk3 is an inseparable specificity on absorption with Jk (a+b−) or Jk (a−b+) and the fact that Jk3 is present on granulocytes but Jk^a and Jk^b are absent from these cells strongly suggest a third (Jk3) specificity.[438] Other specificities may exist in this system. There is recent evidence that the Jk system is coded for on chromosome 2,[439] although previously thought to be coded for on chromosome 7.[440]

Laboratory Studies

Typically the antibody is an IgG antibody which may be of the IgG1 class but is mostly of the IgG3 class.[441] It is frequently capable of binding complement.[442] Many Jk antibodies react better in the antiglobulin phase. Enzyme-treated cells may react better with antibodies against Jk antigens. Because of the in vivo and in vitro lability, as well as the evanescence of the antibodies elicited against this system, it is important to keep good patient records to avoid transfusing potentially dangerous blood. Some Jk^a antibodies react only in the presence of certain substances, such as hydrobenzoic acid esters.[443]

Recently studies using 2M urea determined that the membrane of RBCs from individuals of the Jk (a−b−) phenotype is different from the membrane of normal RBCs. In these experiments, Jk (a−b−) cells, instead of swelling, as normal cells do, crenated and shrank.[444] Since urea is used to lyse RBCs in platelet counts, spuriously high platelet counts may be seen in Jk (a−b−) phenotypes.[444] This resistance to urea lysis can be used to screen large populations of donors to obtain Jk (a−b−) units.[431] Automated instruments such as the Groupamatic-360 are used in blood centers to screen for rare phenotypes[445] such as the Jk (a−b−) or −D− phenotype.

Clinical Aspects

Antibodies to the Kidd system have the reputation of causing severe, sometimes fatal, *delayed* hemolytic transfusion reactions.[446] Classically there is either a very weak or a nondetectable anti-Kidd antibody. Hemolysis may occur up to 7 days after transfusion. These reactions have caused renal damage and death.[447] Furthermore, the reactivity of the antibodies in vitro is deceptively low compared to their hemolytic potential in vivo.

These facts underscore the importance of good, long-term patient record keeping, especially on patients with anti-Kidd antibodies. A history of anti-Kidd antibodies should be respected even when these antibodies are not detectable on subsequent screening. Occasionally "naturally" occurring anti-Jk antibodies have been reported.[448] Like anti-Jk^a or anti-Jk^b, anti-Jk3 produced by Jk (a−b−) may be hemolytic.[431] All Jk antibodies, though rarely, can produce hemolytic disease of the newborn,[449] including anti-Jk3 antibodies.[335] Maternal sensitization to Jk^a has occurred after amniocentesis.[450] Autoantibodies to Jk antigens are rare, less than a dozen having been described in the literature.[451] Three of these have been dependent on neutral aromatic compounds such as the paraben content of the commercial test RBC preservative. All these patients had had viral infections a short time before the appearance of the autoantibody.[451] Therapy with methyldopa[452] and chlorpropamide[453] has likewise been associated with the development of auto-anti-Jk antibodies with development of hemolytic anemia. The cause for anti-Jk^a specificity in the case of chlorpropamide was not identified.[454]

The Kell System

The Kell antigen (K1) was first described by Coombs et al. in 1946,[455] whereas Cellano (k) was described by Levine et al. 3 years later.[456] The genes in the Kell system are codominant. The Kell system has since proved to be of high complexity, with over 15 Kell antigens described to date (Table 5–11). K, k, Kp^a, Kp^b, Js^a, and Js^b are but a few antigens belonging to the Kell system (Fig 5–26). The frequency of these genes is given in Table 5–10.

Biochemistry of the Kell Antigenic System

Because Kell antigens elicit mostly an IgG1 T cell–mediated response characteristic of complex branched antigens such as proteins, the protein nature of Kell antigens had long been suspected.[457] The treatment of Kell-positive cells with papain and dithiothreitol, which destroys the antigen, further suggested the protein nature of the antigen.[458]

More recently, however, it has been proved that at least some, if not all, Kell antigens are associated with a membrane protein. Using radiolabeled anti-

TABLE 5–11.—Kell Antigens*

NUMBER	OTHER NAME	FREQUENCY (%)	COMMENT
K1	K, Kell	9	
K2	k, Cellano	99	
K3	Kp^a, Penney	2	
K4	Kp^b, Rautenberg	>99	
K5	K^o, K^u, Peltz	>99	No cell deformity
K6	Js^a, Sutter	1	
K7	Js^b, Mathews	>99	
K8	Kw	5	
K9	Claas, KL	>99	
K10	Ul^a, Karhula	3	
K11	Coté, K^o-like	>99	Chromosome
K12	Bøc	>99	
K13	Sgro	>99	
K14	San	>99	
K15	Kx	>99	Stabilizing membrane?
K16	Coté-like	>99	
K17	Wk^a, Weeks	<1	
K18		>99	
K19		99	

*From Bryant.[488]

sera against Kell antigens on RBCs, and subjecting the detergent fractions of these cell membranes to SDS-PAGE gels, it has been demonstrated that Kell antigenicity lies on a 93-kilodalton protein. When these fractions are run on gels under reducing conditions, the Kell antigen–bearing protein appears to be associated with a membrane protein aggregate of at least 115 kilodaltons.[459]

Using radiolabeled antisera to Kell antigens, it has been shown that homozygous KK cells bear about 6,100 Kell antigenic sites per cell, whereas heterozygous Kk cells bear about 3,500 sites per cell.[460]

Genetics of the Kell System

Since Kell antigens are most probably proteins, the phenotypic products are probably assembled in a similar way to the model proposed by Rosenfield et al. for the Rh system.[306] Thus, an operon gene may be postulated which turns on the activation of several structural genes lying in sequence—K, k, Kp^a, Kp^b, Js^a, Js^b, etc. Other rare antigens such as Kp^c are low-frequency alleles.[461] The biosynthesis of Kell antigens can be considered in two stages. First, an X^{1}k[462] operon gene located on chromosome X would be responsible for the expression of Kx, a precursor Kell antigen structure; second, this gene would interact in some way to induce Kell genes, located in an autosome to express Kell antigens. An amorphic Ko gene, termed the Ko phenotype, is associated with an absolute absence of Kell antigens but normal Kx on WBCs and increased Kx on RBCs. A suppressor allele X^{2}K results in the lack of expression of Kx antigen and in the weak-

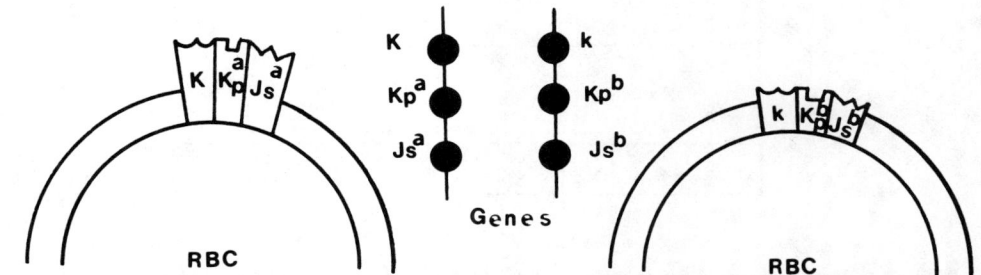

FIG 5–26.—Expression of Kell complex antigens K, Kp, and Js on the RBC membrane resembles expression of Rh D, C and E antigens. That antigens K, Kp, and Js are in effect close to each other has not been demonstrated. The purpose of placing them together in the figure is to denote gene linkage.

ening of the remaining Kell antigens; this is the McLeod phenotype.[463] Other examples of weakened expression of Kell antigens have also been reported (Fig 5–27).[464]

The Kell System at the Laboratory Level

Anti-Kell antibodies account for about two thirds of non-Rh antibodies and therefore are among the more common antibodies, exceeded only by antibodies to the ABO and Rh systems. K1 is about six times less antigenic than the Rh_o (D) antigen.[465] Anti-Kell antibodies to K, k, Kp^a, Kp^b, Js^a, and Js^b are of the IgG class in most cases[466] and therefore are best detected in the antiglobulin phase, although, if they are undiluted, they may react in the saline phase of testing. The majority of anti-Kell antibodies have been of the IgG1 subclass, though IgG4 has occasionally been described.[457] Rarely, IgM antibodies have been documented, especially in the so-called naturally occurring anti-Kell antibodies.[467] Antibodies to K18 are likewise of the IgG1 subclass and can be of the IgG4 subclass; patients with anti-K18 are difficult to transfuse because of the high frequency of K18. These antibodies tend to be hemolytic and must be respected.[468] Kell and para-Kell antigens can be deleted from RBC with bromide-AET, a feature that can be used to produce Ko cells artificially for panels.[469] Kx antigens have been reported on granulocytes as well as RBCs.[462] K1,k antigens, however, are absent from platelets.[275]

Anti-Kell antibodies may produce severe hemolytic transfusion reactions[470] and have resulted in severe cases of hemolytic disease of the newborn.[471] Individuals who are already immunized to Rh_o (D) have a higher propensity to develop anti-Kell antibodies.[472]

Anti-K antibodies are usually produced by homozygous KK individuals, who are rare in the general population. However, when anti-Cellano (k) antibodies are present, transfusion with compatible blood is an extremely difficult endeavor for the blood bank; similarly, patients with anti-K18 antibodies as well as other high-frequency Kell antigens are difficult to transfuse.[468]

Auto-anti-Kell antibodies have been described.[473] The "naturally" occurring anti-Kell antibodies, described above, usually occur in severely septicemic patients.[474] Recently, an acquired K1-like antigen secondary to a severe infection caused by *Streptococcus faesium* was described;[475] cells incubated with supernates from cultures of this bacterium acquired the K1 antigenic determinant. This finding may explain the physiopathology of some naturally occurring anti-Kell antibodies.

Other naturally occurring anti-Kell antibodies caused by infections from *E. coli* O 125:B15[467] or mycobacteria have been documented.[476] Delayed transfusion reactions due to IgG anti-Kell antibodies have been described (e.g., anti-K6).[477] An extremely interesting disease association is that of the Kell antigen and chronic granulomatous disease of children, first described by Giblett et al.[478] The phenotypic product of the X^1k gene is the Kx antigen, and it modifies the expression of Kell antigens. Furthermore, the X^1k gene also codes for a Kx membrane protein (not Kell) which, when lacking, is responsible for the McLeod syndrome, with the development of acanthocytic RBCs and reduced RBC in vivo survival.[479] The lack of this membrane protein is presumably responsible for a progressive disorder of skeletal muscles and high levels of serum creatine phosphokinase in McLeod syndrome patients.[480]

This elevation in CPK results in almost a 200% phosphorylation increase at the RBC membrane. Elevated carbonic anhydrase III has likewise been reported to be elevated in the McLeod syndrome.[481]

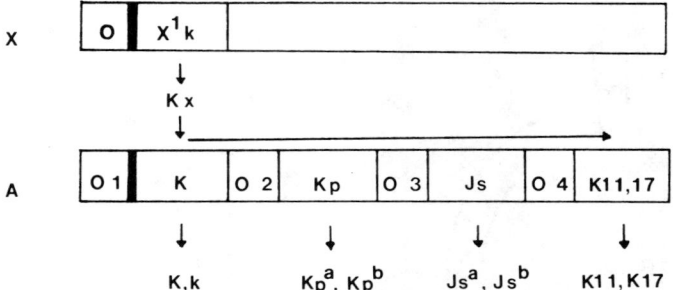

FIG 5–27.—Proposed genetic pathway for the Kell antigenic complex (K, Kp, and Js). An xx block results in weak K, Kp, and Js: no expression of KL precursor substances is identified in this condition. Gene X^14, responsible for the synthesis of Kx, is located on chromosome X. Genes for K, Kp, Js, and other Kell related genes are located on autosome (A).

Different alleles of the X^1k gene are postulated (X^1k to X^4k) according to the expression of Kx phenotypes (Table 5–12).

The lack of Kx antigens on RBCs appears to accompany all cases of the McLeod syndrome, albeit in some cases (X^4k-bearing cells) the antigens may be present on granulocytes but not on RBCs. Leukocyte function may be normal in the absence of Kx antigens, as shown by Densen et al.[482] Thus, the genes responsible for chronic granulomatous disease and X^1k genes, although closely linked, are separate. Kell antigens coded autosomally do not influence RBC membranes; thus Ko individuals usually have normal RBCs.[483] Chronic granulomatous disease may be present without the McLeod syndrome and the McLeod syndrome may be present in the absence of chronic granulomatous disease. Ko subjects produce an anti-K^u antibody that reacts with all cells except Ko cells.[484] McLeod individuals make antibodies to Kx-positive and Km-positive cells (these antibodies used to be called anti-KL antibodies).[485] Ko- and Kx-negative RBCs do not have the Km specificity; thus anti-Km antibodies will react with all cells except Ko and McLeod phenotype cells. Anti-Kx antibodies react strongly with Ko cells which have increased amounts of Kx antigen.[486] McLeod syndrome patients have been described in whom the K1 phenotype was undisturbed.[487]

The Xg System

The Xg system was discovered by Mann et al. in 1962.[489] It is of scientific as well as historical interest because the gene locus appears to be on the short arm of the X chromosome[490] and was the first antigen to be assigned to a specific chromosome.

TABLE 5–12.—CHRONIC GRANULOMATOUS DISEASE: THE MCLEOD SYNDROME AND KELL ANTIGENS*

CGD TYPE†	GENE LINKAGE‡	KX ON WBCs	KX ON RBCs	MCLEOD SYNDROME
I	X^3k	−	+/−	−
II	X^2k	−	−	+
No CGD	X^4k	++	−	+
	K^o	+	+++	−

*From Marsh.[481]
†The Xk gene and the gene responsible for CGD are closely linked but distinct.
‡X^1k gene is normal and associated with routinely seen Kell phenotypes. The presence or absence of autosomally coded Kell antigens are not involved in the physiopathology of CGD or the McLeod syndrome.

The Xg system functions as a hemizygote system in males (XY) and as a dizygote system in females (XX). In females, the Xg genes on X chromosomes do not appear to be inactivated according to the Lyon theory (see Chap. 14). Therefore, Xg^a is expressed phenotypically in the RBCs of all Xg (a+)/ Xg (a−) heterozygous females.[490]

The frequency of the Xg^a phenotype is greater in females than in males (89% frequency versus a 67% frequency).[491]

The progeny of an Xg(a−) female and an Xg(a+) male will produce only Xg(a+) females and Xg(a−) males.

At the laboratory level, the antibody produced against Xg^a is mostly reactive in the antiglobulin phase and is usually of the IgG class, which binds complement.[492] It is not frequently seen as an antibody in transfusion workups. Rarely, anti-Xg^a antibodies may cause febrile transfusion reactions.[493] Recently a linkage between the Xk locus responsible for the McLeod syndrome and the Xg locus has been demonstrated.[494] This finding may explain certain cases of naturally occurring anti-Kell antibodies.

HIGH-FREQUENCY ANTIGENS

The antibodies to the high-incidence antigens described in this section are found on most RBCs. A few of the more interesting high-incidence antigens are described below; many more exist.

Vel Antigen System

The Vel antigen system is a complex system that was initially reported in 1952 by Sussman and Miller.[495] It is now known that the system is independent and not, as formerly thought, part of the P system.[496] Antibodies directed against Vel are sometimes hemolytic in vitro. Several alleles (Vel 1, Vel 2, etc.) have been described. It is possible, however, that these alleles represent modifier genes that regulate the strength of expression of these antigens. Antibodies against the Vel system pose a formidable problem to blood banks, which must find compatible blood for these patients. This is underscored by the initial description of the antibody by Sussman, who presented only 4 of 10,000 negative bloods studied. Anti-Vel antibodies are usually of the IgM class[497] but may react at 37° C in the albumin phase. IgG anti-Vel antibodies have been described.[498]

Gerbich System

Initially discovered by Rosenfield et al.,[499] the anti-Ge antibody reacts with all but exceptional cells. The system is a complex one. Some anti-Ge antibodies react with certain Ge cells but not with others, demonstrating a heterogeneity in the system.[497] Some of these discrepancies occur more frequently in certain Melanesian populations.[500]

Langeris Antigens

Langeris (Lan) antigens were discovered as high-incidence antigens in Holland by van der Hart et al.[501] Lan-negative individuals have been described in the Dutch population in a higher frequency than in other populations. Anti-Lan antibodies have been known to cause mild hemolytic disease of the newborn. These antibodies are usually of the IgG class.[502]

Sid Antigens

The Sid or Sd^a antigen is a high-frequency antigen that exhibits a wide variety of expressions of antigen dosages on RBCs. Individuals that produce anti-Sd^a antibodies are not always negative for the antigen, but may exhibit just a low dosage of it. The antigen was initially reported by Macvie et al.[503] The Sid antigen is secreted in high concentrations in urine and saliva, and 50% of Sd^a-negative patients by RBC typing show positive Sd^a reactions in the urine.[504] The secretion of Sd^a is unrelated to the secretion status of the ABH substances.[503, 504] Sanger et al.[505] demonstrated that the Sd^a antigen and the Cad polyagglutinable antigen are the same but are expressed in different dosages. Anti-Sd^a antibodies are usually of the IgM class and may occur naturally.[503]

En^a Antigens

The En^a antigens were first discovered by Darnborough et al. in 1969 and were thought to represent a single antigenic specificity.[506] En^a-negative cells were noticeable because they lacked membrane sialic acid content, which made them much less mobile in an electrophoretic matrix than normal cells.[507]

It is now known that En^a-negative cells lack MNSs sialoglycoprotein or portions thereof. En^a-negative individuals make a heterogeneous group of antibodies reactive against portions of MNSs sialoglycoprotein (Fig 5–28).[508]

Some examples of anti-En^a represent antibodies to hybrid MNSs sialoglycoproteins. Furthermore, auto anti-En^a antibodies can be inhibited in vitro with MN-SGP.[509]

Transfusion of Patients With Antibodies to High-Incidence Antigens

Patients with antibodies to high-incidence antigens present special problems to the blood bank. The basic strategy to avoid immunizing an individual is to avoid transfusion unless it is absolutely necessary. If transfusion is necessary it should be given in amounts that will allow the patient to tolerate anemia, not in amounts to achieve predesignated hematocrit values.

Should a person become immunized to a high-incidence antigen, there are certain guidelines to follow. Not all antibodies are dangerous, and those which are potentially noxious are not always avid or hemolytic. However, in this section we assume that an antibody to a high-frequency antigen is clinically significant. It should also be mentioned that frozen blood inventories have changed the outlook on transfusion of these cases. Autologous transfusion in elective surgery is one of the best alternatives. Frozen-thawed cells and autologous transfusion are discussed in chapter 9.

ANTIGENS OF LOW INCIDENCE

Antigens of low incidence, or private antigens, may be markers of polymorphism and antigenic individualism of blood as a tissue, like markers present in any other tissue. This individualism has been an obstacle to uncomplicated transplantation. Blood

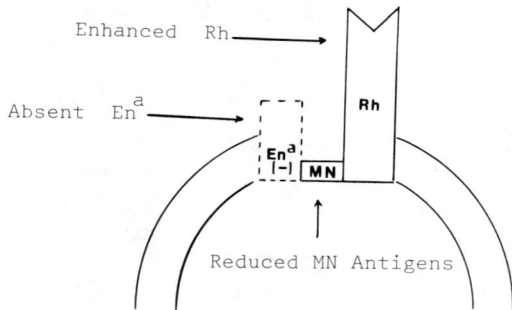

FIG 5–28.—En^a-negative phenotype with resulting enhancement of Rh_o (D) antigens and depressed MN antigens.

transfusion can be thought of as a transplant of a tissue, although the transplant is less complex than with other somatic cells.

In many cases immunization by low-incidence antigens occurs as a result of a previous pregnancy, or when a woman has been transfused with her husband's blood. If the offspring inherits the antigen, hemolytic disease of the newborn may result. Examples of some low-incidence antigens are given below.

The Berrens (Be^a) antigen was initially reported by Davidsohn et al.[510] Like many low-incidence antigens, it was discovered in association with hemolytic disease of the newborn. The Swann (SW^a) antigen was described by Cleghorn.[511] It seems to be associated with the Lutheran system and the secretor gene.[512]

Other antigens of low incidence include antigens of the Good, Radin, Lewis II (unrelated to the Lewis system), Jensen, and Peters systems.

Clinical Significance

Clinically, low-incidence antigens are important in hemolytic disease of the newborn and in cases where a single unit of blood causes immunization and reactions. It is unlikely that another unit with the same antigen would be given to these immunized recipients. For the blood bank, the main problem is to recognize that a low-incidence antigen was responsible for the incompatibility. Once this has been established, finding a compatible unit should not be problematic because it is very unlikely that the antigen will be present in other units.

If an antibody to a low-incidence antigen is responsible for hemolytic disease of the newborn and an exchange transfusion is contemplated, a compatible random donor unit usually meets the requirements for transfusion. When a unique component, such as granulocytes or platelets, is needed, a low-incidence antigen in the donor may cause production of antibodies by the recipient, leading to transfusion reactions. Blood from these donors cannot be used in that recipient.

POLYAGGLUTINATION

The serum of most normal individuals contains IgM isoantibodies, acquired after birth on exposure to bacterial and viral T-like antigens.[513] These antibodies are capable of reacting to most RBCs. These antibodies will agglutinate most RBCs, which, on enzyme proteolysis, reveal otherwise hidden antigenic specificities, termed T antigens (not to be confused with T cell antigens of lymphocytes).[514] This phenomenon is called polyagglutination (Fig 5–29).[515] Polyagglutinability was first described by Hübner in 1925.[516] The term T activation was coined by Friedenreich, who demonstrated that the phenomenon could be produced in vitro by preincubating RBCs with bacterial culture filtrates, then exposing them to normal human serum.[517] Hence its frequently used name, the Hübner-Thomsen-Friedenreich phenomenon.

Today this bacterial filtrate effect is known to be caused, in most cases, by the bacterial neuraminidase content in culture filtrates. Galactosyl moieties are exposed by the cleavage of N-acetylneuraminic acid (NANA). These galactose moieties constitute the T antigenic determinants,[518] which are, in fact, sequences of carbohydrates and amino acids of the MN glycoprotein lying close to the RBC membrane. Thus the remaining β-D-galactoside-N-acetyl-D-galactosamine disaccharide residues on the NH$_2$ terminal portions of glycophorin A and B polypeptide backbones constitute the actual T spec-

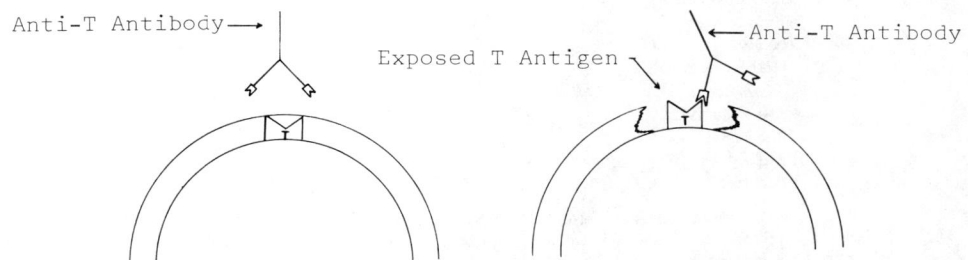

FIG 5–29.—T-polyagglutination. Normally present anti-T isoantibodies attach to the exposed T antigens in digested RBCs.

ificity recognized by peanut agglutinin and by anti-T isoagglutinins.[519]

Several types of T-like activation exist. The better known T activation can be observed both in vitro after bacterial contamination of a sample by a variety of bacteria, or in vivo during sepsis, in which case it is usually transient. T activation is not infrequently seen in septicemia due to *Diplococcus pneumoniae, Clostridium perfringens,* or infection with Vibrio cholerae;[520] viruses such as influenza virus are likewise capable of T exposure.[521] T cryptantigen exposure may occur in hemolytic anemia[522] and in respiratory or bowel diseases of children.[523] T activation may be part of the pathophysiology of the hemolytic uremic syndrome in which septicemia may result in T activation of RBCs, platelets, and the glomerulus.[524]

Tk activation is like T activation in that it may also be associated with sepsis; it is probably caused by bacterial enzymes and it is usually transient. However, it is not caused by a loss of sialic acid from the membrane and therefore reacts positively with polybrene.[525] Tk activation is usually caused by an endobetagalactosidase which exposes a hidden N-acetylglucosamine moiety.[526] Frequently *Bacterioides fragilis* septicemia is the triggering mechanism for Tk activation as a result of the bacterium Tk-producing endogalactosidase.[527]

This type of polyagglutination is often accompanied by reduced H substance, Ii substances, and A substance (when present),[528] probably due to the presence of a bacterial α-fucosidase.[527]

Th polyagglutinability is another form of bacterially induced polyagglutination, probably secondary to bacterial enzyme cleavage of RBC sialoglycoproteins. The lectin *Vicia cretica* selectively agglutinates Th antigens.[529]

Th polyagglutination has been described following septic peritonitis.[530] RBC membrane sialic acid is usually normal, and therefore these cells are reactive with polybrene. VA is another type of polyagglutination. Depression of H substance expression is frequently seen in these cases.[531]

In contrast to T, Tk, and Th polyagglutination, which is caused by bacterial enzyme cleavage, Tn polyagglutination is usually due to an abnormality of stem cell maturation. This results in two populations of cells, some normal RBCs and some Tn-positive RBCs, reacting in a mixed field pattern. The phenomenon is also present on the platelets of these patients, suggesting a stem cell defect.[532] Leukopenia and thrombocytopenia are almost always present in Tn polyagglutination.[533] The abnormality is due to a lack of galactosyl and sialyl transferases,[518] which causes a block of the synthetic pathway from Tn to T formation, with resulting lack of T antigen due to a selective lack of β-3-D-galactosyl transferase.[534] This in turn results in the lack of completion of the carbohydrate moiety of MN-SGP.

TABLE 5–13.—POLYAGGLUTINABILITY*

	TYPE OF POLYAGGLUTINATIONS				
	Microbial, enzymic			Clonal Mutation	Inherited†
REACTIVITY	T	Tk‡	Th§	Tn	Cad
REACTIVITY LECTINS					
Arachis hypogaea	+	+	+	−	−
Dolichos biflorus	−	−	−	+	+
Bandeiraea simplicifolia II	−	+	−	−	−
Salvia sclarea	−	−	−	+	−
Salvia horminum	−	−	−	+	+
Vicia cretica	+	−	+	−	−
Leonurus cardiaca	+/−	−	−	−	+
Hibiscus sabdariffa	+	−	+	+	−
Glycine soja	+	−	−	+	+
OTHER REACTIVITY					
Polybrene	−	+	+	−	+
Anti-MN	+/−	−	−	−	−
Persistence	−	−	−c	+	+

*Data from references 514, 520, 528, 529, 533, 536, and 542–547.
†NOR and HEMPAS are other inherited conditions of polyagglutinability. Cad antisera have anti-Sdª specificity.
‡VA is a Tk-type of polyagglutination.
§Rarely, Th activation may persist indefinitely.[548]

Salvia sclarea is a lectin used to identify Tn-positive cells (Table 5–13). Of concern is the occasional development of a hematologic malignancy such as leukemia in Tn-positive patients. This observation further suggests the clonal origin of this anomaly.[535]

Cad Polyagglutination

Strictly speaking, Cad polyagglutination is not a case of true cryptantigen expression in the same way that acquired polyagglutination is. The Cad phenotype most probably represents a special RBC phenotype in which there is an excessive expression of Sd^a sites per RBC.[536] This view, however, is not accepted by all.[537]

Most sera are capable of agglutinating Cad cells, for isoantibodies against Sd^a are present in the plasma of most normal individuals. Interestingly, the Sd^a phenotype is present in varying strengths (Cad 1, 2, 3, 4), and true Cad polyagglutination may represent the higher Sd^a representation at one end of the Sd^a spectrum. Sd^a antigenic determinants appear to be located on N-acetyl-D-galactosamine residues.[538] Rarely, hemolytic transfusion reactions may occur in individuals with high titers of Sd^a who are transfused with Cad RBCs.[539]

Inherited Dyserythropoiesis

A type I and a type II exist. The type II is termed hereditary erythroblastic multinuclearity (HEMPAS). HEMPAS is of interest in polyagglutination because most normal sera, except the recipient's, possess an IgM, which will agglutinate and/or lyse HEMPAS RBCs.[540] H antigens are deficient in HEMPAS cells. HEMPAS RBCs are agglutinated readily by anti-i.[540] HEMPAS cells show a positive acidified serum test.[541]

Polyagglutination at the Laboratory Level

Most polyagglutination antibodies appear after birth and are present in normal plasma. They are mostly of the IgM type and bind complement. These antibodies produce difficulties in laboratory testing and are recognized when a sample is typed, with resulting agglutination of the patient's cells by all typing antisera, causing a typing discrepancy. The phenomenon can be defined by showing agglutination of patient cells on incubation with several normal AB sera from normal individuals: no agglutination will be seen when patient cells are reacted with cord serum of the same blood type.

The reactivity of different types of polyagglutination with specific lectins is given in Table 5–13.

Clinical Aspects of Polyagglutination

Perhaps the more important clinical aspect of polyagglutination lies in the difficulties caused at the laboratory level by the phenomenon of polyagglutination during typing, screening, and crossmatching. About 1 in 10,000 individuals presents with severe polyagglutination, and about 1 in 200 have a mild variety.[519] The different types of polyagglutination must be defined by special lectins.

The next aspect of clinical importance is the contribution of polyagglutination to hemolysis. During sepsis, however, this type of hemolysis is either not clinically significant or not present in most cases.[519] However, rare cases of severe hemolysis have been documented. The use of washed cells may be justified in these cases.[543]

Two or more types of polyagglutination may be present in the same patient, (e.g., T, Tk, VA in the same patient) due to the presence of various enzymes in the infecting bacterium.[544] Multiple polyagglutinability may coexist with the presence of bacterially induced acquired B antigens.[545]

Finally, Tn activation may flag a case of monoclonality with the potential for the development of leukemia,[546] suggesting that these patients be followed routinely for this eventuality. The exposure of T and Tn antigens by solid tumors is of possible clinical importance, as has been reported by Springer and collaborators.[547]

REFERENCES

1. Issitt P.D., Issitt C.H.: *Applied Blood Group Serology*. Oxner, Calif. Spectra Biologicals, 1975, p. 22.
2. Beattie K.M., Zuelzer W.W.: The frequency and properties of pH-dependent anti-M. *Transfusion* 5:322, 1965.
3. Hughes-Jones N.C., Gardner B., Telford R., et al.: The effect of pH and ionic strength on the reaction of anti-D and erythrocytes. *Immunology* 7:72, 1964.
4. Landsteiner K., van der Scheer J.: On cross reactions of immune sera to azoproteins. *J. Exp. Med.* 63:325, 1936.

5. Landsteiner K.: *The Specificity of Serological Reactions.* Cambridge, Mass., Harvard University Press, 1962.
6. Danielli J.F., Davson H.: A contribution to the theory of permeability of thin films. *J. Cell. Comp. Physiol.* 54:495, 1935.
7. Singer S.J.: The molecular organization of membranes. *Annu. Rev. Biochem.* 43:805, 1974.
8. Hughes R.C.: Glycoproteins as components of cellular membranes. *Prog. Biophys. Mol. Biol.* 26:189, 1973.
9. Marchesi V.T., Tillack T.W., Jackson R.L., et al.: Chemical characterization and surface orientation of the major glycoprotein of the human red cell membrane. *Proc. Natl. Acad. Sci. USA* 69:1445, 1972.
10. Marchesi V.T.: Structure of biological membranes, in Vyas G.N. (ed.): *Membrane Structure and Function of Human Blood Cells.* Washington, D.C., American Association of Blood Banks, 1976, p. 1.
11. Romano E.L., Stolinsky Co., Hughes-Jones N.C.: Distribution and mobility of the A, D and "c" antigens on human red cell membranes: Studies with a gold labelled antiglobulin reagent. *Br. J. Haematol.* 30:507, 1975.
12. Lauf P.K., Joiner C.H.: Increased potassium transport and ouabain binding in human Rh red blood cells. *Blood* 48:457, 1976.
13. Levine P., Tripodi D., Struck J. Jr., et al.: Hemolytic anemia associated with Rh null but not with Bombay blood: A hypothesis based on differing antigenic structures. *Vox Sang.* 24:417, 1973.
14. Marcus D.M., Kundu S.K., Suzuki A.: The P blood group system: Recent progress in immunochemistry and genetics. *Semin. Hematol.* 18:63, 1981.
15. Victoria E.J., Muchmore E.A., Sudora E.J., Masouredis S.P.: The role of antigen mobility in anti-Rh_o (D) induced agglutination. *J. Clin. Invest.* 56:292, 1975.
16. Nicolson G.L., Masouredis S.P., Singer S.J.: Quantitative two-dimensional ultrastructural distribution of Rh_o (D) antigenic sites on human erythrocyte membranes. *Proc. Natl. Acad. Sci. USA* 68:1416, 1971.
17. Economidou J., Hughes-Jones N.C., Gardner B.: Quantitative measurements concerning A and B antigenic sites. *Vox Sang.* 12:321, 1967.
18. Landois L.: *Die Transfusion des Blutes.* Leipzig, Vogel, 1875, p. 185.
19. Landsteiner K.: Über Agglutinationserscheinungen normalen menschlichen Blutes. *Klin. Wochschr.* 14:1132, 1901.
20. Bernstein F.: Ergebnisse einer biostatischen aussamen fassender Betrachtung über die erblichen Blutstrukturen des Menschen. *Klin. Wochenschr.* 3:1495, 1924.
21. Hakamori S., Strycharz G.D.: Investigations on cellular blood-group substances: I. Isolation and chemical composition of blood-groups ABH and Le^b isoantigens of sphingoglycolipid. *Nature Biochem.* 7:1279, 1968.
22. Finne J.: Identification of the blood group ABH-active glycoprotein components of human erythrocyte membrane. *Eur. J. Biochem.* 104:181, 1980.
23. Issitt P.D., Issitt C.H.: *Applied Blood Group Serology,* ed. 2. Oxner, Calif., Spectra Biologicals, 1975, p. 93.
24. Lloyd K.O., Kabat E.A., Rosenfield R.E.: Immunochemical-studies on blood groups: 38. Structures and activities of oligosaccharides produced by alkaline degradation of blood-group Lewis-a substance. Proposed structure of the carbohydrate chains of human blood group A, B, H, Le-a, and Le-b substances. *Biochemistry* 5:1502, 1966.
25. Lloyd K.O., Kabat E.A., Licerio E.: Immunochemical studies on blood groups: XXXV. The activity of fucose-containing oligosaccharides isolated from blood group A, B, and H substances by alkaline degradation. *Biochemistry* 7:2976, 1968.
26. Watkins W.M.: Gene enzyme relationships of the A, B, H, Le blood group genes. *Transfusion* 7:367, 1967.
27. Bhende Y.M., Despande C.K., Bhatia H.M., et al.: A "new" blood group character related to the ABO system. *Lancet* 1:903, 1952.
28. Watkins W.M., Chester M.A., Race C., et al.: Glycosyltransferases in serum from donors from the Bombay Oh phenotype, in *Abstracts.* Washington, D.C., American Association of Blood Banks and International Society of Hematology, 1972, p. 26.
29. Szulman A.E.: The histological distribution of blood group substances A and B in man. *J. Exp. Med.* 111:785, 1960.
30. Szulman A.E.: The ABH antigens in human tissues and secretions during embryonal development. *J. Histochem. Cytochem.* 13:752, 1965.
31. Kools A., Collins J., Aster R.H.: Studies of the ABO antigens of human platelets, abstracted. *Transfusion* 21:615, 1981.
32. Takasaki S., Kobata A.: Chemical characterization and distribution of ABO blood group active glycoprotein in human erythrocyte membrane. *J. Biol. Chem.* 251:3610, 1976.
33. Beattie K.M.: Perspectives on some usual and unusual ABO phenotypes, in Bell C.A. (ed.): *A Seminar on Antigens or Blood Cells and Body Fluids.* Washington, D.C., American Association of Blood Banks, 1980, p. 97.
34. Watkins W.M.: Glycoproteins: Their composition, structure and function, in Gottschalk A. (ed.): *Glycoproteins.* Amsterdam, Elsevier, 1972, 830.
35. Kobata A., Grolman E.F., Ginsburg V.: An enzymatic basis for blood type A in humans. *Arch. Biochem. Biophys.* 124:609, 1968.
36. Kemp T.: Über den Empfindlichkeitsgrad der blutkorperchen gegenüber Isohämagglutininen im Foetalliben und im Kindsalter beim Menschen. *Acta Pathol. Microbiol. Scand.* 7:146, 1930.
37. Grundbacher F.J.: Changes in the human A antigen of erythrocytes with the individual's age. *Nature* 204:192, 1964.
38. Levine P., Tripodi D., Struck J., et al.: Hemolytic

anemia associated with Rh null but not with Bombay blood: A hypothesis based on differing antigenic structures. *Vox Sang.* 24:417, 1973.
39. Economidu J., Hughes-Jones M.C., Gardner B.: Quantitative measurements concerning A and B sites. *Vox Sang.* 12:321, 1967.
40. Topping M.D., Watkins W.M.: Isoelectric points of the human blood group A_1, A_2, and B gene associated glycosyltransferases in ovarian cyst fluids and serum. *Biochem. Biophys. Res. Commun.* 64:89, 1975.
41. Hakomori S., Watanabe K., Laine R.A.: Glycosphingolipids with blood group A, H, and I activity: Their status in group A_1 and A_2 erythrocytes and their changes associated with ontogeny and oncogeny, in Mohr J.F., et al. (eds.): *Human Blood Groups.* Basel, Switzerland, S. Karger, 1977, p. 150.
42. Von Dungern E., Hirszfeld L.: Über gruppenspezifische Strukturen des Blutes: III. *Z. Immun. Forsch.* 8:526, 1911.
43. Mohr J.F., Cunningham R.K., Bates J.F.: Qualitative distinctions between subgroups A_1 and A_2, in Mohr J.F., et al. (eds.): *Human Blood Groups.* Basel, Switzerland, S. Karger, 1977, p. 316.
44. Mollison P.L.: *Blood Transfusion in Clinical Medicine,* ed. 7. Oxford, England, Blackwell Scientific Publications, 1983, p. 71.
45. Race R.R., Sanger R.: *Blood Groups in Man.* Oxford, England, Blackwell Scientific Publications, 1975, p. 50.
46. Mollison P.L.: *Blood Transfusion in Clinical Medicine,* ed. 7. Oxford, England, Scientific Publications, 1983, p. 294.
47. Bird G.W.G.: Relationship of the blood subgroups A_1, A_2 and A_1B, A_2B to haemagglutinins present in the seeds of *Dolichos biflorus. Nature* 170:674, 1952.
48. Race R.R., Sanger R.: *Blood Groups in Man.* Oxford, England, Blackwell Scientific Publications, 1975, p. 13.
49. Taylor G.L., Race R.R., Prior A.M., et al.: Frequency of the isoagglutinin $alpha_1$ in the serum of the sub-groups A_2 and A_2B. *J. Pathol. Bacteriol.* 54:514, 1942.
50. Juel E.: Studies in the subgroups of blood group A: Absorption experiment indicating qualitative differences between subgroup A_1 and A_2. *Acta Pathol. Microbiol. Scand.* 46:251, 1959.
51. Moreno C., Lundblad A., Kabat E.A.: Immunochemical studies on blood groups: LI. A comparative study of A_1 and A_2 blood group glycoproteins with human anti-A. *J. Exp. Med.* 134:439, 1971.
52. Schachter H., Michaels M.A., Tilley C.A., et al.: Qualitative differences in the N-acetyl-D-galactosamine-transferases produced by human A_1 and A_2 genes. *Proc. Natl. Acad. Sci. USA* 70:220, 1973.
53. Friedenreich V.: Eine bisher unbekannte Blutgruppeneigenschaft (A_3). *Z. Immun. Forsch.* 89:409, 1936.
54. Reed T.E.: The frequency and nature of blood group A_3. *Transfusion* 4:457, 1964.
55. Mollison P.: *Blood Transfusion in Clinical Medicine,* ed. 7. Oxford, England, Blackwell Scientific Publications, 1983, p. 272.
56. Mollison P.L.: *Blood Transfusion in Clinical Medicine,* ed. 7. Oxford, England, Blackwell Scientific Publications, 1983, p. 633.
57. Salmon, C., Salmon D., Reviron J.: Étude immunologique et génetique de la variabilité du phenotype A_x. *Nouv. Rev. Fr. Hematol.* 5:275, 1975.
58. Alter A.A., Rosenfield R.E.: The nature of some subtypes of A. *Blood* 23:605, 1964.
59. Salmon C., Borin P., André R.: Le groupe sanguin A_m dans deux generations d'une même famille. *Rev. Hematol.* 13:529, 1958.
60. Landsteiner K., Levine R.: Differentiation of a type of human blood by means of normal animal serum. *J. Immunol.* 18:87, 1930.
61. Race R.R., Sanger R.: *Blood Groups in Man,* ed. 6. Oxford, England, Blackwell Scientific Publications, 1975, pp. 17, 18.
62. Issitt P.D., Issitt C.H.: *Applied Blood Group Serology,* ed. 2. Oxner, Calif., Spectra Biologicals, 1975, p. 81.
63. Lopez M., Benali J., Cartron J.P., et al.: Some notes on the specificity of anti-A_1 reagents. *Vox Sang.* 39:271, 1980.
64. Salmon C., Lopez M., Gerbal A., et al.: Current genetic problems in the ABO blood group systems. *Biomedicine* 18:375, 1973.
65. Race R.R., Sanger R.: *Blood Groups in Man,* ed. 6. Oxford, England, Blackwell Scientific Publications, 1975, p. 19.
66. Zmijewski C.M.: *Immunohematology.* New York, Appleton-Century-Crofts, 1978, p. 55.
67. Fudenberg H.H., Kunkel H.G., Franklin E.C.: High molecular weight antibodies. *Acta Haematol.* 10:522, 1959.
68. Springer G.F., Williamson P., Readler B.L.: Blood group active gram-negative bacteria and higher plants. *Ann. NY Acad. Sci.* 97:104, 1962.
69. Kochwa S., Rosenfield R.E., Tallal L., et al.: Isoagglutinins associated with erythroblastosis. *J. Clin. Invest.* 40:874, 1961.
70. Fong S.W., Oaquandah B.Y., Taylor W.F.: Developmental patterns of ABO isoagglutinins in normal children correlated with the effects of age, sex and maternal isoagglutinins. *Transfusion* 14:551, 1974.
71. Fudenberg H.H., et al. (eds.): *Basic and Clinical Immunology.* Los Altos, Calif., Lange Medical Publications, 1976, p. 39.
72. Witebsky E.: Isolation and purification of blood group A and B substances: Their use in conditioning universal donor blood, in neutralizing anti-Rh sera and in the production of potent grouping sera. *Ann. NY Acad. Sci.* 46:887, 1946.
73. Yokogama M., Fudenberg H.H.: Studies on cross-reacting isoagglutinins. *J. Immunol.* 92:966, 1964.
74. Landsteiner K., Witt D.H.: Observations on the human blood groups: Irregular reactions. Iso-agglu-

tinins in sera of group 4. The factor A_1. *J. Immunol.* 2:221, 1926.
75. Moss W.L.: Studies on isoagglutinins and isohemolysis. *Bull. Johns Hopkins Hosp.* 21:63, 1910.
76. Jones A.R., Kaneli L.: Some properties of cross-reacting antibody of the ABO blood group system. *Blood* 15:395, 1960.
77. Brambell F.W.R., Hemmings W.A., Oakley C.L., et al.: The relative transmission of the fraction of papain hydrolysed homologous gamma globulin from the uterine cavity to the fetal circulation in the rabbit. *Proc. R. Soc. Lond. Biol.* 151:478, 1960.
78. Castella A., LaBarge B.P., Lowenstein K.J., et al.: Auto-anti-A_1 antibody in a patient with metastatic adenocarcinoma. *Transfusion* 23:339, 1983.
79. Ruddle F.H., Creagan R.P.: Parasexual approaches to the genetics of man. *Annu. Rev. Genet.* 9:407, 1975.
80. Renwick J.H., Lawler S.D.: Linkage between the ABO and nail patella syndrome: Clinical and linkage data on family G. *Ann. Hum. Genet.* 20:348, 1956.
81. Weitkamp L.R., Sing C.F, Shreffler D.C., et al.: The genetic linkage relations of adenylate kinase: Further data on the ABO-AK linkage group. *Am. J. Hum. Genet.* 21:600, 1969.
82. Race R.R., Sanger R.: *Blood Groups in Man*, ed. 6. Oxford, England, Blackwell Scientific Publications, 1975, p. 24.
83. Shenkel-Brunner H., Chester M.A., Watkins W.: Alpha-1 fucosyl transferases in human serum from donors of different ABO, secretor and Lewis blood group phenotypes. *Eur. J. Biochem.* 30:269, 1972.
84. Schiff F.: Über gruppenspezifische Serum Präcipitine. *Klin. Wochenschr.* 3:679, 1924.
85. Grubb R.: Observations on the human group system Lewis. *Acta Pathol. Microbiol. Scand.* 28:61, 1951.
86. Trudeau L.R., Judd W.J., Butch S.H., et al.: Is a room temperature crossmatch necessary for the detection of ABO errors? *Transfusion* 23:237, 1983.
87. Huestis D.W., Bove J.R., Bush S.: *Practical Blood Transfusion*. Boston, Little, Brown & Co., 1969, p. 340.
88. Beattie K.M., Zueler W.W.: A serum factor reacting with acriflavin causing an ABO cell group. *Transfusion* 8:254, 1968.
89. Miller W.V. (ed.): *Technical Manual of the American Association of Blood Banks*, ed. 7. Washington, D.C., American Association of Blood Banks, 1977, p. 93.
90. Bird G.W.G.: Observations on the interactions of the erythrocytes of various species with certain seed agglutinins. *Br. J. Exp. Pathol.* 35:252, 1954.
91. Bird G.W.G.: Haemagglutinins in seeds. *Br. Med. Bull.* 15:165, 1959.
92. Bird G.W.G.: Specific agglutinating activity for human red blood cell corpuscles in extracts of *Dolichos biflorus*. *Curr. Sci.* 20:298, 1951.
93. Mäkelä O., Mäkelä P.: Some new blood specific phytagglutinins. *Ann. Med. Exp. Fenn.* 34:402, 1956.
94. Cazal P., Lalaurie M.: Recherches sur quelques phyto-agglutinines spécifiques des groups sanguins ABO. *Acta Haematol.* 8:73, 1952.
95. Voak D., Sacks S., Alderson T., et al.: Monoclonal anti-A from a hybrid myeloma: Evaluation as a blood grouping reagent. *Vox Sang.* 39:134, 1980.
96. Sacks S.H., Lennox E.S.: Monoclonal anti-B as a new blood typing reagent. *Vox Sang.* 40:99, 1981.
97. Messeter L., Brodin T., Chester M.A., et al.: Mouse monoclonal antibodies with anti-A, anti-B, and anti-A,B specificities: Some superior to human polyclonal ABO reagents. *Vox Sang.* 46:185, 1984.
98. Constantoulakis M., Kay H.E.M.: A and B antigens of the human foetal erythrocyte. *Br. J. Haematol.* 8:57, 1962.
99. van Loghem J.J., Dorfmeier H., van der Hart M.: Two A antigens with abnormal serologic properties. *Vox Sang.* 2:16, 1957.
100. Cameron C., Dunsford I., Sickles G.R., et al.: Acquisition of a B-like antigen by red blood cells. *Br. Med. J.* 2:29, 1959.
101. Race R.R., Sanger R.: *Blood Groups in Man*, ed. 6. Oxford, England, Blackwell Scientific Publications, 1975, p. 520.
102. Yamagouchi H., Okuho Y., Tanaka M.: Cis AB bloods found in Japanese families. *Jpn. J. Hum. Genet.* 15:198, 1970.
103. Scherer R., Morarescu R., Ruhenstroth B.: Die spezifische Wirkung der Plasmaproteine bei der blutkorperchen Senkung. *Klin. Wochenschr.* 53:265, 1975.
104. Mollison P.L.: *Blood Transfusion in Clinical Medicine*, ed. 7. Oxford, England, Blackwell Scientific Publications, 1983, p. 57.
105. Bull J.P., Ricketts C., Squire J.R., et al.: Dextran as a plasma substitute. *Lancet* 1:134, 1949.
106. Honig C.L., Bove J.R.: Transfusion-associated fatalities: Review of Bureau of Biologics Reports, 1976–1978. *Transfusion* 20:653, 1980.
107. Schmidt P.J., Kevy S.V.: Sources of error in a hospital blood bank. *Transfusion* 3:198, 1963.
108. Widman F.K. (ed.): *Technical Manual of the American Association of Blood Banks*, ed. 8. Washington, D.C., American Association of Blood Banks, 1981, p. 47.
109. Nevanlinna H.R.: ABO protection in Rh immunization. Read before the 10th Congress of the European Society of Haematology, Strassburg, 1965.
110. Levine M.N., Kuhns W.K., Bolk T.A., et al.: Acquired alteration in the expression of blood groups in a patient with sideroblastic anemia and chronic renal failure. *Transfusion* 24:8, 1984.
111. Sherman L.A., Silberstein L.E., Berkman E.M.: Altered blood group expression in a patient with congenital rubella infection. *Transfusion* 24:267, 1984.
112. Schoentag R., Williams V., Kuhns W.K.: The distribution of blood group substance H and CEA in colorectal carcinoma. *Cancer* 53:503, 1984.
113. Lin F., Liu P.I., McGregor D.H.: Isoantigens A, B, and H in morphologically normal mucosa and

carcinoma of the larynx. *Am. J. Clin. Pathol.* 68:372, 1977.
114. Limas C., Lange P.: Altered reactivity for ABH antigens in transitional cell carcinomas of the urinary bladder. *Cancer* 46:1366, 1980.
115. Giraldo A., Ruby S.G., Humes J.J.: Blood group antigens in urothelium in transitional cell carcinoma. *Ann. Clin. Lab. Sci.* 13:307, 1983.
116. Ockelford P.A., Hill R.S., Nelson H.A., et al.: Serological complications of a major ABO incompatible bone marrow transplantation in a Polynesian with aplastic anemia. *Transfusion* 22:62, 1982.
117. Mangal A.K., Growe G.H., Sinclair M., et al.: Acquired hemolytic anemia due to "auto"-anti-A or "auto"-anti B induced by group O homograft in renal transplant recipients. *Transfusion* 24:201, 1984.
118. Whitsett C.F., Cobb M., Pierce J.A., et al.: Immunological characteristics and clinical significance of anti-H in the A_h phenotype. *Transfusion* 24:164, 1984.
119. Aird I., Bentall H.H.: A relationship between cancer of the stomach and the ABO blood groups. *Br. Med. J.* 1:799, 1953.
120. Mollison P.L.: *Blood Transfusion in Clinical Medicine*, ed. 6. Oxford, England, Blackwell Scientific Publications, 1979, p. 176.
121. Collective Series (1956): An association between blood group A and pernicious anemia. *Br. Med. J.* 2:723, 1976.
122. Roberts J.A.: Some associations between blood groups and disease. *Br. Med. Bull.* 15:129, 1959.
123. Allen T.M., Dawson A.A.: ABO blood groups and ischemic heart disease in men. *Br. Heart J.* 30:377, 1968.
124. Goldstein J., Siviglia G., Hurst R., et al.: Group B erythrocytes enzymatically converted to group O survive normally in A, B and O individuals. *Science* 215:168, 1982.
125. Mourant A.E.: A "new" human blood group antigen of frequent occurrence. *Nature* 158:237, 1946.
126. Sneath J.S., Sneath P.H.A.: Transformation of the Lewis groups of human red cells. *Nature* 176:172, 1955.
127. Rohr T.E., Smith D.F., Zopf D.A., et al.: Le^b active glycolipid in human plasma: Measurement by radioimmunoassay. *Arch. Biochem. Biophys.* 199: 265, 1980.
128. Grubb R.: Correlation between Lewis blood group and secretor character in man. *Nature* 162:933, 1948.
129. Marr A.M.S., Donald A.S.R., Watkins W.M., et al.: Molecular and genetic aspects of human blood group Le^b specificity. *Nature* 215:1345, 1967.
130. Gunson H.H., Latham V.: An agglutinin in serum reacting with cells from Le(a−b−) non-secretor individuals. *Vox Sang.* 22:344, 1972.
131. Mollison P.L.: *Blood Transfusion in Clinical Medicine*, ed. 7, Oxford, England, Blackwell Scientific Publications, 1983, p. 308.
132. Hanfland P., Graham H.A.: Immunochemistry of the Lewis blood group system: Partial characterization of Le^{a-}, Le^{b-} and H-type I (Le^{dH}) blood group active glycosphingolipids from human plasma. *Arch. Biochem. Biophys.* 210:383, 1981.
133. Hirsch H.F., Graham H.A.: Adsorption of Le^c and Le^d from plasma onto red cells. *Transfusion* 20:474, 1979.
134. Mollison P.L.: *Blood Transfusion in Clinical Medicine*, ed. 7. Oxford, England, Blackwell Scientific Publications, 1983, p. 309–311.
135. Bharucha Z.A., Joshi S.R., Bhatia H.M.: Hemolytic disease of the newborn due to anti-Le^b. *Vox Sang.* 41:36, 1981.
136. Cheng M.S.: IgG anti-Le^a in cord serum. *Transfusion* 23:274, 1983.
137. Andresen P.T.: The blood group system L: A new blood group L2. A case of epistasy within the blood groups. *Acta Pathol. Microbiol. Scand.* 25:728, 1948.
138. Brendemoen O.J.: Some factors influencing Rh immunization during pregnancy. *Acta Pathol. Microbiol. Scand.* 31:579, 1952.
139. Hammar L., Mansson S., Rohr T., et al.: Lewis phenotype of erythrocytes and Le^b active glycolipid in serum of pregnant women. *Vox Sang.* 40:27, 1981.
140. Mollison P.L.: *Blood Transfusion in Clinical Medicine*, ed. 7. Oxford, England, Blackwell Scientific Publications, 1983. p. 311.
141. Roy R.B., Wesley R.H., Fitzgerald Z.D.L.: Haemolytic transfusion reaction caused by anti-Le^a. *Vox Sang.* 5:545, 1962.
142. Cooper R.A.: Abnormalities of cell-membrane fluidity in the pathogenesis of disease. *N. Engl. J. Med.* 297:371, 1977.
143. Garraty G., quoted by Mollison P.L.: *Blood Transfusion in Clinical Medicine*, ed. 7. Oxford, England, Blackwell Scientific Publications, 1983, p. 310.
144. Brockhaus M., Magnani J.L., Blaszczyk M., et al.: Monoclonal antibodies directed against the human Le^b blood group antigen. *J. Biol. Chem.* 256:13223, 1981.
145. Messeter L., Brodin T., Chester M.A., et al.: Immunochemical characterization of a monoclonal anti-Le^b blood grouping reagent. *Vox Sang.* 46:66, 1984.
146. Holburn A.M.: IgG anti-Le^a. *Br. J. Haematol.* 27:489, 1974.
147. Waheed A., Kennedy M.S., Gerhan S.: Transfusion significance of Lewis system antibodies: Report on a nationwide survey. *Transfusion* 21:542, 1981.
148. Cutbush M., Giblett E.R., Mollison P.L.: Demonstration of the phenotype Le(a+b+) in infants and in adults. *Br. J. Haematol.* 2:210, 1956.
149. Mollison P.L.: *Blood Transfusion in Clinical Medicine*, ed. 7. Oxford, England, Blackwell Scientific Publications, 1983, p. 638.
150. Oriol R., et al.: The Lewis system and kidney transplantation. *Transplantation* 29:397, 1980.
151. Wiener A.S., Unger L.J., Cohen L., et al.: Type-specific cold auto-antibodies as a cause of acquired haemolytic anemia and haemolytic transfusion reactions: Biologic test with bovine red cells. *Ann. Intern. Med.* 44:221, 1956.

152. Feizi T., Kabat E.A., Vicari G., et al.: Immunochemical studies on blood groups: ILIX. The I antigen complex. Specificity differences among anti-I sera revealed by quantitative precipitin studies. Partial structure of the I determinant specific for one anti-I serum. *J. Immunol.* 106:1578, 1971.
153. Lalezari P., Murphy G.B.: Cold reacting leukocyte agglutinins and their significance, in Curtoni E.S., et al. (eds.): *Histocompatibility Testing.* Copenhagen, Munksgaard, 1967.
154. Shumak K.H., Rachkewich R.A., Crookston M.C., et al.: Antigens of the Ii system on lymphocytes. *Nature New Biol.* 231:148, 1971.
155. Marsh W.L., Nichols M.E., Allen F.H.: Inhibition of anti-I sera by human milk. *Vox Sang.* 18:149, 1970.
156. Testa U., Rochant H., Henri A., et al.: Change in i-antigen expression of erythrocytes during in vivo aging. *Rev. Fr. Transfus. Immunohematol.* 24:299, 1981.
157. Tippett P., Noades J., Sanger R., et al.: Further studies of the I antigen and antibody. *Vox Sang.* 5:107, 1960.
158. Moores P.P., Issitt P.D., Pavone B.G., et al.: Some observations on "Bombay" bloods with comments on evidence for the existence of two different Oh phenotypes. *Transfusion* 15:237, 1975.
159. Wiener, A.S., Moor-Jankowski J., Gordon E.B., et al.: The blood factors I and i in primates including man and in lower species. *Am. J. Phys. Anthropol.* 23:389, 1965.
160. Burnie K.: Ii antigen and antibodies. *Can. J. Med. Technol.* 35:5, 1973.
161. Pittiglio D.H.: *Modern Blood Banking and Transfusion Practices.* New York, F.A. Davis Co., 1983, p. 181.
162. Feizi T.: Immunochemistry of the Ii blood group antigens, in Mohn J.F., Plunkett R.W., Cunningham R.K., et al. (eds.): *Human Blood Groups.* Basel, Switzerland, S. Karger, 1977, p. 164.
163. Marsh W.L., Jensen L., Decary F., et al.: Water soluble blood group substance in secretions of i adults. *Transfusion* 12:222, 1972.
164. Wiener W., Lewis H.B.M., Moores P., et al.: A gene, y, modifying the blood group antigen A. *Vox Sang.* 2:25, 1957.
165. Marsh W.L., Nichols M.E., Ried M.E.: The definition of two I antigen components. *Vox Sang.* 20:209, 1971.
166. Marsh W.L., Jenkins W.J.: Anti-i: A new cold antibody. *Nature* 188:753, 1960.
167. Jenkins W.J., Marsh W.L., Noades, Jean, et al.: The I antigen and antibody. *Vox Sang.* 5:97, 1960.
168. Booth P.B., Jenkins W.J., Marsh W.L.: Anti I^T: A new antibody of the I blood group system occurring in certain melanesian sera. *Br. J. Haematol.* 12:341, 1966.
169. Capra J.D., Dowling P.M., Cook S., et al.: An incomplete cold-reactive gamma G antibody with i specificity in infectious mononucleosis. *Vox Sang.* 16:10, 1969.
170. Mollison P.L.: *Blood Transfusion in Clinical Medicine,* ed. 7. Oxford, England, Blackwell Scientific Publications, 1983, p. 571.
171. Blumberg N., Hicks G., Woll J., et al.: Successful cardiac bypass surgery in the presence of a potent cold agglutinin without exchange. *Transfusion* 23:363, 1983.
172. Klein H.G., Kaltz L.L., McIntosh C.L.: Surgical hypothermia in a patient with a cold agglutinin: Management by plasma exchange. *Transfusion* 20:354, 1980.
173. Duran-Suarez J.R., Trujillo J., Prat I.: An apparent anti-I reacting only in low-ionic-strength solutions. *Transfusion* 24:276, 1984.
174. Marsh W.L.: Anti-i: A cold antibody defining the Ii relationship in human red cells. *Br. J. Haematol.* 7:200, 1961.
175. Shumak K.H., Rachkewich R.A., Greaves M.F.: I and i antigens on normal human T and B lymphocytes and on lymphocytes from patients with chronic lymphocytic leukemia. *Clin. Immunol. Immunopathol.* 4:241, 1975.
176. McGinniss M.H., Schmidt P.J., Carlione P.P.: Close association of I blood group and disease. *Nature* 202:606, 1964.
177. Shumak K.H., Beldotti L.E., Rachkewich R.A.: Diagnosis of haematologic disease using anti-i: I. Disorders with lymphocytosis. *Br. J. Haematol.* 41:399, 1979.
178. Hillman R.S., Giblett E.R.: Red cell membrane alteration associated with "marrow stress." *J. Clin. Invest.* 44:1730, 1965.
179. Crookston J.H., Crookston M.C., Rosse W.F.: Red cell abnormalities in HEMPAS (hereditary erythroblastic multinuclearity with a positive acidified-serum test). *Br. J. Haematol.* 23:83, 1972.
180. Costea N., Yukulis V.J., Heller P.: Inhibition of cold agglutinins (anti-I) by *M. pneumoniae* antigens. *Proc. Soc. Exp. Biol. Med.* 139:476, 1972.
181. Pien F.D., Smith T.F., Taswell H.F., et al.: Cold reactive antibodies in a case of congenital cytomegalovirus infection. *Am. J. Clin. Pathol.* 61:352, 1974.
182. Schmidt P.J., Barile M.F., McGinniss M.H.: Mycoplasma (pleuropneumonia-like organism) and blood groups: I. Associations with neoplastic disease. *Nature* 205:371, 1965.
183. Wexler H., Oppenheim J.D.: Listerial LPS, an endotoxin from a gram-positive bacterium, in Agarwal M.K. (ed.): *Bacterial Endotoxins and Host Response.* Amsterdam, Elsevier-North Holland, 1980, p. 27.
184. Prusanski W., Shumak K.H.: Biologic activity of cold reacting antibodies. *N. Engl. J. Med.* 297:583, 1977.
185. Mollison P.L.: *Blood Transfusion in Clinical Medicine,* ed. 7. Oxford, England, Blackwell Scientific Publications, 1983, pp. 448–449.
186. Rosenfield R.E., et al.: Anti-i, a frequent cold agglutinin in infectious mononucleosis. *Vox Sang.* 10:631, 1965.

187. Roelcke D., Weber M.T.: Simultaneous occurrence of anti-Fl anti-I cold agglutinins in a patient's serum. Vox Sang. 47:122, 1984.
188. Gronemeyer P., Chaplin H., Ghazarian V., et al.: Hemolytic anemia complicating infectious mononucleosis due to the interaction of an IgG cold anti-i and an IgM cold rheumatoid factor. Transfusion 21:715, 1981.
189. Marsh W.L., DePalma H.: Association between the Ii blood group and congenital cataract. Transfusion 22:337, 1982.
190. Landsteiner K., Levine P.: Further observations on individual differences of human blood. Proc. Soc. Exp. Biol. Med. 24:941, 1927.
191. Naiki M., Fong J., Ledeen R., Marcus D.M.: Structure of the human erythrocyte blood group P_1. Biochemistry 14:4831, 1975.
192. Watkins W.M., Morgan W.T.J.: Immunochemical observations on the human blood group P system. J. Immunogenet. 3:15, 1976.
193. Naiki M., Marcus D.M.: An immunochemical study of the human blood group P_1, P and P_K glycosphingolipid antigens. Biochemistry 14:4837, 1975.
194. Roelke D.: Reaction of anti-Gd, anti-Fl, and anti-Sa cold agglutinins with p erythrocytes. Vox Sang. 46:161, 1984.
195. Marcus D.M., Kundu S.K., Suzuki A.: The P blood group system: Recent progress in immunochemistry and genetics. Semin. Hematol. 18:63, 1981.
196. Tippet P.: Chromosomal mapping of the blood group genes. Semin. Hematol. 18:4, 1981.
197. Race R.R., Sanger R.: Blood Groups in Man, ed. 6. Oxford, England. Blackwell Scientific Publications, 1975, p. 140.
198. Levine P., Celano M.J., Falkowski F.: The specificity of the antibody in paroxysmal cold hemoglobinuria (P.C.H.) Transfusion 3:278, 1963.
199. Hinz C.F.: Serologic and physicochemical characterization of Donath-Landsteiner antibodies from six patients. Blood 22:600, 1963.
200. Donath J., Landsteiner K.: Über paroxysmale Hämoglobinurie. Munch. Med. Wochenschr. 51:1590, 1904.
201. Schwarting G.A., Kundu S.K., Marcus D.M., et al.: Reaction of antibodies that cause paroxysmal cold hemoglobinuria (PCH) with globoside and Forssman glycosphingolipids. Blood 53:186, 1979.
202. Levine P., Bobbitt O.B., Waller R.K., et al.: Isoimmunization by a new blood factor in tumor cells. Proc. Soc. Exp. Biol. Med. 77:403, 1951.
203. Levene C., Sela R., Rudolphson Y.: Hemolytic disease of the newborn due to anti-P, P_1, PK (anti-Tja). Transfusion 17:569, 1977.
204. Chandeysson P.L., Flye M.W., Simpkins S.M., et al.: Delayed hemolytic transfusion reaction caused by anti-P_1 antibody. Transfusion 21:77, 1981.
205. Prokop O., Schlesinger D.: Über das Vorkommen von P_1 Blutgruppensubstanz bei einigen, metazoen, insbesondere Ascaris suum und Lumbericus terrestris. Z. Immun. Forsch. 129:344, 1965.
206. Bevan B., Hammond W., Clarke R.L.: Anti P_1 associated with liver-fluke infection. Vox Sang. 16:67, 1970.
207. Venegelen-Tyler V., Nason S.G., Dugan M., et al.: An unusual inhibition of anti-P_1. Transfusion 21:224, 1981.
208. Moureau P.: Les réactions post-transfusionnelles. Rev. Belge. Sci. Méd. 16:258, 1945.
209. Race R.R., Sanger R.: Blood Groups in Man. Oxford, England, Blackwell Scientific Publications, 1975, p. 154.
210. Levine P., Kich E.A.: The rare human isoagglutinin anti-Tja and habitual abortion. Science 120:239, 1954.
211. Cautin G., Lyonnais J.: Anti-P, P_1, PK and early abortion. Transfusion 23:350, 1983.
212. Judd W.J., Steiner E.A., Capps R.D.: Autoagglutinins with apparent anti-P specificity reactive only by low-ionic-strength salt techniques. Transfusion 22:185, 1983.
213. Radermecker M., Brunier M., Francois C., et al.: Anti-P_1 activity in pigeon breeders' serum. Clin. Exp. Immunol. 22:546, 1975.
214. Kallenius G.: Structure of carbohydrate part of receptor on human urothelial cells for pyelonephritogenic Escherichia coli. Lancet 2:604, 1981.
215. Kallenius G., Mollby R., Svenson S.B., et al.: The Pk antigen as receptor for the hemagglutination of pyelonephritic Escherichia coli. FEMS Microbiol. Lett. 7:297, 1980.
216. Landsteiner K., Levine P.: A new agglutinable factor differentiating individual human bloods. Proc. Soc. Exp. Biol. Med. 24:600, 1927.
217. Gedde-Dahl T. Jr., Grimstad A.L., Gunderson S., et al.: A probable crossing over mutation in the MNSs blood group system. Acta Genet. 17:193, 1967.
218. van der Hart M., Bosman H., van Loghem J.J.: Two rare blood group antigens. Vox Sang. 4:108, 1954.
219. Mueller T.J., Dow A.W., Morrison M.: Heterogeneity of the sialoglycoproteins of the normal human erythrocyte membrane. Biochem. Biophys. Res. Commun. 72:94, 1976.
220. Tomita M., Marchesi V.T.: Amino acid sequence and oligosaccharide attachment sites of human erythrocyte glycophorin. Proc. Natl. Acad. Sci. 72:2964, 1975.
221. Lisowska E., Wasniowska K.: Immunochemical characterization of cyanogen bromide degradation products of M and N blood group glycopeptides. Eur. J. Biochem. 88:247, 1978.
222. Lisowska E., Duk M.: Effect of modification of amino groups of human erythrocytes on M, N and Nvg blood group specificities. Vox Sang. 28:392, 1975.
223. Sadler J.E., Paulson J.C., Hill R.L.: The role of sialic acid in the expression of human MN blood group antigens. J. Biol. Chem. 254:2112, 1979.
224. Lisowska E., Kordowicz M.: Specific antibodies for desialized M and N blood group antigens. Vox Sang. 33:164, 1977.

225. Dahr W., Beyreuther K., Steinbach H., et al.: Structure of the Ss blood group antigens: II. A methionine/threonine polymorphism within the N-terminal sequence of the Ss glycoprotein. *Hoppe Seylers Z. Physiol. Chem.* 361:895, 1980.
226. Dahr W., Gielen W., Beyreuther K., et al.: Structure of the Ss blood group antigens: I. Isolation of Ss-active glycopeptides and differentiation of the antigens by modification of methionine. *Hoppe Seylers Z. Physiol. Chem.* 361:145, 1980.
227. Furthmayr H.: Structural comparison of glycophorins and immunochemical analysis of genetic variants. *Nature* 271:519, 1978.
228. Dahr W., Issitt P.D., Moulds J., et al.: Further studies on the membrane glycoprotein defects of S-, s- and En (a-) erythrocytes. *Hoppe Seylers Z. Physiol. Chem.* 359:1217, 1978.
229. Dahr W., Uhlenbruck G., Issitt P.D., et al.: SDS-polyacrylamide gel electrophoretic analysis of the membrane glycoproteins from S- s- U- erythrocytes. *J. Immunogenet.* 2:249, 1975.
230. Dahr W., Uhlenbruck G., Bird G.W.G.: Further characterization of some heterophile agglutinins reacting with alkali-labile carbohydrate chains of human erythrocyte glycoproteins. *Vox Sang.* 28:133, 1975.
231. Anstee D.J., Mawby W.J., Tanner M.J.A.: Abnormal blood group S,s-actine sialoglycoproteins in the membrane of Miltenberger class III, IV and V human erythrocytes. *Biochem. J.* 183:193, 1979.
232. Marquesi V.T.: Structure of biological membranes, in *Membrane Structure and Function of Human Red Cells.* Washington, D.C., American Association of Blood Banks, 1976, p. 1.
233. Levine C., Sela R., Lacser M., et al.: Further examples of human anti-M^e found in sera of Israeli donors. *Vox Sang.* 46:207, 1984.
234. Vengelen-Tyler V., Anstee D.J., Issitt B.G., et al.: Studies on the blood of an Mi^v homozygote. *Transfusion* 21:1, 1981.
235. Judd W.J., Rolih S.D., Dahr W., et al.: Studies on the blood of an $MsHe/MS^u$ proposita and her family: Serological evidence that Henshaw-producing genes do not code for the "N" antigen. *Transfusion* 23:382, 1983.
236. Langley J.W., Issitt P.D., Anstee D.J., et al.: Another individual (J-R) whose red blood cells appear to carry a hybrid MNS,s sialoglycoprotein. *Transfusion* 21:15, 1981.
237. Issitt P.D., Tregellos W.M., Lee C., Wilkinson S.L..: An antibody that recognizes a determinant common to S and s-bearing sialoglycoproteins. *Transfusion* 22:174, 1982.
238. Miceli C., Diekamp U., Sosler S.D.: Heterogeneity of U antibodies. *Transfusion* 23:364, 1983.
239. McKusick V.A.: The anatomy of the human genome. *Am. J. Med.* 69:266, 1980.
240. Landsteiner K., Levine P.: Further observations on individual differences of human blood. *Proc. Soc. Exp. Biol.* NY 24:941, 1927.
241. Mourant A.E.: Dosage effects in the Duffy, S, s, and Rh systems. *Transfusion* 23:361, 1983.
242. Morel P.A.: The erythrocyte blood groups in questions of paternity, in Silver H. (ed.): *Paternity Testing: A Seminar.* Washington, D.C., American Association of Blood Banks, 1900.
243. Boyd W.C.: Estimation of gene frequencies from MNS data. *Science* 118:756, 1953.
244. Adinolfi M., Polley M., Hunter D.A., et al.: Classification of blood group antibodies as beta-2-M or gamma globulin. *Immunology* 5:566, 1962.
245. Kurtz S.R., Ouelle T.R., McMican A., et al.: Survival of MM red cells during hypothermia in two patients with anti-M. *Transfusion* 23:37, 1983.
246. Reid M.E., Ellisor S.S., Barker J.M.: A human allo anti-N enhanced by acid media. *Transfusion* 24:222, 1984.
247. Morel P.A., Bergren M.O., Hill V., et al.: MN specific hemagglutinins of human erythrocytes stored in glucose solutions. *Transfusion* 21:652, 1981.
248. Mollison P.L.: *Blood Transfusion in Clinical Medicine,* ed. 7. Oxford, England, Blackwell Scientific Publications, 1984, pp. 416–417.
249. Stone B., Marsh W.L.: Haemolytic disease of the newborn caused by anti-M. *Br. J. Haematol.* 5:344, 1959.
250. Huestis W.H., Bove J.R., Busch S.: *Practical Blood Transfusion.* Boxton, Little, Brown & Co., 1969, p. 345.
251. Race R.R., Sanger R.: *Blood Groups in Man,* ed. 6. Oxford, England, Blackwell Scientific Publications, 1975, p. 125.
252. Moores P.: Four examples of the S-s-U phenotype in an Indian family. *Vox Sang.* 23:452, 1972.
253. Burki U., Degnan T.J., Rosenfield R.E.: Stillbirth due to anti-U. *Vox Sang.* 9:209, 1964.
254. Lisowska E.: Reaction of erythrocyte mucoproteins with anti-N phytoagglutinins from *Vicia graminea* seeds. *Nature* 198:865, 1963.
255. Allen N.K., Brilliantine L.: A survey of hemagglutinins in various seeds. *J. Immunol.* 102:1295, 1969.
256. Allen R.W., Nunley N., Kimmeth M.E., et al.: Isolation and serological characterization of a monoclonal antibody recognizes the N blood group antigen. *Transfusion* 24:136, 1984.
257. MacPherson C.R., Zartman E.R.: Anti-M antibody as a cause of intrauterine death: A follow-up. *Am. J. Clin. Pathol.* 43:544, 1965.
258. Furlong M.B., Monaghan W.P.: Delayed hemolytic episodes due to anti-M. *Transfusion* 21:45, 1981.
259. Howell E.D., Perkins H.A.: Anti-N-like antibodies in the sera of patients undergoing chronic haemodialysis. *Vox Sang.* 23:291, 1972.
260. Belzer F.O., Kounts S.L., Perkins H.A.: Red cell cold agglutinins as a cause of failure of renal transplantation. *Transplantation* 11:422, 1971.
261. Boettcher B.N.: Specificity and possible origin of anti-N antibodies developed by patients undergoing chronic haemodialysis. *Vox Sang.* 31:408, 1976.
262. Vaisanen V., et al.: Blood group M specific hemagglutinin in pyelonephritogenic *Escherichia coli* (letter). *Lancet* 1:1192, 1982.

263. Kao Y.S., Frank S., DeJongh D.S.: Anti-M in children with acute bacterial infections. *Transfusion* 18:320, 1978.
264. Thomas D.B., Winzler R.J.: Structural studies on human erythrocytes glycoproteins: Alkali-labile tetrasaccharides. *J. Biol. Chem.* 244:5943, 1969.
265. Obeid D., Bird W.G., Wingham J.: Prolonged erythrocyte T-polyagglutination in two children with bowel disorders. *J. Clin. Pathol.* 30:953, 1977.
266. Issitt P.D., Wilkinson S.L.: Anti-Tm is anti-N polypeptide. *Transfusion* 21:493, 1981.
267. Dopp S.L., Islam B.E.: Anti-U and hemolytic disease of the newborn. *Transfusion* 23:273, 1983.
268. Callender S., Race R.R., Paykoc Z.V.: Hypersensitivity to transfused blood. *Br. Med. J.* 2:83, 1945.
269. Crawford M.N., Greenwalt T.J., Sasaki T., et al.: The phenotype Lu(a−b−) together with unconventional Kidd groups in one family. *Transfusion* 1:228, 1961.
270. Race R.R., Sanger R.: *Blood Groups in Man*, ed. 6. Oxford, England, Blackwell Scientific Publications, 1975, p. 261.
271. Crawford M.N., Tipett P., Sanger R.: The antigens Au^a, and P$_1$ of cells of the dominant type of Lu(a−b−). *Vox Sang.* 26:283, 1974.
272. Judson P.A., Anstee D.J.: Comparative effect of trypsin and chymotrypsin on blood group antigens. *Med. Lab. Sci.* 34:1, 1977.
273. Mohr J.: A search for linkage between the Lutheran blood group and other hereditary characters. *Acta Pathol. Microbiol. Scand.* 28:207, 1951.
274. Kissmeyer-Nielsen F.: A further example of anti-Lu^b as a cause of mild hemolytic disease of the newborn. *Vox Sang.* 5:532, 1960.
275. Dunstan R.A., Simpson M.B., Rosse W.F.: Erythrocyte antigens on human platelets: Absence of Rh, Duffy, Kell, Kidd, and Lutheran antigens. *Transfusion* 24:243, 1984.
276. Francais B.J., Hatcher D.E.: Hemolytic disease of the newborn apparently caused by anti-Lu^a. *Transfusion* 1:248, 1961.
277. Knowles R.W. quoted by Mollison P.L.: *Blood Transfusion in Clinical Medicine*, ed. 7. Oxford, England, Blackwell Scientific Publications, 1983, p. 427.
278. Inderbitzen P.E., Windle B.: An example of HDN probably due to anti-Lu^a. *Transfusion* 22:542, 1982.
279. Greenwalt T.J., Sasaki T.: The Lutheran blood groups: A second example of anti-Lu^b, and three further examples of anti-Lu^a. *Blood* 12:998, 1957.
280. Callender S.T., Race R.R.: A serological and genetical study of multiple antibodies formed in response to blood transfusion in a patient with lupus erythematosus diffusus. *Ann. Eugen. (London)* 13:102, 1946.
281. Hackel E., Smolker R.E., Fenske S.A.: Inhibition of anti-Rh and anti-Lutheran antibodies by RNA derivatives. *Vox Sang.* 3:402, 1958.
282. Bretscher M.S.: Major human erythrocyte glycoprotein spans the cell membrane. *Nature New Biol.* 231:229, 1971.
283. Tomita M., Futhmayr H., Marchesi V.T.: Primary structure of human erythrocyte glycophorin A: Isolation and characterization of peptides and complete amino acid sequence. *Biochemistry* 17:4756, 1978.
284. Steane S.M.: Basic membrane biochemistry and its relationship to blood group serology, in Bell C.A. (ed.): *A Seminar on Antigens, On Blood Cells, and Body Fluids*. Washington, D.C., American Association of Blood Banks, 1980, p. 1.
285. Davies D.M., Hall S.J., Graham H.A., et al.: The isolation and partial characterization of Duffy antigens from human red cells (abstract). *Transfusion* 19:638, 1979.
286. Engelfriet C.P., von dem Borne A.E.G., Beckers D., et al.: Immune destruction of red cells, in Bell C.A. (ed.): *A Seminar on Immune-Mediated Cell Destruction*. Washington, D.C., American Association of Blood Banks, 1981, p. 93.
287. Levine P., Stetson R.: An unusual case of intragroup agglutination. *JAMA* 113:126, 1939.
288. Landsteiner K., Wiener A.S.: An agglutinable factor in human blood recognizable by immune sera of rhesus blood. *Proc. Soc. Exp. Biol. Med.* 43:223, 1940.
289. Race R.R.: The Rh genotypes and Fisher's theory. *Blood* 3(suppl. 2):27, 1948.
290. Steinberg A.G.: Evidence for a mutation crossing over at the Rh locus. *Vox Sang.* 10:721, 1965.
291. WHO: Twenty-eighth report of WHO Expert Committee on Biological Standardization. *Technical Report Series*. Geneva, Switzerland, World Health Organization, 1977, p. 610.
292. Wiener A.S.: The Rh-Hr blood types: Serology, genetics and nomenclature. *Trans. NY Acad. Sci.* 13:198, 1951.
293. Rosenfield R.E., Allen F.H., Rubenstein P.: Genetic model for the Rh blood group system. *Proc. Natl. Acad. Sci. USA* 70:1303, 1973.
294. Lauf P.K., Joiner C.H.: Increased potassium transport and ouabain binding in human Rh null red blood cells. *Blood* 48:457, 1976.
295. Plapp F.V., Kowalski M.M., Tilzer L., et al.: Partial purification of Rho (D) antigen from Rh positive and Rh negative erythrocytes. *Proc. Natl. Acad. Sci. USA* 76:2964, 1979.
296. Sinor L.T., Brown P.J., Evans J.P., Plapp F.V.: The Rh antigen specificity of erythrocyte proteolipid. *Transfusion* 24:179, 1984.
297. Moore S., Woodrow C.F., McClelland B.L.: Isolation of membrane components associated with human red cell antigens Rh (D), (c̄) and Fy^a. *Nature* 295:529, 1982.
298. Folkerd E.J., Ellory J.C., Hughes-Jones N.C.: A molecular size determination of Rh (D) antigen by radiation inactivation. *Immunochemistry* 14:529, 1977.
299. Hughes-Jones N.C., Green E.J., Hunt V.A.M.: Loss of Rh antigen activity following the action of phospholipase A2 on red cell. *Vox Sang.* 29:184, 1975.
300. Jameson J.T., Kleeman J.E., Masouredis S.P., et al.: Anti-D prozone and membrane sulfhydryl modification. *Transfusion* 24:130, 1984.

301. Contreras M., Armitage S., Daniels G.L., et al.: Homozygous ·D·. *Vox Sang.* 36:81, 1979.
302. Economidou J., Hughes-Jones N.C., Gardner B.: Quantitative measurements concerning A and B antigen sites. *Vox Sang.* 12:321, 1967.
303. Mollison P.L.: *Blood Transfusion in Clinical Medicine,* ed. 7. Oxford, England, Blackwell Scientific Publications, 1983, p. 511.
304. Rochna E., Hughes-Jones N.C.: The use of purified ^{125}I-labelled anti-gammaglobulin in the determination of the number of D antigen sites on red cells of different phenotypes. *Vox Sang.* 10:675, 1965.
305. Hughes-Jones N.C., Gardner B., Lincoln P.: Observations of the number of available c, D, e and E antigen sites on red cells. *Vox Sang.* 21:210, 1971.
306. Rosenfield R.E., Allen F.H. Jr., Rubenstein P.: Genetic model for the Rh blood-group system: Conjugated operons/repressors/quantitative blood typing. *Proc. Natl. Acad. Sci. USA* 70:1303, 1973.
307. Jacob F., Monod J.: Genetic regulatory mechanisms in the synthesis of proteins. *J. Mol. Biol.* 3:318, 1961.
308. Issitt P.D.: *Serology and Genetics of the Rhesus Blood Group System.* Cincinnati, Montgomery Scientific Publications, 1979, p. 64.
309. Marsh W.L.: Mapping human autosomes: Evidence supporting assignment of rhesus to the short arm of chromosome No. 1. *Science* 183:966, 1974.
310. Weitkamp L.R., Guttormsen S.A., Greendyke R.M.: Genetic linkage between a locus for 6-PGD and the Rh locus: Evaluation of possible heterogeneity in the recombination fraction between sexes and among families. *Am. J. Hum. Genet.* 23:462, 1971.
311. Vos G.H., Vos D., Kirk R.L., et al.: A sample of blood with no detectable Rh antigens. *Lancet* 1:14, 1961.
312. Ishimori T., Hasekura H.: A Japanese with no detectable Rh blood group antigens due to silent Rh alleles or deleted chromosomes. *Transfusion* 7:84, 1967.
313. Levine P., Chelano M.J., Falkowski F., et al.: A second example of ---/--- blood or Rh null. *Nature* 204:892, 1964.
314. Haber G.V., Bastani A., Ardin P.D., et al.: Rh null and pregnancy complicated by anti-"total Rh" ·R· Anti-Rh29(Rh). *Transfusion* 7:389, 1967.
315. Lauf P.K., Joiner C.H.: Increased potassium transport and ouabain binding in human Rh null red blood cells. *Blood* 48:457, 1976.
316. Chown B., Lewis M., Hiroko K., Lowen B.: An unlinked modifier of Rh blood groups: Effects when heterozygous and when homozygous. *Am. J. Hum. Genet.* 24:623, 1972.
317. Race R.R., Sanger R., Selwin J.G.: A possible deletion in a human Rh chromosome: A serological and genetical study. *Br. J. Exp. Pathol.* 32:124, 1951.
318. Issitt P.D., Issitt C.H.: *Applied Blood Group Serology,* ed. 2. Oxner, Calif., Spectra Biologicals, 1979, p. 128.
319. Stratton F., Renton P.H.: Rh genes allelomorphic to D. *Nature* 162:293, 1948.
320. Shapiro M.: The ABO, MN, P and Rh blood group systems in the South African Bantu. *S. Afr. Med. J.* 25:187, 1951.
321. Broman B.: Swedish thoughts on RhD^u nomenclature. *Transfusion* 24:85, 1984.
322. Race R.R., Sanger R. *Blood groups in Man,* ed. 6. Oxford, England. Blackwell Scientific Publications. 1975, p. 195.
323. Rosenfield R.E., Haber G.V., Schroeder R., et al.: Problems in Rh typing as revealed by a single Negro family. *Am. J. Hum. Genet.* 12:147, 1960.
324. Giles G.M., et al.: An Rh gene complex which results in a new antigen detectable by a specific antibody, anti-Rh33. *Vox Sang.* 21:289, 1971.
325. Darnborough J., Dunsford I., Wallace J.A.: The En^a antigen and antibody: A genetical modification of human red cells affecting their blood grouping reactions. *Vox Sang.* 17:241, 1969.
326. Furuhjelm U., Myllyla G., Nevanlinna H.R., et al.: The red cell phenotype En(a−) and Anti-En^a: Serological and physicochemical aspects. *Vox Sang.* 17:256, 1969.
327. Lewis M., Chown B., Kaitas H., et al.: Blood group antigen GO^a and the Rh system. *Transfusion* 7:440, 1967.
328. Levine P., Cellano M., Fenichel R., et al.: A "D"-like antigen in Rhesus red blood cells and in Rh-positive and Rh-negative red cells. *Science* 133:332, 1961.
329. Murray J., Clark E.C.: Production of anti-Rh in guinea pigs from human erythrocytes. *Nature* 169:886, 1952.
330. Swanson J., Matson G.A.: Third example of a human "D-like" antibody or anti-LW. *Transfusion* 4:257, 1964.
331. Levine P., Celano M.J., Vos G.H., et al.: The first human blood ---/---, which lacks the "D-like" antigen. *Nature* 194:304, 1962.
332. Giles C.M.: The LW blood group: A review. *Immunol. Commun.* 9:225, 1980.
333. Swanson J.L., Azar M., Miller J., et al.: Evidence of heterogeneity of LW antigen revealed in family study. *Transfusion* 14:470, 1974.
334. Rosenfield R.E., Haber G.H.: An Rh blood factor rhi (Ce) and its relationship to hr (ce). *Am. J. Hum. Genet.* 10:474, 1958.
335. Rosenfield R.E., Vogel P., Gibbel N., et al.: A 'new' Rh antibody, anti-f. *Br. Med. J.* 1:975, 1953.
336. Stout T.D., Moore B.P.L., Allen F.H. Jr., et al.: A new phenotype D+G− (Rh:1, −12). *Vox Sang.* 8:262, 1963.
337. Race R.R., Sanger R.: *Blood Groups in Man,* ed. 6. Oxford, England, Blackwell Scientific Publications, 1975, p. 302.
338. Issitt P.D., Tessel J.A.: On the incidence of antibodies to the Rh antigens G, rhi (Ce), C and C^G in sera containing anti-CD or anti-C. *Transfusion* 21:412, 1981.

339. Sachs H.W., Reuter W., Tippett P., et al.: An Rh gene complex producing both C^W and c antigen. *Vox Sang.* 35:272, 1978.
340. Svoboda R.K., Van West B., Grumet F.C.: Anti-Rh 41, a new Rh antibody found in association with an abnormal expression of chromosome 1 genetic markers. *Transfusion* 21:150, 1981.
341. Konugres A.A., Holbrook E.R., Corcoran P.A.: Another source of error in red cell typing. *Transfusion* 6:80, 1966.
342. Steiner E., Butch S.H., Carey J.L., et al.: Passive anti-D from intravenous immune serum globulin. *Transfusion* 23:361, 1983.
343. Shirey R.S., Smith B., Sensebrenner L., et al.: Red cell sensitization due to anti-D in antilymphocyte globulin. *Transfusion* 23:396, 1983.
344. Widman F.K. (ed.): *Technical Manual of the American Association of Blood Banks*, ed. 8. Washington, D.C., American Association of Blood Banks, 1981, pp. 137–140.
345. Romans D.G., Tilley C.A., Crookston M.C., et al.: Conversion of incomplete antibodies to direct agglutinins by mild reduction: Evidence for segmental flexibility within the Fc fragment of immunoglobulin G. *Proc. Natl. Acad. Sci. USA* 74:2531, 1977.
346. Lalezari P.: Direct determination of red cell bound antibody specificity. *Br. J. Haematol.* 24:777, 1973.
347. Cohen F., Zuelzer W.W.: Identification of blood group antigens by immunofluorescence and its application to the detection of the transplacental passage of erythrocytes in mother and child. *Vox Sang.* 9:75, 1964.
348. Caren L.D., Bellavance R., Grumet F.C.: Demonstration of gene dosage effects on antigens in the Duffy, Ss, and Rh systems using an enzyme-linked immunoadsorbent assay. *Transfusion* 22:475, 1982.
349. Allen F.H. Jr., Newell J.L.: Naturally occurring anti-Rh antibody. *N. Engl. J. Med.* 259:236, 1958.
350. Naoki K., Uda M., Uchiyama E., et al.: Rh null with naturally occurring antibody. *Transfusion* 24:182, 1984.
351. Krikler S.H., Ferguson D.F., Akabutu J.J., et al.: Transient anti-D in an Rh positive patient with congenital dyserythropoietic anemia, type II. *Transfusion* 24:169, 1984.
352. Mollison P.L.: *Blood Transfusion in Clinical Medicine*, ed. 7. Oxford, England, Blackwell Scientific Publications, 1983, pp. 355–357.
353. Davey M.G., Campbell A.L., James J.: Some consequences of hyperimmunization to the rhesus (D) blood group antigen in man (abstract). *Proc. Austr. Soc. Immunol. Adelaide,* December 1969.
354. Natvig J.B., Kunkel H.G.: Genetic markers of human immunoglobulins: The Gm and Inv systems. *Ser. Haemat.* 1:66, 1968.
355. Adinolfi A., Mollison P.L., Polley M., Rose J.M.: γA blood group antibodies. *J. Exp. Med.* 123:951, 1966.
356. Ayland J., Horton M.A., Tippett P., et al.: Complement binding anti-D made in a D^u variant woman. *Vox Sang.* 34:40, 1978.
357. Raum D.D., Awdeh Z.L., Page P., et al.: MHC determinants of response to Rh immunization. *J. Immunol.* 132:157, 1984.
358. Jakobowicz R., Williams L., Silberman F.: Immunization of Rh negative volunteers by repeated injections of very small amount of Rh positive blood. *Vox Sang.* 23:376, 1972.
359. Schorr J.B., Schorr P.T., Rose F., et al.: The antigenicity of C and E antigens when transfused into Rh-negative (rr) and Rh-positive recipients (abstract), in *Communications of the American Association Blood Banks*. Chicago, 1971.
360. Huestis D.W., Bove J.R., Busch S.: *Practical Blood Transfusion,* ed. 3. Boston, Little, Brown & Co., 1981, p. 280.
361. McBride J.A., O'Hoski P., Barnes C.C., et al.: Rhesus alloimmunization following intensive plasma exchange. *Transfusion* 23:352, 1983.
362. Widman F.K. (ed.): *Technical Manual of the American Association of Blood Banks,* ed. 8. Washington, D.C., American Association of Blood Banks, 1981, p. 401.
363. Sebring E.S., Polesky H.F.: Detection of fetal maternal hemorrhage in Rh immunoglobulin candidates: A rosetting technique using enzyme-treated RhzRhz indicator erythrocytes. *Transfusion* 22:468, 1982.
364. Simonovits I., Timar I., Bajtai G.: Rate of Rh immunization after induced abortion. *Vox Sang.* 38:161, 1980.
365. Mollison P.L.: *Blood Transfusion in Clinical Medicine,* ed. 7. Oxford, England, Blackwell Scientific Publications, 1983, p. 377.
366. Chown B.: Anemia from bleeding of the fetus into the mother's circulation. *Lancet* 1:1213, 1954.
367. Cohen F., Zuelzer W.W., Gustafson D.C., et al.: Mechanisms of iso-immunization: I. The transplacental passage of fetal erythrocytes in homospecific pregnancies. *Blood* 23:621, 1964.
368. Woodrow J.C., Donohoe W.T.A.: Rh-immunization by pregnancy: Results of a summary and their relevance to prophylactic therapy. *Br. Med. J.* 4:139, 1968.
369. Cohen F., Zuelzer W.W.: Mechanisms of isoimmunization: II. Transplacental passage and postnatal survival of fetal erythrocytes in heterospecific pregnancies. *Blood* 30:796, 1967.
370. Widman F.K. (ed.): *Technical Manual of the American Association of Blood Banks,* ed. 8. Washington, D.C., American Association of Blood Banks, 1981, p. 244.
371. Ascari W.O., Levine P., Pollak W.: Incidence of maternal Rh immunization by ABO compatible and incompatible pregnancies. *Br. Med. J.* 1:399, 1969.
372. Mollison P.L.: *Blood Transfusion in Clinical Medicine,* ed. 7. Oxford, England, Blackwell Scientific Publications, 1983, p. 378.

373. Levine P.: Serological factors as possible causes in spontaneous abortions. *J. Hered.* 34:71, 1943.
374. Stern K., Goodman H.S., Berger M.: Experimental isoimmunization to hemo-antigens in man. *J. Immunol.* 87:189, 1961.
375. Stern K.: Multiple differences in red cell antigens and isoimmunization. *Transfusion* 15:179, 1975.
376. Giblett E.R.: Blood group antibodies causing hemolytic disease of the newborn. *Clin. Obstet. Gynecol.* 7:1044, 1964.
377. Mollison P.L.: *Blood Transfusion in Clinical Medicine*, ed. 7. Oxford, England, Blackwell Scientific Publications, 1983, pp. 236–239.
378. Mollison P.L.: *Blood Transfusion in Clinical Medicine*, ed. 7. Oxford, England, Blackwell Scientific Publications, 1983, p. 363.
379. Finn R., Clarke C.A., Donohoe W.T.A., et al.: Experimental studies on the prevention of Rh hemolytic disease. *Br. Med. J.* 1:1486, 1961.
380. Freda V.J., Gorman J.G., Pollack W.: Successful prevention of Rh immunization in man with anti-Rh gamma 2-globulin antibody preparation: A preliminary report. *Transfusion* 4:26, 1964.
381. Mollison P.L., Hughes-Jones N.C., Lindsay M., et al.: Suppression of primary Rh immunization by passively-administered antibody: Experiments in volunteers. *Vox Sang.* 16:421, 1969.
382. Freda V.J., Gorman J.G., Pollack W.L.: Rh factor: Prevention of immunization and clinical trial on mothers. *Science* 151:828, 1966.
383. Pollack W., Ascari W.Q., Kochesky R.J., et al.: Studies on Rh prophylaxis: I. Relationship between doses of anti-Rh and size of antigenic stimulus. *Transfusion* 11:333, 1971.
384. Widman F.K. (ed.): *Technical Manual of the American Association of Blood Banks*, ed. 8. Washington, D.C., American Association of Blood Banks, 1981, p. 256.
385. Pollack W., Ascari W.Q., Crispen J.F., et al.: Studies on Rh prophylaxis: II. Rh immune prophylaxis after transfusion with Rh-positive blood. *Transfusion* 11:340, 1971.
386. Huchet J., Cregut R., Pinon R.: Immunoglobulines anti-D: Efficacité comparée des voies intramusculaire et intra-veineuse. *Rev. Fr. Transfus.* 13:231, 1970.
387. Jouvenceaux A.: Prévention de l'immunization anti-Rh. *Rev. Fr. Transfus.* 14:39, 1971.
388. Mollison P.L.: *Transfusion in Clinical Medicine*, ed. 7. Oxford, England, Blackwell Scientific Publications, 1983, pp. 653–654.
389. Alving B.M., Tankersley D.L., Mason B.L., et al.: Vasoactive enzymes in immunoglobulin preparations, in Alving B.M., Finlayson J.S. (eds.): *Immunoglobulins: Characteristics and Use of Intravenous Preparations.* Washington, D.C., U.S. Government Printing Office, 1979.
390. Finn R., Harper D.T., Stallings S.A., et al.: Transplacental hemorrhage. *Transfusion* 3:114, 1963.
391. Freda V.J., Gorman J.G., Galen R.S., et al.: The threat of Rh immunization from abortions. *Lancet* 2:147, 1970.
392. Mollison P.L.: *Blood Transfusion in Clinical Medicine*, ed. 7. Oxford, England, Blackwell Scientific Publications, 1983, p. 398.
393. LaFerla J.J., Butch S.: Fetal Rh blood group determination in pregnancy termination by dilatation and evacuation. *Transfusion* 23:67, 1983.
394. Bowman J.M., Chown B., Lewis M., et al.: Rh immunization during pregnancy. Antenatal prophylaxis. *Can. Med. Assoc. J.* 118:623, 1978.
395. Davey M.G.: Epidemiology of failures of Rh immunoglobulin and ABO protection, in *Proceedings of a Symposium on Rh Antibody Immunosuppression.* Raritan, N.J., Ortho Research Institute, 1975, p. 13.
396. Widman F.K. (ed.): *Technical Manual of the American Association of Blood Banks*, ed. 8. Washington, D.C., American Association of Blood Banks, 1981, p. 258.
397. Gorman J.G.: *The Role of the Laboratory in Hemolytic Disease of the Newborn.* Philadelphia, Lea & Febiger, 1975, pp. 179, 187.
398. Walker R.H.: Preparation of blood components, in Myhre B.A. (ed.): *Quality Control in the Blood Bank.* Chicago, American Society of Clinical Pathologists, 1973, p. 82.
399. Bierme S.J., Blanc M., Abbal M., et al.: Oral Rh treatment for severely immunized mothers (letter). *Lancet* 1:604, 1979.
400. Bowman J.M., Pollock J.M.: Reversal of Rh alloimmunization: Fact or fancy? *Vox Sang.* 47:209, 1984.
401. Eklund J.R., Nevanlinna H.R., quoted in Mollison P.L.: *Blood Transfusion in Clinical Medicine*, ed. 6. Oxford, England, Blackwell Scientific Publications, 1979, p. 346.
402. Eklund J.R., Nevanlinna H.R.: Rh prevention: A report and analysis of a national programme. *J. Med. Genet.* 10:1, 1973.
403. Woodrow J.C.: Rh immunization and its prevention. *Semin. Hematol.* 3:3, 1970.
404. Mollison P.L.: *Blood Transfusion in Clinical Medicine*, ed. 7. Oxford, England, Blackwell Scientific Publications, 1983, pp. 664–665.
405. Isbister J.P., Ting A., Seeto K.M.: Development of Rh specific maternal autoantibodies following intensive plasmapheresis for Rh immunization during pregnancy. *Vox Sang.* 33:353, 1977.
406. Mollison P.L.: *Blood Transfusion in Clinical Medicine*, ed. 7. Oxford, England, Blackwell Scientific Publications, 1983, pp. 330–401.
407. Issitt P.D.: *Serology and Genetics of the Rhesus Blood Group System.* Montgomery Scientific Publications, 1979, pp. 1–277.
408. Tippett P., Sanger R.: Further observations on subdivisions of the Rh antigen D. *Arztl. Lab.* 23:476, 1977.
409. Cutbush M., Mollison P.L., Parkin D.M.: A new human blood group. *Nature* 165:188, 1950.
410. Albrey J.A., et al.: A new antibody, anti-Fy3, in

the Duffy blood group system. *Vox Sang.* 20:29, 1971.
411. Behzad O., Lee L.L., Gavin J., et al.: A new antierythrocyte antibody in the Duffy system: Anti-Fy4. *Vox Sang.* 24:337, 1973.
412. Colledge K.I., Pezzulich M., Marsh W.L.: Anti-Fy5, an antibody disclosing a probable association between the rhesus and Duffy blood group genes. *Vox Sang.* 24:193, 1973.
413. Davies D.M., Hall S.J., Graham H.A., et al.: The isolation and partial characterization of Duffy antigens from human red cells (abstract). *Transfusion* 19:638, 1979.
414. Masouredis S.P., Sudora E., Mahan L., et al.: Quantitative immunoferritin microassay of Fy^a, Fy^b, Jk^a, U, and Di^b antigen site numbers on human red cells. *Blood* 56:969, 1980.
415. Miller L.H., et al.: Erythrocyte receptors for *(Plasmodium knowlesi)* malaria: The Duffy blood group determinants. *Science* 189:561, 1975.
416. Pasvol G., Wainscoat J.S., Weatherall D.J.: Erythrocytes deficient in glycophorin resist invasion by the malarial parasite *Plasmodium falciparum*. *Nature* 297:64, 1982.
417. Tanner M.J.A., Anstee D.J.: The membrane change in En(a−) human erythrocytes: Absence of the major erythrocyte sialoglycoprotein. *Biochem. J.* 153:271, 1976.
418. Perkins M.E.: Surface proteins of *Plasmodium falciparum* merozoides binding to the erythrocyte receptor, glycophorin. *J. Exp. Med.* 160:788, 1984.
419. Issitt P., Issitt C.: The Duffy blood group system, in *Applied Blood Group Serology*. Oxner, Calif., Spectra Biologicals, 1976, pp. 164–165.
420. Donahue R.P., et al.: Probable assignment of the Duffy blood group to chromosome #1 in man. *Proc. Natl. Acad. Sci. USA* 61:949, 1968.
421. Førre ø., Gaarder P.I., Natvig J.B.: V_H subgroup restriction in human erythrocyte antibodies: Studies of anti-A, anti-B, and anti-Duffy antibodies. *Scand. J. Immunol.* 6:149, 1977.
422. Mollison P.L.: *Blood Transfusion in Clinical Medicine*, ed. 7. Oxford, England, Blackwell Scientific Publications, 1983, p. 408.
423. Williams D., Johnson C.L., Marsh W.L.: Duffy antigen changes on red blood cells stored at low temperature. *Transfusion* 21:357, 1981.
424. Rosenfield R.E., Vogel P.L., Race R.R.: A further example of the human blood group antibody anti-Fy^a. *Rev. Hematol.* 5:315, 1950.
425. Freiesleben E.: Fatal hemolytic transfusion reaction due to anti-Fy^a (Duffy). *Acta Pathol. Microbiol. Scand.* 29:283, 1951.
426. Cutbush M., Mollison P.L.: The Duffy blood group. *Heredity* 4:383, 1950.
427. Geczy A.: A case history of a haemolytic disease of the newborn due to anti-Fy^a. *Vox Sang.* 5:551, 1960.
428. van t' Veer M.B., van Leeuwen I., Haas F.J.L.M., et al.: Red cell auto-antibodies mimicking anti-Fy^b specificity. *Vox Sang.* 47:88, 1984.
429. Allen F.M. Jr., Diamond L.K., Niedziela B.: A new blood group antigen. *Nature* 167:482, 1951.
430. Plaut G., et al.: A new blood-group antibody, anti-Jk^b. *Nature* 171:431, 1953.
431. Woodfield D.G., Douglas R., Smith J., et al: The Jk(a−b−) phenotype in New Zealand polynesians. *Transfusion* 22:276, 1982.
432. Habibi B.: Jk(a−b−) phenotype does exist in caucasians. *Transfusion* 24:184, 1984.
433. Cleghorn T.E.: Unpublished observations, quoted by Race R.R., Sanger R.: *Blood Groups in Man*, ed. 6. Oxford, England, Blackwell Scientific Publications, 1975, p. 365.
434. Marsh W.L., et al.: Kidd blood group antigens of leukocytes and platelets. *Transfusion* 14:378, 1974.
435. Polley M.J., Mollison P.L., Soothhill J.F.: The role of 19S gammaglobulin blood group antibodies in the antiglobulin reaction. *Br. J. Haematol.* 8:149, 1962.
436. Chown B., Lewis M., Kaita H.: The Kidd blood group system in caucasians. *Transfusion* 5:506, 1965.
437. Crawford M., et al.: The phenotype L^u(a−b−) together with unconventional Kidd groups in one family. *Transfusion* 1:228, 1961.
438. Humphrey A.J., Morel P.A.: Further evidence of heterogeneity within the Kidd blood group system. *Transfusion* 16:242, 1976.
439. Lewis M., Kaita H., Philipps S., et al.: Analysis of linkage relationships of Co, J_K, and K with each other and with chromosome 2 loci, ACP1 and Km. *Ann. Hum. Genet.* 46:349, 1982.
440. Keats B.J.B., Morton N.I., Rao D.C.: Possible linkages (lod score over 1.5) and a tentative map of the Jk-Km linkage group. *Cytogenet. Cell. Genet.* 22:304, 1978.
441. Hardman J.T., Beck M.L.: Hemagglutination in capillaries: Correlation with blood group specificity and IgG subclass. *Transfusion* 21:343, 1981.
442. Mollison P.L.: *Blood Transfusion in Clinical Medicine*, ed. 7. Oxford, England, Blackwell Scientific Publications, 1983, pp. 502–503.
443. Halima D., Garraty G., Bueno R.: An apparent anti-J_K^a reacting only in the presence of methyl esters of hydroxybenzoic acid. *Transfusion* 22:521, 1982.
444. Heaton D.C., McLaughlin K.: Jk(a−b−) red cells resist urea lysis. *Transfusion* 22:70, 1982.
445. Okulio Y., Tomita T., Nagao N., et al.: Mass screening donors for −D− and JK(a−b−) using the Groupamatic-360. *Transfusion* 23:362, 1982.
446. Huestis D.W., et al.: The treacherous Kidd antibodies. *Transfusion* 6:513, 1966.
447. Polesky H.F., Bove J.R.: A fatal hemolytic transfusion reaction with acute autohemolysis. *Transfusion* 4:285, 1964.
448. Arcara P.C., O'Connor M.A., Dimmetta R.M.: A family with three J_K(a−b−) members. *Transfusion* 9:282, 1969.
449. Stratton F., Gunson H.H., Rawilson V.: Comple-

ment fixing antibodies in relation to hemolytic disease of the newborn. *Transfusion* 5:216, 1965.
450. Harrison K.L., Popper E.I.: Maternal J_k^a sensitization following amniocentesis and intrauterine transfusion. *Transfusion* 21:90, 1981.
451. Judd W.J., Steiner E.A., Cochran R.K.: Paraben-associated autoanti-JK^a antibodies: Three examples detected using commercially prepared low-ionic-strength saline containing parabens. *Transfusion* 22:31, 1982.
452. Patten E., Beck C.E., Scholl C., et al.: Autoimmune hemolytic anemia with anti-Jk^a specificity in a patient taking Aldomet. *Transfusion* 17:517, 1977.
453. Sosler S.D., Behzad O., Garraty G., et al.: Acute hemolytic anemia due to a chlorpropamide dependent auto anti-JK^a. *Transfusion* 19:641, 1979.
454. Sosler S.D., Behzad O., Garraty G., et al.: Acute hemolytic anemia associated with a chlorpropamide-induced apparent auto-anti-Jk^a. *Transfusion* 24:206, 1984.
455. Coombs R.R.A., Mourant A.E., Race R.R.: Invivo isosentisation of red cells in babies with haemolytic disease. *Lancet* 1:264, 1946.
456. Levine P., Backer M., Wigod M., Ponder R.: A new human hereditary blood property (cellano) present in 99.8% of all bloods. *Science* 109:464, 1949.
457. Hardman J.T., Beck M.L., Pierce S.R.: Capillary IgG subclass determinations relationship to blood group specificity and therapy (abstract). *Proc. Int. Soc. Hematol. (Montreal)* 1980.
458. Branch D.R., Petz L.D.: A new reagent having multiple applications in immunohematology (abstract). *Transfusion* 20:642, 1980.
459. Redman C.M., Marsh W.L., Mueller G.P., et al.: Isolation of Kell-active protein from the red cell membrane. *Transfusion* 24:176, 1984.
460. Hughes-Jones N.C., Gardner B.: The Kell system: Studies with radioactively-labelled anti-K. *Vox Sang.* 21:154, 1971.
461. Kikuchi M., Endo N., Okuho Y., et al.: A Japanese family with two $Kp(a-b-c+)$ members presumed genotype Kp^c/K^o. *Transfusion* 23:254, 1983.
462. Marsh W.L.: Chronic granulomatous disease, the McLeod syndrome, and the Kell blood groups. *Birth Defects* 14:9, 1978.
463. Marsh W.L., Øyen R., Nichols M.E.: Kx antigen, the McLeod phenotype, and chronic granulomatous disease: further studies. *Vox Sang.* 31:356, 1976.
464. Kline W.E., Sullivan C.M., Bowman R.J.: A rare example of weakened expression of the Kell (K_1) antigen. *Vox Sang.* 47:170, 1984.
465. Kornstad L., Heisto H.: The frequency of formation of Kell antibodies in recipients of Kell-positive blood, in *Proceedings of the 6th Congress of the European Society of Haematologists.* Copenhagen, 1957, p. 754.
466. Grove-Rasmussen M., Driesler N., Shaw R.S.: A serologic study of eight samples of anti-Kell serum. *Am. J. Clin. Pathol.* 24:1211, 1954.
467. Marsh W.L., Nichols M.E., Øyen R., et al.: Naturally-occurring anti-Kell stimulated by *E. coli* enterocolitis in a 20-day-old child. *Transfusion* 18:149, 1978.
468. Barrasso C., Baldwin M.L., Drew H., et al.: In vivo survival of K:18 red cells in a recipient with anti-K18. *Transfusion* 23:258, 1983.
469. Moulds J.J., Moulds M.K.: Inactivation of Kell blood group antigens by 2-aminoethylisothiouronium bromide. *Transfusion* 23:274, 1983.
470. Young L.E.: Blood groups and transfusion reactions. *Am. J. Med.* 16:885, 1954.
471. Van Loghem J.J., de Raad H., Van Hattem A.: Erythroblastosis foetalis en de bloedgroep Kell. *Maandschr. Kindergeneesk.* 21:63, 1953.
472. Freda R. quoted in Mollison P.L.: *Blood Transfusion in Clinical Medicine,* ed. 7. Oxford, England, Blackwell Scientific Publications, 1983, p. 238.
473. Viggiano E., Clary N.L., Ballas S.K.: Auto anti-K antibody mimicking an alloantibody. *Transfusion* 22:329, 1982.
474. Judd W.J., Walter W.J., Steiner E.A.: Clinical finding on two patients with naturally occurring anti-Kell agglutinins. *Transfusion* 21:184, 1981.
475. McGinniss M.H., MacLowry J.D., Holland P.V.: Acquisition of K_1-like antigen during terminal sepsis. *Transfusion* 24:28, 1984.
476. Tegoli J., Sausais L., Issitt P.D.: Another example of a "naturally occurring" anti-K_1. *Vox Sang.* 12:305, 1967.
477. Taddie S.J., Barrasso C., Ness P.M.: A delayed transfusion reaction caused by anti-K6. *Transfusion* 22:68, 1982.
478. Giblett E.R., Klebanoff S.J., Pincus S.H., et al.: Kell phenotypes in chronic granulomatous disease: A potential transfusion hazard. *Lancet* 1:1235, 1971.
479. Wimer B.M., Marsh W.L., Taswell H.F., et al.: Haematological changes associated with the McLeod phenotype of the Kell blood group system. *Br. J. Haematol.* 36:219, 1977.
480. Marsh W.L., Marsh N.J., Moore A., et al.: Elevated serum creatine phosphokinase in subjects with McLeod syndrome. *Vox Sang.* 40:403, 1981.
481. Marsh W.L.: Deleted antigens of the Rhesus and Kell blood groups: Associated with cell membrane defects, in Garraty G. (ed.): *Blood Group Antigens and Disease.* Arlington, Va., American Association of Blood Banks, 1983, p. 165.
482. Densen P., Wilkinson-Kroovand S., Mardell G.L., et al.: Kx: Its relationship to chronic granulomatous disease and genetic linkage with Xg. *Blood* 58:34, 1981.
483. Taswell H.F., Lewis J.C., Marsh W.L., et al.: Erythrocyte morphology in genetic defects of the Rh and Kell blood group systems. *Mayo Clin. Proc.* 52:157, 1977.
484. Corcoran P.A., Allen F.H., Lewis M., et al.: A new antibody anti-Ku (anti-Peltz) in the Kell blood group system. *Transfusion* 1:181, 1961.
485. White W., Washington E.D., Sabo B.H., et al.: Anti-Km in a transfused man with McLeod syn-

drome. *Blood Transfus. Immunohematol.* 23:305, 1980.
486. Marsh W.L., Øyen R., Nichols M.E., Allen F.H. Jr.: Chronic granulomatous disease and the Kell groups. *Br. J. Haematol.* 29:247, 1975.
487. Marsh W.L., Schnipper E.F., Johnson C.L., Mueller K.A., Schwartz S.A.: An individual with McLeod syndrome and the Kell blood group antigen K (K1). *Transfusion* 23:336, 1983.
488. Bryant N.J.: *Introduction to Immunohematology,* ed. 2. Philadelphia, W.B. Saunders Co., 1982, p. 394.
489. Mann J.D., Cahan A., Gelb A.G., et al.: A sex-linked blood group. *Lancet* 6:8, 1962.
490. Sparkes R.S., Crist M., Sparkes M.C.: Evidence of autonomous red cell expression of Xg^a antigen in human bone marrow transplantation. *Vox Sang.* 46:119, 1984.
491. Race R.R., Sanger R.: *Blood Groups in Man,* ed. 6. Oxford, England, Blackwell Scientific Publications, 1975, p. 578.
492. Mollison P.L.: *Blood Transfusion in Clinical Medicine,* ed. 7. Oxford, England, Blackwell Scientific Publications, 1983, pp. 428–429.
493. Azar P.M., Saji, H., Yamanaka R., et al.: Anti-Xg^a suspected of causing a transfusion reaction. *Transfusion* 22:340, 1982.
494. Marsh W.L.: Linkage relationship of the Xg and X_k loci. *Cytogenet. Cell Genet.* 22:531, 1978.
495. Sussman L.N., Miller E.B.: Un nouveau facteur sanguin "Vel." *Rev. Hematol.* 7:368, 1952.
496. Race R.R., Sanger R.: *Blood Groups in Man,* ed. 6. Oxford, England, Blackwell Scientific Publications, 1975, p. 415.
497. Cleghorn T.E.: *The Occurrence of Certain Rare Blood Groups in Britain,* thesis. University of Sheffield, 1961, quoted by Race R.R., Sanger R.: *Blood Groups in Man,* ed. 6. Oxford, England, Blackwell Scientific Publications, 1975, p. 415.
498. Drachman D., Lundsgaard A.: Prenatal assessment of blood group antibodies against public antigens: An example of anti-Ve (Vel) in pregnancy. *Scand. J. Haematol.* 7:37, 1970.
499. Rosenfield, R.E., et al.: Ge: A very common red-cell antigen. *Br. J. Haematol.* 6:344, 1960.
500. Booth P.B., McLoughlin K.: The Gerbich blood group system especially in Melanesians. *Vox Sang.* 22:73, 1972.
501. van der Hart M., Mose M., van der Veer M., et al.: Ho and Lan: Two new blood group antigens, Read before the VIII European Congress on Haematology, 1961, quoted by Race R.R., Sanger R.: *Blood Groups in Man,* ed. 6. Oxford, England, Blackwell Scientific Publications, 1975, p. 411.
502. Smith D.S., et al.: Haemolytic disease of the newborn caused by anti-Lan antibody. *Br. Med. J.* 3:90, 1969.
503. Macvie S.J., Morton J.A., Pickles M.M.: The reactions and inheritance of a new blood group antigen, Sd^a. *Vox Sang.* 13:485, 1967.
504. Morton J.A., Pickles M.M., Terry A.M.: The Sd^a blood group antigen in tissue and body fluids. *Vox Sang.* 19:472, 1970.
505. Sanger R., et al.: Plant agglutinin for another blood group. *Lancet* 1:1130, 1971.
506. Darnborough J., Dunsford I., Wallace J.A.: The En^a antigen and antibody: A genetical modification of human red cells affecting their blood grouping reactions. *Vox Sang.* 17:241, 1965.
507. Furuhjelm U., et al.: The red cell phenotype En(a−) and anti-En^a: Serological and physicochemical aspects. *Vox Sang.* 17:256, 1969.
508. Issitt P.D., Wilkinson-Kroovand S., Langley J.W., et al.: Production of allo-anti-En^a by an individual whose red blood cells carry some En^a antigen. *Transfusion* 21:211, 1981.
509. Pavone B.G., Billman R., Bryani J., et al.: An auto-anti-En^a, inhibitable by MN sialoglycoprotein. *Transfusion* 21:25, 1981.
510. Davidsohn I., Stern K., Strauser E.R., et al.: Be, a "new" private blood factor. *Blood* 8:747, 1953.
511. Cleghorn T.E.: A "new" human blood group antigen, Sw^a. *Nature* 184:1324, 1959.
512. Metaxas-Buhler M., Metaxas M.N., Giles C.M: A Swiss family showing inheritance of the Swann antigen with Lu^a. *Vox Sang.* 23:429, 1972.
513. Springer G.F., Tegmeyer H.: Origin of anti-Thomsen-Friedenreich (T) and Tn agglutinins in man and in white leghorn chicks. *Br. J. Haematol.* 47:453, 1981.
514. Prokop O., Uhlenbruch G.: *Human Blood and Serum Groups,* ed. 3. New York, Wiley Interscience, 1969, p. 108.
515. Uhlenbruch G.: Das Studium der Zelloherflache mit Helfe von Enzyme. *Mitt. Max Plank Ges.* 4:227, 1965.
516. Hübner G.: Untersuchungen über Isoagglutination, mit besonderer Berucksichtigung scheinbarer Abweichungen von Gruppenschema. *Z. Immun. Forsch.* 45:223, 1925.
517. Friedenreich V.: *The Thomsem Hemagglutination Phenomenon.* Copenhagen, Levine and Munksgaard, 1930, p. 128.
518. Anstee D.J.: The blood group MNSs-active sialoglycoproteins. *Semin. Hematol.* 18:13, 1981.
519. Rawilson V.I., Stratton F.: Incidence of T activation in a hospital population. *Vox Sang.* 46:306, 1984.
520. Bird G.W.G.: Lectins and red cell polyagglutinability: History, comments and recent developments, in Beck M.L., Judd W.J. (eds.): *Polyagglutination.* Washington, D.C., American Association of Blood Banks, 1980, p. 70.
521. Vaith P., Uhlenbruck G.: The Thomsen agglutination phenomenon: A discovery revisited 50 years later. *Z. Immunitoetsforsch. Immunobiol.* 154:1, 1978.
522. Rickard K.A., Robinson R.J., Worlledge S.M.: Acute acquired haemolytic anaemia associated with polyaagglutination. *Arch. Dis. Child.* 44:102, 1969.
523. Obeid D., Bird G.W.G., Wingham J.: Prolonged erythrocyte T-polyagglutination in two children

with bowel disorders. *J. Clin. Pathol.* 30:953, 1977.
524. Klein P.J., Bulla M., Newman R.A., et al.: Thomsen-Friedenreich antigen in hemolytic uremic syndrome. *Lancet* 2:1024, 1977.
525. Bird G.W.G., Wingham J.: Tk: A new form of red cell polyagglutination. *Br. J. Haematol.* 23:759, 1972.
526. Doinel C., Andreu G., Cartron J.P., et al.: Tk polyagglutination produced in vitro by an endo-beta galactosidase. *Vox Sang.* 38:94, 1980.
527. Inglis G., Bird G.W.G., Mitchell A.A.B., et al.: Effect of *Bacterioides fragilis* in the human erythrocyte membrane: Pathogenesis of Tk polyagglutination. *J. Clin. Pathol.* 28:964, 1975.
528. Inglis G., Bird G.W.G., Mitchell A.A.B., et al.: Tk polyagglutination associated with reduced A and H activity. *Vox Sang.* 35:370, 1978.
529. Bird G.W.G., Wingham J.: *Vicia cretica:* A powerful lectin for T− and Th− but not Tk− or other polyagglutinable erythrocytes. *J. Clin. Pathol.* 34:69, 1981.
530. Bird G.W.G., Wingham J., Beck M.L., et al.: Th: A new form of erythrocyte polyagglutination. *Lancet* 1:1215, 1978.
531. Graninger W., Rameis H., Fisher K., et al.: VA: A new type of erythrocyte polyagglutination characterized by depressed H receptors and associated with hemolytic anemia. I. serological and hematological observations. *Vox Sang.* 32:195, 1977.
532. Cartron J.P., Nurden A.T.: Galactosyl transferase and membrane abnormality in human platelets from Tn-syndrome donor's. *Nature* 282:621, 1979.
533. Bird G.W.G., Shinton N.K., Wingham J.: Persistent mixed field polyagglutination. *Br. J. Haematol.* 21:443, 1971.
534. Cartron J.P., Andrew G., Cartron J., et al.: Demonstration of T-transferase deficiency in Tn-polyagglutinable blood samples. *Eur. J. Biochem.* 92:111, 1978.
535. Ness P.H., Garraty G., Morel P.A.: Tn-polyagglutination preceding acute leukemia (abstract), in *Proceedings of the 30th Annual Meeting of the American Association of Blood Banks.* Atlanta, 1977, p. 6.
536. Sanger R., Gavin J., Tippett P., et al.: Plant agglutinin for another human blood-group. *Lancet* 1:1130, 1971.
537. Bizot M.: Comportement de quelques extraits des gasteropodes terrestres vis-à-vis des substances de specificité Sd^a. *Rev. Fr. Transfus.* 15:371, 1972.
538. Race R.R., Sanger R.: *Blood Groups in Man,* ed. 6. Oxford, England, Blackwell Scientific Publications, 1975, p. 403.
539. Peetermans M.E., Cole-Dergent J.: Haemolytic transfusion reaction due to anti-Sd^a. *Vox Sang.* 18:67, 1970.
540. Worlledge S.M.: Red cell antigens in dyserythropoiesis, in Lewis S.M., Verwilghen R.A.L. (eds.): *Dyserythropoiesis.* New York, Academic Press, 1977, p. 1.
541. Crookston J.H., Crookston M.C.: HEMPAS: Clinical, hematologic, and serologic features, in Salmon C. (ed.): *Blood Groups and Other Red Cell Markers in Health and Disease.* New York, Masson Publishing, 1982, p. 1.
542. Yang E.K.L., Spence L.R., Harding R.Y., et al.: A "new" lectin for detection of T, Tn, and Th polyagglutination. *Transfusion* 22:338, 1982.
543. Judd W.J., Oberman H.A., Flynn S.: Fatal intravascular hemolysis associated with T-polyagglutination. *Transfusion* 22:345, 1982.
544. Bird G.W.G.: Complexity of erythrocyte polyagglutinability, in *Human Blood Groups.* New York, S. Karger, 1977, p. 335.
545. Klarkowski D.B., Ford D.S.: A case of polyagglutination with features of Th and Tk activation associated with an acquired B antigen. *Transfusion* 23:59, 1983.
546. Bird G.W.G., Wingham J., Pippard M.J., et al.: Erythrocyte membrane modifications in malignant disease of myeloid and lymphoreticular tissues. *Br. J. Haematol.* 33:289, 1976.
547. Springer G.F., Desai P.R., Yang H.J., et al.: Carcinoma-associated blood group MN precursor antigens against which all humans possess antibodies. *Clin. Immunol. Immunopathol.* 7:426, 1977.
548. Okubo Y., Seno T., Yamasuchi H.: A persistent type of erythrocyte polyagglutinability Th. *Transfusion* 24:277, 1984.

6

Laboratory Aspects of Blood Banking

THE IMMUNOHEMATOLOGY LABORATORY is unique in a variety of aspects. It is one of the few laboratories which provide a product (blood units, fresh frozen plasma, platelets). These products must be safe and of high quality for safe therapy. However, the risks involved in providing a therapeutic product rather than a laboratory result only make the immunohematology laboratory radically different from other clinical laboratories. The blood bank falls under the jurisdiction of the Food and Drug Administration (FDA), in terms of regulation of therapeutic product quality control, and legally it may be liable for any complication resulting from the transfusion of blood or blood products. These legal liabilities of blood banks are discussed in chapter 18.

Because of the responsibility to provide safe therapeutic products, immunohematology laboratories must comply with certain requirements. The laboratory must be a meticulously clean area so that blood products are not contaminated during laboratory testing. It must also be a well-lit, pleasant, and quiet area, separated from usual laboratory traffic and barred to unauthorized personnel. Technologists whose interpretation relies on somewhat subjective observations must not be distracted. The work area should be uncluttered and ample (3 × 2 feet of benchtop working space per person). The benchtop should be about 30 inches high. White or light-colored Formica surfaces are good for reading agglutination reactions. Neon tube daylight lighting is adequate for laboratory work of this kind.

ANTIGEN-ANTIBODY TESTING IN THE IMMUNOHEMATOLOGY LABORATORY

Chapter 5 reviewed the major antigens that can cause clinical problems in transfusion and described some of the laboratory problems that can arise during antibody testing. This chapter will begin by reviewing general aspects of laboratory testing to promote a better understanding of how antibodies are investigated in the blood bank laboratory.

Antigens of various forms may react with antibodies specifically synthesized against them. The reactivity depends in part on the number of antigen molecules present on the surface of RBCs (e.g., 10,000 Rh antigens or 1 million ABH antigens per RBC). One factor that determines the amount of antigen presented is zygocity, in antigens which exhibit such phenotypic representation (e.g., MN, Rh, etc.).

RBCs of homozygous individuals react much more strongly than RBCs of heterozygous individuals in certain systems (i.e., MM RBCs agglutinate more strongly with anti-M than MN RBCs).

A variety of conditions affect antigen-antibody reactivity in vitro. One of these conditions is the acidity of the incubation medium—certain antibodies react better in a slightly acidified medium. For instance, anti-D antibodies react better in a medium with a pH range between 6.5 and 7.[1] Ionic strength is another condition that affects reactivity to a degree that special low ionic strength solutions have recently been introduced as routine blood bank incubating solutions. In general, slight decrements in the ionic strength of commonly used saline solutions will enhance antibody reactivity.[2] A decrement in ionic strength is achieved by decreasing the percentage of saline from 0.9% to 0.2% and adding glucose to a 7% concentration, thus preserving the osmolarity of the solution. This method has been called a low ionic strength solution (LISS) method. However, the method does have pitfalls; for instance, LISS testing may fail to detect clinically significant antibodies, as demonstrated in one series in which 3 out of 16 cases of anti-Kell antibodies failed to react in this medium.[3]

Antibodies have certain optimal thermal ranges for reacting. Most ABH IgM antibodies react better at cold temperatures and at room temperature, whereas IgG antibodies, such as those elicited against the Rh, Duffy, and some other clinically significant antigens, react better at 37°C.

The speed of centrifugation may also affect laboratory readings. For most purposes, the minimum speed and the minimum time required to produce a well-delineated button of a 5% solution of cells in an immunohematology laboratory test tube are selected for reading routine tests.

The quality of the test cells should be determined by subjecting them to a working centrifugation at 1,000–2,000 rpm for 1 or 2 minutes in a fixed-speed centrifuge.

Other factors determining antigen-antibody reactivity are those that decrease the zeta potential on the surface of cells. High-protein solutions (22%–30% albumin solutions)[4] or treatment of RBCs with enzymes which decrease the membrane sialic acid content[5] bring cells closer together, decreasing the zeta potential and increasing the chance of an antigen-antibody reaction. This improves reactivity in certain antigenic systems, especially those eliciting IgG antibodies (Rh, Duffy, Kell, etc.).

THE COOMBS TEST

The Coombs test, otherwise known as the antiglobulin test, was initially used by Moreschi in 1908[6] and was introduced to blood banking by Coombs et al. in 1945.[7] The principle of the test is that an antibody directed against human serum is capable of bridging the distance between molecules such as IgG or complement, which are bound to RBCs (Fig 6–1) but which by themselves are incapable of bridging the distance between RBCs, to cause agglutination.

In the direct Coombs test, cells are incubated with antiglobulin immediately after a pellet is obtained, and the RBCs are washed with saline. Thus, the only antibody molecules detected by the antihuman serum antibody Coombs reagent are those that have been attached or bound to the patient's RBCs while in the body of the patient. This test is useful for detecting a variety of conditions (e.g., autoimmune hemolytic anemia).

In the classic indirect Coombs test the cells of the patient are incubated in a test tube with the patient's own serum at different temperatures. The cells are then washed to eliminate unbound antibody from the added serum. The anti-human antibody Coombs reagent is then added and incubated with the coated patient's cells. If antibody coating of RBCs is indeed present the RBCs will agglutinate.

The indirect Coombs test has been applied to other types of testing in the blood bank. For instance, if an antiserum of the IgG class is used to detect Kell antigens in order to phenotype a cell putatively positive for Kell antigens, the cells are incubated with the typing antiserum, washed, and reacted with the coated cells. If these cells agglutinate, it can be presumed that the antigen is present on the cells tested. Conversely, if an IgG antibody in the patient's serum is suspected, the serum is incubated with cells of known phenotype. The test cells are then washed and Coombs reagent added. If agglutination is seen it is presumed that antibodies in the patient are of the specificity defined by the prephenotyped RBCs (see subsequent discussion of antibody detection).

Since the Coombs reagent is prepared by injecting whole human serum into goats or rabbits, the reagent will detect coating of cells not only by IgG antibodies but also by other antibody classes, such as IgA, or by nonantibody proteins such as complement, especially C3 and C4. This is especially important when IgM antibodies are searched for, because IgM per se does not remain attached to the RBCs but instead binds complement to the cells and then becomes detached from the cells. The cells therefore react with the Coombs reagent because of complement binding rather than because of IgM binding. In addition, eluates from IgM-mediated antibodies are usually not reactive, because only complement is left on the cell as evidence of IgM antibody attachment to the RBC. This explains the lack of reactivity of eluates in these cases. Nevertheless, antibodies may be detected by patterns of reactivity of the tested cells to which complement has been attached.

It is clear that the Coombs test can be used in various ways to detect immunoglobulin on cell surfaces. Several antibodies, including those directed against Lewis, Duffy, and Kell system antigens, bind complement, but the cells are not lysed. This is because complement activation stops at C3d or C4d, which are detected by the antiglobulin reagent due to its anti-β-globulin specificities.

The quality of the reagent is controlled in the laboratory by coating Rh-positive cells in vitro with anti-D antibody and then testing the reagent at serial dilutions. The highest dilution giving a 1+ reactivity is used for control.

The quality of anticomplement activity is controlled by reacting cells with an antibody known to bind C3b (e.g., anti-Lewis antibodies) and detecting its presence with the antiglobulin antiserum. To coat cells with C4b, the cells are reacted with anti-I and then incubated with the antiglobulin. Alternatively, RBCs can be incubated with normal serum, 10% sucrose, and EDTA.[8] This method yields good results for binding of C3 and C4.

Pitfalls of the Coombs (Antiglobulin) Test

Errors in the Coombs test may stem from direct antibody coating of RBCs or from physicochemical factors that affect agglutination. Some of the more common laboratory pitfalls in the Coombs test are neutralization resulting from residual globulin in a sample which has not been washed properly, contamination of the reagent by globulin as a result of carryover, or expiration of a reagent. All three conditions may produce false negative results. Another less common pitfall causing a false negative Coombs test is elution of antibody from cells. This may result from failure to incubate the cells at the appropriate temperature. Calcium chelating agents such as EDTA and citrate phosphate in dextrose, as well as other substances, may prevent attachment of complement, thus producing false negative results in complement-dependent Coombs testing. Insufficient incubation periods, centrifugation at a lower speed than that required for the test, weak cell suspensions, or failure to add the reagent are also causes of negative results.

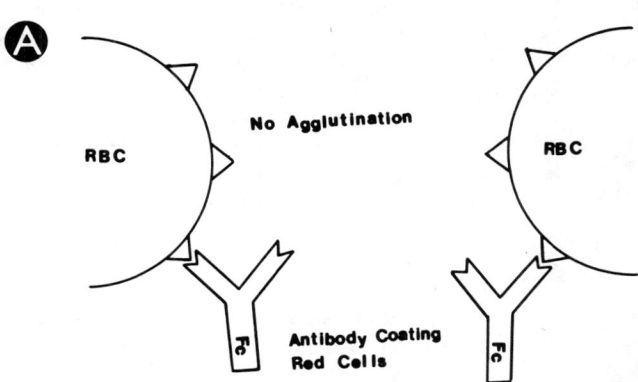

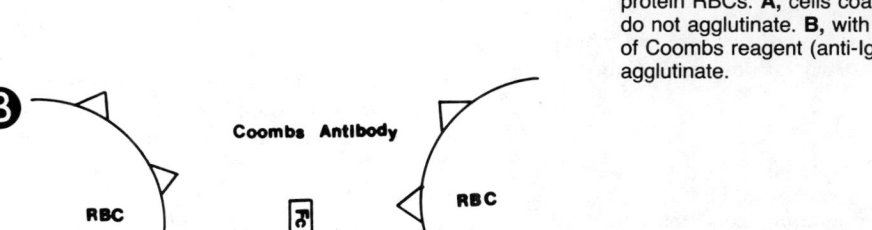

FIG 6–1.—How the Coombs reagent is used for the detection of antibody protein RBCs. **A**, cells coated with IgG do not agglutinate. **B**, with the addition of Coombs reagent (anti-IgG), cells agglutinate.

False positive Coombs tests may be the result of direct antigen-antibody specificities or altered physicochemical phenomena. With respect to the former, there may be specificities in the reagent not related to the antiglobulin specificity. Examples of these are inappropriately absorbed antisera or anti-T activity in a sample which is T-activated due to contamination or other causes (see Chap. 5). Antitransferrin activity may cause false positive reactions with cells coated with this protein. This may be the cause of agglutination of reticulocytes by the Coombs reagent.[9] Naturally occurring cold antibodies (e.g., anti-I or anti-ABH antibodies) present in the sample may cause false positive results. Of course, cells that have been coated in vivo should not be used in indirect Coombs testing, for this in itself will produce a positive test.

Physicochemical factors producing false positive tests include overcentrifugation, high protein content in the serum, or residual fibrin in improperly clotted samples. Silica leached from the glass of containers used for reagent storage and substances leached from metal containers are also capable of producing false positive tests, as is improperly cleaned glassware.

Coombs Panels

The Coombs panel may be made more specific by reacting the cells thought to be coated by immunoglobulins or complement with reagents specific for individual isotypes (e.g., anti-IgG, anti-IgA) as well as with reagents that help distinguish binding of C3 versus C4. This test is a further step in defining which molecules are causing the Coombs reaction. For instance, antibodies which may be predominantly IgA (e.g., some anti-Lu^b antibodies[10]) and which may not be detected with a routine Coombs test can be clarified by using anti-IgA in the Coombs phase.

The Coombs panel may also help pinpoint specific antibodies in patients with multiple antibodies of different isotypes.

Uses of the Coombs Test

The Coombs test is an immensely useful diagnostic test in the immunohematology laboratory. It is commonly used to diagnose hemolytic disease of the newborn,[11] autoimmune hemolytic anemia,[12] and RBC sensitization by pharmacologic agents.[13] These uses will be detailed further in Chapter 10.

It has recently been shown that F(ab)$_2$ fragments agglutinate cells more effectively than do complete immunoglobulins. This finding has potential application to Coombs testing.[14]

A chromogenic enzyme-linked assay has also recently been introduced for Coombs testing. This system is highly sensitive to otherwise undetectable antibodies.[15] In certain cases antibodies are loosely bound to RBCs and may be lost during washing. However, a new method (Graham's method) in which RBCs and serum are separated without washing may be employed.[16]

ANTIBODY DETECTION AND IDENTIFICATION

Antibody Detection

To screen for the presence of significant antibodies frequently found in the population, the serum of the recipient is tested against a pool of RBCs which contains antigens prevalent in donor RBCs. To avoid isoantigen agglutination by anti-A or anti-B in the patient's serum, the test cells must be group O; frequent antigens must be present in at least 30% of the RBCs in the pool of screening cells.[17] Low-incidence antigens often are not represented in these pools. However, D, C, E, c, e, K, Fy^a and Fy^b, M, N, S, s, P, and Lu, Xg should be present. The cells should be homozygous for these antigens, if possible. The screening cell pools may be from up to three recipients, and two or three pools may be used. A single pool may also be used, provided 30% of RBCs contain each antigen present.

Usually screening pools are obtained from commercial sources. Many of the larger companies work with the buyer to solve problems associated with use of their products. They are also under the jurisdiction of the FDA and therefore must comply with strict quality control regulations. Certain aspects must be kept in mind, however—the suspending medium is frequently not known, and the solutions may contain anticoagulants that affect complement binding. It is mandatory, therefore, to follow the instructions provided by the company for use of its products without changing any part of the test protocol.

In addition, the screening test may be incorrectly interpreted if the patient's serum contains antibodies against substances used in the reagents.[18]

If the cells are supplied as a suspension of 25% or more, several washings may be necessary to eliminate the suspending solutions. The expiration date of each reagent is stated on the vial and should be monitored carefully as part of quality control in the laboratory.[19] Screening cells are incubated at various temperatures and may be subjected to certain manipulations, such as enzyme treatment to expose antigens or incubation in high-protein solutions such as albumin to decrease the zeta potential. Cells are usually first incubated at room temperature with the patient's serum. In certain laboratories, however, cold-reacting antibodies are sought at lower temperatures (e.g., 12°C). Samples are then incubated at 37°C, usually in the presence of albumin. Antibodies reacting in this phase are usually of the incomplete or IgG type. After this incubation, the samples are reacted with Coombs reagent. This phase is called the antiglobulin phase of incubation and may detect IgGs which were nonreactive in the albumin phase or may detect binding of complement, for the antiglobulin reagent is capable of detecting both IgG and complement. Many complement-binding antibodies are of the IgM type, although IgG antibodies that bind complement are not infrequent. It is very important that variability in serum to cell ratios be controlled whenever possible.

If the patient's serum reacts with the screening cells at any stage of incubation, a true antibody is likely. An educated guess as to the nature of the antibody reactivity can be made by analyzing the results in each of the incubations performed. For example, if the patient's serum reacts only at cold temperatures, the antibody is probably of the IgM class. However, if the antibody is reactive at 37°C it probably represents an IgG antibody. As another example, if an antibody disappears after incubation with enzymes, it may be an anti-Duffy or an anti-M antibody, for these antibodies are destroyed by proteolytic enzymes. Nevertheless, to identify with assurance the specificity of an antibody, the patient must be studied by antibody identification with the help of an RBC panel (Fig 6–2).

Antibody Identification

RBC Panels

The RBC panel identification test follows essentially the same principles as the antibody screening test. Ordinarily, different cells may be included in the panel. Each cell is phenotyped for the more frequent antigens and the phenotype is recorded on the worksheet provided with the reagent cell vials (Fig 6–2). Cells are selected for inclusion in the panel such that every antigen in the panel has a specific reactivity pattern different from the pattern of agglutination of any other antigen. Special donor cells are used to obtain these differences in patterns of reactivity. Data processing equipment has facilitated selection of cell combinations with adequate antigenic reactivity providing these differential patterns. In a six-cell panel, three cells should exhibit the antigen and three cells should be negative for the antigen to provide a 1:20 probability of identification. A statistical P value less than 1:20 permits excessive random association.[20]

Each cell is group O, to bypass anti-A and anti-B reactivity in the patient's serum. A few drops of the patient's serum are tested individually against each cell, in parallel, in individual tubes. The samples are incubated at different temperatures and finally with antiglobulin. The results are graded and recorded, the reactivity is analyzed, and possible antibodies are considered according to the reactivity patterns. Antigens with the least probable combinations are eliminated.

The next step is to ascertain what antigens could be responsible for the reactivity patterns. Any given selection must be accompanied by positive reactions with the cells giving the specific pattern. Antigens which do not follow the reactivity of the patient's serum agglutination pattern are not responsible for the agglutination and may be crossed out on the patient's panel sheet. All antigens that match the pattern produced by the patient's serum are ruled in as possibly responsible for agglutination of the test cells. Differences in reactivity between cells suggest that multiple antibodies in the patient's sample may be responsible for the positive agglutination pattern. For practical purposes, antigens ruled out as causes of agglutination in a panel must also be absent from the patient's cells, unless there is a possibility of autoimmune hemolytic anemia.

An Approach to Reading RBC Panels.— The results of reacting a patient's serum against each of the cells in an RBC panel can be recorded on a worksheet where the phenotypes of the cells for each of the antigens have been printed. A good method for grading results has been reported by Marsh.[21] In this method, the strength of agglutination is graded from 1 to 12, with 12 being the most reactive.

Once the results are recorded, one can begin the interpretation. Cross out the antigens that are not producing agglutination in any single cell. Start

Red Cell Panel

Patient's Serum

Cell No.	D	C	E	c	e	f	C^w	V	K	k	Kp^a	Kp^b	Js^a	Js^b	Fy^a	Fy^b	Jk^a	Jk^b	Xg^a	Le^a	Le^b	S	s	M	N	P_1	Lu^a	Lu^b		S	Al	Ag	E
1	+	+	o	o	+	o	+	o	o	+	o	+	o	+	+	+	o	+	+	+	o	o	+	o	+	+	o	+					
2	+	+	o	o	+	o	o	o	+	+	o	+	o	+	o	+	+	o	+	o	+	o	+	o	+	+	o	+					
3	+	o	+	+	o	o	o	o	o	+	o	+	o	+	+	+	+	+	+	o	+	o	+	+	+	o	o	+					
4	o	+	o	+	+	+	o	o	o	+	o	+	o	+	+	o	+	o	+	o	+	o	+	+	+	+	o	+					
5	o	o	+	+	+	+	o	o	o	+	o	+	o	+	+	+	o	+	+	o	o	+	+	+	+	+	o	+					
6	o	o	o	+	+	+	o	o	+	+	o	+	o	+	o	+	+	+	+	o	+	o	+	+	+	+	o	+					
7	o	o	o	+	+	+	o	o	o	+	o	+	o	+	o	+	+	+	+	+	o	+	+	+	+	+	o	+					
8	o	o	o	+	+	+	o	o	o	+	o	+	o	+	+	o	+	+	+	o	o	o	+	+	+	+	o	+					
9	o	o	o	+	+	+	o	o	o	+	o	+	o	+	o	o	o	+	+	o	o	o	+	+	+	+	o	+					
10	o	o	o	+	+	+	o	o	o	+	o	+	o	+	+	+	o	+	o	o	+	o	+	o	+	o	o	+					
11	+	+	o	+	+	+	o	o	o	+	o	+	o	+	o	+	+	+	o	+	o	+	o	+	+	o	o	+					
12	o	o	o	+	+	+	o	o	o	+	o	+	+	o	+	o	+	o	+	+	o	o	+	o	+	+	+	+					
13	+	+	+	+	+	o	o	o	o	+	o	+	o	+	o	+	+	+	+	o	+	o	+	+	o	o	+	+					
14	+	+	+	o	+	o	o	o	o	+	o	+	o	+	+	+	+	+	+	+	o	+	o	+	o	o	o	+					
Pt																																	

Comments: — cord cell

A_1

Diagnosis: — A_2

B

FIG 6–2.—Typical RBC panel. The test RBCs are numbered from 1 to 14 on the left-hand side of the panel. Each cell is phenotyped for the antigens listed in the top row of the panel. The right side of the panel is used to record the results of incubating the patient's serum with each of the test cells in saline *(S)* at room temperature, albumin *(Al)* at 37°C, and antiglobulin *(Ag)* at 37°C. A separate column labeled *E* is designated for results of incubating cells after treatment with enzymes. At bottom of panel is a row for autocontrols, labeled *PT* (patient cells). Also at bottom of panel, incubation with cord cells, A_1, A_2, and group B cells is recorded.

with cell 1 and work in an ascending manner, following the numerical sequence of the cells in the panel (Fig 6–3). After all the antigens that could not have produced such a reaction are eliminated, the most probable antibodies remain. In Figure 6–3, the most probable antibody is directed against the D antigen in the Rh system. This assumption is further supported by the fact that the phenotype of the patient is dce.

As mentioned earlier, each antigen and its specific antibody react under special incubation conditions. For instance in Figure 6–4 a cold-reacting antibody in saline agglutinates all the cells in the panel except the cord cells, pointing to the diagnosis of anti-I specificity. In contrast, Figure 6–5 is a representative panel for i specificity, since the only reactive cell is the cord cell. The patient in this case had anti-i antibodies following recovery from infectious mononucleosis (see Chap. 5 for discussion of anti-i antibodies). The panel in Figure 6–6 is characteristic of a cold-reacting antibody with a positive antiglobulin secondary to the binding of complement (anti-Lewis) and a warm-reacting antibody (anti-E). Figures 6–7 and 6–8 show combinations of antibodies frequently found. Figure 6–9 shows reactivity characteristic of that seen in a patient with autoimmune hemolytic anemia of the warm type.

Special Laboratory Techniques

In some cases, antibody specificities cannot be fully elucidated by the use of panels alone. The use of absorption and/or elution procedures may be necessary to further identify certain antibodies or to eliminate unwanted specificities that obscure the more important antibody specificities.

Red Cell Panel

[Figure: Red Cell Panel table with 14 cells tested against antigens D, C, E, c, e, f, Cw, V, K, k, Kpa, Kpb, Jsa, Jsb, Fya, Fyb, Jka, Jkb, Xga, Lea, Leb, S, s, M, N, P1, Lua, Lub, and patient's serum reactions in S, AI, AgE phases. Pt row is blank. Comments: Grading 0 to 4+. Diagnosis: anti-D. Cord cell, A1, A2, B rows blank.]

FIG 6–3.—Typical reactivity of a panel. An anti-D antibody is reacting in all phases of incubation. Note that anti-D antibodies are enhanced by enzymes.

Absorption

Not infrequently, multiply transfused patients or, less frequently, patients worked up in the immunohematology laboratory for the first time have a variety of antibodies to RBC antigens in their serum.

Some specificities, such as those of certain cold antibodies (e.g., anti-I), will not be clinically significant but may become relevant because they cloud specificities of other antibodies (e.g., anti-Kidd or anti-Kell). To eliminate such interference, the serum of the patient may be absorbed with RBCs possessing the unwanted specificities. The absorption procedure may be done indirectly, by absorption of a specificity as a demonstration of an antibody. This may be achieved by eliminating the reactivity of a serum to the specificity of the absorbing antigen. More directly, it may help separate specificities suspected in a panel workup.

The absorption procedure has also been used to eliminate anti-A or anti-B reactivity from sera containing antibodies with useful specificities, which can then be used as reagents.

Absorption Techniques.—Descriptions of the absorption techniques are available in reference textbooks on immunohematology.[22] This section discusses some uses of these techniques.

If a cold antibody is obscuring the laboratory results, the patient's serum can be autoabsorbed with the patient's own cells in the cold (4°–6°C) overnight. This method usually eliminates bothersome antibodies, such as anti-I, and allows further testing of the serum. Occasionally, enzyme-treated cells may have to be used to enhance absorption. Formaldehyde-treated cells may also be used for absorption, for the cells retain antigenic specificity and do not agglutinate.[23] Stroma is sometimes useful for absorption, providing the technique for obtaining stroma does not alter the antigenic specifications under scrutiny.

Absorptions are usually performed at tempera-

Red Cell Panel

Cell No.	D	C	E	c	e	f	C^w	V	K	k	Kp^a	Kp^b	Js^a	Js^b	Fy^a	Fy^b	Jk^a	Jk^b	Xg^a	Le^a	Le^b	S	s	M	N	P_1	Lu^a	Lu^b		Patient's Serum S	AI	Ag	E
1	+	+	o	o	+	o	+	o	o	+	o	+	o	+	+	+	o	+	+	+	o	o	+	o	+	+	o	+		4			
2	+	+	o	o	+	o	o	o	+	+	o	+	o	+	o	+	+	o	+	o	+	o	+	o	+	+	o	+		4			
3	+	o	+	+	o	o	o	o	o	+	o	+	o	+	+	+	+	+	+	o	+	o	+	+	+	o	o	+		4			
4	o	+	o	+	+	+	o	o	o	+	o	+	o	+	+	o	+	o	+	o	+	o	+	+	+	+	o	+		4			
5	o	o	+	+	+	+	o	o	o	+	o	+	o	+	+	+	o	+	+	o	o	+	+	+	+	+	o	+		4			
6	o	o	o	+	+	+	o	o	+	+	o	+	o	+	o	+	+	+	+	o	+	o	+	+	+	+	o	+		4			
7	o	o	o	+	+	+	o	o	o	+	o	+	o	+	o	+	+	+	+	+	o	+	+	+	+	+	o	+		4			
8	o	o	o	+	+	+	o	o	o	+	o	+	o	+	+	o	+	+	+	o	o	o	+	+	+	+	o	+		4			
9	o	o	o	+	+	+	o	o	o	+	o	+	o	+	o	o	o	+	+	o	o	o	+	+	+	+	o	+		4			
10	o	o	o	+	+	+	o	o	o	+	o	+	o	+	+	+	o	+	o	o	+	o	+	o	+	o	o	+		4			
11	+	+	o	+	+	+	o	o	o	+	o	+	o	+	o	+	+	+	o	+	o	+	o	+	+	o	o	+		4			
12	o	o	o	+	+	+	o	o	o	+	o	+	+	o	+	o	+	o	+	+	o	o	+	o	+	+	+	+		4			
13	+	+	+	+	+	o	o	o	o	+	o	+	o	+	o	+	+	+	+	o	+	o	+	+	o	o	+	+		4			
14	+	+	+	o	+	o	o	o	o	+	o	+	o	+	+	+	+	+	+	+	o	+	o	+	o	o	o	+		4			
Pt																														4			

Comments: Grading: 0 to 4+ Hx of Mycoplasmosis	cord cell	0
	A_1	
Diagnosis: anti: I	A_2	
	B	

FIG 6–4.—A typical panel showing anti-I antibodies after mycoplasmal infection. The patient's autocontrol is strongly positive and the cord cells are negative.

tures optimal for removal of antibody. These are the temperatures at which the putative antibody is more reactive (e.g., anti-I at 4°–6°C, warm autoantibodies at 37°C). Sometimes two absorptions will be necessary. However, care must be taken not to overabsorb sera, which could result in the Matuhashi-Ogata phenomenon. In this phenomenon significant specificities not intended to be absorbed out are absorbed from the problem serum.[24] Another testing problem is found when the serum is overdiluted due to residual diluent in the absorbing RBC buttons; significant antibody reactivities are lost when dilution is present.

To absorb out specific antigenic determinants from a serum with a mixture of antibodies, homozygote cells showing strong reactions with the serum are used. To select which cell to use for absorption, one may use prephenotyped cells from panels that have only one of the suspected specificities.

Paradoxically, certain antibody specificities thought to have been absorbed out may reappear. This is thought to be due to dissociation of soluble immune complexes.[25]

Elution

Elution of antibodies from RBCs requires stripping the antibody from coated RBCs without altering the antibody's capacity to react with the antigenic determinants. Elution is used to separate antibodies with significant specificities that may be obscured in a serum with multiple antibodies.

Several methods have been described for antibody elution. The heat method of Landsteiner[26] has been used successfully for several years. The method consists of absorbing the serum with RBCs at room temperature and stripping the antibody by heating the sample to 56°C. A similar method can be used to elute cold antibodies. These are adsorbed at 4°–6°C and then eluted at 37°C.

Eluates can be obtained from stroma, as first demonstrated by Kidd.[27] However, the method has since been modified, and eluates are obtained by stripping the stroma with ether.[28] These methods usually yield hemolyzed samples with significant free hemoglobin. This problem can be bypassed by the use of the low pH method[29] or the digitonin method.[30] The elution of antibodies from RBCs is used to define their specificity by reacting the eluate with cells of known antigenic reactivity. The procedure is extremely helpful in the definition of antibody specificities when multiple antibodies are thought to be causing reactivity. By including certain antigenic reactivities and excluding others, one can make an educated assumption as to the true specificity of such antibodies. Elution may be the only method of demonstrating a clinically significant antibody, especially when the antiglobulin test is negative. Similarly, in hemolytic disease of the newborn, the eluate from the baby's coated cells may be the only sample available for crossmatch for exchange transfusions if a maternal serum sample is unavailable. Thus, elution is useful in several complex conditions or in specialized immunohematology workups.

Neutralization

Neutralization is the use of purified antigens to absorb out a specificity from a serum sample. Since purified antigens are not readily available for many antigens, this method has limited value. However, purified A and B substances, Lewis substances, and other purified antigens may be used to demonstrate the presence of an antibody by the capacity of the specific antigen to neutralize it.

Lectins

Lectins are globular glycoproteins obtained from plants. These molecules have the capacity to combine specifically with certain carbohydrate moieties.[31] The specificity of the binding site on lectins depends on the anomeric configuration of carbohydrates linked to the terminal or subterminal posi-

Red Cell Panel

Cell No.	D	C	E	c	e	f	Cw	V	K	k	Kpa	Kpb	Jsa	Jsb	Fya	Fyb	Jka	Jkb	Xga	Lea	Leb	S	s	M	N	P1	Lua	Lub	Patient's Serum S	AI	Ag	E
1	+	+	o	o	+	o	+	o	o	+	o	+	o	+	+	+	o	+	+	+	o	o	+	o	+	+	o	+	o			
2	+	+	o	o	+	o	o	o	+	+	o	+	o	+	o	+	+	o	+	o	+	o	+	o	+	+	o	+	o			
3	+	o	+	+	o	o	o	o	o	+	o	+	o	+	+	+	+	+	+	o	+	o	+	+	+	o	o	+	o			
4	o	+	o	+	+	+	o	o	o	+	o	+	o	+	+	o	+	o	+	o	+	o	+	+	+	+	o	+	o			
5	o	o	+	+	+	+	o	o	o	+	o	+	o	+	+	+	o	+	+	o	o	+	+	+	+	+	o	+	o			
6	o	o	o	+	+	+	o	o	+	+	o	+	o	+	o	+	+	+	+	o	+	o	+	+	+	+	o	+	o			
7	o	o	o	+	+	+	o	o	o	+	o	+	o	+	o	+	+	+	+	+	o	+	+	+	+	+	o	+	o			
8	o	o	o	+	+	+	o	o	o	+	o	+	o	+	+	o	+	+	+	o	o	o	+	+	+	+	o	+	o			
9	o	o	o	+	+	+	o	o	o	+	o	+	o	+	o	o	o	+	+	o	o	o	+	+	+	+	o	+	o			
10	o	o	o	+	+	+	o	o	o	+	o	+	o	+	+	+	o	+	o	o	+	o	+	o	+	o	o	+	o			
11	+	+	o	+	+	+	o	o	o	+	o	+	o	+	o	+	+	+	o	+	o	+	o	+	+	o	o	+	o			
12	o	o	o	+	+	+	o	o	o	+	o	+	+	o	+	o	+	o	+	+	o	o	+	o	+	+	+	+	o			
13	+	+	+	+	+	o	o	o	o	+	o	+	o	+	o	+	+	+	+	o	+	o	+	+	o	o	+	+	o			
14	+	+	+	o	+	o	o	o	o	+	o	+	o	+	+	+	+	+	+	+	o	+	o	+	o	o	o	+	o			
Pt																																
Comments: Grading: 0 to 4+ Hx of Infectious Mononucleosis																												cord cell	4			
																												A_1				
Diagnosis: anti-i																												A_2				
																												B				

FIG 6–5.—Patient with anti-i antibodies after infectious mononucleosis. Only the cord cells are significantly reactive.

Red Cell Panel

Cell No.	D	C	E	c	e	f	C^w	V	K	k	Kp^a	Kp^b	Js^a	Js^b	Fy^a	Fy^b	Jk^a	Jk^b	Xg^a	Le^a	Le^b	S	s	M	N	P_1	Lu^a	Lu^b		Patient's Serum S	AI	Ag	E
1	+	+	o	o	+	o	+	o	o	+	o	+	o	+	+	+	o	+	+	+	o	o	+	o	+	+	o	+		4	1	4	
2	+	+	o	o	+	o	o	o	+	+	o	+	o	+	o	+	+	o	+	o	+	o	+	o	+	+	o	+		0	0	0	
3	+	o	+	+	o	o	o	o	o	+	o	+	o	+	+	+	+	+	+	o	+	o	+	+	+	o	o	+		0	4	4	
4	o	+	o	+	+	+	o	o	o	+	o	+	o	+	+	o	+	o	+	o	+	o	+	+	+	+	o	+		0	0	0	
5	o	o	+	+	+	+	o	o	o	+	o	+	o	+	+	+	o	+	+	o	o	+	+	+	+	+	o	+		0	4	4	
6	o	o	o	+	+	+	o	o	+	+	o	+	o	+	o	+	+	+	+	o	+	o	+	+	+	+	o	+		0	0	0	
7	o	o	o	+	+	+	o	o	o	+	o	+	o	+	o	+	+	+	+	+	o	+	+	+	+	+	o	+		4	1	4	
8	o	o	o	+	+	+	o	o	o	+	o	+	o	+	+	o	+	+	+	o	o	o	+	+	+	+	o	+		0	0	0	
9	o	o	o	+	+	+	o	o	o	+	o	+	o	+	o	o	o	+	+	o	o	o	+	+	+	+	o	+		0	0	0	
10	o	o	o	+	+	+	o	o	o	+	o	+	o	+	+	+	o	+	o	o	+	o	+	o	+	o	o	+		0	0	0	
11	+	+	o	+	+	+	o	o	o	+	o	+	o	+	o	+	+	+	o	+	o	+	o	+	+	o	o	+		4	1	4	
12	o	o	o	+	+	+	o	o	o	+	o	+	+	o	+	o	+	o	+	+	o	o	+	o	+	+	+	+		4	1	4	
13	+	+	+	+	+	o	o	o	o	+	o	+	o	+	o	+	+	+	+	o	+	o	+	+	o	o	+	+		0	4	4	
14	+	+	+	o	+	o	o	o	o	+	o	+	o	+	+	+	+	+	+	+	o	+	o	+	o	o	o	+		4	4	4	
Pt																														0	0	0	

Comments: Grading: 0 to 4+ — cord cell, A_1, A_2, B

Diagnosis: anti-Le^a & anti-E

other possible: C^w

FIG 6–6.—Red cell panel showing a combination of two antibodies, anti-Le^a, which is mostly reactive in the saline phase, and anti-E, mostly reactive in the 37°C incubation phase. Another possibility that should be excluded by the use of RBCs lacking the antigen is C^w.

tions of carbohydrate moiety N-antigens.[32] Therefore they may be used as agglutinating molecules, which at times are as specific as antibodies. One such example is the *Dolichos biflorus* lectin, which is specific for group A RBCs, although it has a much lower reactivity for group A_2 cells. *Ulex europaeus* is useful in the detection of H substance.[33] *Vicia graminea* exhibits anti-N reactivity,[34] and *Iberis amara,* anti-M reactivity. *Arachis hypogea* has a well-defined anti-T activity, whereas *Salvia sclarea* has anti-Tn reactivity.

These lectins are occasionally used for identification of specific antigenic determinants not easily definable by other means. For instance, in polyagglutination, lectins help define T, Tn, and Cad types of poly-C agglutination (see Table 5–13).

Phenotyping the Multiply Transfused Patient

In certain occasions multiply transfused patients must be phenotyped. The younger autologous cells are separated from the older transfused cells on the basis of density—older cells become denser as they age. The best technique uses phthalate ester gradients, which separate cells on the basis of their different densities. For a full description of the method, see Wallas et al.[35]

Monoclonal Antibodies

A new era of both research and diagnostic immunology was launched by Kohler and Milstein[36] when they showed it was possible to produce monoclonal antibodies by hybridization of immunized mouse cells with mouse plasmacytomas, thereby generating a continuous cell line, a "hybridoma" capable of synthesizing monoclonal antibodies with desired specificities.

The advantage of monoclonal antibodies over polyclonal antibodies is that they are a homogeneous population of molecules, unlike most other antibodies, which are heterogeneous. Furthermore, they recognize a distinct specificity rather than a variety of specificities directed to the multiple sites of an antigen.[37]

In terms of immunohematology research, several monoclonal antibodies have been obtained. For instance, it has been possible to produce monoclonal antibodies against high-frequency antigens present on glycophorin A complexes of RBC membranes.[38] In addition, in practical immunohematology, monoclonal antibodies to group A[39] and group B[40] substances have also been produced, as well as anti-C3 and anti-C4 antibodies, with a potential displacement of polyclonal antibodies currently used in the laboratory.

THE CROSSMATCH

As a test, the crossmatch has recently undergone much scrutiny with the idea of eliminating it. However, the crossmatch still has a definite role in immunohematology practice. It functions as a double-check on completed laboratory testing such as ABO typing, serum screen, and antibody panels, if the patient was found to have RBC antibodies.

Even in the presence of a compatible crossmatch, complete assurance that the cells in any particular unit will survive normally in the transfused host cannot be guaranteed. Thus, in spite of carefully performed laboratory procedures to ensure a safe product, certain units will be hemolyzed in the recipient in the context of a compatible crossmatch. The crossmatch is useful in revealing most major ABO incompatibilities and the presence of many otherwise undetected antibodies in the serum of the recipient.

The crossmatch originally introduced into immunohematology testing by Hectoen[41] was performed in two phases, the minor crossmatch and the major crossmatch. For historical purposes we will review these two phases.

Minor Crossmatch.—In modern blood banking, the minor crossmatch has been completely

Red Cell Panel

Cell No.	D	C	E	c	e	f	C^w	V	K	k	Kp^a	Kp^b	Js^a	Js^b	Fy^a	Fy^b	Jk^a	Jk^b	Xg^a	Le^a	Le^b	S	s	M	N	P_1	Lu^a	Lu^b	Patient's Serum S	Alb	Ag	E
1	+	+	o	o	+	o	+	o	o	+	o	+	o	+	+	+	o	+	+	+	o	o	+	o	+	+	o	+	±	0	±	1
2	+	+	o	o	+	o	o	o	+	+	o	+	o	+	o	+	+	o	+	o	+	o	+	o	+	+	o	+	±	3	3	3
3	+	o	+	+	o	o	o	o	o	+	o	+	o	+	+	+	+	+	+	o	+	o	+	+	+	o	o	+	±	0	±	1
4	o	+	o	+	+	+	o	o	o	+	o	+	o	+	+	o	+	o	+	o	+	o	+	+	+	+	o	+	±	0	±	1
5	o	o	+	+	+	+	o	o	o	+	o	+	o	+	+	+	o	+	+	o	o	+	+	+	+	+	o	+	±	0	±	1
6	o	o	o	+	+	+	o	o	+	+	o	+	o	+	o	+	+	+	+	o	+	o	+	+	+	+	o	+	±	3	3	3
7	o	o	o	+	+	+	o	o	o	+	o	+	o	+	o	+	+	+	+	+	o	+	+	+	+	+	o	+	±	0	±	1
8	o	o	o	+	+	+	o	o	o	+	o	+	o	+	+	o	+	+	+	o	o	o	+	+	+	+	o	+	±	0	±	1
9	o	o	o	+	+	+	o	o	o	+	o	+	o	+	o	o	o	+	+	o	o	o	+	+	+	+	o	+	±	0	±	1
10	o	o	o	+	+	+	o	o	o	+	o	+	o	+	+	+	o	+	o	o	+	o	+	o	+	o	o	+	±	0	±	1
11	+	+	o	+	+	+	o	o	o	+	o	+	o	+	o	+	+	+	o	+	o	+	o	+	+	o	o	+	±	0	±	1
12	o	o	o	+	+	+	o	o	o	+	o	+	+	o	+	o	+	o	+	+	o	o	+	o	+	+	+	+	±	0	±	1
13	+	+	+	+	+	o	o	o	o	+	o	+	o	+	o	+	+	+	+	o	+	o	+	+	o	o	+	+	±	0	±	1
14	+	+	+	o	+	o	o	o	o	+	o	+	o	+	+	+	+	+	+	+	o	+	o	+	o	o	o	+	±	0	±	1
Pt																													±	0	±	1

Comments: Grading: 0 to 4+

Diagnosis: Cold autoantibody and anti-K

	S	Alb	Ag	E
cord cell	±	0	±	1
A_1	±	0	±	1
A_2	±	0	±	1
B	±	0	±	1

FIG 6–7.—Panel showing a weak cold autoantibody reacting with all cells in the saline incubation as well as an anti-K alloantibody reacting in the 37°C incubation.

Red Cell Panel

Cell No.	D	C	E	c	e	f	Cw	V	K	k	Kpa	Kpb	Jsa	Jsb	Lea	Leb	Fya	Fyb	Jka	Jkb	Xga	S	s	M	N	P1	Lua	Lub		S	AI	Ag	E				
1	+	+	0	0	+	0	+	0	0	+	0	+	0	+	+	+	0	+	+	+	0	0	+	0	+	+	0	+		0	3	3	0				
2	+	+	0	0	+	0	0	0	+	+	0	+	0	+	0	+	+	0	+	0	+	0	+	0	+	0	+	+		1	4	4	4				
3	+	0	+	+	0	0	0	0	0	+	0	+	0	+	+	+	+	+	0	+	0	+	+	+	0	0	0	+		1	4	4	3				
4	0	+	0	+	+	+	0	0	0	+	0	+	0	+	+	0	+	0	+	0	+	0	+	+	+	+	0	+		1	4	4	3				
5	0	0	0	+	+	+	0	0	0	+	0	+	0	+	+	+	0	+	+	0	0	+	+	+	+	+	0	+		0	3	3	0				
6	0	0	0	+	+	+	0	0	+	+	0	+	0	+	0	+	+	+	0	+	0	+	+	+	+	+	0	+		1	4	4	4				
7	0	0	0	+	+	+	0	0	0	+	0	+	0	+	0	+	+	+	+	0	+	+	+	+	+	+	0	+		1	4	4	4				
8	0	0	0	+	+	+	0	0	0	+	0	+	0	+	+	0	+	+	+	0	0	0	+	+	+	+	0	+		1	4	4	3				
9	0	0	0	+	+	+	0	0	0	+	0	+	0	+	0	+	0	0	0	+	+	0	0	0	+	+	+	0	+		0	0	0	0				
10	0	0	0	+	+	+	0	0	0	+	0	+	0	+	+	+	0	+	0	0	0	+	0	+	0	+	0	0	+		0	3	3	0				
11	+	+	0	+	+	+	0	0	0	+	0	+	0	+	0	+	+	+	0	+	0	+	0	+	0	+	+	0	0	+		1	4	4	4				
12	0	0	0	+	+	+	0	0	0	+	0	+	+	0	+	0	+	0	+	+	0	0	+	0	+	+	+	+		1	4	4	3				
13	+	+	+	+	+	0	0	0	0	+	0	+	0	+	0	+	+	+	+	0	+	0	+	+	0	0	+	+		1	4	4	4				
14	+	+	+	0	+	0	0	0	0	+	0	+	0	+	+	+	+	+	+	+	0	+	0	+	0	0	0	+		1	4	4	3				
Pt																														0	0	0	0				

Comments: Grading: 0 to 4+
Diagnosis: anti-Fy^a & Jk^a

cord cell
A$_1$
A$_2$
B

FIG 6–8.—Panel showing a combination of two warm antibodies. Cells otherwise positive in the 37°C incubations become negative after treatment with enzymes. This is characteristic of Duffy antigens.

omitted from daily blood sample workups in most blood banks, because donor samples are screened beforehand for the more common antibodies. It is therefore unnecessary to react donor plasma with the patient's cells to demonstrate rare antibodies in the donor's plasma. The presence of a low-incidence antibody in the donor's plasma probably would not cause a transfusion reaction because of the dilution factor of the recipient's plasma volume. It is much more important to simplify blood bank procedures by eliminating this test as an additional source of error than to perform it in the belief that it might reveal some unlikely antibody-antigen interaction.

Major Crossmatch.—The major crossmatch remains important in blood banking practice. The test involves reacting donor cells with the patient's plasma, to emulate in the test tube what would occur in vivo. In addition, other incubations that improve the reactivity of certain antigen-antibody reactions are also performed during a crossmatch. The cells and the plasma are incubated at room temperature in saline, at 37°C, and in the antiglobulin phase. A control with the patient's own cells and plasma is routinely run in parallel.

Common Pitfalls of the Crossmatch Test

Since the crossmatch functions as a double-check on many of the procedures undertaken up to this stage, incompatibility results warrant further investigation. The first item to check is the source of the specimen. The sample should be positively identified and the name of the patient and the hospital number verified. The leading cause of serious incompatibilities is misidentification of the patient sample. If any doubt exists, double-checking the patient's laboratory record is mandatory. The patient's ABO and Rh typings are double-checked. Not infrequently, subgroups of A or B may be the cause of incompatible crossmatch results. The patient's medical history is also important and may indicate the cause of discrepancies. For instance, an incompatible crossmatch may result if the patient has been anticoagulated, has hyperproteinemia (e.g., myeloma), or has received antibiotics.

If the patient has been previously transfused, the blood bank record may be valuable in identifying the cause of crossmatch incompatibilities.

Once identification of the sample has been verified and the patient's clinical and transfusional history has been consulted, the laboratory check should be started. All reagents should be double-checked for reactivity and specificity. The ABO and Rh typings are repeated as well as the screening and, if necessary, the panel workup. The antiglobulin reagent is checked for reactivity and the crossmatch is repeated with a properly checked reagent. Patient samples should not be older than 48 hours, to preserve complement activity[42] as well as to avoid a prolonged lapse between samples, which would allow missing new antibodies developing in the patient.

Some incompatible crossmatches are more than ordinarily difficult to solve. In these cases the potential variables are screened for, some of these variables are detailed in the following sections.

The Patient's Serum

The serum of a patient may be the cause of false results in compatibility testing. The sample from a patient who has increased amount of serum proteins may elicit false agglutination due to rouleaux formation (RBCs aggregated in a "stack of coins" fashion). Diseases such as myeloma and macroglobulinemia are frequently the cause of rouleaux formation.[43] The best way to avoid false agglutination caused by rouleaux is by the saline replacement method. The patient's serum and donor cells are incubated as in the routine crossmatch, then the serum is removed and a drop of saline is added.[44]

Another cause of rouleaux formation is an improperly clotted sample. Patients undergoing anticoagulant therapy frequently have incomplete clotting. If the problem is due to anticoagulation with heparin, which blocks thrombin, the problem may

Red Cell Panel

Cell No.	D	C	E	c	e	f	C^w	V	K	k	Kp^a	Kp^b	Js^a	Js^b	Fy^a	Fy^b	Jk^a	Jk^b	Xg^a	Le^a	Le^b	S	s	M	N	P_1	Lu^a	Lu^b		Patient's Serum S	Al	Ag	E
1	+	+	o	o	+	o	+	o	o	+	o	+	o	+	+	+	o	+	+	+	o	o	+	o	+	+	o	+		0	3	3	3
2	+	+	o	o	+	o	o	o	+	+	o	+	o	+	o	+	+	o	+	o	+	o	+	o	+	+	o	+		0	3	3	3
3	+	o	+	+	o	o	o	o	o	+	o	+	o	+	+	+	+	+	+	o	+	o	+	+	+	o	o	+		0	3	3	3
4	o	+	o	+	+	+	o	o	o	+	o	+	o	+	+	o	+	o	+	o	+	o	+	+	+	+	o	+		0	3	3	3
5	o	o	+	+	+	+	o	o	o	+	o	+	o	+	+	+	o	+	+	o	o	+	+	+	+	+	o	+		0	3	3	3
6	o	o	o	+	+	+	o	o	+	+	o	+	o	+	o	+	+	+	+	o	+	o	+	+	+	+	o	+		0	3	3	3
7	o	o	o	+	+	+	o	o	o	+	o	+	o	+	o	+	+	+	+	+	o	+	+	+	+	+	o	+		0	3	3	3
8	o	o	o	+	+	+	o	o	o	+	o	+	o	+	+	o	+	+	+	o	o	o	+	+	+	+	o	+		0	3	3	3
9	o	o	o	+	+	+	o	o	o	+	o	+	o	+	o	o	o	+	+	o	o	o	+	+	+	+	o	+		0	3	3	3
10	o	o	o	+	+	+	o	o	o	+	o	+	o	+	+	+	o	+	o	o	+	o	+	o	+	o	o	+		0	3	3	3
11	+	+	o	+	+	+	o	o	o	+	o	+	o	+	o	+	+	+	o	+	o	+	o	+	+	o	o	+		0	3	3	3
12	o	o	o	+	+	+	o	o	o	+	o	+	+	o	+	o	+	o	+	+	o	o	+	o	+	+	+	+		0	3	3	3
13	+	+	+	+	+	o	o	o	o	+	o	+	o	+	o	+	+	+	+	o	+	o	+	+	o	o	+	+		0	3	3	3
14	+	+	+	o	+	o	o	o	o	+	o	+	o	+	+	+	+	+	+	+	o	+	o	+	o	o	o	+		0	3	3	3
Pt																														0	3	3	3

Comments: Grading: O to 4+ Hx of SLE		S	Al	Ag	E
	cord cell	0	3	3	3
	A_1	0	3	3	3
Diagnosis: Warm Autoimmune Hemolytic Anemia	A_2	0	3	3	3
	B	0	3	3	3

FIG 6–9.—Panel showing findings typical of a warm autoimmune hemolytic anemia in a patient with systemic lupus erythematosus.

be solved by the addition of protamine sulfate.[45]

Coumadin interferes with factors VII, IX and X, and prothrombin. Samples improperly clotted because of coumadin may be induced to clot by the addition of thrombin to the improperly clotted plasma.[45]

Rarely, a patient's serum reacts against albumin used to promote agglutination. Usually this agglutination reaction occurs because of patient antibodies to stabilizing substances added to albumin reagents, such as caprilate.[46] In the event of such reactivity, caprilate-free albumin solutions should be used in the testing.

Patient serum antibodies against β_2-globulin may also react with albumin preparations contaminated with β_2-globulin.[47] This may also cause false results in tests involving the use of antiglobulin.

Antibodies against antibiotics used in the preservation of panel cells or screening cells may also cause false reactivity.[48] Sometimes antibodies against dyes may cause false or incongruent results, especially in ABO testing. These may be against acriflavin[49] or against yellow tartrazine.[50]

RBC ANTIBODIES

We have reviewed the antibodies to specific antigens individually and their detection through the use of RBC panels. If all units appear to be incompatible at room temperature and a panel shows the presence of an anti-I cold agglutinin, the sample should be absorbed with the patient's own cells in the cold to eliminate the anti-I reactivity. The serum is then tested in the albumin and antiglobulin phases. Absorbed sera can also be used in the crossmatch. Of course, there is the danger of absorbing clinically significant specificities. Cold antibodies may also cause discrepancies in ABO typing, because testing for ABO is performed at room temperature. Alloantibodies such as anti-Lewis and anti-M antibodies cause discrepancies in ABO back typing. Conversely, cold autoantibodies may be a problem in both front and back typing. Washing the patient's cells at 37°C with saline will allow proper ABO and Rh typing. However, if complement has attached to the RBCs, it may obscure the antiglobulin phase of Rh typing. A Coombs panel may help define the type of globulin on RBCs.

In general, cold autoantibodies that do not have a high temperature range can be ignored in transfusion if the patient will not be undergoing procedures, such as open heart surgery, that require inducing hypothermia.

If the patient must be made hypothermic it is advisable to make a temperature range study of the serum to investigate the reactivity of the antibody in the various incubations, to avoid exposing the patient to temperatures at which the antibody becomes clinically significant.

In patients undergoing hypothermia who have circulating antibodies reacting at these temperatures, the surgeon must be informed of the potential danger of hemolysis. The surgical techniques may have to be modified to avoid exposure of the patient to such temperatures. In certain cases, blood warmers and warming blankets may be indicated to prevent transfusion reactions. However, the danger of hemolysis in these patients has been somewhat overrated. Cold alloantibodies with very low temperature ranges can also be ignored in most instances. Patients with circulating anti-Lewis antibodies may have to be transfused with a unit of Le^b-positive plasma to neutralize the antibodies before transfusion of Le^b-positive blood.[51]

Warm Antibodies

Crossmatching blood for recipients with multiple antibodies is one of the most difficult tasks performed by the immunohematology laboratory. Often these patients have been multiply transfused. An accurate patient phenotype is time-saving and may be crucial to the laboratory workup of these cases. This underscores the importance of phenotyping a patient when samples are obtained before the patient has been multiply transfused. Warm alloantibodies and autoantibodies are clinically significant because they react close to or at the patient's normal body temperature.

If an antibody to a high-incidence antigen is present, or if multiple alloantibodies have been produced, the results of the crossmatch may be difficult to interpret, and finding compatible units may be extremely difficult. The presence of warm autoantibodies also creates difficulties in terms of finding compatible units for a recipient. The solution to the problem often entails titration of the patient's serum, absorption-elution studies, and multiple panels. Hemotherapy may have to be curtailed, especially if the hemoglobin of the patient is not too low. Transfusions are considered when the hemoglobin level drops to about 7 or 9 gm/100 ml, but the values at which the patient must be transfused should be determined in each case on an individual basis. It has been recommended that the hemoglobin level not drop below 4.5 gm/100 ml in an adult with chronic blood loss.[52]

If fully compatible blood cannot be found, transfusion of a "least incompatible" unit may have to be considered. This decision is made in consultation with the blood bank director and the treating physician and is a last recourse (for details see Chapter 10). In patients who can tolerate the removal of a unit, autologous transfusion may be the best alternative if elective surgery is contemplated. The technique is detailed further in chapter 9.

INCOMPATIBILITY IN VIVO

The concept that compatibility in vitro is normally but not always followed by good survival of a unit in vivo was reviewed earlier in this chapter. This section addresses the in vivo survival of transfused cells that exhibit varying degrees of incompatibility with the recipient's serum. If the incompatible unit has been inadvertently transfused, an estimate of survival may be achieved by calculating agglutinated versus nonagglutinated cells using antibodies that detect phenotype differences in RBC antigens between the donor and the host (e.g., M and N, or specific antigens in the Rh system), as suggested by the Ashby method.[53]

However, if the information on expected survival of a unit is needed before transfusion, it can be obtained through a ^{51}Cr random labeling release study.[54] A sample of erythrocytes is labeled in vitro, the reaction is stopped with ascorbic acid, and the sample is injected intravenously. After 10–15 minutes a blood sample is taken from the opposite arm and used as the 100% sample, or time zero. Samples are taken at 3, 10, and 60 minutes, and subsequently every 2 days for 14 days. The half-life of ^{51}Cr in RBCs is about 32 days, due to elution of the label from the cell. Typical survival curves are shown in Figure 6–10. If the destruction is intravascular, changes will be seen in the 1-minute sample; if the destruction is extravascular, changes will be seen in the 60-minute sample. Non-complement-binding IgG antibodies produce single-component curves with a constant rate of destruction of cells, whereas IgM antibodies produce two-component curves with an initial accelerated rate followed by a slower rate of destruction.[55] This pattern may

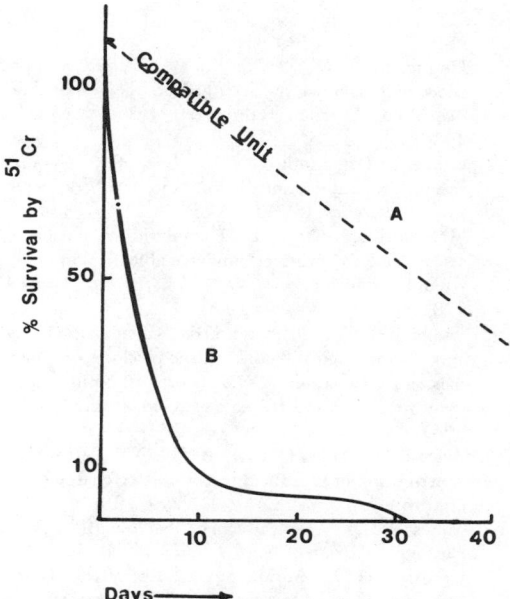

FIG 6–10.—The collapse curve of Mollison after the infusion of Rh$_o$(D)–positive cells into a recipient with anti-D antibodies.

be due to an uneven distribution of antigen, susceptibility of RBCs to lysis, inactivation of complement, or exhaustion of antibody.

Other factors may include trapping and release of RBCs by the liver of complement-coated cells[56] or saturation of immunoglobulin-binding sites on macrophages.[57]

The removal of cells from the circulation may depend on the number of antibody molecules on the RBC, the amount of antibody-binding complement, and the thermal range of the antibody reactivity.

When the antibody produces destruction intravascularly, hemolysis depends on the amount of antibody and complement present. When RBC destruction is extravascular (i.e., in the spleen), hemolysis depends on the amount of antibody and the availability of binding sites on macrophages in the reticuloendothelial system.[58]

In certain instances, the survival of a unit is shortened even though antibodies to an RBC antigen are weak[59] or entirely nondemonstrable. Nondemonstrable antibodies produce the "collapse curve of Mollison" (see Fig 6–10) in ^{51}Cr-labeled cells. Sometimes the "collapse curve" phenomenon is attributable to the presence of a primary immune response.[60]

REFERENCES

1. Hughes-Jones W.C., Gardner B., Telford R.: The effect of pH and ionic strength on the reaction between anti-D and erythrocytes. *Immunology* 7:72, 1964.
2. Moore H.D., Mollison P.L.: Use of a low-ionic strength medium in manual tests for antibody detection. *Transfusion* 16:291, 1976.
3. Molthan L., Strohm P.L.: Hemolytic transfusion reaction due to anti-Kell undetectable in low-ionic-strength solution. *Am. J. Clin. Pathol.* 75:629, 1981.
4. Cameron J.W., Diamond L.K.: Chemical, clinical and immunological studies on the products of human plasma fractionation: XXIX. Serum albumin as a diluent for Rh typing reagents. *J. Clin. Invest.* 24:793, 1945.
5. Eyler E.H., Madoff M.A., Brody O.V., et al. The contribution of sialic acid to the surface charge of the erythrocyte. *J. Biol. Chem.* 237:1992, 1962.
6. Moreschi C.: Neue Tatsachen über die Blutkorperchenagglutination. *Zentralbl. Bakteriol.* 46:49, 1908.
7. Coombs R.R.A., Mourant A.E., Race R.R.: Detection of weak and "incomplete" Rh agglutinins. *Lancet* 2:15, 1945.
8. Jenkins D.E. Jr., Moore W.H., Hartmann R.C.: A rapid method for the production of RBCs in the state "E C4" and "E C43." *Clin. Res.* 19:74, 1971.
9. Jandl J.H.: The agglutination and sequestration of immature red cells. *J. Lab. Clin. Med.* 55:662, 1960.
10. Greenwalt T.J., Saski T.T., Steane E.A.: The Lutheran blood groups: A progress report with observations on the development of the antigens and characteristics of the antibodies. *Transfusion* 7:189, 1967.
11. Coombs R.R.A., Mourant A.E., Race R.R.: In vivo isosensitization of red cells in babies with haemolytic disease. *Lancet* 1:264, 1946.
12. Chaplin H.: Clinical usefulness of specific antiglobulin reagents in autoimmune hemolytic anemias. *Prog. Hematol.* 8:25, 1973.
13. Garraty G., Petz L.D.: Drug-induced hemolytic anemia. *Am. J. Med.* 58:398, 1975.
14. Romans D.G., Dorrington K.J.: Interactions between Fab and Fc regions in liganded immunoglobulin G. *Mol. Immunol.* 16:859, 1979.
15. Leikola J., Perkins H.A.: Enzyme-linked immunoglobulin test: An accurate and simple method to quantify red cell antibodies. *Transfusion* 20:138, 1980.
16. Graham H.A., et al.: A new approach to prepare cells for the Coombs test. *Transfusion* 22:408, 1982.
17. Huestis D.W., Bove J.R., Busch S.: *Practical Blood Transfusion*, ed. 3. Boston, Little, Brown & Co., 1981, p. 423.
18. Watson K.C., Jourliert S.M.: Hemagglutination of cells treated with antibiotics. *Nature* 188:505, 1960.
19. Beattie K.: Control of the antigen-antibody ratio in antibody detection/compatibility tests. *Transfusion* 20:277, 1980.
20. Widman F.K. (ed.): *Technical Manual of the American Association of Blood Banks,* ed. 8. Washington, D.C., American Association of Blood Banks, 1981, p. 185.
21. Marsh W.L.: Scoring of hemagglutination reactions. *Transfusion* 12:352, 1972.
22. Mollison P.L.: *Blood Transfusion in Clinical Medicine,* ed. 7. Oxford, England, Blackwell Scientific Publications, 1983, p. 550.
23. Gold E.R., Lockyer W.J., Tovey G.A.: Use of lyophilized formol-treated cells in blood group serology. *Nature* 182:951. 1958.
24. Ogata T., Matuhasi T.: Problems of specific and crossreactivity of blood group antibodies, in *Proceedings of the 8th Congress of the International Society for Blood Transfusion*. New York, S. Karger, 1962.
25. Crawford, H., Mollison P.L.: Demonstration of multiple antibodies in antiglobulin sera. *Lancet* 2:955, 1951.
26. Landsteiner K., Millen C.P.: Serologic studies on the blood of the primates: II. The blood groups in anthropoid apes. *J. Exp. Med.* 42:853, 1925.
27. Kidd P.: Elution of an incomplete type of antibody from the erythrocytes in acquired hemolytic anemia. *J. Clin. Pathol.* 2:103, 1949.
28. Rubin H.: Antibody elution from red cells. *J. Clin. Pathol.* 16:70, 1963.
29. Rekvig O.P., Hannestad K.: Acid elution of blood group antibodies from intact erythrocytes. *Vox Sang.* 33:280, 1977.
30. Widman F.K., ed.: *Technical Manual of the American Association of Blood Banks,* ed. 8. Washington, D.C., American Association of Blood Banks, 1981, p. 196.
31. Bird G.W.G.: Plant and other agglutinins in the study of some human erythrocyte membrane anomalies. *Ann. NY Acad. Sci.* 234:129. 1974.
32. Bird G.W.G.: Lectins. *Lab. Lore* 9:683, 1981.
33. Cazal P., Lalaurie M.: Recherches sur quelques phytoagglutines spécifiques des groups sanguins, ABO. *Acta Haematol.* 8:73, 1952.
34. Ohensooser F., Silberschmidt K.: Haemagglutinin anti-N in plant seeds. *Nature* 172:914, 1953.
35. Wallas C.H., Tanley P.C., Gorrell L.: Recovery of autologous erythrocytes in transfused patients. *Transfusion* 20:332, 1980.
36. Kohler M., Milstein C.: Continuous cultures of fused cells secreting antibody of predefined specificity. *Nature* 256:495, 1975.
37. Milstein C., et al.: Monoclonal antibodies and cell surface antigens. *Cell Biol. Int. Rep.* 3:1, 1979.
38. Anstee D.J., Edwards P.A.W.: Monoclonal antibodies to human erythrocytes. *Eur. J. Immunol.* 12:228, 1982.
39. Voak D., et al.: Monoclonal anti-A from a hybrid myeloma: Evaluation as a blood group reagent. *Vox Sang.* 39:134, 1980.
40. Sucks S.H., Lenox E.S.: Monoclonal anti-B as a new blood typing reagent. *Vox Sang.* 40:99, 1981.
41. Hectoen L.: Isoagglutination of human corpuscles. *J. Infect. Dis.* 4:297, 1907.

42. Widman F.K. (ed.): *Technical Manual of the American Association of Blood Banks,* ed. 8. Washington, D.C., American Association of Blood Banks, 1981, p. 183.
43. Mollison P.L.: *Blood Transfusion in Clinical Medicine,* ed. 7. Oxford, England, Blackwell Scientific Publications, 1983, p. 478.
44. Grainick M.A.: Rouleaux, in Walker R.H. (ed.): *A Seminar on Problems Encountered in Pre-Transfusion Tests.* Washington, D.C., American Association of Blood Banks, 1972, p. 71.
45. Simmons A.: Coagulation and protein abnormality, in Walker R.H. (ed.): *A Seminar on Problems Encountered in Pre-Transfusion Tests.* Washington, D.C., American Association of Blood Banks, 1972, p. 117.
46. Golde D.W., McGinnis M.G., Holland P.V.: Serum agglutinins to commercially prepared albumin. *Am. J. Clin. Pathol.* 55:655, 1971.
47. Simmons A., Jones J., Hendrix D.: Gamma-globulin contamination of commercial bovine albumin. *Transfusion* 13:142, 1973.
48. Garraty G.: Problems in pre-transfusion tests related to drugs and chemicals. *Am. J. Med. Technol.* 42:209, 1976.
49. Beattie K.M., Ziegler W.W.: A serum factor reacting with acriflavin causing an error in ABO cell grouping. *Transfusion* 8:254, 1968.
50. Jones T.E., Ayrton A.S., Blachman M.S.: Anomalous ABO grouping due to a new serum factor reacting with a reagent colouring material. *Transfusion* 13:150, 1973.
51. Mollison P.L., Polley M.J., Crome P.: Temporary suppression of Lewis blood group antibodies to permit incompatible transfusion. *Lancet* 1:909, 1963.
52. Howarth S., Sharpey-Schaffer E.P.: Low blood pressure phases following hemorrhage. *Lancet* 1:19, 1947.
53. Henry J.B.: *Clinical Diagnosis and Management by Laboratory Methods,* ed. 16. Philadelphia, W.B. Saunders Co., 1979, p. 1013.
54. Dacie J.V.: Autoimmune hemolytic anemia. *Arch. Intern. Med.* 135:1293, 1975.
55. Mollison P.L.: *Blood Transfusion in Clinical Medicine,* ed. 7. Oxford, England, Blackwell Scientific Publications, 1983, pp. 583-585.
56. Mollison P.L.: *Blood Transfusion in Clinical Medicine,* ed. 7. Oxford, England, Blackwell Scientific Publications, 1983, p. 569.
57. LoBuglio A.F., et al.: Red cells coated with immunoglobulin G: Binding and sphering by mononuclear cells in man. *Science* 158:1582, 1967.
58. Mollison P.L.: *Blood Transfusion in Clinical Medicine,* ed. 7. Oxford, England, Blackwell Scientific Publications, 1983, p. 601.
59. Fudenberg H.H., Allen F.H. Jr.: Transfusion reactions in the absence of demonstrable incompatibility. *N. Engl. J. Med.* 256:1180, 1957.
60. Mollison P.L.: *Blood Transfusion in Clinical Medicine,* ed. 7. Oxford, England, Blackwell Scientific Publications, 1983, p. 615.

7

The HLA System

NUCLEATED CELLS have a variety of membrane proteins on their surface. A number of these proteins are embedded in the membrane lipid bilayer and organized in such a way that the portions of the molecules exposed to the immune system may exhibit antigenic determinants capable of stimulating an immune response. One of the more important of these molecular groups is the HLA system (H = human, L = leukocyte, A = first system recognized), otherwise known as the major histocompatibility complex (MHC) in humans and the H2 complex in mice. These two systems are the most widely known in transplantation research. Although mature red blood cells (RBCs) are not nucleated, small amounts of HLA antigens are present on them.[1]

The initial studies which led to the delineation of the HLA antigenic complex were conducted on white blood cells (WBCs) and their agglutinins. This is not surprising, for WBCs are a readily available source of nucleated cells. Leukoagglutinins were first described by Doan in 1926.[2] From subsequent studies the term "histocompatibility antigen" was coined.[3] However, the groundwork for a more formal study of the HLA system was laid by Dausset[4] and further consolidated by van Rood et al.[5]

Two major undertakings in the study of the HLA system have been to standardize methodologies and to create a universally applicable nomenclature that would facilitate comparative studies of the work of different research laboratories. These two goals were achieved by participation in the series of International Histocompatibility Workshops held in the 1960s and 1970s.[6-11]

NOMENCLATURE OF THE HLA SYSTEM

The HLA nomenclature, as it is used today, was derived from the work of the IMIS Terminology Committee of the World Health Organization.[12] The WHO Committee meets after each HLA International Workshop to review the nomenclature of the various antigens.

There are four main loci that code for four major antigenic complexes: HLA-A, HLA-B, HLA-C, and HLA-D. The DR determinant is also a product of the HLA genes and may have similar antigens as HLA-D.[13]

HLA antigens coded for by the A, B, C, and D/DR loci are listed in Table 7–1. The letter "w," as in Bw35, indicates that the specificity remains provisionally identified, except in C antigens, where "w" is preserved to distinguish them from complement nomenclature. This designation is removed once laboratory methods have clearly identified the specificity and the antisera are universally available. The numbers of the HLA-A and HLA-B antigens are not sequential because, although they were previously thought to be one system, they are now regarded as two separate systems; however, the numbers are preserved for historical reasons to avoid confusion. Some HLA antigens are frequently seen

TABLE 7–1.—CURRENTLY ACCEPTED HLA ANTIGENS*

HLA-A	HLA-B	HLA-C	HLA-D	HLA-DR
A1	Bw4	Cw1	Dw1	DR1
A2	B7	Cw2	Dw2	DR2
A3	B8	Cw3	Dw3	DR3
A11	B13	Cw4	Dw4	DR4
Aw23	B14	Cw7	Dw5	DR5
Aw24	B18	Cw8	Dw6	DRw6
A25	B27		Dw7	DR7
A26	Bw35		Dw8	DRw8
A28	B37		Dw9	DRw9
A29	Bw38		Dw10	DRw10
Aw30	Bw39		Dw11	
Aw31	Bw41		Dw12	
Aw32	Bw42			
Aw33	Bw44			
Aw34	Bw45			
Aw36	Bw47			
Aw43	Bw48			
	Bw49			
	Bw50			
	Bw51			
	Bw52			
	Bw53			
	Bw54			
	Bw55			
	Bw56			
	Bw57			
	Bw58			
	Bw59			
	Bw60			
	Bw61			
	Bw62			
	Bw63			

*Based on Hackel and Fisher.[35]

in the population and are termed "public" or supertypic; examples of these antigens are HLA-Bw4 and HLA-Bw6 in the HLA-B series and MT, MB, and DL antigens in the HLA-DR series.

HLA Blanks

Individuals may type with a single phenotypic marker at a locus, for instance HLA-A1. In most cases this is due to homozygosity (e.g., HLA-A1/A1) or to the presence of an as yet undescribed antigen coded for at that locus. An amorphous gene at the same locus may also produce this phenomenon. Finally, a modifying gene may be responsible for suppressing expression of a particular HLA phenotypic product, causing only one allele to be expressed.

Cross-reactivity of Antisera to HLA Antigens

Many polyclonal and monoclonal antisera cross-react with antigens in the HLA system.[14] Table 7–2 lists frequently cross-reacting antisera. These cross-reactivities are grouped into cross-reacting groups. Frequently, cell lysis of typed cells does not occur even though adsorption of the antibody on the cells is present.[4] However, these antibodies can be detected with anti-human Ig.[5] A polyclonal antiserum against HLA antigens frequently has a number of specificities directed against the HLA complex. Epitopes found on several HLA antigens are termed "public," whereas "private" epitopes are distinctive determinants of each HLA antigen.

BIOCHEMISTRY OF THE HLA MOLECULAR COMPLEX

The HLA genes code for a variety of transmembrane glycoproteins which can be grouped into class I and class II proteins. The HLA-A, -B, and -C genes code for class I proteins, which are essentially composed of a 44-kilodalton heavy chain[15] and a 12-kilodalton β_2-microglobulin light chain[16] noncovalently bound to each other (Fig 7–1).[16] Heavy chains are composed of 271 relatively variable amino acid residues. Light chains are nonvariable and homologous to plasma β_2-microglobulin. A high degree of homology exists between class I heavy chains.[17] Up to 87% homology exists between HLA-A and HLA-B antigens. Stretches of lack of homology account for differential antigenic specificity.[18] The α_2 regions of heavy chains are homologous with CH3 domains of Ig heavy chains, suggesting a common paleogene.[19]

The bulk of a class I molecule is extracellular. A short hydrophobic segment in the carboxy-terminal end of the heavy chain is the transmembrane portion of the molecule. A short intracellular segment lies at the end of the carboxy-terminal end of the heavy chain.

The extracellular portion of class I molecules is divided into four domains. Three domains are located on the heavy chain. The most distal, coiled, NH_2 terminus is the $\alpha 1$ domain. Proximal to this domain the heavy chain is looped, forming the $\alpha 2$ domain. Another loop most proximal to the membrane forms the $\alpha 3$ domain. These loops are held

TABLE 7-2.—Cross-reactive Groups in Common HLA Types*

HLA-A	HLA-B
1, 3, 10, 11, w36	7, 27, w42, w54, w55(w22), 256(w22)
2, 28	
w23(9), w24(9)	8, 14, w59(8)
25(10), 26(10), w32, w34(10)	13, w60(40), 61(40)
	w41, w47, w48
	18, w35, w51(5), w52(5), w53
w30, w31, w33	w38(W16), w39(W16)
	w44(12), w45(12)
	w49(W21), w50(W21)
	w46, w57(17), w58(17), w62(15), w63(15)

*Data from Hackel and Fisher. Connecting bars designate strong cross-reactivity.

together by S-S bonds. The $\alpha 1$ and $\alpha 2$ domains are the more antigenic portions of the molecule and are thought to provide epitopic specificity. The $\alpha 3$ domain found in the more constant portion of the molecule is the binding site for the β_2-microglobulin chain. The β_2-microglobulin chain also contains a loop, which constitutes the fourth domain. Most abnormalities in the chemistry of HLA class I antigens have been made by sequencing HLA-A2 and HLA-B7; differences between antigens may be dependent on single amino acid substitutions. Papain cleavage studies of class I molecules which separate heavy from light chains demonstrate that HLA epitope antigenicity is dependent on integrity of the heavy chain and is not related to the light chain.[20]

A new set of antigens, the HT antigens, have likewise been shown to be class I antigens. The genes coding for HT are closely linked with other class I antigens. The HT antigens are thought to be similar to TLQa antigens (see subsequent discussion of the H2 locus of the mouse). These antigens appear on lymphocyte activation.[21]

Class II antigens are coded by HLA-DR genes. The structure of these antigens has been elucidated from studies of class II antigens purified from Raji cells which are phenotypically a B cell line.[22] This is not surprising, for HLA-DR antigens are mostly identified on B cells.

Class II antigens are composed of two chains of similar molecular weight; however, these can be discerned as a heavy 34-kilodalton α chain and a 29-kilodalton β chain composed of 270 amino acids. Like class I antigens, class II antigens have a high degree of amino acid sequence homology even though the sequences may have 10%–90% variability. Unlike class I antigens, both heavy and light chains of class II antigens are heterogeneous, providing polymorphism. Thus, at least two chains and two or possibly three β chains exist. This can result in combinational patterns such as $\alpha 1\beta 2\beta 2$, etc. When one thinks of the HLA-DR antigens as the Ia antigens in humans, this combinational variability provides antigenic diversity and possibly epitope diversity, allowing the antigens to function as a combining site in immune response interactions with effector cells. Unlike class I molecules, the antigenic determinants of class II molecules appear to be predominantly located on the β chain, which has at least three domains, formed by a proximal and a distal loop held in place by disulfide bonds and a free portion containing the NH_2 terminal end of the β chain. The α chain contains a single loop bonded by a disulfide bond and a free NH_2 terminal end. Both chains, like class I chains, have a short hydrophobic transmembrane segment and a short hydrophilic intracellular segment containing the C-terminal end of the molecules.[22]

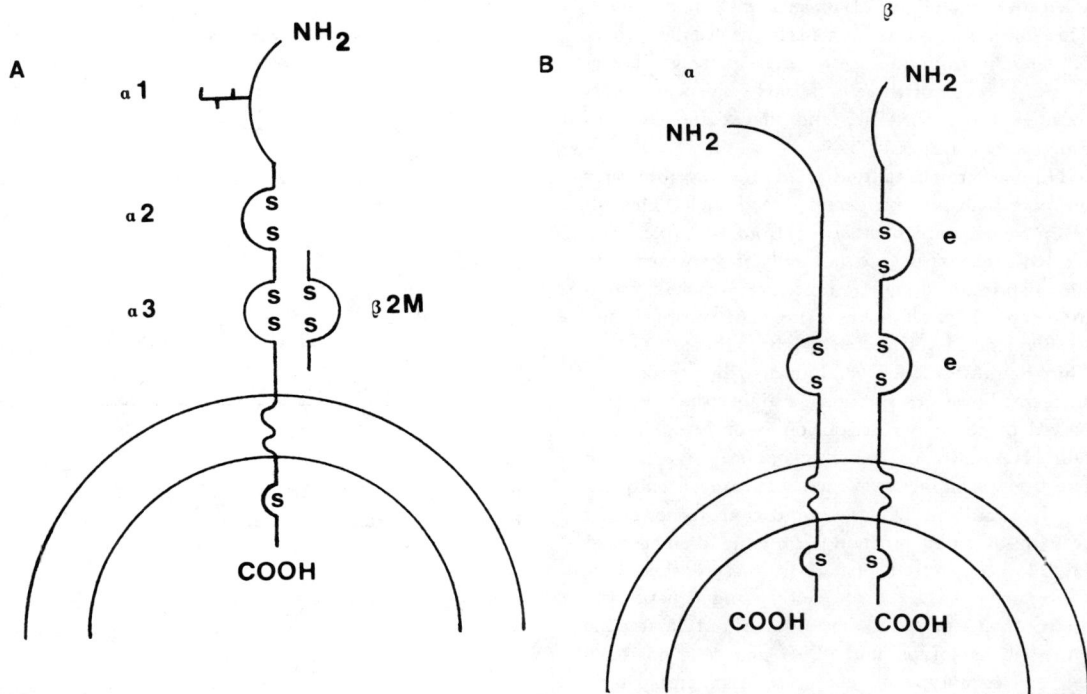

FIG 7–1.—Simplified model of MHC molecules. **A,** class I HLA antigens. The major portion of the molecule is extracellular and contains most of the heavy chain with its three α domains and the β chain with its single loop. A short transmembrane portion anchors the molecule to the cell membrane. Another short segment is intracellular and ends in the C-terminus of the heavy chain. **B,** class II HLA antigens. An α and β chain are defined. The α chain has one loop and the β chain has two loops. The β chain loops one major antigenic determinants or epitopes (e). Like class I antigens, class II antigens have an extracellular portion (the bulk of the molecule), a short transmembrane portion, and an intracellular segment with the C-terminus of each chain.

Class II antigens also reveal supertypic specificities, termed DC, which appear to be identical to MT and MB antigens[23] and cross-react, but are distinct from HLA-DR molecules. The DR antigens are homologous to murine I-E/C antigens, whereas DC1 specificities appear to be the human counterpart of murine I-A antigens.[24] DC and DR antigens may very well be coded by two distinct genes lying close to each other on the short arm of chromosome 6. I-A molecules in man have been recently identified with monoclonal antibodies. They are termed HLA-DS (S for secondary), and are very similar to or the same as DC, MT, and MB antigens. Extrapolating from mouse studies, where I-A antigens are more critical to the immune response than I-E antigens, one can assume that the newly described DS antigens will be highly significant to the study of the immune response in humans.[25] Another gene closely linked to D/DR genes is the secondary B cell antigens gene (SB) whose products are class II molecules, bear structural homology to D/DR gene products, and appear to mediate T cell restriction.[26]

GENETICS OF THE HLA SYSTEM

Megagene Characteristics of the HLA Locus

The HLA locus is an important locus both in the philogeny and in the ontogeny of the immune system. Apart from coding for the Ia genetic products in humans at the HLA-DR27 locus, many other biochemical products important to the immune response are coded for by genes which are in close proximity to HLA genes. The more important ones are given in Table 7–3. Rat-to-rat alloimmunization studies followed by cloning studies have shown a certain homology of MHC antigens across species. This finding suggests that MHC molecules probably share a common ancestor gene preserved across species.[28] Some of these preserved sequences are associated with HLA-Bw6 and may determine immune responsiveness.[29]

Humans are normally diploid and therefore carry no more than two antigens for each allele. The full HLA gene complex inherited from each parent is termed a haplotype and normally is transmitted to the offspring as a genetic unit. Nevertheless, crossing over is possible in the HLA gene complex, and its frequency is estimated at approximately 1%.[29] This should result in a random distribution of HLA antigens; however, a frequency higher than that expected by random distribution is observed in certain HLA antigens, possibly because of a natural selection phenomenon which would eventually result in equilibrium. Large population studies of the crossing-over phenomenon permit the inference that HLA loci are indeed separate from each other. Offspring have a 25% chance of having a haplotype identical to a parent's, a 50% chance of having the same half-haplotype, and a 25% chance of not sharing any haplotype, a fact used in paternity tests (Fig 7–2).

The chromosomal loci for the HLA heavy chain genes are located on the short arm of chromosome 6. This location has been defined by genetic analysis of families as well as by studies with somatic cell hybrids.[30] The β-microglobulin fraction of the HLA molecule, however, is coded for by chromosome 15.[31] In this respect, HLA molecules are similar to immunoglobulins where different subunits of the whole molecule are coded for by unlinked genes. Figure 7–3 shows the arrangement of genes on the short arm of chromosome 6.

The HLA region has been mapped based on the following observations: (1) HLA-A, B, and C gene products are controlled by genes located at a single genetic region;[32] (2) HLA-A and HLA-B are separable by genetic recombination;[33] and (3) HLA-D antigens are coded in an area very close to HLA-A and HLA-B.[34]

The specific locations of the genes, however, have been determined by linkage data, suggesting actual localization of the genes on the short arm of chromosome 6 (see Fig 7–3). The distance between genes can be measured in centimorgans, a measure used by geneticists taking advantage of crossing-over data (see Chap. 14).

TABLE 7–3.—ASSIGNMENT OF GENES ASSOCIATED WITH THE IMMUNE SYSTEM, OTHER THAN HLA GENES LOCATED IN CHROMOSOME 6*

Confirmed:
Factor B (properdin pathway)
C2
C4F
C4S
Provisional:
CR1
CR2
Monkey red blood cell receptor (MRRC)
Plasminogen activator (PLA)
P blood group

Linkage Disequilibrium

The gene frequency of a given antigen trait is calculated by the formula $GF = 1 - \sqrt{1 - AF}$, where GF is the gene frequency and AF is the antigen frequency. When expected frequencies are calculated based on population studies, the distance between genes can be calculated if one assumes that linkage exists where crossing over is observed.

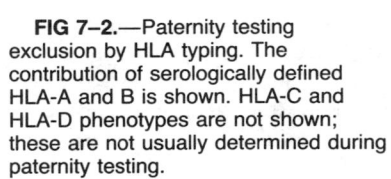

FIG 7–2.—Paternity testing exclusion by HLA typing. The contribution of serologically defined HLA-A and B is shown. HLA-C and HLA-D phenotypes are not shown; these are not usually determined during paternity testing.

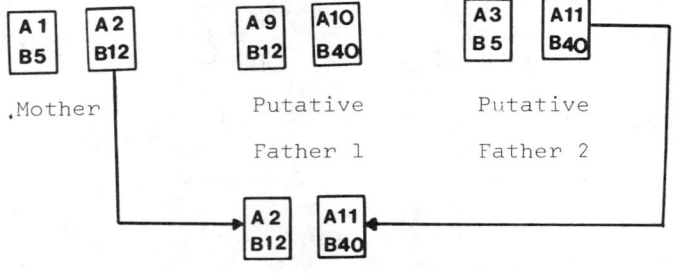

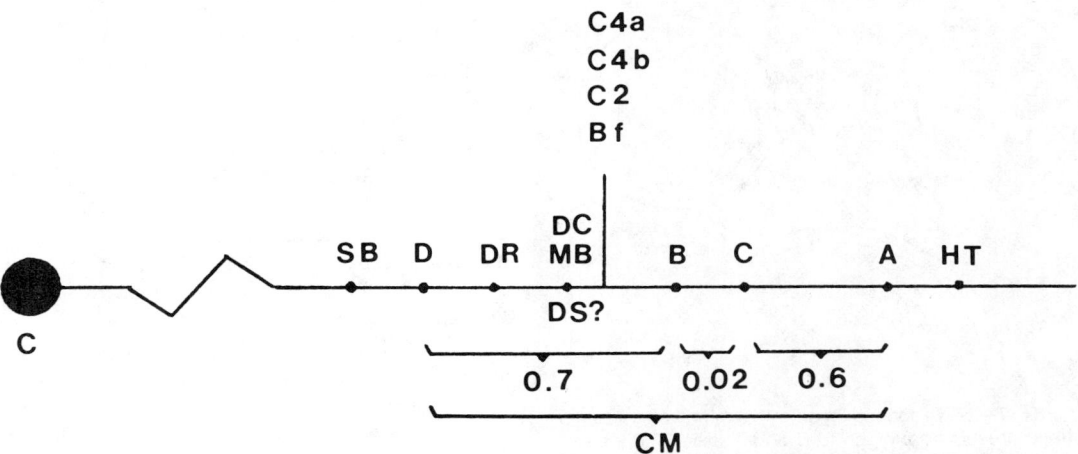

FIG 7–3.—Proposed display of HLA genes on the short arm of chromosome 6. The distance between genes is measured in centimorgans (CM), which is also a measure of the probability of crossing-over. The components of complement C2, C4, and Bf are coded for by genes located between HLA-D and HLA-DR genes and HLA-B genes. SB genes are thought to be closest to the centromere (Left side, C).

However, certain HLA alleles are more often linked together in certain populations than would be expected from population statistical analysis. For instance, HLA-A1 ($GF_1 = 0.138$) and HLA-B8 ($GF_2 = 0.090$) would have an expected combined GF of 0.0124 [calculated from $(GF_1)(GF_2)$]; however, the actual GF of the A1/B8 haplotype is 0.0609 (more than four times the expected combined GF in caucasians). The linkage disequilibrium $\Delta = OF - EF$, where OF is the observed frequency and EF is the expected frequency. Thus, in the above example, $\Delta = 0.0604 - 0.0124 = 0.0485$.[35]

In summary, linkage disequilibrium provides the statistical data that suggest that two gene loci occur close together in a fashion not attributable to random distribution. However, the linkage disequilibrium existing between two genes may suggest a natural selection pressure tending to equilibrium. Evidence of linkage disequilibrium is a sensitive measure of natural selection.[36]

IMMUNOBIOLOGY OF THE HLA SYSTEM

Although initial interest in the HLA system stemmed from its role in transplantation, today it is acknowledged to have a major significance in the interaction of various aspects of the immune response, not restricted to transplantation. The observation that different strains of animals in the same species may respond differently to the same antigen was probably the first indication of a genetic mechanism that determines immune responsiveness. Although the interactions of the various cells in the immune system are complex and far from being fully understood, there is some knowledge as to why this intraspecies difference in immune responsiveness should exist.[37] In other words, there are good responders and nonresponders to a specific antigenic stimulus.

It has been shown in vitro that macrophages are needed for the mounting of a proper immune response.[38] Macrophages participate in the immune response, modifying or presenting antigens to the immune system. This function affects both specific antigen recognition by T cells as well as spatial presentation of antigen to these cells. T cells are capable of cooperating with macrophages via membrane receptors which are coded for by the HLA-D and DR genes in humans (Fig 7–4) and by the I region of the H2 complex in mice (Fig 7–5).[39] A dual recognition molecular complex is probably associated in some way on the membrane. This system may be responsible for the elimination of self-reacting clones in the development of tolerance,[40] and is responsible for mixed lymphocyte culture (MLC) responses,[41] which are discussed later in this chapter. T cytotoxic killer cells result from MLCs; during these reactions class II proteins function as the stimulator molecule, whereas class I proteins are the target antigens during killing of foreign cells.

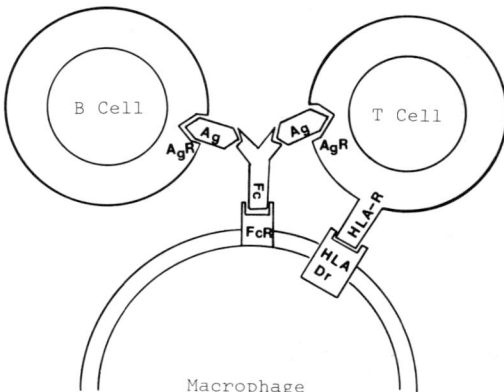

FIG 7–4.—Proposed model showing a macrophage presenting antigen to B and T cells. The interaction of T cells and macrophages is mediated both by antigen receptors and by the HLA-DR genes.

However, the recognition of the class I proteins is highly specific and can be used to recognize "split" specificities within the same HLA antigen (e.g., HLA-B5 splits).[42] Thus T cell clones can be used to study epitope subspecificity within HLA-antigen determinants.

The Major Histocompatibility Region of the Mouse

A great deal has been learned about histocompatibility from the MHC region of the mouse, termed the H2 region. A simplified map of this complex is given in Figure 7–5.

The gene products manifested as cell membrane molecules were first noted to have a role in the immune response by McDevitt et al.[43] The genes coding for these products are called Ir genes (immune response genes), and the products are called Ia products. As in the human HLA complex, these products interact in a dual-signal fashion to stimulate T cells. Although anti-idiotypic antibodies are also involved in immunoregulation of antibody formation, it is clear that the MHC dual-system recognition plays a major role in determining immune responsiveness to a particular antigen.

The HLA-D, DR locus is considered to be the human counterpart to the Ia subregion of the mouse MHC complex. The products of the MHC locus have been shown to have some bearing on whether suppressor effects on T cells are enhanced or suppressed during the immune response, both in mice, through products of the I-J subregion of the Ia region of the mouse MHC,[44] and in man, through HLA-D products.[45] This genetically regulated immunoregulation shows a specific influence of MHC products on suppressor T cell subpopulations.

The TLQa region in the mouse is located distal to the centromere in chromosome 17. It is considered separate from the H2 complex but is thought to code for differentiation antigens. As mentioned above, it is believed that a region similar to that of the mouse exists in humans. The products have been called HT antigens and they appear to be associated with β-microglobulin.[46]

Both the K/O region of the H2 complex of the mouse encoding the CD antigens and the TLQa region are instrumental in the development of helper T cells and cytoxic T cells. As reviewed in chapter 4, helper T cells bear Ly-1 antigens and suppressor T cells bear Ly-1,2 antigens.[47] It is quite possible that these antigens interact in some way with the MHC to deliver their functions.

LABORATORY IDENTIFICATION OF HLA ANTIGENS

HLA-A, B, and C are detected by cytotoxicity microtiter assays. The National Institutes of Health method, developed by Terasaki et al.,[48] is widely used. In this method granulocyte samples with RBCs are separated on Ficoll-Hypaque. The donor panel is selected from about 60 individuals in a random population. If the majority of the population is caucasian, individuals from other populations (black or Oriental) may have to be used to recruit specificities not found in the majority of the population.

Polyclonal antisera are obtained from multiparous women or multiply transfused individuals who have developed antibodies against HLA antigens. Donors of cells and sera are made available to donate via a donor file when reagent samples are needed. Recently, monoclonal antisera to HLA antigens have become available, and will very likely replace polyclonal antisera in HLA testing for they circumvent cross-reactivity. However, the production of epitope-specific anti-HLA monoclonal antibodies has not been an easy task because of the low immunogenicity of the epitopes. Patient cells and typing serum are incubated in microtiter wells in the presence of complement, washed, and stained for viability with a vital stain. Percent killing is assessed to determine cytotoxicity. HLA-D antigens

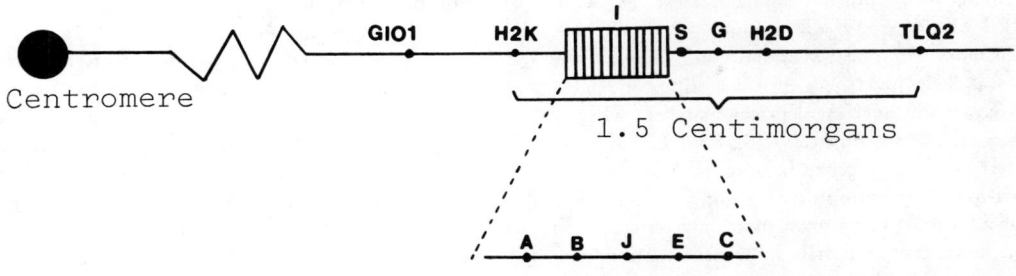

FIG 7-5.—Location of the H2 histocompatibility complex of the mouse on chromosome 17. The I region of the H2 complex is shown in expanded form below; it is composed of genes A, B, J, E, and C. The distance between genes is measured in centimorgans (see Fig 7-3 for the location of HLA histocompatibility genes in humans).

are typed by an MLC assay. In this method, the stimulating cell of known phenotype is treated with mitomycin or some other agent that prevents cell division. The patient's cells are not treated, allowing them to divide when stimulated. Division is measured by ^{3}H-thymidine incorporation into the DNA of the dividing cells. The method is discussed in detail by O'Leary et al.[49]

Another sensitive method to define antigens in the HLA-D locus is the primed lymphocyte defined test.[50] The HLA-DR antigens can be detected by serologic testing.

HLA AND TRANSPLANTATION

HLA and Kidney Transplantation

Most studies on HLA and transplantation have been undertaken in patients who have received kidney allografts. Transplantation workups involve two phases, pretransplantation workup and posttransplantation workup, or follow-up.

Pretransplantation Workup

The pretransplantation workup entails determining the presence or absence of antigens capable of producing an immune response or potentially harmful antibodies to antigens in the transplanted organ. Most HLA workups include an initial blood typing and grouping, for donor and recipient must be ABO compatible.[51] One such study is the complement-dependent cytotoxicity crossmatch, in which patient serum is reacted against donor lymphocytes. This can be considered a screening test, along with the non-complement-fixing HLA antibody assessment test, which is also significant. Screening tests are useful, but hyperacute rejections have occurred in the face of a negative cytotoxic crossmatch.[52] This suggests that other antigens are significant in the rejection process. Furthermore, siblings receiving a kidney with identical HLA matching have shown good survival only if they are maintained with immunosuppressive therapy.

Following the serologic typing of both the donor and the recipient, the HLA-A and HLA-B phenotypes are compared and graded as outlined below (Table 7-4):[54]

A match: no HLA antigen difference.

B match: no donor antigen mismatch, but not all recipient antigens detected on donor.

C match: one donor antigen different from recipient.

D match: two donor antigens different from recipient.

E match: three or four donor antigens different from recipient.

F match: ABO incompatibility or a positive cytotoxic crossmatch.

This type of matching is most useful in related individuals. In unrelated transplants, the relevance

TABLE 7-4.—SURVIVAL 1 YEAR AFTER RENAL TRANSPLANTATION

| MATCHED | % SURVIVAL | |
HLA-A and B	Related	Cadaver*
Identical	90–95	75
One haplotype	70–80	55
Neither haplotype	50–60	45

*Data from Dausset et al.,[53] representing European experience.

of this matching procedure is not clear, as far as survival of the transplanted kidney is concerned. For instance, in one series, survival of a kidney graft was 80% in HLA-identical siblings and 61% in parent-to-child HLA-identical matches, whereas cadaver transplant survival with no HLA identity resulted in 2-year survival in only 40% of cases.[55]

Cell-mediated immunity testing is a relatively recent addition to pretransplantation testing. Good results have been reported in transplantation outcome when these tests are negative,[56] but not all the study series using this approach concur with this assessment.[57] However, it is thought that negative results on both serologic and cellular testing should improve graft survival outcome. Matching for HLA-DR antigens has recently been shown by Ting and Morris to be of significance in cadaver kidney renal allografts.[58] These workers showed that donor and recipient had to share at least two DR antigens for optimal graft survival.

Several other tests to assess immune responsiveness have been suggested. These include (1) skin testing with chlorodinitrobenzene,[59] (2) lymphocyte responsiveness to phytohemagglutinin,[60] and (3) the presence of lymphocytotoxins.[61]

Transplantation Follow-Up

Posttransplantation immunologic monitoring is difficult to carry out because most patients are immunosuppressed and many develop infections, making data difficult to interpret. However, crossmatching of patient serum with donor cells and MLC culture of donor and recipient cells are useful in predicting transplantation outcome. The detection of B cell antibodies in transplant recipients has been correlated with good graft survival.[62]

Blood Transfusion Before Renal Transplantation

The paradoxic finding that kidney transplant survival is better after transfusion of blood was first reported by Dossetor et al. in 1967[63] and subsequently by other authors in retrospective series[64] and prospective series.[61]

The specific reasons for better allograft survival in patients with a history of prior transfusion have not been fully elucidated. However, a selection process may be at play, for these patients are not transplanted in the face of a positive WBC stimulation test. Transfusions may thus unmask potentially immunizing donor alloantigens which can be screened for in other donors. Nevertheless, other factors must be at play in the protective role of pretransplant blood transfusion.

The protective effect of pretransplant transfusion is so important that deliberate transfusions are recommended before transplantation with a cadaver kidney.[65] Whole blood, unmodified, has a tendency to induce the production of unwanted cytotoxic antibodies; therefore, granulocyte-poor blood seems to be the preferred component. Frozen thawed blood has a lesser protective effect.[65] A suggested protocol involves transfusing patients with up to 250 ml of whole blood every 2 weeks, from 8 weeks to 2 weeks prior to transplantation. Transfusions are withheld in the 2 weeks prior to transplantation.[65]

Bone Marrow Transplants and HLA Matching

Potential recipients of a bone marrow transplant are patients with bone marrow aplasia or patients with leukemia who have undergone radical treatment for the disease, with development of secondary bone marrow suppression.[66] As a rule, these patients are difficult to treat because of the threat of secondary infection. The propensity for infection to develop stems from compromise of both cellular and humoral defense mechanisms. Bone marrow transplantation has been developed in recent years to restore defense mechanisms in such patients. Unlike other tissues used as grafts, however, donor bone marrow contains lymphoid cells which are immunocompetent and therefore capable of mounting an immune response against the host tissues, causing graft-versus-host disease (GVHD).[67] GVHD occurs in up to 50% of bone marrow transplants.[68] Obviously, the best source of marrow would be an identical twin, but in lieu of this, marrow from siblings with identical HLA haplotypes and both a negative MLC and a negative cytotoxic crossmatch may have to be used. A last recourse is marrow from unrelated donors with identical HLA haplotypes and a negative WBC crossmatch. This kind of transplantation has a much lower success rate than transplantation with HLA-matched related donors, suggesting, as mentioned earlier, that other antigenic determinants not fully described today are involved in the rejection process (Table 7–5).[69]

Patients are pretreated with total body irradiation to eliminate remaining host immunocompetent cells. The bone marrow is obtained from the donor under sterile conditions by multiple bone marrow aspiration. After filtering to eliminate large cell

TABLE 7–5.—SOME CHARACTERISTICS OF RENAL AND BONE MARROW (BM) TRANSPLANTS

ORGAN	TRANSFUSION	ABO COMPATIBILITY	MHC CROSSMATCH	HLA IDENTITY	GVHD
Kidney	Recommended	Required	Must be negative	Recommended	May be present
BM	Not recommended	Not required	May not be negative	Required*	Often present

*Studies are underway to determine if this is an absolute requirement.

clumps, the anticoagulated marrow is transfused intravenously into the recipient. Apart from GVHD, the major complications of bone marrow transplant are infection and severe bleeding secondary to thrombocytopenia.

The WBC count will be very low initially but will increase steadily if the graft is successful. Blasts in leukemic patients should be searched for. Their presence indicates relapse of the disease (see Chap. 2).

HLA TYPING IN PLATELET TRANSFUSION THERAPY

The use of platelets in the treatment of leukemics and other patients with bleeding secondary to thrombocytopenia has revolutionized therapy for such diseases. The general protocol for the use of platelets is discussed in chapter 8. However, some of the guidelines for HLA typing of platelets are given here.[70]

Patients are usually treated initially with pooled ABO-compatible random donor platelets. The development of antibodies in these patients eventually produces a refractory state, and platelet counts do not increase further. The next choice is to use platelets from a compatible single random donor. Generally a refractory state develops after therapy with this type of platelet concentrate as well. The use of HLA-matched platelets should then be considered.

Significance of HLA Antigens on Platelets

The expression of HLA antigens on platelets is variable and is restricted to certain HLA specificities, such as HLA-B12. The variability in HLA antigen expression will differ when HLA-B12 is accompanied in the haplotype by specific HLA-A genes. If HLA-A11 is found in the haplotype, B12 expression will be enhanced, whereas if HLA-A2, A3, or A28 is present, HLA-B12 expression will be decreased.[71] Matching for the HLA-C locus on platelets does not appear to determine posttransfusion platelet survival. This lack of significance is probably due to the fact that HLA-C antigens are not represented strongly on platelets.[72] The significance of HLA expression on platelets is underlined by the observation that HLA matching is considerably more important to subsequent posttransfusion platelet survival than ABO matching of platelets.[73] However, ABO-incompatible platelets tend to have a decreased survival when compared to ABO-HLA-compatible platelets.[74] Continued platelet therapy eventually results in a refractory state secondary to anti-HLA antibodies produced by the host.[75] Recent studies show that it is the WBCs contaminating platelet units which are largely responsible for the development of anti-HLA antibodies.[76] It should be noted, however, that 30% of patients are nonresponders and do not develop anti-HLA antibodies during platelet therapy;[77] in these patients, selecting for compatible HLA platelets may be an unnecessary expense. Furthermore, many patients needing platelet transfusion therapy are immunocompromised and will not have a significant response to allogeneic platelet antigens.[78]

Clinical Response to Platelet Therapy

One-hour and 24-hour postinfusion platelet counts must be performed, and can help assess alloimmunization.[79] Usually, alloimmunized recipients will show progressively lower postinfusion increases in the platelet count. Febrile reactions to incompatible platelet units and granulocytopenia are also seen in alloimmunized recipients of platelets.[80]

It is crucial that one distinguish a refractory state to platelet transfusion due to alloimmunization from failure to obtain an increment in the platelet count due to other causes (e.g., infection, splenomegaly, DIC, chemotherapy) so that adequate therapy may be carried out. Assessment of alloimmunization can be achieved by performing a lymphocytotoxicity crossmatch, as well as by assessing platelet-associated antibodies using radioimmunoassays, enzyme-linked immunoassays, or immunofluorescence. With these tests it is possible to reduce platelet transfusion failures to almost 7%, according to some workers.[81]

HLA MATCHING FOR GRANULOCYTE TRANSFUSIONS

The transfusion of granulocytes has recently become part of the therapeutic armory for marrow-suppressed individuals.[82] The general tendency is not to transfuse patients until they have counts of 1,000μl or less.

Although granulocytes from random donors have proved useful, HLA-matched granulocytes are preferred by some authors because of the better posttransfusion granulocyte survival.[83] However, better posttransfusional granulocyte survival does not equate increased clinical usefulness in all cases.[84] It appears that HLA matching of granulocytes is critical only in patients who are already alloimmunized to HLA antigens and in whom a poor response to granulocytes can be anticipated.[85] Furthermore, migration and phagocytosis by granulocytes are hindered by alloantibody coating.[86] Laboratory tests to help predict granulocyte posttransfusion survival are currently under study.[87] The protocol for granulocyte use is discussed in chapter 8. Because of the amount of RBC contamination in granulocyte units, ABO and Rh compatibility as well as a negative RBC crossmatch are mandatory.

As with all other transplanted tissues, tissue-specific antigens have been described for granulocytes[88] and may induce antibody stimulation.

HLA IN PATERNITY TESTING

The usefulness of HLA typing in paternity testing is now uncontested.[88] The probability of paternity exclusion by HLA typing alone without using any other system surpasses the 85% cumulative chance of direct exclusion.

The usefulness of this system stems from its polymorphism, its pattern of inheritance, its antigen frequencies of less than 50%, and the accuracy of testing. An example of a paternity exclusion using HLA testing is shown in Figure 7–2.[89, 90]

HLA AND DISEASE

Disease develops as the result of (1) molecular interactions at various levels of the genome, (2) the expression of genome products, and (3) their interaction with the environment. However, these very complex interactions are more often than not incompletely understood. The MHC as a polymorphic array of membrane markers is a logical turf for exploring the relationship between such factors and susceptibility to certain diseases. That some individuals are more prone to disease than others because of inherited factors is an ancient notion in medicine, but it was not until recently that scientific evidence has been adduced.

Pioneer work in this field was the demonstration of a higher incidence of gastric carcinoma in group A individuals in the ABO system.[91] However, disease associations related to the HLA system were suggested initially by work done on the H2 complex of the mouse[92] and its correlation with susceptibility to leukemia.[93] Soon thereafter, similar associations were reported in the HLA system at the HLA-B locus.[94]

Selection of Samples

HLA disease associations are arrived at by statistical analysis. The following parameters must be defined: (1) statistical dependence, (2) strength of association, and (3) pattern of distribution in family studies. The selection of samples is important to avoid comparison of dissimilar groups when linkage is tested for or biased comparisons in populations where certain phenotypes are more frequent. One must avoid type I statistical errors (false conclusion of association) or type II errors (failure to detect an association). The disease population sample should be similar to the control sample to avoid type I errors.[95]

Statistical Evaluation

Studies of HLA and disease associations are based on statistical analysis of populations using Lod scores.[94] This statistical treatment of data compares the correlation between the probability that a given trait will appear at random and the probability that a given trait will be link-expressed (at a defined recombinant fraction H). The calculation is set up as a logarithm of the ratio of these two values and is called a Lod score. If the Lod score exceeds 3, link-

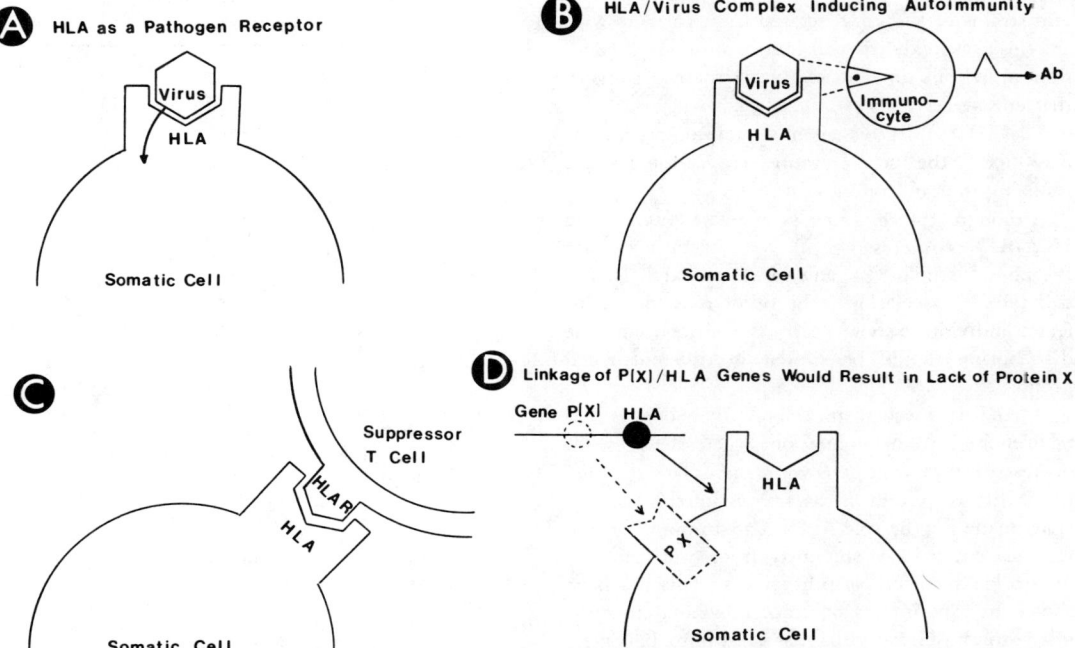

FIG 7–6.—Proposed theories of the correlation of the HLA histocompatibility complex and disease. **A**, the HLA complex functions as a direct receptor for a viral particle, allowing the particle to enter the cell. **B**, the HLA complex and the viral particle modify the configuration of the HLA molecule, which becomes non-self. Immunocytes then produce autoantibodies against HLA-type antigens. **C**, the HLA molecular complex interacts with the HLA system, stimulating a clone of suppressor T cells, resulting in the lack of antibodies against a disease-causing antigen or inducing the stimulation of helper T cells, which induce the production of a clone whose autoantibodies would be directed against HLA antigens. **D**, purported linkage of a P(x) gene and a specific HLA antigen results in the absence or presence of protein x responsible for disease.

age is present. If values are below -2, linkage is excluded.

Possible associations are also studied by 2×2 contingency tables,[96] as described in chapter 14. These data produce relative risk (RR) values, where $RR = (a \times d) / (b \times c)$, using the entries in the 2×2 contingency table. Detailed examples have been provided by Rubinstein.[95]

In assessing RR values, one should remember that gene frequencies tend to vary in the population, which affects the numerical RR value significantly. To circumvent this problem, a δ (delta) measurement is used. In recessive traits $\delta = 2D'$ and in dominant traits $\delta = D'$, where $D' = D/D_{max}$. In this ratio D is the actual linkage disequilibrium and D_{max} is the maximal value of D in a certain population.[97] The actual value of δ is $(FAD - FAP)/(1 - FAP)$, where FAD is the diseased population and FAP is the control population. Since HLA antigens segregate as a haplotype, other HLA antigens in the haplotype may also be of significance to linkage. This concept introduces further complexity to the calculations, which are then termed three-locus linkage studies.[98]

A haplotype relative risk (HRR) has been proposed and is expressed as $Dh = \dfrac{O - E}{E}$, where O indicates observed and E indicates expected frequencies. Dh is the haplodelta value using delta as proposed above.[99]

Possible Mechanisms of Disease Susceptibility

Just how the HLA system is associated with susceptibility to disease is speculative. Some possibilities are outlined below and illustrated in Figure 7–6.

1. The HLA molecules may be direct membrane receptors for a virus or other infective agent. One possible case where this mechanism is at work is the well-known association between ankylosing spon-

dylitis and HLA-B27. It has been shown that certain strains of *Klebsiella* isolated from patients with ankylosing spondylitis will induce antibody production in rabbits innoculated with these organisms that cross-react with HLA-B27.[100]

The HLA infective agent's molecular complex may modify the "self" immune recognition system, resulting in autoimmune disease.

Although the relation between *Klebsiella* and HLA-B27 is interesting, it does not fully explain the physiopathology of ankylosing spondylitis. For this type of association to be valid, most of the affected individuals should carry the antigen, and the distribution should be similar in different racial groups.[95]

2. Another mechanism, a more likely one, is that of immune system modulation, where the presence or absence of an antigen would modulate the susceptibility to certain diseases. Most of the assumptions made for the role of HLA in immune system responsiveness have stemmed from work in the mouse H2 histocompatibility locus. This has been shown in experiments on mice in which susceptibility to the Gross virus was shown to be determined by at least three genes, only one of which was associated with the H2 complex.[92]

Ia molecules in the mouse have been shown to modulate T cell responses; these antigens are products of I-A and I-E subloci of the Ir gene and may exert their influence in three ways: (1) by inducing clonal deletion of antigen reactive cells, (2) by regulating antigen presentation, or (3) by regulating T helper or T suppressor cells. These findings can be extrapolated to humans, where HLA-DR products function as Ir gene products. Evidence for the role of HLA-DR antigens and immune regulation has accumulated in recent years. IgE reaginic responses to ragweed antigens or the failure to respond to them appears to be linked to the HLA-Dw2/DR2 antigens.[101] Type I diabetes is more often found in patients bearing DR3 and DR4 phenotypes.[102]

Individuals bearing HLA-DR3 antigens have a greater propensity to develop circulating antibodies than individuals not bearing this phenotype, and their B cells appear to be more prone to be stimulated into antibody production, probably due to a decreased suppressor T cell function.[103] Furthermore, many individuals bearing HLA-B8/DRw3 show a diminished capacity to clear antibody-coated RBCs from the circulation, possibly due to Fc receptor abnormalities.[104]

The DR4 phenotype is often associated with in vitro T cell reactivity to denatured collagen, which may have some bearing on the physiopathology of

TABLE 7–6.—EXAMPLES OF HLA-DISEASE ASSOCIATIONS

DISEASE	HLA ANTIGEN	RR*
Allergic:		
Hay fever (Ra5)[114]	Dw2	65
Asthma[115]	MB3	18.5
Atopic dermatitis[116]	A2, Bw35, Cw4†	Variable
Autoimmune:		
Cutaneous SLE[117]	DR3	67.1
Scleroderma[118]	A9, DR3	12.18
Sjögren's syndrome[119]	DR3	9.72
Pemphigus[120]	A10, A26	12.25
Graves' disease[121]	DR3	Variable
Hashimoto's[122]	DR3, DR5	5.71, 3.1
Neoplasia:		
Cervical Ca.[123]	Aw31	6.4
Endometrial Ca.[123]	Aw23	13
Hepatocarcinoma[124]	B12	3.23
B cell lymphoma[125]	Aw33	...
Burkitt's lymphoma[107]	DR7	3.3
Kaposi in AIDS[106]	DR5	5.6
Other:		
Insulin-dependent diabetes[126]	DR3, DR4	3.4, 1.26
Chronic active hepatitis[102]	B8, DR3	13.8, 17
Primary biliary cirrhosis[127]	DR3	7.6
Multiple sclerosis[102]	DR3	3.9

*Most data are from caucasian populations.
†As a haplotype.

autoimmune-mediated arthritis.[105] Kaposi's sarcoma in AIDS patients is often associated with the DR5 phenotype,[106] and Burkitt's lymphoma with HLA-DR7[107] (Tables 7–6 and 7–7).

3. A gene that would facilitate or be directly responsible for a disease may be in close proximity, and therefore linked, to an HLA antigen. It is thought that these "susceptibility" genes arise as point mutations. Examples of these disease associations are complement deficiencies arising from gene deletions. It is known, for instance, that genes coding for C2 are closely associated with the HLA megagene stretch.[108] Other examples of diseases not associated with immunity are the 21-hydroxylase-deficiency gene associated with adrenal hyperplasia,[105] and the gene responsible for hemochromatosis which appears to be linked to HLA-A3 (RR > 8).[109]

Categories of Disease Associations and HLA Phenotype

The main categories of disease associations are as follows:

1. Known or suspected hereditary element (e.g., HLA-B27 and ankylosing spondylitis).[110]

TABLE 7-7.—HLA-Disease Associations

DISEASE	HLA ASSOCIATION	PHENOTYPE IN CAUCASIANS (%)	PHENOTYPE IN CAUCASIAN PTS. (%)
Ankylosing spondylitis[128]	HLA-B27	10	85
Rheumatoid arthritis[128]	HLA-Dw4	12	12
Multiple sclerosis[129]	HLA-A3	23	40
Juvenile diabetes[130]	HLA-B8, HLA-B15	1.3 combined	7.3
Idiopathic hemochromatosis[131]	HLA-A3	23	69
HB$_s$Ag-negative chronic active hepatitis[132]	HLA-B8	22	Variable
Dermatitis herpetiformis[133]	HLA-B8	22	Variable
Acute leukemia and Hodgkins's disease[134]	HLA-A2	50	Variable

2. Malignant diseases (e.g., leukemia and HLA-A2 and HLA-B12 haplotypes).[111]
3. Diseases with possible immunologic etiology (e.g., HLA-B8 and dermatitis herpetiformis).[112]

These associations have been defined by statistical analysis of large populations. Such analysis yields a suggestion of incidence and association of HLA type with a particular disease. However, it does not imply that the association is clear-cut or straightforward in every case. At present, only a few diseases can be shown to be associated with a particular HLA type with any degree of confidence (see Table 7–6). Of interest in RBC antigen studies is the recent discovery that Bg antigens, which are associated with the HLA system, may be increased in strength in certain cases of anemia.[113]

Evidently the physiopathology of most HLA-disease associations is much more complex than single HLA antigen associations. It is therefore difficult to make conclusive assumptions about etiology of disease and defined HLA linkage or disease susceptibility and the HLA system at the present time.

REFERENCES

1. Nordhagen R., Aas M.: Association between HLA and red cell antigens. *Vox Sang.* 35:319, 1978.
2. Doan C.A.: The recognition of a biologic differentiation in the white blood cells. *JAMA* 86:1593, 1926.
3. Snell G.D.: Reference and methods for the study of histocompatibility genes. *J. Genet.* 49:87, 1948.
4. Dausset J.: Iso-leuco-anticorps. *Acta Haematol.* 20:156, 1958.
5. van Rood J.J., van Leeuwen A., Ernisse J.G.: Leucocyte antibodies in sera of pregnant women. *Vox Sang.* 4:427, 1959.
6. van Rood J.J., cited by Bodmer W.F. (ed.): The HLA system: Introduction. *Br. Med. Bull.* 34:215, 1978.
7. Curtoni E.S., Mattiuz P.L., Tosi R.M., cited by Bodmer W.F. (ed.): The HLA system: Introduction. *Br. Med. Bull.* 34:214, 1978.
8. Terasaki P.O., cited by Bodmer W.F. (ed.): The HLA system: Introduction. *Br. Med. Bull.* 34:214, 1978.
9. Dausset J., Colombani J., cited by Bodmer W.F. (ed.): The HLA system: Introduction. *Br. Med. Bull.* 34:215, 1978.
10. Kissmeyer-Nielsen F., cited by Bodmer W.F. (ed.): The HLA system: Introduction. *Br. Med. Bull.* 34:216, 1978.
11. Bodmer W.F., Batchelor J.R., Bodmer J.C., et al., cited by Bodmer W.F. (ed.): The HLA system: Introduction. *Br. Med. Bull.* 34:216, 1978.
12. WHO-IMIS Terminology Committee: Nomenclature for factors of the HL-A System. *Transplant. Proc.* 8:109, 1976.
13. Bradley B.A., Festenstein H., cited by Bodmer W.F., Bodmer J.G. (eds.): The HLA system. *Br. Med. Bull.* 34:203, 1978.
14. Mittal K.K., Terasaki P.I.: Crossreactivity in the HL-A system. *Tissue Antigens* 2:94, 1972.

15. Springer T.A., Strominger J.L., Mann D.L.: Formal purification of detergent-solubilized HL-A antigen and its cleavage by papain. *Proc. Natl. Acad. Sci. USA* 71:1539, 1974.
16. Cresswell P., Springer T., Strominger J.L., et al.: Immunological identity of the small subunit of HL-A antigens and β2-microglobulin and its turnover on the cell membrane. *Proc. Natl. Acad. Sci. USA* 71:2123, 1974.
17. Strominger J.L., Orr H.T., Parham P., et al.: An evaluation of the significance of amino acid sequence homologies in human histocompatibility antigens (HLA-A and HLA-B) with immunoglobulins and other proteins, using relatively short sequences. *Scand. J. Immunol.* 11:573, 1980.
18. Orr H.T., Strominger J.L.: Towards a structural definition of serological specificity: The HLA system in the biology and function of the major histocompatibility complex, in *Proceedings of the 33rd Annual Meeting of the American Association of Blood Banks*. Washington, D.C., American Association of Blood Banks, 1980, p. 9.
19. Orr H.T., Lancet D., Robb R.J., et al.: The heavy chain of human histocompatibility antigen HLA-B7 contains an immunoglobulin-like region. *Nature* 282:266, 1979.
20. Nakamuro K., Tanigaki N., Pressman D.: Isolation of HL-A 33,000-dalton fragments carrying high HL-A alloantigenic activity. *Transplantation* 19:431, 1975.
21. Gazit E., Terhost C., Mahorey R.J., et al.: Alloantigens of the human T(HT) genetic region of the HLA linkage group. *Hum. Immunol.* 1:97, 1980.
22. Larhammer D., Wiman K., Schenning L., et al.: Evolutionary relationship between HLA-DR antigen β-chains, HLA-A, -B, -C antigen subunits and immunoglobulin chains. *Scand. J. Immunol.* 14:617, 1981.
23. Tanigaki N., Tosi R.: The genetic control of human Ia alloantigens: A three loci model derived from the immunochemical analysis of "supertypic" specificities. *Immunol. Rev.* 66:5, 1982.
24. Shackelford D.A., Kaufman J.F., Korman A.J., et al.: HLA-DR antigens: Structure, separation of subpopulation, gene cloning and function. *Immunol. Rev.* 66:133, 1982.
25. Goyert S.M., Shively J.E., Silver J.: Biochemical characterization of a second family of human Ia molecules, HLA-DS equivalent to murine I-A subregion molecules. *J. Exp. Med.* 156-550, 1982.
26. Shaw S., Pollack M.S., Payne S.M., et al.: HLA-linked B cell alloantigens of a new segregant series: Population and family studies of the SB antigens. *Hum. Immunol.* 1:177, 1980.
27. Ferrone S., Allison J.P., Pellegrino M.A.: Human DR (Ia-like antigens): Biological and molecular profile. *Contemp. Top. Mol. Immunol.* 7:239, 1978.
28. Boyd H.C., Smilek D.E., Spielman R.S., et al.: Monoclonal rat anti-MHC alloantibodies detect HLA-linked polymorphisms in humans. *Immunogenetics* 12:313, 1981.
29. Cavalli-Sforza L.L., Bodmer W.F.: *The Genetics of Human Populations*. San Francisco, W.H. Freeman, 1971, p. 55.
30. Van Someren H., Westerveld A., Hagmeijer A., et al.: Human antigen and enzyme markers in man-Chinese hamster somatic cell hybrids: Evidence for syntony between the HL-A, PGM3, ME1, and IPO-B loci. *Proc. Natl. Acad. Sci. USA* 71:962, 1974.
31. Goodfellow P.N., Jones E.A., Van Heyningen V., et al.: The beta-2-microglobulin gene is on chromosome 15 and not in the HLA region. *Nature* 254:267, 1975.
32. Cepellini R.: Old and new facts and speculations about transplantation antigens of man. *Prog. Immunol.* 1:973, 1971.
33. Kissmeyer-Nielsen F., Svejgaard A., Ahrous S., et al.: Crossing over within the HLA system. *Nature* 224:75, 1969.
34. Bach F.H., Amos D.B.: Hu-1: Major histocompatibility locus in man. *Science* 156:1506, 1967.
35. Hackel E., Fisher R.A.: Theoretical aspects of HLA: Genetics and biology, in Hackel E., Mallory D.C. (eds.): *Theoretical Aspects of HLA*. Washington, D.C., American Association of Blood Banks, 1982, p. 1.
36. Lewontin R.C.: *The Genetic Basis of Evolutionary Change*. New York, Columbia University Press, 1974.
37. Benacerraf B., McDevitt H.O.: Histocompatibility immune response genes. *Science* 175:273, 1972.
38. Waldron J.A. Jr., Horn R.G., Rosenthal A.S.: Antigen-induced proliferation of guinea pig lymphocytes in vitro: Obligatory role of macrophages in the recognition of antigen by immune T-lymphocytes. *J. Immunol.* 111:58, 1973.
39. Thomas D.W., Yamashita U., Shevach E.M.: The role of Ia antigens in T-cell activation. *Immunol. Rev.* 35:97, 1977.
40. Jerne N.K.: The somatic generation of immune recognition. *Eur. J. Immunol.* 1:1, 1971.
41. Benacerraf B.: Role of MHC gene products in immune regulation. *Science* 212:1229, 1981.
42. Robinson M., Moreen H.J., Amos D.B.: Target antigen of cell mediated lympholysis: Discrimination of HLA subtypes by cytotoxic lymphocytes. *J. Immunol.* 121:1486, 1978.
43. McDevitt H.O., Deak B.D., Shreffler C., et al.: Genetic control of the immune response mapping of the IR-1 locus. *J. Exp. Med.* 135:1259, 1972.
44. Tada T., Taniguchi M., Okumura K.: Regulation of antibody response by antigen specific T-cell factors bearing T-region determinants. *Prog. Immunol.* 3:369, 1977.
45. Engleman E.G., McDevitt H.O.: A suppressor T cell of the mixed lymphocyte reaction specific for the HLA-D region in man. *J. Clin. Invest.* 61:828, 1978.
46. Guzit E., Terhorst C., Yunis E.J.: The human "T" genetic region of the HLA linkage groups in a poly-

morphism detected on lectin activated lymphocytes. *Nature* 284:275, 1980.
47. Kisielow P., Hirst J.A., Shika H., et al.: Ly antigens as markers for functionally distinct subpopulations of thymus-derived lymphocytes of the mouse. *Nature* 253:219, 1975.
48. Terasaki P., McClelland J.D., Park M.S., et al.: Microdroplet lymphocyte cytotoxicity test, in *Manual of Tissue Typing Techniques*. Washington, D.C., Dept. of Health, Education and Welfare, publication No. (NIH) 74, 545, 1973, p. 54.
49. O'Leary J., Reinsmoen N., Yunis E.J.: Mixed lymphocyte reaction, in Rose N.R., Friedman H. (eds.): *Manual of Clinical Immunology*. American Society for Microbiology, 1976, p. 820.
50. Sheehy M.J., Sondel P.M., Bach M.L., et al.: LD (lymphocyte-defined) typing: A rapid assay with primed lymphocytes. *Science* 188:1308, 1975.
51. Rappoport F.T., Dausset J., Legrand L., et al.: Erythrocytes in human transplantation: Effects of pre-treatment with ABO group-specific antigens. *J. Clin. Invest.* 47:2206, 1968.
52. Williams G.M., DePlanque B., Lower R., et al.: Antibodies and human transplant rejection. *Ann. Surg.* 170:603, 1969.
53. Dausset J., Hori J., Busson M., et al.: Serologically defined HL-A antigens and long-term survival of cadaver kidney transplants: A joint analysis of 918 cases performed by France transplant and the London transplant group. *N. Engl. J. Med.* 290:979, 1974.
54. Opelz G., Mickey M.R., Terasaki P.I.: HL-A and kidney transplants: Re-examination. *Transplantation* 17:371, 1974.
55. Opelz G.: Histocompatibility testing in renal transplantation. *Urology Suppl.* 9:72, 1977.
56. Botha J.R., Myburgh J.A., Smit J.A., et al.: Crossmatching assays of cell-mediated immunity for transplant patients. *S. Afr. Med. J.* 50:1275, 1976.
57. Stiller C.R., Sinclair N.R., Abrahams S., et al.: Anti-donor immune responses in prediction of transplant rejection. *N. Engl. J. Med.* 294:978, 1976.
58. Ting A., Morris P.J.: Powerful effect of HL-DR matching on survival of cadaveric renal allografts. *Lancet* 2:282, 1980.
59. Rolley R.T., Sterioff S., Parks L.C., et al.: Delayed cutaneous hypersensitivity and human renal allotransplantation. *Transplant. Proc.* 9:81, 1977.
60. Jones A.R., Bewick M., Vaughan R.W., et al.: Transformation of lymphocytes from patients awaiting cadaver renal transplants. *Lancet* 2:529, 1976.
61. Opelz G., Terasaki P.I.: Prolongation effect of blood transfusions on kidney graft survival. *Transplantation* 22:380, 1976.
62. Ettenger R.B., Terasaki P.I., Ting A., et al.: Anti-B lymphocytotoxins in renal-allograft rejection. *N. Engl. J. Med.* 295:305, 1976.
63. Dossetor J.B., MacKinnon K.J., Gault M.H., et al.: Cadaver kidney transplants. *Transplantation Suppl.* 5:844, 1967.
64. Festenstein H., Sachs J.A., Pegrum G.D., et al.: Influence of HLA matching and blood transfusion on outcome of 502 London Transplant Group renal graft recipients. *Lancet* 1:157, 1976.
65. Perkins H.A.: Transplantation, in Hackel E., Mallory D. (eds.): *Theoretical Aspects of HLA: A Technical Workshop*. Washington, D.C., American Association of Blood Banks, 1982, p. 129.
66. Thomas E.D.: Bone marrow transplantation for aplastic anemia or acute leukemia. *Scand. J. Urol. Nephrol. Suppl.* 42:6, 1977.
67. Elkins W.L.: Cellular immunology and the pathogenesis of graft-versus-host reaction. *Prog. Allergy* 15:78, 1971.
68. van Bekkum D.W.: Bone marrow transplantation. *Transplant. Proc.* 9:174, 1977.
69. Parkman R., Rosen F., Rappaport T., et al.: Detection of genetically determined histocompatibility antigen differences between HL-A identical and MLC non-reactive siblings. *Transplantation* 21:110, 1976.
70. Slichter S.J.: Controversies in platelet transfusion therapy. *Annu. Rev. Med.* 31:509, 1980.
71. Moore S.B.: HLA and blood component therapy, in Hackel E., Mallory D. (eds.): *Theoretical Aspects of HLA*. Washington, D.C., American Association of Blood Banks, 1982, p. 81.
72. Mueller-Eckhart G., Hauck M., Kayser W., et al.: HLA-C antigens on platelets. *Tissue Antigens* 16:91, 1980.
73. Lohrman H.P., Bull M.I., DeHer J.A., et al.: Platelet transfusion from HLA compatible unrelated donors to alloimmunized platelets. *Ann. Intern. Med.* 80:9, 1974.
74. Duquesnoy R.J., Anderson A.J., Tomasuolo P.A., et al.: ABO compatibility and platelet transfusions of alloimmunized thrombocytopenic patients. *Blood* 54:595, 1979.
75. Yankee, R.A., Graff R.S., Dawlings R., et al: Selection of unrelated compatible platelet donors by lymphocyte HLA matching. *N. Engl. J. Med.* 288:760, 1973.
76. Eernisse J.G., Brand A.: Prevention of platelet refractoriness due to HLA antibodies by administration of leukocyte-poor blood components. *Exp. Hematol.* 9:77, 1981.
77. Howard J.E., Perkins H.A.: The natural history of alloimmunization to platelets. *Transfusion* 18:496, 1978.
78. Dutcher J.P., Schiffer C.A., Aisner J., et al.: Longterm followup of patients with leukemia receiving platelet transfusions: Identification of a large group of patients who do not become alloimmunized. *Blood* 58:1007, 1981.
79. Daly P.A., Schiffer C.A., Aisner J., et al.: Platelet transfusion therapy: One hour posttransfusion increments are valuable in predicting the need for HLA-matched preparations. *JAMA* 243:435, 1980.
80. Herzig R.H., Poplack D.G., Yankee R.A.: Prolonged granulocytopenia from incompatible platelet transfusions. *N. Engl. J. Med.* 290:1120, 1974.

81. Myers T.J., Kim B.K., Steiner M., et al.: Selection of donor platelets for alloimmunized patients using a platelet-associated IgG assay. *Blood* 58:444, 1980.
82. Herzig R.H., Herzig G.P., Graw R.G., et al.: Successful granulocyte transfusion therapy for gram-negative septicemia. *N. Engl. J. Med.* 196:701, 1977.
83. McCullough J., Wood N., Weiblen B.J., et al.: The role of histocompatibility testing in granulocyte transfusion, in *The Granulocyte: Function and Clinical Utilization. Prog. Clin. Biol. Res.* 13:321, 1977.
84. McCredie K.B., Hester J.P., Freireich E.J., et al.: Platelet and leukocyte transfusions in acute leukemia. *Hum. Pathol.* 5:699, 1974.
85. Dahlke M.B., Keashen M.A., Alavi J.B., et al.: Response to granulocyte transfusions in the alloimmunized patient. *Transfusion* 20:555, 1980.
86. Nusbacher J., MacPherson J.L., Gore I. Jr., et al.: Inhibition of granulocyte erythrophagocytosis by HLA antisera. *Blood* 53:350, 1979.
87. Verheught F.W.A., von Dem Borne A.E.G.Kr., Decary F., et al.: The detection of granulocyte alloantibodies with a direct immunofluorescence test. *Br. J. Haemat.* 36:533, 1977.
88. Lalezari P., Thalenfeld B., Weinstein W.J.: The third neutrophil antigen, in Terasaki P.I. (ed.): *Histocompatibility Testing.* Copenhagen, Munksgaard, 1970, p. 319.
89. Jeannet M., Hassig H., Bernheim J.: Use of the HLA-A system in disputed paternity cases. *Vox Sang.* 23:197, 1972.
90. Soulier J.P., Prou-Wartelle Q., Muller J.Y.: Paternity research using HL-A system. *Haematologia* 8:249, 1974.
91. Aird I., Bentall H.A., Rolients J.A.F.: A relationship between cancer of the stomach and the ABO blood groups. *Br. Med. J.* 1:799, 1953.
92. Lilly F., Boyse E.A., Old L.J.: Genetic basis of susceptibility to viral leukaemogenesis. *Lancet* 2:1207, 1964.
93. Kourilski F.M., Dausset J., Feingold N., et al.: Leucocyte groups and acute leukemia. *JNCI* 41:81, 1968.
94. Haldone J.B.S., Smith C.A.B.: A new estimate of linkage between the genes for colour blindness and haemophilia in man. *Am. Eugen.* 14:10, 1947.
95. Rubinstein P.: HLA disease associations: In search of meaning, in Hackel E., Mallory D. (eds.): *Theoretical Aspects of HLA: A Technical Workshop.* Arlington, Va., American Association of Blood Banks, 1982, p. 103.
96. Jersild C., Dupont B., Fog T., et al.: Histocompatibility determinants in multiple sclerosis. *Transplant. Rev.* 22:148, 1975.
97. Bengtsson B.O., Thomson G.: Measuring the strength of association between HLA and disease. *Tissue Antigens* 18:356, 1981.
98. Thompson G., Bodmer W.F.: HLA haplotype associations with disease. *Tissue Antigens* 13:91, 1979.
99. Rubinstein P., Walker M., Carpenter C., et al.: Genetics of HLA-disease associations: The use of haplotype relative risk (HRR) and haplo-delta (Dh) estimates. *Hum. Immunol.* 3:384, 1981.
100. Geczy A.F., Yap J.: A survey of isolates of *Klebsiella pneumoniae* which cross-react with HL-A-B27-associated cell-surface structure on the lymphocytes of patients with ankylosing spondylitis. *J. Rheumatol.* 9:97, 1982.
101. Marsh D.G., Chase G.A., Friedhoff L.R., et al.: Association of HLA antigens and total serum immunoglobulin E level with allergic response and failure to respond to ragweed allergen Ra3. *Proc. Natl. Acad. Sci. USA* 76:2903, 1979.
102. Braun W.F.: HLA and disease: A comprehensive review. Boca Raton, Fla., CRC Press, Inc., 1979, p. 1.
103. Ambinder J.M., Chiorazzi N., Gibofsky A., et al.: Special characteristics of cellular immune function in normal individuals of the HLA-DR3 type. *Clin. Immunol. Immunopathol.* 23:269, 1982.
104. Lawley T.J., Hall R.P., Fauci A.S., et al.: Defective Fc-receptor functions associated with the HLA-B8/DRW3 haplotype: Studies in patients with dermatitis herpetiformis and normal subjects. *N. Engl. J. Med.* 304:185, 1981.
105. Zmijewski C.M.: HLA and disease. *CRC Crit. Rev. Clin. Lab. Sci.* 20:285, 1984.
106. Friedman-Kein A., Laubenstein L.J., Rubinstein P., et al.: Disseminated Kaposi sarcoma in homosexual men. *Ann. Intern. Med.* 96:693, 1982.
107. Jones E.H., Biggar R.J., Nkrumah F.K., et al.: Study of the HLA system in Burkitt's lymphoma. *Hum. Immunol.* 1:207, 1980.
108. Awdeh Z.L., Raum D., Alper C.A.: Major histocompatibility complex (MHC) linked complement haplotypes (complotypes) (abstract). *Fed. Proc.* 40:1066, 1981.
109. Simon M., Bourel M., Genetet B., et al.: Idiopathic hemochromatosis: Demonstration of recessive transmission and early detection by family HLA typing. *N. Engl. J. Med.* 297:1017, 1977.
110. Brewerton D.A., Hart F.D., Nicholls A., et al.: Ankylosing spondylitis and HL-A27. *Lancet* 1:904, 1973.
111. Svejgaard A., Platz R., Ryder L.P., et al.: HL-A and disease associations: A survey. *Transplant. Rev.* 22:3, 1975.
112. Barneston R., Heading R.C., White A.G.: HL-B8 and dermatitis herpetiformis, letter. *Lancet* 2:1027, 1973.
113. Morton J.A., Pickles M.M., Turner J.E., et al.: Changes in red cell Bg antigens in haematological disease. *Immunol. Commun.* 9:173, 1980.
114. Marsh D.G., Hsu S.H., Roebber M., et al.: HLA-Dw2 a genetic marker for human immune response to short ragweed pollen allergen Ra5: I. Response resulting primarily from natural antigen exposure. *J. Exp. Med.* 155:1439, 1982.
115. Nakai Y., Kano T., Moriuchi J., et al.: Association between the MB system and asthma in the Japanese. *Hum. Immunol.* 4:265, 1982.

116. Schultz L.F., Grummet N., Vose P.: HLA antigen in atopic dermatitis: A family study. *Dermatologica* 160:17, 1979.
117. Sontheimer R.D., Stastny P., Gilliam J.N.: Human histocompatibility antigen associations in subacute cutaneous lupus erythematosus. *J. Clin. Immunol.* 67:312, 1980.
118. Ercilla M.G., Arriaga F., Gratacos M.R., et al.: HLA antigens and scleroderma. *Arch. Dermatol. Res.* 271:381, 1981.
119. Ryder L.P., Anderson E., Svejgaard, Eds.: *HLA Diseases Registry,* ed. 3. Copenhagen, Munksgaard, 1979, p. 1.
120. David M., Zamier R., Segal R., et al.: HLA antigens in Jews with pemphigus vulgaris. *Dermatologica* 163:326, 1981.
121. McKenna R., Kearns M., Sugrue D., et al.: HLA and hyperthyroidism in Ireland. *Tissue Antigens* 19:97, 1982.
122. Farid N.R., Sampson L., Moens H., et al.: The association of goitrous autoimmune thyroiditis with HLA-DR5. *Tissue Antigens* 17:265, 1981.
123. Sniecinski I., Haley J., Morgan-Byrne J., et al.: Histocompatibility-antigen distribution in patients with cervical and endometrial carcinomas. *Gynecol. Oncol.* 11:68, 1981.
124. Zervas J., Karvountzis G., Theodoropoulous G.: HLA antigens in hepatocellular carcinoma. *Gastroenterology* 79:601, 1980.
125. van den Tweel J.G., Dugas D.J., Loon J., et al.: HLA typing in non-Hodgkin's lymphomas: Comparative study in caucasoids, Mexican-Americans and negroids. *Tissue Antigens* 20:364, 1982.
126. Barbosa J., Chern M.M., Reinsmoen N., et al.: HLA-Dw antigens in unrelated juvenile, insulin-dependent diabetics. *Tissue Antigens* 14:426, 1979.
127. Ercilla G., Pares A., Arriaga F., et al.: Primary biliary cirrhosis associated with HLA-DRw3. *Tissue Antigens* 14:499, 1979.
128. Batchelor J.R., Morris P.J., in Bodmer W.F., Bodmer J.G., Batchelor J.R., et al. (eds.): *Histocompatibility Testing: Report of the Seventh International Histocompatibility Workshop and Conference.* Copenhagen, Munksgaard, 1977, p. 205.
129. Naito S., Namerow N., Mickey M.R., et al.: Multiple sclerosis: Association with HL-A3. *Tissue Antigens* 2:1, 1972.
130. Thomsen M., Platz P., Andersen O.O., et al.: MLC typing in juvenile diabetes mellitus and idiopathic Addison's disease. *Transplant. Rev.* 22:125, 1975.
131. Bomford A., Eddleston A.L., Kennedy L.A., et al.: Histocompatibility antigens as markers of abnormal iron metabolism in patients with idiopathic haemochromatosis and their relatives. *Lancet* 1:327, 1977.
132. MacKay I.R., Morris P.J.: Association of autoimmune active chronic hepatitis with HL-A1, 8. *Lancet* 2:793, 1972.
133. Gebhard R.L., Katz S.I., Marks J., et al.: HL-A antigen type and small-intestinal disease in dermatitis herpetiformis. *Lancet* 2:760, 1973.
134. Hannia R., Lawler S., Oliver R.T.D.: The HLA system in acute leukemia and Hodgkin's disease. *Br. Med. Bull.* 34:212, 1978.

8

Components and Fractions

SINCE THE FIRST human-to-human blood transfusion, a great deal has been learned about storage and preservation techniques and the better utilization of blood as a therapeutic agent.

Banked blood is separated into components and stored and delivered in this form to redress more efficaciously homeostatic imbalances created by loss of volume, oxygen-carrying capacity, and coagulation factors. The ability to separate blood into its components has resulted from development of techniques for anticoagulating blood[1] and centrifuging it within a system of interconnected sterile plastic bags. These techniques enable blood banks to separate blood components relatively easily and cheaply.

DONOR SELECTION

Blood cannot be manufactured artificially. Therefore, blood supplies must be obtained by voluntary donation. About 3% of the population volunteer blood. Their reasons are various, but altruistic motives prevail.[2] The use of blood from paid donors is not encouraged, because such donors often have a higher risk of transmitting disease.[3] For example, the net risk of transmitting hepatitis from paid donors is up to 10 times higher than when blood from voluntary donors is used.[4]

The voluntary donor comes to the donor room a healthy individual and should leave in the same state. A donor program depends on recruiting new donors and maintaining a pool of previous donors. Donors are more likely to donate again if they are received courteously and appreciation is expressed for their contribution.

Donors are advised to eat a regular meal 2–3 hours before donating. The donor room should be pleasant and impeccably clean. A separate room or area should be designated for interviews and physical examination. A blood bank physician must be available for questions regarding acceptability of donors and to treat donor reactions. Nurses or technical personnel trained in donor procedures are qualified to screen donors, perform phlebotomies, collect and process blood units, and perform other laboratory procedures associated with screening, such as blood typing and determining hematocrit.

Medical History

Recording a good but succinct donor clinical history is of paramount importance for obtaining safe components for transfusion. The history can be recorded on a card bearing all of the initial relevant information, such as name, age, sex, address, license number, or other identifying number. The reverse of the card may bear the consent form. The donor should be 18 years old to donate without a written permission from a parent or guardian. Donors may donate at age 17 with written permission from a parent or guardian. Persons may donate until their 66th birthday. Exceptions to the older age limit may be made at the discretion of the blood bank physician.

The occupation of the donor should be noted,

and persons that operate aircraft or are employed in other hazardous professions must be informed they cannot resume activities for at least 72 hours.

One should inquire about previous donations and history of reactions to donation, if any. There must be an interval of at least 8 weeks between donations, and no more than five donations a year are allowed. Pregnant women should not donate blood during pregnancy and for 6 weeks after delivery. The donor should be free of systemic infections of all sorts. A history of hepatitis of any sort is a cause for permanent rejection, as is a history of jaundice of any etiology. Relatives of persons who had hepatitis and who were in close contact with these persons must wait until 6 months after exposure and are accepted after this period only if they are symptom free. Persons receiving hepatitis immune globulin are deferred 9 months after the last injection.[5] A person donating a unit which results in transmission of hepatitis is permanently excluded. If, however, the unit is only one of several units that have been given in the course of 6 months to a patient who develops hepatitis, the donor is not excluded from future donation. Drug addiction is cause for permanent rejection. Tattoos and skin grafts warrant a 6-month deferment.

A history of sexual promiscuity in male homosexuals is associated with a higher incidence of hepatitis B,[6] as well as a higher incidence of a recently described syndrome—acquired immunodeficiency syndrome (AIDS).[7,8] Nonhomosexual Haitians who have recently immigrated to the United States have also presented with a higher incidence of AIDS,[9] as have individuals immigrating from Zaire to Europe.[10] However, many of these individuals were later found to belong to other high risk groups for AIDS. Of special interest to the blood banking community, hemophiliacs receiving blood products have been reported to develop the disease.[11] Because of the high mortality from AIDS, it may be necessary to screen the donor population for persons at risk of transmitting the disease (see Chap. 13).[12]

Donors who have traveled to malarial areas may not contribute for 6 months; if they have taken antimalarial drugs they may not contribute for 3 years. If they have had malaria they must wait at least 3 years after recovery or after cessation of therapy. Monoclonal antisera to the parasite may provide a screening test in endemic areas.[13]

Patients with active tuberculosis may not contribute, and those with a history of tuberculosis must be evaluated by a blood bank physician for acceptability. Persons with a positive purified protein derivative test (PPD) may be accepted for donation. Patients with a history of brucellosis, typhus, or other disease with a hematologic phase may donate after a 2-year symptom-free period without medication.[14] Syphilis is rarely transmitted by blood products that have been refrigerated more than 96 hours.[15] However, patients who have had syphilis are permanently rejected.[16] Units positive on the rapid plasma reagin (RPR) or VDRL test are rejected. Infected units of platelets stored at room temperature could potentially transmit syphilis. By the time the syphilis test result has become positive, the disease is no longer hematogenous, a fact that has made the AABB drop the requirement for donor screening for syphilis.[17]

Chagas' disease may also be transmitted by blood,[18] and patients with a history of this disease are rejected.

Cytomegalovirus infection secondary to massive transfusions[19] has been reported as a complication of open heart surgery, resulting in a mononucleosis-like syndrome. However, the infection in donors is usually subclinical, making screening for this disease impractical, except in selected neonatal transfusions.[20]

Patients exposed to measles, German measles, chickenpox, or mumps through contact with an infected individual should wait at least 3 weeks after exposure to ensure absence of disease before donating blood. Vaccination against any of these diseases as well as vaccination for polio, yellow fever, and influenza warrants a 2- to 3-week wait (except for German measles vaccination which warrants a 1-month wait[21]) because the vaccines contain live virus. Persons immunized against rabies must wait at least a year before donation.[22] Patients on medications other than vitamins, contraceptives, or replacement hormones may not donate until the drug is discontinued, and only after a physician clears the screening. Donors who have taken aspirin should wait 48 hours if they are to donate platelets.

An excellent guideline for drugs that may cause rejection of a donor is given by Milam.[23] Patients who have undergone major surgery or received transfusions of any component or plasma fraction except albumin cannot donate for 6 months and until healing is complete, if they have undergone minor surgery (e.g., appendectomy or tonsillectomy). Oral surgery warrants a 72-hour deferment. Acutely ill patients are deferred until they are no longer sick.

Chronic diseases of the kidney, liver, stomach, respiratory system, or cardiovascular system are cause for rejection (e.g., rheumatic or coronary heart disease; essential hypertension). Metabolic diseases such as diabetes are cause for rejection because affected persons are prone to infections and may be taking medication. Patients with gout can donate if they are not taking medication. Carcinomas that have the potential to metastasize are reason for permanent rejection. Examples of these are lymphomas, melanoma, and colonic carcinoma. Benign tumors are usually not a cause for rejection.

Autoimmune disease, including systemic lupus erythematosus (SLE), rheumatoid arthritis, and dermatitis herpetiformis, are cause for permanent rejection, as are asthma and severe allergic conditions. The IgE responsible for allergies present in the donated plasma can be transfused to patients.[24] These antibodies will then produce a transient allergic reaction to antigens the person is not intrinsically allergic to.

Patients with gastrointestinal disorders such as chronic ulcerative colitis and peptic ulcer who want to donate should be screened by the blood bank physician. If the disease is not active, they can usually be accepted for donation. Patients with a history of seizures are permanently rejected, because they may convulse during or after donation.[25]

Anemic patients are not accepted. Patients with polycythemia are not accepted and their therapeutic bleedings should not be used for transfusion. Any patient with a bleeding tendency is not acceptable.

Donor Physical Examination

Donor physical examination should be conducted in a special area affording adequate privacy for this purpose. The donor should appear healthy. Blood pressure should be between 50 and 100 mm Hg diastolic and between 90 and 180 mm Hg systolic. The pulse should be regular and between 50 and 100 beats per minute. The chest should be auscultated for murmurs, rales, etc. Hemoglobin can be measured in the blood bank by the Phillips–Van Slyke method[26] and should be no less than 12.5 gm/100 ml in females (it is tested using copper sulfate at a specific gravity of 1.053), and no less than 13.5 gm/100 for males (tested by the same method at a specific gravity of 1.055). The hematocrit should be no less than 41% for males and no less than 38% for females.[27]

The temperature of the donor should not be above 37.5° C (99.5° F). Donors should be weighed before donation. As a rule, a donor may donate 10% of the total blood volume. The total blood volume can be calculated by multiplying the body weight in kilograms by 77 in men and by 67 in women. This generally means that no more than 450 ± 45 ml of blood should be taken, plus 30 ml for samples.[21] In rare cases, donors weighing less than 100 pounds (45 kg) may have to have blood drawn (if they have a special phenotype, or for autologous transfusion). Exceptional cases are evaluated by the blood bank physician. In these persons, the amount of anticoagulant may have to be reduced according to the following formulas:[28]

Volume to be drawn = body weight (kg) × 450/110.

Volume of anticoagulant = normal volume of anticoagulant × volume to be drawn/450.

The usual amount of citrate phosphate in dextrose (CPD) anticoagulant in a bag is 63 ml.

In general, complex laboratory screening for donors discourages donations and is to be avoided.[29]

THE DONATION

The donor signs a consent form that includes a brief explanation of the process and lists some of the potential complications. An explanation of the donation process and its side effects should be repeated verbally. Donors may need to be reassured, especially those donating blood for the first time. The donor is asked to recline in a comfortable donor chair, and the arm from which the unit is to be drawn is inspected to make sure no cutaneous infections or other lesions are present. A pressure cuff is applied above the venipuncture site and inflated to 50–60 mm Hg of pressure. An adequate vein is selected in the antecubital space by palpation. The venipuncture site is prepared with a detergent scrub for at least 30 seconds, spanning an area at least 1½ inches in diameter. Soap is removed with 70% ethanol and a tincture of iodine is applied to the scrubbed area, working from the center to the periphery. Detergent scrubs are available commercially in disposable packages. The aseptic area is no longer palpated. Although it is not recommendable to have a novice draw blood from a donor, a reference which deals with a good venipuncture technique for those who seek it is the article by Linke and Henry.[30] Not more than two venipunctures should be made in an attempt to draw a unit. The venipuncture is usually made with a 16-gauge needle and the blood is collected in appropriate containers. These are mixed, usually automatically, with a mixer-scale which signals the completion of collection with a sound and a light. In lieu of this device, collection bags may be weighed manually with a scale. A normal collection should not last more than 10 minutes. The final container should weigh 425–475 gm, minus the bag weight and including the anticoagulant. That is, it should contain 405–500 ml (1 ml of blood weighs approximately 1.050 gm). The tubing is clamped, sealed, and cut. A good, aseptic unit-drawing technique will ensure uncontaminated units most of the time. All containers (component bags, segments, sample tubes, etc.) are checked for appropriate numbering and identifications. The needle is removed carefully and antiseptically with sterile gauze. Pressure on the venipuncture site is applied with gauze. The donor lifts his or her arm to reduce venous return, and with the opposite hand continues applying pressure with the gauze on the venipuncture site until hemostasis is complete.

Care of the Donor after Donation

The donor is encouraged to drink fluids if he or she feels inclined to do so. A 15-minute rest in the donor chair is advised. After this, the donor is allowed to sit up and then stand. After another 15–20 minutes, the donor is thanked and allowed to leave if he or she feels well.

Adverse Reactions to Donation

One of the more common reactions to donation is a vasovagal reaction, caused in many cases by apprehension, the sight of blood, and blood volume changes. These reactions may be slight, moderate, or severe.[31] Reaction is manifested by dizziness, diaphoresis, and pallor, but may result in nausea, vomiting and even fainting (syncope). Syncope is the most common of the severe reactions.[32] Rarely, vascular collapse and shock are seen. A slowing down of the pulse (to 30–60 beats per minute) is probably the best single indicator of a vasovagal episode,[33] in contrast to the rapid pulse observed in hypovolemic shock.[34] Cardiogenic shock may be manifested by a rapid or slow pulse.[35] Syncope or fainting is directly related to the volume of blood withdrawn from the donor (fainting was seen in 8.5% of donors giving 440 ml, which is the usual donation,[36] and in 100% of persons giving 1,500 ml experimentally).[37] Hyperexcitability and twitching probably result from respiratory alkalosis in very anxious patients who hyperventilate.

Treatment of Donor Reactions.—Severe donor reactions are medical emergencies. These are rare but do occur, and donor room personnel should be prepared to deal with such episodes. At the first sign of a donor reaction, the donation is stopped by clamping the tubing, but the needle is left in the vein.

All donor room personnel should be trained in cardiopulmonary resuscitation (CPR).[38] Essentially, an adequate airway, regular breathing, and circulation must be established. Infusion of saline may be required to restore volume; 300–500 cc can be given rapidly via the phlebotomy line. The patient should be placed in a modified Trendelenburg position to improve cerebral blood flow. Constricting belts and garments are removed or loosened. While resuscitation is started, the hospital emergency team should be contacted (the telephone number of the emergency team should be visibly posted in the donor room). If medications used in emergencies are to be stored in the donor room, these must be in date. Some medications that are useful to have on hand in the donor room medicine cabinet include epinephrine, caffeine sodium benzoate for hypotensive episodes, trimethobenzamide (Tigan) as an antiemetic, a barbiturate (Amytal) for convulsive episodes, an antihistamine (Benadryl), an oxygen tank, and disposable syringes.[39] Medications can be administered only by the blood bank physician or other treating physician.

Muscle twitching due to hyperventilatory respiratory alkalosis can be controlled by allowing the donor to rebreathe exhaled air into a paper bag. In these cases oxygen is *not* indicated because PCO_2 is already low and decreasing it will depress the respiratory center further.

If the donor has seizures, the most important point is to prevent self-inflicted injury. Sodium phenytoin or phenobarbital may be indicated but should be administered only by a physician. Maintaining an adequate airway is essential to prevent hypoxia in these patients, by placing a soft object that cannot be swallowed between the teeth. This is not easily achieved and should not be attempted once the jaw is set into tonic spasms for fear of breaking the patient's teeth.

Air embolism is rarely seen today with the use of plastic containers, but it was frequent when blood was collected in glass bottles.[40] Treatment of air embolism includes raising the lower extremities of the recumbent patient as the patient lies on his or her left side.[41]

PREPARATION, STORAGE AND USE OF COMPONENTS

Once the unit has been obtained from the donor, it can be stored either as whole blood or separated into components. At this point, it is appropriate to consider some aspects of anticoagulants.

Anticoagulants

As with many other discoveries in science, it is difficult to tell who was responsible for first describing the use of citrate as a safe anticoagulant, but the merit is closely linked with the names of two investigators, Agote and Hustin.[42]

Disodium citrate is the acidic salt of sodium citrate and is widely used as an anticoagulant in blood units (e.g., acid citrate in dextrose (ACD) and CPD). It is used as 1.7%–2% solution in dextrose 2.5% in water as a anticoagulant preservative solution. Citrate chelates calcium, which is essential for coagulation. The amount of citrate is in excess of the total calcium present in a unit as a measure to prevent clot formation. Acid citrate was initially used to prevent carmelization or yellow discoloration of the units,[43] but was later shown to improve survival of the stored cells as well as the nonacid citrate. Subsequently CPD solutions were introduced. The rationale for using CPD is that phosphate ions present in the solution supply the adenosine phosphate pool necessary for synthesis of adenosine triphosphate (ATP) essential to the glycolytic metabolism of RBCs. The dextrose in the solution also contributes to the metabolic needs of the RBCs in the unit, allowing preservation of cells in storage with a viability of at least 70% of cells for up to 21 days.[44]

The oxygen transport function of RBCs is decreased during storage due to a drop in levels of 2,3-diphosphoglycerate (2,3-DPG), but it may be restored by 50% within 24 hours after transfusion.[45] ATP levels also drop after 21 days of storage to about 86%.[46] These observations prompted studies on the possibility of restoring some of these metabolites by adding substances such as adenine to the CPD solution.[47] The addition of adenine allows prolongation of storage to 35 days[48] and is not toxic at the dosage usually found in CPD-adenine (CPD-A1)-preserved units.[49] The FDA[50] and the American Association of Blood Banks (AABB)[51] currently accept storage of units preserved with CPD-A1 for 35 days. It is of interest that CPD-A1-preserved RBCs survive better in units containing more plasma (whole blood) than units with less plasma (packed cells).[52] CPD-A2, a solution with twice as much adenine and glucose, has been developed and extends viability of RBCs to 49 days; however, it is not yet FDA approved.[53] RBC membrane vesiculations has been found in units stored for long periods in CPD-A1.[54]

Heparin has also been used as an anticoagulant. About 1,500 units of heparin will anticoagulate one unit of blood. Heparin had occasionally been suggested as an anticoagulant in transfusions when it was feared that CPD would produce lowering of the pH. Currently the AABB does not accept heparin as a good anticoagulant for plasma.[55] EDTA, another calcium-chelating substance, is not used as an anticoagulant because it damages platelets.[56]

Preparation, Storage, and Indications for Whole Blood

Whole blood is obtained by drawing a unit into a collecting bag containing 63 ml of CPD anticoagulant (14 ml/100 ml of blood is usually an adequate amount of CPD[57] or CPD-A1[58] to anticoagulate a unit of blood). The freshest unit of whole blood is usually more than 24 hours old by the time it is ready for use, due to inventory storage as well as because of the time required for hepatitis testing, HTLV-III testing, RPR testing, typing, and screening. This delay causes a virtually complete loss of platelet viability.[59] By 24 hours after collection the factor VIII level has decreased to 40% of the level of a freshly drawn unit.[60] The half-life of factor V also decreases with storage; it is calculated to be approximately 14 days.[61] Antithrombin III levels are usually preserved in stored blood,[62] as are levels of fibronectin.[63] Whole blood units are stored in the liquid state at 1°–6° C.[64] An important aspect of unit storage is the "storage lesion," reflected in a variety of metabolic changes that result in damage to the membranes of stored RBCs. An important change is the decrease in production of ATP.[65] This decrement in metabolic input eventually results in loss of lipid structures vital to the membranes of RBCs. Ca^{++} ion equilibrium is lost, with subsequent formation of microvesicles.[66]

Damage to RBC membranes, if severe enough, allows escape of potassium into the stored plasma, where potassium reaches 7 times its normal plasma value by the 28th day of storage.[65] These changes result in actual cell attrition from the unit, with a drop in the hematocrit and an increment in the level of hemoglobin in the supernatant plasma.[67]

Oxygen dissociation curves are shifted to the left on prolonged storage.[68] This shift to the left produces an increased binding of oxygen by the hemoglobin molecule,[69] impairing oxygen release to the tissues. It has been shown that the increase in binding is dependent on the concentration of 2,3-DPG. 2,3-DPG inhibits binding of oxygen to a certain extent; therefore, if 2,3-DPG decreases, oxygen binding increases. In stored units RBCs have decreased amounts of 2,3-DPG, falling to 37% of normal levels after 28 days of storage in the liquid state.[70] Normal values of 2,3-DPG are restored in vivo 24 hours after transfusion.[69]

Stored whole blood, therefore, contains both unwanted elements (e.g., increased potassium) and a decrement in important clotting factors (e.g., factors VIII and V) as well as a lack of functional platelets. We must also remember the net benefit of transfusing 1 unit of blood. A unit of blood increases the hematocrit of an adult 70-kg patient only about 3%.[71] Hemoglobin increases by about 1 gm/100 ml in a 70-kg patient who initially had a blood volume of 5,300 ml, 24 hours after transfusion of 1 unit of blood.[72]

If one weighs the benefits versus the drawbacks of transfusing whole blood, the indications for whole blood transfusion are relatively few. One such indication is massive bleeding. Here, the initial transfusions are geared to restore a volume deficit as well as the oxygen-carrying capacity of RBCs. A further discussion on transfusion of whole blood is given in the section on transfusion practices in chapter 18.

Packed Cells

The RBC component obtained by differential centrifugation of a unit of whole blood after the platelet-rich plasma has been separated constitutes a unit of packed cells.

If a unit of blood is collected in a system of multiple polyvinyl chloride bags, such as shown in Figure 8-1, the components can be separated by centrifugation without a technologist entering the system, thus preventing contamination. These plastic bags have revolutionized blood storage and allowed centrifugation of units with minimal complications. Leaching of di-2-ethyl phthalate from the plastic bags has not caused major toxic effects,[73] although an inhibition effect on lymphocytes by phthalate has been documented.[74]

Platelet-rich plasma and packed cells are separated by spinning the blood at a low speed (2,500 rpm for 3 minutes in an RC-3 Sorval centrifuge) and expressing the platelet-rich plasma out of the unit.[75] With this method, a unit of packed cells is obtained which has an expiration time comparable to any other unit because the transfer container system has not been entered. However, units may be packed, to eliminate unnecessary plasma, after they have been stored within date as whole blood. These units have a 24-hour expiration time, because they have been entered to separate the plasma and therefore are considered potentially exposed to contamination.

The advantages of using packed RBCs versus whole blood have been extensively reviewed elsewhere;[76] a few are summarized here. The oxygen-carrying capacity of a unit of packed cells is the same as that of a unit of whole blood, but the volume of packed cells is half that of a unit of whole blood. Thus, a patient's circulation is less overloaded, and a greater dose of RBCs may be administered. This becomes critical in anemic patients who do not tolerate volume increases very well, such as those in renal failure or heart failure. Furthermore, one is transfusing less unnecessary plasma, poor in clotting factors and rich in potentially toxic potassium and ammonium. This rationale is now accepted, as shown by a trend in the United States toward using more packed cells (70%) and less whole blood (30%).[77]

One disadvantage to using packed RBCs is the slower rate at which they flow through an infusion line. This can be remedied by infusing 50 ml of saline into the packed cells via a Y connector to decrease rheologic resistance and improve flow.[78] With this method a unit can be transfused at an improved maximum rate of 5 minutes, as compared to the 10–15 minutes required to transfuse a unit to which saline has not been added.

Leukocyte-Poor RBCs

Most of the WBCs in a stored unit of blood are not viable by 24 hours and usually serve only to

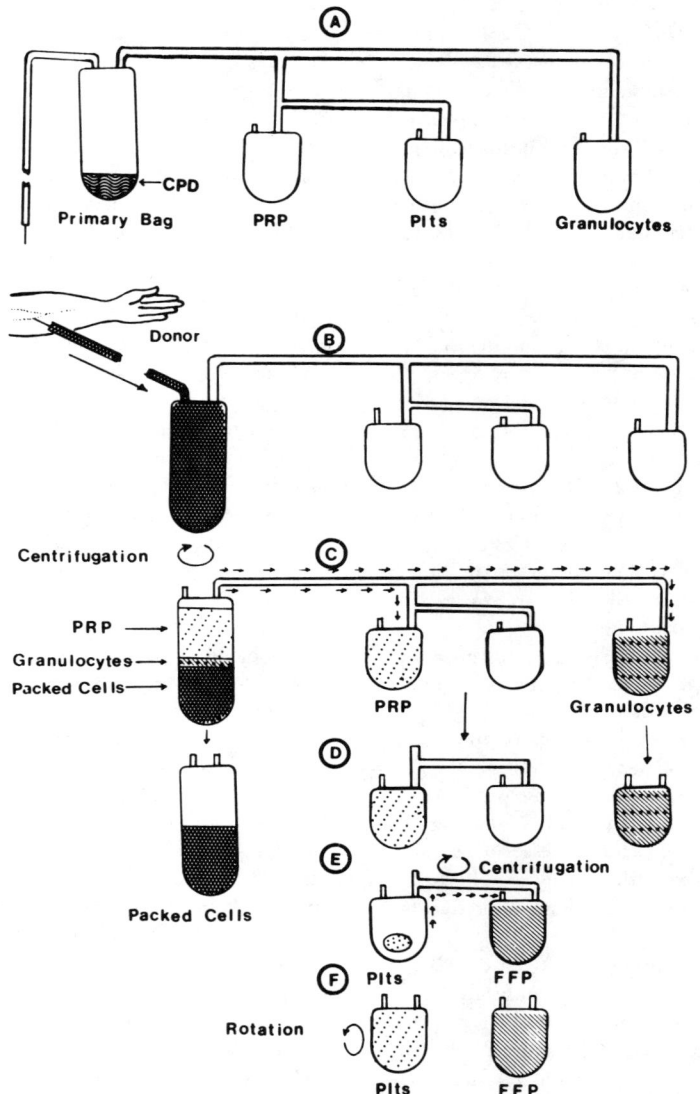

FIG 8–1.—How components are obtained from a unit of whole blood by differential centrifugation. *A,* the empty differential centrifugation bag system with a main primary bag *(left)* containing the appropriate amount of citrate dextrose in phosphate (CDP) for anticoagulation. Two satellite bags are seen, one for platelet-rich plasma *(PRP),* another for the collection of platelets *(Plts).* A satellite bag for granulocytes is seen at right. *B,* collection from a vein in the antecubital portion of the arm. *C,* the first centrifugation step and separation of the collected whole blood into components—first the PRP layer, then the granulocyte or Buffy coat layer, and finally the packed cell layer. This primary bag is put into an expression clamp and the fluid is collected from the top of the bag by layers *(small arrows).* The top of the PRP collection bag is clamped proximally to the connection with the satellite bag. *D, left,* the primary bag with packed cells is shown separate from the collection system. *Center,* the PRP and Plts bags are shown adjoining each other but separate from the main collection system. *Right,* a separated unit of granulocytes is seen. *E,* the second centrifugation step, which results in a unit of platelets and a unit of FFP, which is the supernate plasma expressed from the original PRP bag into the FFP bag. *F,* the platelet bag undergoing rotation. *Right,* a separate bag of FFP.

immunize the transfused recipients. Immunization frequently results in febrile transfusion reactions,[79] which are caused mainly by antibodies formed against HLA and granulocyte-specific antigens.[80] It has been recommended that patients who develop febrile reactions to transfusion due to the formation of HLA antibodies receive leukocyte-poor units. In one study, the incidence of febrile transfusion reactions was decreased by 77% when microaggregate filters were used.[81]

A common method used to eliminate granulocytes from a unit is differential centrifugation. Up to 85% of the granulocytes can be removed with this method. However, 20% or more of the RBCs in the unit are lost as well.[82] These units can be prepared by inverted centrifugation of the unit at 4,100 rpm in a Sorval RC-3 centrifuge (Fig 8–2).[83] Then the packed cells are drained into a transfer bag from below without disturbing the supernatant Buffy coat, which is left behind.

If this method is combined with microaggregate

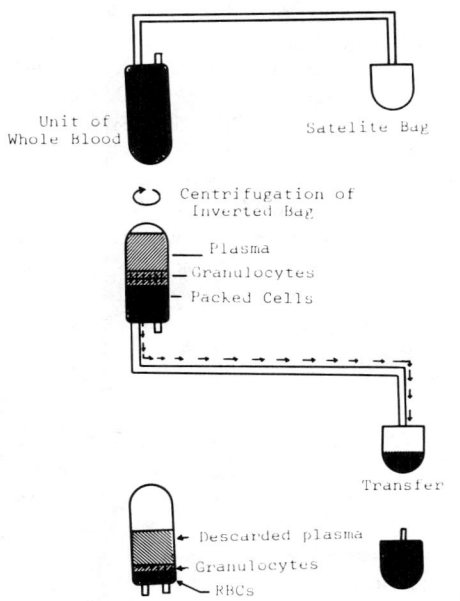

FIG 8–2.—Preparation of granulocyte-poor units by inverted centrifugation. *Top,* a unit of whole blood with adjacent satellite bag. The unit is centrifuged inverted so the ports of entry are facing downward. Three layers are formed: the topmost layer is plasma, the middle layer is the Buffy coat, and the bottom layer is packed cells. The packed cells are transferred to the smaller satellite bags *(center, small arrows);* the plasma, Buffy coat, and remaining RBCs are discarded *(bottom).*

filtration, up to 96% of the WBCs may be removed, but the loss of RBCs increases to 35%.[84] Screen filters retain only 1%–3% WBCs, whereas depth filters retain 20%–62% WBCs.[85] Leukocyte absorption filters can remove up to 98% WBCs.[86] When the Buffy coat is removed in an integral transfer container system, the unit will have a normal expiration time (21–35 days, depending on the anticoagulant used). However, if the removal of granulocytes requires entering the bag in any way, expiration time is 24 hours at 4°–6° C. Should febrile reactions persist after units have been treated by any of these methods, frozen-thawed cells may be considered. Freezing and deglycerolizing eliminates up to 97%–99% of the WBCs in a unit.[87] This removes by far the most WBCs and is the method of choice when a radical elimination of WBCs is desired. However, it is costly and time-consuming, and the unit has an expiration time of 24 hours stored at 4°–6° C. Nevertheless, with the newer cell washers it is possible to remove up to 93% of the WBCs from a unit of blood, preserving a mean of 82% of the original RBCs in the unit.[88]

Frozen-Thawed Blood

The ability to store blood in the frozen state has improved storage of special units for remarkable lengths of time (up to 3 years, according to AABB standards).[89]

Freezing RBCs with the help of cryoprotective agents such as glycerol stemmed from research conducted on freezing sperm cells.[90] The technique was applied to preserve rabbit RBCs[91] and subsequently was tested on human RBCs.[92] It has been shown that freezing damage is not due to direct damage from crystal formation within the cells but to osmotic damage. Hyperosmolar fluids are formed secondary to water exclusion due to ice formation on freezing.[93] These solutions produce denaturation of membrane lipoprotein complexes vital to the cell membrane integrity.[94]

Certain substances can be used as cryoprotecting agents (CPA). Glycerol is one of the more useful CPAs, for it reduces ice crystal formation. Glycerol acts as an osmolar "buffer" for the cell, inducing gradual changes in osmolarity, and thus permitting cells to be frozen and thawed with reduced damage to the membrane structures.[95] Another advantage of glycerol as a CPA is that it is not toxic to humans at relatively high concentrations.[96] For these reasons, glycerol has become the CPA of choice for cryopreservation of RBCs. Nevertheless, cells cryopreserved with glycerol must be washed with saline solutions of decreasing osmolarity to rid them of the internalized glycerol, which otherwise would cause osmotic hemolysis. Optimal removal is about 98% of the glycerol and prevents osmotic lysis.[97]

Processing Units for Frozen Storage.—Units collected in CPD or CPDA-1 should be less than 6 days old[98] and packed to a hematocrit of 85%–90%. Two methods are currently popular for glycerolizing units: a low-glycerol method[99] and a high-glycerol method.[79] In the low-glycerol method, 35% glycerol is slowly added to a unit at room temperature to achieve a final concentration of 14%. The unit is then immersed directly into liquid nitrogen ($-196°$ C) and stored in liquid nitrogen vapor phase ($-150°$ C).[100] This method is more widely used in European countries. The major drawback is that storage of large quantities of blood in liquid nitrogen is both extremely cumbersome and expensive.

The high-glycerol method has more to recommend it than the low-glycerol method. In this method, units are frozen on addition of 57% glycerol in two stages to allow equilibration targeted to achieve a final concentration of 40%. The cells are frozen by placing them directly into a $-80°$ C mechanical freezer. The machinery is less cumbersome and less expensive to maintain than liquid nitrogen. Another advantage to using the high-glycerol method is that temperature variations are less critical because RBCs tolerate changes better at this concentration of the cryoprotectant,[101] thus allowing transportation of these units on dry ice.[102]

As mentioned above, the FDA accepts storage of frozen blood for up to 3 years. It is appropriate to note here that frozen RBC units have been shown to be effective for after 7 years of storage.[103]

Thawing.—Thawing is performed by immersing the unit in its storage container into a 37° C water bath for about 10 minutes. The units should not be warmed above 38° C.

Deglycerolization

Deglycerolization is best achieved by mechanical methods. Of the several systems available, the Haemonetics model 17 and the IBM model 2991 are among the more popular. Both systems employ approximately three wash solutions of NaCl, decreasing from 12% to 1.6%, and finishing with a solution of 0.8% NaCl plus 2% glucose with sodium phosphate (25 mEq/L).[104] The agglomeration method is another possibility but is not very popular, as it gives only a 70%–80% postthaw RBC yield.[105] All the above mentioned methods are open methods and potentially expose the unit to bacterial contamination; thus the units have a 24-hour expiration time.[106] However, units stored experimentally for up to 11 days were safely transfused to patients and no bacterial growth was demonstrated.[107] Frozen-thawed cells are usually issued at a 70% hematocrit, but they may be stored at a hematocrit of 40% and then centrifuged to a hematocrit of 70% to eliminate hemolyzed plasma.[108] As inadequately deglycerolyzed cells will hemolyse in vivo, quality control monitoring using 0.7% NaCl is recommended.[109]

Physiology of Frozen Deglycerolized Cells

With good processing practices, the postthaw recovery of viable RBCs should be about 80% of the thawed cells[104] and the posttransfusional survival should be about 90% in well-processed units with a minimal standard of at least 70% viable RBCs 24 hours posttransfusion.[110] This may result in an overall 30%–40% attrition of cells—10% is lost in processing of the frozen deglycerolized unit and 10%–15% is lost to reticuloendothelial system removal of damaged cells 24 hours after transfusion.[111]

Both ATP levels and 2,3-DPG levels in RBCs from deglycerolized units are comparable to those found before freezing, even after 31 months of storage.[112]

Uses of Frozen, Deglycerolized RBCs

Freezing RBCs has dramatically changed the possibilities of storing units with rare phenotypes for prolonged times. Another use for frozen units is autologous transfusion. Some patients tolerate or accept only their own blood for transfusion (e.g., patients with an antibody to a high-incidence antigent), where compatible blood would otherwise be difficult or impossible to obtain. These patients can predeposit their own blood into frozen storage and thus accumulate units, allowing them to undergo elective surgery requiring several units of blood.[113]

Deglycerolizing cells is sometimes referred to as the "purification" of RBC concentrates.[114] In the course of washing RBCs several times to eliminate the glycerol, the unit is cleared of its plasma, most granulocytes (98%), and most platelets, as well as cell debris. It is therefore the component of choice when one wants to provide plasma-free RBCs and granulocyte-free RBCs. There are very specific indications for using this type of unit. One indication is in patients with anti-IgA antibodies, who may develop anaphylaxis if they receive plasma. Frozen-thawed RBCs can be safely given to such individuals[115] because these units are free of most of the plasma containing the antigen, namely plasma IgA. Another specific indication for using frozen-thawed units is in patients with paroxysmal nocturnal hemoglobinuria, a disease characterized by RBCs with an abnormal susceptibility to plasma complement components; these components of complement are probably activated by antibodies against WBCs.[116] It is advisable to transfuse these patients with deglycerolized cells, which are free of most of the complement-containing plasma as well as 98% free of granulocytes.[117] Patients with thalassemia who need transfusions of "younger" RBCs (neocytes) benefit from frozen-thawed units which, because of the freezing protocols requiring blood no older than 6 days, contain a greater percentage of young RBCs.[118] These patients also undergo transfusion quite frequently and therefore develop febrile reactions quite often, which justifies the use of this granulocyte-poor product.

Whether deglycerolized RBC transfusions carry a reduced risk of transmitting hepatitis had been controversial. Evidence that this was the case was given in the literature.[119] In vitro removal of HB_sAg was suggested and apparently depended on the concentration of glycerol.[120] However, recent studies on a series of over 24,000 transfusions demonstrated that frozen-thawed units *were not* significantly capable of reducing the risk of hepatitis when compared with nonfrozen units.[121] Even though the findings were criticized by certain investigations because the studies were not prospective,[122] it is now believed that the transmission of hepatitis cannot be significantly decreased by use of frozen-thawed units.

Another use for frozen-thawed units is to prevent the transmission of cytomegalovirus (CMV) infection through transfusion. The risk of a postperfusion syndrome developing secondary to CMV infection after open heart surgery is approximately 21%–38%.[123] This risk can be decreased by using deglycerolized cells,[124] which seem to survive as well as nonfrozen units during bypass pump trauma.[125] Again, the decision to use deglycerolized cells must be weighed against such factors as cost-effectiveness, personnel time consumption, and expiration time of these products. A more relevant indication for eliminating CMV from blood products is in the transfusion of neonates, where frozen-thawed units screened for CMV must be used.[20] Another definite indication for frozen-thawed cells is to help decrease the WBC content of RBC units. As mentioned above, removal of the buffy coat from an RBC unit results in a decrease in the number of febrile transfusion reactions,[126] which are caused by host anti-HLA antibodies.[127] Sensitivity occurs in about 25% of patients receiving whole blood, whereas only 5%–10% become sensitized when frozen-thawed cells are used.[128]

The method that most effectively removes WBCs from a unit of whole blood is the freezing and deglycerolizing method used for frozen-thawed units. As many as 98% of the WBCs are removed by this method.[129]

Frozen-thawed RBCs should also be used to decrease the potential of inducing graft-versus-host disease (GVHD) in immunosuppressed patients. These units should be irradiated as well. GVHD has also been seen in babies receiving frozen-thawed cells in intrauterine transfusions and thought to be due to the immature immunocompetence of the conceptus.[129] Blood transfusions should be avoided in candidates for bone marrow transplantation. However, the use of frozen-thawed cells in transplant candidates who do need transfusions has been advocated.[130] Frozen-thawed units are not recommended for cadaver kidney transplant patients.[131] It is possible that the beneficial effect of transfusion on renal graft recipients is the result of induced unresponsiveness secondary to the WBC content of the transfused blood units.[132]

FRESH FROZEN PLASMA

Fresh frozen plasma (FFP) is a byproduct of the differential centrifugation of a freshly drawn unit of whole blood in a multiple-bag system (see Fig 8–1). It is obtained after platelets have been separated from platelet-rich plasma, which in turn has been obtained from a unit of whole blood anticoagulated with CPD (heparin is not acceptable).[133] FFP is obtained from platelet-rich plasma by centrifugation at 4,100 rpm in an RC-3 centrifuge for 5 minutes[134] at room temperature within 6 hours of collection of the unit.[135] FFP must be stored at $-30°$ C, although $-18°$ C is acceptable to the

FDA.[136] It should be noted, however, that storage at $-18°$ C results in greater deterioration of certain clotting factors.[137] Storage under these conditions is acceptable for up to 12 months.[138] FFP units are brittle in the frozen state and should be handled carefully and stored in cardboard boxes to avoid breakage. Units of plasma are thawed in a water bath at 37° C for transfusion. The unit should be placed in a plastic bag to avoid wetting of the portals of entry and thus potential contamination of the portals by the unsterile water in the water bath. Ingestion of oral contraceptives or carotenoids by the donor may discolor the plasma.[139]

Clinical Use of FFP

Most of the clinical indications for FFP are to restore clotting factors, not to restore volume. FFP has the advantage that all the procoagulants are present at physiologic levels, that is, at levels comparable to those found when the unit was obtained from the donor. This is in contrast to plasma stored in the liquid state, which loses significant amounts of labile clotting factors—50% of factor V by 2 weeks of storage and 50% of factor VIII by 24 hours of storage.[140] The loss of factor V in a unit is not clinically significant until levels drop to 15% of normal.[140] However, the factor VIII loss may be of concern, especially in massive transfusion. The effects of massive transfusion should not be overemphasized, for most of the 30% of patients receiving an average of 30 units of blood who will have increased bleeding, will bleed from dilutional thrombocytopenia and only 10% from disseminated intravascular coagulation.[141] FFP is therefore recommended mainly in patients with clotting deficiencies who can tolerate, without complications, significant increments in volume on transfusion.

FFP units must be ABO compatible and given through a transfusion filter[140] within 24 hours after thawing if stored refrigerated in a blood bank refrigerator.[142]

CRYOPRECIPITATE

Preparation

Cryoprecipitate is a component of plasma obtained by thawing a unit of FFP in the cold under controlled conditions. CPD-anticoagulated units of FFP are a suitable source of cryoprecipitate. However, the initial unit from which the FFP unit was obtained must have an integral transfer bag to avoid an open system and thus potentially contaminate the unit.[143] The unit of blood from which the plasma destined for the preparation of cryoprecipitate is extracted must be placed in the cold as soon as possible (within a few hours).[144] Freezing should be achieved as quickly as possible, and, once frozen, the plasma must not be stored for more than 3 months if cryoprecipitate is to be obtained from it. Storage temperature must be $-18°$ C or $-30°$ C,[145] although the colder temperature ($-30°$) appears to be better for the preservation of clotting factors.[146] Fifteen percent higher levels of factor VIII are found in CPD plasma units as compared to ACD units.[147] Once a unit has been selected for the preparation of cryoprecipitate, it should be placed in a refrigerator at 1°–6° C to thaw slowly overnight (approximately 18 hours). Once the plasma has softened to a mushy "crushed ice" consistency, the unit with its attached integral transfer bags is then centrifuged with a hard spin at 4,100 rpm for 5 minutes.[145] The unit is then placed on a plasma expressor clamp and about 90% of the volume is removed. The residual ice in the unit serves as a sieve and the thicker, tenacious cryoprecipitate will remain behind. The residual volume, about 3 ml, contains the cryoglobulins.[148]

One unit of antihemophilic factor is defined as the relative factor VIII activity found in 1 ml of normal fresh human plasma. The mean procoagulant content in 1 unit of cryoprecipitate is 110 ± 50. Donors can be screened for optimal levels of factor VIII in their plasma. Exercise will increase the yield of factor VIII from a particular donor.[149] DDAVP is a synthetic derivative of vasopressin which will increase the yield of factor VIII in plasma twofold;[150] it has been given to donors prior to donation to improve factor VIII levels. Each bag of cryoprecipitate contains about 30%–50% of factor VIII of the original unit of FFP.[143] In addition, the unit contains 40%–75% of the original content of von Willebrand's factor VIII, and 23% of the original content of fibrinogen (factor I) (i.e., 250 mg/bag).[151] About 30% of factor XIII is also present in a unit of cryoprecipitate.[151] After infusion of cryoprecipitate, a biphasic curve is observed. The first drop in factor VIII levels occurs within the first 6 hours and is very steep (i.e., to 50% of the value seen immediately after infusion). This initial drop is interpreted as a redistribution from the intravascular space to the extravascular space. In the following 18 hours factor VIII levels drop more slowly and gradually. This drop probably represents true biologic half-life or utilization of AHF.[152] The in vivo activity of factor VIII measured after infusion should be 90–100 units per bag infused.[148]

There appears to be better recovery of AHF from units from type AB donors rather than from type O donors.[153] Cryoprecipitate units are thawed at 37° C for use. They are then pooled and kept at room temperature until no longer than 6 hours before transfusion.[154]

Clinical Uses

To calculate the dosage of cryoprecipitate to be given, one must first determine the plasma volume and the starting factor VIII level in the patient's plasma. An example is given below.

An 8-year-old hemophiliac boy weighs 30 kg and has 1% factor VIII activity in his plasma. How many bags of cryoprecipitate should be given to reach a 50% level of factor VIII?

Plasma volume = 45 × 30 kg = 1,350 ml

Since the average bag contains about 90 units of factor VIII, 1,350/90 = 15 bags of cryoprecipitate should be given to reach a 50% level of factor VIII activity.

Cryoprecipitate has revolutionized treatment of hemophilia A, von Willebrand's disease, and hypofibrinogenemia of various causes. This mode of therapy stemmed from the finding by Pool that precipitated cryoglobulins in a thawed unit of FFP contained up to 50% of the factor VIII present in a unit of plasma.[155] Pool et al. also found that the cryoprecipitate could be used effectively in the treatment of hemophilia A, which is caused by a factor VIII molecular defect. However, most hemophilia centers today use factor VIII concentrates unless cryoprecipitate is more convenient (e.g., for treating mild hemophilia in a hospitalized patient). Although cryoprecipitate is less expensive, lyophilized concentrates are more convenient for home therapy because, due to its large volume, cryoprecipitate is more cumbersome to transport and store. Furthermore, if large amounts of factor VIII are needed, the volume of cryoprecipitate may overload the circulatory system. The dose is determined by the levels of factor VIII needed in different clinical situations, some of which are described below.[156]

1. Minor hemorrhage requires a 30% level of factor VIII, achieved by giving 15 units/kg of body weight.

2. Major hemorrhage due to trauma requires 50% factor VIII levels, achieved by giving doses of 25 units/kg of body weight.

3. Surgery or life-threatening bleeding requires 80% factor VIII levels, achieved by infusing 40 units/kg of body weight.

The dosage in units is calculated by the following formula:

Units of factor VIII = .05 × body weight (kg) × desired increase in factor VIII (% of total)

If cryoprecipitate is chosen as therapy for hemophilia A, a continuous infusion is given until bleeding is controlled. This may require several days of treatment.

Cryoprecipitate is the component used to treat von Willebrand's disease, an ailment which does not respond properly to lyophilized factor VIII concentrates.[157] Likewise, in conditions where fibrinogen is depleted (e.g., disseminated intravascular coagulation), cryoprecipitate may provide sufficient concentration of fibrinogen (250 mg per bag)[158] in a smaller volume (3 ml per bag) than a unit of FFP (250 ml per bag). Lyophilized fibrinogen preparations are no longer used owing to the high risk of hepatitis they carry. The half-life of factor VIII is so short that a new dose is usually necessary every 12 hours. Most the the time cryoprecipitate is given as multiple-bag pools. Since the volume in each bag is only 3 ml and the material is highly viscous, it can be recovered by rinsing the inside of the bags with saline. A total volume of 250 cc of saline solution may be used. Care must be exercised not to contaminate the product.[148] Cryoprecipitate has also been used successfully to correct the coagulopathy observed in uremics[159] and in the treatment of antithrombin deficiency.[160]

Complications

Certain complications can result from the use of cryoprecipitate. The most common is a rash, resulting from plasma protein sensitivity. A dreaded complication is anaphylaxis in IgA-deficient patients who have developed anti-IgA antibodies. Many patients undergoing prolonged treatment for hemophilia develop hepatitis, and most patients eventually develop anti-HB_sAg antibodies. A potential complication which group A or B recipients of cryoprecipitate may develop is hemolysis from ABO-incompatible plasma.[161] The development of factor VIII antibodies acting as coagulation inhibitors is a complication of chronic therapy in hemophiliacs. These inhibitors may appear in up to 15%

of hemophiliacs receiving replacement therapy.[162] Some of these antibodies may produce severe reactions when the patient is exposed to factor VIII infusions.[163] Units of FFP, cryoprecipitate, and other components all carry the same risk of transmitting AIDS as a unit of blood.

PLATELETS

Platelets, which were reviewed in more detail in Chapter 2, are discoid structures with three main components: the peripheral zone, the cytosol, and the organelles. The peripheral zone is responsible mainly for platelet adhesiveness, the cytosol is the site of the microtubules and microfilaments and is associated with platelet contractility, and the organelles are the recipients of secretory products of platelets. Among the organelles, the dense granules are of primary importance to the hemostatic physiology of platelets. Analysis has shown these granules to contain ATP, ADP and serotonin, as well as many other substances important to the hemostatic function of platelets.[164]

Platelet Unit Preparation

Two methods are currently available, a manual method and an automated method. Each is reviewed below.

Manual Method

Platelet concentrates can be obtained from freshly drawn units of whole blood. Units from donors who have ingested aspirin within 48 hours should not be used as a source of platelets.[165] Units of whole blood are collected in an integral plastic bag system and separated into components within 4 hours. Platelet-rich plasma is separated first from units of whole blood by centrifuging the units at room temperature using a light spin (2,500 rpm in an RC-3 centrifuge) for 3 minutes. The platelet-rich plasma is expressed into a satellite bag and this bag is centrifuged at high speed (4,100 rpm in an RC-3 centrifuge) at room temperature for 5 minutes. The plasma is then expressed into a satellite bag and used as FFP (see Fig 8–1). The remaining platelet button is then resuspended in a residual plasma volume of approximately 50 cc.[166] Platelet survival is increased if platelets are stored at 22° C rather than 4° C.[167] These units are stored under continuous rotation in special 22° C platelet incubators. It has been found that platelets are capable of converting all the glucose and glycogen content of the suspending plasma into lactate after 72 hours of storage at room temperature.[168] It is therefore necessary to preserve the residual 50 cc of plasma in the unit and to promote oxygen exchange via constant agitation. Platelet units must not reach pH levels below 6, as this results in damage to and loss of viability of these cells. Furthermore, the pH must be above 6 after 72 hours of collection, an FDA[169] and an AABB standard.[170] Each unit must contain a minimum of 5.5×10^{10} platelets in at least 75% of the units.[170] All units must be screened for HB_sAg and HTLV-III before transfusion. This testing may cut into the expiration time of the unit. New polyolefin containers which permit a better gas exchange are now available, allowing a 5-day storage of platelets.[171, 172]

Automated Methods

The preparation of single donor units by mechanized means will be discussed here briefly; details of apheresis are discussed in chapter 9.

At least two machines are currently in vogue: the Haemonetics model 30, which separates components in a discontinuous flow, and the modified IBM Cell Separator, which uses a continuous flow. In the Haemonetics model 30, the tubing and the centrifuge bowl are disposable. Via a system of peristaltic pumps, blood from the donor enters the machine at a rate of about 20 ml/minute.[173] As the blood leaves the donor, it is anticoagulated with ACD solution and directed to the centrifuge bowl. A volume of blood enters the bowl (which varies in capacity). It is then separated by the centrifugal force generated by the spinning bowl. The topmost layer is plasma (Fig 8–3). Below this is a platelet layer and then a granulocyte layer. RBCs lie at the lower portion of the bowl. When separation is adequate, the plasma is drawn off, permitting collection of the next layer, the platelet layer. The RBCs and the plasma are then shifted to a reservoir and reinfused to the patient by gravity. During reinfusion platelets are not collected, and therefore the system is called discontinuous-flow platelet apheresis. The processing of one volume is termed a "pass" or "cycle" through the machine. Eight cycles yield approximately 5×10^{11} platelets.[174] The number is calculated as follows: Platelet count/cu mm $\times$ 1,000 $\times$ volume of platelet concentrate (ml) = number of platelets in platelet concentrate.

The AABB recommends that 75% of the units contain at least 3×10^{11} platelets,[175] that they do not attain pH values below 6, and, if stored at 22°

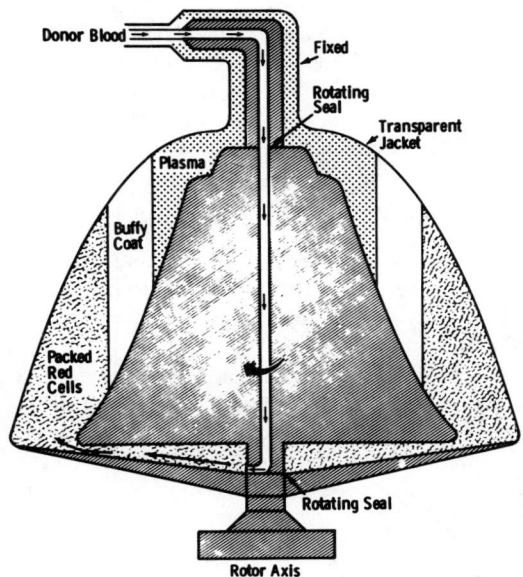

FIG 8–3.—Sagittal section of the modified Latham bowl. The donor blood enters through the centermost portion of the portal of entry of the Latham bowl. As the blood enters the bowl through the lower portion, it is separated by the centrifugal force created by the rotating core. The upper and lower portion of this core create a rotating seal by apposition of surfaces. The space between the transparent jacket and the core is filled by the separated components—the packed cells, the Buffy coat band, and the plasma band. Components are collected sequentially; plasma is collected first since it is the uppermost layer, then the Buffy coat, and, if necessary, the RBCs. These components are drawn off through the outermost channel surrounding the collecting tube *(dotted area* at top of figure).

C, that they be under continuous gentle rotation.[176] These units have an expiration time of 24 hours because the systems are considered open systems and potentially exposed to contamination, even though platelet viability seems to be preserved for 48 hours if stored in a 2,000-ml volume of plasma at 22° C.[177]

Use of Platelets in Clinical Practice

Platelets are used to correct documented thrombocytopenia. This fact should be stressed when unwarranted requests are received by the blood bank. A good reason to be cautious when issuing units of platelets is that every unit of platelets carries the same risk of transmitting hepatitis or AIDS as a unit of blood, and because of its RBC contaminant (which should be no greater than 0.5 ml of RBCs in a properly prepared unit[178]). A unit of platelets is capable of immunizing recipients, especially against Rh antigens. Furthermore, platelets are cell fragments with a surrounding cell membrane and as such carry HLA antigens. These antigens eventually may immunize the recipient, which explains most cases of a refractory stage in platelet therapy. Recent studies have shown, however, that it is the granulocytes present in platelet concentrates which are mostly responsible for immunization against HLA antigens, not the platelets per se.[179] Although therapy with platelets was reported about 70 years ago by Duke,[180] it was not until the past two decades that the use of platelets became practical, owing to the ability to separate these corpuscles and concentrate them in small volumes of plasma by using an integral satellite plastic bag collection system.[181] Patients with blood dyscrasias leading to bleeding disorders and oncology patients with a bleeding tendency, who would have succumbed in the past to a hemorrhagic episode, today can be treated and their lives prolonged by the use of platelet transfusion therapy.

There are two basic causes of thrombocytopenia: increased destruction and decreased production of platelets. These two causes may be combined in single disease entities. Examples of increased destruction are disseminated intravascular coagulation and immune-mediated thrombocytopenia. Decreased production of platelets is seen in bone marrow replacement by tumor or in bone marrow aplasia. Details on etiology and therapy of thrombocytopenias are given in chapter 2. Thrombocytopenias may also be induced by drugs of various sorts. There is no general rule or protocol for the transfusion of platelet concentrates. However, certain facts must be kept in mind in order to use this component appropriately.

Platelets as well as any other type of therapy should be given as part of a carefully planned therapeutic strategy. For instance, a patient with DIC may need immediate therapy with platelets as part of the lifesaving therapy, whereas a patient who is chronically thrombocytopenic may tolerate low thrombocyte counts without a major threat to life. Nevertheless, there are certain guidelines which must be used to assess the need for platelet therapy. Experience has shown that the risk of hemorrhage increases when the platelet count drops below 100,000/cu mm.[182] Spontaneous bleeding does not usually occur until the count is in the vicinity of 20,000/cu mm.[183] Nevertheless, acute drops in the thrombocyte count may be associated with spontaneous bleeding at levels of 50,000/cu mm or more.[184]

It is recommended that a platelet count be done before transfusing platelets. However, a number of patients will have clinical bleeding in spite of relatively high platelet counts, due to poor platelet function. It is therefore useful to obtain a template bleeding time (TBT), which gives a more accurate assessment of the potential to bleed than a platelet count by itself. Ideally, both tests should be performed before instituting replacement therapy with platelets.[185] Bleeding times greater than 15 minutes indicate severe thrombocytopenia and warrant correction by platelet infusion. The TBT test may be difficult to perform in certain patients, especially those with multiple intravenous lines in place or extensive skin lesions. Emergencies may require replacement before these tests can be performed. Other platelet tests are not a reliable method of assessing a tendency to hemorrhage. The main information source, apart from the TBT result and the platelet count, remains the clinical history. Thus, petechiae, gum bleeding, menorrhagia, and other evidence of a bleeding tendency should alert the clinician to an underlying thrombocytopenia and or platelet dysfunction.

In tertiary care centers the major use of platelet transfusions is in patients with hematologic dyscrasias, advanced carcinomatosis, and open heart surgery. In most oncology clinic patients, the thrombocytopenia is usually secondary to chemotherapy, which in many cases has a marrow-suppressive effect. Thrombocytopenia can also result from bone marrow replacement. It is important that the blood banker and the hematologist or the oncologist cooperate in planning platelet therapy for these chronic users. This will permit early HLA typing and planning of a replacement support strategy. Since platelets are usually in short supply, survival of these patients often depends on an adequate therapeutic plan.

Calculation of Dosage for Platelet Therapy

Platelets are usually given in doses of 5 pooled units to increase the count of an average 70-kg adult to hemostatic levels.[186] The calculation for dose, regardless of the size of the individual, is as follows: One unit of platelets containing 0.7×10^{11} should increase the platelet count of a 70-kg adult by about 10,000 $\mu l/m^2$. A 70-kg adult has a body surface area of approximately 1.70 m^2. Therefore, 1 unit will increase the platelet count by about 5,000–10,000/μl.[187] Another way to calculate dosage is n units of platelets to be transfused = 0.1 unit/kg of body weight. The therapeutic effectiveness should be calculated by using the following formula:

$$\triangle P = (fPc) - (iPc)(bsa)/n$$

where $\triangle P$ = increment in platelet count, fPc = final platelet count, iPc = initial platelet count, bsa = body surface area, and n = number of platelets given $\times 10^{11}$.

Single donor platelets are usually given through a 170-μ filter and infusion set. However, some investigators suggest using microaggregate filters to eliminate possible microaggregate infusion,[188] though this practice does not completely eliminate granulocytes.[189]

Single Donor and HLA-Matched Platelets

Leukemic patients as well as other patients on chronic platelet replacement therapy eventually develop antibodies to histocompatibility antigens, thereby becoming refractory to platelet therapy with random donor platelets, which have been shown to carry these antigens.[190] However, only HLA-A and HLA-B antigens have been found on platelets; HLA-C and HLA-D antigens have not been demonstrated.[191,192] Most cases of poor response to platelet therapy are due to anti-HLA antigens.[193] Other antigens, called platelet-specific antigens, have been incriminated in posttransfusion thrombocytopenia. Auto-platelet-specific antibodies have not been shown to be directly responsible for lack of response to platelet transfusion; however, as some recipients do not respond to HLA-matched platelets, antibodies to these antigens may very well play a role in this development of a refractory state.[194] Nevertheless, antiplatelet antibodies have been documented as causative of autoimmune thrombocytopenia.[194] Three platelet-specific antigen systems have been described. PlA1 and PlA2,[195] PlE1 and PlE2,[196] ZW, and KO a and b.[197] The likelihood of developing antibodies against platelets increases dramatically with the number of previous transfusions received by the patient. With the demonstration that patients can become refractory to platelet therapy with random donor units, it became evident that HLA matching was necessary for better platelet therapy response.[193] Antibodies to platelets were found in an increasing proportion of patients, in relation to the number of transfusions as follows: after 10 transfusions, 5% were immunized, and after 100 transfusions, 80% were immunized.[198] About 30% of patients receive platelets and do not become immunized against them.[199]

HLA-Matched Platelets

Therapy with platelets is first attempted with random units. In centers where a platelet crossmatch test is available, it should be performed once it is evident that the patient has become refractory to random unit transfusion. However, platelet crossmatches require a radiolabeled immunoassay or a comparatively sensitive method, not usually available to the average blood bank. A possible alternative is to use a single random donor as a source of platelets if an automated apheresis machine is available. ABO-compatible units should be given whenever possible, for ABH antigens are present on platelets,[200] and decreased platelet survival curves have been noted in patients receiving ABO-incompatible units.[201] The Rh typing should be respected in situations when Rh immunization may severely compromise a patient (e.g., Rh-negative young woman of childbearing age). Although platelets do not have Rh antigens,[202] platelet units are contaminated with amounts of RBCs potentially capable of immunizing a patient.[203] Patients who require platelets frequently are immunosuppressed and are not as readily immunized as immunocompetent recipients, averaging less than 10% of Rh-negative persons transfused with Rh-positive platelets.[204]

We have said that recipients are usually immunized against HLA antigens after chronic platelet transfusions. Furthermore, patients previously refractory to random donor platelets who are then given HLA-matched platelets have a better platelet survival time.[205] However, finding an "A" match for recipients is a difficult task. It has therefore been necessary to use B and C matches, where donors lack one antigen which the recipient possesses (see Chap. 7). Using B matches, the survival is comparable to A matches in platelet transfusions.[205] Poor matches, such as C and D matches, have less good results, but as many as 35% of patients will respond adequately.[206]

In platelet transfusions, HLA compatibility is more important than ABO compatibility. Thus, if a donor with a good match is found who is ABO incompatible, the HLA matching takes priority over the ABO matching. Large donor pools should exist for purposes of recruiting appropriate donors. The HLA typing information is recorded in data processing units and matched by computer. Clearly, complex backup systems are needed which are best handled in a large blood collecting facility such as a regional blood center.[206] Therapy for a chronic platelet user must be planned carefully and HLA typing performed before initiating transfusion of blood or components. HLA typing should also be done before chemotherapy is instituted.

Interestingly, HLA2-negative patients frequently respond better to HLA-mismatched platelets than HLA2-positive patients.[206] In spite of transfusion with A-matched platelets, about 25% of patients will develop a refractory state to transfusion with these HLA-matched thrombocytes.[204] This may well be the result of immunization to platelet-specific antibodies.[207] However, HLA antigen representation on platelets is quite variable.[208] HLA sensitization is thought to be produced mainly by contaminant WBCs in the platelet units. Methods involving centrifugation of platelets at low speeds (1,000 rpm) and passing the supernate through cotton filters have been developed to reduce the WBC content of platelet units, thus reducing the immunization potential.[209]

Other Reasons for a Poor Response to Platelets

Patients receiving platelets are frequently receiving chemotherapy for a variety of neoplastic diseases. Most chemotherapeutic drugs are potentially toxic to the bone marrow, and some directly affect platelet survival. Other drugs such as acetaminophen[210] and methicillin[211] may adversely affect platelet survival as well.

Other conditions that adversely affect platelet survival are splenomegaly[212] and fever.[213] In addition to random donor units and HLA-matched platelets, other platelet preparations are available. The ideal platelet preparation for an alloimmunized recipient is frozen units, which can be stored and transfused after thawing when the need for platelets is present. However, the technology to freeze platelets is still in the experimental stages. Platelets have been successfully frozen using dimethyl sulfoxide (DMSO) as cryoprotectant and transfused with acceptable results.[214] About 50%–65% in vivo recovery can be obtained using frozen-thawed platelets.[215] With new methods, however, and using a controlled freezing rate, platelet concentrates frozen in DMSO will yield up to 85% viable platelets, using nonfrozen units as 100%-viability controls.[216] The use of frozen-thawed platelets may result in inactivation of potentially engraftable cells in immunosuppressed patients. However, no work in this field is available to date. Irradiated platelets should be used in very immunosuppressed patients to avoid GVHD.[217]

Monocyte-free platelet concentrate preparations can be prepared by centrifuging pooled platelets at 700 rpm for 3 minutes.[218] Patients who have severe allergic reactions to plasma and who require platelet transfusions may respond to therapy without allergic reactions if given washed platelets.[219]

Platelet Therapy in Special Clinical Situations

Hematology and oncology clinic patients often are treated with medications that can produce severe thrombocytopenia. Spontaneous bleeding usually occurs when the platelet count has gradually fallen to below 20,000/cu mm. One must remember, however, that spontaneous bleeding may sometimes occur into a vital organ (e.g., CNS), so it has been suggested that these patients be treated prophylactically when platelet levels reach dangerously low levels.[220] This guideline can be followed whenever it seems appropriate, but a strict protocol cannot be delineated, because patients bleed at platelet values significantly lower or higher than those stated. A TBT test is a better gauge of bleeding tendency and should be performed concomitantly with platelet counts when monitoring these patients.

Myeloproliferative disorders per se may cause bleeding due to platelet malfunction in the presence of a normal or increased platelet count, such as occurs in polycythemia vera[221] and acute myelogenous leukemia.[222] Bleeding may be corrected with chemotherapy.

Other hematologic diseases that produce thrombocytopenia but for which platelet therapy is not routinely indicated are diseases with increased destruction of platelets [e.g., idiopathic thrombocytopenic purpura (ITP)].[223] In ITP, platelet survival is very short, usually due to the presence of platelet anti-PL antibodies. Steroids may improve survival, but only in certain cases. Most physicians prefer not to expose these patients to platelet transfusions whenever possible. Nevertheless, platelet transfusions may have to be given during surgery (e.g., splenectomy) in an attempt to improve hemostasis. During splenectomy, platelets are given after the splenic pedicle is clamped.[224] If bleeding persists postoperatively, a slow continuous infusion of platelets may be attempted, followed by a large dose of platelets. This supposedly "mops up" antibody and permits the second platelet pool to be hemostatically effective.[225] A bleeding diathesis due to platelet malfunction with normal platelet counts may be seen in other disorders, such as uremia[226] or myeloma.[227] Platelet function improves after dialysis in uremic patients and after plasmapheresis in patients with myeloma.

A major surgical complication of modern surgery is the thrombocytopenia resulting from cardiopulmonary bypass. The platelet count often drops dramatically once the patient's blood is subjected to extracorporeal circulation;[228] this drop is probably associated with damage to the platelets in the oxygenator.[229] One can expect a normal platelet count to drop to levels below 150,000/cu mm but rarely below 100,000/cu mm. At these values it is unlikely that massive hemorrhage would occur, and other causes for bleeding, such as improper mechanical hemostasis due to poor surgical technique,[230] must be sought. A platelet count and a TBT help establish the true etiology of post-open heart surgery hemorrhage. Another factor to remember is that these patients are heparinized, and bleed more readily until the heparin effect has been reversed with protamine and the patient has been taken off bypass. This type of bleeding is more rationally corrected by the use of FFP than platelets.

It should be evident that treating patients who have postsurgical thrombocytopenia with platelets in the face of platelet counts higher than 60,000/µl is in most cases geared to treat the inexperienced surgeon, not the patient. Platelet counts lower than 50,000/µl in patients who initially had normal platelet counts may indicate the presence of DIC if protamine was used to reverse the heparin affect. A coagulation profile should be performed in these cases. Abnormally functioning platelets may be present in these patients due to the appearance of fibrin split products, a complication also frequently found in patients with severe liver disease.[231] Some of these patients bleed so severely that they require massive transfusion. These patients may have a bleeding diathesis in spite of a normal platelet count or platelet counts that do not explain spontaneous bleeding (e.g., 100,000/µl), due to the presence of inactive platelets present in stored blood.[232] A TBT helps resolve the cause of bleeding and should be performed in these cases.

Complications Resulting From Platelet Transfusions

The practice of storing platelets at room temperature may give rise to significant bacterial growth in as many as 3.6% of platelet concentrates.[233] This warrants constant monitoring of the quality of platelet concentrate preparation, and culturing residual contents of platelet concentrate when severe chills and fever have been reported following a platelet concentrate transfusion. Another aspect to keep in mind is that donors are no longer required by the AABB standards to be screened for syphilis by laboratory methods.[234] One of the causes for low probability of transmission of spirochetes through blood components is the low storage temperature of the components (4°–6° C). These temperatures are incompatible with viable spirochetes after 72 hours.[235] Although platelets are now required to be stored at room temperature, there have not been reports of cases of posttransfusional syphilis, which has been in itself a rare complication of transfusion.[236] The more frequent reactions to platelet transfusion are urticarial reactions due to plasma protein sensitivity.[237] Severe anaphylactic reactions to platelet concentrates may occasionally occur in IgA-deficient patients who have developed anti-IgA antibodies.[238] This reaction must be differentiated from the severe pulmonary edema secondary to pulmonary infiltration due to leukoagglutinins.[239] Theoretically, hemolysis may occur if patients are transfused with incompatible plasma, which may be abundant in platelet concentrates (up to 250 cc, if five platelet concentrates are pooled). In one series, a direct positive antiglobulin was seen, but severe hemolysis was not documented in any of the patients who received several platelet concentrates with ABO incompatible units. This complication could be more severe in children who have a smaller blood volume.[240] We have developed a centrifugation method whereby the pool is centrifuged at 4,100 rpm for 7 minutes to decrease the plasma volume, and platelets are resuspended with gentle rotation at room temperature for approximately 60 minutes before transfusion, making sure the platelet button is fully resuspended in approximately 50 cc of plasma (personal observation). Other authors have likewise achieved good posttransfusion platelet viability after plasma volume reduction.[241]

GRANULOCYTES

Granulocytes are given to infected immunosuppressed patients in whom a trial of triple antibiotic therapy has not succeeded. Often clinicians are unaware of the therapeutic reasons for using granulocytes, the dosage, or the expiration time of this component. It is therefore sometimes necessary to educate users in the indications, as well as the counterindications for granulocyte therapy. This section describes methods of preparing granulocyte units, indications for therapy, protocols, and possible complications.

Preleukapheresis Testing

Donors must be ABO compatible with recipients.[242] A crossmatch is also necessary, for granulocyte units are heavily contaminated with RBCs, and RBC-mediated transfusion reactions may occur if incompatible units are used.

Prepheresis testing of donors for HBsAg and HTLV-III is mandatory[243] and should be repeated every 6 months. RPR testing is also suggested. All general criteria for blood donations apply to cytapheresis donations, except that donors for cytapheresis may donate every 48 hours, but no more than 250 ml of RBCs should be lost in a period of 8 weeks.[242] The extracorporeal blood volume must not be greater than 15% of the estimated total blood volume.[242] Hemoglobin should not drop below 10 gm/100 ml and the platelet count should be greater than $150,000/\mu l$.[244] The bleeding time should be normal in all apheresis donors.[243]

The need for HLA histocompatibility matching between granulocyte donor and recipient has been the subject of some debate. However, granulocyte transfusions in which donor and recipient have been HLA matched appear to yield better results in terms of granulocyte recovery after transfusion.[245] An increase in the peripheral count after granulocyte transfusion is not a good parameter by which to judge the success of transfusion because 45% of the transfused granulocytes are marginated or migrate to the extravascular space on transfusion.[246] Therefore, evaluation of successful therapy on the basis of increments in peripheral counts is a futile exercise. Furthermore, many transfused granulocytes in bona fide neutropenic patients migrate to the sites of infection, as has been demonstrated experimentally in rabbits.[247] On the other hand, more than 60% of patients with leukemia[248] and most patients with aplastic anemia develop WBC antibodies a few weeks after transfusion therapy is initiated. In canine experiments, infected neutropenic dogs alloimmunized to granulocytes and then transfused with granulocytes had a poorer prognosis than dogs not alloimmunized to WBCs.[249]

From these observations, it is evident that alloimmunized recipients should receive HLA-matched granulocytes if possible. Siblings, so long as they are ABO compatible, are a good source of granulocytes even when an A or B match cannot be obtained, because theoretically they may share non-HLA antigens, improving the granulocyte survival. A WBC crossmatch using leukocyte stimulation may be attempted, if the test is available, to predict response to transfusion. A major point in favor of transfusions with HLA-matched granulocytes is that they are associated with a reduced incidence of febrile reactions. Some WBC-induced reactions may be severe and even life-threatening.

The effectiveness of granulocyte transfusions is substantially reduced when the patient's serum contains antibodies against granulocytes.[250]

Preparation of Granulocyte Units

Granulocyte units may be obtained by manual or automated methods. Each is described below.

Manual Methods

Granulocyte units are collected from freshly drawn units of blood. The units are prepared by separating the Buffy coat of the unit into a satellite bag of an integral plastic bag system composed of four bags (the main collection bag and three satellite bags). The satellite bags are distributed as follows. Platelet-rich plasma (PRP) is collected after a slow spin (2,400 rpm in an RC-3 centrifuge) into satellite bag 1. The PRP is then centrifuged, and FFP is collected into an adjacent satellite bag 2, leaving the platelets in the original satellite bag. Once the PRP has been extracted from the original collection bag, granulocytes are then collected into the remaining empty satellite bag 3 and separated (see Fig 8-1). Even though the AABB standards allow up to 24 hours' storage,[251] granulocyte units should be transfused within 6-8 hours after collection if the half-life viability of the granulocytes is to be preserved.[252] Granulocytes stored at 1°-6° C have a decreased chemotactic ability.[253] Random donor granulocyte units, and other types of units of granulocytes (i.e., HLA-matched units), are heavily contaminated with RBCs and require a crossmatch to avoid RBC-mediated transfusion reactions. And unlike other apheresis products (e.g., platelets) obtained by automated methods, granulocytes can be stored at 4°-6° C without any major lessening of their function.[254] The total number of granulocytes per unit is about 4×10^9.

Automated Methods

Three major methods for granulocyte collection have been used: Continuous-flow centrifugation (CFC), intermittent-flow centrifugation (IFC), and continuous-flow filtration (CFF).

The first two have yielded adequate and functional granulocytes.[255] CFF yields virtually nonfunctional granulocytes[256, 257] which are deformed and degranulated,[258] and CFF has therefore fallen into disuse in most medical centers. Since the machinery used for leukapheresis is the same as that used for other apheresis procedures, the reader is referred to chapter 9 for further details on the procedure. The following discussion focuses on methods of increasing granulocyte yields from donors, rather than on the details of cytapheresis.

Both CFC[254, 259] and IFC[260] give good granulocyte survival results, even though cells are subjected to higher centrifugal forces and for a longer time during IFC cytapheresis.[261]

The Leukocyte Donor

Granulocyte donors should meet the general donor criteria acceptable to inspecting agencies such as the AABB.[262] A carefully prepared consent form should be available to the donor, explaining the procedure in detail and outlining its risks and complications. Donors should not undergo leukapheresis more than four times in 7 consecutive days, and not more than once every 48 hours.[263] Apart from general donor requirements, individuals donating by cytapheresis should have a platelet count greater than 150,000/cu mm and a normal PT and PTT. These values should be reviewed before each procedure, because the platelet count may fall by 20% after each procedure, and the hematocrit may fall by 3%.[252] Loss of blood is anticipated and may be up to 150 ml per granulocyte donation.[252]

When granulocytes are given therapeutically, the higher the dose, the more effective the treatment.[264] To ensure the highest yields, standards have been set for units of granulocytes obtained by automated methods. At least 75% of the units must contain 7×10^9 granulocytes. Donors stimulated with steroids must yield units containing at least 1×10^{10} in 75% of the units.[265]

Increments in Granulocyte Yield

The granulocyte yield can be increased by prolonging the cytapheresis procedure, by adding substances that improve separation, or by stimulating intravascular granulocyte levels.

In the first case the run may be prolonged, allowing the "dwell time" to increase, using up to 60 ml/minute rates in CFC procedures.[266]

In the second case, a better separation of cells is produced by infusing a substance into the donor that causes rouleaux formation. This allows WBCs to float to the top layer and erythrocytes to aggregate at the bottom of the cytapheresis bowl. Several dextrans have been used successfully for this purpose, but hydroxyethyl starch (HES) is currently the material of choice[267] because it is less antigenic than dextran. HES is supplied as a 6% solution in saline (MW 450,000). It is considered to be an inert, nontoxic, nonallergenic substance.[268] However, elimination of HES from the donor's body is slow. Eighty percent is eliminated in the first 8 days, but small amounts remain for several months,[269] and long-term effects are unknown. Usually 500 ml of HES with a total concentration of citrate of 1.85% is given slowly through the collection infusion line during the procedure.

The third method takes advantage of certain drug actions that will increase the granulocyte count. Corticosteroids[270] and etiocholanolone[271] will increase the WBC count up to twice the normal count. Corticosteroids given orally are much more popular than etiocholanolone because the latter produces a flu-like syndrome in the donor.[266] The most frequently used steroid is dexamethasone, 4 mg/sq m given orally 6–12 hours before the procedure, and then 4 mg/sq m given intravenously immediately before the donation.[272]

HES and dexamethasone have synergistic effects and, if used in combination in a donor undergoing apheresis with IFC instrumentation, can produce 6 cycle units containing a total of almost 2×10^{10} granulocytes.[272] Making the donor exercise before the procedure also increases granulocyte counts and is recommended in addition to giving the medications to improve granulocyte yields.

Use of Cells From Donors With Chronic Myelogenous Leukemia

Although leukocytes from individuals with chronic myelogenous leukemia are functionally defective,[273] this deficiency is compensated for by the large number of cells obtainable from these patients. The therapeutic efficacy of chronic myelogenous leukemia granulocytes has been demonstrated in infected neutropenic individuals.[274] Potential engraftment of leukemic cells into recipients of chronic myelogenous leukemia granulocytes has been reported in very immunosuppressed patients. This engraftment however, is short-lived, lasting at most 2 months.[275] Rarely, permanent engraftment has been reported in patients receiving these cells after total body irradiation for a bone marrow graft.[276] Other disadvantages are found when granulocytes from persons with chronic granulocytic leukemia are used. A major complication is the transmission of toxoplasmosis[277] as well as other diseases (cytomegalovirus) to the recipient. Another major drawback to using donors with chronic granulocytic leukemia is that these patients are in short supply and are not often able to tolerate the procedure. If these patients are the only available granulocyte donors, they should be used.

Indications and Criteria for Granulocyte Transfusions

Patients who receive chemotherapy for the treatment of leukemia as well as other neoplastic diseases eventually develop severe granulocytopenia. These patients are extremely prone to infections by a variety of opportunistic bacteria, especially gram-negative bacteria,[278] fungi, and viruses. It is suggested that treatment with granulocytes be given as soon as possible to these patients. A 48-hour trial with a triple antibiotic therapy is a reasonable period to elicit a response to multiple antibiotic therapy.[274] Nevertheless, certain workers recommend initiating granulocyte therapy sooner.[279] For instance, beginning granulocyte therapy in febrile neutropenic patients (with fever of 39° C or greater and a WBC count lower than 500/μl) who fail to improve clinically after 24 hours of treatment with a triple antibiotic schedule (e.g., cephalothin, 50 mg/kg/day q8h; gentamicin, 7 mg/kg/day q8h; and carbenicillin, 500 mg/kg/day q4h). Antibiotic therapy is continued for at least 5 days during treatment. Most centers strive for a total dose of granulocytes of at least 1×10^{10} cells.[280] Such units are given daily for at least 4 days.[281] Therapy is continued until clinical improvement (absence of fever for 24 hours) is noted.[279] The granulocytes may be discontinued if fever is absent for 5 days and cultures are negative. If random donor single granulocyte units obtained from freshly separated Buffy coats are used, then units are given in pools of 2 units each. If a given pool contains granulocytes that induce a febrile reaction in the recipient, the infusion can be interrupted and another pool of 2 units transfused. Regardless of the source of granulocytes, the units should be irradiated to avoid engraftment of lymphocytes with potential GVHD, especially units to be given to candidates for bone marrow transplantation and who are therefore severely immunosuppressed.[282] All granulocyte units, but especially units for bone marrow transplant candidates, should be irradiated with 1,500 rad before transfusion to abrogate lymphocyte division and potential engraftment of incompatible lymphocytes.[282] It has been shown that potential bone marrow transplant recipients can be protected with granulocyte transfusion prophylaxis with units prepared in this manner as an adjunct to antibiotic prophylaxis.[282] Prophylactic granulocyte transfusions in acute leukemia have not modified the outcome in these patients and therefore are not recommended.[283]

Complications of Granulocyte Transfusions

As was mentioned above, granulocyte transfusions may cause RBC incompatibility reactions because of the substantial RBC contamination present in granulocyte units, in addition to the reactions attributable to WBCs and plasma. Reactions related to granulocytes may appear clinically in two forms. The more frequent form manifests with fever and chills during the transfusion. It is also the most frequent reaction to transfusions in the overall population of transfused patients and is seen in 1%–3% of transfusion reactions.[284] This type of reaction has been attributed largely to alloimmunization against HLA antigens present on granulocytes as well as on platelets.[285] Fever appearing after the transfusion of chronic granulocytic leukemia granulocyte units may be caused by the infusion of pyrogenic debris present in these units due to damaged cells which release lysosome enzymes.[286] The presence of similar pyrogens may explain why up to 15% of patients receiving filtration leukapheresis WBCs, which are severely damaged by the filtration collection process, react with chills and fever, in contrast to only 5% of patients receiving CFC granulocyte units.[287] It is obvious that procedures that produce less damage to cells are associated with a lower incidence of febrile transfusion reactions. Furthermore, selection of HLA-matched granulocytes for patients who are significantly alloimmunized will prevent reactions caused by antibodies to histocompatible antigens. Most patients can be premedicated with Tylenol before granulocyte transfusions to prevent fever and related symptoms. Urticarial reactions may be very frequent as well.[288] These reactions are IgE-mediated reactions and are usually secondary to sensitivity to plasma proteins.[289] Premedication with Benadryl is indicated in subsequent transfusions.[288] Severe anaphylactoid reactions to plasma have been reported but are rare.[290] Most of these reactions are due to anti-IgA antibodies in IgA-deficient individuals.[290] Washing units of granulocytes with saline may be attempted if IgA-deficient donors cannot be obtained. However, such manipulation of granulocytes is discouraged because of the inherent fragility of granulocytes. The second, less frequent type of granulocyte reaction appears as pulmonary edema. This is a rather alarming reaction and is manifested clinically by the acute appearance of cyanosis, dyspnea, and wheezing. Rales may be heard on auscultation, and a chest x-ray film reveals the pulmonary infiltrates. Pulmonary edema is produced by leukoagglutinins, which cause clumping of granulocytes in the capillary circulation of the lungs.[291] Interestingly, patients may develop pulmonary edema after infusion of plasma obtained from donors with high levels of leukoagglutinins.[292] This type of reaction should be kept in mind if patients have not previously had leukoagglutinins in their plasma. For other details on reactions to transfusion see chapter 11.

Complications Resulting From Granulocyte Donation

Cytapheresis is not an entirely benign procedure, and deaths have occurred during therapeutic apheresis.[293] It is a good practice to review the indications for granulocyte transfusion before asking patients or normal donors to undergo a procedure that may be harmful. On the other hand, the more common reactions are usually not severe. Symptoms resulting from hypovolemia are perhaps the most disagreeable of these reactions. These are more frequent in persons undergoing cytapheresis with the continuous-flow machines, where the extracorporeal volume of blood may reach up to 650 ml,[294] whereas only half that volume is in extracorporeal circulation in discontinuous centrifugation techniques. Citrate toxicity is also frequently found in donors undergoing CFC or DFC. Citrate toxicity is manifested by circumoral numbness or a tingling sensation at the tips of the fingers. More severe complications include postcytapheresis thrombocytopenia, with platelet count drops of up to 50,000/ μl per procedure,[295] and hemorrhage from excessive anticoagulation, especially when heparin has been used.[296] If donors are to be premedicated with steroids, extreme care must be exercised in selecting them to ensure that they will tolerate the procedure without major complications. A history of a bleeding ulcer or other potential counterindication to steroid therapy should be carefully sought in these donors. Embolism is not frequently reported as a complication, but it may be triggered during leukapheresis. In DFC the bowl may trap platelets and form clots. Overload and potential long-term complications from HES are potential problems stemming from the use of this rouleaux-inducing agent. Rarer leukocyte donor reactions include seizures, dyspnea, and hemolysis.[297] Absolute decrements in lymphocyte counts (up to 23%), both in T cells (23%) and B cells (up to 46% of the count), have been reported in healthy cytapheresis donors.[298]

PLASMA FRACTIONS

Plasma fractions are obtained by the biochemical separation of plasma pools. As such they are available commercially only from centers where large volumes of plasma are processed. The blood bank may be involved in the storage and issuing of such fractions. The more frequently used fractions are factor VIII and factor IX concentrates, albumin, and γ-globulin.

Factor VIII Concentrates

Since it is difficult to obtain a uniform product when preparing cryoprecipitate, the use of lyophilized factor VIII concentrates has become more popular. Furthermore, when large concentrations of factor VIII are needed, the dosage can be achieved only with these lyophilized concentrates. Concentrates may contain up to 40 units/ml.[299] The concentration is stated on the label of the vials and the product is accompanied by diluent for transfusion. Factor VIII concentrates are prepared from pools of cryoprecipitate as the starting material.[300] The pooled cryoprecipitate is then chromatographed to yield fractions rich in factor VIII.[301]

Factor VIII is a 1- to 2-million-dalton molecular weight[302] globulin which runs as an α-globulin[303] on electrophoresis. It has a carbohydrate moiety essential for its coagulant activity,[304] which can be destroyed by glycolytic enzymes.

At least three measurable properties are identified in the factor VIII molecule: its coagulant activity (VIII AHF), its antigenic activity, assessed by antibodies raised in rabbits (VIII AGN), and the capacity of factor VIII to support aggregation of platelets induced by the antibiotic ristocetin, namely von Willebrand's factor VIII (or F VIII vW). When factor VIII is separated via molecular sieves two fractions are recognized, a low molecular weight fraction, which contains the coagulant activity,[305] and a high molecular weight fraction, which contains both the antigenic activity plus the factor VIII vW activity.[305] The presence of these components may explain why factor VIII lyophilized concentrates lack factor VIII vW properties but preserve factor VIII procoagulant activity.[306] It is for this reason that patients with von Willebrand's disease must receive cryoprecipitate as replacement therapy instead of factor VIII lyophilized concentrates. A more detailed discussion on clotting factors is given in Chapter 3.

Replacement Therapy With Factor VIII Concentrates

Factor VIII concentrates are used to treat hemophilia A. The following formula is used to calculate the dose of factor VIII required:[307]

$$PV(.05 \times bw) \times DI = \text{units of AHF}$$

where PV = plasma volume, bw = body weight in grams, and DI = desired increase.

The concentration of the product in numbers of factor VIII units is stated on the label and in the instructions. Therapy schedules and protocols vary according to different authorities. However, a practical protocol is the following.[299] For all surgery the plasma level is brought to 100% 1 hour before surgery (50 units/kg). After minor surgery the plasma level is kept above 60% for the first 4 days and above 20% for the following 4 days. After major surgery the plasma level is similarly kept above 60% for the first 4 days but in the following 4 days levels of 40% are recommended.

Orthopedic surgery and trauma require bringing plasma levels to 100% immediately and maintaining levels of 80% the first 4 days, 40% the following 4 days, and 20% during ambulation if bleeding persists.[299]

Complications From Factor VIII Concentrates

About 7% of hemophilic patients eventually develop factor VIII antibodies.[308] These are usually IgG4 antibodies that act as blocking antibodies or inhibitors that attach to the procoagulant active site.[309] These patients represent a challenge to the hematologist because they become refractory to therapy. Factor IX concentrates have been used to override the effect of these inhibitors.[310] ϵ-Aminocaproic acid (EACA) has also been used to override inhibitor effects but should be used with great caution, lest thrombosis develop.[311] It has recently become possible to prepare porcine factor VIII fractions; this product appears to be substantially less antigenic than the earlier preparations and may be therapeutic for patients who have developed anti-AHF antibodies.[312] Extensive plasma exchange has likewise been of help in one case.[313]

A major risk with factor VIII replacement therapy is the development of hepatitis. The increased risk of acquiring viral hepatitis from fractions of plasma pools has been documented since 1960.[314] This risk is evidently proportional to the size of the pool of plasma from which factor VIII has been obtained. Research using preparations of factor VIII heated to 60° C to eliminate HBV transmission has yielded promising results.[315]

AIDS as a result of therapy with factor VIII concentrates is a recently described, ominous complication of this type of therapy.[11] See chapter 13.

A less common complication, but one to keep in mind, is hemolysis of the patient's RBCs from the transfused anti-A and anti-B, frequently contaminating these AHF concentrates.[316] Fortunately, RBC hemolysis is rare. It occurs most often during administration of massive doses of AHF.

Recently it was shown that treatment with factor VIII concentrates as well as immunoglobulin fractions may result in unfavorable reactions such as wheezing, chest tightness, and hypotension, some instances of which are attributable to the kallikrein content of these preparations.[317]

Factor IX Concentrates (The Prothrombin Complex)

Factors II, VII, IX, and X belong to the prothrombin complex. These procoagulants are all synthesized in the liver[318] and are dependent on vitamin K.[319] Vitamin K is involved not in the actual synthesis of the proteins but in their postsynthetic modification into biologically active procoagulants within liver cells.[320] The prothrombin complex factors (factors II, VII, IX, and X) all run in the α and β regions, although some investigators have also found activity running with the albumin band.[321] However, Most workers agree that factor IX runs in the $\alpha 1$ band on electrophoresis.[321] The molecular weight of factor IX has been calculated to be about 80,000 daltons.[322] Barium sulfate selectively removes the prothrombin complex factors from plasma; this process is carboxylation dependent.[323] Coumadin competes in vivo with vitamin K, bringing about a deficiency of prothrombin complex factors.[324] Commercially available factor IX concentrates contain all of the prothrombin factors (i.e., factors II, VII, IX, X). These concentrates and concentrates of factor VIII are initially separated from plasma by the Cohn fractionation method.[325] Cohn fraction I, containing fibrinogen and factor VIII, is separated first by cold alcohol precipitation. The supernate contains the prothrombin complex, which must be further purified via chromatography on DEAE-cellulose.[326] This method probably gives purer yields than methods that extract the prothrombin complex from Cohn fraction III after removing the lipoprotein from this fraction.[325]

Clinical Uses of Factor IX Concentrates

Although commercially available lyophilized factor IX is used mostly for hemophilia B therapy, it may be used for other factor deficiencies, such as deficiencies of factors II, VII, and X, as well as to override factor VIII deficiencies, as mentioned earlier.[310]

Therapy schedules are prepared in the same way as for factor VIII deficiencies.[299] The dosage is calculated as follows: 1 unit of factor IX per kilogram of body weight increases the plasma factor IX level by 1%. A good therapy regimen to follow is given below:[299]

1. Hematoma, 5–10 units/kg of body weight
2. Hemarthrosis, 10–20 units/kg of body weight
3. Hematuria or GI bleeding, 40 units/kg of body weight ÷ 3.

4. Trauma, surgery, CNS, retroperitoneal or retropharyngeal hemorrhage, 50 units/kg of body weight.

5. Dental procedures, EACA (Amicar), 100 mg/kg 4 hours before surgery.

Complications of Therapy With Factor IX Concentrates

Inhibitors may develop, albeit this occurs less frequently than in factor VIII therapy. About 1%–3% of patients have this complication, manifested in the production by recipients of monoclonal IgG κ antibodies against factor IX.[326] The inhibitors to factor VIII can be expressed in Bethesda units to assess their level in plasma.[327] It may be possible similarly to assess inhibitors to factor IX.

Unlike factor VIII concentrates, factor IX concentrates do not appear to contain significant amounts of ABH antibodies.[328]

A major complication of factor IX therapy is the high risk of posttransfusion hepatitis.[329] The risk of hepatitis appears to be greater with use of factor IX concentrates than with use of factor VIII concentrates.[299] It is not possible to remove all viral particles chemically, and more aggressive separation procedures yield products which fail to retain procoagulant activity.[330] Nevertheless, third-generation testing for hepatitis as well as careful screening of donors has resulted in an 80% reduction in the incidence of hepatitis B from these products.[299] Solid phase anti-HB$_S$Ag antibodies may provide HBV-free factor concentrates in the future. As is the case with factor VIII concentrates, AIDS has likewise been reported as a serious complication of factor IX therapy. See chapter 13.

The development of hypercoagulability with subsequent thrombosis is another feared complication from the use of factor IX concentrates.[331, 332] It is recommended that patients with hepatic damage or vascular disease be carefully evaluated before being treated with factor IX concentrates.[333] Concomitant infusion of subcutaneous heparin (5,000 units/12 hours) has been recommended in patients receiving these preparations, especially hemophilia B patients undergoing elective surgery.[307]

Fibrinogen

Fibrinogen is a major constituent of plasma. It is present at levels of 200–400 mg/100 ml of plasma. It has a molecular weight of about 340,000 daltons and is composed of three pairs of polypeptide chains, α, β, and γ, joined by disulfide bonds.[334]

Fibrinogen is activated by thrombin during the clotting cascade. This enzyme splits fibrinogen at the arginyl-glycyl bonds at the N-terminal ends, producing fibrinopeptides A and B.

Fibrinogen deficiencies can be seen in a variety of diseases (e.g., liver damage and DIC). Lyophilized fibrinogen concentrate is no longer used in clinical practice because of the high associated risk of transmitting hepatitis.[335] In lieu of lyophilized concentrates, cryoprecipitate is now recommended as a good source of fibrinogen.[336]

Albumin

Albumin is the most abundant of the plasma proteins, constituting about 55% of the plasma proteins.[337] It is obtained from fraction V on Cohn fractionation. Albumin is a 69,000-dalton molecular weight protein that is synthesized in the liver and contains 610 amino acids arranged in a single polypeptide chain that is folded upon itself.[337] The major function of this protein is to preserve the intravascular oncotic pressure of plasma; it also functions as a carrier of various substances in blood. During its preparation albumin withstands heating at 60° C for 10 hours, which is the basis for the loss of infectivity by HBV from this fraction.[338–340] Plasma protein fraction (PPF) is a less purified fraction[341] which contains 92% albumin.[342] Both salt-poor albumin (the purer form) and PPF do not carry the risk of transmitting hepatitis.[340] Albumin preparations of the PPF type may contain prekallikrein and kallikrein substances which are responsible for nonimmunologically mediated vasoactive reactions, especially if large amounts of PPF are given rapidly.[343]

Albumin is available as a 5% solution (normal serum albumin-5, NSA-5) with an oncotic pressure similar to plasma,[344] and as a 25% solution (NSA-25), which has a high oncotic pressure and must not be given intravenously to dehydrated patients.[345] Conversely, albumin may be used to treat edema as long as the edema is not caused by heart failure, in which case the intravascular volume is already increased.

Albumin has been successfully used as a volume expander in hemorrhage and trauma to correct hypovolemic shock[346] and in extensively burned patients to restore protein loss.[347] Albumin does have an advantage over FFP in that it does not carry the risk of transmitting hepatitis. However, the use of colloid solutions has been abused in recent years, to the extent of producing shortages of supplies and excessive monetary expenditure. In one study, the use of albumin generated greater costs than the overall use of antibiotics.[348] This excessive expenditure is a burden on medical care costs and exploits indigent donor populations.[349]

Most of the albumin used in a large hospital is for replacement of blood loss in surgery.[350] Early experiments on dogs showed that a blood volume loss of up to 60% could be corrected with plasma.[351] Albumin can be used to restore blood volume because it has sufficient oncotic pressure, due to its protein content.[352] Subsequently experiments on rabbits showed that PPF was as effective in restoring blood volume,[353] and in humans it was safe as a substitute for plasma in burn patients, but 30% greater volumes were required.[354] However, recent studies on albumin replacement have shown that these colloidal solutions may induce fluid shifts to the pulmonary interstitium, with subsequent overload on the myocardium.[355] These findings suggest that albumin solutions should be used in combination with diuretics and probably should not be given in massive doses to patients with renal, pulmonary, or cardiac compromise. Patients resuscitated with crystalloid solutions have dryer lungs and improved pulmonary function than patients who receive albumin.[356] This implies that an attempt to use crystalloids should precede any decision to use colloids. However, replacement with crystalloid solutions requires three times the volume of colloid replacement,[357, 358] and vast replacement of blood volume with crystalloid solutions in patients with renal compromise may be unwise because of the potential of causing severe pulmonary edema.[359] The question then arises as to when to start transfusing blood or components after starting crystalloids. It is not possible to establish a single protocol applicable to patients, because each patient reacts differently and one surgeon's philosophy on the subject may differ from another's. In principle, it is thought that patients with good renal, cardiac, and pulmonary function who had a normal hematocrit initially and who have lost blood can have up to 25% of their total blood volume replaced exclusively with crystalloid solutions.[360] Losses of up to 70% of the blood volume can be managed exclusively with packed RBCs and crystalloids.[361]

The treatment of burn patients is a special case in replacement therapy. Crystalloid is given in the first 24 hours for burns covering greater than 15% of body surface area in adults or 10% of body surface area in children.[362] After the first 24 hours colloids are started to maintain a plasma albumin level of at least 2.5 gm/100 ml.[363] It has been shown that burn patients do better with FFP as replacement, probably because of its γ-globulin content.[364] Patients with 20%–40% surface area burns who receive plasma do better than those who receive crystalloid.[365] It appears that burn patients require the oncotic pressure to preserve their intravascular volume.[365]

Patients made hypoproteinemic because of nutritional deprivation must not be treated with intravenous albumin for any length of time.[366] Albumin catabolizes slowly[367] and lacks certain essential amino acids that are better supplied by amino acid supplements.[363]

The administration of albumin, especially as PPF, may be complicated by severe vasoactive reactions,[363, 368] and therefore its use is not entirely risk-free. Anaphylactoid reactions to albumin have also been reported.[369] Antibodies to albumin may cause blocking of factor IX activity,[321] and in some cases these antibodies may cause confusion during laboratory testing,[370] due to false positive reactions on the direct Coombs test.

Immunoglobulins

Immunoglobulins are glycoproteins composed of about 90% polypeptide and about 10%–20% carbohydrate and comprise about 20% of the total plasma protein. On electrophoresis immunoglobulins migrate mostly in the γ zone, but some migrate in the β zone.[371] Immunoglobulins contain the antibody activity of sera. A more detailed description of the classes and subclasses of immunoglobulins (IgG, IgM, IgA, IgD, and IgE) is given in chapter 4.

γ-Globulins can be purified by modification of the Cohn fractionation method and are separated mostly in Cohn fraction II.[372] The preparation process includes heating at 60° C, which eliminates infectivity by HBV. Preparations for clinical use are given intramuscularly or intravenously. Intravenous injections of preparations available in this country used to cause reactions in the recipient. These reactions were presumably due to IgG aggregation and complement activation.[373] These reactions do not occur if the immunoglobulin preparation is manufactured at pH 4.[374]

Use of Immunoglobulin Preparations

Immunoglobulin preparations are used in the prophylaxis of infectious diseases caused by bacteria (e.g., diphtheria)[375] or viruses (e.g., hepatitis, measles, rubella). The value of immune serum globulin (ISG) in the prevention of viral hepatitis A has been proved.[376] The protecting dose for individuals who have been in contact with patients who have viral hepatitis A up to 14 days post exposure is 0.02–0.04 ml/kg of a 16.5% solution given intramuscularly.[377]

Although passive-active immunization may be achieved via ISG against viral hepatitis B,[378] the use of hepatitis B immune globulin (HBIG) is recommended,[379] not ISG. The recommended dose of HBIG is 0.6 ml/kg within 6 days of exposure; the dose may be repeated 1 month later.[377] More details on the protocol for use is given in chapter 16. Passive immunization against measles within 6 days of exposure can also be achieved with special hyperimmune γ-globulin fractions obtained from plasma pools of immunized donors. However, large doses are needed (450 mg).[380] Zoster and vaccinia immune globulin can be obtained from specialized centers such as the Centers for Disease Control in Atlanta.[377] Tetanus immune globulin can be given prophylactically in a dose of 250 units.[381] The use of immunoglobulin fractions to prevent immunization against the Rh(D) antigen is discussed in detail in chapters 5 and 16. Immune globulin fractions can also be used in replacement therapy for patients with congenital or acquired hypogammaglobulinemia. Patients with levels of less than 2 gm/L should receive replacement therapy. Initially a bolus of 0.25 gm/kg is given, then 0.025 gm/kg/week is given as a maintenance dose.[382]

Other Products Used as Plasma Expanders

Dextrans

Dextrans are polysaccharides produced by bacteria, usually *Leuconostoc mesenteroides* and *dextranicum*, using a sucrose substrate. These substances are composed of chains of D-glucose molecules linked in α-D (1–6) linkages. These chains differ only in chain length or branching, which determines their molecular weight.[383] Uniform preparations are not available, so mean molecular weight estimates of these products are given by the manufacturers.[384]

Clinical dextrans are available at different molecular weights (40,000, 70,000, or 110,000 daltons). Ideally these substitutes should not weigh less than 70,000 daltons to prevent rapid elimination via the kidney,[385] or more than 100,000 daltons to prevent rouleaux formation.[386] The presence of rouleaux may cause confusion and difficulty in immunohematologic testing. Dextran 40 is available as a 10% solution, while Dextran 70 and Dextran 110 are available as 6% solutions. Usually Dextran 40 is used for acute correction of volume, as it is eliminated faster than Dextran 110, which is intended for prolonged plasma expansion.[387]

Dextran continues to be the preferred plasma expander in surgical situations where the oxygen-carrying capacity is not excessively compromised.[388] However, complications from its use have been documented. Frequently an increment in the bleeding time is observed, presumably caused by the effect of dextran on platelet function.[389] If given in DIC it may complicate the coagulopathy by producing a drop in the platelet count and an increment in fibrin split products.[390] Nevertheless, because of its effect on platelets, it may help prevent deep vein thrombosis in the postoperative care of patients.[391] Another potential complication with the use of dextran is that it may produce anaphylactoid reactions,[392] even in subjects never before exposed to this medication.[393]

Hydroxyethyl Starch

Hydroxyethyl starch (HES) is a modified starch which resists digestion by serum amylase.[394] The molecular weight varies from 65,000 to 450,000 daltons. HES has advantages over dextran in that it produces less compromise to platelet function[394] and is less antigenic,[371] therefore causing fewer allergic reactions.[369] Nevertheless, it may be found in tissues long after infusion.

Gelatin

Gelatin (MW 25,000–45,000 daltons) has been used commercially as a plasma expander since 1951.[395, 396] In Europe it has been used successfully and is available as a 4% solution through the Swiss Red Cross under the commercial name of Physiogel. These preparations, obtained from animal collagen, are heat-treated to modify and diminish antigenicity, but allergic reactions, though rare, do occur.[392] The FDA has not yet approved the use of this plasma expander in the United States. The major use for intravenous infusion of gelatin solutions is in the short-term correction of volume loss, because the renal threshold for gelatin is low and the gelatin is therefore eliminated via the kidney within a short time.[397] Since adequate oncotic pressure is preserved only for 4 hours, gelatin solutions are not recommended for diseases causing chronic oncotic derangements. Compared to dextran, gelatin does not increase the bleeding time, but like dextran it will induce rouleaux formation.[398] Gelatin may have a place in short-term plasma volume expansion. However, the decision to use gelatin regularly to combat volume losses must await further experience and possibly a critical comparison with the currently available plasma expanders.[399]

Substitutes for Blood

Artificial Oxygen Carriers

There is, to date, no substitute for blood. However, a great deal of research effort has been invested in attempting to produce a substance, artificially, or semiartificially, which will emulate blood in its vital function of carrying oxygen to tissues and ridding tissues of CO_2.

Blood can maintain vital functions even at a hematocrit as low as 6%, without the need of additional oxygen carriers;[400] therefore substitute replacement is probably not necessary until hematocrit levels fall below 6%. In the face of increasing blood demands, the need for artificial oxygen carriers is understated. The ideal oxygen carrier should be (1) nontoxic, (2) noninfectious, (3) nonantigenic, (4) similar to blood in its oxygen-carrying and oxygen off-loading properties, (5) not be retained for extensive periods of time, and (6) produced from readily available raw materials.

None of the currently studied oxygen carriers possesses all of these attributes. Three different types of oxygen carriers have been extensively studied:[400] stroma-free hemoglobin, perfluorochemicals, and synthetic chelates. The first two have been extensively studied, and are reviewed here in some detail.

Stroma-Free Hemoglobin

The misconception that hemoglobin produces renal damage has long been dispelled; stroma in hemolysates has been shown to be the major factor responsible for damage consecutive to hemolysate transfusions.[401] Stroma-free hemoglobin (SFH) was the first artificial oxygen carrier produced.[399] RBC hemoglobin obtained by controlled freeze-thawing and from which cell stroma has been eliminated by filtration[402] is safe for transfusion, as shown with bloodless rats (Hct. 0–1%) kept alive with continuous infusions of SFH in high oxygen saturation environments.[403] Other mammals with a lower metabolic rate, such as cats[404] and baboons,[405] are capable of surviving in ambient air with these infusions. However, the half-life of SFH is about 3.5 hours, making it clinically useless.[406]

In order to improve their circulating half-life, SFH preparations have been modified by cross-linking to large molecular weight polymers such as dextran.[407] Hemoglobin complexed in this manner has a better half-life, but its oxygen off-loading capacity is drastically decreased when compared to SFH.[408] In order to improve off-loading, hemoglobin has been modified by pyridoxylation and polymerization, yielding a product with a 1.32 oxygen binding coefficient and a torr (an oxygen off-load measure) of 16; normal RBCs have a torr of 24.[409] Three main disadvantages of SFH are (1) it degrades on long-term storage at 4° C to methemoglobin (40% loss after 1 year);[410] (2) it may transmit hepatitis,[411] and its potential for transmitting AIDS is unknown; and (3) current preparations do not equate RBC off-loading properties. Complications from the use of SFH preparations result from the presence in these solutions of endotoxins[412] and from inappropriate perfusion, with subsequent axonal swelling and perivascular edema.[413]

Should some of the listed drawbacks be circumvented, SF solutions would hold significant therapeutic promise.

Perfluorocarbons

Perfluorocarbons are synthetic compounds similar to hydrocarbons[414] in which hydrogen atoms have been replaced by fluoride atoms (Fig 8–4).[415] Perfluorocarbons have been selected because they are inert, nontoxic, and can dissolve greater amounts of oxygen than other fluids at comparable pressures. However, diffusion of CO_2, N_2, and O_2 through these fluids, under physiologic conditions, is no greater than water,[416] limiting their clinical useful-

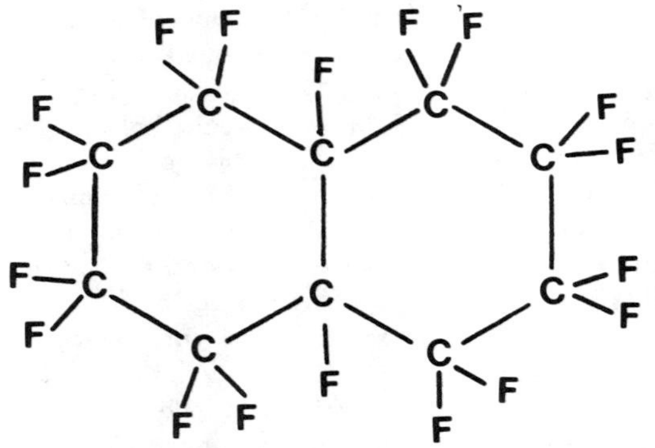

FIG 8–4.—Structure of perfluorodecalin. Note the fluoride atoms linked to the free carbon radicals. These fluorinated radicals may each potentially bind a molecule of oxygen.

ness. The advantage of perfluorocarbons over saline, however, is that perfluorocarbons transport oxygen more effectively. When perfluorocarbons are equilibrated with 100% oxygen, they dissolve 10% more oxygen than packed RBCs. At a higher Pa_{O_2}, the increment in oxygen saturation of perfluorocarbons increases linearly and surpasses that of RBCs. At a P_{O_2} of 100 mm Hg, RBC hemoglobin saturation reaches a plateau. However, at a P_{O_2} of 650–760 mm Hg, perfluorodecalin far surpasses the oxygen saturation of RBCs.[400] However, oxygen at these concentrations is toxic to both experimental animals and humans, causing the adult respiratory distress syndrome and retrolental fibroplasia.[417]

Perfluorodecalin is the safest perfluorocarbon because of its short retention in tissues.[418] Unmodified, perfluorochemicals are insoluble in water, and when used intravenously they have a tendency to induce embolism[419] due to interaction between the perfluorocarbon with platelets[420] and clotting factors.[421] To avoid these thrombotic phenomena, perfluorochemicals are sonicated to produce 2-μ or smaller particles by emulsification with albumin.[415]

In addition, substances such as HES or gelatin are added to supply oncotic pressure.[400] It is known that mice can tolerate complete submersion in perfluorodecalin, so long as oxygen is bubbled into the perfluorocarbon solution.[422] However, these animals will likewise survive complete submersion in saline if the solution is under hyperbaric oxygen.[423] Experimental animals have been replaced with perfluorochemicals to 0–1% hematocrit and maintained alive with supplemental oxygen. However, the best results have been obtained in animals in which 80% of the blood volume was replaced with the oxygen carrier, rather than total replacement.[424] A commercial preparation Fluosol-DA (Green-Cross Corp., Osaka, Japan) containing Pluronic-60 (a perfluorocarbon) stabilized with yolk phospholipids has been extensively tested and has proved relatively nontoxic to humans.[425] These studies proved Fluosol-DA was tolerated by humans. However, in a controlled clinical study, Fluosol given at a dosage of 20 ml/kg of body weight to severely anemic patients receiving low supplemental oxygen (101 ± 25 mm Hg) functioned only as a volume expander. At oxygen concentrations above 300 mm Hg, Fluosol could carry 0.8% oxygen per volume.[426] However, at similarly low hematocrits, plasma is likewise capable of transporting and off-loading oxygen.[427]

These findings have prevented FDA approval of these compounds under their current formulation.[428] In a series of 22 patients, 15 patients with acute anemia were treated with crystalloid and 100% oxygen by mask. Seven patients who could not be stabilized were given 60% oxygen by mask and transfused with Fluosol. Five of these seven patients died despite receiving Fluosol within 2 days of Fluosol infusion. One of the two survivors received blood transfusions following Fluosol.[428] It should be noted, however, that in this series only 4%–5% fluorocrits (those allowed by the FDA) were used. Evidently more work lies ahead before a clinically useful artificial oxygen carrier is fully developed. Other potential uses of perfluorocarbons may be in the treatment of myocardial infarction, as these fluids could be used to perfuse hypoxic areas by diffusion through occlusive thrombi.[429] These substances may also prove useful in perfusion of organs stored for transplantation.[430] Perfluorocarbons, though inert, are not completely devoid of toxic effects. Endothelial swelling in microcapillaries,[431] the development of foamy macrophages, and altered immune system responsiveness[432] are some of the known toxic effects of these substances. Other potential complications are coagulopathies with a resulting bleeding diathesis.[433] However, surprisingly little bleeding is observed experimentally, probably due to a tighter closure of vessels during vasospasm.

Newer Components

It is currently possible to rejuvenate RBCs that have expired by restoring ATP and 2,3-DPG to the cells. This is done by adding a solution enriched with inosine, adenine, pyruvate, and phosphate.[434, 435]

Bone marrow has been successfully frozen in DMSO and retrieved from the frozen state;[436] likewise, peripheral blood stem cells have been isolated, frozen, and retrieved from the frozen state.[437] These techniques offer possibilities to bone marrow transplant candidates who may need these cells during spells of neutropenia (e.g., leukemics under treatment).[436, 437] Granulocytes have been preserved for up to 8 months in the frozen state with up to 77% in vivo recovery and 77% bactericidal activity.[438] Neocytes, or young RBCs, can be prepared with automated RBC separators; these cells survive longer and therefore can reduce transfusion requirements for the multitransfused patient. These preparations, however, contain substantial numbers of immunocompetent cells.[439]

BONE MARROW TRANSPLANTATION

Blood bankers can expect to be involved in bone marrow transplantation in the near future, as transplantation groups become more numerous in this country; by the end of 1980 more than 1,000 patients had undergone bone marrow transplantation.[440] Bone marrow transplantation has become a reality in terms of attempting cures for leukemia and aplastic anemia.[441]

Definition and Scientific Rationale

Donor bone marrow hemopoietic cells transfused to an irradiated marrow recipient home in to the bone marrow of the recipient, developing and maturing in these sites if the donor cells are histocompatible.[441]

The development of bone marrow transplantation as a viable choice for therapy of patients who have lost the capacity to produce hemopoietic cells, because of therapeutic bone marrow ablation or aplasia, has been possible owing to better and more accurate methods for typing and matching potential donors for these patients. This has resulted from the understanding of the major histocompatibility system. This subject is reviewed in detail in chapter 7, but we will very briefly go over the salient points.

The products of the HLA genes are antigens termed HLA-A, B, C, and D. Each of the genes coding for these products have a large number of alleles, thus making the HLA system an extremely polymorphic one. Serologically defined antigens are HLA-A, B, and C. HLA-D is defined by MLC cultures; HLA-DR is serologically defined.

Lymphocytes from the peripheral blood of donors are used to detect these antigens. Serologic antigens are detected by lymphocyte death (cytotoxicity). HLA-D is defined by radioactive measurement of DNA synthesis through radioactive thymidine uptake. ABO matching in bone marrow transplantation is important but not critical in the way it is for solid organ transplant.[442] For instance, in one series of 12 cases of patients who received ABO-incompatible, HLA-compatible bone marrow cells, the incidence of GVHD and survival were comparable to what was seen in recipients of ABO-compatible transplanted marrow.[443] Nevertheless, extensive plasmapheresis and exchange with AB plasma is performed before the procedure to avoid hemolytic transfusion reactions from the contaminating RBCs in the bone marrow cell suspensions, rather than to avoid destruction of the lymphocytes by the isoantibodies present in incompatible plasma.[443] For practical purposes, most bone marrow donors have been siblings. There is a 25% chance that a sibling is HLA-compatible in HLA-A, B, C, and D.[441] However, donors who are not siblings and who are compatible at HLA loci have been successfully used in bone marrow transplantation.[444]

Compatible matched donors are confirmed by mixed lymphocyte cultures (MLC). Despite all these tests, transplant rejection may occur, because of minor loci mismatches which are always possible, except in identical twin transplants.

Contrary to renal transplantation, previous blood transfusions significantly reduce the successful outcome of bone marrow transplantation.[445] This fact is underscored by the finding that survival of patients falls to 65% in patients with aplastic anemia who received nonirradiated granulocyte units, and to 45% in multitransfused patients.[446]

Prior Treatment and Bone Marrow Engraftment for Patients With Leukemia

Supralethal whole body radiation (1,000 rad, midpoint tissue dose) is given to eliminate tumor cells, and produce immunosuppression of the recipient prior to engraftment.[447] Multiple aspirations of the anterior and posterior iliac crests are performed on the donor in the surgical suite. The marrow is collected in heparinized tissue culture medium and filtered to obtain 4×10^8 cells per kilogram of body weight. The suspension is then infused intravenously.[448] Patients are placed in conventional protective isolation and covered against infection with oral antibiotics (Nystatin, Vancomycin, Polymixin B), for existing flora, and Cotrimoxazole for pneumocystis.

Febrile episodes are considered to be evidence of infection. Patients are treated with carbenicillin and aminoglycoside antibiotics.[449]

Evidence of engraftment is monitored by the following: (1) karyotype analysis of peripheral blood, (2) RBC antigen and isoenzyme phenotyping, and (3) rising blood cell counts. WBC counts and bone marrow cellularity can be expected to rise in 10–30 days, whereas platelets may not appear for 20–100 days after transplant.[450]

Indications for Bone Marrow Transplantation

The two major indications for bone marrow transplantation are attempted cure of acute leukemia, and the treatment of aplastic anemia. Other indications are severe combined immunodeficiency syndrome[451] and thalassemia.[440]

Bone Marrow Transplantation in Acute Leukemia

Cyclophosphamide followed by total body irradiation with 1,000 rad is the most effective method (to date) of killing leukemic cells, due to penetration of privileged sites such as the CNS and the testicle.

In one series, 100 patients, 54 with AML and 46 with ALL, were treated with cyclophosphamide followed by irradiation and bone marrow grafting. About 20% of ALL patients were alive 2–5 years after transplantation, without recurrence or antileukemic treatment, whereas 15% of AML patients were alive 2–5 years after bone marrow transplantation.[441]

This mortality rate was not considered high because these patients were end-stage leukemics. If patients are treated during their first remission, however, up to two thirds may experience long-term survival.[452] The major complications in these patients are (1) rejection of the graft, which occurs in about 30% of cases;[453] (2) GVHD, which is severe in 50% of the cases;[441] (3) recurrent leukemia (Table 8–1); and (4) severe infections, which have caused death in 15% of cases[453] (pneumonia was seen in 63% of the cases).[454] Patients with severe GVHD appear to have a similar recurrence rate as leukemics and patients with mild GVHD.[441] When a bone marrow transplant recipient receives bone marrow from an identical twin, the survival rate may exceed 60%. Deaths in these cases is usually from infection prior to marrow recovery or from leukemic recurrence; GVHD does not occur in these cases.[455] GVHD can be improved by the use of antithymocyte globulin (ATG), but patients eventually develop immunodeficiency as a result of this treatment and die from interstitial pneumonia,[441, 456] thus making the use of ATG not advisable.[456]

This type of pneumonia is brought on by CMV, herpes virus, and *Pneumocystis carinii* infections due to immunosuppression.[457] Open lung biopsy is usually necessary for confirmatory diagnosis. Due to failure of ATG to prevent GVHD, a combination of posttransplantation use of methotrexate and glucocorticoids has been used successfully.[457]

Bone Marrow Transplantation in Aplastic Anemia

Without the benefit of bone marrow transplantation, patients develop fatal infections and bleeding. Only 10% of patients are alive more than 2 years from the time of diagnosis. If a patient with bone marrow aplasia receives a bone marrow transplant within 30 days of the diagnosis, the chances of survival are 70%; the figure drops to 50% if the transplant is received after this period.[458]

Like leukemics, patients with aplastic anemia are treated with cyclophosphamide, followed by total body irradiation, and then transfused with histocompatible hemopoietic cells.

The most frequent cause of transplant failure is graft rejection, which occurred in 21 of 68 patients in one series.[459] GVHD will develop in 65% of such patients.[460] Death is most often due to severe GVHD, manifested by dermatitis with epidermolysis, severe diarrhea, and hepatitis. Autologous recovery after rejection has been documented.[461] This is thought to be due to the effect of chemotherapy on the etiology of aplastic anemia.

Some criteria must be followed before a bone marrow transplant is contemplated in a patient with aplastic anemia:[462] the marrow must be decreased to 25% of normal, or 50% of normal with less than 30% hemopoietic cells; the patient should be anemic, with less than 1% reticulocytes, a granulocyte count below 500/µl, and a platelet count below 20,000; and a bone marrow aspiration should indicate more than 70% nonmyeloid cells.

Blood Bank Support in Patients Receiving Bone Marrow Transplantation

Blood and blood components are critical for survival in the 2–3 weeks following transplantation.

TABLE 8–1.—COMPLICATIONS IN PATIENTS WITH END-STAGE LEUKEMIA TREATED WITH BONE MARROW TRANSPLANT*

DISEASE	NO. OF PTS.	NO. WITH GVHD	NO. WITH RECURRENT LEUKEMIA
ALL	46	36	16
AML	54	41	13

*Data from Blume et al.[457]

The patient does not produce hemopoietic cells and must therefore receive the necessary elements to provide oxygen-carrying capacity and hemostasis.

Blood transfusions may be taken from compatible family members to reduce the number of donors and thus the potential for viral infections. Screening for CMV may be necessary. Frequent platelet transfusions are given to maintain the platelet count above 20,000/mm^3. Platelets can be from random donors; if the patient does not respond to these units, HLA-matched units may have to be used.[441] Granulocytes may be necessary for treatment of infections. These should be HLA matched.[441] Nevertheless, granulocyte transfusions increase the number of overall transfusions, with the subsequent development of interstitial pneumonia, usually caused by CMV.[463]

All components must be exposed to 1,500 rad in order to inactivate lymphocytes, which otherwise might engraft and lead to the development of GVHD.[441]

Engrafted immunocompetent cells are capable of producing antiplatelet and antigranulocyte antibodies responsible in part for posttransplantation thrombocytopenia and granulocytopenia.[464] Isohemagglutinins of graft origin have also been documented in liver transplant recipients. These antibodies may cause hemolysis.[465] This complication has also been reported after bone marrow transplantation.[466] However, ABO incompatibility and Rh-incompatibility do not appear to influence bone marrow outcome.[467]

REFERENCES

1. Hustin A.: Principe d'une nouvelle méthode de transfusion muqueuse. *J. Med. Brux.* 2:436, 1914.
2. London P., Hemphil B.M.: The motivations of blood donors. *Transfusion* 4:449, 1965.
3. Kunin C.M.: Serum hepatitis from whole blood: Incidence and relation to source of blood. *Am. J. Med. Sci* 237:293, 1959.
4. Allen J.F., Dawson D., Syaman W.A., et al.: Blood transfusions and serum hepatitis. *Ann. Surg.* 150:455, 1959.
5. Schmidt P.J. (ed.): *Standards for Blood Banks and Transfusion Services,* ed. 11. Arlington, Va., American Association of Blood Banks, 1984, p. 5.
6. Szmuness W., Stevens C.E., Harley E.J., et al.: Hepatitis B vaccine: Demonstration of efficacy in a controlled clinical trial in a high-risk population in the United States. *N. Engl. J. Med.* 303:833, 1980.
7. Centers for Disease Control: *Pneumocystis* pneumonia—Los Angeles. *MMWR* 30:250, 1981.
8. Peter J.B.: Acquired immune deficiency syndrome: A new medical mystery. *Diagn. Med.* 6:25, 1983.
9. Centers for Disease Control: Opportunistic infections and Kaposi's sarcoma in Haitians in the United States. *MMWR* 31:353, 1982.
10. Offenstadt G., Pinta P., Hericord P., et al.: Multiple opportunistic infection due to AIDS in a previously healthy black woman from Zaire. *N. Engl. J. Med.* 308:775, 1983.
11. Centers for Disease Control: *Pneumocystis carinii* pneumonia among persons with hemophilia A. *MMWR* 31:365, 1982.
12. Check W.A.: Preventing AIDS transmission: Should blood donors be screened? *JAMA* 249:567, 1983.
13. Soulier J.P.: Diseases transmissible by blood transfusion. *Vox Sang.* 47:1, 1984.
14. Huestis D.W., Bove J.R., Busch S.: *Practical Blood Transfusion,* ed. 2. Boston, Little, Brown & Co., 1976, p. 38.
15. van der Sluis J.J., Onvlee P.C., Kothe H.A., et al.: Transfusion syphilis, survival of *Treponema pallidum* in donor blood: I. Report of an orientating study. *Vox Sang.* 47:197, 1984.
16. Code of Federal Regulations, Food and Drugs, 21, part 640.5, 1979 revision. Washington, D.C., U.S. Government Printing Office, p. 115.
17. Widman F.K. (ed.): *Technical Manual of the American Association of Blood Banks,* ed. 8. Washington, D.C., AABB 1981, p. 318.
18. Rohwedder R.W.: Infeccion chagásica en dadores de sangre y las probabilidades de transmitirla por medio de la transfusión. *Bul. Chil. Parisitol.* 24:88, 1969.
19. Foster K.M.: Post-transfusion mononucleosis. *Aust. Ann. Med.* 15:305, 1966.
20. Yeager A.S., Grumet F.C., Hafleigh E.B., et al.: Prevention of transfusion-acquired cytomegalovirus infections in newborn infants. *J. Pediatr.* 98:281, 1981.
21. Schmidt P. (ed.): *Standards for Blood Banks and Transfusion Services,* ed. 11. Arlington, Va., American Association of Blood Banks, 1984, p. 4.
22. Widman F.K. (ed.): *Technical Manual of the American Association of Blood Banks,* ed. 7. Washington, D.C., American Association of Blood Banks, 1977, p. 6.
23. Milam J.D.: Donor selection, in Dawson R.B., Fletcher J.L. (eds.): *Donor Room Procedures: A Technical Workshop.* Washington, D.C., American Association of Blood Banks, 1977, p. 8.
24. Mollison P.L.: *Blood Transfusion in Clinical Medicine,* ed. 7. Oxford, England, Blackwell Scientific Publications, 1983, pp. 745–746.

25. Widman F.K. (ed.): *Technical Manual of the American Association of Blood Banks,* ed. 8. Washington, D.C., American Association of Blood Banks, 1981, pp. 6–7.
26. Allred S.: Quality control in the donor room, in Dawson R.B., Fletcher J.L. (eds.): *Donor Room Procedures: A Technical Workshop.* Washington, D.C., American Association of Blood Banks, 1977, p. 44.
27. Schmidt P. (ed.): *Standards for Blood Banks and Transfusion Services,* ed. 11. Arlington, Va., American Association of Blood Banks, 1984, p. 3.
28. Miller W.V. (ed.): *Technical Manual of the American Association of Blood Banks,* ed. 7. Washington, D.C., American Association of Blood Banks, 1977, p. 272.
29. Bove J.R., Davey M., de Wit C.D., et al.: Should the blood donor examination be used to screen for clinically hidden diseases and risk factors as a part of preventive medicine? *Vox Sang.* 47:379, 1984.
30. Linke G.E., Henry B.H.: Clinical pathology/laboratory medicine purposes and practice, in Henry J.B. (ed.): *Todd-Sanford-Davidsohn, Clinical Diagnosis and Management by Laboratory Methods,* ed. 17. Philadelphia, W.B. Saunders Co., 1984, p. 6.
31. Roekel I.: Donor reactions, in Dawson R.B., Fletcher J.L. (eds.): *Donor Room Procedures: A Technical Workshop.* Washington, D.C., American Association of Blood Banks, 1977, p. 24.
32. Logic J.R., Johnson S.A., Smith J.J.: Cardiovascular and hematologic responses to phlebotomy in blood donors. *Transfusion* 3:83, 1963.
33. Mollison P.L.: *Blood Transfusion in Clinical Medicine,* ed. 7. Oxford, England, Blackwell Scientific Publications, 1983, p. 137.
34. Beecher H.K., Simeone F.A.: The internal state of the severely wounded man on entry to the most forward hospital. *Surgery* 22:672, 1947.
35. Miller R.H.: *Textbook of Basic Emergency Medicine,* ed. 2. St. Louis, C.V. Mosby Co., 1980, p. 88.
36. Poles F.C., Boycott M.: Syncope in blood donors. *Lancet* 2:531, 1942.
37. Howarth S., Sharpey-Schafer E.P.: Low blood pressure phases following hemorrhage. *Lancet* 1:10, 1947.
38. Standards and guidelines for cardiopulmonary resuscitation (CPR) and emergency cardiac care (ECC). *JAMA* 244:453, 1980.
39. Huestis D.W., Bove J.R., Busch S.: *Practical Blood Transfusion,* ed. 3. Boston, Little, Brown & Co., 1981, p. 49.
40. Mollison P.L.: *Blood Transfusion in Clinical Medicine,* ed. 7. Oxford, England, Blackwell Scientific Publications, 1983, pp. 5–6.
41. Mollison P.L.: *Blood Transfusion in Clinical Medicine,* ed. 7. Oxford, England, Blackwell Scientific Publications, 1983, pp. 754–755.
42. Rosenfield R.: Early 20th century origins of modern blood transfusion therapy. *Mt. Sinai J. Med.* 41:626, 1974.
43. Loutit J.F., Mollison P.L., Young I.M.: Citric acid-sodium citrate-glucose mixtures for blood storage. *J. Exp. Physiol.* 32:183, 1943.
44. Beuther E.: The maintenance of red cell function during liquid storage, in Schmidt P.J. (ed.): *Progress in Transfusion and Transplantation.* Washington, D.C., American Association of Blood Banks, 1972, p. 285.
45. Valeri C.R., Hirsch N.M.: Restoration in vivo of erythrocyte adenosine triphosphate, 2,3-diphosphoglycerate, potassium ion and sodium ion concentrations following the transfusion of acid-citrate-dextrose-stored human red blood cells. *J. Lab. Clin. Med.* 73:722, 1969.
46. Dawson R.B., Kocholaty W.F., Gray J.L.: Hemoglobin function and 2,3-DPG levels of blood stored at 4° C in ACD and CPD: pH effect. *Transfusion* 10:200, 1970.
47. Shields C.E.: Comparison studies of whole blood stored in ACD and CPD with adenine. *Transfusion* 8:1, 1968.
48. Valeri C.R.: Metabolic regeneration of depleted erythrocytes and their frozen storage, in Grenwalt T.J., Jamieson G.A. (eds.): *The Human Red Cell In Vitro.* New York, Grune & Stratton, 1974, p. 281.
49. Okerblom O., deVerdier C.H., Finnson M., et al.: Further studies on the effect of adenine in blood preservation. *Transfusion* 7:1, 1967.
50. Code of Federal Regulations 21, Food and Drugs, Parts 600 to 1299, 1979, p. 118.
51. Schmidt P.J. (ed.): *Standards for Blood Banks and Transfusion Services,* ed. 11. Arlington, Va., American Association of Blood Banks, 1984, pp. 16–17.
52. Widman F.K. (ed.): *Technical Manual of the American Association of Blood Banks,* ed. 8. Washington, D.C., AABB, 1981, pp. 52–53.
53. Sohmer P.R., Moore G.L., Beutler E., et al.: In vivo viability of red blood cells stored in CPDA-2. *Transfusion* 22:479, 1982.
54. Greenwalt T.J., Bryan D.J., Dumaswala J.: Erythrocyte membrane vesiculation and changes in membrane composition during storage in citrate-phosphate-dextrose-adenine-1. *Vox Sang.* 47:261, 1984.
55. Schmidt P.J. (ed.): *Standards for Blood Banks and Transfusion Services,* ed. 11. Arlington, Va., American Association of Blood Banks, 1984, p. 10.
56. Mollison P.L.: *Blood Transfusion in Clinical Medicine,* ed. 7. Oxford, England, Blackwell Scientific Publications, 1983, p. 34.
57. Huestis D.W., Bove J.R., Busch S.: *Practical Blood Transfusion,* ed. 3. Boston, Little, Brown & Co., 1981, p. 57.
58. Zuck T.: *Proceedings of Workshop on Adenine and Red Cell Preservation.* Washington, D.C., Department of Health, Education and Welfare, 1976, pp. 1–74.
59. Baldini M., Costea N., Dameshek W.: The validity of stored human platelets. *Blood* 16:1669, 1960.
60. Slichter S.J., Counts R.B., Henderson R., et al.: Preparation of cryoprecipitated factor VIII concentrates. *Transfusion* 16:616, 1976.
61. Caggiano V.: Red blood cell transfusions, in Silver H.S. (ed.): *Blood, Blood Components and Derivatives*

in Transfusion Therapy: A Technical Workshop. Washington, D.C., American Association of Blood Banks, 1980, p. 14.
62. Lundsgaard-Hauser P., Ehrengruber E., Frei E., et al.: Antithrombin III and related parameters in surgical patients receiving blood components. *Vox Sang.* 46:19, 1984.
63. Snyder E.L., Ferri P.M., Mosher D.F.: Fibronectin in liquid and frozen stored blood components. *Transfusion* 24:53, 1984.
64. Widman F.K. (ed.): *Technical Manual of the American Association of Blood Banks,* ed. 8. Washington, D.C., American Association of Blood Banks, 1981, pp. 54–55.
65. Hardin A.R., Weed R.I., Reed C.C.: Changes in physical properties of stored erythrocytes: Relationship to survival in vivo. *Transfusion* 9:229, 1969.
66. Allan D., Billah M.M., Finean J.B., et al.: Release of diacylglycerol-enriched vesicles from erythrocytes with increased intracellular (Ca^{2+}). *Nature* 261:58, 1976.
67. Bailey D.N., Bove J.R.: Chemical and hematological changes in stored CPD blood. *Transfusion* 15:244, 1975.
68. Valtis D.J., Kennedy A.C.: Defective gas-transport function of stored red blood cells. *Lancet* 1:119, 1954.
69. Chanutin A., Curnish R.R.: Effect of organic and inorganic phosphates on the oxygen equilibrium of human erythrocytes. *Arch. Biochem. Biophys.* 121:96, 1967.
70. Chanutin A., Curnish R.R.: The effect of adenosine, inosine and adenine on the concentrations of organic phosphate and an electrophoretic component (B) of human red cells during storage of blood in acid-citrate-dextrose and citrate-phosphate-dextrose. *Transfusion* 5:254, 1965.
71. Borucki D.T. (ed.): *Blood Component Therapy: A Physician's Handbook,* ed. 3. Washington, D.C., American Association of Blood Banks, 1981, pp. 2–4.
72. Widman F.K. (ed.): *Technical Manual of the American Association of Blood Banks,* ed. 8. Washington, D.C., American Association of Blood Banks, 1981, p. 267.
73. Jaeger R.J., Rubin R.J.: Migration of phthalate ester plasticizer from polyvinyl chloride blood bags into stored human blood and its localization in human tissues. *N. Engl. J. Med.* 287:1114, 1972.
74. Turner J.H., Petricciani J.D., Crouch M.L., et al.: An evaluation of the effects of diethylhexyl phthalate (DEHP) on mitotically capable cells in blood packs. *Transfusion* 14:560, 1974.
75. Widman F.K. (ed.): *Technical Manual of the American Association of Blood Banks,* ed. 8. Washington, D.C., American Association of Blood banks, 1981, pp. 47–48.
76. Westphal R.G.: Rational alternatives to the use of whole blood. *Ann. Intern. Med.* 76:987, 1972.
77. Caggiano V.: Red blood cell transfusions, in Silver H. (ed.): *Blood, Blood Components, and Derivatives in Transfusion Therapy: A Technical Workshop.* Washington, D.C., American Association of Blood Banks, 1980, pp. 1–28.
78. Caggiano V.: Red blood cell transfusions, in Silver H. (ed.): *Blood, Blood Components and Derivatives in Transfusion Therapy: A Technical Workshop.* Washington, D.C., American Association of Blood Banks, 1980, p. 7.
79. McCord R.G., Myhre B.A.: A method for rapid and thorough workup of febrile and allergic transfusion reactions. *Lab. Med.* 9:39, 1978.
80. Thulstrup H.: The influence of leukocyte and thrombocyte incompatibility on non-haemolytic transfusion reaction: A retrospective study. *Vox Sang.* 21:233, 1971.
81. Wenz, B.: Microaggregate filtration and the febrile transfusion reaction: A comparative study. *Transfusion* 23:95, 1983.
82. Tenczar F.J.: Comparison of inverted centrifugation, saline washing and dextran sedimentation in the preparation of leukocyte-poor red cells. *Transfusion* 13:183, 1973.
83. Widman F.K. (ed.): *Technical Manual of the American Association of Blood Banks,* ed. 8. Washington, D.C., American Association of Blood Banks, 1981, p. 411.
84. Halterman R.H., Grumet F.C., Watson L., et al.: Comparison of methods for the preparation of leukocyte-poor blood. *Transfusion* 12:23, 1972.
85. Snyder E.L., Root R.K., Hezzey A., et al.: Effect of microaggregate blood filtration on granulocyte concentrates in vitro. *Transfusion* 23:25, 1983.
86. Mijovic V., Brozovic A.S., Hughes B., et al.: Leukocyte-depleted blood: A comparison of filtration techniques. *Transfusion* 23:30, 1983.
87. Meryman H.T., Hornblower M.: A method for freezing and washing red blood cells using a high glycerol concentration. *Transfusion* 12:145, 1972.
88. Bryant L.R., Holland L., Corkern S., et al.: Optimal leukocyte removal from refrigerated blood with the IBM 2991 blood cell processor. *Transfusion* 18:469, 1978.
89. Schmidt P.J.: *Standards for Blood Banks and Transfusion Services,* ed. 11. Arlington, Va., American Association of Blood Banks, 1984, p. 17.
90. Polge C., Smith A.U., Parkes A.S.: Revival of spermatozoa after vitrification and dehydration at low temperature. *Nature* 164:666, 1949.
91. Smith A.U.: Prevention of haemolysis during freezing and thawing of red blood cells. *Lancet* 2:910, 1950.
92. Mollison P.L., Sloviter H.A.: Successful transfusion of previously frozen human red cells. *Lancet* 2:862, 1951.
93. Lovelock J.E.: The haemolysis of human blood cells by freezing and thawing. *Biochim. Biophys. Acta* 10:414, 1954.
94. Lovelock J.E.: The denaturation of lipid protein complexes as cause of damage by freezing. *Proc. R. Soc. Lond.* 147:427, 1957.
95. Lovelock J.E.: The mechanism of the protective ac-

tion of glycerol against haemolysis by freezing and thawing. *Biochim. Biophys. Acta* 11:28, 1953.
96. Sloviter H.A., Smart C.R., Moss N.H.: The intravenous administration of glycerol to humans. *Surg. Forum* 9:55, 1957.
97. Mollison P.L.: *Blood Transfusion in Clinical Medicine*, ed. 7. Oxford, England, Blackwell Scientific Publications, 1983, pp. 153–154.
98. Valeri C.R.: Factors influencing the 24-hour post-transfusion survival and the oxygen transport function of previously frozen red cells preserved with 40% W/V glycerol and frozen at 80C. *Transfusion* 14:1, 1974.
99. Rowe A.W.: Preservation of blood by the low glycerol rapid freeze process, in Guy R.L. (ed.): *Red Cell Freezing: A Technical Workshop*. Washington, D.C., American Association of Blood Banks, 1973, p. 55.
100. Widman F.K. (ed.): *Technical Manual of the American Association of Blood Banks*, ed. 8. Washington, D.C., American Association of Blood Banks, 1981, pp. 60–61.
101. Meryman H.T.: A high glycerol red cell freezing method, in Guy R.L. (ed.): *Red Blood Cell Freezing: A Technical Workshop*. Washington, D.C., American Association of Blood Banks, 1973, p. 73.
102. McPeak D.W., Camp F.R. Jr.: Frozen blood shipping. *Milit. Med.* 140:468, 1975.
103. Valeri C.R., Szymanski I.O., Runk A.H.: Therapeutic effectiveness of homologous erythrocyte transfusions following frozen storage at −80C for up to seven years. *Transfusion* 10:1020, 1970.
104. Widman F.K. (ed.): *Technical Manual of the American Association of Blood Banks*, ed. 8. Washington, D.C., American Association of Blood Banks, 1981, pp. 61–63.
105. Widman F.K. (ed.): *Technical Manual of the American Association of Blood Banks*, ed. 8. Washington, D.C., American Association of Blood Banks, 1981, pp. 408–409.
106. Widman F.K. (ed.): *Technical Manual of the American Association of Blood Banks*, ed. 8. Washington, D.C., American Association of Blood Banks, 1981, p. 62.
107. Tullis J.L., Ketchel M.M., Pyle H.M., et al.: Studies on the in vivo survival of glycerolized and frozen human red cells. *JAMA* 168:300, 1958.
108. Valeri C.R.: Discussion in Greep J.A. (ed.): *Clinical Uses of Frozen Thawed Red Blood Cells*. New York, Alan R. Liss, Inc., 1976, p. 121.
109. Meryman H.T., Hornblower M.: Quality control of deglycerolized red blood cells. *Transfusion* 21:235, 1981.
110. Szymansky I.O., Valeri C.R.: Automated differential agglutination technique to measure red cell survival: II. Survival in vivo of preserved red cells. *Transfusion* 8:74, 1968.
111. Huestis D.W., Bove J.R., Busch S.: *Practical Blood Transfusion*, ed. 3. Boston, Little, Brown & Co., 1981, p. 64.
112. O'Brien T.G., Watkins E. Jr.: Gas-exchange dynamics of glycerolyzed frozen blood. *J. Thorac. Cardiovas. Surg.* 40:611, 1960.
113. Umlas J.: Routine use of previously frozen erythrocytes in a community teaching hospital, in Dawson R.B. (ed.): *Clinical and Practical Aspects of the Use of Frozen Blood: A Technical Workshop*. Washington, D.C., American Association of Blood Banks, 1977, p. 103.
114. Croweley J.P., Valeri C.R.: The purification of red cells for transfusion by freeze preservation and washing: I. The mechanism of leukocyte removal from washed freeze-preserved red cells. *Transfusion* 14:188, 1974.
115. Miller W.V., Holland P.V., Sugarboker E., et al.: Anaphylactic reactions to IgA: A difficult transfusion problem. *Am. J. Clin. Pathol.* 54:618, 1970.
116. Yap P.L., Pryde E.A.D., McClelland D.B.L.: IgA content of frozen-thawed-washed red blood cells and blood products measured by radioimmunoassay. *Transfusion* 22:36, 1982.
117. Sirchia G., Ferrone S., Mercuriali F.: Leucocyte antigen-antibody reaction and lysis of paroxysmal nocturnal hemoglobinuria erythrocytes. *Blood* 36:335, 1970.
118. Propper R.D., Button L.N., Nathan D.G.: New approaches to the transfusion management of thalassemia. *Blood* 55:55, 1980.
119. Carr J.B., deQuesada A.M., Shires D.L.: Decreased incidence of transfusion hepatitis after exclusive transfusion with reconstituted frozen erythrocytes. *Ann. Intern. Med.* 78:693, 1973.
120. Contreras T.J., Valeri C.R.: Removal of HBsAg from blood in vitro: I. Effects of washing alone, glycerol addition and removal, and glycerolyzation, freezing and washing. *Transfusion* 16:594, 1976.
121. Haugen R.K.: Hepatitis after the transfusion of frozen red cells and washed red cells. *N. Engl. J. Med.* 301:393, 1979.
122. Goldfinger D.: Hepatitis after frozen or washed red cells. *N. Engl. J. Med.* 305:581, 1980.
123. Randall J.L., Plotkin S.: Herpes virus opportunism, in Prier J.E., Friedman H.F. (eds.): *Opportunistic Pathogens*. Baltimore, University Park Press, 1974, p. 261.
124. Land D.M.: Transfusion and perfusion-associated cytomegalovirus and Epstein-Barr virus infections: Current understanding and investigation, in Grenwalt T.J., Jameson G.A. (eds.): *Transmissible Disease and Blood Transfusion*. Washington, D.C., American National Red Cross, 6th Science Symposium, 1974.
125. Valeri C.R., Bougas J.A., Telarico L., et al.: Behavior of previously frozen erythrocytes used during open heart surgery. *Transfusion* 10:238, 1970.
126. Brittingham T.E., Chaplin H. Jr.: Febrile transfusion reactions caused by sensitivity to donor leukocytes and platelets. *JAMA* 165:819, 1957.
127. Polesky H.F.: Frozen deglycerolized versus washed red cells in transplantation and HLA sensitization, in Dawson R.B. (ed.): *Clinical and Practical Aspects of the Use of Frozen Blood: A Technical Workshop*.

Washington, D.C., American Association of Blood Banks, 1977, p. 113.
128. Perkins H.A.: HLA antigens and blood transfusion: Effects on renal transplants. *Transplant. Proc.* 1C(suppl. 1):220, 1977.
129. Umlas J.: Routine use of previously frozen erythrocytes in a community teaching hospital, in Dawson R.B. (ed.): *Clinical and Practical Aspects of the Use of Frozen Blood: A Technical Workshop.* Washington, D.C., American Association of Blood Banks, 1977, p. 105.
130. Kevy S.V., Jacobson M., Button L.: *Clinical Uses of Frozen-Thawed Red Blood Cells.* New York, Alan R. Liss, Inc., 1976, p. 89.
131. Opelz G., Terasaki P.I., Graver B., et al.: Blood transfusions and renal transplantation. *Transplant Proc.* 11:1889, 1979.
132. Opelz G., Graver B., Terasaki P.I.: Induction of high kidney graft survival rate by multiple transfusion. *Lancet* 1:1223, 1981.
133. Widman F.K. (ed.): *Technical Manual of the American Association of Blood Banks,* ed. 8. Washington, D.C., American Association of Blood Banks, 1981, p. 43.
134. Widman F.K. (ed.): *Technical Manual of the American Association of Blood Banks,* ed. 8. Washington, D.C., American Association of Blood Banks, 1981, pp. 43–45.
135. Schmidt P.J. (ed.): *Standards for Blood Banks and Transfusion Services,* ed. 11. Arlington, Va., American Association of Blood Banks, 1984, p. 10.
136. Rules and Regulations. Federal Register vol. 35, No. 172, Sept. 3, 1970, p. 13990.
137. Anstall H.B., Grove-Rasmussen M., Shaw R.S.: Optimal conditions for storage of fresh frozen plasma. *Transfusion* 1:87, 1961.
138. Widman F.K. (ed.): *Technical Manual of the American Association of Blood Banks,* ed. 8. Washington, D.C., American Association of Blood Banks, 1981, pp. 43–45.
139. Bareford D., Cumberbatch M., Torey L.D.: Plasma discolouration due to sun-tanning aids. *Vox Sang.* 46:180, 1984.
140. Slichter S.J., Counts R.B., Henderson R., et al.: Preparation of cryoprecipitated factor VIII concentrates. *Transfusion* 16:616, 1976.
141. Sherman L.: Alterations in hemostasis during massive transfusion, in Nusbacher J. (ed.): *Massive Transfusion 1978.* Washington, D.C., American Association of Blood Banks, 1981, pp. 43–45.
142. Schmidt P.J. (ed.): *Standards for Blood Banks and Transfusion Services,* ed. 11. Arlington, Va., American Association of Blood Banks, 1984, p. 31.
143. Pool J.G., Shannon A.F.: Production of high potency concentrates of anti-hemophilic globulin in a closed bag system. *N. Engl. J. Med.* 273:1443, 1965.
144. Kasper C.K., et al.: Determinants of factor VIII recovery in cryoprecipitate. *Transfusion* 15:312, 1975.
145. Widman F.K. (ed.): *Technical Manual of the Association of American Blood Banks,* ed. 8. Washington, D.C., American Association of Blood Banks, 1981, pp. 45–46.
146. Anstall H.B., Grove-Rasmussen M., Shaw R.S.: Optimal conditions for storage of fresh frozen plasma. *Transfusion* 1:87, 1961.
147. Vermeer C.: Contributions to the optimal use of human blood: VIII. Stability of blood coagulation factor VIII during collection and storage of whole blood and plasma. *Vox Sang.* 31:55, 1976.
148. Walker R.H.: Preparation of blood components, in Myhre B.A. (ed.): *Quality Control in the Blood Bank.* Chicago, American Society of Clinical Pathologists, 1973, p. 61.
149. van Gastel C.J., Sixma J.J., Borst-Eilers E., et al.: Preparation and infusion of cryoprecipitate from exercised donors. *Br. J. Haematol.* 25:461, 1973.
150. Nilsson I.M., Walter H., Mikaelsson M., et al.: Factor VIII concentrate prepared from DDAVP-stimulated blood donor plasma. *Scand. J. Haematol.* 22:42, 1979.
151. Snyder E.L. (ed.): *Blood Transfusion Therapy: A Physicians Handbook.* Arlington, Va., American Association of Blood Banks, 1983, p. 23.
152. Cederbaum A.I.: The appropriate use of plasma and plasma components in clinical medicine, in Silver H. (ed.): *Blood, Blood Components and Derivatives in Transfusion Therapy: A Technical Workshop.* Washington, D.C., American Association of Blood Banks, 1980, p. 110.
153. Triantaphyllopoulos D.C., McGarry B.J.: Cryoprecipitate and blood groups. *Lancet* 2:203, 1979.
154. Widman F.K. (ed.): *Technical Manual of the American Association of Blood Banks,* ed. 8. Washington, D.C., American Association of Blood Banks, 1981, p. 45.
155. Pool J.G., Heshgold E.J., Pappenhagen A.R.: High potency antihemophilic factor concentrate, prepared from cryoglobulin precipitate. *Nature* 203:312, 1964.
156. Kasper C.K.: Management of hemophiliacs for surgical operation, in McCullough N.C. III (ed.): *Comprehensive Management of Musculoskeletal Disorders in Hemophilia.* Washington, D.C., National Academy of Sciences, 1973, p. 140.
157. Chediak J.R., Telfer M.C., Green D.: Platelet function and immunologic parameters in von Willebrand's disease following cryoprecipitate and factor VIII concentrate infusion. *Am. J. Med.* 62:369, 1977.
158. Lewis, J.H., Hasiba U., Spero J.A.: The management of specific coagulation factor deficiencies, in Dawson R.B. (ed.): *Hemostasis for Blood Bankers: A Technical Workshop.* Washington, D.C., American Association of Blood Banks, 1977, p. 41.
159. Janson P.A., Jubelirer S.J., Weinstein M.J., et al.: Treatment of the bleeding tendency in uremia with cryoprecipitate. *N. Engl. J. Med.* 303:1318, 1980.
160. Mintz P.D., Blatt P.M., Kuhns W.J., et al.: An-

tithrombin III in fresh frozen plasma, cryoprecipitate, and cryoprecipitate-depleted plasma. *Transfusion* 19:597, 1979.
161. Orringer E.P., Koury M.J., Blatt P.M., et al.: Hemolysis caused by factor VIII concentrates. *Arch. Intern. Med.* 136:1018, 1976.
162. Weiss A.E.: Circulating inhibitors in hemophilia A and B: Epidemiology and methods of detection, in Brinkhous K.M., Kemker H.C. (eds.): *Handbook of Hemophilia*. New York, American Elsevier Publishing Co., 1975, chap. 42.
163. Allain J.P., Frommel D.: Antibodies to factor VIII: Patterns of immune response to factor VIII in hemophilia A. *Blood* 47:973, 1976.
164. Marcus A.J., Zucker-Franklin D., Safier L.B., et al.: Studies on human platelet granules and membranes. *J. Clin. Invest.* 45:14, 1966.
165. Widman F.K. (ed.): *Technical Manual of the American Association of Blood Banks*, ed. 8. Washington, D.C., American Association of Blood Banks, 1981, pp. 4–5.
166. Widman F.K. (ed.): *Technical Manual of the American Association of Blood Banks*, ed. 8. Washington, D.C., American Association of Blood Banks, 1981, p. 47.
167. Filip D.J., Aster R.H.: Relative hemostatic effectiveness of human platelets stored at 4C and at 22C. *J. Lab. Clin. Med.* 91:618, 1978.
168. Murphy S.: Platelet metabolism, morphology, and function during storage for transfusion, in Mallory D. McG. (ed.): *Platelet Physiology and Transfusion: A Technical Workshop*. Washington, D.C., American Association of Blood Banks, 1978, p. 7.
169. Code of Federal Regulations, Title 21, Food and Drugs, Parts 640.20–640.26.
170. Schmidt P.J. (ed.): *Standards for Blood Banks and Transfusion Services*, ed. 11. Arlington, Va., American Association of Blood Banks, 1984, p. 11.
171. Murphy S., Holme S.: Improved platelet preservation in a new container, abstracted. *Transfusion* 20:624, 1980.
172. Rock G., Sherring V.A., Tittley P.: Five-day storage of platelet concentrates. *Transfusion* 24:147, 1984.
173. McCullough J., Undis J., Allen J.W.: Platelet production and inventory management, in Mallory D. McG. (ed.): *Platelet Physiology and Transfusion: A Technical Workshop*. Washington, D.C., American Association of Blood Banks, 1978, p. 27.
174. Olson P.R., Cox C., McCullough J.: Laboratory and clinical effects of the infusion of ACD solution during platelet pheresis. *Vox Sang.* 33:79, 1977.
175. Widman F.K. (ed.): *Technical Manual of the American Association of Blood Banks*, ed. 8. Washington, D.C., American Association of Blood Banks, 1981, p. 360.
176. Schmidt P.J. (ed.): *Standards for Blood Banks and Transfusion Services*, ed. 11. Arlington, Va., American Association of Blood Banks, 1984, pp. 11, 21.
177. Rock G.A., Blanchette V.S., Wong S.C.: Storage of platelets collected by apheresis. *Transfusion* 23:99, 1983.
178. Walker R.H.: Preparation of blood components, in Myhre B.A. (ed.): *Quality Control in the Blood Bank (ASCP Commission on Continuing Education Council on Immunohematology)*. Chicago, American Society of Clinical Pathologists, 1973, p. 82.
179. Class F.H.J., Smeenk R.J., Schmidt R., et al.: Alloimmunization against the MHC antigens after platelet transfusions is due to contaminating leukocytes in the platelet suspension. *Exp. Hematol.* 9:84, 1981.
180. Duke W.W.: Relationship of blood platelets to hemorrhagic disease: Description of method for determining bleeding time and coagulation time and report of cases of hemorrhagic disease relieved by transfusion. *JAMA* 55:1185, 1910.
181. Kliman A., Gaydos L.A., Schroeder L.R., et al.: Repeated plasmapheresis of blood donors as a source of platelets. *Blood* 18:303, 1961.
182. Hersh E.M., Bodey G.P., Nies B.A., et al.: Causes of death in acute leukemia: A ten year study of 414 patients from 1954–1963. *JAMA* 193:105, 1965.
183. Gaydos L.A., Freireich E.J., Mantel N.: The quantitative relation between platelet count and hemorrhage in patients with acute leukemia. *N. Engl. J. Med.* 266:905, 1962.
184. Shulman N.R., Watkins S.P. Jr., Itscoitz S.B., et al.: Evidence that the spleen retains the youngest and hemostatically most effective platelets. *Trans. Assoc. Am. Physicians* 81:302, 1968.
185. Harker L.A., Slichter S.J.: The bleeding time as a screening test for evaluation of platelet function. *N. Engl. J. Med.* 287:155, 1972.
186. Aisner J.: Clinical use of platelet transfusions for patients with cancer, in Schiffer C.J. (ed.): *Platelet Physiology and Transfusion: A Technical Workshop*. Washington, D.C., American Association of Blood Banks, 1978, p. 42.
187. Snyder E.L. (ed.): *Blood Transfusion Therapy: A Physician's Handbook*. Washington, D.C., American Association of Blood Banks, 1984, p. 15.
188. Snyder E.L., Grum P., Cooper-Smith, M., et al.: Transfusion of platelets through microaggregate filters. *Anaesthesiology* 51(suppl. S):205, 1979.
189. Medeiros L.J., Szik W.H.: Failure of microaggregate blood filter to produce leukocyte-poor platelet concentrates (letter). *Vox Sang.* 47:191, 1984.
190. Colombane J.: Blood platelets in HL-A serology. *Transplant Proc.* 3:1078, 1971.
191. Duquesnoy R.J., Filip D.J., Tomasulo P.A., et al.: Role of HLA-C matching in histocompatible platelet transfusion therapy of alloimmunized thrombocytopenic patients. *Transplant. Proc.* 9:1827, 1977.
192. van Rood J.J., van Leeuwen A., Keuning J.J., et al.: The serological recognition of the human MLC determinants using a modified cytotoxicity technique. *Tissue Antigens* 5:73, 1975.
193. Yankee R.A., Graff K.S., Dowling R., et al.: Selection of unrelated compatible platelet donors by

lymphocyte HL-A matching. *N. Engl. J. Med.* 288:760, 1973.
194. Silvergleid A.J.: Clinical platelet transfusions, in Silver H. (ed.): *Components and Derivatives in Transfusion Therapy: A Technical Workshop.* Washington, D.C., American Association of Blood Banks, 1980, p. 56.
195. Shulman N.R., Aster R.H., Leitner A., et al.: Immunoreactions involving platelets: V. Posttransfusion purpura due to a complement-fixing antibody against a genetically controlled platelet antigen. A proposed mechanism for thrombocytopenia and its relevance in autoimmunity. *J. Clin. Invest.* 40:1597, 1961.
196. Svejgaard A.: Isoantigenic systems of human blood platelets: A survey. *Semin. Hematol.* 2:5, 1979.
197. van Der Weerdt C.M., et al.: The ZW blood group system in platelets. *Vox Sang.* 8:513, 1963.
198. Shulman N.R.: Immunological considerations attending platelet transfusion. *Transfusion* 6:39, 1966.
199. Howard J.E., Perkins H.A.: The natural history of alloimmunization to platelets. *Transfusion* 18:496, 1978.
200. Duquesnoy R.J., Anderson A.J., Tomasulo P.A., et al.; ABO compatibility and platelet transfusion of allimmunized thrombocytopenic patients. *Blood* 54:595, 1979.
201. Baldini M., Costea N., Ebbe S.: Studies on the antigenic structure of blood platelets, in *Proceedings of the Congress of the European Society of Hematologists.* Vienna, European Society of Haematologists, 1962, p. 378.
202. Gurevitch J., Nelken D.: Studies on platelet antigens: III. Rh-Hr antigens in platelets. *Vox Sang.* 2:342, 1957.
203. Stern K., Davidson I., Masartis L.: Experimental studies on Rh immunization. *Am. J. Clin. Pathol.* 26:833, 1956.
204. Goldfinger D., McGuiniss M.H.: Rh-incompatible platelet transfusions: Risks and consequences of sensitizing immunosuppressed patients. *N. Engl. J. Med.* 284:942, 1971.
205. Lohrmann H.P., Bull M.I., Decter J.A., et al.: Platelet transfusion from HL-A compatible unrelated donors to alloimmunized patients. *Ann. Intern. Med.* 80:9, 1974.
206. Tomasulo P.A.: Management of the alloimmunized patient with HLA-matched platelets, in Mallory D. McG. (ed.): *Platelet Physiology and Transfusion: A Technical Workshop.* Washington, D.C., American Association of Blood Banks, 1978, p. 69.
207. Wu K.K., Thompson J.S., Koepke J.A., et al.: Heterogeneity of antibody response to human platelet transfusion. *J. Clin. Invest.* 58:432, 1976.
208. Liebert M., Aster R.H.: Expression of HLA-B12 on platelets on lymphocytes and in serum: A quantitative study. *Tissue Antigens* 9:199, 1977.
209. Brand A., et al.: Platelet immunology with special regard to platelet transfusion therapy. Amsterdam, Excerpta Medica, International Congress Series No. 415, 1978, p. 639.
210. Eisner E.V., Shahidi N.T.: Immune thrombocytopenia due to a drug metabolite. *N. Engl. J. Med.* 187:376, 1972.
211. Schiffer C.A., Weinstein J.H., Wiernik P.H.: Methicillin-associated thrombocytopenia. *Ann. Intern. Med.* 85:338, 1976.
212. Harker L.A.: The role of the spleen in thrombokinetics. *J. Lab. Clin. Med.* 77:247, 1971.
213. Hester J.P., McCredie K.B., Freireich E.J.: Platelet replacement therapy: A clinical assessment, in Greenwalt T.J., Jamieson G.A. (eds.): *The Blood Platelet in Transfusion Therapy.* New York, Alan R. Liss, Inc., 1978, p. 281.
214. Valeri C.R.: Hemostatic effectiveness of liquid preserved and previously frozen human platelets. *N. Engl. J. Med.* 290:353, 1974.
215. Schiffer C.A., Aisner J., Wiernick P.H.: Frozen autologous platelet transfusion for patients with leukemia. *N. Engl. J. Med.* 299:7, 1978.
216. Lazarus H.M., Kaniecki-Green E.A., Warm S.E., et al.: Therapeutic effectiveness of frozen platelet concentrates for transfusion. *Blood* 57:243, 1981.
217. Cohen D., Weinstein H., Mihm M., et al.: Nonfatal graft-versus-host disease occurring after transfusion with leukocytes and platelets obtained from normal donors. *Blood* 53:1053, 1979.
218. Herzig R.H., Herzig G.P., Bull M.I., et al.: Correction of poor platelet transfusion responses with leukocyte-poor HLA-matched platelet concentrates. *Blood* 46:743, 1975.
219. Silvergleid A.J., Hafleigh E.B., Haralim M.A.: Clinical value of washed platelet concentrates in patients with non-hemolytic transfusion reactions. *Transfusion* 17:33, 1976.
220. Higby D.J., Cohen E., Holland J.F., et al.: The prophylactic treatment of thrombocytopenic leukemic patients with platelets: A double blind study. *Transfusion* 14:440, 1974.
221. Cardamone J.M., Edson J.R., McArthur J.R., et al.: Abnormalities of platelet function in the myeloproliferative disorders. *JAMA* 221:270, 1972.
222. Sultan Y., Caen J.P.: Platelet dysfunction in preleukemic states and in various types of leukemia. *Ann. NY Acad. Sci.* 201:300, 1972.
223. Wintrobe M.M., Lee G.R., Boggs D.R., et al.: *Clinical Hematology,* ed. 8. Philadelphia, Lea & Febiger, 1981, p. 516.
224. Bergin J.J., Zuck T.F., Miller R.E.: Compelling splenectomy in medically compromised patients. *Ann. Surg.* 178:761, 1973.
225. Nagasama T., Kim B.K., Baldini M.G.: Temporary suppression of circulating anti-platelet alloantibodies by the massive infusion of fresh, stored, or lyophilized platelets. *Transfusion* 18:429, 1978.
226. Rabiner S.F.: Uremic bleeding. *Prog. Hemost. Thromb.* 1:233, 1972.
227. Lackner H.: Hemostatic abnormalities associated with dysproteinemias. *Semin. Hematol.* 10:125, 1973.

228. Bick R.L.: Alterations of hemostasis associated with cardiopulmonary bypass: Pathophysiology, prevention, diagnosis, and management. *Semin. Thromb. Hemost.* 3:59, 1976.
229. Dutton R.C., Edmunds L.H. Jr., Hutchinson J.C., et al.: Platelet aggregate emboli produced in patients during cardiopulmonary bypass with membrane and bubble oxygenators and blood filters. *J. Thorac. Cardiovasc. Surg.* 67:258, 1974.
230. Dieter R.A., Jr., Neville W.E., Pifarre R., et al.: Preoperative coagulation profiles and post hemodilution cardiopulmonary bypass hemorrhage. *Am. J. Surg.* 121:689, 1971.
231. Thomas D.P.: Abnormalities of platelet aggregation in patients with alcoholic cirrhosis. *Ann. NY Acad. Sci.* 201:243, 1972.
232. Krevans J.R., Jackson D.P.: Hemorrhagic disorder following massive whole blood transfusions. *JAMA* 159:171, 1955.
233. Cunningham M., Cash J.K.: Bacterial contamination of platelet concentrates stored at 20 C. *J. Clin. Pathol.* 26:401, 1973.
234. Snyder P.J. (ed.): *Standards for Blood Banks and Transfusion Services,* ed. 11. Arlington, Va., American Association of Blood Banks, 1984, pp. 12–13.
235. Widman F.K. (ed.): *Technical Manual of the American Association of Blood Banks,* ed. 8. Washington, D.C., American Association of Blood Banks, 1981, pp. 316–318.
236. Chambers R.W., Foley H.T., Schmidt P.J.: Transmission of syphilis by fresh blood components. *Transfusion* 9:32, 1969.
237. Widman F.K. (ed.): *Technical Manual of the American Association of Blood Banks,* ed. 8. Washington, D.C., American Association of Blood Banks, 1981, pp. 311–316.
238. Vyas F.N., Perkins H.A., Fudenberg H.H.: Anaphylactoid transfusion reactions associated with anti-IgA. *Lancet* 2:312, 1968.
239. Ward H.N.: Pulmonary infiltrates associated with leukoagglutinin transfusion reactions. *Ann. Intern. Med.* 73:689, 1970.
240. Silvergleid A.J.: Clinical platelet transfusions, in Silver H. (ed.): *Components and Derivatives in Transfusion Therapy: A Technical Workshop.* Washington, D.C., American Association of Blood Banks, 1980, p. 63.
241. Moroff G., Friedman A., Robkin-Kline L. et al.: Reduction of the volume of stored platelet concentrates for use in neonatal patients. *Transfusion* 24:144, 1984.
242. Schmidt P.J. (ed.): *Standards for Blood Banks and Transfusion Services,* ed. 11. American Association of Blood Banks, Arlington, Va., 1984, p. 26.
243. Schmidt P.J. (ed.): *Standards for Blood Banks and Transfusion Services,* ed. 11. American Association of Blood Banks, Arlington, Va., 1984, p. 5.
244. McCullough J.J.: Introduction to granulocyte function and donor selection for granulocyte transfusions, in Cohen E., Dawson R.B. (eds.): *Leukapheresis and Granulocyte Transfusions: A Technical Workshop.* Washington, D.C., American Association of Blood Banks, 1975, pp. 1–7.
245. Higby D.J., Mishler J.M., Cohen E., et al.: Increased elevation of peripheral leukocyte counts by infusion of histocompatible granulocytes. *Vox Sang.* 27:186, 1974.
246. Cartwright G.E., Athens J.W., Wintrobe M.M.: The kinetics of granulopoiesis in normal man. *Blood* 24:780, 1964.
247. Rosenshein M., Price T., Dale D.: Neutropenia, inflammation and the kinetics of transfused neutrophils. *Clin. Res.* 26:507a, 1978.
248. Tejada F., Bias W.B., Santos G.W., et al.: Immunologic response of patients with acute leukemia to platelet transfusions. *Blood* 42:405, 1973.
249. Westrick M.A., Dobelak-Fehir K.M., Epstein R.B.: The effect of prior whole blood transfusion on subsequent granulocyte support in leukopenic dogs. *Transfusion* 17:611, 1977.
250. Dahlke M.B., Keashen M.A., Alavi J.B., et al.: Response to granulocyte transfusions in the alloimmunized patient. *Transfusion* 20:555, 1980.
251. Schmidt P.J. (ed): *Standards for Blood Banks and Transfusion Services,* ed. 11. Arlington, Va., American Association of Blood Banks, 1984, p. 18.
252. McCullough J.J.: Introduction to granulocyte function and donor selection for granulocyte transfusions, in Cohen E., Dawson R.B. (eds.): *Leukapheresis and Granulocyte Transfusions: A Technical Workshop.* Washington, D.C., American Association of Blood Banks, 1975, p. 1.
253. McCullough J., Weiblen B.J., Fine D.: Effects of storage of granulocytes on their fate in vivo. *Transfusion* 23:20, 1983.
254. Glasser L.: Effect of storage on normal neutrophils collected by discontinuous-flow centrifugation leukapheresis. *Blood* 50:1145, 1977.
255. Price T.H.: Neutrophil transfusion: In vivo function of neutrophils collected using cell separators. *Transfusion* 23:504, 1983.
256. Price T.H., Dale D.C.: Neutrophil transfusion: The effect of collection technique and storage on in vivo chemotaxis. *Blood* 50(suppl. 1):309, 1977.
257. Klock J.C., Boyles J., Bainton D.F., et al.: Nylon-fiber-induced neutrophil fragmentation. *Blood* 54:1216, 1979.
258. Higby D.J.: Filtration leukapheresis: A review, in Cohen E., Dawson B. (eds.): *Leukapheresis and Granulocyte Transfusion.* Washington, D.C., American Association of Blood Banks, 1975, p. 71.
259. Graw R.G. Jr., Herzig G., Perry S., et al.: Normal granulocyte transfusion therapy: Treatment of septicemia due to gram-negative bacteria. *N. Engl. J. Med.* 287:367, 1972.
260. Glasser L.: Discontinuous flow centrifugation leukapheresis and neutrophil function. *Transfusion* 17:513, 1977.
261. Glasser L.: Functional considerations of granulocyte

concentrates used for clinical transfusions. *Transfusion* 19:1, 1979.
262. Widman F.K. (ed.): *Technical Manual of the American Association of Blood Banks*, ed. 8. Washington, D.C., American Association of Blood Banks, 1981, pp. 1–15.
263. Schmidt P.J. (ed): *Standards for Blood Banks and Transfusion Services*, ed. 11. Arlington, Va., American Association of Blood Banks, 1984, pp. 21–22.
264. Freireich E.J., Levin R.H., Whang J., et al.: The function and fate of transfused leukocytes from donors with chronic myelocytic leukemia in leukopenic recipients. *Ann. NY Acad. Sci.* 113:1081, 1964.
265. Schmidt P.J. (ed.): *Standards for Blood Banks and Transfusion Services*, ed. 11. Arlington, Va., American Association of Blood Banks, 1984, p. 11.
266. Nusbacher J.: Controlling the leukapheresis process, in Cohen E., Dawson R.B. (eds.): *Leukapheresis and Granulocyte Transfusions: A Technical Workshop*. Washington, D.C., American Association of Blood Banks, 1975, p. 53.
267. McCredie K.B., Bodey G.P., Burgess M.A., et al.: Increased granulocyte collection using the blood cell separation and the addition of etiocholanolone and hydroxyethyl starch. *Transfusion* 14:357, 1974.
268. Maurer P., Berardinelli B.: Immunologic studies with hydroxyethyl starch (HES): A proposed plasma expander. *Transfusion* 8:265, 1968.
269. Mishler J.M.: Hydroxyethyl starch as an adjunct to leukocyte separation by centrifugal means: Review of safety and efficacy. *Transfusion* 15:449, 1975.
270. Nusbacher J., et al.: Leukapheresis: The effect of a single high oral dose of prednisone on granulocyte mobilization, yield and function. *Transfusion* 13:366, 1973.
271. Wolff S.M., Kimball H.R., Perry S., et al.: The biological properties of etiocholanolone. *Ann. Intern. Med.* 67:1268, 1967.
272. Huestis D.W.: Granulocyte collection with the Haemonetics system: Normal and leukemic donors (Arizona Medical Center), in Cohen E., Dawson R.B. (eds.): *Leukapheresis and Granulocyte Transfusions: A Technical Workshop*. Washington, D.C., American Association of Blood Banks, 1975, p. 37.
273. El-Maalem H., Fletcher J.: Defective neutrophil function in chronic granulocytic leukaemia. *Br. J. Haematol.* 34:95, 1976.
274. Lowenthal R.M., Grossman L., Goldman J.L., et al.: Granulocyte transfusions in treatment of infections in patients with acute leukemia and aplastic anemia. *Lancet* 1:353, 1975.
275. Morse E.E., Freireich E.J., Carbone P.P., et al.: The transfusion of leukocytes from donors with chronic myelocytic leukemia to patients with leukopenia. *Transfusion* 78:183, 1966.
276. Graw R.G., Jr., Buckner C.D., Whang-Peng J., et al.: Complications of bone marrow transplantation: Graft-versus-host disease resulting from chronic-myelogenous-leukemia leukocyte transfusions. *Lancet* 2:338, 1970.

277. Seigel S.E., Lunde M.N., Gelderman A.H., et al: Transmission of toxoplasmosis by leukocyte transfusion. *Blood* 37:388, 1971.
278. Herzig R.H., Herzig G.P., Graw R.G. Jr., et al.: Successful granulocyte transfusion therapy for gram-negative septicemia: A prospectively randomized controlled study. *N. Engl. J. Med.* 296:701, 1977.
279. Hershko C., Naparstek E., Eldor A., et al.: Granulocyte transfusion therapy: A clinical trial in patients with acute leukemia and sepsis. *Vox Sang.* 34:129, 1978.
280. Nusbacher J., MacPherson J.: A comparison of techniques for leukapheresis and plateletpheresis, in Nusbacher J., Berkman E.M. (eds.): *Fundamentals of a Pheresis Program: A Technical Workshop*. Washington, D.C., American Association of Blood Banks, 1979, pp. 49–54.
281. Mollison P.L.: *Blood Transfusion in Clinical Medicine*, ed. 7. Oxford, England, Blackwell Scientific Publications, 1983, pp. 171–172.
282. Clift R.A., Sanders J.E., Thomas E.D., et al.: Granulocyte transfusions for the prevention of infection in patients receiving bone-marrow transplants. *N. Engl. J. Med.* 298:1052, 1978.
283. Ford J.M., Cullen M.M., Roberts L.M., et el.: Prophylactic granulocyte transfusions: Results of a randomized controlled trial in patients with acute myelogenous leukemia. *Transfusion* 22:311, 1982.
284. Ahrons S., Kissmeyer-Nielsen F.: Serological investigations of 1358 transfusion reactions in 74,000 transfusions. *Dan. Med. Bull.* 15:257, 1968.
285. Polesky H.F.: Clinical problems with HLA sensitization, in *Clinical Uses of Frozen-Thawed Red Blood Cells*. New York, Alan R. Liss, Inc., 1976, pp. 141–155.
286. Donald J., Higby M.D.: Granulocyte transfusions, in Silver H. (ed.): *Blood, Blood Components and Derivatives in Transfusion Therapy: A Technical Workshop*. Washington, D.C., American Association of Blood Banks, 1980, p. 29.
287. Buchholz D.H., Houx J.L.: Survey of filtration leukapheresis. *Exp. Hematol.* 7(suppl. 4):1-10, 1979.
288. Stephen C.R., Martin R.C., Bourgeois-Gavardin M.: Antihistaminic drugs in treatment of non-hemolytic transfusion reactions. *JAMA* 158:525, 1955.
289. Mollison P.L.: *Blood Transfusion in Clinical Medicine*, ed. 7. Oxford, England, Blackwell Scientific Publications, 1983, p. 738-739.
290. Bjerrum D.J., Jersild C.: Class-specific anti-IgA associated with severe anaphylactic transfusion reactions in a patient with pernicious anemia. *Vox Sang.* 21:411, 1971.
291. Ward H.N.: Pulmonary infiltrates associated with leukoagglutinin transfusion reactions. *Ann. Intern. Med.* 73:689, 1970.
292. Kernoff P.B.A., Durrant I.J., Rizza C.R., et al.: Severe allergic pulmonary oedema after plasma transfusion. *Br. J. Haematol.* 23:777, 1972.
293. Huestis D.W., Thomas S.F.: Presently available plasmapheresis technics, in Berkman E.M., Umlas

J. (eds.): *Therapeutic Hemapheresis: A Technical Workshop.* Washington, D.C., American Association of Blood Banks, 1980, p. 1.
294. Widman F.K. (ed.): *Technical Manual of the American Association of Blood Banks,* ed. 8. Washington, D.C., American Association of Blood Banks, 1981, pp. 30-32.
295. Graw R.G., et al.: Leukocyte and platelet collection from normal donors with the continuous-flow blood cell separator. *Transfusion* 11:94, 1971.
296. Nusbacher J.: Controlling the leukapheresis process (Rochester Regional Red Cross Blood Center), in Cohen E., Dawson R.B. (eds.): *Leukapheresis and Granulocyte Transfusions: A Technical Workshop.* Washington, D.C., American Association of Blood Banks, 1975, p. 53.
297. Higby D.J.: Granulocyte transfusions, in Silver H. (ed): *Blood, Blood Components and Derivatives in Transfusion Therapy: A Technical Workshop.* Washington, D.C., American Association of Blood Banks, 1980, p. 29.
298. Senhauser D.A., Westphal R.G., Bohman J.E., et al.: Immune system changes in cytapheresis donors. *Transfusion* 22:302, 1982.
299. Hilgartner M.W.: The management of hemophilia, in Mallory D. McG. (ed.): *Hemophilia: A Technical Workshop.* Washington, D.C., American Association of Blood Banks, 1978, p. 17.
300. Biggs R.: *Human Blood Coagulation, Haemostasis and Thrombosis,* ed. 2. Oxford, England, Blackwell Scientific Publications, 1976.
301. Kekwick R.A., Wolf P.: A concentrate of human antihaemophilic factor: Its use in six cases of haemophilia. *Lancet* 1:647, 1957.
302. Hershgold E.J., et al.: Native and purified factor VIII: Molecular and electron microscopical properties and a comparison with hemophilic plasma. *Fed. Proc.* 26:488, 1967.
303. Bidwell E., Dike G.W.R., Denson K.W.E.: Experiments with factor VIII separated from fibrinogen by electrophoresis in free buffer film. *Br. J. Haematol.* 12:583, 1966.
304. Austen D.E.G., Bidwell E.: Carbohydrate structure of factor VIII. *Thromb. Diath. Haemorrh.* 28:464, 1972.
305. Weiss H.J., Hoyer L.W.: Von Willebrand factor: Dissociation from antihemophilic factor procoagulant activity. *Science* 182:1149, 1973.
306. Green D., Potter E.V.: Failure of AHF concentrates to control bleeding in von Willebrand's disease. *Am. J. Med.* 60:357, 1976.
307. Cederbaum A.I.: The appropriate use of plasma and plasma components in clinical medicine, in Silver H. (ed.): *Blood, Blood Components and Derivatives in Transfusion Therapy: A Technical Workshop.* Washington, D.C., American Association of Blood Banks, 1980, p. 105.
308. Biggs R.: Jaundice and antibodies directed against factors VIII and IX in patients treated for haemophilia and Christmas disease in the United Kingdom. *Br. J. Haematol.* 26:313, 1974.

309. Biggs R., Bidwell E.: A method for the study of antihaemophilic globulin inhibitors with reference to 6 cases. *Br. J. Haematol.* 5:379, 1959.
310. Menache D., Guillin M.C.: The use of factor IX concentrates for patients with conditions other than factor IX deficiency. *Br. J. Haematol.* 31(suppl.):247, 1975.
311. Walsh P.N., Rizza C.R., Matthews J.M., et al.: Epsilon-amino caproic acid therapy for dental extractions in haemophilia and Christmas disease: A double blind controlled trial. *Br. J. Haematol.* 20:463, 1971.
312. Kernoff P.B.A., et al.: Clinical experience with polyelectrolyte fractioned porcine factor VIII concentrate in the treatment of haemophiliacs with antibodies to factor VIII (abstract). *Br. J. Haematol.* 49:131, 1981.
313. Sultan N.Y., Maisonneuve P., Bismuth A., et al.: Successful management of a patient with an acquired factor VIII inhibitor. *Transfusion* 23:61, 1983.
314. Anderson H., et al.: The clinical use of dried fibrinogen (human) and the risk of transmitting hepatitis by its administration. *Transfusion* 6:234, 1960.
315. Gerety R.J., Aronson D.L.: Plasma derivatives and viral hepatitis. *Transfusion* 22:347, 1982.
316. Rosati L.A., Barnes B., Oberman H.A., et al.: Hemolytic anemia due to anti-A in concentrated antihemophilic factor preparations. *Transfusion* 10:139, 1970.
317. Alving B.M., et al.: Vasoactive enzymes in immunoglobulin preparations, in Alving B.M., Finlayson J.S. (eds.): *Immunoglobulins: Characteristics and Use of Intravenous Preparations.* Washington, D.C., U.S. Government Printing Office, 1979.
318. Anderson G.F., Barhart M.I.: Intracellular localization of prothrombin. *Proc. Soc. Exp. Biol. Med.* 116:1, 1964.
319. Biggs R.: *Human Blood Coagulation, Haemostasis and Thrombosis.* Oxford, England, Blackwell Scientific Publications, 1976, p. 275.
320. Davie E.W., Fujikawa K.: Basic mechanisms in blood coagulation. *Annu. Rev. Biochem.* 44:799, 1975.
321. Biggs R.: *Human Blood Coagulation, Haemostasis and Thrombosis.* Oxford, England, Blackwell Scientific Publications, 1976, p. 277.
322. Aronson D.L., Preiss J.W., Mosesson M.W.: Molecular weights of factor VIII (AHF) and factor IX (PTC) by electron irradiation. *Thromb. Diath. Haemorrh.* 8:270, 1962.
323. Erslen A.J., Gabuzda G.T.: *Pathophysiology of Blood,* ed. 2. Philadelphia, W.B. Saunders Co., 1979, p. 177.
324. Cohn E.J., et al.: A system for the separation into fractions of the protein and lipoprotein components of biological tissues and fluids. *J. Am. Chem. Soc.* 68:459, 1946.
325. Casillas G., Simonetti C., Pavlovsky A.: Chromatographic behavior of clotting factors. *Br. J. Haematol.* 16:363, 1969.

326. Gilchrist G.S., Ekert H., Shanbrom E., et al.: Evaluation of a new concentrate for the treatment of factor IX deficiency. *N. Engl. J. Med.* 280:291, 1969.
327. Shapiro S.S., Hutlin M.: Acquired inhibitors of the blood coagulation factors. *Semin. Thromb. Hemostas.* 1:336, 1975.
328. Kasper C.K., Aledort L., Aronson D., et al.: A more uniform measurement of factor VIII inhibitors. *Thromb. Diath. Haemorrh.* 34:612, 1975.
329. Langdell R.D.: Safety and efficacy of blood products, in Mallory D. McG. (ed.): *Hemophilia: A Technical Workshop.* Washington, D.C., American Association of Blood Banks, 1978, p. 43.
330. Johnson A.J., Newman J.: Removal or concentration of hepatitis-associated antigen (HAA) from human plasma fractions. *Fed. Proc.* 31:654, 1972.
331. Brozovic M., quoted by Biggs R.: *Human Blood Coagulation, Haemostasis and Thrombosis,* ed. 2. Oxford, England, Blackwell Scientific Publications, 1976, p. 300.
332. Kasper C.K.: Postoperative thrombosis in hemophilia B. *N. Engl. J. Med.* 289:160, 1973.
333. Menache D.: Clinical use of factor IX concentrates. *Thromb. Diath. Haemorrh.* 33:600, 1975.
334. Marder V.J., Budzinsky A.Z.: Fibrinogen and its derivatives: Hereditary and acquired abnormalities. *Schweiz. Med. Worchenschr.* 104:1338, 1974.
335. Bove J.R.: Fibrinogen: Is the benefit worth the risk? *Transfusion* 18:129, 1975.
336. Ness P.M., Perkins H.A.: Cryoprecipitate as a reliable source of fibrinogen replacement. *JAMA* 241:1698, 1979.
337. Harper H.A.: *Review of Physiological Chemistry,* ed. 16. Los Altos, Calif., Lange Medical Publications, 1975, pp. 199–210.
338. Cohn E.J.: Blood proteins and their therapeutic value. *Science* 101:54, 1945.
339. Gellis S.S., et al.: Chemical, clinical, and immunological studies on the products of human plasma fractionation. *J. Clin. Invest.* 27:239, 1948.
340. Hoofnagle J.H., Barker L.F., Thiel J., et al.: Hepatitis B virus and hepatitis B surface antigen in human albumin products. *Transfusion* 1:141, 1976.
341. Hink J.H. Jr., Hidalgo J., Seeberg V.P., et al.: Preparation and properties of a heat treated human plasma protein fraction. *Vox Sang.* 2:174, 1957.
342. Mollison P.L.: *Blood Transfusion in Clinical Medicine,* ed. 7. Oxford, England, Blackwell Scientific Publications, 1983, p. 179.
343. Vandongen R., Gordon R.D.: Generation and survival of angiotensin in non-refrigerated plasma: An explanation for presence of pressor material in human plasma protein solutions used clinically. *Transfusion* 9:205, 1969.
344. Uses of blood and components. *Med. Lett. Drug. Ther.* 14(24):89, 1972.
345. Wintrobe M.M., Lee G.R., Boggs D.R., et al.: *Clinical hematology,* ed. 8. Philadelphia, Lea & Febiger, 1981, p. 519.
346. Gutierrez V.S., Berman I.R., Soloway H.B., et al.: Relationship of hypoproteinemia and prolonged mechanical ventilation to the development of pulmonary insufficiency in shock. *Ann. Surg.* 171:385, 1970.
347. Hoyle C.L., McCall D.C., Danford R.O., et al.: Renal function during the early post-burn period: A comparison of colloid versus non-colloid-containing balanced salt solution. *Ann. Surg.* 169:404, 1969.
348. Silver H.: Normal serum albumin and plasma protein fraction, in Silver H. (ed.): *Blood, Blood Components and Derivatives in Transfusion Therapy: A Technical Workshop.* Washington, D.C., American Association of Blood Banks, 1980, p. 89.
349. International Forum: Can a national all-voluntary blood transfusion service by adequate blood component therapy cover actual and future needs of albumin? *Vox Sang.* 31:225, 1976.
350. Alexander M.R., Ambre J.J., Liskow B.I., et al.: Therapeutic use of albumin. *JAMA* 241:2527, 1979.
351. Magladery J.W., Solandt D.Y., Best C.H.: Serum and plasma in treatment of haemorrhage in experimental animals. *Br. Med. J.* 2:248, 1940.
352. Heyl J.T., Gibson J.G. II, Janeway C.A.: Studies on the plasma proteins: V. The effect of concentrated solutions of human and bovine serum albumin on blood volume after acute blood loss in man. *J. Clin. Invest.* 22:763, 1943.
353. Farrow S.P.: *Effects of infusion of various colloid solutions upon the circulatory volumes of rabbits,* thesis. University of Birmingham, England, 1967.
354. Watson J.S., Walker C.C., Sanders R.: A comparison between dried plasma and plasma protein fraction in the resuscitation of burn patients. *Burns* 3:108, 1977.
355. Weaver D.W., Ledgerwood A.M., Lucas C.E., et al.: Pulmonary effects of albumin resuscitation for severe hypovolemic shock. *Arch. Surg.* 113:387, 1978.
356. Collins J.A., Braitberg A., Butcher R.H. Jr.: Changes in lung and body weight and lung water content in rats treated for hemorrhage with various fluids. *Surgery* 73:401, 1973.
357. Stodel W.E., et al.: The effect of various resuscitative regimens on hemorrhagic shock in puppies. *J. Pediatr. Surg.* 12:809, 1977.
358. Mollison P.L.: *Blood Transfusion in Clinical Medicine,* ed. 7. Oxford, England, Blackwell Scientific Publications, 1983, pp. 46–47.
359. Mills M., McFee A.S., Boisch B.I.: The post-resuscitation wet lung syndrome, abstracted. *Ann. Thorac. Surg.* 3:182, 1967.
360. Rush B.F.: Volume replacement: When, what and how much? in Schumer W., Nyhus L.M. (eds.): *Treatment of Shock: Principles and Practice.* Philadelphia, Lea & Febiger, 1974.
361. Mayer K.: Crystalloids versus colloid, in Silver H. (ed.): *Blood, Blood Components and Derivatives, in*

Transfusion Therapy: A Technical Workshop. Washington, D.C., American Association of Blood Banks, 1980, p. 97.
362. Bull J.P.: Shock caused by burns and its treatment. *Br. Med. Bull.* 10:9, 1954.
363. Tullis J.L.: Albumin: 1. Background and use. 2. Guidelines for clinical use. *JAMA* 237:355, 460, 1977.
364. Markley K., Bocanegra M., Bazan A., et al.: Clinical evaluation of saline solution therapy in burn shock: II. Comparison of plasma therapy with saline solution therapy. *JAMA* 170:1633, 1959.
365. Davies J.W.L.: Blood volume changes in patients with burns treated with either colloid or saline solutions. *Clin. Sci.* 26:429, 1964.
366. Davison A.M.: The use of albumin concentrates in hypoproteinemic state. *Clin. Hematol.* 5:135, 1976.
367. Tullis J.L.: Albumin: 2. Guidelines for clinical use. *JAMA* 237:460, 1977.
368. Bland J.H.L., Laver M.B., Lowenstein E.: Vasodilator effect of commercial 5% plasma protein fraction solutions. *JAMA* 224:1721, 1973.
369. Ring J., Messmer K.: Incidence and severity of anaphylactoid reactions to colloid volume substitutes. *Lancet* 1:466, 1977.
370. Case J.: Albumin autoagglutinating phenomenon as a factor contributing to false positive reactions when typing with rapid slide-test reagents. *Vox Sang.* 30:441, 1976.
371. Fudenberg H.H., et al.: *Basic and Clinical Immunology.* Los Altos, Calif. Lange Medical Publications, 1976, p. 15.
372. Fudenberg H.H., et al.: *Basic and Clinical Immunology.* Los Altos, Calif., Lange Medical Publications, 1976, p. 617.
373. Barandun S., Kistler P., Jeunet F., et al.: Intravenous administration of human gamma-globulin. *Vox Sang.* 7:157, 1962.
374. Hassig A.: Prophylaxis and therapy with human immunoglobulin preparations. *Bibl. Haematol.* 29, part 2, p. 551.
375. Mollison P.L.: *Blood Transfusion in Clinical Medicine,* ed. 7. Oxford, England, Blackwell Scientific Publications, 1983, pp. 189-190.
376. Pollack T.M., Reid D.: Immunoglobulin for the prevention of infectious hepatitis in persons working overseas. *Lancet* 1:281, 1969.
377. Snyder E.L.: *Blood Transfusion Therapy: A Physicians Handbook.* Washington, D.C., American Association of Blood Banks, 1983, pp. 33-34.
378. Hoofnagle J.H., Seeff L.B., Bales Z.B., et al.: Passive-active immunity from hepatitis B immune globulin. *Ann. Intern. Med.* 91:813, 1979.
379. Mosley J.W.: Hepatitis B immune globulin: Some progress and some problems. *Ann. Intern. Med.* 91:914, 1979.
380. Kekwick R.A., Mackay M.E.: The separation of protein fractions from human plasma with ether. Special Reproduction Series of the Medical Research Council (London), No. 286, 1954, p. 58.
381. Ellis M.: Human antitetanus serum in the treatment of tetanus. *Br. Med. J.* 1:1123, 1963.
382. Mollison P.L.: *Blood Transfusion in Clinical Medicine,* ed. 7. Oxford, England, Blackwell Scientific Publications, 1983, p. 190.
383. Windholz M. (ed.): *The Merck Index: An Encyclopedia of Chemicals and Drugs,* ed. 9. Rahway N.J., Merck & Co., 1976, p. 2900.
384. Mollison P.L.: *Blood Transfusion in Clinical Medicine,* ed 7. Oxford, England, Blackwell Scientific Publications, 1983, p. 58.
385. Arturson G., Wallenius G.: The renal clearance of dextran of different molecular sizes in normal humans. *Scand. J. Clin. Lab. Invest.* 16:81, 1964.
386. Shires T.G.: Shock, in Schwartz S.I., et al. (eds.): *Principles of Surgery,* ed. 3. New York, McGraw-Hill Book Co., 1979, pp. 165-166.
387. Mollison P.L.: *Blood Transfusion in Clinical Medicine,* ed 7. Oxford, England, Blackwell Scientific Publications, 1983, pp. 58-59.
388. Shires T.G., Camizaro P.C., Carrico J.C.: Shock, in Schwartz S.I., et al. (eds.): *Principles of Surgery,* ed 3. McGraw-Hill Book Co., New York, 1979, p. 165.
389. Langdell R.D., Adelson E., Furth F.W., et al.: Dextran and prolonged bleeding time: Results of a 60-gram, one-liter infusion given to one hundred and sixty-three normal human subjects. *JAMA* 162:346, 1958.
390. Moriau M., Rodhain J., Noel H., et al.: Comparative effects of dextrans, gelatin and stable plasma protein solution (SPPS) on the experimental disseminated intravascular coagulation (DIC). *Vox Sang.* 27:411, 1974.
391. Bonnar J., Walsh, J.: Prevention of thrombosis after pelvic surgery by British Dextran 70. *Lancet* 1:614, 1972.
392. Lorenz W., Doenicke A., Messmer K., et al.: Histamine release of human subjects by modified gelatin (Haemaceel) and dextran: An explanation for anaphylactoid reactions observed under clinical conditions? *Br. J. Anaesth.* 48:151, 1976.
393. Kabat E.A., Berg D.: Dextran: An antigen in man. *J. Immunol.* 70:514, 1953.
394. Mishler J.M., et al.: Leukapheresis: Increased efficiency of collection by the use of hydroxyethyl starch and dexamethasone, in Goldman J.M., Lowenthal R.M. (eds.): *Leucocytes: Separation, Collection and Transfusion.* New York, Academic Press, 1975.
395. Karlson K.E., Garzon A.A., Shaftan G.W., et al.: Increased blood loss associated with administration of certain plasma expanders: Dextran 75, Dextran 40 and hydroxyethyl starch. *Surgery* 62:670, 1967.
396. Campbell D.H., et al.: The preparation and properties of a modified gelatin (oxypolygelatin) as an oncotic substitute for serum albumin. *Tex. Rep. Biol. Med.* 9:235, 1951.
397. Lundsgaard-Hansen P., Tschirren B.: Modified fluid gelatin as a plasma substitute, in Jameson G.A., Greenwalt T.J. (eds.): *Blood Substitutes and*

Plasma Expanders. New York, Alan R. Liss, 1978, pp. 227-257.
398. Rudowsky W., Kostrzewska E.: Aspects of treatment: Blood substitutes. Ann. R. Coll. Surg. Engl. 58:115, 1976.
399. Silver H.: Special products for hemotherapy, in Silver H. (ed.): Blood, Blood Components and Derivatives in Transfusion Therapy: A Technical Workshop. Washington, D.C., American Association of Blood Banks, 1980, p. 133.
400. Geyer R.P.: Substitutes for blood and its components, in Jamieson G.A., Greenwalt T.J. (eds.): Blood Substitutes and Plasma Expanders. Prog. Clin. Biol. Res. 19:191, 1978.
401. Palani C.K., DeWoskin E., Moss G.S.: Scope and limitations of stroma-free hemoglobin solution as an oxygen-carrying blood substitute. Surg. Clin. North Am. 55:3, 1975.
402. Moss G.S., DeWoskin R., Rosen A.L., et al.: Transport of oxygen and carbon dioxide by hemoglobin-saline solution in the red cell primate, in Jamieson G.A., Greenwalt T.J. (eds.): Blood Substitutes and Plasma Expanders. Prog. Clin. Biol. Res. 19:191, 1978.
403. Geyer R.P.: The design of artificial blood substitutes, in Ariens E.J. (ed.): Drug Design. New York, Academic Press, 1976, vol. 3, pp. 1-58.
404. Amberson W.R., et al.: On the use of Ringer-Locke solutions containing hemoglobin as a substitute for normal blood in mammals. J. Cell. Comp. Physiol. 5:359, 1934.
405. Moss G.S., DeWoskin R., Rosen A.L., et al.: Transport of oxygen and carbon dioxide by hemoglobin-saline solution in the red cell-free primate. Surg. Gynecol. Obstet. 142:357, 1976.
406. DeVenuto F., Zuck T.F., Zegna A.I., et al.: Characteristics of stroma-free hemoglobin prepared by crystallization. J. Lab. Clin. Med. 89:509, 1977.
407. Tam S.C., Blumenstein J., Wong J.T.F.: Soluble dextran-hemoglobin complex as a potential substitute. Proc. Natl. Acad. Sci. USA 73:2128, 1976.
408. Blumenstein J., Tam S.C., Chang J.E., et al.: Experimental transfusion of dextran-hemoglobin, in Jamieson G.A., Greenwalt T.J. (eds.): Blood Substitutes and Plasma Expanders. Prog. Clin. Biol. Res. 19:205, 1978.
409. Sehgal L.R., Rosen A.L., Gould S.A., et al.: Preparation and in vitro characteristics of polymerized pyridoxylated hemoglobin. Transfusion 23:158, 1983.
410. Kramlová M., Přístoupil T.I., Ulrych S., et al.: Stroma-free haemoglobin solution for infusion changes during storage. Haematologia 10:365, 1976.
411. Mollison P.L.: Blood Transfusion in Clinical Medicine, ed. 7. Oxford, England, Blackwell Scientific Publications, 1983, pp. 63-64.
412. Greenburg G.: Hemoglobin solutions: New life for old blood. Diagn. Med. 4:19, 1981.
413. Schuschereba S.T., Friedman H.I., DeVenuto F., et al.: Morphologic effects on the retina of massive exchange transfusions with stroma-free hemoglobin solutions. Lab. Invest. 48:339, 1983.

414. Geyer R.P.: Substitutes for blood: Experimental and practical considerations, in Myhre B.A. (ed.): A Seminar on Blood Components: Ex Unum Pluribus. Washington, D.C., American Association of Blood Banks, 1977, p. 75.
415. Sloviter A.H.: Perfluorocompounds as artificial erythrocytes. Fed. Proc. 34:1484, 1975.
416. O'Brien R.N., Langlais A.J., Seufert W.D.: Diffusion coefficients of respiratory gases in a perfluorocarbon liquid. Science 217:153, 1982.
417. Robins S.L., Cotran R.S.: Pathologic Basis of Disease, ed. 2. Philadelphia, W.B. Saunders, 1979, p. 541.
418. Yocoyama K., Yamanouchi K., Watanabe M., et al.: Preparation of prefluorodecalin emulsion and approach to the red cell substitute. Fed. Proc. 34:1478, 1975.
419. Rice C.L., Moss G.S.: Blood and blood substitutes: Current practice. Adv. Surg. 13:93-114, 1979.
420. Lau P., Shankar V.S., Mayer L.L., et al.: Coagulation defects in rabbits after infusion of dispersed fluorochemicals. Transfusion 15:432, 1975.
421. Sloviter H.A., quoted by Silver H.: Special products for hemotherapy, in Silver H. (ed.): Blood, Blood Components and Derivatives in Transfusion Therapy: A Technical Workshop. Washington, D.C., American Association of Blood Banks, 1980, p. 133.
422. Clark L.C. Jr., Gollan F.: Survival of mammals breathing organic liquids equilibrated with oxygen at atmospheric pressure. Science 152:1755, 1966.
423. Kylstra J.A., Paganelli C.V., Lanphier E.H.: Pulmonary gas exchange in dogs ventilated with hyperbarically oxygenated liquid. J. Appl. Physiol. 21:177, 1966.
424. Geyer R.P.: Fluorocarbon-polyol artificial blood substitutes. N. Engl. J. Med. 289:1077, 1973.
425. Ohyanagy H., Toshima K., Naito R., et al.: Clinical studies of perfluorochemical blood substitutes: Safety of Fluosol-DA (20%) in normal human volunteers. Clin. Ther. 2:306, 1979.
426. Tremper K.K., Friedman A.E., Levine E.M., et al.: The preoperative treatment of severely anemic patients with a perfluorochemical oxygen-transport fluid, Fluosol-DA. N. Engl. J. Med. 307:277, 1982.
427. Cowart V.S.: Blood substitutes: Two ways to get there. JAMA 249:159, 1983.
428. Marwick C.: FDA committee questions Fluosol efficacy; US approval not imminent. JAMA 250:2585, 1983.
429. Glogar D.H., Kloher R.A., Muller J., et al.: Fluorocarbons reduce myocardial ischemic damage after coronary occlusion. Science 211:1439, 1981.
430. Hall C.A., Rappazzo M.E.: Organ perfusion with fluorocarbon, in Jamieson G.A., Greenwalt T.J. (eds.): Blood Substitutes and Plasma Expanders. Prog. Clin. Biol. Res. 19:41, 1978.
431. Nanney L., Fink L.M., Virmani R.: Morphologic demonstration of perfluorocarbon retention in liver, spleen, lung and kidney of rabbits. Lab. Invest. 48:62A, 1983.

432. Shah K.H., Yamamura Y., Usuba A.: Immunopathologic changes by artificial blood perfluorochemicals. *Lab. Invest.* 48:62A, 1983.
433. Silver H.: Special products for hemotherapy, in Silver H. (ed.): *Blood, Blood Components and Derivatives in Transfusion Therapy: A Technical Workshop.* Washington, D.C., American Association of Blood Banks, 1980, p. 133.
434. Valeri C.R., Zaroulis C.G.: Rejuvenation and freezing of outdated stored human cells. *N. Engl. J. Med.* 287:1307, 1972.
435. Hamasaki N., Hirota-Chigita C.: Acid-citrate-dextrose-phosphoenolpyruvate medium as a rejuvenant for blood storage. *Transfusion* 23:1, 1983.
436. Goldman J.M., Th'ng K.H., Park D.S., et al.: Collection, cryopreservation, and subsequent viability of haemopoietic stem cells intended for treatment of chronic granulocytic leukaemia in blast-cell transformation. *Br. J. Haematol.* 40:185, 1978.
437. Goldman J.M., Catovsky D., Hows J., et al.: Cryopreserved peripheral blood cells functioning as autografts in patients with chronic granulocytic leukaemia in transformation. *Br. Med. J.* 1:1310, 1979.
438. Richman C.H.: Prolonged cryopreservation of human granulocytes. *Transfusion* 23:508, 1983.
439. Marcus R.E., Knott L.J.: CFU-GM and T cell subsets in young red cell collections. *Transfusion* 24:379, 1984.
440. Blume K.G.: Marrow transplantation, in Williams W., et al. (eds.): *Hematology,* ed. 3. New York, McGraw-Hill Book Co., 1983, p. 1584.
441. Thomas D.E.: Marrow transplantation for acute leukemia, in Perkins H.A. (ed.): *Human Bone Marrow Transplantation.* Washington, D.C., American Association of Blood Banks, 1976, p. 3.
442. Perkins, H.A.: HLA-The major histocompatibility complex, in Perkins H.A. (ed.): *Human Bone Marrow Transplantation.* Washington, D.C., American Association of Blood Banks, 1976, p. 3.
443. Hershko C., Gale R.P., Ho W., et al.: ABH antigens and bone-marrow transplantation. *Br. J. Haematol.* 44:65, 1980.
444. Hansen J.A., Clift R.A., Thomas E.D., et al.: Transplantation of marrow from an unrelated donor to a patient with acute leukemia. *N. Engl. J. Med.* 303:565, 1980.
445. Storb R., Thomas E.D., Buckner C.D., et al.: Allogeneic marrow grafting for treatment of aplastic anemia. *Blood* 43:157, 1974.
446. Storb R., Thomas E.D., Buckner C.D., et al.: Marrow transplantation in thirty "untransfused" patients with severe aplastic anemia. *Ann. Intern. Med.* 92:30, 1980.
447. Thomas E.D., Storb R., Clift R.A., et al.: Bone marrow transplantation. *N. Engl. J. Med.* 292:895, 1975.
448. Thomas E.D., Storb R.: Technique for human marrow grafting. *Blood* 36:507, 1970.
449. Gale R.P., Sarna G.: A cytoreductive conditioning for bone marrow transplantation in resistant leukemia (SCARI), in Perkins H.A. (ed.): *Human Bone Marrow Transplantation.* Washington, D.C., American Association of Blood Banks, 1976, p. 55.
450. Goldman S.F., Niethammer D., Flad H.D., et al.: Hemopoietic and lymphopoietic split chimerism in severe combined immunodeficiency disease (SCID). *Transplant. Proc.* 11:225, 1979.
451. Thomas E.D., Buckner C.D., Clift R.A., et al.: Marrow transplantation for acute non-lymphoblastic leukemia in first remission. *N. Engl. J. Med.* 301:597, 1979.
452. Santos G.W., et al.: HLA-identical marrow transplants in aplastic anemia, acute leukemia, and lymphosarcoma employing cyclophosphamide, in Perkins H.A. (ed.): *Human Bone Marrow Transplantation.* Washington D.C., American Association of Blood Banks, 1976, p. 63.
453. Neiman P.E., Einstein A.B., Thomas E.D., et al.: Interstitial pneumonia and cytomegalovirus infection as complications of human marrow transplantation. *Transplantation* 15:478, 1973.
454. Fefer A., et al.: Bone marrow transplantation for hematologic neoplasia in 16 patients with identical twins. *N. Engl. J. Med.* 290:1389, 1974.
455. Doney K.C., Weiden P.L.: Failure of early administration of antithymocyte globulin to lessen graft-versus-host disease in human allogeneic marrow transplant recipients. *Transplantation* 31:141, 1981.
456. Neiman P., Wasserman P.B., Wentworth B.B., et al.: Interstitial pneumonia and cytomegalovirus infection as complications of human marrow transplantation. *Transplantation* 15:478, 1973.
457. Blume K.G., Beutler E., Bross K.J., et al.: Bone marrow ablation and allogeneic marrow transplantation in acute leukemia. *N. Engl. J. Med.* 302:1041, 1980.
458. Camitta E., Thomas E.D., Nathan D.G., et al.: Severe aplastic anemia: A prospective study on the effect of early marrow transplantation on acute mortality. *Blood* 48:63, 1976.
459. Storb R.: Aplastic anemia treated by allogeneic marrow transplantation: The Seattle experience, in Perkins H.A. (ed.): *Human Bone Marrow Transplantation.* Washington, D.C., American Association of Blood Banks, 1976, p. 35.
460. Gale R.P.: Bone marrow transplantation in severe aplastic anemia, in Perkins H.A. (ed.): *Human Bone Marrow Transplantation.* Washington D.C., American Association of Blood Banks, 1976, p. 47.
461. Gmur J., et al.: Autologous hematologic recovery from aplastic anemia following high dose cyclophosphamide and HLA-matched allogeneic bone marrow transplantation. *Acta Haematol.* 62:20, 1979.
462. Camitta B.M., Thomas E.D., Nathan D.G., et al.: A prospective study of androgens and bone marrow transplantation for treatment of severe aplastic anemia. *Blood* 53:504, 1979.
463. Winston D.J., Ho W.G., Young L.S., et al.: Prophylactic granulocyte transfusions during human bone marrow transplantation. *Am. J. Med.* 68:893, 1980.

464. Minchinton R.M., Waters A.H., Malpas J.S., et al.: Platelet- and granulocyte-specific antibodies after allogeneic and autologous bone marrow grafts. *Vox Sang.* 46:125, 1984.
465. Ramsey G., Nusbacher J., Starzl T.E., et al.: Isohemagglutinins of graft origin after ABO unmatched liver transplantation. *N. Engl. J. Med.* 311:1167, 1984.
466. Ockelford P.A., Hill R.S., Nelson L., et al.: Serologic complications of a major ABO incompatible bone marrow transplantation in a Polynesian with aplastic anemia. *Transfusion* 22:62, 1982.
467. Lasky L.C., Warkentin P.I., Kersey J.H., et al.: Hemotherapy in patients undergoing blood group incompatible bone marrow transplantation. *Transfusion* 23:277, 1983.

9

Apheresis Techniques and Autotransfusion

DONOR APHERESIS

APHERESIS entails withdrawing blood from a donor, separating out and retaining certain components (plasma, leukocytes, platelets, etc.), and retransfusing the remainder into the donor. Both manual and automated methods are available. Apheresis holds great promise for therapeutic purposes as more and more applications are discovered and adopted. It is the responsibility of the blood bank director to review with the treating physician not familiar with the procedure the indications for apheresis in individual patients as well as the potential complications of the procedure. Most apheresis procedures are undertaken at blood centers (about 56%), the remainder in hospitals.[1]

There are two major systems for processing cells: the continuous flow centrifugation (CFC) system and the discontinuous flow centrifugation system (Fig 9–1). (Filtration leukapheresis, a third possibility, will not be discussed in this chapter for it is infrequently used.) Both the CFC and the DFC systems function on the same principle. A centrifugal force is created by a conical central piece, which rotates on its axis. This freely rotating piece is usually harnessed in a transparent, disposable plastic shield (see Fig 8–3). On production of a centrifugal force, the cells aggregate at the bottom part of the bowl and the plasma becomes the supernate. It is then possible to separate the components according to density. The plasma is separated first, then the platelets and/or granulocytes, and finally the red blood cells (RBCs). Each separation method is described individually below.

Discontinuous Flow Centrifugation System

One of the more frequently used machines that functions on the DFC principle is the Haemonetics model 30. The prototype of this machine, which uses the Latham bowl principle, was designed by Cohn in 1951 and subsequently perfected by Tullis.[2,3] All parts of the machine that come in contact with blood components are disposable, which minimizes possible infection of the patient or donor. The central core of the disposable bowl in DFC machines rotates, creating a centrifugal field in which whole blood is separated into components. Sterility is maintained via a rotary seal.[4] Blood enters the bowl through a central tube that traverses the bowl and allows filling from below (see Fig 9–1). As the blood separates into components, the lighter plasma collects at the top and is drawn off through an exit portal at the top of the bowl leading to a receptacle bag for this component. If platelet or white blood cell (WBC) separation is desired, the platelets and the granulocytes can be separated by allowing the pink band that contains these components to rise to the top of the bowl; then the components are drawn off through a different exit portal into separate collecting bags. Enriched platelet or granulocyte bands can thus be prepared. The two bowl sizes most frequently used in the Haemonetics model 30 are a 375-ml capacity bowl and a smaller 225-ml capacity bowl. The 225-ml bowl appears to be better for collecting platelets than the larger one.[5] Before entering the centrifugation bowl, blood is drawn from the donor by a peristal-

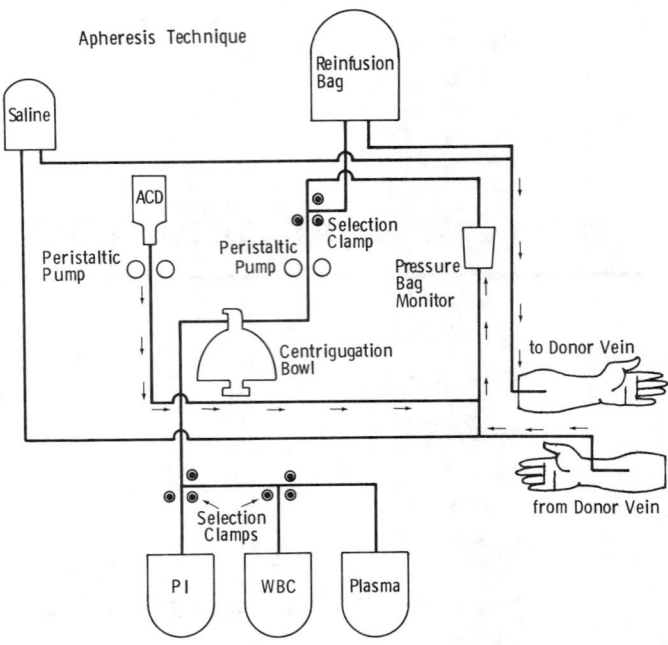

FIG 9–1.—The Haemonetics system for performing hemapheresis. Collection starts from an arm vein, shown at the lower right. The collection flow is shown by *arrows*. The collecting pressure is gauged by the pressure bag monitor. Blood is collected into the same line where acid-citrate-dextrose (ACD) anticoagulant is slowly added, with the aid of a peristaltic pump. Blood then is collected into the reinfusion bag *(top)* via a peristaltic pump and transported into the Latham centrifugation bowl *(center)*. Once the components have been separated, the blood is drawn off into satellite bags *(bottom)*. The collection bag situated labeled *Pl* is used for collection of platelets. The bag labeled *WBC* is used to collect granulocytes, and the remaining bag is used to collect plasma. Residual packed cells after centrifugation are pumped back into the reinfusion bag *(top)* and by gravity are returned to the donor vein.

tic pump system, which infuses an anticoagulant into the tubing. The anticoagulant solution, usually acid-citrate-dextrose (ACD), prevents clotting of the blood within the system during centrifugation.[1]

Heparin has been used to anticoagulate donors; however, these donors must be monitored with the thrombin time dilution test.[6] Usually 10,000 units of heparin by continuous infusion are necessary to anticoagulate donors.[6]

Since automated blood processing is largely used for separation of plasma, platelets, or granulocytes, the anticoagulated packed cells are usually returned by emptying the residual packed cell content in the bowl to the donor. This process is achieved by the peristaltic pumps in the pheresis machine, which force the packed cells into a reservoir bag located at the highest point of the apheresis machine. The blood collected in the reinfusion bag is returned to the donor by gravity.

The method is considered discontinuous because only one volume at a time is centrifuged, and a lag time for reinfusion is required. However, DFC apheresis runs can be shortened if a two-arm vein system is employed. With this system, blood in the reservoir is reinfused at the same time a second bowl fill-up is being processed. The extracorporeal volume per run may be as high as 750 ml using the large bowl and 450 ml using the small bowl,[7] an aspect that must be considered when calculating the volume that can be safely removed from any particular patient on each run.

In DFC platelet units, WBC contamination is quite frequent; to avoid this, a surge flow technique has been developed. With this method, an additional pump produces a surge flow that forces platelets to the top of the RBC band.[8]

Continuous Flow Centrifugation

The main blood cell separator used for CFC apheresis is the IBM model 2997 (Fig 9–2). This machine utilizes a hoop-like separation module system. The modules are disposable. The moving portals of entry have a rotary ceramic seal. Separation takes place in a space formed by a rigid hollow plastic belt within which blood separates. The blood components are separated by rotation and are collected from within the top part of the belt into collection bags, in contrast to the upward displacement mechanism of the DFC system. In this way, continuous collection is possible.[9, 10]

The Celltrifuge II machine (Fenwall Laboratories, Deerfield, Ill.) uses a "jumprope" principle, obviating the rotary seal mechanism used in the other machines (Haemonetics model 30 and IBM 2997). CFC cell separators have advantages over the DFC machines in that the cycle time is shorter and the extracorporeal volume is small, ranging from 255 to 280 ml in the IBM 2997 and in the Aminco model (Fig 9–3). Blood is drawn at a rate of 40–50 ml/minute. Granulocytes are separated by setting the centrifuge speed at 450 g.[10] Even though CFC systems have definite advantages over DFC systems, the equipment is more complex and therefore more prone to breakdown. Furthermore, CFC cell separators are less easy to transport than the Haemonetics model 30, and in the case of the IBM 2997 separator, the machine is significantly more expensive.

Donor Selection

Donors for apheresis should be screened by a qualified apheresis nurse, and a physician should be available for consultation. Donor selection criteria are the same as for blood donor selection (see Chap. 8). However, special attention to certain details are necessary due to the peculiarities of the procedure.

Calculation of Blood Volume Changes

The apheresis donor will undergo vascular volume changes to which he or she must adapt via

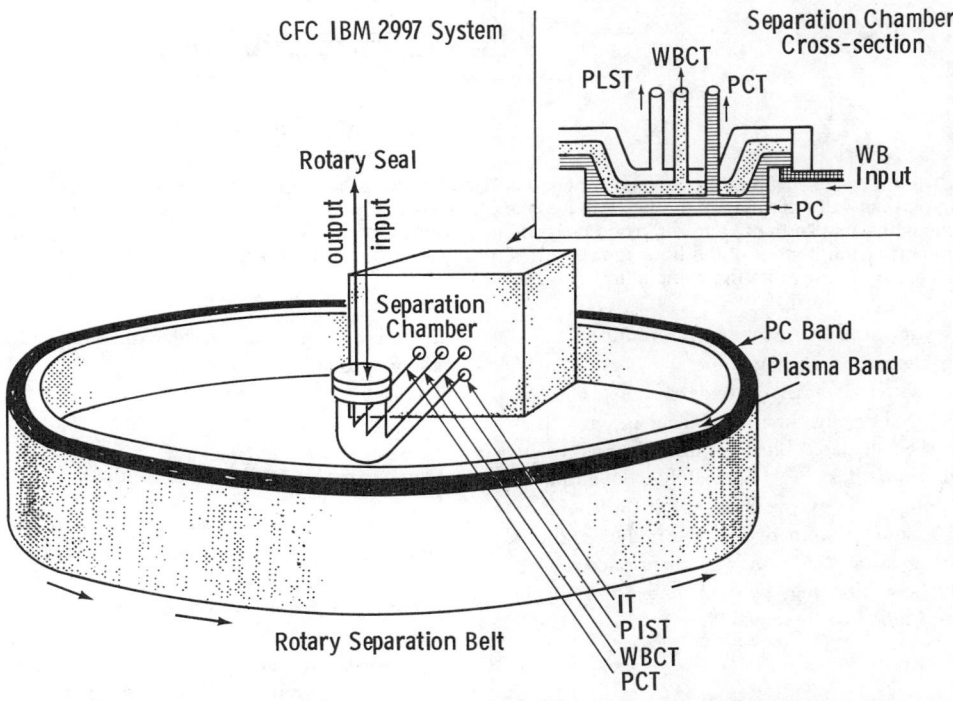

FIG 9–2.—Continuous flow centrifugation system provided by the 2997 IBM machine. The blood enters in the central area of the system and sterility is preserved by a ceramic rotary seal. The blood penetrates the separation chamber via the input tube *(IT)* (*insert* shows cross section of the separation chamber). The blood enters the chamber by the whole blood input tube *(WB)*. Then the blood penetrates the rotary separation belt *(bottom)*. The rotating belt creates a centrifugal force which separates the blood into components *(center plasma band)*. Packed cells are found in the outermost portion of the belt *(PC band)*. Once the blood is separated, it is collected in the separation chamber (see *insert*). Packed cells *(PC)* are collected by the packed cell tube *(PCT)*. The middle layer of granulocytes is collected via the white blood cell tube *(WBCT)*. Platelets and plasma can be collected by the tube lying in the outermost portion *(PLST)*.

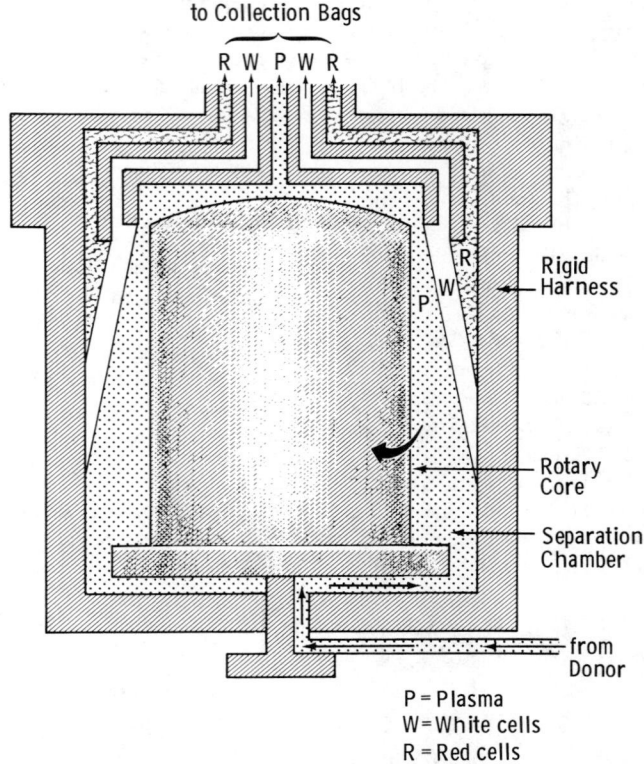

FIG 9–3.—Cross section of the Aminco continuous flow centrifugation rotor. Components are drawn off through different ports of exit at the top of the bowl. Plasma is collected at the innermost portion of the bowl. Granulocytes are found in the middle band, and red blood cells in the outermost band. The blood is fed into the system through an entry port at the bottom of the bowl *(arrows)*. The rotary core, as in the Latham Bowl, creates the centrifugal force necessary to separate the components.

homeostatic mechanisms. It is important to calculate what extracorporeal volume the donor can afford to lose on the basis of body weight. The volume removed at any time should not be more than 12% of the calculated blood volume (just as for autologous donations).[11] A normal blood volume in men is approximately the body weight in kilograms times 77, and in women it is the body weight in kilograms times 67.[12] As was mentioned above, different bowl sizes may be used, depending on the volume of blood to be removed.

Donor Medical History

A detailed medical questionnaire must be prepared with an emphasis on any history of bleeding tendency, hematomata, and so forth. These questions are particularly significant if heparin is to be employed during the procedure. Current menstrual flow, bleeding ulcer, or hematuria are reasons for donor disqualification.[10]

Reactions to Infused Materials

Since heparin is prepared from bovine and porcine tissues, allergy to products from these animals should be investigated.[13]

Some donors must receive special agents to increase granulocyte counts or to improve separation of cells. A substance frequently used to improve the separation of granulocytes during cytapheresis is hydroxyethyl starch (HES). This substance is described in more detail in chapter 8. However, some characteristics of HES will be discussed here in the context of granulocyte donation. HES is known to cause coagulation abnormalities, rouleaux formation, and progressive intravascular expansion, and it persists in the body for prolonged periods, stored in tissues.[14] In experiments in vitro, HES appears to affect clotting mostly due to a plasma dilution;[15] however, in vivo complex hemostatic mechanisms are at play, and bleeding may be related to platelet dysfunction secondary to HES. It should be noted, however, that platelets obtained by mechanical platelet apheresis, both with HES and in the absence of HES, have abnormal epinephrine curves. Nevertheless, these abnormalities were less severe in donors receiving HES; furthermore, glycogen platelet granules are less numerous in platelets from HES donors.[16] In addition, donors receiving HES may have abnormal typing and crossmatching results, especially if HES exceeds 30%. This problem is resolved by a saline replacement technique during crossmatching.[17] HES levels can be monitored by electrophoresis of a serum sample and staining of the bands by PAS.[18] This method, however, may be somewhat cumbersome to institute in the blood bank laboratory for routine testing of HES. Anaphylactoid reactions to HES are occasionally observed in granulocyte donors pretreated with HES; these reactions, though rare, may mimic an anginal attack, with chest pain and difficulty in breathing.[19]

It is therefore necessary to ascertain first whether the donor reacted adversely to past apheresis procedures and then whether the donor has ever had an allergic reaction to any of the medications employed during the procedure. A possible substitute which does not have many of the disadvantages of HES is modified fluid gelatin,[14] although allergic reactions may also be present with gelatin infusions, and may even be more common than with other substitutes.[20] Other much less frequent reactions to HES have been reported, such as lichen planus and erythema multiforme. Erythema multiforme may develop following the use of HES in previously healthy donors who were exposed to HES in previous donations.[21] Similarly, lichen planus has occasionally developed in granulocyte donors receiving HES.[22] However, the single case reported in the literature is difficult to interpret and not statistically significant.[23] One way to avoid some of the adverse effects of HES is to use the proposed low-dose HES method, which has proved to be adequate for leukocyte collection. Using this method, the rate of elimination of HES is increased and the side effects minimized, when compared to standard HES dosage.[24]

Platelets must not be drawn for platelet concentrates if donors have taken aspirin in the preceding 48 hours,[25] due to the negative effect of salicylates on platelet aggregation secondary to acetylation of platelet cyclo-oxygenase.[26] Salicylates may also adversely affect granulocyte function,[27] a fact that should be considered when one is screening donors for granulocytes.

Preapheresis Laboratory Testing

An apheresis donor must meet all the requirements of blood donation. Selection tests include ABO and Rh testing, RBC antibody screening, and hepatitis HB_sAg testing. Donors used to donate platelets or granulocytes can be tested for HLA typing and leukocyte or platelet crossmatching in specialized institutions. Hemoglobin and hematocrit values must be within the ranges required for blood donation (see Chap. 8). The donor platelet count should not be less than 150,000 μl[13] and the plasma protein concentration must not be below 6.0 gm/100 ml.[28]

Donors who donate via apheresis separators on a regular schedule must have their weight checked at every apheresis episode and undergo protein electrophoresis, and these laboratory data should be reviewed at least every 4 months to detect possible adverse effects from the donations.[28] A coagulation profile is routinely done on all donors prior to apheresis and must be within normal limits before the procedure is initiated.

Effects of Apheresis on the Donor and Frequency of Donation

Apheresis depletes donors of both cellular elements and intravascular fluid. The elements depleted depend on what component is separated from the blood during the procedure as well as on losses inherent to the procedure (i.e., loss of whole blood from pretesting and residual blood trapped in the apheresis tubing). The total blood loss during each procedure will determine the frequency of donation. For example, if it is impossible to return the donor's packed cells, because of breakage of tubing or for some other technical reason, deferral of donation for 8 weeks is mandatory. The same waiting period is likewise recommended if donors have recently donated a unit of blood.[28] Blood test samples and residual blood lost at each procedure should not exceed 25 ml of packed cells or 50 ml of whole blood. The volume of blood removed must not exceed 500 ml per cycle, and plasma from no more than 1,000 ml of blood should be retained per each procedure for every 48 hours. During plasmapheresis, plasma from no more than 2,000 ml of blood should be retained over a 7-day period.[28] This rule is based on the observation that even during plateletpheresis, up to 17% of the total plasma protein may be depleted.[29] When patients undergo vigorous exchange (e.g., one-and-a-half plasma volume exchange), replacement of fluid with 5% albumin is recommended. Using half saline and half albumin as replacement in these cases is not recommended, because colloid osmotic pressure may reach 10–12 mm Hg, a level at which pulmonary edema is likely.[30] Furthermore, replacement fluid in plasma exchange is best undertaken with albumin rather than fresh frozen plasma (FFP), for FFP, in addition to carrying the risk of hepatitis, may also lead to a greater incidence of complement activation as well as urticarial reactions.[31] The total annual loss of RBCs should not exceed 2,000 ml of whole blood.[13] These rules can be modified during therapeutic or normal donor plasmapheresis or cytapheresis, but the decision to do so must be made by a qualified physician. Changes in certain physiologic parameters have been observed in donors undergoing leukapheresis with CFC technology. Hemoglobin values may drop by 8% during each procedure, and drops in platelet counts of up to 30,000/cu mm have been observed.[32] These changes may be falsely greater if HES is used to improve separation, mostly due to hemodilution.[33]

Intensive therapeutic plasma exchange (in 17 patients) as is used for reduction of immune complexes results in 25%–50% reduction in fibrinogen, and in factors II, V, VII, VIII, IX, X, XI, XII, and Fletcher factor. However, the PT and APTT usually do not change significantly. Most clotting factors except fibrinogen return to normal after 48 hours. Complement components C3 and C4 can fall by as much as 40% after each exchange and may fall by 50% after three exchanges.[34]

In general, granulocyte counts will not decrease significantly,[35] probably because of entry of extravascular granulocyte pools into the intravascular space. Counts may actually increase by 610 granulocytes/µl using the DFC method for plateletpheresis.[36] In one series, intensive plateletpheresis (10 weekly donations) produced a decrement in the number of lymphocytes, and B cells were significantly decreased in 50% of the donors.[37] In another series, normal donors undergoing cytapheresis had a 23% lower mean lymphocyte count, a 25% lower T cell count, and a 46% lower B cell count. A 27% lower mean immunoglobulin level and a 14% lower mean IgG level were also noted.[38] If heparin is used during any of these procedures, coagulation profiles must be performed before and after apheresis.[32] About 40% of collecting facilities use a twice-weekly schedule for granulocyte donation.[1]

Donor Management

Automated apheresis is not always an innocuous procedure. Donors must sign a detailed consent form before undergoing the procedure. In this consent form, potential complications are discussed. The consent form must be reviewed by the donor with the nurse or physician conducting the screening.

A light meal is recommended before the procedure. Diuretic beverages, such as coffee or tea, are curtailed to avoid having to interrupt the procedure too often. An explanation of the procedure and reassurance prior to starting apheresis helps reduce anxiety and vasovagal reactions, which may result in syncope.[39] Apheresis personnel should ideally be registered nurses who have been especially trained for this procedure. An apheresis worksheet is prepared by the institution where apheresis is performed, and should have a space for recording laboratory test values especially relevant to the procedure, such as hemoglobin, hematocrit, WBC count, platelet count, and coagulation profiles (e.g., thrombin, prothrombin, and partial thromboplastin times) before and after the procedure. Fluid volume removed from the donor as well as fluid infused are recorded. An area in the worksheet for remarks is useful for recording reactions experienced during the procedure.

Donor Reactions

Donor reactions to apheresis occur in approximately 5% of cases.[40] When donor reactions manifest during the procedure, it may be necessary to terminate the procedure. Minor reactions to the anticoagulant or pain at the collection/infusion site can be relieved during the procedure by a temporary interruption of the run. However, significant reactions warrant complete interruption of the procedure and, if feasible, return of blood and plasma to the donor before the procedure is terminated.

Donor reactions can generally be classified as mild, moderate, or severe.

Mild Reactions

Mild reactions are those that do not jeopardize donor welfare and safety to any significant degree. They constitute 94% of the reactions.[1] These reactions include slight hyperventilation, nausea, chills, and dizziness. Many of these reactions are anxiety induced and may be relieved by temporarily suspending the run, distracting the attention of the donor from the procedure, and providing reassurance. The decision to suspend the procedure is a matter of clinical judgment and is best made by the blood bank physician or, in his or her absence, by the apheresis nurse. Mild reactions may become severe, in which case the procedure is terminated. The apheresis procedure cannot resume until mild reactions are under control and the donor is willing to proceed. Measures to correct mild reactions include placing cold compresses behind the head or on the forehead, loosening tight clothing, lowering the donor's head, and raising the donor's lower extremities. Donors who are vomiting are placed in a sitting position.

Paresthesias are not uncommon mild donor reactions. They are thought to be due to transient hypocalcemia induced by calcium-chelating anticoagulants.[41] The duration depends on the rate of reinfusion as well as on the rate of citrate metabolism in the donor.[42] Symptoms should subside in a few minutes. Drinking a glass of milk before apheresis purportedly prevents or minimizes paresthesias during donation. Intravenous calcium injection is not necessary in most of these reactions.[43] Decreasing the reinfusion rate will prevent the appearance of these unpleasant symptoms in most cases. Conversely, reinfusion of citrated blood at rates greater than 1.5 mg/kg/minute may produce paresthesia symptoms in many cases.[44] Chills, muscle twitching, or cramps may also be related to mild hypocalcemia. However, chilliness alone may be due to low room temperature. Other minor, transient reactions seen during CFC for leukapheresis such as perineal or perianal burning are usually due to sensitivity to heparin or dexamethasone.[43]

Anxious donors often hyperventilate, causing respiratory alkalosis and tetany. Hyperventilation is remedied by having the donor rebreathe exhaled CO^2 into a paper bag.

Severe Reactions

Moderate and severe reactions respectively make up 6% and 0.5% of all reactions.[1] In all severe apheresis donor reactions, the apheresis room physician should be notified. Severe hypovolemic reactions often occur when the total extracorporeal volume exceeds 15%–20% of the donor's total volume.[45] However, the threshold varies, depending on the physiologic and hemodynamic status of each donor. Hypovolemia is more frequently seen in donors apheresed with the Haemonetics machine, which draws a greater extracorporeal volume (> 500 cc), than with CFC machines, which draw a smaller extracorporeal volume. When hypovolemic reactions are present, the best management is to stop the procedure and reinfuse as much of the blood volume as is possible. Intravenous saline infusions may be necessary, and notification of the blood bank physician is recommended in all cases. Although mild vasovagal reactions often subside, they may instead progress and produce fainting (syncope). The procedure must be stopped and the donor's extremities raised by tilting the apheresis chair. Reinfusion of the removed volume may not be critical if blood pressure is adequate. Syncope was found to be the most frequent severe reaction to apheresis in one series.[46] Occasionally donors who are premedicated to obtain higher yields of granulocytes may react adversely to these medications. Reactions to HES are very rare. In one large series, 0.03% had mild hypotensive episodes, 0.05% had wheezing, and 0.006% had severe hypotension.[47] Other adverse effects to HES were discussed above.

Rarely, massive clotting in the apheresis bowl may be present, especially in DFC software.[48] Platelet fibrin aggregates may also appear (personal observation). Hemolysis due to kinks in the tubing may be observed.[49]

Other rare but serious complications found during filtration leukapheresis include priapism[50] and abdominal pain. Abdominal pain is seen most often in female donors and simulates menstrual cramps; this reaction can be prevented by giving dexamethasone.[51] Cramps may also be caused by administration of heparin to premenstrual donors.[52] Air embolism is a potentially serious but rare hazard of apheresis. Care should be taken before each run to purge the system of trapped air with priming solutions. If a significant amount of air does enter the system, the procedure is immediately stopped and the donor is placed on his or her left side with the body elevated at the extremities and lowered at the head to prevent a right ventricular "air lock" at the ventricular outlet.[53] This maneuver displaces air away from the ventricular outlet. It is impossible to predict in any given case what amount of air will be dangerous. Studies in dogs indicate that about 200 ml is a lethal dose,[53] but as little as 40 ml has been lethal.[53] Cyanosis, mill-wheel murmur in the precordium, and a marked increase in venous pressure are signs that air embolism has occurred.[54] Air embolism during apheresis is extremely rare.

Special Uses and Storage Procedures for Apheresis Products

Donor plasmapheresis is used mostly for the acquisition of plasma products, such as albumin and factor VIII and factor IX concentrates. Single donor plasmapheresis has been used to obtain high-FVIII-titer cryoprecipitate, as well as for reducing the risk of hepatitis and AIDS in hemophiliacs.[55] Another use of donor apheresis is providing platelets, usually HLA-matched platelets. Less frequently platelet-pheresis is done to provide maternal platelets in neonatal thrombocytopenia (see Chap. 16, on pediatric blood banking). If prolonged storage of apheresis platelets is anticipated (i.e., 48 hours or less), these are best collected into fairly large quantities of plasma (e.g., a 2,000-ml bag rather than a 300-ml bag) to better preserve viability and function. In addition, these platelets are best preserved at 22°–25° C with rotation.[56] This procedure is possible if platelets have been collected using a closed system. Large amounts of ABO-incompatible plasma in units obtained by apheresis must be reduced by differential centrifugation immediately prior to infusion. Hemolytic reactions due to infusion of ABO-incompatible plasma in such units have been reported.[57] Another application of donor apheresis is to obtain granulocytes for transfusion. Most institutions preserve these units at 22°–25° C; other facilities, however, continue to store these units at 4° C.[1] Functionally, granulocytes obtained by cytapheresis using the Fenwall CS-3000 or the IBM 2997 machines are normal, as compared to controls.[58] Less frequent applications of cytapheresis include obtaining erythroid progenitor cells[59] as well as other special cell populations such as lymphocytes and monocytes (see Chap. 8).

THERAPEUTIC APHERESIS

One of the more difficult problems the blood bank physician encounters is evaluating if the need for therapeutic plasmapheresis is truly indicated.

There are few definite indications for therapeutic apheresis. Other uses remain in the realm of clinical experimentation and should be evaluated as such. Since the procedure is not innocuous, documentation that a certain application of apheresis for a particular disease has been successful is recommendable. If, however, reports of success in treating such disease by apheresis are not available, the procedure must be considered experimental, and evaluated by a human subjects committee.

A consent form containing a short explanation of the procedure must be reviewed and signed by the patient before the apheresis treatment is initiated. A physical examination and appropriate laboratory tests are performed prior to the procedure and a worksheet is prepared to monitor each session. These forms differ slightly from forms used for apheresis donation. A space is usually provided for a short clinical history, an explanation of why the treatment has been selected, and a list of parameters to be monitored during the treatment.

A consent form must be signed by the patient or legal guardian and possible complications reviewed carefully, preferably by a blood bank physician. The blood bank physician must evaluate the general status of the patient before accepting him or her as a subject for what may prove to be a potentially harmful procedure. The therapeutic apheresis worksheet is slightly different from the donor worksheet. A space for the treating physician to give a short clinical history of the patient is very useful. The rationale for using apheresis as a therapeutic tool, expected parameters of improvement, and expected duration of the overall treatment should be recorded on the worksheet. Blood type and hematologic and immunologic parameters before and after apheresis must be recorded, as well as the input and output of fluids.

Therapeutic apheresis procedures can be used to remove plasma, platelets, blood cells, and other selected substances and selected cell populations.

Therapeutic Plasmapheresis

Plasmapheresis is of therapeutic value only if the causes or symptoms of the disease are related to a factor present in the patient's plasma. During therapeutic plasmapheresis the putative factor can be removed by retrieval of plasma, followed by return to the patient of his or her own cellular elements. However, this form of therapy is of little use if the noxious plasma factor is produced faster than it can be removed. Conditions influencing synthesis/removal rates include (1) rate of synthesis of the toxin, (2) rate of removal, (3) extravascular volume of the noxious factor, and (4) catabolic rate of the noxious factor.

Intravascular substances, which are not distributed in the extravascular space, are more accessible to removal than substances that shift in and out of the extravascular space.

If the substance is isolated in the intravascular space and the replacing fluid does not contain this substance, the impact of removal can be calculated by formulas 1, 2, and 3:

$$(1) \quad \frac{Y}{Y_o} = e^{-x}$$

where Y is the measured concentration of the substance to be removed, Y_o is the starting concentration of the substance, e is the constant (2.71828), and x is the volume of plasma exchanged per pass. Discontinuous exchanges are calculated as follows:

$$(2) \quad \frac{Y}{Y_o} = \left(\frac{V - \Delta X}{V}\right)^n$$

$$(3) \quad \frac{Y}{Y_o} = \left(\frac{V}{V + \Delta X}\right)^n$$

where V is the plasma volume, $[X]$ is the amount of volume exchanged per pass, and n is the number of passes. Formula 2 calculates exchange before replacement, formula 3 calculates exchange after replacements. Expected results per exchange are shown in Table 9–1.

Although no set parameters have been established regarding the duration and the size of a plasma exchange, an accepted protocol is to remove 1.5 times the plasma volume twice a week for 2 weeks and then once weekly[60] until the desired plasma value target is achieved. Typically patients will tolerate the procedure for about 5 hours without any major difficulty, but one may have to stop the procedure earlier in patients with lower tolerance. The success of the procedure is higher in diseases where the presence of the noxious substance is transient (e.g., acute hemolysis). The procedure is usually of transient benefit only in patients with chronic plasma elevations of the noxious substance (for example, in patients with dysproteinemias such as myeloma). These aspects must be considered in weighing the advantages versus the disadvantages of therapeutic apheresis before subjecting patients to a potentially dangerous procedure.

In one study, where no more than 9 L of plasma was removed per week during plasma exchange, 0.4% of the patients had serious post-plasma exchange complications. These ranged from myocardial infarction and pulmonary embolism to unexplained death.[61]

Therapeutic plasmapheresis has been used for two main types of diseases, those in which a particular protein causes a hyperviscosity syndrome and those in which a circulating substance causes damage to tissues.

Plasmapheresis for Treating Hyperviscosity Syndromes

The hyperviscosity syndrome is seen almost exclusively in malignant gammopathies such as Waldenström's macroglobulinemia and malignant myeloma.

An increment in γ-globulins to the extent seen in macroglobulinemia or myeloma may bring about an increase in the viscosity of plasma. Dangerous side effects of hyperviscosity include vascular impairment, with damage to tissues supplied by the impaired vessels. When serum viscosity is greater than 4 times the viscosity of water, clinically significant hyperviscosity is considered to be present. Although diseases associated with hyperviscosity are primarily treated with chemotherapy, acute reductions in serum hyperviscosity are often necessary and can be achieved via automated plasmapheresis.[62] No other therapy decreases serum viscosity as effectively and as rapidly as plasmapheresis, which makes it a universally accepted therapeutic modality.[63] Patients with paraproteinemias suffering from the hyperviscosity syndrome and who are treated by plasmapheresis should be monitored with serum viscosity tests. This test is useful to determine serum paraprotein levels at which patients become asymptomatic.[64] The clinical improvement of vascular insufficiency in these diseases is correlated with a decrease to below 4 times the viscosity of water. Abnormal clotting[65] and renal failure[66] may also improve after a partial exchange. A one-plasma

TABLE 9–1.—% OF NOXIOUS SUBSTANCES REMOVED AFTER CONTINUOUS PLASMA EXCHANGE*

NO. OF VOLUMES EXCHANGED	% SUBSTANCE REMOVED
1	63.2
2	86.5
3	95

*Adapted from Tullis.[2]

volume exchange (2–3 L of plasma) may be necessary to improve symptoms. This volume exchange can be repeated every other day. Patients usually tolerate replacement with crystalloid after a one-half plasma volume exchange and are routinely given 5% albumin as replacement after 1.5 L has been exchanged. To avoid the risk of hepatitis and allergic reactions, fresh frozen plasma (FFP) should be curtailed until a coagulopathy from decrement of plasma clotting factors is proved on a coagulation profile. Plasmapheresis can be discontinued when the serum viscosity is below 4 poise. Clotting parameters may be altered after a one-plasma volume exchange and may require replacement with FFP,[60] especially in patients who are already hemostatically compromised.[67] Complement components will also be decreased during extensive plasma exchange with albumin replacement alone.[1, 68] The use of FFP to replenish complement stores may be justified after very aggressive plasmapheresis.

Electrolyte levels do not usually suffer dramatic changes during plasma exchange, because of effective body electrolyte homeostatic mechanisms.[60] However, levels of ionized calcium may drop to 1.25 mEq/L and citrate levels may reach 2.3 m/L during rapid exchanges; nevertheless, calcium values usually return to normal within 15 minutes after the procedure is concluded.[69] In most cases, these ion changes do not require intravenous replacement.[60]

Plasmapheresis in Diseases With Circulating Immune Complexes

Certain autoimmune disorders such as systemic lupus erythematosus, rapidly progressive glomerulonephritis, myasthenia gravis, and rheumatoid arthritis cause the appearance of immune complexes (IC), which are thought to be responsible for most of the tissue damage observed in these diseases.

Circulating IC can be reduced by partial plasma exchange and presumably improve the outcome in some of these diseases.[1] Although apheresis treatment for these diseases has a place in therapy, results may be quite variable and difficult to interpret. Measurement of IC in the clinical laboratory has been uneven and does not always correlate with evolution, severity, or duration of disease.[70] In one series only 50% of patients treated with plasmapheresis for systemic lupus erythematosus showed improvement. Of this group, all had demonstrable DNA anti-DNA complexes;[71] however, in another series improvement was seen after the exchange even in the absence of circulating IC.[72] Improvement has been demonstrated by morphological evidence of removal of IC from the glomerular tuft and by improvement in renal function.[73] Nevertheless, such a correlation has not been found by all workers. Improvement in these cases is thought to be due to "unblocking" of splenic macrophage Fc receptors secondary to removal of IC by the apheresis procedure. This removal would explain improvement despite relatively high circulating IC levels.[70] Short-term improvement in rapidly progressive glomerulonephritis associated with pulmonary hemorrhage (Goodpasture's syndrome) has been demonstrated in some cases after using a combination of corticosteroids, cyclophosphamide, and partial plasma exchange.[74–76] Patients already in renal failure did not improve on this protocol.[77] Improvement was manifested by disappearance of pulmonary hemorrhages and an overall increase in short-term patient survival, from 50% to 80%, when both plasmapheresis and immunosuppressive therapy were used simultaneously.[63] However, both long-term renal function improvement and overall patient survival were unpredictable. Control studies using plasma exchange alone have not been conducted, and the full role of partial plasma exchange remains to be determined.

Partial plasma exchange has also been used as adjunct therapy in myasthenia gravis (MG) in a small group of patients. Improvement was purportedly shown by a decrease in the required dosage of anticholinesterase drugs.[78] In this study it was suggested that care be taken when replacing these patients with FFP, for they tend to form anaphylactoid antibodies to infused FFP more frequently than patients plasmapheresed for other diseases.[78] It is difficult to evaluate the precise role of plasmapheresis in patients with MG in most of the reported series, because these patients were receiving other immunosuppressive therapy concomitantly with the plasmapheresis treatment.[79, 80] Only one truly controlled prospective study has been undertaken to assess treatment of MG by plasmapheresis.[81] In addition, uniform success in the treatment of MG using plasmapheresis and immunosuppression has not been documented to date.[81] Because only short-term improvement has been achieved using plasmapheresis to treat this disease, and because it is an expensive procedure, it is recommended that partial exchange be used only during crises, and only after other conventional therapeutic measures have failed.[82] A 2-L plasma exchange, daily for 5 consecutive days, employing albumin as replacement fluid, has been recommended as a good protocol. This protocol can be repeated after 2–3 weeks.[83] It must be stressed here that some of these patients are acutely ill and may not be able to tolerate the procedure, so careful consideration must be given to some of the disadvantages of apheresis when planning to treat these patients by plasma exchange.

Rheumatoid arthritis has been treated by partial plasma exchange, but only as an adjunct to gold salts and penicillamine.[84] Plasmapheresis in the treatment of rheumatoid arthritis should probably be reserved to increase effectiveness of standard therapy when patients become unresponsive to it.[85]

Other diseases in which plasmapheresis has been used successfully for short-term improvement are Raynaud's disease,[86] Crohn's disease,[87] and multiple sclerosis.[88] Less frequent indications for plasmapheresis are (1) to decrease plasma volume in order to replenish procoagulants,[89] and (2) to eliminate protein-bound nondialyzable toxins such as α-amanitin in mushroom poisoning.[90] Diseases in which plasmapheresis has proved to be of doubtful benefit to the patient and the beneficial effects are mostly anecdotal are pemphigus vulgaris,[91] asthma,[92] and carcinomatosis.[93] See Table 9–2 for other applications of apheresis.

Diseases in which plasmapheresis is usually of no benefit include hepatic coma[94] and chronic idiopathic thrombocytopenic purpura.[95] However, intensive plasma exchange has been used successfully (with remission of 9–24 months) to treat acute immune thrombocytopenic purpura (ITP) refractory to steroids. No benefit was seen in this study for patients with chronic ITP.[96] Plasma exchange to treat thrombotic thrombocytopenic purpura (TTP) has been employed and reported to be successful. In most studies, serum antiplatelet IgG and circulatory IC as revealed by C1q levels were used to assess successful plasma exchange therapy for TTP. However, most reports of improvement of TTP by plasma exchange are anecdotal and represent single case studies not controlled prospectively. Furthermore, most of these studies only report those cases of TTP in which plasma exchange proved to be suc-

TABLE 9–2.—Applications of Therapeutic Plasmapheresis

DISEASE	CLINICAL USEFULNESS*	SUBSTANCE REMOVED†	TREATMENT‡	EXCHANGE PROTOCOL	REFERENCE
HEMATOLOGIC					
Paraproteinemia, Waldenström's	A	IgM			62
Paraproteinemia, myeloma	A	IgG	P		66
TTP	A	IC	P, S		97
Refractory ITP	C	IgG	P		96
Posttransfusion purpura	A	IgG	P, S		154
Autoimmune hemolytic anemia	C	IgG	P		155
Factor VIII inhibitors	C	IgG (IgG4)	P		156
Pure erythrocyte aplasia	E	?			157
RENAL					
Goodpasture's syndrome	A	Anti-GBM IgG	P		74
Refractory progressive SLE	C	Non-anti-GBM, IgG, IC	P, CT	3/wk, 2 wk	70
Rapidly progressive glomerulonephritis	C	IC			158
NEUROLOGIC					
Myasthenia gravis	A	IgG + CI	P, S	3/wk, 2 wk	79
Multiple sclerosis	E	IgG + CI			88
Amyotrophic lateral sclerosis	C	IC? + CI			159
Guillain-Barré syndrome	C	IC + CI			160
OTHER					
Polymyositis	C	IC			161
Thyrotoxicosis	A	TH			162
Protein-bound poisons	A	PP			90
Carcinomatosis	E	IgG4?			93
Systemic vasculitis	C	Ig			163
Familial hypercholesterolemia	C	LP			164
Rheumatoid arthritis	C	IC	P, O		84

*A, accepted; C, controversial; E, experimental.
†GBM, glomerular basement membrane; IC, immune complex; CI, cellular immunity; PP, plasma protein; LP, lipoprotein.
‡P, plasma/exchange; S, steroids; CT, cytotoxic therapy; O, other.

cessful.[97] Therefore, the use of extensive plasmapheresis in this disease remains investigational and by no means should be considered the standard mode of therapy for TTP until controlled prospective studies are undertaken.

Hazards and Costs of Therapeutic Plasmapheresis

Therapeutic apheresis, like donor apheresis, is not an innocuous procedure. Minor donor complications (e.g., vasovagal reactions, citrate toxicity, hematomata) were reviewed earlier and are applicable to patients undergoing therapeutic apheresis. More serious complications include formation of thromboemboli[29, 30, 68] and hemolysis.[49] A hemostatic imbalance is theoretically possible by large volume replacement with albumin infusions, which lack procoagulants.[67] Prolonged plasmapheresis may produce dangerous thrombocytopenia and potentially low levels of lipoproteins, leading to the development of atherosclerosis.[98] The most disturbing results of therapeutic plasmapheresis are the five reported deaths that occurred during plasma exchange. Two of these deaths occurred in patients who were in good clinical condition before the procedure.[99]

Another serious consideration is that plasmapheresis is an expensive procedure. The total cost of an apheresis treatment may reach $20,000.[100]

Experimental Plasmapheresis Techniques

Experimentally, it has been possible to separate substances from plasma on a selective basis. However, there are two major drawbacks: (1) embolization of adsorbing material, and (2) thrombocytopenia from platelet aggregation and adhesion to the adsorbent material.[101] The adsorbing material is encased in a column which is connected on-line to the return tubing. Plasma is then pumped through the column and back into the patient via the return tubing.

Activated charcoal-coated glass beads have been used to adsorb bile acids from plasma of severely icteric patients to relieve pruritus. These columns remove approximately 590 ± 206 μmoles of bile acids, resulting in a 65% drop in the skin bile acid concentration.[102] Plasma cholesterol levels in hypercholesterolemic patients can be lowered via heparin-agarose columns,[103] and IgG has been selectively removed with protein A columns in myeloma and autoimmune hemolytic anemia, with promising results.[101] DNA-trapping charcoal columns have been devised to adsorb DNA/anti-DNA IC in patients with SLE on an experimental basis, with promising results.[104] Protein A filters have been used to "unblock" IgG antibodies experimentally to treat disseminated carcinomatosis in dogs.[101] This method was also applied to a patient, with reportedly good results.[105]

Similarly, immunoadsorption using protein "A" sepharose columns has been used effectively in dogs for the selective removal of IgG.[106]

It should be noted that these columns are to date unavailable commercially and the procedures strictly experimental. Furthermore, most reports are anecdotal and not statistically significant. In most of these cases other treatment was given concomitantly and the purportedly beneficial results have not been critically compared with plasma exchange alone. However, the idea of using filters which clear the autologous plasma from pathogenic material is appealing in that the risk of transmitting hepatitis from extraneous FFP,[107] as well as the risk of immunization to other antigens present in extraneous FFP, is obviated by reinfusion of the patient's own plasma.[100] Nevertheless, the dangers of therapeutic plasmapheresis are present with this treatment modality, in addition to the previously mentioned thrombocytopenia, potential embolization of adsorbent material, and potential patient reactions from activation of complement.[103]

Therapeutic Cytapheresis

Selective cytapheresis has been used to remove a variety of unwanted cells from whole blood in patients with diseases caused by neoplastic and non-neoplastic cells. Although cytapheresis has been used to treat both acute and chronic diseases, its most successful application has been in the treatment of diseases in which an acute reduction of cell numbers is required. No other therapy will reduce these usually neoplastic cell populations as fast as selective cytapheresis, making it the procedure of choice in certain cases.[108]

Automated erythrocytapheresis has been used successfully in sickle cell disease to exchange sickle cells and for normal RBCs in sickle cell crises.[109]

Therapeutic plateletpheresis is frequently used prophylactically to prevent thrombosis in the acute management of both primary thrombocytosis and in polycythemia vera when the platelet count exceeds 1 million/μl.[110] A 6-hour automated apheresis run can decrease the platelet count by 50%. Chronic plateletpheresis for these patients has produced controversial results and therefore is not recommended.[108]

Leukostasis secondary to very high WBC counts may be complicated by thrombosis in patients with chronic granulocytic leukemia. Leukapheresis has been used successfully to decrease counts acutely as a temporizing measure until chemotherapy reduces the WBC count for more prolonged periods of time.[111] Therapeutic leukapheresis has been used similarly in acute myelocytic and promyelocytic leukemia.[108] The procedure dramatically alleviates symptoms for short periods of time. Long-term leukapheresis for patients with chronic granulocytic leukemia has not yielded satisfactory results;[108] this was demonstrated in a prospective study in which intensive chronic leukapheresis was employed as the sole therapeutic modality. This treatment failed to improve survival of patients with chronic myelogenous leukemia as compared to controls who received chemotherapy alone.[112] Nevertheless, intensive leukapheresis has proved to be of some benefit in chronic lymphocytic leukemia.[113] Isolated reports of improvement in hairy cell leukemia after intensive leukapheresis have also been published.[114,115] Intensive leukocytapheresis has been used to induce remissions in the pancytopenic phase of hairy cell leukemia, prolonging remission and thereby reducing the patient's transfusion requirements.[115] Leukapheresis has likewise been successfully employed to reduce leukostasis in patients suffering hairy cell leukemia and exhibiting counts greater than $5 \times 10^6/\mu l$.[116] Similarly, leukapheresis has helped improve the clinical states of skin lesions in patients with the Sézary syndrome.[117,118] However, reports on leukapheresis for treating the latter two diseases were isolated and not prospectively controlled; they must therefore be considered anecdotal. Lymphocytapheresis has been used successfully, albeit experimentally, in a few patients as adjunctive therapy for autoimmune diseases such as rheumatoid arthritis.[119] The long-term effect of cytapheresis in these diseases is not known.

MANAGEMENT TECHNIQUES FOR AN APHERESIS PROGRAM

Facilities

Blood banks with hemapheresis facilities for donors or patients should ideally have an area specially designated for these procedures; if possible, the donor apheresis area should be separate from the patient apheresis area. The same criteria for a blood donor room apply to the apheresis room. This room should be pleasant and provide privacy for the donor or patient undergoing the procedure. Approximately 300 sq ft of floor space per patient or apheresis machine is adequate.[120] Apheresis procedures may last 6 hours or longer, so the apheresis chair should be designed for maximum comfort.

Personnel

Ideally, apheresis machines should be operated by registered nurses with special training in apheresis techniques. Laboratory technicians, too, have often proved to be good apheresis managers.[120] A year's experience in an active apheresis department (two or more apheresis procedures scheduled at least once daily) is desirable before a nurse or technician can be considered adequately trained in apheresis. Personality, attitude, and motivation of nurses in this area are of paramount importance to good donor and patient care. In active apheresis programs, scheduled chart reviews and scheduled therapeutic and replacement sessions are mandatory. The blood bank physician is responsible for reviewing general preapheresis laboratory testing as well as HLA testing and analysis of parameters to evaluate therapeutic effectiveness of the procedure (e.g., serum viscosity in Waldenström's microglobulinemia).

Donor Recruitment

In large facilities, donor recruiters must be educated in hemapheresis donor procedures in order to convey both the importance of this type of donation and the details of the procedure to prospective donors to the general blood donor pool.

Apheresis Control

The only way to prevent abuse of the apheresis facility and overloading of the nursing staff is by establishing priorities for use of apheresis machines and criteria for extent and duration of therapy. A predefined and publicly known apheresis room schedule is vital. Most apheresis procedures for clinical indications are elective and can be scheduled in advance; "emergency" apheresis must not be allowed to become the rule. Contingency plans for emergencies can be covered on an overtime and "on call" basis, and usually can be triaged according to the severity of the disease. In exceptional cases elective procedures can be cancelled to provide for emergency cases. The decision on what constitutes an emergency is made by the blood bank director in consultation with the treating physician. Emergency cases or severely ill patients who must undergo hemapheresis are best handled in intensive care units or in emergency rooms, not in donor rooms or apheresis rooms, because adequate equipment and personnel to treat emergencies are usually not immediately available.

In scheduling donors, the apheresis room physician must preplan with the treating physicians the needs of patients for granulocyte or platelet support. Usually patients receiving aggressive chemotherapy for leukemia will become markedly thrombocytopenic and neutropenic by the first week and will remain so for 2–3 weeks after chemotherapy. It is recommendable to plan for platelet and granulocyte support during this period.[121] HLA-matched platelets can be obtained from single donors and a computerized file maintained. A part of preapheresis planning is to obtain patient samples for HLA matching as soon as possible.

The fiscal administration of an apheresis program is of utmost importance in today's prospective payment health care environment. The cost of the procedure includes surgical supplies (disposable bowl, tubing, syringes, etc.), laboratory testing of donor samples and blood products, preapheresis and postapheresis testing, and nursing staff expenses. The average cost of a 6-hour run varies between $300 and $400, depending on the time of day and the day of the week in which the procedure is scheduled, because of personnel overtime expenses.

AUTOLOGOUS TRANSFUSION

If blood is viewed as a tissue transplant, the most compatible match is the patient's own blood. Each patient can donate only a certain amount of blood at a time without developing hypovolemic anemia. A variety of strategies have been designed to cope with this problem while providing the patient with the alternative of autologous transfusion. Autologous transfusion is advantageous because there is virtually no risk of immunization to RBC, WBC, or platelet antigens or to plasma proteins. Errors in typing and crossmatching can be completely eliminated (presuming adequate identification of the unit has been adhered to), and the risks of transmitting hepatitis or other blood-borne infections to the recipient are significantly minimized.[122]

Screening Patients for Predeposit Phlebotomy

The phlebotomy procedure must not jeopardize the general condition of the patient. The major question the physician should ask himself or herself is whether it is safer for the patient to give blood or to receive it.[123] It is always advisable for a physician to be available on the premises, both to assist in the procedure, should blood volume decrease in a compromised patient resulting in complications, and to adjudicate departures from standard criteria for blood donation. The customary age and weight criteria may have to be adjusted, depending on the case at hand. Usually children with sufficiently large veins can tolerate the procedure adequately.[124] No more than 450 ± 45 ml or the equivalent of 12% of the calculated blood volume, whichever is lower, should be drawn at any one time.[124]

To calculate the amount of anticoagulant removed from the collection bag for collections smaller than 40 ml in patients weighing less than 110 pounds, the following formula is used:[124]

$$\text{Residual anticoagulant (ml)} = V_1 \left(\frac{VB}{450}\right)$$

where V_1 = citrate-phosphate-dextrose in a 450-ml collection bag and VB = patient weight in pounds × 450, divided by 110.

The hemoglobin value should be greater than 11 gm/100 ml and the hematocrit greater than 34%.[124] Although hemoglobin production may be increased up to 5 times in normal donors receiving supplementary iron who undergo frequent phlebotomy,[125] it is unwise for a patient to donate more frequently than every 4 days.[124] This rate is partially based on the observation that at least 72 hours are required to recover intravascular proteins completely in normal donors.[126] Iron supplementation in autologous transfusion programs is strongly suggested for patients who need to be drawn frequently[127] and is started several days before the first phlebotomy,[128] with 70 mg of elemental iron each day.[127] Patients can safely donate 4–5 predeposit phlebotomy units of blood if they are in relatively good physical condition and can tolerate the procedure provided 4- to 5-day intervals are observed between donations.[128] Although most studies have been performed on patients in relatively optimal physical condition, studies have also shown satisfactory results in patients scheduled for elective open heart surgery.[129] This by no means precludes careful evaluation and selection of patients for autologous transfusion. Before any predeposit autologous transfusion is performed, a consent form describing the advantages and potential hazards of the procedure must be signed by the patient. The patient must also sign the label on the unit and the collection bag after it is drawn but before it is separated from the phlebotomy line. This practice ensures positive identification of the unit. Units for autologous transfusion are labeled "for autologous use only" and are kept on a separate shelf in the blood bank refrigerator. Under no circumstances should these units be used for other patients unless the blood bank physician explicitly permits it.

Current Methods for Autologous Transfusion

There are two main types of autologous transfusion: predeposit autologous transfusion[130] and intraoperative autologous transfusion.[131] Each is described below.

Predeposit Autologous Transfusion

In predeposit autologous transfusion, donor criteria may be modified by the blood bank and the treating physicians, provided each case is individually evaluated to decide the safest strategy. The choice of type of deposit transfusion is between liquid storage predeposit autologous transfusion (LSPAT) and frozen storage predeposit autologous transfusion (FSPAT).[128]

Liquid Storage Predeposit Autologous Transfusion (LSPAT).—The storage of blood predeposited by this method can be in the amount of 1–2 units for minor surgery or up to 5–6 units. When more than 2 units are necessary, the "leapfrog" technique is recommended.[124] A calendar of 29 days is prepared. On day 1, 1 unit is withdrawn. On day 8 units 2 and 3 are withdrawn and unit 1 is reinfused. On day 15, units 4 and 5 are withdrawn and unit 2 is reinfused. On day 22, units 6 and 7 are withdrawn and unit 3 is reinfused. Finally, on day 29, units 8 and 9 are withdrawn and unit 4 is reinfused. In this way, units 5 to 9 are available for surgery. Units 8 and 9 will be fresh, units 6 and 7 will be 1 week old, and unit 5 will be 2 weeks old.[124] By use of a Y-set connector a single vein technique is possible whereby the same line through which blood is withdrawn is used to infuse the older unit.[124] These dates can be modified accordingly for CPD-A.

The major advantages of liquid storage over frozen storage are that blood is immediately available, it does not have the short expiration time of frozen-thawed cells (24 hours) after thawing, it is less costly than frozen-thawed units, and the equipment to store and produce liquid units is readily available in most blood banks.

Patients with a history of hepatitis must not predeposit blood in the frozen state because the washing procedure exposes blood bank technologists to a high risk of hepatitis.[129] Another indication for liquid versus frozen storage is in patients with sickle cell anemia, in whom glycerolization with routine glycerolizing solutions is contraindicated because glycerol is not properly washed from these units.[132, 133]

One disadvantage of liquid storage is that it produces increments in plasma potassium content, lactate, ammonia, and hemoglobin levels, as well as a drop in pH.[134] When prolonged storage is warranted or when storage time is unpredictable it is better to glycerolize and freeze units.

Somewhat different techniques for liquid storage are used when intraoperative hemodilution is contemplated. Hemodilution is the artificial production of low hemoglobin levels to induce vasoconstriction, decrease viscosity, and thus improve organ flow perfusion, thereby reducing the need for transfusion of units withdrawn immediately before surgery.[135] In patients who are to undergo hemodilution, certain authors suggest that volumes of up to 2,000 ml of blood be withdrawn at the time patients receive replacement with dextran or albumin, until the hematocrit is lowered to about 25%.[136] This method allows loss of up to 2,000 ml during surgery. However, most clinicians prefer not to replace more than 1,000 ml of blood with colloid or crystalloid.[135] Withdrawal and replacement for hemodilution should be done when the patient is in the operating room, to minimize possible mistakes in identification of the unit.

Frozen Storage Predeposit Autologous Transfusion (FSPAT).—Frozen storage of RBCs has revolutionized autologous transfusion, especially for elective surgery, and its use is ideal for patients who lack high-incidence antigens and have developed antibodies to most units, or who have produced multiple antibodies. Screening of donors should follow other donor screening standards. If units are acceptable, they can be used by other recipients in case the patient does not use them.[137] Patients with rare phenotypes are encouraged to predeposit units for autologous transfusion, should they ever need transfusions. It is not unlikely that some of these units will be available for other patients if the units are acceptable. The strategy for thawing units depends on the estimated needs during the procedure. If the procedure calls for few units, about half the autologous units available can be thawed just before surgery. More units are then thawed according to need. This tactic minimizes unnecessary outdating and deglycerolizing expenditure. However, if the anticipated needs are great and supplies of autologous units are low, it may be necessary to infuse homologous units first and finish the procedure with autologous units, so autologous cells will be more abundant once hemostasis is achieved.[137] For more details on frozen-thawed blood, see chapter 8.

Clinical Uses of Predeposit Autologous Transfusions

Perhaps the most important use of predeposit autologous transfusion is in patients with antibodies that preclude transfusion of homologous blood and who intend to undergo elective surgery.[123] However, other patients who don't have positive screens are also participating in predeposit programs (e.g., in orthopedic surgery). As stated above, predeposit autologous transfusion precludes sensitization and minimizes infection of the patient donor. Although autologous transfusions have traditionally been used in elective surgery with small needs, it has also been successfully used in cardiovascular surgery.[138, 139]

Patients with defective cells who require autologous transfusions are best handled by liquid storage, but in certain cases, frozen predeposit may have to be used to meet prolonged storage requirements (e.g., in patients with the S/A trait who may need frozen predeposited cells, deglycerolizing solutions have been modified).[137]

Autologous transfusions have been used, albeit less frequently, for other clinical situations in which patients tend to become sensitized to plasma proteins (e.g., IgA-deficient individuals with anti-IgA antibodies). Another potential use for autologous transfusion is in patients who for religious reasons cannot accept homologous transfusions but can accept autologous transfusions.[140]

Intraoperative RBC Salvage

The first attempt at intraoperative blood salvage was performed by Blundell in 1818;[141] however, the first successful intraoperative blood salvage using anticoagulated blood with sodium phosphate was undertaken by John Duncan in 1886.[142] Nevertheless, these methods remained rudimentary until the work of Wilson and Taswell,[143] who introduced a version of the Latham bowl to salvage blood intraoperatively in a variety of procedures.

There are two basic types of intraoperative cell salvage systems. In one system the blood is aspirated from the surgical field and anticoagulated in the aspiration tubing. The blood is then filtered through microaggregate filters and collected in a reservoir prior to reinfusion into the patient. The second system employs an automated cell washer which is almost identical in principle to the blood cell separators reviewed earlier in this chapter. The blood is aspirated from the field, simultaneously anticoagulated, and pumped into the blood processor's centrifuge bowl. In the bowl it is washed with saline and reinfused into the patient.

Filtration Method

Several filtration systems are commercially available. Two of the more popular ones are reviewed below.

The Bentley ATS-100 autotransfuser and the Sorenson ATS system both use microaggregate filters to eliminate particulate material sucked from the surgical field. The Bentley device uses a peristaltic pump and the Sorenson device uses wall vaccuum to force the blood through the filter. Both systems require anticoagulation, either in vivo or of the blood as it enters the tubing. The two systems are relatively inexpensive and the blood is immediately available. A disturbing feature of the product obtained by these methods is the presence in the filtrate of thromboplastinic substances, muscle debris, fat globules, and tissue enzymes, which are capable of triggering disseminated intravascular coagulation.[144] However, in the experience of some authors, this does not occur. It has been shown, for instance, that blood collected from the mediastinum during open heart surgery does not clot, due to defibrination. This inhibition of clotting may be due to inhibition by antithrombin III of activated clotting factors.[145] Although it was initially thought that reinfused salvaged mediastinal blood would improve clotting,[146] these same authors later showed that platelets in this fluid have expended their β-thromboglobulin and no longer promote hemostasis.[147] It is recommended by these authors that blood obtained during trauma surgery be anticoagulated, washed, and filtered of debris before infusion.[148]

Blood contaminated with fat or bacteria is to be avoided, for current washing procedures do not eliminate these harmful contaminants.[148] Other complications include bleeding due to systemic anticoagulation, and the low hematocrit and high free hemoglobin of the filtered product.[142]

Intraoperative Automated RBC Salvage

One of the more popular machines is the Haemonetics Cell Saver. This machine operates on the same principle as the Haemonetics model 30. If a hospital has a Haemonetics model 30, it can be adapted for cell saving. The system retrieves blood from the surgical field, and after initial filtration the fluid enters the bowl, where the RBCs are washed with saline. The advantage of this system is that the patient receives only washed, packed RBCs which are almost free of tissue debris and free hemoglobin, thus minimizing the risk of disseminated intravascular coagulation and fat emboli. A disadvantage to this system is the length of the washing procedure (about 20 minutes before the patient can get 300–500 cc of packed cells). In addition, the machine costs about $9,000, occupies operating room floor space, and requires an additional person in the surgical suite to operate it, though sometimes anesthesia personnel undertake this responsibility. However, intraoperative cell salvage, along with priming the cardiopulmonary bypass machine with crystalloid solutions rather than blood,[149] has resulted in reductions of up to 25% in blood use in open heart surgery,[150] although not all workers have achieved such results.[151, 152] Differences in heparin dosage may account for the differences in blood use in these cases.[150–152]

Contraindications to Intraoperative Blood Salvage

Definite contraindications to blood salvage exist during certain types of surgery. For instance, most abdominal surgery, where the potential for spilling intestinal contents exists, is an absolute contraindication to any type of intraoperative RBC salvage. This contraindication is also true for grossly contaminated wounds,[149] cancer surgery, and in general any kind of surgery producing extensive tissue crushing or debris that is capable of releasing highly thromboplastic material (e.g., brain tissue).[153]

REFERENCES

1. French J.E., Solomon J.M., Fratantoni J.C.: Survey on the current use of leukapheresis and the collection of granulocyte concentrates. *Transfusion* 22:220, 1982.
2. Tullis J.L.: Separation and purification of leukocytes and platelets. *Blood* 7:891, 1952.
3. Tullis J.L., Tinch R.J., Baudanza P., et al.: Plateletpheresis in a disposable system. *Transfusion* 7:232, 1971.
4. *Owner's Operating and Maintenance Manual: Model 30 Cell Separator Blood Processor*. Braintree, Mass., Haemonetics Corp., 1978, p. 6.1.
5. Nusbacher J., Sher M.L., MacPherson J.L.: Plateletpheresis using the Haemonetics Model 30 cell separator. *Vox Sang.* 33:9, 1977.
6. Morales M., Pizzuto J., Reyna Ma., et al.: Use of heparin for cytapheresis and plasmapheresis in a continuous flow centrifuge. *Transfusion* 22:384, 1982.
7. Nusbacher J., MacPherson M.S.: A comparison of techniques for leukapheresis and plateletpheresis, in Nusbacher J., Berkman E.M. (eds.): *Fundamentals of a Pheresis Program: A Technical Workshop*. Washington, D.C., American Association of Blood Banks, 1979, p. 49.
8. Hogge D.E., Schiffer C.A.: Collection of platelets depleted of red cells and white cells with the 'surge pump" adaptation of a blood cell separator. *Transfusion* 23:177, 1983.
9. Hester J.P., Kellogg R.M., Mulzet A.P., et al.: Principles of blood separation and component extraction in a disposable continuous-flow single-stage channel. *Blood* 54:254, 1979.
10. Wuertz E.M.: Blood collection by pheresis, in Dawson R.B., Fletcher J.L. (eds.).: *Donor Room Procedures: A Technical Workshop*. Washington, D.C., American Association of Blood Banks, 1981, p. 67.
11. Widman F.K. (ed.): *Technical Manual of the American Association of Blood Banks*, ed. 8. Washington, D.C., American Association of Blood Banks, 1981, pp. 344–345.
12. Borucki D.T. (ed.): *Blood Component Therapy: A Physician's Handbook*, ed. 3. Washington, D.C., American Association of Blood Banks, 1981, p. 6.
13. Katz A.J.: Donor selection for pheresis donation, in Nusbacher J., Berkman E.M. (eds.): *Fundamentals of a Pheresis Program: A Technical Workshop*. Washington, D.C., American Association of Blood Banks, 1979, p. 35.
14. Rock G., Wise P., Kardish R., et al.: Modified fluid gelatin in leukapheresis: Accumulation and persistence in the body. *Transfusion* 24:68, 1984.

15. Strauss R.G., Smith-Floss A.M.: Review of the effects of hydroxyethyl starch on the blood coagulation system. *Transfusion* 21:299, 1981.
16. Maguire L.C., Henriksen R.A., Strauss R.G., et al.: Function and morphology of platelets produced for transfusion by intermitent-flow-centrifugation plateletpheresis or combined platelet-leukapheresis. *Transfusion* 21:118, 1981.
17. Daniels M.J., Strauss R.G., Smith-Floss A.M.: Effects of hydroxyethyl starch on erythrocyte typing and blood crossmatching. *Transfusion* 22:226, 1982.
18. Trivedi S.M., Humphrey R.L., Braine H.G., et al.: Hydroxyethyl starch serum levels in leukapheresis measured by modified periodic acid-Schiff staining technique. *Transfusion* 24:260, 1984.
19. Dutcher J.P., Aisner J., Hogge D.E., et al.: Donor reaction to hydroxyethyl starch during granulocytapheresis. *Transfusion* 24:66, 1984.
20. Mollison P.L.: *Blood Transfusion in Clinical Medicine,* 7 ed. Oxford, England, Blackwell Scientific Publications, 1983, p. 62.
21. Klein R.E., Mogollon G.: Erythema multiforme following infusion of hydroxyethyl starch. *Transfusion* 24:166, 1984.
22. Bode U., Deisseroth A.B.: Donor toxicity in granulocyte collections: Association of lichen planus with the use of hydroxyethyl starch leukapheresis. *Transfusion* 21:83, 1981.
23. Newman R.S., Barr R.J., Ocariz J.A., et al.: Does hydroxyethyl starch cause lichen planus? Lichen planus in a long time routine blood donor never exposed to hydroxyethyl starch. *Transfusion* 23:531, 1983.
24. Szymanski I.O., Teno R.A., Gandhi J.G., et al.: Studies on low-dose hydroxyethyl starch leukapheresis: Rate of elimination of HES in vivo and function of the harvested granulocytes in vitro. *Vox Sang.* 47:325, 1984.
25. Widman F.K. (ed.): *Technical Manual of the American Association of Blood Banks,* ed. 8. Washington, D.C., American Association of Blood Banks, 1981, p. 5.
26. Burch J.W., Stanford N., Majerus P.W.: Inhibition of platelet prostaglandin synthetase by oral aspirin. *J. Clin. Invest.* 61:314, 1978.
27. Spagnuollo P.J., Ellner J.J.: Salicylate blockade of granulocyte adherence and the inflammatory response to experimental peritonitis. *Blood* 53:1018, 1979.
28. Oberman H.L. (ed.): *Standards for Blood Banks and Transfusion Services,* ed. 10. Washington, D.C., American Association of Blood Banks, 1981, pp. 19–27.
29. Reiss R.F., Katz A.J.: Statewide support of thrombocytopenic donors with ABO matched single donor platelets. *Transfusion* 16:312, 1976.
30. Lasky L.C., Finnerty E.P., Genis L., et al.: Protein and colloid osmotic pressure changes with albumin and/or saline replacement during plasma exchange. *Transfusion* 24:256, 1984.
31. Rosenkvist J., Berkowicz A., Holsφe E., et al.: Plasma exchange in myasthenia gravis complicated with complement activation and urticarial reactions using FFP as replacement solution. *Vox Sang.* 46:13, 1984.
32. McCullough J., Fortuny I.E.: Laboratory evaluation of normal donors undergoing leukapheresis on the continuous flow centrifuge. *Transfusion* 13:394, 1973.
33. McCredie K.B., Freireich E.J., Hester J.P., et al.: Increased granulocyte collection with the blood cell separator and the addition of etiocholanolone and hydroxyethyl starch. *Transfusion* 14:357, 1974.
34. Volkin R.L., Starz T.W., Winkelstein A., et al.: Changes in coagulation factors, complement, immunoglobulins, and immune complex concentrations with plasma exchange. *Transfusion* 22:54, 1982.
35. Graw R.G.Jr., Herzig G.P., Eisel R.J., et al.: Leukocyte and platelet collection from normal donors with the continuous-flow blood cell separator. *Transfusion* 11:94, 1971.
36. Nusbacher J., Scher M.L., MacPherson J.L.: Plateletpheresis using the Haemonetics Model 30 Cell Separator. *Vox Sang.* 33:9, 1977.
37. Koepke J.A., Parks W.M., Goeken J.A., et al.: The safety of weekly plateletpheresis: Effect on the donor's lymphocyte population. *Transfusion* 21:59, 1981.
38. Senhauser D.A., Westphal R.G., Bohman J.E., et al.: Immune system changes in cytapheresis donors. *Transfusion* 22:302, 1982.
39. Engle G.L.: *Fainting.* Springfield, Ill., Charles C Thomas, Publisher, 1962, p. 16.
40. MacPherson J.L., Nusbacher J., Bennett J.M.: The acquisition of granulocytes by leukapheresis. *Transfusion* 16:221, 1976.
41. Szymanski O.: Ionized calcium during plateletpheresis. *Transfusion* 18:701, 1978.
42. Ladenson J.H., Miller W.V., Sherman L.A.: The relationship between physical symptoms, ECG, free calcium and other blood chemistries in reinfusion with citrated blood. *Transfusion* 18:670, 1978.
43. Kotmas L.K.: Pheresis donor reactions and complications: Prevention, recognition and management, in Nusbacher J., Berkman E.M. (eds.): *Fundamentals of a Pheresis Program: A Technical Work Shop.* Washington, D.C., American Association of Blood Banks, 1979, p. 63.
44. Olson P.R., Cox C., McCullough J.: Laboratory and clinical effects of the infusion of ACD solution during plateletpheresis. *Vox Sang.* 33:79, 1977.
45. Ebert R.V., Stead E.A. Jr., Gibson J.G.: Response of normal subjects to acute blood loss. *Arch. Intern. Med.* 68:578, 1941.
46. Huestis D.W., White R.F., Price M.J., et al.: Use of hydroxyethyl starch to improve granulocyte collection in the Latham blood processor. *Transfusion* 15:559, 1975.
47. Ring J., Messmer K.: Incidence and severity of anaphylactoid reactions to colloid volume substitutes. *Lancet* 1:466, 1977.
48. Drescher W.P., Shih N., Hess K., et al.: Massive

extracorporeal blood clotting during discontinuous-flow leukapheresis. *Transfusion* 18:89, 1978.
49. Howard J.E., Perkins H.A.: Lysis of donor RBC during plateletpheresis with a blood processor. *JAMA* 236:289, 1976.
50. Dahlke M.D., Shah S.L., Sherwood W.C., et al.: Priapism during filtration leukapheresis. *Transfusion* 19:482, 1979.
51. Wiltbank T.B., Nusbacher J., Higby D.J., et al.: Abdominal pain in donors during filtration leukapheresis. *Transfusion* 17:159, 1977.
52. Higby D.J.: Filtration leukapheresis: A review, in *Leukapheresis and Granulocyte Transfusions: A Technical Workshop*. Washington, D.C., American Association of Blood Banks, 1975, p. 69.
53. Durant T.M., Oppenheimer M.J., Lynch P.R., et al.: Body position in relation to venous air embolism: A roentgenologic study. *Am. J. Med. Sci.* 227:509, 1954.
54. Nicholson M.J., Crehan J.P.: Emergency treatment of air embolism. *Curr. Res. Anesth.* 35:634, 1956.
55. McLeod B.C., Scott P.J.: Use of "single donor" factor VIII from plasma exchange donation. *JAMA* 252:2726, 1984.
56. Rock G.A., Blanchette V.S., Wong S.C.: Storage of platelets collected by apheresis. *Transfusion* 23:99, 1983.
57. Conway L.P., Scott E.P.: Acute hemolytic transfusion reaction due to ABO incompatible plasma in platelet apheresis concentrate. *Transfusion* 24:416, 1984.
58. Price T.H.: Neutrophil transfusion: In vivo function of neutrophils collected using cell separators. *Transfusion* 23:504, 1983.
59. Barr R.D., Stevens C.A., Koekebakker M., et al.: Collection of erythroid progenitor cells by cytapheresis and plasmapheresis of peripheral blood normal donors. *Transfusion* 22:388, 1982.
60. Chopeck M., McCullough J.: Protein and biochemical changes during plasma exchange, in *Therapeutic Hemapheresis: A Technical Workshop*. Washington, D.C., American Association of Blood Banks, 1980, p. 16.
61. Ziselman E.M., Bongiovanni M.B., Wurzel H.A.: The complications of therapeutic plasma exchange. *Vox Sang.* 46:270, 1984.
62. Lawson N.S., Nosanchuk J.S., Oberman H.A., et al.: Therapeutic plasma pheresis in treatment of patients with Waldenström's macroglobulinemia. *Transfusion* 8:174, 1968.
63. Blumberg N., Katz A.J.: Partial plasma exchange: Diseases in which it is of reported efficacy, in Berkman E.M., Umlas J. (eds.): *Therapeutic Hemapheresis: A Technical Workshop*. Washington, D.C., American Association of Blood Banks, 1980, p. 79.
64. Beck J.R., Quinn B.M., Meier F.A., et al.: Hyperviscosity syndrome in paraproteinemia managed by plasma exchange; monitored by serum tests. *Transfusion* 22:51, 1982.
65. Ibister J.P., Biggs J.C., Penny R.: Experience with large volume plasmapheresis in malignant paraproteinemia and immune disorders. *Aust. NZJ. Med.* 8:154, 1978.
66. Misiani R., Remuzzi G., Bertani T., et al.: Plasmapheresis in the treatment of acute renal failure in multiple myeloma. *Am. J. Med.* 66:684, 1979.
67. Flaum M.A., Cuneo R.A., Appelbaum, et al.: The hemostatic imbalance of plasma exchange transfusion. *Blood* 54:694, 1979.
68. Keller A.J., Urbaniak S.J.: Intensive plasma exchange on the cell separator: Effects on serum immunoglobulins and complement components. *Br. J. Haematol.* 38:531, 1978.
69. Denlinger J.K., Nahrwood M.L., Gibbs P.S., et al.: Hypocalcemia during rapid blood transfusion in anaesthesized man. *Br. J. Anaesth.* 48:995, 1976.
70. Plasma exchange in SLE (editorial). *Lancet* 1 688, 1980.
71. Jones J.V., Bucknall R.C., Cumming R.H., et al.: Plasmapheresis in the management of systemic lupus erythematosus. *Lancet* 1:709, 1976.
72. Hubbard H.C., Portnoy B.: Systemic lupus erythematosus, in pregnancy treated with plasmapheresis. *Br. J. Dermatol.* 101:87, 1979.
73. Moran C.J., Parry J.F., Mowbray J., et al.: Plasmapheresis in systemic lupus erythematosus. *Br. Med. J.* 4:1573, 1977.
74. Lockwood C.M., Rees A.J., Pearson T.A., et al.: Immunosuppression and plasma-exchange in the treatment of Goodpasture's syndrome. *Lancet* 1:711, 1976.
75. Erickson S.B., Kurtz S.B., Donadio J.V., et al.: Use of combined plasmapheresis and immunosuppression in the treatment of Goodpasture's syndrome. *Mayo Clin. Proc.* 54:714, 1979.
76. Munk Z.M., Skamene E.: Goodpasture's syndrome: Effects of plasmapheresis. *Clin. Exp. Immunol.* 36:244, 1979.
77. Lockwood C.M., Peters D.K.: The treatment of Goodpasture's syndrome and glomerulonephritis. *Plasma Ther.* 1:19, 1979.
78. Dau P.C., Lindstrom J.M., Cassel C.K., et al.: Plasmapheresis and immunosuppressive drug therapy in myasthenia gravis. *N. Engl. J. Med.* 297:1134, 1977.
79. Pinching A.J., Peters D.K., Newsom J.D.: Remission of myasthenia gravis following plasma exchange. *Lancet* 2:1373, 1976.
80. Behan P.O., Shakir R.A., Simpson J.A., et al.: Plasma exchange combined immunosuppressive therapy in myasthenia gravis. *Lancet* 1:438, 1979.
81. Kornfeld P., Ambinder E.P., Papatestas A.E., et al.: Plasmapheresis in myasthenia gravis: Controlled study. *Lancet* 2:629, 1979.
82. Plasmapheresis for myasthenia gravis (editorial). *Med. Lett.* 21:64, 1979.
83. Pinching A.J., Peters D.K., Newson-Davis J.: Plasma exchange in the investigation and treatment of myasthenia gravis. *Plasma Ther.* 1:29, 1979.
84. Wallace D.J., Goldfinger D., Lowe D., et al.: Plasmapheresis and lymphoplasmapheresis in the management of rheumatoid arthritis. *Arthritis Rheum.* 22:703, 1979.

85. Wallace D.J., Goldfinger D., Brachman M., et al.: Therapeutic apheresis in the management of rheumatoid arthritis (RA). *Clin. Res.* 28:77a, 1980.
86. Dodds A.J., O'Reilly M.J.G., Yates C.J.P., et al.: Haemorrhoealogical response to plasma exchange in Raynaud's syndrome. *Br. Med. J.* 2:1186, 1979.
87. Holdstock G.E., Fisher J.A., Hamblin T.J., et al.: Plasmapheresis in Crohn's disease. *Digestion* 19:197, 1979.
88. Schauf C.L., Stetoski D.A., Davis F.A., et al.: Concerning the application of plasmapheresis to multiple sclerosis. *Plasma Ther.* 1:33, 1979.
89. Laningham J.E.T.: Partial plasma exchange, an adjunct therapy to complex clinical problems. *Transfusion* 17:547, 1977.
90. Mercuriali F., Sirchia G.: Plasma exchange for mushroom poisoning. *Transfusion* 17:644, 1977.
91. Auerbach R., Bystryn J.C.: Plasmapheresis and immunosuppressive therapy. *Arch. Dermatol.* 115:728, 1979.
92. Muers M.F., Dawkins K.D.: Plasmapheresis in severe asthma. *Lancet* 2:260, 1978.
93. Israel L., Edelstein R., Mannoni P., et al.: Plasmapheresis in patients with disseminated cancer: Clinical results and correlation with changes in serum protein. The concept of "nonspecific blocking factors." *Cancer* 40:3146, 1977.
94. Redeker A.G., Yamahiro H.S.: Controlled trial of exchange transfusion therapy in fulminant hepatitis. *Lancet* 1:3, 1973.
95. Buskard N.A.: Failure of plasma exchange to improve immune thrombocytopenia. *Blood* 54:108a, 1979.
96. Blanchette V.S., Hogan V.A., McCombie N.E., et al.: Intensive plasma exchange therapy in ten patients with idiopathic thrombocytopenic purpura. *Transfusion* 24:388, 1984.
97. CoFrancesco E., Pogliani E., Salvatore M., Polli E.E.: Demonstration of immune complexes in thrombotic thrombocytopenic purpura: Failure to respond to plasma exchange (letter). *Transfusion* 22:540, 1982.
98. Lundsgaard-Hansen P.: Intensive plasmapheresis as a risk factor for arteriosclerotic cardiovascular disease? *Vox Sang.* 33:1, 1977.
99. Bove J.R., quoted by Huestis D.W., Thomas S.F.: Presently available plasmapheresis technics, in Berkman E.M., Umlas J. (eds.): *Therapeutic hemapheresis: A Technical Workshop.* Washington, D.C., American Association of Blood Banks, 1980, p. 1.
100. Keesey J.: Caution on plasmapheresis for myasthenia gravis. *N. Engl. J. Med.* 298:1029, 1978.
101. Pineda A.A.: Therapeutic plasmapheresis: New techniques and applications, in Berkman E.M., Umlas J. (eds.): *Therapeutic Hemapheresis: A Technical Workshop.* Washington, D.C., American Association of Blood Banks, 1980, p. 139.
102. Lauterburg B.H., Dickson E.R., Pineda A.A., et al.: Removal of bile acids and bilirubin by plasma perfusion of U.S.P.D. charcoal coated glass beads. *J. Lab. Clin. Med.* 94:585, 1979.
103. Burgstaler E.A., Pineda A.A., Ellefson R.D.: Removal of plasma lipoproteins from circulating blood with a heparin-agarose column. *Mayo Clin. Proc.* 55:180, 1980.
104. Terman D.S., Buffaloe G., Mattioli C., et al.: Extracorporeal immunoadsorption: Initial experience in human systemic lupus erythematosus. *Lancet* 2:824, 1979.
105. Bansal S.C., Bansal B.R., Thomas H.L., et al.: Exvivo removal of serum IgG in a patient with colon carcinoma: Some biochemical, immunological and histological observations. *Cancer* 42:1, 1978.
106. Branda R.F., Klausner J.S., Miller W.J., et al.: Specific removal of antibodies with an immune-absorption system. *Transfusion* 24:157, 1984.
107. Grindon A.J.: Partial plasma exchange: A critical review, in Berkman E.M., Umlas J. (eds.): *Therapeutic Hemapheresis: A Technical Workshop.* Washington, D.C., American Association of Blood Banks, 1980, p. 97.
108. Goldfinger D.: Clinical applications of therapeutic cytapheresis, in Berkman E.M., Umlas J. (eds.): *Therapeutic Hemapheresis: A Technical Workshop.* Washington, D.C., American Association of Blood Banks, 1980, p. 65.
109. Kleinman S., Thompson-Breton R., Goldfinger D., et al.: Exchange red blood cell pheresis in the management of complications of sickle cell anemia. *Plasma Ther.* 1:27, 1980.
110. Pineda A.A., Brzica S.M. Jr., Taswell H.F.: Continuous and semi-continuous-flow centrifugation systems: Therapeutic applications, with plasma-, platelet-, lympha-, and eosinapheresis. *Transfusion* 17:407, 1977.
111. Lowenthal R.M., Buskard N.A., Goldman J.M., et al.: Intensive leukapheresis as initial therapy for chronic granulocytic leukemia. *Blood* 46:835, 1975.
112. Hester J.P., McCredie K.B., Freireich E.J.: Response to chronic leukapheresis and survival of chronic myelogenous leukemia patients. *Transfusion* 22:305, 1982.
113. Cooper I.A., Ding J.C., Adams P.B.: Intensive leukapheresis in the management of cytopenias in patients with chronic lymphocytic leukemia (CLL) and lymphocytic lymphoma. *Am. J. Hematol.* 6:387, 1979.
114. Fay J.W., Moore J.O., Logue J.L., et al.: Leukapheresis therapy of leukemia reticuloendotheliosis (hairy cell leukemia). *Blood* 54:747, 1979.
115. Choundhury A.M., Bhoopalam N.B., Hoffstadter L.K.: Effect of intense leukocytapheresis in pancytopenic phase of hairy cell leukemia. *Transfusion* 23:526, 1983.
116. Worsley A., Cuttner J., Gordon R., et al.: Therapeutic leukapheresis in a patient with hairy cell leukemia presenting with a white count greater than 500,000 µl. *Transfusion* 22:308, 1982.
117. Edelson R., Facktor M., Andrews A., et al.: Successful management of the Sézary syndrome: Mobilization and removal of extravascular neoplastic T

cells by leukapheresis. *Engl. J. Med.* 291:293, 1974.
118. Decaro J.H., Novoa J.E., de Anda G., et al.: Leukapheresis in a patient with Sézary syndrome. *Vox Sang.* 47:276, 1984.
119. Tenenbaum J., Urowitz M.B., Keystone E.C., et al.: Leukapheresis in severe rheumatoid arthritis. *Ann. Rheum. Dis.* 38:40, 1979.
120. Wright S.K.: The organization of a hospital-based hemapheresis center, in Nusbacher J., Berkman E.M. (eds.): *Fundamentals of a Pheresis Program: A Technical Workshop.* Washington, D.C., American Association of Blood Banks, 1979, p. 1.
121. McElligott M.C.: Organization of a pheresis program in a regional blood center, in Nusbacher J., Berkman E.M. (eds.): *Fundamentals of Pheresis Program: A Technical Workshop.* Washington, D.C., American Association of Blood Banks, 1979, p. 23.
122. Mollison P.L.: *Blood Transfusion in Clinical Medicine,* ed. 7. Oxford, England, Blackwell Scientific Publications, 1979.
123. Milles G., Langston H.T., Dalessandro W.: *Autologous Transfusions.* Springfield, Ill., Charles C Thomas, Publisher, 1971.
124. Widman F.K. (ed.): *Technical Manual of the American Association of Blood Banks,* ed. 8. Washington, D.C., American Association of Blood Banks, 1981, p. 342.
125. Hamstra R.D., Block M.H.: Erythropoiesis in response to blood loss in man. *J. Appl. Physiol.* 27:503, 1969.
126. Adamson J., Hillman R.S.: Blood volume and plasma protein replacement following acute blood loss in normal man. *JAMA* 205:609, 1968.
127. Zuck T.F., Bergin J.J.: Adequacy of oral iron, to support erythropoiesis during intensive phlebotomy for autologous transfusion, in *XIII International Transfusion Congress.* Washington, D.C., 1972, p. 53.
128. Zuck T.F.: Donor response to predeposit autologous transfusion phlebotomy, in Dawson R.B. (ed.): *Autologous Transfusions: A Technical Workshop.* Washington, D.C., American Association of Blood Banks, 1976, p. 51.
129. Silver H.: Banked and fresh autologous blood in cardiopulmonary bypass surgery. *Transfusion* 15:600, 1975.
130. Newman M.M., Hamstra R.D., Block M.H.: Use of banked autologous blood in elective surgery. *JAMA* 218:861, 1971.
131. Duncan L.E., Klebanoff G., Rogers W.: A clinical experience with intraoperative autotransfusion. *Ann. Surg.* 180:296, 1974.
132. Ascari W.Q., Jolly P.C., Thomas P.A.: Autologous blood transfusion in pulmonary surgery. *Transfusion* 8:111, 1968.
133. Rivers S.L., Liles B.: Problems associated with freezing and thawing of red cells containing A-S hemoglobin. *Transfusion* 13:356, 1973.
134. Bailey D.N., Bove J.R.: Chemical and hematological changes in stored CPD blood. *Transfusion* 15:244, 1975.
135. Mollison P.L.: *Blood Transfusion in Clinical Medicine,* ed. 7. Oxford, England, Blackwell Scientific Publications, 1983, p. 48.
136. Messmer K.: Hemodilution. *Surg. Clin. North Am.* 55:659, 1975.
137. Huggins C.: Autologous transfusion preservation of blood by freezing, in Dawson R.B. (ed.): *Autologous Transfusions: A Technical Workshop.* Washington, D.C., American Association of Blood Banks, 1976, p. 27.
138. Cuello L., Vazquez E., Perez V., Raffucci F.L.: Autologous blood transfusion in cardiovascular surgery. *Transfusion* 7:309, 1967.
139. Cove H., Matloff J., Sacks H.J., et al.: Autologous blood transfusion in coronary artery bypass surgery. *Transfusion* 16:245, 1976.
140. Cooley D.A., Crawford E.J., Howell J.F., et al.: Open heart surgery in Jehova's Witnesses. *Am. J. Cardiol.* 13:779, 1964.
141. Blundell J.: Experiments on the transfusion of blood. *Medico. Chi. Trans.* 9:56, 1818.
142. Gilcher R.D.: Autologous transfusion blood salvage, in Dawson R.B. (ed.): *Autologous Transfusions: A Technical Workshop.* Washington, D.C., American Association of Blood Banks, 1976.
143. Wilson J., Taswell H.F.: Autotransfusion: Historical review and preliminary report on a new method. *Mayo Clin. Proc.* 43:26, 1968.
144. Reul G.J., Cooley D.A., Sandiford F.M., et al.: Experience with autotransfusion in the surgical management of trauma. *Surgery* 76:546, 1974.
145. Hauer J.M., Thurer R.L., Kruskall M., et al.: An abbreviated pathway for thrombin activation: Studies of defibrinogenated mediastinal blood (abstract). *Blood* 58:218, 1981.
146. Schaff H.V., Hauer J.M., Bell W.R., et al.: Retransfusion of shed mediastinal blood following cardiac surgery: A prospective study. *J. Thorac. Cardiovasc. Surg.* 75:4, 1978.
147. Hauer J.M., Thurer R.L., Weintraub R.M.: Platelet function in shed mediastinal blood following cardiac surgery (abstract), in *Proceedings of the Joint Congress, International Society of Haematologists and International Society of Blood Transfusion.* Budapest, Hungary, 1982.
148. Hauer J.M., Thurer R.L.: Controversies in autotransfusion. *Vox Sang.* 46:8, 1984.
149. Moran J.M., Babka R., Silberman S., et al.: Immediate centrifugation of oxygenator contents after cardiopulmonary bypass. *J. Thorac. Cardiovasc. Surg.* 76:510, 1978.
150. Tector A.J., Gabriel R.P., Malericka W.E., et al.: Reduction of blood usage in open heart surgery. *Chest* 70:4, 1976.
151. Pliam M.B., McGoon D.C., Trahan S.: Failure of transfusion of autologous whole blood to reduce banked-blood requirements in open-heart surgical patients. *J. Thorac. Cardiovasc. Surg.* 70:2, 1975.
152. Sherman M.M., Dobnik D.B., Dennis R.C., et al.:

Autologous blood transfusion during cardiopulmonary bypass. *Chest* 70:5, 1976.
153. Yaw P.B., Sentany M., Link W.J., et al.: Tumor cells carried through autotransfusion: Contra-indication to intraoperative blood recovery? *JAMA* 231:490, 1975.
154. Abramson N.E., Eisenberg P.D., Aster R.H.: Posttransfusion purpura: Immunologic aspects and therapy. *N. Engl. J. Med.* 291:1163, 1974.
155. Besa E.C., Ray P.K., Swami P.K., et al.: Specific immune adsorption of IgG antibody in a patient with chronic lymphocytic leukemia and autoimmune hemolytic anemia. *Am. J. Med.* 71:1035, 1981.
156. Wensley R.T., Stevens R.F., Burn A.M., et al.: Plasma exchange and human factor VIII concentrate in managing haemophilia A with factor VIII inhibitors. *Br. Med. J.* 281:1388, 1980.
157. Messner H.A., Fauser A.A., Curtis J.E., et al.: Control of pure red cell aplasia by repeated plasmapheresis. *Blood* 54:71a, 1979.
158. Lockwood C.M.: Plasma exchange in nephritis. *Plasma Ther.* 2:227, 1981.
159. Valbonesi M., Garelli S., Mosconi L., et al.: Plasma exchange in the management of selected neurological diseases. *Plasma Ther.* 2:13, 1981.
160. Ropper A.H.: Management of Guillain-Barré syndrome, in Ropper A.H., Kennedy S.K., Servas N.T. (eds.): *Neurological and Neurosurgical Intensive Care*. Baltimore, University Park Press, 1983, pp. 163–174.
161. Dau P.: The role of plasma exchange in treatment of idiopathic polymyocitis. *Prog. Clin. Biol. Res.* 106:223, 1982.
162. Dandona P., Marshall N.J., Bidey S.P., et al.: Successful treatment of exophthalmos and pretibial myxoedema with plasmapheresis. *Br. Med. J.* 1:374, 1979.
163. Geltman D., Khon R.W., Gorovic P., et al.: The effect of combination therapy (steroids, immunosuppressives and plasmapheresis) on five mixed cryoglobulinemia patients with renal, neurologic, and vascular involvement. *Arthritis Rheum.* 24:1121, 1981.
164. Lupien P.J., Murjani S., Lou M., et al.: Removal of cholesterol from blood by affinity binding to heparin-agarose: Evaluation of treatment in homozygous familial hypercholesterolemia. *Pediatr. Res.* 14:113, 1980.

10

Immune Hemolysis

THE DESTRUCTION of red blood cells (RBCs) mediated by RBC-antibody coating is termed immune hemolysis. Various types of immune hemolysis exist (Table 10–1). This chapter discusses only the autoimmune hemolytic anemias and the immune–mediated anemias secondary to drugs.

AUTOIMMUNE HEMOLYTIC ANEMIA

Autoimmune hemolytic anemia (AHA) is an uncommon but not rare disease that is estimated to occur in 1 per 80,000 population.[1,2] Most patients are over age 40, but the disease has been seen in infants[3] and may also be seen in the very old, in whom it may follow a fulminant course.[2] In older patients the age distribution has been found to correlate with the age distribution of lymphoproliferative disorders, whereas in younger patients it correlates with the incidence of other autoimmune diseases (e.g., SLE). AHA is more common in females than it is in males.

There are two important features that characterize AHA: (1) a shortened RBC survival time (less than 100–150 days) and (2) evidence of an immune response capable of destroying autologous RBCs, as evidenced by demonstrating RBC coating with immunoglobulin or complement (positive direct Coombs test or other evidence of complement coating). Two main types of AHA can be identified on the basis of laboratory studies: warm-type AHA and cold-type AHA, depending on the reactivity of the antibodies in vitro. About 7.3% of patients with autoimmune antibodies to RBCs have combined cold- and warm-reacting autoantibodies.[4]

Warm-Type Autoimmune Hemolytic Anemia

The majority of cases of AHA are mediated by warm-antibody RBC coating (80%–90% of all cases).[5] The etiology of warm idiopathic AHA remains unknown.[6] However, it is often found in association with other autoimmune disorders such as SLE.[7] Like NZB mice, which exhibit a "lupus-like" syndrome and a high propensity to develop autoimmune hemolysis, patients with SLE may have a genetic predisposition to developing autoantibodies against RBCs and other tissues.[7] It has been proposed that these animals have a B cell imbalance, making B cells polyclonally activated during fetal development. T cell help activation may likewise take place in these instances.

Pathophysiology

In over 80% of AHA cases, IgG and complement coat the RBCs.[8] IgG alone is found in about 36% of cases,[8] and complement alone in 10% of cases.[8] However, binding of RBC isoantibodies per se does not cause direct red cell damage;[9] neither does IgG binding to RBCs.[10]

It is now thought that IgM binding induces binding of complement, which may, in itself, cause destruction of the RBC, or leave C3b attached to the RBC, which is then picked up by macrophages

TABLE 10–1.—IMMUNE HEMOLYSIS*

TYPE	ONSET	SEVERITY	THERAPY	PROGNOSIS
AUTOIMMUNE HEMOLYTIC ANEMIA				
Warm type	Occasionally acute	May be severe	Steroids	Fair
Idiopathic			Splenectomy	
Secondary to:			Immunosuppression	
Other immune disorders (e.g., SLE, RA, ulcerative colitis)				
Neoplasms: CLL; lymphoproliferative disorders; ovarian teratomas				
Infections				
Cold agglutinin syndrome	Insidious	Mild to moderate	Avoid cold	Usually good
Idiopathic			Chlorambucil	
Secondary to:				
Infections (e.g., *Mycoplasma*, IM, other)				
Neoplasms: lymphoproliferative diseases				
PAROXYSMAL COLD HEMOGLOBINURIA	Acute with hemoglobinuria	Moderate	Steroids? Transfusions	Excellent
Idiopathic				
Secondary to infection (viral, syphilis)				
DRUG-INDUCED	Subacute or acute	Moderate to severe	Stop drug	Excellent
HEMOLYSIS DUE TO RBC ALLOIMMUNIZATION	Acute or subacute	Moderate to severe	Steroids	Variable
Transfusion			Prophylactic	
HDN	Chronic until birth			

*Data from Petz and Garraty.[1]

possessing receptors for C3b. Conversely, coating of RBC by IgG induces macrophage pickup and phagocytosis via FcR present on these phagocytic cells.[11]

RBCs coated with non-complement-binding IgG have been shown to adhere to monocytes in vitro.[12] This adherence of IgG-coated RBCs to monocytic phagocytes leads to cytotoxicity and eventually phagocytosis of the coated RBCs.[13]

This adherence and phagocytosis is dependent on the Fc portion of the binding IgG, as demonstrated both by the blocking of binding if the system is saturated with IgG[11] and by failure of adherence to occur if RBCs are coated with F(ab')$_2$ fragments of coating antibodies.[14] In addition, there is evidence that IgG1 and especially IgG3 are involved in RBC hemolysis, whereas IgG2 and IgG4 are not.[11]

In vivo studies transfusing chromium-labeled RBCs[15] have shown that RBCs coated with IgG tend to lodge in the spleen, whereas RBCs coated with complement tend to be trapped in the liver.

Stasis in the spleen tends to promote adherence of IgG-coated RBCs to macrophages in this organ.[11]

In addition, as the number of IgG-sensitized RBCs increases, the likelihood of splenic sequestration of these cells increases.[16] It appears that binding of coated RBCs by macrophages is via Fc receptors.

Fc and Complement Receptors on Macrophages

Many developments have taken place in the study and understanding of macrophages since they were first described by Metchnikoff.[17] The macrophage was described only as a phagocytic cell; it is now known to be involved in several other functions in the immune process. The newer discoveries include knowledge that macrophages participate in a crucial manner in the sensitization of lymphocytes[18] and the regulation of lymphocyte responses.[14] It has been shown that membrane-bound antigen is more immunogenic and that antigen presentation by macrophages to T cells is mediated by type II MHC glycoproteins, although class I molecules may likewise be involved in the antigen presentation process.[18] This macrophage-dependent activation of antigen-specific T cells requires both antigen and a soluble monokine, interleukin I (IL-1).[19] Other functions of macrophages include tumor cytolysis[20] and parasite cytolysis.[21]

We now know that the probable origin of macrophage precursors (promonocytes) is the bone marrow. These precursor cells are thought to become circulating blood monocytes which then become fixed tissue macrophages in definite target organs (e.g., peritoneum or lung).[22] The idea that mature macrophages divide locally to supply the tissue macrophage population has been sustained by some authors,[23] although the evidence for bone marrow supply to provide tissue macrophages appears to be more conclusive.[22] The mechanism by which these phenomena occur is not known. Certain high molecular weight substances (23,000 MW) have been shown to induce maturation of bone marrow stem cells to monocytes.[24]

Monocytes and macrophages have been shown to display receptors for the Fc portion of IgG as well as for third component of complement.[25] At least two Fc receptors exist on murine monocytes and macrophages; one site binds IgG2a and is trypsin sensitive, and another is trypsin resistant and binds IgG1 and IgG2b immune complexes.[26] Monoclonal antibodies have been obtained against the FcR, and appear to bind to a 60,000-dalton protein[27] on the surface of macrophages. It appears that the IgG2a receptor site binds to the sequences between C2 and C3 domains of the Fc portion of immunoglobulins, whereas IgG2b binds to the C2 domain.[28] Several receptors for complement have been identified, among which are C1qr, the three receptors to C3 (CR1, CR2 and CR3), as well as receptors for factor H and soluble factors C3a and C4a.[29] Of great interest is CR1, which is critical to C3b binding by macrophages and appears to be a 250,000-dalton glycoprotein.[30] FcR and CR are critical to one of the main functions of macrophages, that is, their role in antigen presentation to other immunocytes. An important role of these receptors is in phagocytosis, where C3b receptors are involved in binding of particles coated with C3b but are not directly involved in internalization of coated particles.[31] Instead, internalization appears to be mediated by Fc receptors.[32]

Other investigators have shown that receptors for C3b and C3bi promote phagocytosis but do not promote the release of oxygen from human phagocytes.[33] Monocytes and macrophages are capable of capping and patching. This phenomenon occurs when two receptors and ligand complexes are linked by antibody, causing them to precipitate in the membrane.[34] It has been demonstrated that after ligand binding to receptors, the complexes are translocated to specific regions of macrophages. This allows macrophages to maintain integrity of membrane transport systems during removal of cell surface by phagocytosis. FcR and CR tend to move away from the cell uropod, whereas FcR and CR complexes move toward the uropod.[35]

The macrophage cell family is viewed today not as a single class of cells but as a variety of cells with subspecialized populations which would perform different functions (such as presenting antigen to B and T cells, storing antigen, or becoming cytolytic to tumors), not only from tissue to tissue but within tissues as well. Subpopulations of cells in terms of surface FcR and CR have been observed in macrophages from the peritoneum and other organs after separation by density gradients.[36,37] Likewise, macrophages separated on density gradients exhibit other differences; for instance, alveolar macrophages exhibit variability in the development of Fc receptors after in vivo stimulation with Freunds adjuvant.[38] Recently, authors have shown differences in subpopulations of human monocytes separated by elutriation. Denser cells had a higher content of peroxidase activity than lighter cells.[39] It has been shown that heterogeneity in terms of surface receptors such as HLA-DR exist in monocytes.[40] It has recently been shown by Todd et al. (personal communication) that alveolar macrophages, which are rarely contaminated by monocytes, bear only M02 and not M01. M01 is a monoclonal antibody capable of detecting C3bi receptors on promonocytes and monocytes,[41] and M02 is capable of detecting a macromolecule characteristic of tissue macrophages. The molecules these monoclonal antibodies detect are biochemically distinct.[42] It has been shown that M01 binds to the receptor for C3bi (CR3), and that M02 binds to a 60,000-dalton protein with no apparent relation to C3b but specific to macrophages.

Recently, investigators have shown that T cell proliferation induction as well as T cell inhibition may be mediated by macrophages in specific cases. These are also functions that may differ with a variety of macrophage subpopulations.

For instance, it has been shown that peripheral blood monocytes have a greater accessory cell function than alveolar macrophage in T cell proliferation studies.[43] The role that these receptors have in terms of monocyte migration patterns needs to be clarified, as well as how these receptors are involved in the homing mechanisms of these cells. In AHA, erythrocytes which are coated with complement alone, such as is seen in coating by cold antibodies, are trapped in the liver, whereas RBCs coated by

IgG tend to be trapped by the splenic macrophages.[44] It is possible that under stimulated circumstances, macrophages in tissues display different receptors on their surface. This has been observed in monocytes of patients with AHA, in whom the proportion of FcR varies.[45] These findings suggest not only that individual cells redistribute their surface receptors but that under pathologic circumstances, the subpopulations may be altered in these disease states. Therefore, in AHA, activated Kupffer cells and spleen macrophages may develop different Fc and CR surface receptors than would normal individuals. If subpopulations of FcR- and CR-bearing cells are altered during disease, the stimulus for population shifts could be initiated in the bone marrow. In other studies, it has been shown that patients with SLE have monocytes bearing an increased number of FcR,[46] although other authors have found decreased available FcR in these patients.[47] In addition, Fc receptors on monocytoid cells are cell cycle dependent[47] and double from G1 to G2+M.[48]

Just how monocytic phagocytes mature from monocytoid cells to mature macrophages and migrate to tissues is not known and may very well be unrelated to FcR or CR; however, a turnover of cells from the bone marrow to distant sites has been demonstrated by tracing labeled populations of macrophages.[49] This label has been traced to specialized endothelium of certain target organs (e.g., liver and spleen).[49] Thus, the endothelial cell surface may be involved in monocyte migration. However, the correlation of capacity to migrate with expression of surface immunoglobulin, complement receptors or endothelial cell surface was not assessed in these studies.

The Hemolytic Process

It is evident from coating of RBC by anti-Rh antibodies of the IgG class that complement is not essential for cell lysis. The lysis in these cases appears to be mediated by the interaction of the Fc portion of the antibody molecule and the FcR on macrophages.[50] On interaction, a second message appears to be delivered to the cytoplasm, and a complex array of intracellular reactions takes place. Activation of macrophage membranes takes place, and the lamellipodium is projected to the adherent erythrocyte. This portion of the phagocytic cell is organelle-free and much more adherent. Subsequently, the whole or a portion of the RBC is ingested, producing complete lysis or spherocytes, respectively.[51] Phagocytosis is not essential for cell destruction; monocytes, for instance, are capable of lysing cells by concentrating lysosomes at the point of RBC adherence. Lymphocytes, by a poorly understood membrane mechanism, can likewise lyse sensitized RBCs.[52]

Three important factors are responsible for greater or lesser lytic activity: (1) The number of antigenic sites on a cell (ABH sites number in the millions, whereas Rh sites number in the thousands). (2) The affinity or capacity of IgG antibodies to bind complement (IgG1 and IgG3 have a greater affinity than do IgG2 or IgG4). (3) The affinity of the FcR for Fc on the phagocytic cell differs (granulocyte FcR has a lower affinity for monomeric Fc than does the macrophage FcR).[51] Furthermore, aggregated Fc molecules have a higher affinity for the Fc receptors, a fact that may involve antigen mobility on the surface of RBCs. It has recently been shown that lymphocytes may be directly cytotoxic to RBCs without the mediation of complement.[52] This mechanism is also thought to contribute to RBC lysis in AHA.

Clinical and Laboratory Aspects

Onset of warm AHA is usually slow, but some cases of AHA manifest with the acute onset of icterus. The usual symptoms of anemia are found—pallor, asthenia, and jaundice (39% of cases).[53] Splenomegaly is not infrequent (50% of cases); if it is severe, the diagnosis of lymphoma should be entertained and evidence of it sought. In addition, AHA may appear following chemotherapy or radiotherapy for lymphoma.[54] If AHA is mild, a positive Coombs test may be the only abnormal finding. Reticulocytes are elevated in moderate cases (10%–20%) and in severe cases may reach 50%–80%. A corrected reticulocyte count (normal, 0.5%–1.5%) can be calculated as follows: .05 (5% reticulocytes) = 150,000 reticulocytes/μl, divided by a normal value of 50,000 = 3; this means that a patient with a reticulocyte count of 5% has a threefold increase in RBC production.

The hemoglobin is less than 7 gm/dl in about 50% of the cases[55] and the hematocrit may likewise be very decreased (10%–20%). The finding of spherocytes is helpful in the diagnosis when hereditary spherocytosis has been ruled out. Erythroid hyperplasia is frequently seen in bone marrow biopsy specimens. Leukocytosis during active hemolysis is usually present, although leukopenia has been reported in AHA.

Indirect serum bilirubin levels are usually elevated and vary from 0.8 to 8.6 mg/dl in most cases.[53] However, hemoglobinemia is not frequently seen. Serum haptoglobin (an α_2-glycoprotein) is complexed with hemoglobin; if the catabolic rate of this complex increases, the rate of synthesis cannot keep up with the catabolic rate; hence normal levels (50–150 mg/dl) will drop in relation to the severity of hemolysis.

Serum lactic dehydrogenase is likewise elevated in AHA and is used as an indication of the severity of hemolysis.

Autoagglutination of anticoagulated samples is a useful finding; it may be more marked for cold agglutinins. The tube of anticoagulated blood is tilted and granular clumps are seen sliding on the side of the tube.

Monocytic erythrophagocytosis is occasionally found. Thrombocytopenia may be present in up to 13% of cases (Evans' syndrome)[56] and appears to be immune–mediated.[57] Several cases of Evans' syndrome present with decreased immunoglobulin levels, accompanied by decreased T4/T8 ratios.[58]

Hemoglobinemia may be seen in certain cases of AHA, but it is not a constant finding.

Red Cell Survival Studies

The more frequently used method is to take a sample of RBCs, label them with $Na_2{}^{51}CrO_4$, and inject them, using no more than 0.5 µCi/kg of body weight. The $T_{50}Cr$ value is then calculated. This value is the point at which survival of tagged cells falls to 50% of the initial value, measured 10 minutes after injection to allow mixing.[59] $T_{50}Cr$ values are considered normal if survival is 25 days or more. If the survival is 23 days, the destruction is twice normal (i.e., 2% per day rather than 1% per day). Survival in AHA may drop to 15 days or lower in severe cases. Marked deviations from normal are more reliable than small changes; hence the test is used to predict survival of a transfused unit rather than to determine the diagnosis of AHA. In addition, ^{51}Cr studies are useful to determine localization of organ site of destruction of RBCs. ^{51}Cr studies are also useful to help diagnose AHA when a Coombs test is negative. In most cases, serologic testing will help determine the prognosis of survival of a unit (in vivo compatibility); however, in complicated cases, such as in the presence of a high incidence antibody, when obtaining a unit is close to impossible, ^{51}Cr studies may help predict if transfusion with a unit positive for the antigen will have optimal survival in vivo.[59]

Three main patterns of RBC destruction can be identified by ^{51}Cr labeling:

1. Intravascular (e.g., due to isoantibodies, anti-A, etc.).[60]
2. Extravascular intrasplenic (e.g., non-complement-binding IgG antibody).[61]
3. Extravascular intrahepatic (e.g., complement-binding IgG or IgM antibody).[62]

The classic example of intravascular hemolysis is that seen in ABO-incompatible transfusion reactions, in which the complement-mediated lysis is usually quite brisk. Cells that are not immediately destroyed are picked up by macrophages bearing receptors for such complement components as C3b, C3d, C4b, C5, and C1q.[63]

Macrophages bearing receptors for complement are probably responsible for intrahepatic lysis. Therefore, it is not surprising that IgM-inducing complement coating of cells will be removed by the liver.[64] This uptake of coated RBCs with complement (C3b) does not lead to phagocytosis in all cases, and many cells are returned to the circulation after being picked up by the liver macrophages,[65] as has been shown in vitro when C3b-coated cells[65] provided only a weak stimulus for ingestion.[66]

A two-signal message for phagocytosis has been postulated in which Fc receptor sites plus C3b receptor sites are required for adequate phagocytosis. IgM does not seem to be efficient in performing this opsonizing function.[67]

The C3b inactivation system is apparently the mechanism for the release of RBCs trapped by macrophages. This enzyme system cleaves C3b to C3c and C3d, which may actually protect RBCs coated by these complement bypass products (Fig 10–1).[63]

In classic IgG-mediated autoimmune hemolysis, the destruction of coated RBCs occurs mainly in the extravascular space in the spleen sinusoids. Splenic macrophages possess IgG Fc receptors as well as C3b receptors,[69] and therefore cells coated with IgG and complement are more apt to be trapped by splenic macrophages.[70] This is further corroborated by in vitro studies with RBCs tagged by a radiolabel.[65] Most of the radioactivity was detected in the spleen.

Although phagocytosis is an important function of macrophages, it is not the sole process responsible for the pathogenesis of AHA. Macrophages also have an important role in the presentation of antigens to other cells of the immune system, the B and T cells.[71, 72]

It is possible that these functions as well as T cell suppressor functions may be altered in idiopathic AHA and in hemolysis induced by methyldopa.[73]

These are some of the possible mechanisms in-

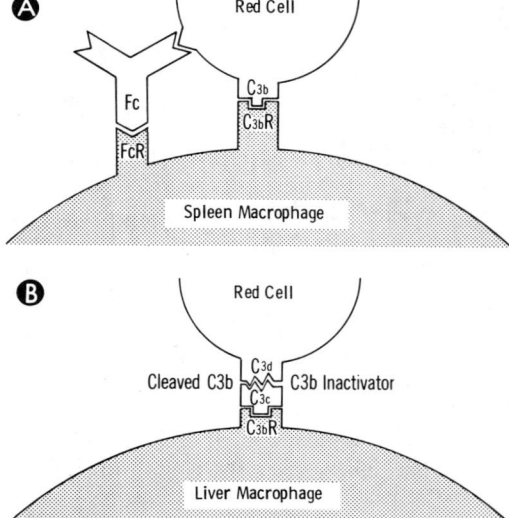

FIG 10–1.—Mechanism of trapping by splenic and liver macrophages coated with immunoglobulin or complement, or both. **A,** red cell coated with immunoglobulin and complement trapped by splenic macrophage possessing both FcR and CR1 (C3bR). **B,** red cell coated with complement trapped by Kupffer cell bearing C3bR. C3 may then be cleaved by C3b inactivator, releasing red cells coated with C3d.

volved in the pathogenesis of autoimmune hemolysis. Just how antibody formation against "self" antigens is triggered is far from elucidated.

Drawbacks of In Vivo Compatibility Testing.—Patients with AHA are more susceptible to RBC alloimmunization than other patients; therefore, this type of testing should be reserved for severely anemic patients for whom transfusion has been prescribed. The test is performed immediately before the transfusion to avoid further alloimmunization against the selected unit.

These patients often have anti-e antibodies and frequently develop anti-Rh core antibodies,[74, 75] making future transfusions difficult.

Other specificities of autoantibodies to RBC antigens have also been described, including anti-Kell, anti-Kidd, and Xg^a antibodies.[76, 77]

Interestingly, sera of some patients with warm AHA will react against Rh null cells. These may have anti-En^a specificities[78] or anti-Wr^b specificities.[79] Occasionally a positive antiglobulin test may be a result of malarial infection.[80]

It should be noted that some cases of AHA have arisen as a consequence of transfusion.[81, 82]

Management of patients with AHA may be further complicated by the appearance of alloantibodies. The chance of this occurring may be increased after transfusion, which is another good reason to avoid transfusing these patients whenever possible.

Monocyte in Vitro Assay.—An in vitro assay using the patient's own monocytes has recently been introduced to assess survival of potentially transfusable cells. Lysis by monocytes is often mediated by IgG3 antibodies not detected by the routine Coombs test. Coating by IgG2 and IgG4 usually does not result in hemolysis.[83] Some lysis occurring on these assays is actually caused by K lymphocytes rather than by monocytes, and does not require complement.[84]

Immunohematology Laboratory Workup

Warm antibodies are, for the most part, of the IgG class. Although these "incomplete" antibodies rarely cause direct agglutination, they may do so if RBCs are suspended in albumin. IgG antibodies very rarely produce in vitro lysis, though auto-anti-P antibodies seen in PCH will cause in vitro lysis. More commonly, IgG antibodies sensitize cells which can then be agglutinated with Coombs reagent, which reacts against IgG, IgM, IgA and complement, by bridging the distance that cannot be bridged by IgG alone under certain conditions. It has been suggested that IgG will agglutinate cells which are suspended in albumin or have been treated with trypsin because they have a decreased zeta potential.[85] However, this theory does not provide a satisfactory explanation for the increased reactivity of cells with antibody using LISS solutions. Other workers believe that the repellant forces on RBCs are due to hydration of sialic acid residues on RBC membranes.[86]

It is very possible that the two mechanisms intervene during cell agglutination of albumin-suspended RBCs by IgG.

Monospecific antisera can be used to identify the sensitizing antibody. Further precision can be achieved with monoclonal antibodies directed against specific Ig classes.

If the direct Coombs test is positive, the type of antibody or other protein coating the cells should be identified (i.e., IgG or complement). Phenotyping the patient's RBCs can be attempted by heat elution for 30 minutes at 45° C.[87] The specificity of the antibody coating the cells can be identified by eluting it from the RBCs with other methods.[88] The digitonin method or ether elution method can be used to release the antibody from RBCs[89] and tested against an RBC panel (see Chap. 6). RBC panels can be enzyme treated to optimize reactions of antibodies such as Rh and Kidd; antigens such as M, N, S, and Duffy are destroyed by this procedure. Most warm autoantibodies can be subclassified as follows: (1) Antibodies reacting with anti-IgG alone are most frequent and predominantly of the IgG1 subclass. (2) Antibodies reacting with anti-IgG and anti-C3 or C4. These antibodies are not frequently seen in SLE.[90, 91] (3) Antibodies reacting with anti-C3 or anti-C4, or both anti-C3 and C4, are the least frequent of the three types.

Some cases of warm AHA escape detection (approximately 2%)[91] by the Coombs test and must be studied by more sensitive methods.[92] Normally, RBCs have fewer than 35 molecules of IgG bound per cell. In the majority of Coombs-positive AHA cases, at least 500 molecules are present on the RBC surface, which is the lower level of sensitivity for the Coombs reagent.[91] Nevertheless, Coombs-negative AHA cases reveal that RBCs are coated with 65–470 molecules of IgG per cell, below the range of detectability by a routine Coombs test.[93]

The antibodies in some of these AHA samples may prove to be both anti-IgG and anticomplement antibodies rather than anticomplement only. The clonality of lymphocytes responsible for the production of the antibody is restricted, but lymphocytes are rarely monoclonal in both the IgG alone and the IgG plus complement groups.[94] The pattern of reactivity (IgG, IgG plus C, or C alone) tends to remain unchanged throughout the course of the disease, although it may vary in a few cases.

Most autoantibodies causing AHA have specificity for the Rh system. Many actually may start as anti-e antibodies and later develop into antibodies against precursors or core antigens of the Rh molecular complex.[95] Antibodies to core antigens have specificities for all RBCs, although certain cases of AHA described recently have been associated exclusively with IgA antibodies against the Rh system.[96] However, most IgA antibodies seen in AHA are usually associated with IgG and/or complement.[76]

Drug Therapy for AHA

Steroid therapy of animals, following IV transfusion of radiolabeled IgG-coated RBCs, resulted in decreased clearance of coated cells.[97] This favorable response has likewise been observed in most patients with AHA.[98] Steroids are given orally in the form of prednisone at high doses (60–80 mg/day) and continued for 2 weeks as the hematocrit improves. This dose is tapered weekly, first to 30 mg/day for 1 week and then to 5 mg/week if the hematocrit improves. The duration of the treatment is usually 2 months. Remissions are usually complete in the first episode, but relapses are frequent. Complete remissions are seen in 20% of cases; 10% of patients do not respond to steroid therapy.[1, 2]

It appears that steroid therapy, rather than act as immune suppressant of antibody synthesis, acts by inhibiting RES phagocytic functions.[99] About two thirds of AHA cases refractory to steroids benefit from a splenectomy, by showing temporary or permanent remission.[100] The rationale of removing the spleen is that in doing so the main site of RBC sequestration is eliminated, as well as a major site of antibody synthesis.[101] Scanning of the spleen after ^{51}Cr labeling of RBCs cannot be used as a reliable guide for helping decide on performing a splenectomy.[55] If both steroid therapy and splenectomy fail, immunosuppressive drug therapy may be attempted using cyclophosphamide, 60 mg/m^2. Immunosuppressive therapy has been successful in some of these refractory cases and is indicated when both these procedures have failed, or the patient is a poor splenectomy risk.[102]

Blood Transfusion in AHA

Blood transfusion to patients with AHA demands close cooperation between clinicians and the blood bank. The decision to transfuse blood to a patient with AHA is not an easy one, and the procedure should be undertaken with extreme caution. The hematocrit may be low enough to prompt the treating clinician to order blood; however, the blood bank personnel usually find incompatible crossmatches.

It should be remembered, however, that the anemia of AHA is progressive over a relatively long period of time in most cases. This allows patients to compensate at relatively low hematocrits. Double-blind studies have shown that most patients will tolerate hemoglobin levels above 8 gm/dl fairly well.[103] These patients will remain stable if hemoglobin levels remain at 8–10 gm/dl and patients are kept at rest. Nevertheless, those patients experiencing angina or circulatory failure will require transfusion, as will severely anemic patients (5–8 gm/dl of hemoglobin). It is wise in the vast majority of AHA cases to withhold transfusion until such time as the patient is moderately to severely symptomatic, because (1) the hematocrit and hemoglobin increment is very transient,[98] (2) the transfusion may occasionally result in catastrophic renal failure,[104] and (3) the patient is very frequently alloimmunized to transfused blood, decreasing the chance to obtain a compatible unit during angina or another emergency. If transfusion is decided on, it is usually undertaken with the least incompatible unit, though some authors do not believe there is a net benefit in this practice.[98]

Prognosis of AHA

The prognosis of AHA depends on underlying disorders (e.g., SLE, lymphoma). Morbidity may be high, and mortality may reach 15%–25%.[105]

Cold Autoimmune Hemolytic Anemia

The term "cold autoimmune hemolytic anemia" applies to conditions where autoimmune antibodies against RBC antigens and reactive at low temperatures arise in a host. These antibodies characteristically exhibit their highest reactivity in vitro between 0° and 5° C and readily bind complement. In vivo, however, these antibodies are capable of binding complement at higher temperatures but usually at temperatures below 37° C. Cold-type AHA constitutes about 10%–20% of AHA cases[106] and can be found mainly in two forms: cold agglutinin disease (CAD), or paroxysmal cold hemoglobinuria (PCH).

Cold Agglutinin Disease

CAD can be idiopathic or secondary to infections (especially *Mycoplasma pneumoniae* or infectious mononucleosis) or a lymphoproliferative disease such as lymphoma. Cold agglutinin disease is the more common of the cold-type AHA. The disease is usually more frequent in females[107] and has a peak incidence in the fifth and sixth decades of life,[108] although it has occasionally been seen in children.[3]

Pathogenesis.—Cold agglutinin production may be induced transiently as a result of infections with *M. pneumoniae (MP)*[109] or infectious mononucleosis (IM).[110] Most patients with *M. pneumoniae* infections develop high-titer cold agglutinins; however, few of these patients develop overt hemolysis,[111] although evidence of cell damage with decreased RBC survival is often present.[109] Similarly, cold agglutinins will be present in over 60% of cases of IM, but these patients rarely develop anemia.[112] Antibodies elicited against MP though unreactive with the organism, do cross-react with lipopolysaccharide fractions of the mycoplasma[113] and have, for the most part, anti-I specificity.[114] It is thought, however, that antibodies in IM are probably due to de novo expression of "i" antigens on lymphocytes during certain stages of cell development, often expressed during IM infection. Cold agglutinins in IM possess anti-i specificity in up to 50% of cases.[115] Since adults possess small amounts of "i" antigen, it is possible this is the reason anemia is usually mild in IM.

Pathophysiology of Anemia in CAD.—Antibodies in CAD are usually complement-binding antibodies of the IgM κ type, though some examples of IgM λ have been described.[116] IgM κ antibodies are usually of Ii specificity, whereas IgM λ are not. IgA κ cold agglutinins have been reported, but the specificity has been to Pr_1 antigens.[117]

IgM itself is capable of activating complement and may readily induce intravascular hemolysis such as occurs in isoantibody sensitization during ABO-incompatible transfusions. If hemolysis does not occur intravascularly, RBC survival may be decreased to 2–20 days.[118] However, antibodies do not appear to produce damage on their own[60] in the absence of complement. In addition, C1 appears to enhance binding of antibody to RBC antigens.[119] Even though IgM is much more efficient in binding complement than is IgG, at least 60 molecules of IgM per RBC are required to initiate immune clearance, whereas only 1.4 molecules of IgG per RBC are required for clearance.[70] If cells are not immediately destroyed intravascularly by the complete activation of the complement sequence, RBCs will remain coated with C3b after IgM has eluted. Thus cold agglutinins which do not induce immediate hemolysis do so through attachment of C3b on RBCs. IgM coating of RBCs in vivo usually elutes from the cell after binding[120] complement; subsequently, complement remains firmly attached to RBCs. Few monocytes and macrophages possess receptors for IgM, but many have receptors for C3b. At least 550 molecules of C3b are required for RBC clearance, which usually takes place in the liver.[68] C3b-coated RBCs, which are trapped by the RES, are sometimes incompletely phagocytized; these may break away, presumably due to the action of C3b inactivator, which cleaves C3b to C3c and C3d, explaining the reappearance of C-coated RBCs as circulating C3d-coated RBCs.[121] C3d-coated RBCs have a practically normal survival. In addition, cells sensitized to C3 before progression to C3b are likewise not phagocytized.[122] C3d competes for C3b binding sites and eventually may prevent lysis by complement.[123] As was mentioned above, C3b-coated RBCs usually are entrapped and may be destroyed in the liver by Kupffer cells.[15] Phagocytosis of coated RBCs by macrophages is probably achieved mostly via complement receptors on the phagocytic cell membrane. Several receptors for complement have been identified using monoclonal antibodies. These receptors were described earlier in the section on warm AHA.

Clinical Findings.—Most symptomatology in CAD is associated with anemia and acrocyanosis, which may develop acutely on exposure to cold temperatures, as occurs in cases of mycoplasma during the second or third week of illness[76] and resolves in about 2 weeks. Nevertheless, clinically detectable hemolysis occurring as a result of MP infections is not a frequent event; approximately 51 cases had been reported in the world literature up to 1978.[124] Hemolytic anemia due to cold antibodies, appearing as a consequence of IM, is likewise not a frequent event (1 in 1,000 cases of IM).[110] Anemia, however, may appear over a prolonged period of time. The symptoms are usually less severe in IM than in infections with *Mycoplasma*.[109] However, CAD secondary to infection may develop very rapidly and is occasionally fatal.[124] Hemoglobinuria may occur and be brought on after exposure to cold, but usually is not accompanied by fever or renal failure.[108] Acrocyanosis is a common finding and affects the tips of most fingers, causing gangrene in some cases,[125] unlike Raynaud's syndrome due to collagen disease, where the distribution of acrocyanosis is uneven. Acrocyanosis appears to be the result of both RBC agglutination and cryoprecipitation of plasma proteins in the small vessels of the extremities where blood temperature may be as low as 28°–31° C and well within the thermal range of reactivity of these cold agglutinins.[126] IgA cold agglutinins, usually monoclonal in character, do not bind complement and therefore do not produce hemolysis, but they do cause acrocyanosis.[127] Hepatosplenomegaly may be present in certain cases.[108] Unlike CAD associated with lymphoproliferative diseases, the anemia present in patients with *Mycoplasma* infections and infectious mononucleosis is usually self-limited. CAD associated with lymphoproliferative disorders is seen in older patients. The severity of the anemia, acrocyanosis, and skin ulcerations is usually increased during the colder months and tends to improve on warming. Hemoglobinuria may likewise be present in CAD secondary to malignancy and is more frequently seen during the winter. Diseases often associated with this type of CAD are lymphoma, reticulum cell sarcoma, and Waldenström's macroglobulinemia. Acrocyanosis without hemolytic anemia points to the diagnosis of a myeloma, not infrequently of the IgA class.

Laboratory Findings.—Anemia is usually not as severe as in warm-type AHA, and hemoglobin values may range from 7.4 gm/dl to 9 mg/dl, rarely dropping below these levels.[108] The hematocrit may drop to 10%–13%. The hemolysis varies, depending on the etiology as well as on the degree of exposure to cold.[90] Reticulocytosis is present in amounts proportional to the degree of hemolysis. Spherocytosis is usually less severe than in warm-type AHA. Polychromasia may be present. The mean RBC volume may be read as falsely high in automatic aperture counters due to autoagglutination. High mean corpuscular hemoglobin and mean corpuscular hemoglobin concentrations help define the diagnosis in these cases.[128]

Blood Bank Studies.—Autoagglutination may be the first evidence that a cold agglutination is present and is usually detected when the specimen reaches room temperature. Autoagglutination will disperse on warming. Most cold agglutinins are of the IgM class and frequently bear κ light chains if induced by *Mycoplasma,* but bear λ light chains if induced by IM.[129] These antibodies usually exhibit specificities to Ii RBC antigens, though anti-Pr_1 specificities have likewise been described. These specificities are located on the 26 amino terminal residues of α and δ sialoglycoproteins.[130] Cold antibodies due to MP or IM are polyclonal, whereas those associated with lymphoproliferative disorders are monoclonal or oligoclonal[131] and may be detected as monoclonal peaks on electrophoresis.[132] Usually these monoclonal IgM antibodies are IgM κ, whereas 20% of those found in macroglobulinemia are IgM λ.[133] Pathologic cold agglutinins will agglutinate cells at 0°–4° C at titers of 1 × 10^6 or more; commonly, however, titers are 1:1,000. Normal individuals, including newborns, have low-titer cold agglutinins (1:32 or lower).[134] Titers greater than 1:64 at room temperature are considered pathologic. Usually, the reactivity of these antibodies decreases on incubation at temperatures greater than 31° C,[135] although the thermal range may vary, with a few antibodies reacting better at higher temperatures. Cold agglutinins usually react better with enzyme-treated cells.[136] Identification of the specificity of pathologic cold agglutinins must be attempted. A direct Coombs test, antibody identification with a panel, and eluates of RBC samples preincubated in the cold and eluted in the warm must be performed. Cold agglutinin titers are prepared by doubling dilutions at 4° C, room temperature, 30° C and 37° C to define the thermal range. Incubations at 30° C with albumin must also be performed, for they correlate better with the actual in vivo reactivity.[137] Further identification of the type of protein that coats the RBCs must be obtained. Polyclonal and monoclonal antibodies against human immunoglobulins and complement are commercially available for this purpose. The vast majority of cases, however, are identified as complement which has been attached by IgM no longer present on the RBCs. Though most cold agglutinins have been of the IgM class, both IgA[138, 139] and IgG[140] antibodies have been identified; many of these have Pr reactivity and are protease sensitive.[139]

Therapy of CAD AHA.—The therapy and outcome of CAD will depend on the underlying disease. Patients with CAD secondary to MP or infectious mononucleosis usually respond well to supportive therapy. Transfusion is reserved for patients with severe anemia and should be supplied in the form of washed cells to avoid the transfusion of additional sources of complement. Keeping the patient warm, with special attention to the extremities, is of paramount importance. In CAD secondary to MP treatment with antibiotics (e.g., tetracyclines, or erythromycin) is usually effective. Steroids have not been successful in the treatment of CAD due to *Mycoplasma*[90] but appear to be successful in severe cases of CAD secondary to IM.[141] Steroids do not appear to be indicated for idiopathic CAD or CAD secondary to a lymphoproliferative disorder.[90] Immunosuppressive therapy has been attempted successfully in certain severe intractable cases using chlorambucil.[142] Splenectomy is very rarely indicated. If anemia is very severe, transfusions may be necessary. Blood warmers may be necessary in these cases. To obtain compatible blood units, samples may be autoabsorbed overnight at 4°–6° C. Crossmatching must be performed in the warm (37° C) in severe cases, where the antibody is of high titer and conflicts with the crossmatch tests.[143] Plasmapheresis has been utilized successfully in few cases,[144] but permanent improvement cannot be expected using this therapeutic modality.[145] CAD associated with a lymphoproliferative disorder usually follows a smoldering course, and the outcome is determined more by the development of the malignancy than by the autoimmune hemolytic anemia per se.

Paroxysmal Cold Hemoglobinuria

Paroxysmal cold hemoglobinuria (PCH) is a relatively rare cause of autoimmune hemolysis (7%–10% of cases of AHA).[146] Although the disease was fully described in the mid-19th century, the actual serology was described by Donath and Landsteiner at the turn of the century.[147] These authors described a biphasic, cold reactive autoantibody capable of binding complement in the cold, and lysing the cells on warming. Characteristically, the disease was associated with congenital and tertiary syphilis in the past, but with the advent of the control of endemic syphilis, PCH is now seen most frequently in association with viral respiratory diseases, measles, and chicken pox,[148] and therefore today the disease is more frequent in children. Other causes of PCH are IM[149] and infection by *M. pneumoniae*.[150]

Pathophysiology.—The Donath-Landsteiner antibody (D-L) is usually an IgG3 biphasic cold agglutinin[151] which binds C1q to RBCs[152] at lower temperatures (most probably in surface capillaries near the skin, where the body temperature is lower) and then on warming, the antibody elutes off, leaving C3 attached to the RBC. Complement then proceeds to activation of C9, causing hemolysis.[153] The antibody will, in addition to binding complement, cause agglutination of RBCs.[154]

Clinical Manifestations.—The classic description of PCH associated with lues revealed that patients who are exposed to cold temperatures develop muscular pain, backache, headaches, chills, and fever minutes to hours after exposure. Characteristically, the first urine passed after the hemolytic episode is hemoglobinuric. Nevertheless, patients with the D-L antibody which developed after viral syndromes infrequently develop paroxysmal hemoglobinuria, and in contrast to syphilis-induced PCH it is transient. Both findings have prompted certain authors to question the validity of the term PCH for viral-induced PCH.[155] Other symptoms of PCH are acrocyanosis and unusual susceptibility to frostbite. Urticaria triggered by exposure to cold is also seen in these patients.

Laboratory Findings.—In classic PCH, the hematocrit and hemoglobin may drop dramatically. Hemoglobinuria, as in other types of hemolysis, will appear on saturation of haptoglobin. Other hematologic findings will be similar to other types of hemolysis (splenocytes, schistocytes, polychromatophilic cells). Evidence of erythrophagocytosis is frequently seen. Leukopenia followed by leukocytosis is also present.

Blood Bank Serology.—The direct Coombs test will be positive due to coating by complement. However, in order to detect the IgG responsible for the hemolytic process, incubations must be performed in the cold (12°–15° C). The Donath-Landsteiner test can be performed. The patient's serum is incubated in the cold (4° C) in the presence of a fresh source of complement, and then warmed to 37° C.[156] In the majority of cases of PCH, the antibody reacts to determinants on the P antigen.[157] This specificity is restricted to P, for most D-L antibodies will not react with P^K or pp cells.[158] Rarely, cold anti-p antibodies have been documented,[159] and occasionally D-L antibodies have been reported to react against H-I specificities.[160] Rarely, biphasic anti-I agglutinins may be seen after *Mycoplasma* infections.[150] Anti-i antibodies arising as a consequence of IM exhibit a biphasic behavior in vitro.[161] Consistently, D-L antibodies are inhibited by globoside, which shares specificities with Forssman antigens present in a variety of tissues as well as organisms.[162]

Management of PCH.—Treatment is usually geared to the underlying disease (e.g., antibiotic therapy for syphilis). Patients are instructed to avoid exposure to cold if possible. The value of steroids has not been fully assessed in PCH; in a few cases, splenectomy has proved helpful but the data are anecdotal,[163] and splenectomy should probably be reserved for refractory cases. Antihistaminics may be given to treat cold-induced urticaria.

Transfusion should probably be with P-negative units, though P-positive units have been given without major complications.[155] Today, most cases of viral-induced PCH are self-limited and require only supportive treatment. Certain cases of syphilis-induced PCH will revert after antibiotic therapy.[164]

DRUG-INDUCED IMMUNE HEMOLYSIS

About 12%–18% of all cases of AHA are caused by drugs.[90] However, the disease is not frequent; of all drug-induced blood disorders, in one series 50% were thrombocytopenia, 25% granulocytopenia, and 5% hemolytic anemia.[165]

The diagnosis of AHA induced by drugs is important because in most cases the outcome is good and the disease can be easily prevented or treated. The first description of damage to blood cells by a drug was provided by Ackroyd, who pioneered the study of the possible role of drugs in the pathogenesis of immune hemolysis.[166]

Pathogenesis of Drug-Induced AHA

Four main mechanisms are recognized in drug-induced AHA in the blood bank laboratory:

1. A hapten (usually a small molecular weight drug) and the RBC membrane produces a complex capable of stimulating an immune response (Fig 10–2,A).
2. A soluble immune complex consisting of the drug plus antibody is formed. This complex then attaches to the RBC, which is destroyed as an innocent bystander (Fig 10–2,B).
3. The drug produces damage to the RBC membrane, which then permits absorption of immunoglobulins and other proteins onto the cell (Fig 10–2,C).
4. The drug may cause an autoimmune type of anemia indistinguishable from idiopathic autoimmune hemolysis (Fig 10–2,D).

Examples of the different mechanisms of drug-mediated immune hemolysis are given in Table 10–2.

Conjugation Between a Haptenic Drug and the RBC

Haptens are characteristically small molecules (MW < 500 daltons) which, on their own, are incapable of stimulating an immune response; however, when coupled with high molecular weight proteins, haptens induce antibody formation. The prototype for this type of drug reaction is penicillin,[186] and the reaction usually occurs when the antibiotic is given frequently intravenously and at high doses (e.g., 10 million units/day for 1 week).[186] Usually, patients developing hemolytic anemia due to penicillin do not have other reactions to penicillin.

Penicillin is likewise capable of binding to plasma proteins, inducing soluble immune complexes.[187] When penicillin acts as a hapten, it is bound by high affinity bonds (probably covalent) to

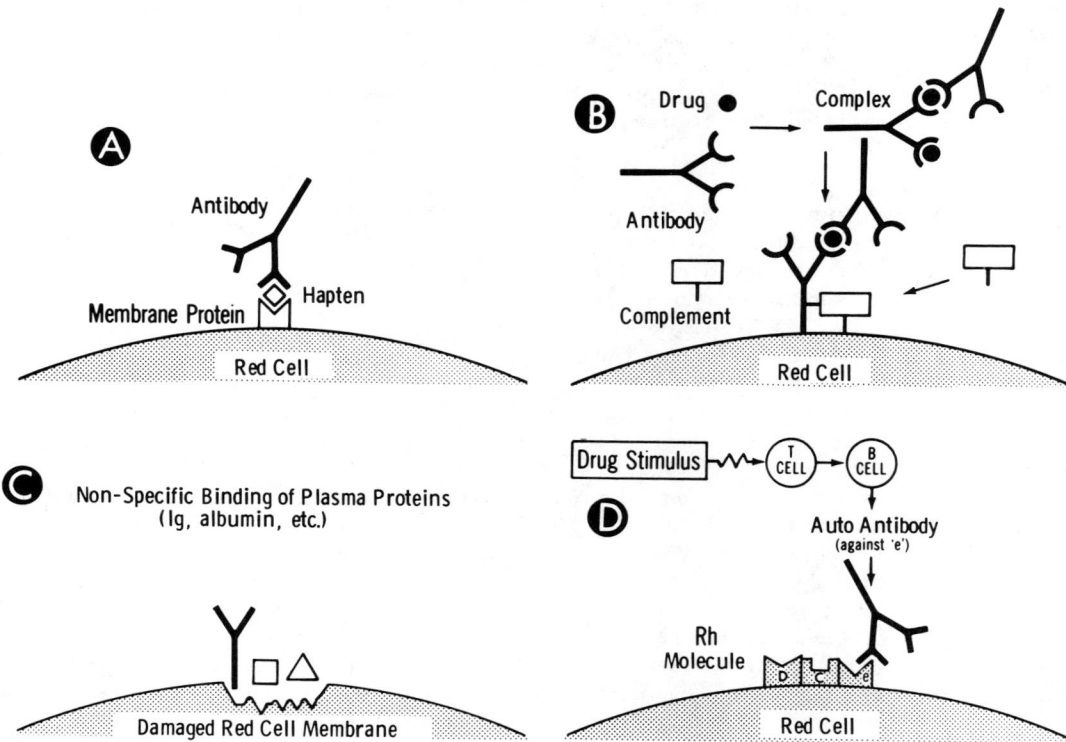

FIG 10–2.—Mechanisms of immune hemolysis caused by drugs. **A,** drug acts as a hapten, and hapten-antihapten interaction takes place. **B,** drug-anti-drug immune complexes form in the soluble phase and secondarily attach to RBCs which are innocent bystanders. **C,** damage or alteration of red cell membrane surface with secondary nonspecific binding of plasma proteins (e.g., IgG, IgA, IgM, albumin, fibrinogen). **D,** drug, through a stimulus, inhibits suppressor T cells, allowing "forbidden" T helper cell clones to stimulate B cells in the production of autoantibodies (e.g.,anti-e).

membrane moieties.[188] About 30% of patients receiving high-dose penicillin therapy exhibit RBC coating with this hapten, 3% of these patients develop a positive Coombs test.[189] Most normal individuals exhibit IgM antibodies against determinants present in penicillin (> 90%),[190] such as the bencyl penicilloyl group (BPO).[191] Conversely, hemolytic antipenicillin antibodies are non-complement-binding IgG antibodies, and though sometimes directed against the BPO group,[192] are usually directed against other penicillin specificities.[193] In few cases, penicillin will induce coating with complement in addition to IgG.[194] Other drugs that cause a similar hapten coating of cells are cephalosporin,[195] though this drug usually causes a positive Coombs via the fourth mechanism listed in Table 10–2, and carbromal.[170] Interestingly, cephalosporins possess cross-reactive epitopes with penicillin.[196] As in most other cases of immune hemolytic anemia, where cells are coated with IgG, this type of drug-mediated immune hemolysis causes predominantly splenic sequestration of sensitized RBCs.[197] Hemolysis may be brisk, and reticulocytes are usually present. Spherocytes are rare.[198] The laboratory investigation of AHA due to a membrane-bound hapten should first exclude any other cause of a positive direct Coombs test result. A history of taking high-dose penicillin or other antibiotic is helpful.

In the laboratory, this type of drug-induced hemolysis is suspected after finding a positive Coombs test in patients receiving the drug. The diagnosis is arrived at by incubating normal RBCs with 40 mg/ml penicillin or other suspect antibiotic at pH 9.6 in barbital buffer to coat RBCs with the drug,[199] followed by washing and incubating with the patient's serum or RBC eluate. The cells should react only with drug-coated cells. Sera usually react at titers of 1:1,000. Treatment is prophylactic, by interrupting penicillin therapy or other causative agent. Transfusion is indicated if

TABLE 10–2.—Some Known Mechanisms and Examples of Drug-Induced Immune Hemolysis

MECHANISM	DRUG	ANTIBODY	COMPLEMENT	SITE OF DESTRUCTION	REFERENCE
Membrane bound hapten (MB)	Penicillin, tetracyclines	IgG	Occasional	Spleen	167, 168
	Cephalosporins				169
	Carbromal				170
	Cisplatin				171
Plasma-bound hapten (PB)	Quinidine	Occasional	Consistent	Intravascular	172
	Phenacetin	IgG		Liver	173
	Chlorpropamide				174
	Rifampin				175
	Sulfonamides				176
	Antihistamine				177
	Stibophen				178
	Thiazides				179
Combined (MB/PB)	Streptomycin	IgG	Consistent	Combined	180
Nonspecific membrane damage		IgG, IgA		Multiple	181
Decreased T cell suppression	α-Methyldopa	IgG	Rarely	Spleen	182
	Levodopa				183
	Mefenamic acid				184
	Procainamide				185

hemolysis is severe, in the acute stages. Steroids may be indicated in severe cases.[197]

Immune Complex Mechanism

This type of immune hemolysis has also been termed "innocent bystander-type hemolysis." Although infrequent in incidence, it is the mechanism attributed to the widest variety of drugs implicated in drug-induced immune hemolysis.[199] Antibodies against the drug are presumably formed when the drug hapten is complexed with a plasma protein inducing formation of IgM or IgG antibodies against the drug. These antibodies, in the presence of the drug, may form soluble immune complexes (IC) capable of binding complement and activating it to C3b at a site remote from the RBCs,[199] which then attach to CR1, the receptor for C3b on RBCs.[200] This RBC receptor for C3b constitutes one of the body's mechanisms for trapping circulating IC for disposal by the RES. However, it is thought that actual attachment of IC to cell membranes with subsequent activation and attachment of complement at the RB membrane occurs more frequently,[199] as has been shown for drug-induced immune thrombocytopenias[201] and subsequently proposed as the mechanism for this type of drug-induced immune hemolysis.[202] Recently, reports that these antibodies may also be of the IgG class have been published, and IgG antibodies may be even more common than IgM antibodies in reactions to quinidine.[203] Complement coating of RBCs is a constant finding in this type of drug-mediated immune hemolysis. IgG may be detected in some of these cases on laboratory testing.[203] Since IC elute on binding complement, other cells may be damaged by the same IC, thus requiring relatively small concentrations of antibody.[202] In addition, unlike penicillin-induced reactions, a relatively small amount of the drug is needed to cause the reaction.[204] Of interest is that many of the drugs that cause hemolysis due to IC formation may also cause thrombocytopenia.[203] However, the mechanism of platelet lysis may be different, for platelets possess IgG Fc receptors.[205] It has been observed recently that drug-induced hemolysis of this type produces attachment of IC to specific RBC structures. For instance, in an IC-type streptomycin reaction, there was specific attachment of high affinity to M and Rh_o (D) antigens;[206] thus this mechanism is a combined hapten-like bond of streptomycin to the RBC membrane, with the subsequent production of an IgG antibody capable of binding complement.[206] In another example of IC binding to RBC antigens, a reaction to glafenin in which the IC specificity was against "e" was described.[207] Rifampin, which induces antibody formation in up to 30% of patients,[208] has stimulated the formation of IC which appeared to bind to I-positive cells.[209]

Clinically, these patients frequently develop acute intravascular hemolysis (about 80% of the cases[198]), with the complication of renal failure (in up to 50% of cases[210]), and DIC, which may terminate fatally.[178]

The laboratory diagnosis is based on demonstrating the capacity of the patient's serum to hemolyze RBCs in the presence of the drug. The problem serum is incubated with the drug at 1 mg/ml concentrations with the patient's serum (pH 7) and a fresh source of complement at 37° C, with normal group O cells. Hemolysis, agglutination, a positive Coombs test, and complement coating is then sought.[199] Treatment consists in discontinuing the offending drug immediately and treating DIC and renal failure if present. Plasmapheresis and exchange transfusion may be warranted.[179] Blood transfusion before exchange may be hazardous due to the nonspecific ability of the patient's serum to hemolyze transfused cells.

Nonspecific Adsorption of Plasma Proteins

Cephalosporins are, to date, the only drugs known to produce a positive DAT by this mechanism. The drug acts by modifying RBC membranes to allow nonspecific protein adsorption on RBCs. Less than 5% of patients receiving these drugs develop a positive direct Coombs test[196] and even less frequently do cephalosporins induce hemolytic anemia; four cases of hemolysis due to cephalosporins have been described in the literature.[211] Nevertheless, none of these cases was induced by nonspecific adsorption.[212] A variety of proteins adsorb onto the surface of RBCs in this type of drug-induced positive direct Coombs test, notably IgG, IgA, IgM, C3, and C4, but also other proteins such as fibrinogen, α_1-antitrypsin, and α_2-macroglobulin.[189] Since the proteins bound to the RBC have done so nonspecifically, and since the binding is not immunologically mediated, the eluates obtained from RBCs will be negative.[199] The main significance of this type of drug-induced positive DAT is its capacity to interfere with crossmatching tests.

Drug-induced Immune Hemolysis Via Suppressor T Cell Inhibition

The main drug in this category is α-methyldopa (Aldomet).[182] This type of drug-induced immune hemolysis is by far the most frequent form of all drug-induced immune hemolytic anemias, accounting for about 80% of cases. Aldomet also accounts for about 11% of all cases of warm AHA.[198] It is followed in frequency by penicillin-induced hemolysis, which is substantially less frequent.[213] About 15%–20% of patients receiving Aldomet for 3–6 months will develop a positive DAT;[214] however, only 1% of these patients will actually develop hemolysis.[215] Unlike other drug-induced immune hemolysis, methyldopa induces the formation of antibodies directed against normal RBCs, agglutinating them in the absence of the drug. These findings make methyldopa immune hemolysis similar to idiopathic autoimmune hemolysis.[199]

Pathogenesis

The pathogenesis of Aldomet-induced AHA remains unclear. Several hypotheses have been advanced to explain the induction of these antibodies. One theory assumes that methyldopa alters the Rh locus during erythrocyte development, based on the fact that Aldomet-induced antibodies react for the most part against Rh specificities.[216] However, the lack of appreciable binding of methyldopa to RBCs in vitro, plus the finding of non-Rh specificities such as Wr^b,[217] do not support this hypothesis. Other authors propose that methyldopa in its quinone form induces IgG aggregation with nonspecific IgG adherence to RBCs;[218] however, this does not explain the consistent specificity of Aldomet antibodies for Rh antigens. The more probable mechanism is that Aldomet induces the stimulation of "forbidden" B cell clones against specific RBC antigens.[219] Recently, strong evidence has been brought forth demonstrating that both in vivo and in vitro, methyldopa inhibits suppressor T cells.[220] It has been postulated that methyldopa causes a persistent elevation of intracellular T cell cyclic AMP, which directly inhibits suppressor T cells,[182] leading to unregulated autoantibody by "forbidden" B cell clones. These responses may very well be regulated by HLA-DR antigens.[181] The B cell clones will not only produce antibodies against RBCs, but against other tissue antigens as well, suggesting other autoimmune disease. Examples of these antibodies are antinuclear antibodies, rheumatoid factors, and anti-gastric mucosa antibodies.[221] Clinically, Aldomet-induced AHA is indistinguishable from idiopathic warm AHA, except for the clinical history of Aldomet intake. The anemia develops in a gradual manner. Acute hemolysis has not been reported in this type of drug-induced AHA. The development of antibodies is dose-related; thus a positive DAT develops in 11% of patients taking 1 gm/day or less, in 20% of those taking up to 2 gm/day, and in 36% of patients taking over 2 gm/day.[214]

The direct antiglobulin test usually becomes negative after 1–24 months of discontinuing the drug.[222]

Laboratory Testing

A strongly reactive positive Coombs test is consistently found in all cases due to coating of RBCs by IgG1.[223] Free and bound IgG are routinely found, and both the free serum antibody as well as eluates of the RBC-bound antibody are reactive with normal RBCs. In the vast majority of cases of Aldomet-induced AHA the antibody reacted with Rh antigens. In a series of 13 cases, the Rh antibody specificities of Aldomet-induced AHA were as follows: 6 had anti-e, 5 had anti-D, and 2 had anti-c specificity.[7] In some cases, anti-Rh core antibodies are also seen[224] and are heterogeneous, suggesting polyclonality.[224] As was mentioned above, specificities other than the Rh may be exhibited by Aldomet-induced antibodies, such as Wr^b [217] and anti-Jk^a.[225]

About 17% of Aldomet-induced AHA cases have complement coating in addition to the IgG, but coating by IgG is, in contrast to idiopathic AHA, an invariable finding in Aldomet-induced AHA.[226] Unlike idiopathic AHA, the patient's serum will not lyse enzyme-treated RBCs in Aldomet-induced AHA.[226] Therapy in most cases consists of eliminating Aldomet from the therapeutic schedules of patients developing hemolytic anemia, although the development of a positive Coombs test does not preclude continuation of therapy. Steroid therapy may be indicated in severe Aldomet-induced hemolytic anemias.[227] Blood transfusions are occasionally necessary, and on diagnosis of Aldomet-induced positive DAT, the finding may have to be ignored and blood given.

Occasionally deaths from Aldomet-induced AHA have been reported.[228]

Other Drugs Producing "Aldomet"-Type AHA

Some drugs closely related to α-methyldopa, such as Levodopa, have caused a similar type of AHA.[183] Mefenanic acid,[184] procainamide,[185] Dilantin,[229] and chlorpromazine[215] may likewise cause AHA similar to that caused by Aldomet.

REFERENCES

1. Petz L.D., Garraty G.: *Acquired Immune Hemolytic Anemias*, ed. 1. New York, Churchill Livingstone, 1980, p. 28.
2. Swisher S.N.: Acquired hemolytic disease. *Postgrad. Med.* 40:378, 1966.
3. Habibi B., Homberg J.C., Schaison G., et al.: Autoimmune hemolytic anemia in children: A review of 80 cases. *Am. J. Med.* 56:61, 1974.
4. Sokal R.J., Hewitt S., Stamps B.K.: Autoimmune haemolysis: An 18-year study of 865 cases referred to a regional transfusion center. *Br. Med. J.* 1:2023, 1981.
5. Bell C.A., Zwicker H., Sacks H.J.: Autoimmune hemolytic anemia: Routine serologic evaluation in a general hospital population. *Am. J. Clin. Pathol.* 60:903, 1973.
6. Talal N.: Tolerance and autoimmunity, in Parker C.W. (ed.): *Clinical Immunology*. Philadelphia, W.B. Saunders Co., 1980, p. 86.
7. Brown D.L., Dacie J.V., Worlledge S.: Autoallergic blood diseases, in Lachman P.J., Peters D.K. (eds.): *Clinical Aspects of Immunology*, ed. 4. Oxford, England, Blackwell Scientific Publications, 1982, pp. 762, 763.
8. Mollison P.L.: *Blood Transfusion in Clinical Medicine*, ed. 7. Oxford, England, Blackwell Scientific Publications, 1983, p. 458.
9. Pale K.J., Mirevova L., Bradek V., et al.: The effect of anti-A antibody on red cell phosphates and adenosine triphosphate activity in vitro. *Scand. J. Haematol.* 5:191, 1968.
10. von dem Borne A.E.G., Engelfriet C.P., DoBeckers D., et al.: Autoimmune hemolytic anaemia: IV. Biochemical studies of red cells from patients with autoimmune haemolytic anaemia with incomplete warm auto-antibodies. *Clin. Exp. Immunol.* 8:377, 1971.
11. Engelfriet C.P., von dem Borne A.E.G., DoBeckers F.W., et al.: Immune destruction of red cells, in Bell C.A. (ed.): *A Seminar on Immune-Mediated Cell Destruction*. Washington, D.C., American Association of Blood Banks, 1981, p. 93.
12. Huber H., Douglas S.D., Fudenberg H.H.: The IgG receptor, an immunological marker for the characterization of mononuclear cells. *Immunology* 17:7, 1969.
13. Abramson N., LoBuglio A.F., Jandl J.H., et al.: The interaction between human monocytes and red cells: Binding characteristics. *J. Exp. Med.* 132:1191, 1970.
14. von dem Borne A.E.G., Engelfriet C.P.: Mechanisms of red cell destruction by non-complement binding IgG antibodies: The essential role in vivo of the Fc part of IgG. *Br. J. Haematol.* 36:467, 1977.
15. Schreiber A.D., Frank M.M.: The role of antibody

and complement in the clearance and destruction of erythrocytes: I. In vivo effect of IgG and IgM complement fixing sites. *J. Clin. Invest.* 51:575, 1972.
16. LoBuglio A.F., Cotran R.S., Jandl J.H.: Red cells coated with immunoglobulin G: Binding and sphering by mononuclear cells in man. *Science* 158:1582, 1967.
17. Metchnikoff E.: *Immunity in Infectious Diseases.* Cambridge, England, University Press, 1905.
18. Unanue E.R., Beller D.I., Lu C.Y., et al.: Antigen presentation: Comments on its regulation and mechanism. *J. Immunol.* 132:1, 1984.
19. DeFreitas E.C., Chesnut R.W., Grey H.M., et al.: Macrophage-dependent activation of antigen-specific T cells requires antigen and a soluble monokine. *J. Immunol.* 131:23, 1983.
20. Johnson J.W., Marino P.A., Schreiber R.D., et al.: Sequential activation of murine mononuclear phagocytes for tumor cytolysis: Differential expression of markers by macrophages in the several stages of development. *J. Immunol.* 131:1038, 1983.
21. Shepherd V.L., Stahl P.D., Bernd P., et al.: Receptor-mediated entry of β-glucuronidase into the parasitophorous vacuoles of macrophages infected with *Leishmania mexicana amazonensis. J. Exp. Med.* 157:1471, 1983.
22. Van Furth R., in Forster O., Landy M. (eds.): *Heterogeneity of Mononuclear Phagocytes.* New York, Academic Press, 1981, p. 3.
23. DeBakker J.M., Daems W.Th., in Forster O., Landy M. (eds.): *Heterogeneity of Mononuclear Phagocytes.* New York, Academic Press, 1981, p. 11.
24. Burgues A.W., Camarkis J., Metcalf D.: Purification and properties of colony stimulating factor from mouse lung-conditioned medium. *J. Biol. Chem.* 252:1998, 1977.
25. Arend W.P., Ragsdale C.G., in Forster O., Landy M. (eds.): *Heterogeneity of Mononuclear Phagocytes.* New York, Academic Press, 1981, p. 150.
26. Unkeless J.: The presence of two Fc receptors on mouse macrophages: Evidence from a variant cell line and differential trypsin sensitivity. *J. Exp. Med.* 145:931, 1977.
27. Kulczycki A. Jr., Hempstead B.L., Hofmann S.L., et al.: The cell surface receptor for immunoglobulin E: II. Properties of the purified biologically active ε receptors. *J. Biol. Chem.* 254:3194, 1979.
28. Davies D.R., Metzger H.: Structural basis of antibody function. *Annu. Rev. Immunol.* 1:87, 1983.
29. Fearon D.T., Wong W.W.: Complement ligand-receptor interactions that mediate biological responses. *Annu. Rev. Immunol.* 1:243, 1983.
30. Fearon D.T.: Regulation of the amplification C3 convertase of human complement by an inhibitory protein isolated from human erythrocyte membranes. *Proc. Natl. Acad. Sci. USA* 76:5867, 1979.
31. Newman S.L., Johnson R.B. Jr.: Role of binding through C3b and IgG in polymorphonuclear function: Studies with trypsin generated C3b. *J. Immunol.* 123:1839, 1979.
32. Ehlenberger A.G., Nussenzweig V.: The role of membrane receptors for C3b and C3d in phagocytosis. *J. Exp. Med.* 145:357, 1977.
33. Wright S.D., Silverstein S.C.: Receptors for C3b and C3bi promote phagocytosis but not the release of toxic oxygen from human phagocytes. *J. Exp. Med.* 158:2016, 1983.
34. Young-Karlan B.R., Ashman R.F.: Order of events leading to surface immunoglobulin capping: Analysis of a transmembrane signal. *J. Immunol.* 127:1177, 1981.
35. Oliver J.M., Berlin R.D.: Cytoskeleton-membrane interaction and remodeling of the cell surface during phagocytosis and chemotaxis. *Adv. Exp. Med. Biol.* 155:113, 1982.
36. Walker W.S., in Nelson D.S. (ed.): *Immunobiology of the Macrophage.* New York, Academic Press, 1976, p. 99.
37. Rhodes J.R.: Macrophage heterogeneity in receptor activity: The activation of macrophage Fc receptor function in vivo and in vitro. *J. Immunol.* 114:976, 1975.
38. Arend W.P., Manik M.: The macrophage receptor for IgG: Number and affinity of binding sites. *J. Immunol.* 110:1455, 1973.
39. Akiyama Y., Miller P.J., Thurman J.B., et al.: Characterization of a human blood monocyte subset with low peroxidase activity. *J. Clin. Invest.* 72:1093, 1983.
40. Raff H.V., Stobo J.D., in Forster O., Landy M. (eds.): *Heterogeneity of Mononuclear Phagocytes.* New York, Academic Press, 1981, p. 68.
41. Todd R.F. III, Nadler L.M., Schlossman S.F.: Antigens on human monocytes identified by monoclonal antibodies. *J. Immunol.* 126:1435, 1981.
42. Todd R.F. III, Schlossman S.F.: Analysis of antigenic determinants on human monocytes and macrophages. *Blood* 59:775, 1982.
43. Toews G.B., Vial W.C., Dunn M.M., et al.: The accessory cell function of human alveolar macrophages in specific T cell proliferation. *J. Immunol.* 132:181, 1984.
44. Frank M.M., in *Seminar on Laboratory Management of Hemolysis.* Washington, D.C., American Association of Blood Banks, 1979, pp. 29–43.
45. Fries L.F., Brickman C.M., Frank M.M.: Monocyte receptors for the Fc portion of IgG increase in number in auto-immune hemolytic anemia and other hemolytic states and are decreased by glucocorticoid therapy. *J. Immunol.* 131:1240, 1983.
46. Fries L.F., Mullins W.W., Cho K.R., et al.: Monocyte receptors for the Fc portion of IgG are increased in systemic lupus erythematosus. *J. Immunol.* 132:695, 1984.
47. Katayama S., Chia D., Knutson D.W., et al.: Decreased Fc receptor avidity and degradative function of monocytes from patients with systemic lupus erythematosus. *J. Immunol.* 131:217, 1983.
48. Gandour D.M., Walker W.S.: Macrophage cell cycling: Influence on Fc receptors and antibody-dependent phagocytosis. *J. Immunol.* 130:1108, 1983.
49. Mauer A.M., Athens J.W., Aschenbrucker H., et

al.: Leukokinetic studies: II. A method for labeling granulocytes in vitro with radioactive diisopropylphosphate (DFP32). *J. Clin. Invest.* 39:1481, 1960.
50. Rosse W.F.: Philip Levine Award Lecture: The lysis of erythrocytes by incomplete antibodies. *Am. J. Clin. Pathol.* 77:5, 1982.
51. Rosse W.F., deBoisfleury A., Bessis M.: The interaction of phagocytic and red cells modified by immune reactions: Comparison of antibody and complement-coated red cells. *Blood Cells* 1:345, 1975.
52. Kurlander R.J., Rosse W.F.: Lymphocyte mediated lysis of antibody coated human red cells in the presence of human serum. *Blood* 53:1197, 1979.
53. Pirofsky B.: *Autoimmunization and the Autoimmune Hemolytic Anemias.* Baltimore, Williams & Wilkins Co., 1969, p. 1.
54. Lewis F.B., Schwartz R.S., Dameshek W.: X-radiation and alkylating agents as possible "trigger" mechanisms in the autoimmune complications of malignant lymphoproliferative disease. *Clin. Exp. Immunol.* 1:3, 1966.
55. Allgood J.W., Chaplin H.: Idiopathic acquired autoimmune hemolytic anemia. *Am. J. Med.* 43:254, 1967.
56. Dacie J.V., Worlledge S.M.: Autoallergic blood diseases, in Gell P.G.H., Coombs R.R.A., Lachman P.J. (eds.): *Clinical Aspects of Immunology,* ed. 3. Oxford, England, Blackwell Scientific Publications, 1975, p. 1149.
57. Zucker-Franklin D., Karpatkin S.: Red cell and platelet fragmentation in idiopathic autoimmune thrombocytopenia purpura. *N. Engl. J. Med.* 297:517, 1977.
58. Wang W., Herrod H., Pui C.H., et al.: Immunoregulatory abnormalities in Evans syndrome. *Am. J. Hematol.* 15:381, 1983.
59. Mollison P.L.: Determination of red cell survival using ^{51}Cr, in Bell C.A. (ed.): *A Seminar on Immune-Mediated Cell Destruction.* Washington, D.C. American Association of Blood Banks, 1981, p. 45.
60. Jandl J.H., Jones A.R., Castle W.B.: The destruction of red cells by antibodies in man: I. Observations on the sequestration and lysis of red cells altered by immune mechanisms. *J. Clin. Invest.* 36:1428, 1957.
61. Hughes-Jones N.C., Mollison P.L., Veall N.: Removal of incompatible red cells by the spleen. *Br. J. Haematol.* 11:461, 1965.
62. Brown D.L., Lachman P.J., Dacie J.V.: The in vivo behavior of complement coated red cells: Studies in C6-deficient, C3-depleted and normal rabbits. *Clin. Exp. Immunol.* 7:401, 1970.
63. Lay W.H., Nussenzweig V.: Receptors for complement on leukocytes. *J. Exp. Med.* 128:991, 1968.
64. Brown D.L., Lachman P.J., Dacie J.V.: The in vivo behavior of complement coated red cells: Studies in C6-deficient, C3-depleted and normal rabbits. *Clin. Exp. Immunol.* 7:401, 1970.
65. Schreiber A.D., Frank M.M.: The role of antibody and complement in the immune clearance and destruction of erythrocytes: In vivo effects of IgG and IgM complement fixing sites. *J. Clin. Invest.* 51:575, 1972.
66. Mantovani B., Rabbinovitch M., Nussenzweig V.: Phagocytosis of immune complexes by macrophages: Different roles of the macrophage receptor sites for complement (C3) and for immunoglobulin (IgG). *J. Exp. Med.* 135:780, 1972.
67. Frank M.M.: Mechanisms of cell destruction in immune hemolytic anemia, in Barns A. Jr. (ed.): *A Seminar on Laboratory Management of Hemolysis.* Washington, D.C., American Association of Blood Banks, 1979, p. 35.
68. Jaffe C.J., Atkinson J.P., Frank M.M.: The role of complement in the clearance of cold agglutinin sensitized erythrocytes in man. *J. Clin. Invest.* 58:942, 1976.
69. Hallgren R., Sjöstrom P., Bill A.: The uptake of IgG and IgM coated sheep erythrocytes in perfused rabbit liver. *Immunology* 34:347, 1978.
70. Schreiber A.D., Frank M.M.: The role of antibody and complement in immune clearance and destruction of erythrocytes: II. Molecular nature of IgG and IgM complement fixing sites and effects of their interaction with serum. *J. Clin. Invest.* 51:583, 1972.
71. Unanue E.R., Cerrotini J.C.: The immunogenicity of antigen bound to the plasma membrane of macrophages. *J. Exp. Med.* 131:711, 1970.
72. Lee S.T., Paraskevas F.: Macrophage-T cell interactions: I. The uptake by T cells of Fc receptors released from macrophages. *Cell. Immunol.* 40:141, 1978.
73. Kirtland H.H., Horwitz D.A., Mohler D.N.: Inhibition of suppressor "T" cell function by methyldopa: A proposed cause of autoimmune hemolytic anemia. *Blood* 52:151, 1978.
74. Adams J., Moore V.K., Issitt P.D.: Autoimmune hemolytic anemia caused by anti-D. *Transfusion* 13:214, 1972.
75. Issitt P.D., Issitt C.H.: *Applied Blood Group Serology,* ed. 2, Oxnard, California, Spectra Biologicals, 1975, p. 300.
76. Dacie J.V.: *The Hemolytic Anemias, Congenital and Acquired: Part II. The Autoimmune Hemolytic Anemias,* ed. 2. New York, Grune & Stratton, 1962
77. Yokoyama M., Eith D.T., Bowman M.: The first example of auto-anti-Xg^a. *Vox Sang.* 12:138, 1967.
78. Dacie J.V.: Autoimmune hemolytic anemia. *Arch. Intern. Med.* 135:1293, 1975.
79. Issitt P.D., Pavone B.G., Goldfinger D. et al.: Anti Wr^b, and other antibodies responsible for positive direct antiglobulin tests in 150 individuals. *Br. J. Haematol.* 34:5, 1976.
80. Abdalla S., Weatherall D.J.: The direct antiglobulin test in *P. falciparum* malaria. *Br. J. Haematol.* 51:415, 1982.
81. Dameshek W., Levine P.: Isoimmunization with Rh factor in acquired hemolytic anemia. *N. Engl. J. Med.* 228:641, 1943.
82. Fudenberg H.H., Rosenfield R.E., Wasserman L.R.: Unusual specificity of auto antibody in au-

toimmune hemolytic anemia. *J. Mt. Sinai Hosp.* 25:324, 1958.
83. Engelfriet C.P., von dem Borne A.E.G., Do Beckers F.W., et al.: Immune destruction of red cells, in Bell C.A. (ed.): *A Seminar on Immune-Mediated Cell Destruction.* Washington, D.C., American Association of Blood Banks, 1981, p. 93.
84. Urbaniak S.J.: ADCC (K-cell) lysis of human erythrocytes sensitized with Rhesus alloantibodies: I. Investigation of in vitro culture variables. *Br. J. Haematol.* 42:303, 1979.
85. Pollack W., Reckel R.P.: A reappraisal of the forces involved in hemagglutination. *Int. Arch. Allergy Appl. Immunol.* 54:29, 1977.
86. Steane E.A., Greenwalt T.J.: Red cell agglutination, in Mohn J.F., Pluckett R.W., Cunningham R.K., et al. (eds.): *Human Blood Groups: Proceedings of the 5th International Convocation of Immunology.* New York, S. Karger, 1977, pp. 36–43.
87. Petz L.D., Garraty G.: *Acquired Immune Hemolytic Anemias.* New York, Churchill Livingstone, 1980, p. 160.
88. Rubin H.: Antibody elution from red cells. *J. Clin. Pathol.* 16:70, 1963.
89. Jenkins D.E. Jr., Moore W.H.: A rapid method for the preparation of high potency auto and alloantibody eluates. *Transfusion* 17:110, 1977.
90. Dacie J.V., Worlledge S.M.: Autoimmune hemolytic anemias. *Prog. Hematol.* 6:82, 1969.
91. Rubin H.: Autoimmune hemolytic anemias: Warm and cold antibody types. *Am. J. Clin. Pathol.* 68:638, 1977.
92. Gilliland B.C.: Coombs-negative immune hemolytic anemia. *Semin. Hematol.* 13:267, 1976.
93. Gilliland B.C., Baxter E., Evans R.S.: Red cell antibodies in acquired hemolytic anemia with negative antiglobulin serum tests. *N. Engl. J. Med.* 285:252, 1971.
94. Engelfriet C.P., von dem Borne A.E.G., Do Beckers F.W., et al.: Autoimmune haemolytic anemia: Serological and immunochemical characteristics of the autoantibodies; mechanisms of cell destruction. *Semin. Hematol.* 7:328, 1974.
95. Wiener A.S., Gordon E.B., Gullop C.: Studies on autoantibodies in human sera. *J. Immunol.* 71:58, 1953.
96. Sturgeon P., Smith L.E., Chun H.M.T., et al.: Autoimmune hemolytic anemia associated exclusively with IgA of Rh specificity. *Transfusion* 19:324, 1979.
97. Atkinson J.P., Schreiber A.D., Frank M.M.: Effects of corticosteroids and splenectomy on the immune clearance and destruction of erythrocytes. *J. Clin. Invest.* 52:1509, 1973.
98. Pirofsky B.: Clinical aspects of autoimmune hemolytic anemia. *Semin. Hematol.* 13:251, 1976.
99. Forget B.G.: Hemolytic anemias: Congenital and acquired. *Hosp. Practice* April 1980, p. 67.
100. Bowdler A.J.: The role of the spleen and splenectomy in autoimmune hemolytic disease. *Semin. Hematol.* 13:335, 1976.
101. Pirofsky B., Bardona E.J.: Autoimmune hemolytic anemia: II. Therapeutic aspects *Semin. Hematol.* 7:376, 1974.
102. Murphy S., LoBuglio A.F.: Drug therapy of autoimmune hemolytic anemia. *Semin. Hematol.* 13:323, 1976.
103. Elwood P.C., Waters W.E., Green W.J., et al.: Symptoms and circulating haemoglobin level. *J. Chron. Dis.* 21:615, 1969.
104. Bell C.A., Zwicker H., Sacks H.J.: Autoimmune hemolytic anemia. *Am. J. Clin. Pathol.* 60:903, 1973.
105. Silverstein M.N., Gomes M.R., Elveback L.R., et al.: Idiopathic acquired hemolytic anemia: Survival in 117 cases. *Arch. Intern. Med.* 129:85, 1972.
106. Eyster M.E., Jenkins M.E., Jenkins D.E. Jr.: Erythrocyte coating substances in patients with positive direct antiglobulin reactions: Correlation of γG globulin and complement coating with underlying disease overt hemolysis and response to therapy. *Am. J. Med.* 46:360, 1969.
107. Dausset J., Colombani J.: The serology and the prognosis of 128 cases of autoimmune hemolytic anemia. *Blood* 14:1280, 1959.
108. Schubothe H.: The cold hemagglutinin disease. *Semin. Hematol.* 3:27, 1965.
109. Feizi T.: Cold agglutinins: The direct Coombs test and serum immunoglobulins in *Mycoplasma* pneumonial infection. *Ann. NY Acad. Sci.* 143:801, 1967.
110. Worlledge S.M., Dacie J.V.: Haemolytic and other anemias in infectious mononucleosis, in Carler R.L., Penman H.G. (eds.): *Infectious Mononucleosis.* Oxford, England, Blackwell Scientific Publications, 1969, p. 389.
111. Jacobson L.B., Longstreth G.F., Edington T.S.: Clinical and immunological features of transient cold agglutinin hemolytic anemia. *Am. J. Med.* 54:514, 1973.
112. Hossaini A.A.: Anti-I in infectious mononucleosis. *Am. J. Clin. Pathol.* 53:198, 1970.
113. Costea N., Yakulis V.J., Heller P.: Inhibition of cold agglutinins (anti-I) by *M. pneumoniae* antigens. *Proc. Soc. Exp. Biol. Med.* 139:476, 1972.
114. Feizi T., Kabat E.A., Vicari G., et al.: Blood Groups: XLIX. The I antigen complex. Specificity differences among anti-I sera revealed by quantitative precipitin studies; partial structure of the I determinant specific for one anti-I serum. *J. Immunol.* 106:1578, 1971.
115. Rosenfield R.E., Schmidt P.J., Calvo R.C., et al.: Anti-I, a frequent cold agglutinin in infectious mononucleosis. *Vox Sang.* 10:631, 1965.
116. Roelcke D., Ebert W., Feizi T.: Studies on the specificities of two IgM lambda cold agglutinins. *Immunology* 27:879, 1974.
117. Garraty G., Petz L.D., Brodsky I., et al.: An IgA high-titer cold agglutinin with an unusual blood group specificity within the Pr complex. *Vox Sang.* 25:32, 1973.
118. Mollison P.L.: *Blood Transfusions in Clinical Medi-*

119. Rosse W.F., Borsos T., Rapp H.J.: Cold reacting antibodies: The enhancement of antibody fixation by the first component of complement (C'1a). *J. Immunol.* 100:259, 1968.
120. Petz L.D., Garraty G.: *Acquired Immune Hemolytic Anemias.* New York, Churchill Livingstone, 1980, p. 126.
121. Rubin H.: Autoimmune hemolytic anemias: Warm and cold antibody types. *Am. J. Clin. Pathol.* 68:638, 1977.
122. Bianco C., Griffin F.M., Silverstein S.C.: Studies of the macrophage complement receptor. *J. Exp. Med.* 141:1278, 1975.
123. Engelfriet C.P., von dem Borne A.E.G., Do Beckers F.W., et al.: Autoimmune hemolytic anemias: V. Studies on the resistance against complement hemolysis of the red cells of patients with chronic cold agglutinin disease. *Clin. Exp. Immunol.* 11:255, 1972.
124. Tanowitz H.B., Robbins N., Leidich N.: Hemolytic anemia associated with severe *Mycoplasma pneumoniae* pneumonia. *NY State J. Med.* 78:2231, 1978.
125. Gaddy C.G., Powell L.W. Jr.: Raynaud's syndrome associated with idiopathic cryoglobulinemia and cold agglutinins: Report of a case and discussion of classification of cryoglobulinemia. *Arch. Intern. Med.* 102:468, 1958.
126. Logue G.L., Rosse W.F., Gockerman J.P.: Measurement of the third component of complement bound to red blood cells in patients with the cold agglutinin syndrome. *J. Clin. Invest.* 52:493, 1973.
127. Tonthat H., Rochant H., Henry A., et al.: A new case of monoclonal IgA Kappa cold agglutinin with anti-Prld specificity in a patient with persistent HB antigen cirrhosis. *Vox Sang.* 30:464, 1976.
128. Hattersby P.G., Gerard P.W., Caggiano V., et al.: Erroneous values on the model S Coulter counter due to high titer cold autoagglutinins. *Am. J. Clin. Pathol.* 55:442, 1971.
129. Pruzanski W., Shumak K.H.: Biologic reactivity of cold reacting autoantibodies. *N. Engl. J. Med.* 297:538 and 583, 1977.
130. Anstee D.J.: Blood group MNSs-active sialoglycoproteins of the human erythrocyte membrane, in Sander S.G., Nusbacher J., Schanfield M.S. (eds.): *Immunobiology of the Erythrocyte. Prog. Clin. Biol. Res.* 43:67, 1980.
131. MacKenzie M.R., Fudenberg H.H.: Macroglobulinemia: An analysis of forty patients. *Blood* 39:874, 1972.
132. Christenson W.N., Dacie J.V., Croucher B.E.E., et al.: Electrophoretic studies on sera containing high titer cold haemagglutinins: Identification of the antibody as the cause of an abnormal $\gamma 1$ peak. *Br. J. Haematol.* 3:153, 1957.
133. Harboe M.: Cold autoagglutinins. *Vox Sang.* 20:289, 1971.
134. Adinolfi M.: Anti-I antibody in normal newborn infants. *Immunology* 9:43, 1965.
135. Dacie J.V.: *The Haemolytic Anemias, Congenital and Acquired: Part II. The Autoimmune Hemolytic Anemias,* ed. 2. London, Churchill, 1962, p. 462.
136. Evans R.S., Turner E., Bingham M.: Studies with radioiodinated cold agglutinins of few patients *Am. J. Med.* 38:378, 1965.
137. Race R.R., Sanger R.: *Blood Groups in Man,* ed. 6. Oxford, England, Blackwell Scientific Publications, 1975, p. 447.
138. Roelcke D., Dorow W.: Besonderheiten der Reaction Sweise mit Plasmacytomgamma "A"-Paraprotein identischen Kalteagglutinins. *Klin. Wochenschr.* 46:126, 1968.
139. Roelcke D.: Cold agglutination: Antibodies and antigens. *Clin. Immunol. Immunopathol.* 2:266, 1974.
140. Mygind K., Ahrons S.: IgG cold agglutinins and first trimester abortion. *Vox Sang.* 23:552, 1973.
141. Tonkin A.M., Mond H.G., Alford F.P., et al.: Severe acute haemolytic anaemia complicating infectious mononucleosis. *Med. J. Aust.* 2:1048, 1973.
142. Schwartz R., Damesheck W.: The treatment of autoimmune hemolytic anemia with 6-mercaptopurine and thioguanine. *Blood* 19:483, 1962.
143. Widman F.K. (ed.): *Technical Manual,* ed. 8. Washington, D.C., American Association of Blood Banks, 1981, p. 226.
144. Taft E.G., Propp R.P., Sullivan S.A.: Plasma exchange for cold agglutinin hemolytic anemia. *Transfusion* 17:173, 1977.
145. Rosenfield R.E., Jagathambal K.: Transfusion therapy for autoimmune hemolytic anemia. *Semin. Hematol.* 13:311, 1976.
146. Petz L.D., Garraty G.: *Acquired Immune Hemolytic Anemias.* New York, Churchill Livingstone, 1980, p. 54.
147. Donath J., Landsteiner K.: Über paroxysmale Hemoglobinurie. *Munch. Med. Wochenschr.* 51:1590, 1904.
148. Worlledge S.M., Rousso C.: Studies of the serology of paroxysmal cold haemoglobinuria (P.C.H.) with special reference to its relationship with F blood group system. *Vox Sang.* 10:293, 1965.
149. Wishart M.M., Davey M.G.: Infectious mononucleosis complicated by acute haemolytic anaemias with a positive Donath Landsteiner reaction. *J. Clin. Pathol.* 26:332, 1973.
150. Bell C.A., Swicker H., Rosenbaum D.L.: Paroxysmal cold hemoglobinuria (P.C.H.) following *Mycoplasma* infection: anti-I specificity of the biphasic hemolysin. *Transfusion* 13:138, 1973.
151. Hinz C.F. Jr.: Serologic and physicochemical characterization of the Donath-Landsteiner antibodies from 6 patients. *Blood* 22:600, 1963.
152. Hinz C.F. Jr., Mollner A.M.: Studies on immune hemolysis: III. Role of 11s component initiating the Donath-Landsteiner reaction. *J. Immunol.* 91:512, 1964.
153. Hinz C.F. Jr., Picken M.E., Lepow I.H.: Studies on immune human hemolysis: The Donath-Land-

steiner reaction as a model system for studying the mechanism of action of complement and the role of CI and CII esterase. *J. Exp. Med.* 113:193, 1961.
154. Knapp T.: The laboratory investigation of three cases of paroxysmal cold haemoglobinuria. *Can. J. Med. Technol.* 26:172, 1964.
155. Wollach B., Heddle N., Barr R.D., et al.: Transient Donath-Landsteiner haemolytic anaemia. *Br. J. Haematol.* 48:425, 1981.
156. Widman F.K.: *Technical Manual,* ed. 8. Washington, D.C., American Association of Blood Banks, 1981, p. 227.
157. Levine P., Celano M.J., Falkowski F.: The specificity of the antibody in paroxysmal cold hemoglobinuria (PCH). *Transfusion* 3:278, 1963.
158. Worlledge S.M., Rousso C.: Studies of the serology of paroxysmal cold hemoglobinuria (PCH) with special reference to its relationship with "P" blood group system. *Vox Sang.* 10:293, 1965.
159. Schwarting G.A., Marcus D.M., Metaxas M.N.: Identification of sialosyl paragloboside as the erythrocyte receptor for "anti-P" antibody. *Vox Sang.* 32:257, 1977.
160. Weiner W., Gordon E.G., Rowe D.: A Donath-Landsteiner antibody. *Vox Sang.* 9:684, 1964.
161. Mollison P.L.: *Blood Transfusions in Clinical Medicine,* ed. 7. Oxford, England, Blackwell Scientific Publications, 1983, p. 454.
162. Schwarting G.A., Kindu S.K., Markers D.M.: Reaction of antibodies that cause paroxysmal cold hemoglobinuria (PCH) with globoside and Forssman glycosphingolipids. *Blood* 53:186, 1979.
163. Petz L.D., Garraty G.: *Acquired Immune Hemolytic Anemias.* New York, Churchill Livingstone, 1980, p. 428.
164. Banov C.H.: Paroxysmal cold hemoglobinuria: Apparent remission after splenectomy. *JAMA* 174:1974, 1960.
165. Danielson D., Douglas S.W., Herzog P., et al.: Drug induced blood disorders. *JAMA* 252:3257, 1984.
166. Ackroyd J.E.: The pathogenesis of thrombocytopenic purpura due to hypersensitivity to Sedormid (allylisopropyl-acetylcarbamide). *Clin. Sci.* 7:249, 1949.
167. White J.M., Brown D.L., Hepner G.W., et al.: Penicillin induced hemolytic anemia. *Br. Med. J.* 3:26, 1968.
168. Wenz B., Klein R.L., Lalezari P.: Tetracycline-induced immune hemolytic anemia. *Transfusion* 14:265, 1974.
169. Rubin R.N., Burka E.R.: Anticephalothin: Antibody and Coombs' positive hemolytic anemia. *Ann. Intern. Med.* 86:64, 1977.
170. Stephanini M., Johnson N.L.: Positive anti-human globulin test in patients receiving carbromal. *Am. J. Med. Sci.* 259:49, 1970.
171. Getaz P.E., Beckley S., Fitzpatrick J., et al.: Cisplatin-induced hemolysis. *N. Engl. J. Med.* 302:334, 1980.
172. Ballas S.K., Caro J.F., Miguel O.: Quinidine-induced hemolytic anemia: Immunohematologic characterization. *Transfusion* 18:215, 1978.
173. Bird G.W.G., Eeles G.H., Litchfield J.A., et al.: Haemolytic anemia with antibodies to tolbutamide and phenacetin. *Br. Med. J.* 1:728, 1972.
174. Logue G.L., Boyd A.E., Rosse W.F.: Chlorpropamide-induced immune hemolytic anemia. *N. Engl. J. Med.* 283:900, 1970.
175. Poole G., Stradling P., Worlledge S.: Potentially serious side effects of high-dose twice-weekly rifampin. *Br. Med. J.* 3:343, 1971.
176. Tajima H.: Clinical studies on hemolytic anemia: I. Autoimmune hemolytic anemia. *Acta Haematol. Jpn.* 23:188, 1960.
177. Bengtsson U., Ahlstedt S., Aurell M., et al.: Antazoline-induced immune haemolytic anaemia, haemoglobinuria and acute renal failure. *Acta Med. Scand.* 198:223, 1975.
178. Weiss H.J., Berger R.E., Tice A.D., et al.: Fatal disseminated intravascular coagulation and hemolytic anemia following stibophen therapy. *Am. J. Med. Sci.* 264:375, 1972.
179. Garraty G., Houston M., Petz L.D., et al.: Acute immune intravascular hemolysis due to hydrochlorothiazide. *Am. J. Clin. Pathol.* 76:73, 1981.
180. Wintrobe M.M.: *Clinical Hematology,* ed. 8. Philadelphia, Lea & Febiger, 1981, p. 944.
181. Molthan L., Reidenberg M.H., Eichman M.F.: Positive direct Coombs' tests due to cephalothin. *N. Engl. J. Med.* 277:123, 1967.
182. Kirtland H.H., Mohler D.N., Horwitz D.A.: Methyldopa inhibition of suppressor lymphocyte function: A proposed cause of acute immune hemolytic anemia. *N. Engl. J. Med.* 302:825, 1980.
183. Lindstrom F.D., Lieden G., Engstrom M.S.: Dose related levodopa-induced hemolytic anaemia. *Ann. Intern. Med.* 86:298, 1977.
184. Farid N.R., Johnson R.J., Low W.T.: Haemolytic reaction to mefenamic acid. *Lancet* 2:382, 1971.
185. Kleinman S., Nelson R., Smith L., et al.: Positive direct antiglobulin tests and immune hemolytic anemia in patients receiving procainamide. *N. Engl. J. Med.* 311:809, 1984.
186. Petz L.D., Fudenberg H.H.: Coombs-positive hemolytic anemia caused by penicillin administration. *N. Engl. J. Med.* 274:171, 1966.
187. DeWeck A.L.: Studies on penicillin hypersensitivity: I. The specificity of rabbit "anti-penicillin" antibodies. *Int. Arch. Allergy Appl. Immunol.* 21:20, 1962.
188. Thiel J.A., Mitchell S., Parker C.W.: Specificity of hemagglutination reactions in human and experimental penicillin hypersensitivity. *J. Allergy* 35:399, 1967.
189. Spath P., Garraty G., Petz L.D.: Studies on the immune response to penicillin and cephalothin in humans: II. Immunohematologic reactions to cephalothin administration. *J. Immunol.* 107:860, 1971.
190. Garraty G., Petz L.D.: Drug-induced immune hemolytic anemia. *Am. J. Med.* 58:398, 1975.
191. Levine B.B., Ovary Z.: Studies on the mechanism

191. of the formation of the penicillin antigen: III. The N-CD-alpha-benzyl penicilloyl group as an antigenic determinant responsible for hypersensitivity to penicillin G. *J. Exp. Med.* 114:875, 1961.
192. Levine B., Redmond A.: Immunochemical mechanisms of penicillin induced Coombs' positivity and hemolytic anemia in man. *Int. Arch. Allergy Appl. Immunol.* 1:594, 1967.
193. White J.M., Brown D.L., Hepner G.W., et al.: Penicillin induced hemolytic anemia. *Br. Med. J.* 3:26, 1968.
194. Funicella T., Weinger R.S., Moake J.L., et al.: Penicillin-induced immune hemolytic anemia associated with circulatory immune complexes. *Am. J. Hematol.* 3:219, 1977.
195. Grainick H.R., Wright L.D., McGuinniss M.H.: Coombs' positive reactions associated with sodium cephalothin therapy. *JAMA* 199:725, 1967.
196. Petz L.D.: Immunologic cross reactivity between penicillins and cephalosporins: A review. *J. Infect. Dis.* 137:574, 1978.
197. Nesmith L.W., Davis J.W.: Hemolytic anemia caused by penicillin. *JAMA* 203:27, 1968.
198. Worlledge S.M.: Immune drug induced hemolytic anemias. *Semin. Hematol.* 6:181, 1969.
199. Garraty G.: Laboratory investigation of drug-induced immune hemolytic anemia, supplement, in Bell C.A. (ed.): *A Seminar on Laboratory Management of Hemolysis.* Washington, D.C., American Association of Blood Banks, 1979, pp. 1–19.
200. Fearon D.T.: Identification of the membrane glycoprotein that is the C3b receptor of the human erythrocyte, polymorphonuclear leukocyte, B lymphocyte and monocyte. *J. Exp. Med.* 152:20, 1980.
201. Miescher P.A., Gorestein F.: Mechanisms of immunogenic platelet damage, in Johnson S.A., Monto R.W., Rebuck J.W., et al. (eds.): *Blood Platelets.* London, Churchill, 1961, p. 671.
202. Croft J.D., Swisher S.N., Gilliland B.C., et al.: Coombs' test positivity induced by drugs: Mechanisms of immunologic reactions and red cell destruction. *Ann. Intern. Med.* 68:176, 1968.
203. Zeigler Z., Shadduck R.K., Winkelstein A., et al.: Immune hemolytic anemia and thrombocytopenia secondary to quinidine: In vitro studies of the quinidine dependent red cell and platelet antibodies. *Blood* 53:396, 1979.
204. Petz L.D., Garraty G.: *Acquired Immune Hemolytic Anemias.* New York, Churchill Livingstone, 1980, p. 273.
205. Henson P.M., Spiegelberg H.L.: Release of serotonin from human platelets induced by aggregated immunoglobulins of different classes and subclasses. *J. Clin. Invest.* 52:1282, 1973.
206. Martinez I., Letona J., Barbolla L., et al.: Immune haemolytic anaemia in renal failure induced by streptomycin. *Br. J. Haematol.* 35:561, 1977.
207. Goudeman M., Salmon C., quoted by Mollison P.L.: *Blood Transfusion in Clinical Medicine,* ed. 7. Oxford, England, Blackwell Scientific Publications, 1983, pp. 461–462.
208. Lakshmminayaran S., Sahn S.A., Hudson L.D.: Massive haemolysis caused by rifampin. *Br. Med. J.* 2:282, 1973.
209. Duran-Suarez J.R., Martin-Vega C., Argelagues E., et al.: Red cell I antigen as immune complex receptor in drug induced hemolytic anemias. *Vox Sang.* 41:313, 1981.
210. Lay W.H.: Drug-induced haemolytic reaction due to antibodies against the erythrocyte/dipyrone complex. *Vox Sang.* 11:601, 1966.
211. Jeannet M., Block A., Dayer J.M., et al.: Cephalothin-induced immune haemolytic anaemia. *Acta Haematol.* 55:109, 1976.
212. Petz L.D., Garraty G.: *Acquired Immune Hemolytic Anemias.* New York, Churchill Livingstone, 1980, p. 284.
213. Mollison P.L.: *Blood Transfusions in Clinical Medicine,* ed. 7. Oxford, England, Blackwell Scientific Publications, 1983, p. 462.
214. Carstairs K.C., Breckenridge A., Dollery C.T., et al.: Incidence of a positive direct Coombs' test in patients on α-methyldopa. *Lancet* 2:133, 1966.
215. Worlledge S.M.: Immune drug-induced hemolytic anemias. *Semin. Hematol.* 10:327, 1973.
216. LoBuglio A.F., Jandl J.H.: The nature of the alpha-methyldopa red cell antibody. *N. Engl. J. Med.* 276:658, 1967.
217. Issitt P.D., Pavone P.G., Goldfinger D., et al.: Anti-Wr[b] and other autoantibodies responsible for positive direct antiglobulin tests in 150 individuals. *Br. J. Haematol.* 34:5, 1976.
218. Gottlieb A.J., Wurzel H.A.: Protein-quinone interaction: In vitro induction of direct antiglobulin reactions with methyldopa. *Blood* 43:85, 1974.
219. Dameshek W.: Alpha-methyldopa red-cell antibody: Cross-reaction or forbidden clones? *N. Engl. J. Med.* 276:1382, 1967.
220. Kirtland H.H., Horwitz D.A., Mohler D.N.: Inhibition of suppressor T-cell function by methyldopa: A proposed cause of autoimmune hemolytic anemia. *Blood* 52:151, 1978.
221. Worlledge S.M.: Auto antibody formation associated with methyldopa (Aldomet) therapy. *Br. J. Haematol.* 16:5, 1969.
222. Ewing D.J., Hughes C.J., Wardle D.F.: Methyldopa-induced autoimmune haemolytic anaemia: A report of two further cases. *Guys Hosp. Rep.* 117:111, 1968.
223. van Der Menten F.W., van Der Hart M., Fleer A., et al.: The role of adherence to human mononuclear phagocytes in the destruction of red cells sensitized with non-complement binding IgG antibodies. *Br. J. Haematol.* 38:541, 1978.
224. Bakemeier R.F., Leddy J.D.: Erythrocyte autoantibody associated with alpha-methyldopa: Heterogeneity of structure and specificity. *Blood* 32:1, 1968.
225. Patten, E., Beck C.E., Scholl C., et al.: Autoimmune hemolytic anemia with anti-JK[a] specificity in a patient taking Aldomet. *Transfusion* 17:517, 1977.
226. Petz L.D., Garraty G.: *Acquired Immune Hemolytic*

Anemias. New York, Churchill Livingstone, 1980, pp. 290–291.
227. Surveyor I., Evans B., Saunders K.C., et al.: Autoimmune hemolytic anemia complicating methyldopa therapy. *Postgrad. Med. J.* 44:438, 1968.
228. deGruchy G.C.: *Drug-induced Blood Disorders.* Oxford, England, Blackwell Scientific Publications, 1975, p. 1.
229. Schwartz R.S., Costea N.: Autoimmune hemolytic anemia: Clinical correlations and biological implications. *Semin. Hematol.* 3:2, 1966.

Transfusion Reactions

It was by observing transfusion reactions that early health professionals learned to be cautious in the use of blood as a therapeutic modality. Treating a patient's hematocrit, rather than considering carefully the true need for transfusion, is a poor transfusion practice. This chapter discusses the more important reactions to transfusion of blood and blood products. Hemolytic transfusion reactions are analyzed first, because of their ominous implications. The (usually) less severe reactions are discussed second.

HEMOLYTIC TRANSFUSION REACTIONS

No matter what their etiology or degree, hemolytic transfusion reactions are always a source of concern, for it is these reactions that are responsible for most red cell transfusion-related deaths. Hemolytic transfusion reactions may be divided into two groups: immune-mediated hemolysis and non-immune mediated hemolysis.

Immune Mediated Hemolytic Transfusion Reactions

Although a more detailed history of transfusions is given in chapter 1, a brief account of the first attempt to transfuse blood to humans is relevant here in that it resulted in a fatal hemolytic transfusion reaction. As related in chapter 1, the first transfusion was undertaken by Denis, a French physician, in 1667. Nine ounces of lamb's blood were given intravenously to a patient reportedly suffering from what was termed "luetic madness." This description of this first hemolytic transfusion reaction is classic, leaving little to be added. In Denis' words: "The first infusion of blood produced no detectable symptoms. The second time, however, his arm became hot, the pulse rose, sweat burst out over his forehead, he complained of pain in the kidneys and was sick at the bottom of his stomach. The urine was very dark, in fact, black." After the third transfusion the patient died.[1]

Following these experiments, the transfusion of blood was banned for almost 150 years.[2] Although Blundell, a British obstetrician, was successful in transfusing patients with human blood in the 19th century,[3] it was not until Landsteiner's discovery of ABO blood groups at the turn of the century[4] that the fatality from transfusion reactions decreased sufficiently for the transfusion of blood to become a routine practice.

Epidemiology of Immune Mediated Hemolytic Transfusion Reactions

Hemolytic transfusion reactions occur in as many as 1 in 14,000 transfusions.[5] These reactions tend to occur more frequently in older age groups, perhaps reflecting the type of surgery performed on these patients—especially cardiovascular surgery, which accounted for 25% of the cases in one series.[6] Furthermore, these reactions tend to occur in individuals who not only received a large number of units, but who were previously immunized. About 86% of cases occur during surgery or in the emergency room.[6]

Pathophysiology of Immune Mediated Hemolytic Transfusion Reactions

Immune–mediated destruction of transfused red blood cells (RBCs) occurs when the host's plasma contains circulatory antibodies against antigens present on transfused RBCs, or, less frequently, when incompatible plasma is transfused. RBC destruction can occur intravascularly or extravascularly.[7] Reactions leading to intravascular hemolysis are by far the most dreaded (see Chapter 10).

Transfusion Reactions Leading to Intravascular Hemolysis

The vast majority of fatal hemolytic transfusion reactions are due to the transfusion of ABO-incompatible blood, accounting for about 86% of deaths from incompatible transfusion in one series.[8] These reactions are mostly due to intravascular hemolysis caused by activation of the classical pathway of complement. Intravascular hemolysis of RBCs due to activation of the alternative pathway has not to date been documented.

IgM antibodies against other than ABO antigen systems (such as Jk, Vel, and Tj^a) have occasionally been responsible for severe intravascular hemolysis.[9] In addition, not all IgM antibodies against RBC antigens are hemolytic. For instance, antibodies against the MN and Rh systems of the IgM class, are seldom hemolytic, and antibodies against Lewis antigens, which are routinely of the IgM class, usually produce only a mild and relatively slow type of hemolysis.[10] Presumably these antibodies do not produce brisk intravascular hemolysis, due to entrapment by the reticuloendothelial system (RES) of RBCs, before activation of complement and subsequent RBC hemolysis can occur.[11]

The potential development of antibodies secondary to sensitization by RBCs is a deterrant against indiscriminate transfusion. Indeed, the risk of forming alloantibodies against transfused RBCs increases with multiple transfusions. In one series, 15 of 131 multiply transfused patients developed IgG alloantibodies.[12]

Mechanisms of RBC Damage

Although the precise mechanisms whereby complement produces RBC membrane damage are not fully understood, some parts of the puzzle have been elucidated. A detailed description of complement activation is given in chapters 4 and 10; however, a summary is given here for completeness.

RBCs must first be sensitized by antibody. The most effective antibody to produce complement binding is IgM. Usually a single molecule of IgM is sufficient to bind complement.[13] IgG is likewise capable of binding complement. IgG3 and IgG1 are particularly capable of binding complement, though IgG2 has been reported to be capable of binding complement, albeit less efficiently. IgG4 is not known to bind complement.[14] Two IgG Fc fragments must be attached to the cell at a distance no greater than 400 Å to be able to bind C1q.[15, 16] C1q attaches to immune complexes composed of two or more Fc fragments. Two other components form C1, namely C1r and C1s. C1r, a proenzyme, cleaves C1s, C1s cleaves C4 into C4a and C4b and cleaves C2 into C2a and C2b. C2a, now termed C2b, combines with C4b to form C4b2b, termed C3b convertase. C3b convertase cleaves C3 into C3a, an anaphylatoxin, and C3b. C3b combines with C4b2a (now termed C4b2b) to form C5 convertase (C4b2a3b, now termed C4b2b3b), which cleaves C5 into C5a and C5b. C5a functions as an anaphylatoxin and may have a role in vasodilation during hemolysis. C5b is the lytic unit binding C6C7 and C8 plus six Cq units onto the RBC membrane.[17] It has been shown that the C5–C9 complex is a cylindrically shaped macromolecule that penetrates the membrane bilayer.[18] These findings give support to the model for cell lysis by complement originally proposed by Mayer, whereby holes ranging from 8 to 10 nm in size are produced.[19, 20] These membrane defects allow ions to enter the RBCs rapidly, producing osmotic destruction of the cells.

Another mechanism for clearance of IgM-coated RBCs or RBCs coated with C3b complement components is trapping by macrophages in the liver. Liver macrophages may not possess many Fc receptors for this Ig class,[21] but they do possess receptors for the complement fragments coating the cells.[22] However, some of these cells tend to reappear in the circulation due to conversion of C3b to C3d, which causes release of coated RBCs from liver macrophages (see Fig 10–1). Furthermore, a second signal appears to be necessary for C3b-coated RBCs to be ingested by macrophages.[23]

A second explanation for the reappearance of coated RBCs is that they have been partially engulfed by macrophages and then converted into spherocytes by resealing of the membrane.[24]

Extravascular immune hemolysis usually occurs when RBCs are coated with IgG.[9] Receptors for IgG1 and IgG3 have been demonstrated on monocytes[21] and on splenic tissue macrophages.[25] These cells are thought to capture the sensitized RBCs and destroy them in the extravascular space in the spleen.[26] It must be kept in mind that most alloantibodies (e.g., those of the Rh, Kell, and Duffy systems) destroy cells extravascularly.[9] Direct attack by cytotoxic killer cells has been proposed as another mechanism of extravascular RBC destruction,[27] but this mechanism has not been completely demonstrated. Extravascular hemolysis has been shown to be an extremely efficient system for hemolysis, reaching volumes of up to 400 cc of coated RBCs per 24 hours,[28] which explains the very decreased survival of incompatible RBCs coated with IgG in patients with high antibody titers.

Once intravascular hemolysis occurs, the major complication in severe hemolytic reactions is disseminated intravascular coagulation (DIC),[29] which was fully described in chapter 3. Although the mechanisms by which intravascular hemolysis produces DIC are not completely understood, some interesting facts that will help clarify the physiopathology of this complication of hemolytic transfusion reactions are reviewed below.

RBC stroma by itself is a relatively weak procoagulant; however, it will trigger severe DIC experimentally in animals with a depressed RES function.[30] It has been shown that the most likely substance in erythrocyte stroma to produce this procoagulant effect is a phospholipid with platelet factor 3–like activity named erythrocytin.[31] However, the mechanism by which DIC is triggered cannot be solely attributed to the release of RBC stroma. Conditions such as massive hemolysis secondary to ingestion of fava beans do not routinely produce DIC and may in fact produce elevation of fibrinogen, factor V, and factor VIII levels.[32] Intravascular lysis of RBCs induced by the intravenous (IV) administration of water to rabbits has also failed to produce DIC.[33] Nevertheless, paroxysmal nocturnal hemoglobinuria[34] and malaria[35] have been complicated by DIC.

The fact remains, however, that both in humans[36,37] and in animals[38] the transfusion of incompatible blood frequently results in DIC. It is possible that the RES is blocked by immune complexes composed of circulating antibodies complexed with RBC antigens, allowing RBC stroma to become more prone to triggering DIC. Furthermore, it has shown that antigen-antibody complexes are capable of triggering the coagulation cascade.[39]

The primary procoagulant target in DIC is fibrinogen. Both thrombin and plasmin act on fibrinogen. Thrombin produces fibrin monomers that polymerize to form fibrin strands. Plasmin, however, produces fibrin degradation products and also digests factors V and VIII. The RES traps and eliminates both circulating fibrin and fibrin split products,[40] but if the RES is blocked (for example, by immune complexes), the development of bilateral renal cortical necrosis is much more likely to occur.[41]

Bilateral cortical necrosis with fibrin deposition in the renal microcapillaries is the mechanism by which renal damage is produced in experimental hemolytic transfusion reactions.[42] This lesion is also the main pathologic finding in kidneys of patients who have severe hemolytic reactions.[43] Even using current therapy, bilateral cortical necrosis still carries a 50% mortality.[44] The misconception that stroma-free hemoglobin is responsible for the renal damage observed in hemolytic reactions has led to inappropriate therapy for hemolytic transfusion reactions.[45] In fact, stroma-free hemoglobin has been used safely as a plasma expander[46] without evidence of renal damage,[47] and as a blood substitute,[48] with similar results. The second major complication of DIC triggered by acute hemolytic transfusion reactions is the development of a bleeding diathesis caused by consumption of hemostatic factors.[49] The resulting hemostatic defect in this disorder is manifested by thrombocytopenia, hypofibrinogenemia, and decreased levels of factors VIII and V. Factors XI, X, and IX may also be decreased in DIC.[50]

Clinical Findings in Intravascular Immune Hemolytic Reactions

A severe hemolytic transfusion reaction in a conscious patient may start with pain and burning at the infusion site. Severe back pain, substernal tightness, dyspnea, and a feeling of impending doom have been described by survivors of such reactions. The patient frequently has hemoglobinuria (50% of fatal cases).[8] If the reaction is severe the patient may progress rapidly into shock, with prolonged and marked hypotension in 50% of cases.[8] Hypotension is a harbinger of severe hemolytic transfusion reactions.[6] Vomiting and diarrhea may also be present. In severe cases gastrointestinal or genitourinary bleeding is present, and in postoperative patients, oozing from surgical wounds and venipuncture sites is not uncommon. Often the only sign that a transfusion reaction has taken place in an anesthetized patient is increased bleeding and/or hypotension, and frequently hemoglobinuria. Many times the reaction will be very mild, with backache, fever, and chills.[51] In one series, fever was the most frequent presenting symptom.[6] Even if the symptoms are mild, the transfusion must be stopped. Symptoms and signs will usually be less severe if the antibody titer is low (for example, in immunosuppressed patients and infants).

Laboratory Findings

As soon as a hemolytic transfusion reaction is suspected, the laboratory workup is started. Clotted and anticoagulated patient blood samples are sent to the blood bank, along with the remainder of the untransfused unit and a fresh sample of urine. In the blood bank, the following tests are routinely performed on transfusion reaction specimens:[52, 53]

1. A thorough clerical check.
2. Repeated ABO, Rh, and screening on pretransfusion and posttransfusion samples of recipient.
3. Repeated ABO, Rh, and screening of donor segment.
4. Check for mixed field reactions on peripheral blood by retyping and by direct Coombs test; 95% of these cases also have a positive result on the indirect Coombs test.[6]
5. Repeated crossmatch, major and minor.
6. Observe for serum hemolysis.
7. Spin urine sample, check for hemoglobinuria versus hematuria; look for casts.

About 32% of patients with fatal immune hemolytic transfusion reactions had DIC in one series.[8] However, this finding was present in only 4% of overall IHTR.[6] Clotting studies must be performed in severe immune hemolytic transfusion reactions to rule out DIC. Some of these clotting studies are usually performed outside the blood bank. Therefore, anticoagulated samples and a clotted sample must be obtained in addition to the blood bank transfusion reaction workup samples and sent to the coagulation laboratory for the hematology tests listed below:[54]

1. A peripheral smear is done to look for decreased numbers of platelets and schistocytes as evidence of DIC.

2. A small friable clot is usually present in DIC, especially if fibrinogen levels are below 75 mg/ml.
3. The prothrombin time (PT) is usually less than 40%; the activated partial thromboplastin time (PTT) may be prolonged to 100 seconds (normal, 47 seconds); the thrombin time (TT) is likewise prolonged.
4. Fibrinogen levels and fibrin split products.
5. Bleeding time.

The development of DIC in immune hemolytic transfusion reactions often depends on the causative antibody (e.g., immune hemolytic transfusion reaction is more frequent in ABO-incompatible transfusion reactions than in reactions secondary to Kell or Jk antibodies[6]). Clinical chemistry tests on serum samples must also be performed for hemoglobinemia and free hemoglobin; for instance, free hemoglobin was found in 21 of 24 cases in one series,[6] and the indirect bilirubin level was elevated in 32 of 40 cases of HTR.[6] In addition, decreased haptoglobin levels and decreased hemopexin levels are seen in these cases. The serum lactic dehydrogenase (LDH) level may be elevated.

A urine sample will show hemoglobinuria when hemolysis elevates the plasma hemoglobin above 125–150 mg/100 ml.[55]

Prevention and Treatment of Intravascular Immune Hemolytic Transfusion Reactions

In a recent nationwide review of 70 transfusion-associated fatalities, 44 were hemolytic. Clerical errors were to blame in 33 of 37 cases. This made clerical errors responsible for 89% of the cases of fatal acute hemolysis studied.[8] The error was clarified in 37 cases. Errors initiated in the blood bank accounted for 35% of cases in the same study.[8] Of these, 69% were clerical mistakes and 31% were technical serologic errors. Sixty-five percent of the fatalities were caused by errors outside the blood bank, in the wards or surgical suites. Blood sample collection and identification mistakes accounted for 19% of all fatalities. In 46% of cases, units were properly identified but given to the wrong person.[8] This study clearly showed that true prevention can be exercised in these types of transfusion reactions.

A good clerical staff is of paramount importance. These individuals must be trained with the specific goals of heightening attention to detail and providing a thorough understanding of the transfusion process. The nursing and medical staffs in a hospital must be routinely trained in transfusion practices. The paper work required to process a unit must be designed to help avoid mistakes by making each step clear and functional. The number of individuals handling a unit of blood should be as small as possible. All identification should be rechecked as a unit is being prepared for transfusion. This includes positive correlation of the unit numbers and transfusion slip numbers, and especially positive identification of the patient's name and number on the wrist band. Patients should verbally identify themselves if they are able to do so. Anesthetized, comatose, or obtunded patients must be carefully identified via their wrist band identification.

The transfusion team consists of two people, both knowledgeable in the theory and practice of transfusion. A specially trained transfusion team is the ideal solution, but in many hospitals it is economically unfeasible. The two individuals performing a transfusion should be either physicians or registered nurses.

The laboratory technologist must not be overworked; a tired technologist is an invitation to disaster. Only experienced technologists should perform crossmatching, and the techniques should be simplified as much as possible to avoid confusion. Unauthorized personnel should be banned from the laboratory area, for they distract technologists who are in the process of crossmatching or typing patients, often on a "stat" basis.

In institutions where strict transfusion-practice guidelines are carefully observed, clerical errors accounted for 51% of immune hemolytic transfusion reactions.[6] In the same study, antibodies not detectable in the pretransfusion sample accounted for about 49% of the cases. The antibodies detected after these reactions occurred in the following order of frequency: Jk > Rh,(E); Fy^a; Rh,(D) > A$_1$ or Le. Failure to recognize an antibody that was present in the pretransfusion sample occurred in 15 of all 47 cases presented in this study. The frequency of these antibodies was as follows: K > Fy^a > Rh,(E) or Rh,(c) or Le. Donor antibodies present in plasma, not detected in the pretransfusion workup, were found after the transfusion reaction in 3 cases. Failure to complete the crossmatch was responsible for 3 cases, and 2 cases were due to hemolytic anti-A,B present in group O plasma during massive transfusion with group O blood. In this institution, only one of 47 immune hemolytic transfusion reactions was due to transfusion of ABO-incompatible blood.[56] Since fatal accidents are almost always due to clerical error, they can be avoided if the above-mentioned simple but crucial guidelines are followed. Fortunately, fatal errors are quite rare (approximately 1 in 18,000 transfusions).[57] The practice of retyping the patient at the bedside immediately before transfusion, as is done in other countries, has proved to be an excellent practice as a prevention against ABO-incompatible transfusions.[58]

Treatment of Intravascular Immune Hemolytic Transfusion Reactions

Therapy of acute immune mediated hemolytic transfusion reactions has undergone a major reassessment, mainly due to the ideas promulgated by Goldfinger.[45, 59] As stated earlier, the pathophysiology of renal damage in incompatible transfusions is mostly secondary to DIC, probably initiated by immune complexes,[59, 60] and perpetrated by blocking of RES by immune complexes. The idea that tubular necrosis is caused by hemoglobin plugging has never been proved, and the supporting data are not based on sound scientific evidence.[45, 59, 61] It should therefore be dispelled from the modern medical approach to the treatment of hemolytic transfusion reactions.[45, 59] After the vascular insult, an impaired cortical blood flow leads to decreased glomerular filtration, with resulting renal insufficiency.[45, 59] The use of heparin has been advocated in the early phases of severe immune mediated intravascular hemolytic reactions, but only when there is no doubt that the reaction is a major one (usually caused by 200 ml or more of incompatible blood, although it may be triggered by smaller volumes) and with documented hemoglobinemia.[59, 62] Heparin has also been used successfully experimentally in dogs.[38] Conclusive evidence of DIC (e.g., low fibrinogen, low platelet count, prolonged PT, PTT, and TT) should be present before heparin is given. Heparin should be used cautiously and is not recommended in most patients with a preexisting bleeding tendency (e.g., DIC due to obstetric complication, or in the immediate postoperative period). A hematology consult is advisable before instituting such therapy. Failures of heparin therapy in acute hemolytic reactions probably stem from it being given too late.[45, 59] The immediate infusion of 50–100 mg of sodium heparin followed by the slow infusion of about 300 mg of heparin over 24 hours has been advocated.[63] Heparin is not recommended when active bleeding is present; this is a frequent occurrence, especially when the transfusion mistake is noticed at an advanced stage.

Although therapy with mannitol has been the traditional approach to preventing renal failure in hemolytic transfusion reactions, a true improvement has not been documented either experimentally[64] or in clinical practice,[65] and therefore the use of mannitol in these cases is no longer recommended.[45] Instead, diuretics that improve cortical flow, such as ethacrinic acid[66] and furosemide,[67] are a more logical approach to the therapy of renal damage produced by hypoperfusion of the renal cortex. These diuretics should only be used in the fully hydrated patient and with caution, for they may be toxic.[59] Perhaps the most important aspect of therapy in these reactions is to avoid renal hypoperfusion by preventing hypovolemic shock. This is best achieved by full hydration with IV fluids and combatting shock.[59] In addition to full hydration, treating shock with α-adrenergic blocking agents may also help to prevent cortical intravascular fibrin deposition.[59,68]

Management Scheme for Acute Hemolytic Reactions

An algorithm for the management of acute hemolytic transfusion reactions is given in Figure 11-1. These steps must be followed:

1. Stop the transfusion immediately. Keep the line open with IV saline.
2. Take samples of clotted and anticoagulated blood for blood bank and coagulation laboratory workup.
3. Take a urine sample.
4. Start aggressive IV hydration and furosemide IV (80–120 mg).
5. Based on coagulation laboratory results and on clinical status, consider heparin and fresh frozen plasma (FFP) therapy.
6. Follow-up renal output and coagulation parameters.
7. Get renal consult for possible dialysis if renal failure ensues.
8. Do not use heparin if significant bleeding is present (e.g., in obstetric cases where denuded surface bleeding is a hazard).

Prognosis of Immune Hemolytic Transfusion Reactions

According to one study, about 15% of patients with immune hemolytic transfusion reactions do not develop significant complications. About 34% develop oliguria, and 13% develop anuria, which is of bad prognosis—less than 10% of these patients survive. These authors report 17%–40% mortality from immune hemolytic transfusion reactions.[6] Other authors report a similar mortality.[69] Ninety percent of the deaths reported nationwide were from transfusions of ABO-incompatible blood.[8]

Non-ABO Hemolytic Reactions

Non-ABO-incompatible transfusions accounted for about 10% of deaths from hemolytic transfusion reactions in a series of 44 fatal reactions.[8] Anti-Kell and anti-Jk^a antibodies are the most frequently lethal antibodies in this group of reactions.[69] Most non-ABO antibodies are of the IgG type, although IgM antibodies not directed to ABH antigens can, though rarely, be involved in fatal hemolysis (i.e., anti-M and anti-P antibodies).[8]

Delayed Transfusion Reactions

Most antibodies causing delayed immune hemolytic transfusion reactions occur as a result of secondary immune responses. However, on occasion these reactions may be the result of what would seem a primary immune response, as has been described in a case of anti-C.[70]

Delayed transfusion reactions occur due to a sudden rise in antibody stimulated by transfusion and triggered by antigens not present on the patient's RBCs. They occur 3–5 days after the transfusion, prior to which there is usually no evidence of a reaction. Typically the patient becomes jaundiced and occasionally may have hemoglobinuria.[71] Renal failure is rare.[72] In general, delayed hemolysis is a rare event. Usually non-ABO antibodies of the IgG type capable of binding complement are responsible for these reactions, usually causing mixed field agglutination. These reactions usually disappear after 2 weeks,[73] though a recent report claims that C3d coating may prevail well beyond this period of time in most cases of delayed immune hemolytic transfusion reaction, and that the coating by complement is much stronger than previously thought.[74] Delayed immune hemolytic transfusion reactions have been fatal on occasion, albeit this is a rare event. In one series, 2 of 44 fatal hemolytic transfusion reactions were of the delayed type;[8] of these, 1 involved anti-c antibody and the other involved an anti-c plus anti-E antibody.

In an extensive review of delayed hemolytic reactions, 44% of the antibodies found were against

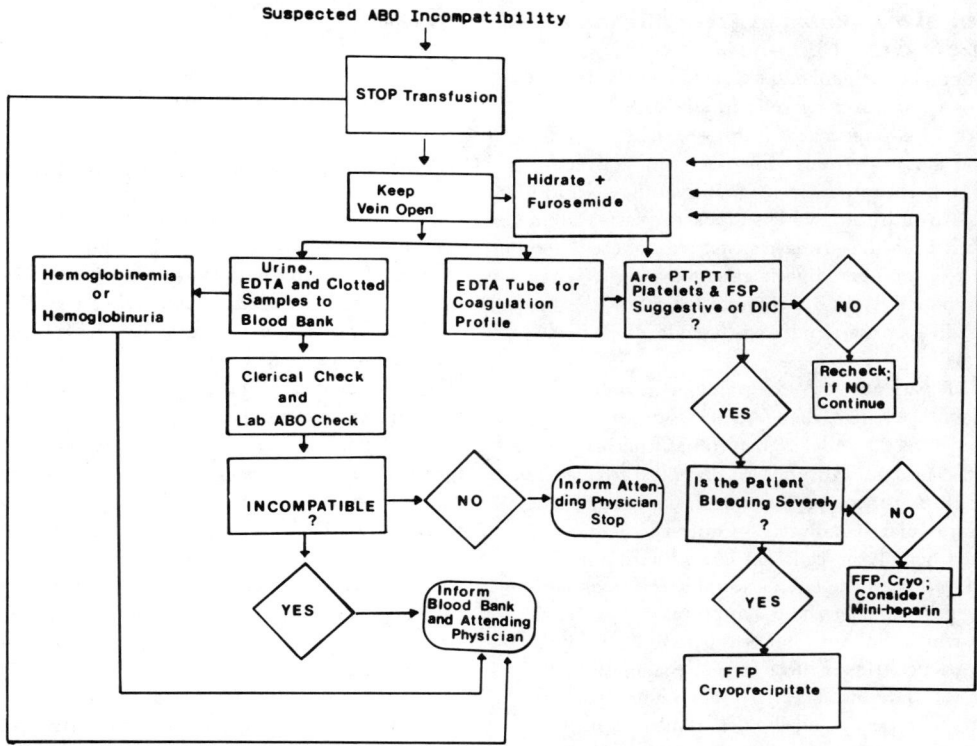

FIG 11–1.—Algorithm for management of immune hemolytic transfusion reactions.

the Rh system; of these, 52% were anti-E and 37% were anti-c. Antibodies against the Kidd system were found in 33% of the delayed transfusion reactions in the same series.[75] Typically anti-Jk antibodies, which are often evanescent, are difficult to detect and are therefore potentially dangerous.[76] In many of these cases, it is the good recordkeeping in the blood bank which will save a patient from a transfusion reaction. Antibodies against Kell, Duffy, and Lutheran systems were found in the remainder of these cases.[75] Occasionally anti-MNSs antibodies have been found in delayed immune hemolytic transfusion reactions.[75, 77] Since these antibodies are usually difficult to demonstrate by routine methods in these cases, an in vitro monocyte assay may be indicated to prove anti-MNSs specificity.[77] Anti-p[78] and anti-K6[79] antibodies have likewise been responsible for delayed immune hemolytic transfusion reactions in rare cases. It is thought that with improved methodology for detection of antibodies in pretransfusion testing, the number of cases of delayed immune hemolytic transfusion reactions reported will increase.[56]

Extravascular Hemolysis

Most clinically significant antibodies are of the IgG class and react at 37° C. The RBCs sensitized by IgG antibodies are destroyed mostly extravascularly in the RES. This occurs mainly in the spleen, where macrophages possess Fc receptors for IgG. The receptors for Fc recognize sequences on Fc located in the carboxyl terminus of the IgG molecule.[80] These RBCs may be totally engulfed by macrophages, or a portion of the RBC may be "pinched off" and resealed by these phagocytic cells, converting erythrocytes into fairly rigid spherocytes[81] that are more prone to lysis when they percolate through the fine-channel mesh of the spleen.[82]

In splenectomized patients extravascular hemolysis may be delayed and emulate a delayed immune hemolytic transfusion reaction, as was shown in a splenectomized patient with a pretransfusion anti-Fy antibody and who was transfused with Fy-incompatible blood. This patient probably would have reacted in a more immediate manner had the spleen been present.[83]

Clinical Symptoms in Predominantly Extravascular Hemolysis

Hemoglobin liberated by the destruction of RBCs is catabolized by cells in the RES.[84] In the RES, protoporphyrin rings are separated from the iron and globin portions of hemoglobin, converting protoporphyrin into biliverdin. Biliverdin is rapidly reduced to bilirubin, which binds to plasma albumin.[84] Bilirubin is thus transported to the liver, where it is conjugated with glucuronic acid. When this catabolic system is saturated, bilirubin levels in serum will increase rapidly and jaundice will be apparent.

Not all patients with extravascular hemolysis become jaundiced. It is therefore necessary to measure bilirubin levels in order to determine whether there is excess plasma bilirubin.[85] Fever is frequently present during incompatible transfusions that result in extravascular hemolysis.[86] Contrary to immune mediated hemolysis, cells not coated with antibodies removed from the circulation due to freeze damage do not produce these symptoms.[87] IgG antibodies which do not produce hemolysis in vitro usually do not trigger intravascular coagulation, except in very rare instances.[63] In one report, patients with these types of antibodies resulting in DIC were treated successfully with heparin.[63]

Management of Hemolytic Transfusion Reactions Due to Extravascular Hemolysis

Transfusion should be stopped immediately and the transfusion line kept open with saline. Usually coagulation studies are not necessary unless clinical evidence of a coagulopathy is present. Clotted and anticoagulated blood samples and urine samples are sent to the blood bank for analysis. Serum hemolysis is almost universally absent in cases of extravascular hemolysis.

Treatment of these reactions is mostly symptomatic. Urinary output should be monitored for early detection of renal shutdown, an unlikely occurrence.

Survival of Transfused Cells in Patients Without Detectable Antibodies

This topic is analyzed in detail in chapter 10. A short note is relevant here because some cases of shortened RBC survival are seen in patients with a negative antibody screen. Although antibodies are nondetectable by routine procedures in these cases, a chromium survival study will show a "collapse" curve revealing the existence of antibodies,[88] albeit undetectable by routine laboratory methods that are present on RBCs, and are responsible for short post-transfusion survival of RBCs.

Reactions Due to Incompatible Plasma

Plasma of many group O donors (about 40%[89,90]) contains warm-reacting (37° C) anti-A_1 antibodies capable of reacting with host cells in transfused A_2 patients. The reaction is noted because of short RBC survival or rarely because of a frank hemolytic transfusion reaction with development of anemia and subsequent death of the patient.[91] Attempts are made to screen these dangerous group O donors out of the donor population, especially when group O blood is to be used as an out-of-group substitute. These reactions have also been observed in hemophiliacs receiving large amounts of ABO-incompatible plasma[92] or factor VIII concentrates.[93] In addition, patients receiving abundant ABO-incompatible plasma in plateletapheresis units have likewise reacted with a hemolytic transfusion reaction to these units.[94]

Reactions due to transfused plasma containing antibodies other than anti-A or anti-B have likewise been described; of these, anti-Kell antibodies can be particularly dangerous.[95]

Other Causes of Hemolytic Transfusion Reactions

Sudden massive hemolysis has been reported in patients receiving FFP who are concomitantly suffering from severe clostridial sepsis with T activation of their RBCs. In these cases the anti-T present in donor plasma was presumably responsible for the hemolytic transfusion reaction.[96]

Non-Antibody-Mediated Hemolysis

A variety of patients develop hemolysis or hemoglobinemia in the absence of immune mediated hemolysis; the more important types are reviewed below.

Paroxysmal Nocturnal Hemoglobinuria

Paroxysmal nocturnal hemoglobinuria (PNH) is very probably a myeloproliferative disease. The syndrome frequently precedes the development of leukemia.[97] RBCs in PNH are abnormally sensitive to serum complement (see Chap. 2).[98] How complement is activated in these patients is not entirely clear. It is known that the RBC membrane has a low content of cholinesterase and that the decrement parallels the severity of the disease.[99] Interestingly, only a few of these patients develop renal shutdown, despite severe hemolysis.[100] PNH can be diagnosed at the laboratory level by performing the Ham test or acid serum hemolysis test.[101] Affected patients usually react to transfusions of whole blood with chills, fever, and delayed hemoglobinemia.[102] It is possible that some of these reactions are due to antileukocyte antibodies which may trigger hemolysis.[103] For this reason, PNH patients should be transfused with granulocyte-poor units, preferably frozen-thawed units, lacking both plasma and granulocytes.

Other RBC Deficiencies Causing Hemolysis

Other diseases of RBCs causing hemolysis concern mostly donors but may affect recipients. For instance, donors with glucose-6-phosphate dehydrogenase (G6PD) deficiency may have to be screened for the G6PD deficiency if the units are stored in citrate-phosphate-dextrose adenine, because cells from these donors have a shortened survival when stored in this anticoagulant.[104]

Donors with sickle cell trait may not donate if their cells are to be frozen, because the RBCs tend to gelate or hemolyze when they are washed after frozen storage.[105] Furthermore, sickle cell trait cells may sickle in a baby's circulation after exchange transfusion.[106] A method for freezing sickle cells has been developed, and is mentioned in Chapter 8.

RBC Hemolysis Due to Physical Agents

Osmotic Shock to RBCs

RBCs should not be mixed with other solutions. However, if it becomes necessary, the only crystalloid solution that is compatible with blood is saline.

It has been shown that 5% dextrose is capable of hemolyzing RBCs.[107] Cells exposed to 5% dextrose swell to 170%–180% of their size. These cells lose potassium and are rapidly hemolyzed. The reason for hemolysis, other than making the cells hypertonic, has not been fully clarified.[108] Osmotic shock is also incurred when distilled water is given IV by accident or when it enters the circulation after having been used for irrigation in patients post prostatectomy. Humans tolerate volumes of up to 100 ml of distilled water without complications. However, 300–900 ml will produce severe hemolysis in most cases, and volumes above 1.5 L are likely to produce renal shutdown and death.[108]

Heating or Freezing

Blood may hemolyze if it is warmed to 50° C or more. If large volumes of blood heated in this way are transfused, renal shutdown may be induced.[108] RBCs heated to 41° C may not be grossly hemolyzed, but their posttransfusion survival is dramatically reduced.[109] Blood may be frozen accidentally by inadvertent storage of units in freezers. When the units thaw, they hemolyze for lack of a cryoprotective agent. Units frozen and thawed in this way appear purple in color, which alerts physicians or nurses that a unit is hemolyzed.[108]

Other Causes of Hemolysis

Contaminated units will occasionally show hemolysis, which may be discovered on transfusion by the appearance of hemoglobinemia. Another frequent cause of hemolysis in hospitals where cardiac surgery is performed is that caused by the pump-oxygenator.[108] More frequent, however, is intraoperative hemolysis produced by vaccum suction.[110]

IMMUNE MEDIATED NONHEMOLYTIC TRANSFUSION REACTIONS

The reported overall frequency of reactions to transfused blood and blood components varies from 3%[111] to 7%.[112] Ninety percent of these reactions are nonhemolytic. Nonhemolytic reactions may be against formed elements or against plasma. These reactions will be reviewed according to the most likely cause.

Reactions Against WBCs

Reactions against leukocytes are the most frequent of the reported reactions to transfused components (e.g., whole blood, packed cells, platelets, and granulocytes). These reactions usually appear as febrile reactions which may or may not be accompanied by a flu-like syndrome. Fever due to incompatible RBCs or to pyrogens in an infected unit must be ruled out. In one series, 191 recipients reacted to transfusion with nonhemolytic reactions in a group of 5030 recipients. About 10% of these 191 patients had multiple reactions. Another 10% were reported as having "severe" reactions. Some 84.4% of those having a reaction had had previous transfusions. About 64% of patients had anti-HLA antibodies when tested for B cell reactivity.[113] In another study of 49 febrile reactions, 65% of patients had leukoagglutinins in their plasma.[114] Most patients who had febrile reactions did not have further reactions after receiving leukocyte-poor RBC units.[115] The reactions may be caused by lysis of donor granulocytes via host cytotoxic antibodies plus complement or by the reaction of infused antibodies against the recipient's WBCs.[116] Antibodies in these cases are usually of the IgG class.[116] In about 37% of cases anti-HLA antibodies are detected;[117] in the remainder, antibodies against granulocyte-specific antigens are detected.[118] Interestingly, antibodies against platelet-specific antigens are usually of the IgM class.[116]

The development of anti-HLA antibodies apparently depends on the transfusion schedule.[119] In addition, the chance of developing leukoagglutinins appears to increase with the frequency of transfusion.[120] Transfusion of 5–10 units of components containing granulocytes frequently produces immunization.[121]

The so-called naturally occurring isoimmunization occurs very rarely.[122] However, maternal immunization by fetal leukocytes is frequent.[123] Up to 25% of women will become immunized against leukocytes during their first pregnancy and about 55% will do so over the course of multiple pregnancies.[124] These IgG antibodies do not cross the placenta,[125] whereas antibodies specific to granulocytes do cross the placenta and cause neutropenia of the newborn.[125] It is possible that anti-HLA antibodies are of the IgG2 or IgG4 class, which do not cross the placenta, whereas specific granulocyte antibodies may be of the IgG1 or IgG3 class, which do cross the placenta.

Although granulocytes are known to be immunogenic, other HLA-bearing formed blood elements such as lymphocytes and platelets are also capable of immunizing a recipient.[126] Solid tissue grafts containing these cells (e.g., kidney grafts) can likewise produce immunization.[127] Donor plasma containing leukoagglutinins may bring about a febrile reaction in patients receiving such a unit.[128]

A leukocyte reaction should be suspected when a patient develops fever during or after a transfusion. However, since hemolytic reactions can manifest clinically with fever, all febrile reactions must be investigated as transfusion reactions. Transfusion is immediately stopped and the transfusion workup started. Once RBC incompatibility has been ruled out, one must try to determine whether the reaction was caused by WBCs. Clinically, fever of a leukocyte reaction characteristically appears 30 minutes to 2 hours after transfusion is started. It is usually accompanied by shaking chills and disappears after 2–24 hours, depending on the severity of the event.[129] At the laboratory level, once RBC antibodies have been ruled out, leukoagglutinins may be sought, although this test is not routinely performed. Some laboratories, however, do offer it, and it has proved useful in the study of febrile reactions.[125] A leukoagglutinin screen is used for detecting anti-granulocyte-specific antibodies.[130] Another useful test for demonstrating antibodies is the lymphocytotoxicity test, in which cell killing by antiserum and complement is measured.[125] This test is primarily used for detecting anti-HLA antibodies.[130] It should be noted that the predictive value of these laboratory tests has not been universally accepted and their use has not yielded a net decrease in granulocyte reactions.[131]

Management of Febrile Reactions

All febrile reactions warrant stopping the transfusion. A transfusion reaction investigation must be conducted lest a hemolytic transfusion reaction be missed. Some hemolytic reactions may appear initially as febrile reactions. Fever can be treated symptomatically, preferably with a non-aspirin-containing antipyretic agent such as acetaminophen. Febrile reactions can be prevented in multiply transfused patients by transfusing leukocyte-poor units. About 85% of patients will not react to subsequent units and 15% will have repeated reactions. Therefore, the accepted procedure is to start leukocyte-poor units after repeated febrile transfusion reactions have occurred.[132] Buffy coat–poor units obtained by differential centrifugation are used initially. If reactions persist, removal of the Buffy coat by centrifugation and filtration with microaggregate filters will remove close to 90% of the granulocytes. In one study, microaggregate filtration reduced the incidence of febrile reactions by 77%.[133] In another study, the incidence of non-HTR was reduced from 0.49% to 0.21% using saline-washed RBCs.[134] However, the routine use of this method would more than double the cost per unit of blood.[135] Nevertheless, the best units for patients who have had multiple severe febrile or allergic transfusion reactions are washed cells or frozen-thawed cells, which contain little plasma and less than 2% residual WBCs.[136] Patients who have had severe reactions to granulocytes in blood or blood components can be premedicated with antipyretics[137] and/or corticosteroids.[118] Antihistaminics have not proved to be of value in treating these reactions.[138]

Pulmonary Infiltrates Due to Leukoagglutinins

On occasion, patients receiving blood or blood components will experience severe dyspnea and cyanosis and present with acute pulmonary edema; x-ray examination reveals bilateral hilar pulmonary infiltrates. Assuming no overload has occurred, leukoagglutinins can be considered the cause of such reactions. The reaction is thought to be caused by agglutination of WBCs and entrapment of the agglutinates in the alveolar capillaries.[139] These reactions can also be triggered by transfused plasma that contains leukoagglutinins in high titer.[140] Plasma that has been implicated in severe reactions of this sort has often been obtained from multiparous women. Once such donors have been identified, they should subsequently not donate plasma for transfusion.[141] Reactions to leukoagglutinins may be life-threatening in patients who are already compromised. Treatment includes IV administration of corticosteroids and epinephrine.[116]

Granulocyte transfusion produces immunization and febrile reactions much more frequently than transfusion of any other component. These reactions are probably related to the content of damaged cells that have released pyrogenic material as well as the fact that granulocytes transfused into patients receiving random donor granulocyte units have been obtained from a number of different donors, often 12 or more.[112] Granulocyte units may also produce severe pulmonary edema,[142] as described above.

Graft-versus-Host Disease

Graft-versus-host disease (GVHD) is a rare complication of transfusion. GVHD was discussed in the section on granulocytes in chapter 8 but will be reviewed here briefly as a disease that may occur after transfusion of blood or blood components.

Engraftment of transfused lymphocytes occurs almost exclusively in immunosuppressed individuals.[143] GVHD in such patients is frequently fatal. Recent reports indicate that GVHD may, at times, be caused by an abnormal clone of cytotoxic suppressor T cells.[144] Units of components containing viable lymphocytes must be irradiated with approximately 2,000 rads to inhibit mitosis of these cells before the units can be transfused into immunosuppressed individuals.

Untoward Reactions to Platelet Transfusions

As mentioned earlier, units of platelets may be contaminated with granulocytes and may also possess HLA antigens; therefore, febrile reactions are not uncommon in patients receiving these components on a long-term basis. Other complications of platelet sensitization are present as well. An important complication is the poor survival of transfused platelets on sensitization.[145] Transfusion of selected HLA-matched platelets results in improved post-transfusion counts and improved platelet survival in the circulation.[146] If a patient has antibodies against one HLA marker, transfusion of platelets from donors negative for that marker will bypass the refractory state.[147] Often anti-HLA sensitization by platelet infusion is a result of leukocyte contamination of platelet units. By reducing numbers of contaminant WBCs in a unit of platelets, refractory responses can be mitigated.[148] Refractory response to platelet infusion may disappear altogether if a transfusion-free interval is possible.[149] Anti-Pl^{A1} antibodies are platelet-specific antibodies usually found in neonatal thrombocytopenia;[150] rarely, these antibodies complicate transfusions, resulting in posttransfusion purpura.[150] Posttransfusion thrombocytopenia is usually seen in multiparous middle-aged women.[151] Thrombocytopenia in these cases may last 10–60 days.

Sensitization to Rh antigens by Rh-positive platelet units was discussed in chapter 8. ABO compatibility must be enforced if multiple units of platelets are used. Lack of ABO compatibility between donor platelet plasma and recipient red cells has resulted in severe hemolytic transfusion reactions from the large volume of ABO-incompatible plasma contained in pooled platelets.[152]

TRANSFUSION REACTIONS CAUSED BY PLASMA PROTEIN SENSITIVITY

Transfusion reaction against plasma is the next most common reaction after febrile transfusion reaction. In some series, reaction to transfused plasma has been present in 3% of all recipients.[153] These reactions can be grouped in terms of their clinical severity or in terms of the causative protein. Two main types are recognized according to clinical severity: minor reactions and severe reactions. Most minor reactions to plasma are manifested clinically by hives, urticaria, and wheals. Most such reactions are due to sensitization to γ-globulins.[116] Major reactions are infrequent—1 per 20,000, in one series.[116] However, these reactions may be life-threatening, especially when transfused IgA in plasma triggers anaphylaxis in an IgA-deficient recipient with circulating anti-IgA antibodies.[154] Nevertheless, not all patients with anti-IgA antibodies develop anaphylaxis. As many as 3% of urticarial plasma transfusion reactions are associated with anti-IgA antibodies.[155]

The following section considers reactions to the different plasma proteins by the type of protein inducing the reaction.

Anti-IgG Antibodies

Antibodies against IgG are usually directed against the Gm portion of the γ heavy chain[156] or against hidden portions of the molecule, revealed by IgG pepsin digests.[157] It was the discovery of these antibodies that allowed the study of IgG polymorphism. Different anti-IgG antibody specificities can recognize differences in single amino acid substitutions. Four determinants are discernible in subclass IgG1, whereas 12 are discernible in IgG3, one in IgG2, and none in IgG4.[158, 159] The function of these allotypes is unknown; however, homozygous G3m(b) individuals have higher levels of IgG3 than heterozygotes.[160] Gm allotype distribution differs in various racial groups; for example, Gm1 is present in all blacks, whereas 35%–65% of whites lack it.[161] Antibodies against Gm allotypes may appear as autoantibodies in patients with rheumatoid arthritis, called rheumatoid agglutinators (Raggs)[160] or may occur in multiparous women or multiply transfused individuals, called serum normal agglutinators (Scraggs).[162]

In rheumatoid arthritis, rheumatoid factor (RF) may be directed against various portions of the IgG molecule. Usually RF antibodies are of the IgM class and may act as cryoglobulins, although antibodies of the IgG class are not infrequent. The deposition of IgM anti-IgG complexes presumably causes some of the pathology found in rheumatoid arthritis.[163] Patients with rheumatoid arthritis produce a variety of antibodies against the IgG molecule; these may be non-species-specific or species-specific.[163]

Anti-Gm antibodies have been found in up to 70% of multiply transfused pediatric patients,[164] but adults may be more difficult to immunize against Gm by transfusion.[165] So-called natural anti-Gm antibodies have been described in non-transfused, multiparous patients. These antibodies are probably acquired in utero from immunization by maternal Gm proteins.[166] Milgrom antibodies are a special variety of anti-Gm antibodies specific for certain Rh antibodies. Milgrom antibodies are very rare in the normal population (0.5%).[167]

Reactions to Injected IgG

Injection of IgG-containing products (e.g., plasma, γ-globulin) may cause febrile[168] or urticarial reactions[169] or may produce severe anaphylactic reactions in hypogammaglobulinemic patients. These reactions may be occasionally produced against Gm antigens[168] and must be differentiated from reactions produced by anti-IgA antibodies by assaying anti-IgA levels in patient blood samples. However, most reactions seen in hypogammaglobulinemic patients have not been directly associated with anti-Ig antibodies[170] and may be caused by other types of antibodies. The actual immune responsiveness or nonresponsiveness to Gm stimulus may be linked to specific Ir genes, as has been shown in animals[171] and humans[172] for other antigens.

Other Reactions to Plasma

Following infusion of plasma, a serum sickness-type of reaction has been described in patients with anti-IgG antibodies.[173]

Mild reactions to IgG, such as urticaria and hives, may be handled with Benadryl. Treatment for IgG-induced anaphylaxis is the same as that given below for IgA.[159, 174]

Prevention of Plasma Reactions

In patients with a history of mild reactions, premedication with Benadryl is sufficient; patients with more severe reactions to IgG require avoiding transfusion of plasma or components when possible. For instance, if the patient needs blood, frozen-thawed cells should be used; if the patient needs platelets, the platelets should be washed (see Chap.

8). γ-Globulin injections should be avoided if possible in these patients. If components are desperately needed, premedication with steroids and Benadryl may be attempted, but in patients prone to severe reactions, there is no assurance, even with premedication, that severe reactions will not occur.

The serum sickness type of reaction due to anti-Gm antibodies discussed above is not a frequent occurrence, but it may be present in immunized patients receiving γ-globulin.[175] Severe anaphylactic reactions secondary to IV infusion of γ-globulin are more common than after IM injection; patients develop tachycardia, tachypnea, and hypotension in these cases.[176] Reactions after IV injection of γ-globulin are presumably caused by aggregated IgGs in immunoglobulin suspensions, which activate complement with subsequent release of vasoactive substances. Complement activation by these aggregates occurs because of the proximate Fc fragments in aggregates that allow binding of C1q with subsequent activation of other complement components, and anaphylatoxin release. Because of these reactions, the FDA had not licensed IV preparations of γ-globulin for use in this country. However, preparations for IV first developed in Europe are currently used in the United States. Studies using IV γ-globulin[177] have shown that preparations with a high protein content (300 mg) cause reactions, while preparations containing lower concentration (12 mg) of protein do not cause reactions.[178]

Reactions to IgA

There are two IgA heavy chain allotype markers, IgA2m1 and IgA2m2. IgA1 does not seem to have any allotypes, or else they are very rare.[160] Only about 2% of caucasians lack the A2m1 marker, whereas 50% of blacks lack the A2m1 allotype.[161] Patients who have normal serum IgA levels and react to IgA are probably reacting to the allotype they lack; these patients usually produce low-titer antibodies. However, individuals with a total lack of IgA produce high-titered (e.g., 1:1,000 or more) class-specific anti-IgA antibodies against all types of IgA.[179] These antibodies are usually of the IgG class, although IgE has by no means been ruled out in all studies. Both antiallotypic antibodies as well as polyspecific antibodies directed against all types of IgA are capable of producing severe life-threatening anaphylactic reactions.[116, 154]

The diagnosis of IgA deficiency is usually done by sensitive radioimmunoassay (RIA) techniques. This test permits distinguishing a true deficiency from a low IgA plasma level. If simple immunodiffusion techniques are employed, about 49% fewer subjects with IgA deficiency are detected than when RIA is used.[179] About 25% of truly IgA-deficient individuals will produce anti-IgA antibodies.[180] Most of these individuals do not have a history of transfusion or pregnancy.[180] Intrauterine immunization of the fetus may explain discrepancies in immunization history. This mechanism, however, has only been proved in one case.[181] The overall incidence of IgA deficiency is about 1 in 700[182] to 1 in 800[179] normal individuals. Clinically, IgA reactions may be mild or very severe. Anaphylactic reactions are characterized by marked hypotension, wheezing bronchospasm, and laryngeal edema.[183, 184] The severity of the reactions is apparently in direct relation to the anti-IgA antibody titer. Titers less than 256, by hemagglutination test, only rarely lead to severe reactions.[185] Intramuscular injections of immunoglobulin, as used in the prevention of hepatitis or for Rh immunization, contain small amounts of IgA and have occasionally caused severe anaphylactic reactions.[186, 187] Of all the immunoglobulins, IgA has been implicated in most of the severe reactions. In one study, 89% of specimens from patients who had anaphylactoid reactions contained anti-IgA antibodies,[188] in contrast to the extremely low incidence of anti-IgG antibodies.[189] However, recent studies of posttransfusion anaphylaxis do not reveal that anti-IgA antibodies are the dominant cause of anaphylaxis.[190] Conversely, not all patients with anti-IgA antibodies will have reactions, as shown in a study in which 16% of a population of multiply transfused patients had anti-IgA antibodies but no history of transfusion reactions.[189] It is quite possible that the response to alloimmunization is controlled by the Ir genes, as has been demonstrated experimentally in mice.[191]

Whether anti-IgA antibodies are oligoclonal or polyclonal probably does not bear on either the titer or the severity of reactions.[192]

Management of Anaphylaxis Due to Anti-IgA Antibodies[177]

1. Stop the transfusion immediately.
2. Establish an airway.
3. Restore volume with saline IV.
4. Give epinephrine solution, 0.4–1 ml of 1:1,000, IM; repeat in 5–10 minutes. If necessary, give aqueous diphenhydramine hydrochloride, 5–20 mg.

Prevention of Anaphylactic Reactions to Plasma Secondary to Anti-IgA Antibodies

All patients who have had anaphylactoid reactions during transfusion must be studied by RIA for the presence or absence of IgA, anti-IgA antibodies (class-specific antibodies or alloantibodies), and possibly for anti-Gm antibodies if the other tests are negative. Once the presence of anti-IgA antibodies has been established, no plasma products should be given further, if possible. If plasma products must be given, IgA-deficient plasma from IgA-deficient donors may be obtained from the American Red Cross and other institutions with large donor files.

If these patients require blood, IgA-deficient units should be used. If they are not available, frozen-thawed units may be used but should be transfused slowly and by a team of nurses and physicians prepared to treat anaphylaxis. Premedication with steroids and antihistaminics is recommended but may not prevent a reaction. Units washed six times with modern cell washers may alternatively be given.[193]

Other Antibodies to Immunoglobulins

Anti-IgM antibodies have been described in about 4% of multiparous women and in about 7% of multiply transfused individuals.[194] The incidence of anti-IgM antibodies in immunodeficient patients is much higher.[195] About 30% of patients with anti-IgM antibodies have urticaria and fever, but a direct correlation between these antibodies and urticarial reactions has not been demonstrated.[196] Anti-Km antibodies to the light chain of the Km allotype also exist; these were previously known as Inv determinants.[197] The clinical significance of these antibodies is not known.

Reactions Due to IgE

Although IgE levels may be elevated in multiply transfused patients, the role of IgE in transfusion reactions is not easy to evaluate because it is extremely difficult to measure its concentration accurately.[198] Normal values for IgE are 250 ng/ml and about 700 ng/ml in severely allergic individuals.[199] Apparently these high levels of IgE can be observed in allergic transfusion reactions.[200] The clinical role of antibodies against IgE has not been reported.

Patients with atopic allergies may have urticarial reactions if they receive components or fractions consisting of pooled sera, presumably because of the binding of atopens to mast cells sensitized with IgE specific for these antigens.[201] Conversely, transfusion of plasma from patients with atopic allergy produces symptoms in nonallergic patients receiving sensitized plasma.[202]

Antibodies to Lipoproteins

Allotypes of lipoproteins have been designated Ag antigens. Ten such allotypes have been described.[203] Multiply transfused individuals often have anti-Ag antibodies.[204] These patients will likewise often develop febrile reactions;[205] however, they also have circulating leukoagglutinins, which are the more probable cause of such reactions.

NON-IMMUNE-MEDIATED, NONHEMOLYTIC TRANSFUSION REACTIONS TO BLOOD

So far this chapter has dealt with immune-mediated reactions and some nonimmune causes of hemolysis. Many reactions to transfusions are not mediated by the immune system. Other reactions to transfusion that may compromise the patient and are related to transfusion, but are not caused by antibodies, will be reviewed.

Transfusion of Cold Blood

In practice, the transfusion of cold blood is not of great significance, unless the rate of transfusion is very rapid and the volume of blood transfused is high (> 4 units in an adult).[206] The massive transfusion of ice-cold blood is a dangerous practice, as has been shown by Boyan et al.[207, 208] In their studies, 48% of a group of 24 patients had cardiac arrest on transfusion of 6 units of cold blood at rates of 50 ml/minute or more. More than 80% of patients had cardiac arrest on transfusion of 12 units at rates over 100 ml/minute. Conversely, only 3% of patients had cardiac arrest on massive transfusion of warmed blood. Cardiac arrhythmias have also been documented following transfusion of cold blood.[209] Some of the reasons cited for this effect are increased cardiac output, and oxygen consumption from decrements of less than 1° C, as well as increased oxygen affinity of hemoglobin at decreased temperatures.[210] For these reasons, blood warmers have been recommended in massive blood transfusion.[211] Water bath heat exchanges are preferred to microwave heaters because of the potential for hemolysis when microwaves are used.[211] Special precautions are taken during exchange transfusions in babies, in whom transfusion of 1 unit of cold blood may be hazardous.[206]

Minor complications of transfusion of a few units of cold blood include pain at the infusion site due to venospasm[212] and chills due to lowering of body temperature.

Circulatory Overload

When blood or plasma is transfused rapidly into a normal individual, expected effects include a transient rise in the venous pressure and a decrease of the lungs' vital capacity due to accumulation of the added fluid in the respiratory venous capillary bed.[213] By 24 hours after transfusion, the intravascular blood volume has usually dropped to pretransfusion levels.[214] Most transfusion sets deliver about 15 drops/ml. The usual rate of transfusion for 1 unit of blood is about 60 drops/minute, which allows transfusion of 1 unit (500 ml) in 2 hours. Transfusing the same volume at 200 drops/minute takes 35 minutes.[215] Severely anemic patients must be transfused very slowly (1 unit of packed cells over 4–6 hours) to avoid pulmonary edema.[216]

The main clinical symptoms of circulatory overload are associated with pulmonary edema and include dry cough, chest tightness, jugular vein engorgement, and headache. If transfusion is continued, transudate fluid filters into alveoli, producing audible crepitation and rales. This constitutes a medical emergency and the following measures are taken:[215]

1. Transfusion must be stopped immediately.
2. Furosemide may be necessary (40 mg IV).
3. The patient must be propped up.
4. Close observation for 12 hours is warranted.

This syndrome should not be confused with the syndrome found in patients who have undergone bypass with postoperative hypoxia; in such patients the syndrome is caused by interstitial infiltration by immature plasma cells, suggesting an immune-mediated phenomenon.[217] Overload can be prevented by monitoring central venous pressure in patients receiving massive blood transfusion.[217]

Reactions From Toxic Substances in Blood and Blood Component Units

Citrate Toxicity

Citrate is a relatively nontoxic substance, but if it is infused rapidly it may bind ionized calcium in sufficient amounts to produce cardiac conduction system compromise and even death.[218] The severity of citrate toxicity depends on the rate at which blood stored in CPD is infused, as has been shown experimentally by Collins.[219] Rates of less than 1.5 ml/kg/5 minutes do not produce citrate toxicity in normal animals, whereas rates above 1.5 ml/kg/5 minutes produce decreased cardiac output and death due to depression of ionized calcium. An increment in potassium content (i.e., in older units) has a synergistic effect with the low ionized calcium levels, further compromising recipients.[220] In addition, hypothermia may also potentiate the synergism between high potassium and low ionized calcium levels.[219] Another factor that can increase citrate toxicity is impaired liver function. It is therefore a good practice to treat patients with liver failure who need RBCs with packed cells.[221]

The margin of safety of citrate dosage is very narrow (0.06 mmoles of citrate/kg/minute for 20 minutes may be lethal, whereas 0.04 mmoles/kg/minute is a safe dose) as has been shown in animal experiments.[222] However, in adults, only massive transfusions (e.g., 14 units[223]) are capable of inducing significant ionized calcium changes. Such changes may be manifested as ECG QT segment prolongation.[223] Citrate toxicity is probably more dangerous in infants undergoing exchange transfusion. The citrate level may reach up to 100 mg/100 ml after 1 unit exchange[224] and provoke ECG ST segment prolongations.[225] These changes can be prevented by giving 10% calcium gluconate via a different vein from that used for transfusion.[225] Nevertheless, deaths from calcium overload have been reported in the pediatric population[226] subsequent to calcium gluconate therapy, and therefore its use must be undertaken with extreme caution. Some investigators are totally opposed to its use in these infants.[227]

Acid Load in Banked Blood

Although massive transfusion of banked blood into young healthy recruits has not produced clinically significant acidosis, this has not been the case in pH-compromised individuals.[227] The concern for such complications secondary to decreased pH has been supported by experiments with animals which showed increased mortality when animals were transfused with acidified blood: 86% of animals that received bicarbonate to combat acidosis survived ACD blood unit transfusions.[228] A better survival was likewise shown in patients who received 50 mEq of bicarbonate for every 5 ACD units.[229] When CPD units are used, this complication probably results only after many more units are transfused.[227]

Transfusional Hyperkalemia and Ammonium Load

It has been calculated that a unit of packed cells contains 1–2 mEq of potassium.[230] This amount is potentially significant in pediatric exchange transfusions.[231] However, it may not be truly significant in massive transfusion unless units are close to expiration[227] or the patient is hyperkalemic already (i.e., has massive tissue injury).[232] Potassium toxicity, as mentioned earlier, is potentiated by low pH and citrate toxicity. This combination has been shown experimentally to be very dangerous: rabbits transfused with blood containing high potassium and citrate levels had a 79% mortality, compared to a 10% mortality in animals treated with blood lacking these elements.[233]

Ammonium levels, like potassium levels, increase in stored blood, from 100 μg/100 ml in fresh blood to 900 μg/100 ml in 21-day-old blood. These levels are undesirable in patients with liver failure.[234]

Air Embolism

Air embolism is very rare since the use of bottles for blood transfusion was discontinued.[235] In the event that large amounts of air are introduced into the venous system, turning the patient on his or her side and lifting the lower extremities has proved to decrease mortality from air embolism.[236]

Microaggregates

Microaggregates of leukocytes and platelets routinely form in stored blood. These aggregates may be as large as 200 μ in diameter.[237] These microaggregates are known to find their way into alveolar capillaries and cause pulmonary microembolism,[238] which was thought to cause pulmonary insufficiency[239] during massive transfusion. However, recent data obtained both experimentally in animals[240] and clinically in patients[241] show that these microaggregates do not appear to pose a major threat during massive transfusion. It is believed that most of the pathologic changes seen in lungs of individuals who have been massively transfused are more likely due to underlying shock than to microaggregate emboli.[242] Furthermore, some studies have not found significant differences in the pulmonary function of patients receiving blood through standard 170-μ filters versus microaggregate filters.[243] However, certain authors do suggest that such aggregates may be significant in rapid transfusions of more than 5 units.[244] To eliminate large aggregates from transfused blood, early workers advocated the use of 170-μ filters, which are now required for all transfusions.[245]

Recently, a variety of microaggregate filters have been introduced in transfusion therapy.[237] These filters trap microaggregates larger than 20–40 μ, depending on the type of filter used. Three basic types of filters are available: screen filters, depth filters, and filters combining screen plus artificial mesh to provide filtration.

Screen filters usually trap aggregates larger than 40 μ, but only small volumes of residual blood are trapped in the filter, and the rate of infusion is faster.[246] These considerations are important in massive transfusions.

Mesh filters or depth filters trap more blood in the filter (about 20% of a unit of packed cells) but screen particles larger than 20 μ. Flushing these filters should be avoided, because both microaggregates and other thrombogenic or potentially immunogenic material are transfused into the recipient.[247]

As more and more units are transfused through the same filter, the screening filtration rate (SFR) of the filter decreases dramatically.[237] This decrease in SFR is due to the trapping of granulocyte debris and platelet aggregates.[247] The use of microaggregate filters decreases the number of granulocytes and lymphocytes transfused;[247] therefore, these filters can be used as adjunctive prevention in febrile reactions.[247] The efficiency of a filter can be improved by production of larger aggregates in the units by centrifugation of the units at high speed before filtration.[248, 249]

In normal individuals, the pulmonary capillaries function as a filter of venous blood. However, in patients undergoing cardiopulmonary surgery, the lungs are bypassed, eliminating this filtration effect. The systemic capillaries must then clear the circulation from microaggregate debris. Such capillaries include CNS, myocardial, and renal capillaries, making them prone to blockage. Microemboli have been reported in the CNS[250] and the myocardium[251] of patients subjected to massive transfusion during bypass surgery.

In summary, microfiltration has a role both in massive transfusions during open heart surgery (especially if older blood—for example, 3-week-old blood—is used[252]) and in the prevention of febrile reactions,[247] especially if filters are combined with other leukocyte-depleting procedures (e.g., inverted centrifugation). One must remember, however, that using microfiltration on a large scale increases the cost of each unit transfused. Therefore, one must weigh the net advantages of microfiltration against the additional cost of transfusion.

Other Particulate Material Transfused Via Blood Transfusion

Some substances from plastic bag containers are leached into the suspending plasma due to the effect of plasma lipase. The main substance originating from plastic is mono-2-ethylhexylphthalate (MEHP).[253] The clinical significance of this substance is not yet known, but it has been found to accumulate in adipose tissues for extended periods of time.

INFECTIONS TRANSMITTED BY BLOOD AND BLOOD COMPONENT TRANSFUSION

Blood obtained from apparently healthy donors can transmit disease if donors are carriers of infection or have subclinical infection.

The following section reviews some of the infections (other than hepatitis, which is reviewed in chapter 12 and AIDS, which is reviewed in Chapter 13) that can be transmitted by transfusion of blood and blood components, including viral, bacterial, and parasitic infections.

Viral Infections Transmitted by Blood Transfusion

Though viral hepatitis and AIDS are the most important infections transmitted by blood, other viruses are capable of being transmitted by blood and blood product transfusion. The most prevalent is cytomegalovirus (CMV) infection. CMV has proved to be the etiologic agent of the postperfusion syndrome.[254] It occurs in 3%–10% of cases following open heart surgery.[255] CMV is characterized by the development of fever, splenomegaly, and atypical lymphocytes[256] in patients who were transfused with relatively fresh blood during open heart surgery. The CMV virus, which frequently infects WBCs, is present in about 12% of the donor population.[257] It is therefore not surprising that patients who are immunosuppressed and receive granulocytes frequently develop CMV infections. These infections are more severe than in post-open heart surgery patients and are characterized by fever, hepatosplenomegaly, thrombocytopenia, and hemolytic anemia.[258] CMV infection occasionally mimics hepatitis,[259] producing elevated transaminase levels and jaundice. Other viruses such as herpes virus and the Epstein-Barr virus (EBV) produce a similar syndrome but much less frequently.[259] EBV infection by transfusion has been seen when patients develop infectious mononucleosis after transfusion. The transmission of infectious mononucleosis by transfusion is infrequent[260] but has been reported in patients receiving blood components. The transmission of EBV is not surprising, because it can be found in donor WBCs years after infection.[261] However, recipients do not become infected, owing to the 95% prevalence of protective antibodies in the general population.[259] In a few cases EBV has been the causative agent of the postperfusion syndrome.[262, 263] EBV infection is of concern in perinatal transfusion (see Chap. 16).

Other viruses likewise can be transmitted by transfusion. Arboviruses and "slow" viruses of the nervous system are potentially transmissible via transfusion.[264] Since the incubation period is so long, however, the correlation of transfusion with these diseases is usually very difficult to make. Rocky Mountain spotted fever is potentially transmissible for it remains in host lymph nodes for long periods of time. However, the disease has not been reported to be transmitted by transfusion.[255] As mentioned above, a recently described viral disease that can be transmitted via transfusion is the acquired immunodeficiency syndrome, now known to be caused by the HTLV virus (see Chap. 13).

Bacterial Disease Transmitted by Blood or Blood Component Transfusion

Part of the daily quality control program of a blood bank is the inspection of blood units for possible contamination. One should look for the following:

1. Purplish discoloration of the blood in the container.
2. Presence of clots.[265]
3. Hemoglobin in the plasma due to hemolysis (although hemolysis may be absent in up to 25% of cases).[265]
4. Presence of gas in the unit.

Contaminated units are discarded by autoclaving and incinerating.

The major cause for contamination of units is a poorly prepared venipuncture site at the time of donation. Strict quality control must be exercised in the donor room, with asepsis maintained during preparation of donor venipuncture site and during venipuncture procedure.

About 2% of units of freshly drawn blood are contaminated with bacteria.[265] Many bacteria may contaminate freshly drawn blood units; the more frequent ones are staphylococci and diphtheroids, but fortunately most of these bacteria do not appear to tolerate refrigeration beyond 4 days.[266] Unlike gram-negative bacteria, gram-positive bacteria do not seem to thrive under cold temperatures; this explains why most cases of contamination are caused for the most part by gram-negative organisms.[267] Gram-negative bacteria that are capable of growing at cold temperatures (psychrophilic) have been shown to be of the *Pseudomonas,* coliform, and *Achromobacter* species.[268] On the other hand, if the unit is contaminated with mesophilic organisms capable of growing at warm temperatures, and if the unit is allowed to remain at warm temperatures for 24 hours, organisms may multiply and reach dangerous levels.[265] Some of these bacteria utilize citrate as a source of carbon, thereby depleting citrate; this induces clotting within units. Patients receiving contaminated blood may develop cough, diarrhea, flushing of the skin, very high fever, DIC,[269] vascular collapse, shock, and death.[270] In a series of 28 patients who had transfusion reactions from contaminated blood, 58% died from the transfusion.[271] Of these, 6 patients died from DIC.[271] It has been recently reported that contamination of units of blood with *Yersinia enterocolitica* may cause very severe, sometimes fatal reactions.[272] Transfusion should be stopped immediately if such reactions occur. The patient may present with bacterial shock, or "warm shock," in which the skin is flushed and warm but the patient is hypotensive. This type of shock is usually caused by gram-negative endotoxins.[273] Differential diagnosis between "warm shock" due to a contaminated unit and a major incompatible transfusion reaction may be difficult to make if hemolysis and hemoglobinuria are present. A negative Coombs test should help in the diagnosis. Laboratory diagnosis is obtained by culturing a sample of blood from the bag and a blood sample from the patient. The treatment of endotoxic shock depends on the severity of the case and on the causative agent. Volume replacement with crystalloid, vasopressors, IV steroids, and antibiotics may be necessary.[273]

Salmonella,[274] *Brucella,*[275] and *Clostridium*[276] are organisms which have all been implicated in infection via transfusion of infected units. If there is a history of *Brucella* or *Salmonella* infection, donors must be permanently excluded from the donor pool due to the chronicity of these infections.

Syphilis

Syphilis was a major transfusion problem in the past.[277] However, refrigeration of units,[278] screening of donors,[279] and antibiotic treatment of severely ill patients[277] have made posttransfusion syphilis almost an extinct entity. Spirochetes do not survive beyond 72 hours when refrigerated at 4°–6° C.[278] The FDA still requires blood donors to be screened for syphilis, but the AABB does not. Syphilis may be a consideration in the use of platelets that have been stored at room temperature,[255] although no instances of syphilis transmitted by this component have been reported since storage of platelets at room temperature became a requirement. It must be noted, however, that syphilis is usually transmitted in the seronegative phase, and donors with positive antibodies are usually at a stage where syphilis is not transmitted.[280] It has been documented that up to 20% of platelet concentrates stored at room temperature are contaminated with other types of bacteria,[281] which emphasizes the potential risks of failing to screen donors or failing to observe asepsis during venipuncture.

Only one case of posttransfusion syphilis (out of a series of 1 million transfusions) has been documented recently; it was secondary to the transfusion of relatively fresh blood.[282] The disease is manifested as secondary syphilis with lymphadenopathy, flu-like syndrome, and a generalized skin rash. Diagnosis is proved by fluorescent treponemal antibody testing and the fluorescent treponemal antibody-absorbed test.

Treatment consists of benzathine penicillin G or procaine penicillin G with 2% aluminum monoestearate, 1.2 million units injected in each buttock.

Tetracycline, 40 gm/day, or erythromycin, 40 gm/day, is given for 2 weeks to patients allergic to penicillin.[283] It must be remembered that transient seroconversion is possible with transfusion of seropositive plasma, but the positive serology usually does not last more than 20 days.[277]

Relapsing fever, another spirochetal disease, has rarely been transmitted by transfusion.[284]

Transfusion Reactions Due to Pyrogens

Some patients develop fever on transfusion. Although the units received may be sterile, bacterial pyrogens, usually lipopolysaccharides, may be responsible for the fever.[285] Pyrogens are not a frequent cause of febrile transfusion reactions.

Parasitic Diseases Transmitted by Blood Transfusion

Perhaps the more important of the blood-borne parasites are the plasmodia. Plasmodia are not endemic in the United States, but they do represent a world health problem. In a review of world incidence, over 1,000 cases of posttransfusion malaria were reported since 1950.[255] In the United States the problem became significant during military conflicts in endemic areas. Ten cases were reported in the United States during the 1960s. Another potential source of infected donors is the immigrant arriving to the United States from an endemic area.[255] Cases of posttransfusion malaria were reported in patients receiving blood from veterans of the Vietnam War, 1964–1971.[286]

As shown in a review of 2,000 cases, blood stored at 4°–6° C for up to 2 weeks was infective, but in most cases the blood had been stored at 4°–6° C for less than 5 days.[287] Screening peripheral smears of donors is of little value in preventing the transmission of malaria because negative smears may be present in units contaminated with up to half a million parasites.[288] The indirect fluorescent antibody test, however, is more sensitive and may be of use in screening donors in endemic areas.[286] The difficulty of screening donors with laboratory methods underscores the importance of obtaining a good clinical history during donor screening. Furthermore, freezing and thawing blood will not eliminate infectivity.[289] Following AABB donor screening standards should help exclude potentially infected donors. Asymptomatic travelers who have been to endemic malarial areas (as listed by the Malaria Program, Centers for Disease Control, U.S. Department of Health and Human Services) and who have not taken antimalarial drugs may be accepted as donors 6 months after their return to the United States.[290] Persons who have taken antimalarial drugs must wait 3 years. Immigrants from endemic areas must also wait 3 years before being accepted as blood donors.[290]

In considering whether one should accept donors who have had malaria, it is useful to remember that donors may be asymptomatic.[291] Factors to keep in mind during donor screening are:

1. *Plasmodium falciparum* is usually eliminated in 1 year, but may be harbored in the host for 2–3 years.
2. *Plasmodium vivax* may be found up to 3 years after onset and is responsible for 20% of cases of posttransfusion malaria.[287]
3. *Plasmodium ovale* may be found up to 4 years after onset.
4. *Plasmodium malariae* infection has been reported to relapse 10–46 years after onset. This parasite is responsible for 50% of cases of posttransfusion malaria.[287]

Individuals who have had malaria probably should not be considered for donation of RBCs. Fresh frozen plasma has not been known to transmit malaria.[279] Chloroquine given to donors 2 days before donation has helped to prevent malaria transmission via transfusion in endemic countries.[287] Prophylaxis with chloroquine (600 mg) for the recipient 24 hours before transfusion followed by 300 mg/week for 1 month has also helped in these countries.[287] For more details on screening for donors, see chapter 8.

Treatment of Patients With Posttransfusional Malaria

Most malarial parasitic infections can be treated by giving 1,500 mg of chloroquine over 3 days or amodiaquine base for the same period.[259] For *P. falciparum* infections the treatment is different than for other forms: chloroquine, 640 mg 3 times a day for 10 days, pyrimethamine, 25 mg, 2 times a day for 3 days, and sulfadiazine, 500 mg every 6 hours for 5 days.[259]

Other Parasites Transmitted by Transfusion

Babesiosis is another RBC parasitic infection that can be transmitted by transfusion. The disease is found in the United States and is transmitted by ticks. No chemotherapy is available. Exchange blood transfusions have been attempted in severe cases.[292] Babesiosis tends to have a worse prognosis in splenectomized individuals.[259]

Nonmalarial Parasites Transmitted via Transfusion

Following are descriptions of some infections caused by transfusion of blood or blood components contaminated with nonplasmodial parasites.

Chagas' Disease

Chagas' disease is caused by *Trypanosoma cruzi* and is usually transmitted by a triatoma or "kissing-bug." It is prevalent in Southern Mexico and Central and South America. In certain countries in South America as many as 20% of blood donors have a positive serology for Chagas' disease.[293] As many as 12% of recipients of blood serologically positive for *Trypanosoma cruzi* will develop the disease.[293] The parasite survives well in refrigerated blood and can therefore be transmitted by transfusion. The parasite has remained viable for 3 weeks in units kept at 4°–6° C; however, the blood is considered to be infective the first week after donation.[284] The disease manifests with splenomegaly, lymphadenopathy, and hepatomegaly. A complement fixation test (the Machado-Guerreiro test) is used for diagnosis, but results may be negative in the first months of infection.[294] There is also rapid hemagglutination test suitable for blood banks.[295]

Treatment with Nifurtimox, a nitrofuran, is effective in the acute stages of Chagas' disease, but overall the treatment for Chagas' disease has not been satisfactory.[296] Nifurtimox is highly toxic, mutagenic, and carcinogenic. These aspects should be weighed against the effects of the parasite in chronic cases with cardiomyopathy. It has been shown experimentally that the addition of crystal violet to a unit of blood will kill the parasite but will not affect the RBCs.[297] This method of treatment of the units awaits extensive clinical trials.

African Trypanosomiasis and Kala-azar

Trypanosomiasis and kala-azar are rare in the United States and have never been reported as a result of transfusion. In endemic areas they have been reported as a complication of blood transfusion, but even in endemic areas they are not frequently seen as a complication of transfusion.[298] Only children have been victims of posttransfusional kala-azar and African trypanosomiasis.[299]

Filariasis

Patients with filariasis transmit the filarial stage of the organism. However, the disease, which is caused only by the adult worm stage of the parasite, requires an intermediate insect host for its maturation. Therefore, patients with filariasis may transmit the parasite, converting the recipient into a carrier, but do not develop lymphatic disease.[259] The transfusion recipients of these parasites may harbor them for many years.[300] The filariae remain viable in refrigerated blood for up to 2 weeks.[301] Donors with this type of parasitemia should be excluded because some recipients have developed allergic reactions to the parasite.[302]

Toxoplasmosis

Toxoplasmosis has not been reported as a posttransfusional complication in recipients of blood who are otherwise healthy. However, leukemics who receive multiple transfusions or transfusions of granulocytes and who may be immunocompromised have developed toxoplasmosis after transfusion of infected blood or granulocyte units.[303] One such patient developed fatal toxoplasmosis after granulocyte transfusions.[304]

The disease, which is caused by *Toxoplasma gondii*, may be carried by asymptomatic donors. The parasite remains viable in refrigerated blood up to 50 days.[303] Persons with a positive test for toxoplasmosis should not be accepted as donors of granulocytes.[304] These donors may be screened by an indirect fluorescent antibody test.[305] Encephalitis, pneumonitis, and myocarditis may develop in the recipient. Pyrimethamine, 25 mg/day for 1 month, plus trisulfapyrimadine, 6 gm/day for 1 month, plus folinic acid, 6 mg/day for 1 month, is the treatment of choice for this disease.[306]

INCOMPATIBLE IV FLUIDS

Not infrequently the question of what solutions can be injected into a unit, or what solutions can be run along the same infusion line as blood, arises during the transfusion of a blood unit. Blood bank personnel should be prepared to answer these questions. In essence:

1. No medications are to be injected into a unit (e.g., Benadryl, steroids, etc.).[307]

2. No solutions other than saline should be run along the same line as blood or blood products.

3. Whenever possible, a special line for transfu-

sion of blood and components should be available.

Exceptions to these rules should be made in consultation with the blood bank physician. For instance, if packed cells are to be reconstituted with FFP, this is better done in the blood bank, where aseptic techniques are routinely observed. For all practical purposes, solutions other than sodium chloride injection (USP, 0.9%) must not be used along with RBCs or added to RBCs.[307] To increase the rheology of packed cells which are otherwise running too slowly, back-infusion of about 50 ml of saline into the unit can be employed.[308] Cryoprecipitate can be rinsed from the walls of the cryoprecipitate bags and pooled in a transfer bag by the addition of 20–30 cc of saline. This procedure is usually performed in the blood bank.

As was mentioned above, several commonly used IV solutions are incompatible with blood and have deleterious effects when transfused with blood. Aqueous dextrose (5% dextrose) has been known for a long time to cause hemolysis of RBCs, presenting clinically as hemolytic transfusion reactions.[309] In vitro dextrose solutions of 5%, 10%, and 25% will cause both clumping and hemolysis.[309] The infusion of blood through a set where dextrose 5% in water was infused may cause phlebitis due to hemolysis.[310] Ninety percent of cases of hemoglobinuria reported to a blood bank in a large medical center during 1979 were caused by incompatible solutions.[311] When lactated Ringer's solution is given in combination with blood, clots may form due to recalcification of plasma by the calcium content in the Ringer's solution.[308] This finding has also been demonstrated in vitro. The addition of Ringer's solution to blood causes clumping and clotting.[312]

OTHER COMPLICATIONS OF TRANSFUSION

Other complications of transfusion include hemochromatosis and thrombophlebitis, each of which is described below.

Hemochromatosis

Multiply transfused patients may eventually develop hemochromatosis.[313] Hepatomegaly, skin pigmentation, and diabetes may (rarely) develop from chronic iron overload secondary to transfusion.[314] Patients with hyperplastic bone marrow anemia (e.g., as seen in thalassemia) develop hemochromatosis and liver damage more frequently than those with hypoplastic marrow.[315] Desferrioxamine, an iron chelating agent, has been used as treatment for iron overload in thalassemia with limited success,[316] unless the therapy is given as a constant infusion over long periods of time.[317]

Thrombophlebitis

Venous infusion lasting more than 12 hours tends to produce thrombophlebitis.[318] After 48 hours septic phlebitis may develop.[319] It is therefore a good practice to change infusion sites every 8 hours.[320] Plastics are universally used in infusion sets, for they are less likely to produce phlebitis than rubber.[318]

REPORTABLE CASES IN THE UNITED STATES

Transfusion-associated fatalities in the United States must be reported to the Bureau of Biologics. Cases of infectious hepatitis transmitted via transfusion as well as other serious infections (e.g., brucellosis, *Salmonella* infection, and malaria) should also be reported.[321] All units of blood found to be positive for hepatitis, syphilis, or some other transmissible disease must be reported to the physician of the patient who received such a unit and also to the FDA.[321] Cases of AIDS must likewise be reported to the Bureau of Biologics.

REFERENCES

1. Denis J.: A letter concerning a new way of curing sundry diseases of transfusion of blood. *Philos. Trans. R. Soc. Lond.* [Biol.] 2:489, 1667.
2. Zmijewsky C.M.: *Immunohematology,* ed. 3. New York, Appleton-Century-Crofts, 1978, p. 9.
3. Blundell J.: Successful case of transfusion. *Lancet* 1:431, 1829.
4. Landsteiner K.: Über Agglutinationserscheinungen normalen menschlicher Blutes. *Wien. Klin. Wochenschr.* 14:1132, 1901.
5. Baker R.J., Moinichen S.L., Nyhus L.M.: Transfusion reaction: A reappraisal of surgical incidence and significance. *Ann. Surg.* 169:684, 1969.
6. Taswell H.F., Pineda A.A., Moore S.B.: Hemo-

lytic transfusion reactions: Frequency and clinical laboratory aspects, in Bell C.A., (ed.): *A Seminar on Immune-Mediated Cell Destruction.* Washington, D.C., American Association of Blood Banks, 1981, p. 71.
7. Fairley N.H.: The fate of extracorpuscular circulating haemoglobin. *Br. Med. J.* 2:213, 1940.
8. Honig C.L., Bove J.R.: Transfusion-associated fatalities: Review of Bureau of Biologics Reports 1976–1978. *Tranfusion* 20:653, 1980.
9. Petz L.D., Garraty G.: *Acquired Immune Hemolytic Anemias.* New York, Churchill Livingstone, 1980, pp. 110–138.
10. Mollison P.L.: *Blood Transfusion in Clinical Medicine,* ed. 7. Oxford, England, Blackwell Scientific Publications, 1983, pp. 574–575.
11. Mollison P.L.: *Blood Transfusion in Clinical Medicine,* ed. 7. Oxford, England, Blackwell Scientific Publications, 1983, pp. 627–628.
12. Rouault C.L., et al., quoted by Mollison P.L.: *Blood Transfusion in Clinical Medicine,* ed. 7. Oxford, England, Blackwell Scientific Publications, 1983, p. 534.
13. Borsos T., Rapp H.J.: Hemolysis titration based on fixation of the activated first component of complement: Evidence that one molecule of hemolysin suffices to sensitize an erythrocyte. *J. Immunol.* 95:559, 1965.
14. Augener W., Grey H.M., Cooper N.R., et al.: The reaction of monomeric and aggregated immunoglobulins with C1. *Immunochemistry* 8:1011, 1971.
15. Frank M.M., Dourmaskin R.R., Humphrey J.H.: Observations on the mechanisms of immune hemolysis: Importance of immunoglobulin class and source of complement on the extent of damage. *J. Immunol.* 104:1502, 1970.
16. Hughes-Jones N.C.: Binding of C1q, in Pollack W., et al. (eds.): *An International Symposium on "The Nature and Significance of Complement Activation."* Raritan, N.J., Ortho Research Institute of Medical Sciences, 1976, p. 3.
17. Müller-Eberhard H.J.: Complement. *Annu. Rev. Biochem.* 44:697, 1975.
18. Bhaki S., Tranum-Jensen J.: Molecular nature of the complement lesion. *Proc. Natl. Acad. Sci. USA* 75:5655, 1978.
19. Borsos T., Dourmaskin R.R., Humphrey J.H.: Lesions in erythrocyte membranes caused by immune haemolysis. *Nature* 202:251, 1964.
20. Mayer M.M.: Mechanisms of cytolysis by complement. *Proc. Natl. Acad. Sci. USA* 69:2954, 1972.
21. Abramson N., Gelfand E.W., Jandl J.L., et al.: The interaction between human monocytes and red cells: Specificity of IgG subclasses and IgG fragments. *J. Exp. Med.* 132:1207, 1970.
22. Atkinson J.P., Frank M.M.: Studies on in vivo effects of antibody. *J. Clin. Invest.* 54:339, 1974.
23. Frank M.M.: Mechanism of cell destruction in immunohemolytic anemia, in Bell C.A. (ed.): *A Seminar on Laboratory Management of Hemolysis.* Washington, D.C., American Association of Blood Banks, 1979, pp. 29–43.
24. Cooper R.A.: Loss of membrane components in the pathogenesis of antibody-induced spherocytosis. *J. Clin. Invest.* 51:16, 1972.
·25. Nelson D.S.: *Macrophages and Immunity.* Amsterdam, North Holland, 1969, p. 235.
26. Jandl J.H.: Mechanisms of antibody-induced red cell destruction. *Semin. Hematol.* 9:35, 1965.
27. Hinz C.F. Jr., Chickosky J.F.: Lymphocyte cytotoxicity for human erythrocytes, in Schwarz M.R. (ed.): *Leukocyte Culture Conference.* Seattle, University of Washington, 1972.
28. Mollison P.L.: *Blood Transfusion in Clinical Medicine,* ed. 7. Oxford, England, Blackwell Scientific Publications, 1983, pp. 564–567.
29. Ingram G.I.C.: The bleeding complications of blood tranfusion. *Transfusion* 5:1, 1965.
30. Rabiner S.F., Friedman L.H.: The role of intravascular haemolysis and the reticulo-endothelial system in the production of the hypercoagulable state. *Br. J. Haematol.* 14:105, 1968.
31. Quick A.J.: Influence of erythrocytes on the coagulation of blood. *Am. J. Med. Sci.* 239:101, 1960.
32. Mannucci P.M., Lobina C.F., Caocci L., et al.: Effect on blood coagulation of massive intravascular hemolysis. *Blood* 33:207, 1969.
33. Slaastad R.A., Eika C.: Failure to trigger intravascular coagulation by water induced haemolysis in rabbits. *Scand. J. Haematol.* 11:217, 1973.
34. Newcomp T.F., Gardner F.H.: Thrombin generation in paroxysmal nocturnal hemoglobinuria. *Br. J. Haematol.* 9:84, 1963.
35. Denis L.H., Eichelberger J.W., Inman M.M., et al.: Depletion of coagulation factors in drug-resistant *Plasmodium falciparum* malaria. *Blood* 29:713, 1967.
36. Krevans J.R., Jackson D.P., Conley C.L., et al.: The nature of the hemorrhagic disorder accompanying hemolytic transfusion reactions in man. *Blood* 12:834, 1957.
37. Djaldetti M., Amir J., Shaklai M., et al.: Haemorrhagic diathesis following transfusion of incompatible blood. *Scand. J. Haematol.* 10:197, 1973.
38. Takaki A., Kato S., Takeda H., et al.: The role of disseminated intravascular coagulation in shock induced by transfusion of human blood in dogs. *Transfusion* 19:404, 1979.
39. Robbins J., Stetson C.A., Jr.: An effect of antigen-antibody interaction on blood coagulation. *J. Exp. Med.* 109:1, 1959.
40. Gans H., Lowman J.T.: The uptake of fibrin and fibrin-degradation products by the isolated perfused rat liver. *Blood* 29:526, 1967.
41. Rodriguez-Erdmann F.: Pathogenesis of bilateral renal cortical necrosis: Its production by means of exogenous fibrin. *Arch. Pathol.* 79:615, 1965.
42. Hardaway R.M., McKay D.G., Wahle G.H. Jr., et al.: Pathologic study of intravascular coagulation

following incompatible blood transfusion in dogs: I. Intravenous injection of incompatible blood. *Am. J. Surg.* 91:24, 1956.
43. Wahle G.H. Jr., Muirhead E.E.: Bilateral renal cortical necrosis in a child, associated with an incompatible blood transfusion. *Texas Med. J.* 49:770, 1953.
44. Bluemle L.W. Jr., Webster G.D. Jr., Elkington J.R.: Acute tubular necrosis: Analysis of one hundred cases with respect to mortality, complications and treatment with and without dialysis. *Arch. Intern. Med.* 104:180, 1959.
45. Goldfinger D.: Complications of hemolytic transfusion reactions: Pathogenesis and therapy, in Dawson R.B. (ed.): *New Approaches to Transfusion Reactions: A Technical Workshop.* Washington, D.C., American Association of Blood Banks, 1974.
46. Rabiner S.F., Helbert J.R., Lopas H., et al.: Evaluation of a stroma-free hemoglobin solution for use as a plasma expander. *J. Exp. Med.* 126:1127, 1967.
47. Relihan M., Litwin M.S.: Effects of stroma-free hemoglobin solution on clearance rate and renal function. *Surgery* 71:395, 1972.
48. Palani C.K., DeWoskin E., Moss J.S.: Scope and limitations of stroma-free hemoglobin solution as an oxygen-carrying blood substitute. *Surg. Clin. North Am.* 55:3, 1975.
49. Gerrits W.B.J.: Fibrinogen and its derivatives in intravascular coagulation. *Neth. J. Med.* 18:31, 1975.
50. Rapaport S.I., Tatter D., Coeur-Barron N., et al.: *Pseudomonas* septicemia with intravascular clotting leading to the generalized Shwartzman reaction. *N. Engl. J. Med.* 271:80, 1964.
51. Young L.E., Platzer R.F., Yuile C.L., et al.: Recovery of group O recipient after transfusion of two liters of group A blood. *Am. J. Clin. Pathol.* 17:777, 1947.
52. Huestis D.W., Bove J.R., Busch S.: *Practical Blood Transfusion,* ed. 3. Boston, Little, Brown & Co., 1981, pp. 265–267.
53. Widman F.K. (ed.): *Technical Manual,* ed. 8. Washington, D.C., American Association of Blood Banks, 1981, p. 305.
54. Deykin D.: The clinical challenge of disseminated intravascular coagulation. *N. Engl. J. Med.* 283:636, 1970.
55. Mollison P.L.: *Blood Transfusion in Clinical Medicine,* ed. 7. Oxford, England, Blackwell Scientific Publications, 1983, p. 630.
56. Moore S.B., Taswell H.F., Pineda A.A., et al.: Delayed hemolytic transfusion reactions: Evidence of the need for an improved pretransfusion compatibility test. *Am. J. Clin. Pathol.* 74:94, 1980.
57. Mayer K.: A different view of transfusion safety: Type and screen, transfusion of Coombs incompatible cells, fatal transfusion-induced graft versus host disease, in Polesky H.F., Walker R.H. (eds.): *Safety in Transfusion Practices.* Skokie, Ill., American College of Pathologists, 1982.
58. Gelabert A., quoted by Mollison P.L.: *Blood Transfusion in Clinical Medicine,* ed. 7. Oxford, England, Blackwell Scientific Publications, 1983, p. 651.
59. Goldfinger D.: Acute hemolytic transfusion reactions: A fresh look at pathogenesis and considerations regarding therapy. *Transfusion* 17:85, 1977.
60. Kaplan A.P., Gigli I., Austen K.F.: Immunologic activation of Hageman factor and its relationship to fibrinolysis, bradykinin generation and complement. *J. Clin. Invest.* 50:51a, 1971.
61. Emmanouel D.S., Katz A.I.: Acute renal failure in obstetric septic shock: Current views on pathogenesis and management. *Am. J. Obstet. Gynecol.* 117:145, 1973.
62. Greenwalt T.J.: Pathogenesis and management of hemolytic transfusion reactions. *Semin. Hematol.* 18:84, 1981.
63. Rock R.C., Bove J.R., Nemerson Y.: Heparin treatment of intravascular coagulation accompanying hemolytic transfusion reactions. *Transfusion* 9:57, 1969.
64. Shumacker H.B. Jr., et al.: Osmotic diuresis and experimental renal ischemia. *Surgery* 55:687, 1964.
65. Atik B., Manale B., Pearson J.: Prevention of acute renal failure: Hemodynamic observations of transfusion reactions. *JAMA* 183:455, 1963.
66. Hook H.B., Blatt A.H., Brody M.J., et al.: Effects of several saluretic-diuretic agents on renal hemodynamics. *J. Pharmacol. Exp. Ther.* 154:667, 1966.
67. Ludens J.H., Heitz D.C., Brody M.J., et al.: Differential effect of furosemide on renal and limb blood flows in the conscious dog. *J. Pharmacol Exp. Ther.* 171:300, 1970.
68. Muller-Berghaus G., Davidson E., McKay D.G.: Prevention of the generalized Shwartzman reaction in pregnant rats by alpha-adrenergic blockade: Effects on the coagulation mechanism. *Obstet. Gynecol.* 30:774, 1967.
69. Pineda A.A., Brzica S.M. Jr., Taswell H.F.: Hemolytic transfusion reaction: Recent experience in a large blood bank. *Mayo Clin. Proc.* 53:378, 1978.
70. Patten E., Reddi C.R., Riglin H., Edwards J.: Delayed hemolytic transfusion reaction caused by a primary immune response. *Transfusion* 22:248, 1982.
71. Mollison P.L.: *Blood Transfusion in Clinical Medicine,* ed. 7. Oxford, England, Blackwell Scientific Publications, 1983, pp. 661–662.
72. Meltz D.J., David D.S., Bertles J.F., et al.: Delayed haemolytic transfusion reaction with renal failure. *Lancet* 1:1348, 1971.
73. Chaplin H. Jr.: The implication of red cell-bound complement in delayed hemolytic reactions (editorial). *Transfusion* 24:185, 1984.
74. Salama A., Mueller-Eckhart C.: Delayed hemolytic transfusion reactions: Evidence for complement activation involving allogeneic and autologous red cells. *Transfusion* 24:188, 1984.
75. Howard P.L.: Delayed hemolytic transfusion reactions. *Ann. Clin. Lab. Sci.* 3:13, 1973.

76. Widman F.K. (ed.): *Technical Manual of the American Association of Blood Banks*, ed. 8. Washington, D.C., American Association of Blood Banks, 1981, pp. 155–156.
77. Alperin J.B., Riglin H., Branch D.R., et al.: Anti-M causing delayed hemolytic transfusion reaction. *Transfusion* 23:322, 1983.
78. Chandeysson P.L., Flye M., Simpkins S.M., et al.: Delayed hemolytic transfusion reaction caused by anti-P_1 antibody. *Transfusion* 21:77, 1981.
79. Taddie S.J., Barrasso C., Ness P.M.: A delayed transfusion reaction caused by anti-K6. *Transfusion* 22:68, 1982.
80. Yasmeen D., Ellerson J.R., Dorrington K.J., et al.: Evidence for the domain hypothesis: Location of the site of cytophilic activity toward guinea pig macrophages in the CH_3 homology region of human immunoglobulin G. *J. Immunol.* 110:1706, 1973.
81. Brown D.L., Nelson D.A.: Surface microfragmentation of red cells as a mechanism for complement-mediated immune spherocytosis. *Br. J. Haematol.* 24:301, 1973.
82. Mohandas N., de Boisfleury A.: Antibody-induced spherocytic anemia: I. Changes in red cell deformity. *Blood Cells* 3:187, 1977.
83. Boyland I.P., Mufti G.J., Hamblin T.J.: Delayed hemolytic transfusion reaction caused by anti-Fy^b in a splenectomized patient (letter). *Transfusion* 22:402, 1982.
84. Zymmerman H.J.: Evaluation of the function and integrity of the liver, in Henry J.B. (ed.): *Clinical Diagnosis and Management by Laboratory Methods*, ed. 16. Philadelphia, W.B. Saunders Co., 1979, p. 305.
85. Mollison P.L.: *Blood Transfusion in Clinical Medicine*, ed. 7. Oxford, England, Blackwell Scientific Publications, 1983, pp. 653–654.
86. Jandl J.H., Kaplan M.E.: The destruction of red cells by antibodies in man: III. Quantitative factors influencing the patterns of hemolysis in vivo. *J. Clin. Invest.* 39:1145, 1960.
87. Chaplin H. Jr., Crawford H., Cutbush M., et al.: The preservation of red cells at $-79°$ C. *Clin. Sci.* 15:27, 1956.
88. Mollison P.L.: *Blood Transfusion in Clinical Medicine*, ed. 7. Oxford, England, Blackwell Scientific Publications, 1983, p. 613.
89. Aubert E.F., Boorman K.E., Dodd B.E., et al.: The universal donor with high titer iso-agglutinins: The effect of anti-A iso-agglutinins on recipients of group A. *Br. Med. J.* 1:659, 1942.
90. Ervin D.M., Young L.E.: Dangerous universal donors: I. Observations on destruction of recipients of A cells after transfusion of group O blood containing high titer of A antibodies of immune type not easily neutralizable by soluble A substance. *Blood* 5:61, 1950.
91. Grove-Rasmussen M., Shaw R.S., Marceau E.: Hemolytic transfusion reaction in a group A patient receiving group O blood containing immune anti-A antibodies in high titer. *Am. J. Clin. Pathol.* 23:838, 1953.
92. Delmas-Marsalet Y., Parquet-Gernez A., Bauters F., et al.: Anémies hemolytiques dues à la plasmathérapie chez les hémophiles. *Rev. Fr. Transfus.* 12:351, 1969.
93. Tamagnini G.P., Dormandy K.M., Ellis D., et al.: Factor VIII concentrate on haemophilia (letter). *Lancet* 2:188, 1975.
94. Conway L.T., Scott E.P.: Acute hemolytic transfusion reaction due to ABO incompatible plasma in a platelet apheresis concentrate. *Transfusion* 24:413, 1984.
95. Zettner A., Bove J.R.: Hemolytic transfusion reaction due to interdonor incompatibility. *Transfusion* 3:48, 1963.
96. Judd W.J., Oberman H., Flynn S.: Fatal intravascular hemolysis associated with T-polyagglutination (letter). *Transfusion* 22:345, 1982.
97. Dameshek W.: Paroxysmal nocturnal hemoglobinuria: A "candidate" myeloproliferative disorder? *Blood* 33:263, 1969.
98. Rosse W.F., Dacie J.V.: Immune hemolysis of normal human and paroxysmal nocturnal hemoglobinuria (PNH) red blood cells: I. The sensitivity of PNH red cells to lysis by complement and specific antibody. *J. Clin. Invest.* 45:736, 1966.
99. Metz J., Bradlow B.A., Lewis S.M., et al.: The acetyl cholinesterase activity of the erythrocytes in paroxysmal nocturnal hemoglobinuria in relation to the severity of the disease. *Br. J. Haematol.* 6:372, 1960.
100. Ross J.F.: Hemoglobinemia and hemoglobinurias. *N. Engl. J. Med.* 233:732, 1945.
101. Dacie J.V., Richardson N.: The influence of pH on in vitro haemolysis in nocturnal haemoglobinuria. *J. Pathol.* 55:375, 1943.
102. Crosby W.H., Stefanini M.: Pathogenesis of the plasma transfusion reaction with especial reference to the blood coagulation system. *J. Lab. Clin. Med.* 40:374, 1952.
103. Sirchia G., Ferrone S., Mercuriali F.: Leukocyte antigen-antibody reaction and lysis of paroxysmal nocturnal hemoglobinuria erythrocytes. *Blood* 36:334, 1970.
104. Orlina A.R., Josephson A.M., McDonald B.J.: The poststorage viability of glucose-6-phosphate dehydrogenase deficient erythrocytes. *J. Lab. Clin. Med.* 75:930, 1970.
105. Meryman H.T., Hornblower M.: Freezing and deglycerolizing sickle trait red blood cells. *Transfusion* 16:627, 1976.
106. Veiga S., Vaithianathan T.: Massive intravascular sickling after exchange transfusion with sickle cell trait blood. *Transfusion* 3:387, 1963.
107. DeCesare W.R., Bove J.R., Ebaugh F.G. Jr.: The mechanism of the effect of iso- and hyperosmolar dextrose-saline solutions on in-vivo survival of human erythrocytes. *Transfusion* 4:237, 1964.
108. Mollison P.L.: *Blood Transfusion in Clinical Medicine*,

ed. 7. Oxford, England, Blackwell Scientific Publications, 1983, p. 640.
109. Karle H.: Destruction of erythrocytes during experimental fever: Quantitative aspects. *Br. J. Haematol.* 16:409, 1964.
110. Wallace H.W., Blakemore W.S.: Intravascular and extravascular hemolysis accompanying extracorporeal circulation. *Circulation* 42:521, 1970.
111. Ahrons S., Kissmeyer-Nielsen F.: Serological investigations of 1,358 transfusion reactions in 74,000 transfusions. *Dan. Med. Bull.* 15:257, 1968.
112. Barton J.C.: Nonhemolytic noninfectious transfusion reactions. *Semin. Hematol.* 18:95, 1981.
113. Decary F., Ferver P., Gianedoni L., et al.: An investigation of nonhemolytic transfusion reactions. *Vox Sang.* 46:277, 1984.
114. Payne R.: The association of febrile transfusion reactions with leuko-agglutinins. *Vox Sang.* 2:233, 1957.
115. Greenwalt T.J., Gajewski M., McKenna J.L.: A new method for preparing Buffy coat-poor blood. *Transfusion* 2:221, 1962.
116. Grumet F.C., Yankee R.A.: Non-red cell reactions, in Dawson R.B. (ed.): *New Approaches to Transfusion Reactions: A Technical Workshop*. Washington D.C., American Association of Blood Banks, 1974, p. 39.
117. Heinrich D., Mueller-Eckhardt C., Stier W.: The specificity of leukocyte and platelet alloantibodies in sera of patients with non-hemolytic transfusion reactions: Absorption and elution studies. *Vox Sang.* 25:442, 1973.
118. Leverenz S., Ihle R., Frick G.: HL-A system und Transfusionreaktionen: 2. Mitteilung. *Dtsch. Ges. Wesen.* 30:1688, 1975.
119. Curlone E.S., Scudiller G., Mattrusz P.L., et al.: Anti-HLA antibody evolution in recipients of planned transfusions. *Tissue Antigens* 2:415, 1972.
120. Leverenz S., Ihle R., Frick G.: HL-A-System und Transfusionreaktionen: 1. Mitteilung. *Dtsch. Ges. Wesen.* 29:1546, 1974.
121. Gleichmann H., Breininger J.: Over 95% sensitization against allogeneic leukocytes following single massive blood transfusion. *Vox Sang.* 28:66, 1975.
122. Collins Z.V., Arnold P.F., Peetoom F., et al.: A naturally occurring monospecific anti-HL-Ag isoantibody. *Tissue Antigens* 3:358, 1973.
123. Rodey E.G., Kunicki J., Anderson J., et al.: Procurement and identification of HL-A lymphocytotoxic antibodies in sera of non-pregnant multiparous blood donors. *Transfusion* 14:167, 1974.
124. Goodman H.S., Masiatis L.: Analysis of the isoimmune response to leukocytes: I. Maternal cytotoxic leukocytes isoantibodies formed during the first pregnancy. *Vox Sang.* 16:97, 1967.
125. Zmijewski C.M.: *Immunohematology,* ed. 3. New York, Appleton-Century-Crofts, 1978, pp. 243–297.
126. Perkins H.A., Payne R., Ferguson J., et al.: Nonhemolytic febrile transfusion reactions: Quantitative effects of blood components with emphasis on isoantigenic incompatibility of leukocytes. *Vox Sang.* 11:578, 1966.
127. Walford R.L., Gallagher R., Sjaarda J.R.: Serologic typing of human lymphocytes with immune serum obtained after homografting. *Science* 144:868, 1964.
128. Brittingham T.E.: Immunologic studies on leukocytes. *Vox Sang.* 2:242, 1957.
129. Brittingham T.E., Chaplin H.: Febrile transfusion reactions caused by sensitivity to donor leukocytes and platelets. *JAMA* 165:819, 1957.
130. Mollison P.L.: *Blood Transfusion in Clinical Medicine,* ed. 7. Oxford, England, Blackwell Scientific Publications, 1983, pp. 733–734.
131. Ungerlieder R.S., Applebaum F.R., Trapani R.J., et al.: Lack of predictive value of anti-leukocyte antibody screening in granulocyte transfusion therapy. *Transfusion* 19:90, 1979.
132. Walker R.H., quoted by Mollison P.L.: *Blood Transfusion in Clinical Medicine,* ed. 7. Oxford, England, Blackwell Scientific Publications, 1977, p. 627.
133. Wenz B.: Microaggregate blood filtration and the febrile transfusion reaction: A comparative study. *Transfusion* 23:95, 1983.
134. Goldfinger D., Lowe C.: Prevention of adverse reactions to blood transfusion by the administration of saline washed red blood cells. *Transfusion* 21:277, 1981.
135. Westphal R.: Washed RBC to prevent transfusion reactions (letter). *Transfusion* 22:82, 1982.
136. Meryman H.T., Hornblower M.: A method for freezing and washing red blood cells using a high glycerol concentration. *Transfusion* 12:145, 1972.
137. Jandl J.H., Tomlinson A.S.: The destruction of red cells by antibodies in man: II. Pyrogenic, leukocytic and dermal responses to immune hemolysis. *J. Clin. Invest.* 37:1202: 1958.
138. Hobsley M.: Chlorfeniramine maleate in prophylaxis of pyrexial reactions during blood transfusions. *Lancet* 1:497, 1958.
139. Ward H.N.: Pulmonary infiltrates associated with leukoagglutinin transfusion reactions. *Ann. Intern. Med.* 73:689, 1970.
140. Kernoff P.B.A., Durrant I.J., Rigga C.R., et al.: Severe allergic pulmonary oedema after plasma transfusion. *Br. J. Haematol.* 23:777, 1972.
141. Chaplin H., quoted by Mollison P.L.: *Blood Transfusion in Clinical Medicine,* ed. 7. Oxford, England, Blackwell Scientific Publications, 1983, p. 744.
142. Greenwalt T.J., Perry S.: Preservation and utilization of the components of blood, in Brown E.B., Moore C.V. (eds.): *Progress in Hematology*. New York, Grune & Stratton, 1969, pp. 148–180.
143. Graw R.G. Jr., Buchner C.D., Whang-Peng J.: Complications of bone marrow transplantation graft versus host disease resulting from chronic myelogenous leukaemia leukocyte transfusions. *Lancet* 2:338, 1970.
144. Reinherz E.L., Parkman R., Rapaport J., et al.:

Aberrations of suppressor T cells in human graft versus host disease. *N. Engl. J. Med.* 300:1061, 1979.
145. Hirsch E.O., Gardner F.H.: The transfusion of human blood platelets. *J. Lab. Clin. Med.* 39:556, 1952.
146. Yankee R.A., Grumet F.C., Rogentine G.N.: Platelet transfusion therapy: The selection of compatible platelet donors for refractory patients by lymphocyte HL-A typing. *N. Engl. J. Med.* 281:1208, 1969.
147. Duquesnoy R.J., Filip D.J., Aster R.H.: Influence of HLA-A$_2$ on the effectiveness of platelet transfusions in alloimmunized thrombocytopenic patients. *Blood* 50:407, 1977.
148. Herzig R.H., Herzig G.P., Bull M.I., et al.: Correction of poor platelet transfusion responses with leukocyte-poor HL-A-matched platelet concentrates. *Blood* 46:743, 1975.
149. Gockerman J.P., Bowman R.P., Conrad M.E.: Detection of platelet isoantibodies by ^{3}H serotonin platelet release and its clinical application to the problem of platelet maching. *J. Clin. Invest.* 55:75, 1975.
150. Shulman N.R., Aster R.H., Leitner A., et al.: Platelet and leukocyte isoantigens and their antibodies: Serologic, physiological and clinical studies, in Brown E.B., Moore C.V. (eds.): *Progress in Hematology*. New York, Grune & Stratton, 1964, pp. 222–304.
151. Ziegler Z., Murphy S., Gardner F.H.: Post-transfusion purpura: A heterogeneous syndrome. *Blood* 45:529, 1975.
152. Mollison P.L.: *Blood Transfusion in Clinical Medicine*, ed. 7. Oxford, England, Blackwell Scientific Publications, 1983, p. 636.
153. Stephen C.R., Martin R.C., Bourgeois-Gavardin M.: Antihistaminic drugs in treatment of nonhemolytic transfusion reactions. *JAMA* 158:525, 1955.
154. Leikola J., Koistinen J., Lehtinen M., et al.: IgA-induced anaphylactic transfusion reactions: A report of four cases. *Blood* 42:111, 1973.
155. Homburger H.A.: Measurement of anti-IgA antibodies by a two-site immunoradiometric assay. *Transfusion* 21:38, 1981.
156. Van Loghem E., De Lange G., Koistinen J.: The first isoallotype of human IgA proteins. *Scand. J. Immunol.* 5:11, 1976.
157. Osterland C.K., Harboe M., Kunkel H.G.: Anti-gamma-globulin factors in human sera revealed by enzymatic splitting of anti-Rh antibodies. *Vox Sang.* 8:133, 1963.
158. World Health Organization: Review of the notation for the allotypic and related markers of human immunoglobulins: Amended report of WHO meeting, 1974. *J. Immunol.* 117:1056, 1976.
159. Natvig J.B., Kunkel H.G.: Human immunoglobulins: Classes, subclasses, genetic variants and idiotypes. *Adv. Immunol.* 16:1, 1973.
160. Schanfield M.S.: Genetic markers of immunoglobulins, in Fundenberg H.H., et al. (eds.): *Basic and Clinical Immunology*. Los Altos, Calif., Lange Medical Publications, 1978, pp. 59–65.
161. Grubb R.: *The Genetic Markers of Human Immunoglobulins*. New York, Springer-Verlag, 1970, p. 11.
162. Fudenberg H.H., Fudenberg B.R.: Antibody to hereditary human gamma-globulin (Gm) factor resulting from maternal-fetal incompatibility. *Science* 145:170, 1964.
163. Sell S.: *Immunology, Immunopathology and Immunity*, ed. 3. New York, Harper & Row, 1980, p. 266.
164. Allen J.C., Kunkel H.G.: Antibodies to genetic types of gamma-globulin after multiple transfusions. *Science* 139:418, 1963.
165. Auerswald V.W., Bodis-Wollner I., Kiesewetter E., et al.: Zur Frage der Antikorperbildung erwachsener gegen Gm nach wiederholter parenteraler Zufuhr von homologem Gammaglobulin. *Wien. Med. Wochenschr.* 117:1006, 1967.
166. Grubb R.: *The Genetic Markers of Human Immunoglobulins*. New York, Springer-Verlag, 1970, p. 42.
167. Milgrom F., Dubiski S., Wozniczko G.: Human sera with "anti-antibody." *Vox Sang.* 1:172, 1956.
168. Barton J.C.: Nonhemolytic, noninfectious transfusion reactions, in Conrad M.E. (ed.): *Transfusion Problems in Hematology*. *Semin. Hematol.* 18:101, 1981.
169. Medical Research Council: Hypogammaglobulinemia in the United Kingdom: Report of a Medical Research Working Party. *Lancet* 1:163, 1969.
170. Caldera L.H., Ropars C., Griscelli C., et al.: Anticorps anti-immunoglobulines chez les sujets atteints de déficit immunitaire: Intérêt dans les réactions d'intolérance aux injections thérapeutiques de gammaglobulines. *Rev. Fr. Transfus.* 16:393, 1973.
171. Benacerraf B., McDevitt H.O.: Histocompatibility-linked immune response genes. *Science* 175:273, 1972.
172. Levine B., Stember R., Fotino M.: Ragweed hay fever: Genetic control and linkage to HL-A haplotypes. *Science* 178:1201, 1972.
173. Avoy D.R.: Delayed serum sickness-like transfusion reactions in a multiply transfused patient. *Vox Sang.* 41:239, 1981.
174. Kelly J.F., Patterson R.: Anaphylaxis: Course, mechanisms and treatment. *JAMA* 227:1431, 1974.
175. Mowbray J.F., quoted by Mollison P.L.: *Blood Transfusion in Clinical Medicine*, ed. 7. Oxford, England, Blackwell Scientific Publications, 1983, pp. 727–728.
176. Barandun S., Kistler P., Jeunet F., et al.: Intravenous injection of human gamma-globulin. *Vox Sang.* 7:157, 1962.
177. Malgras J., Hauptmann G., Zorn J.J., et al.: Mesure del'activité anticomplémentaire des préparations de gamma-globulines injectables par voie intra-veineuse. *Rev. Fr. Transfus.* 13:173, 1970.
178. Vyas G.N., Holmdahl L., Perkins H.A., et al.: Serological specificity of human anti-IgA and its significance in transfusion. *Blood* 34:573, 1969.

179. Koistinen J.: Selective IgA deficiency in blood donors. *Vox Sang.* 29:192, 1975.
180. Vyas G.N., Perkins H.A., Yang Y.M., et al.: Healthy blood donors with selective absence of immunoglobulin A: Prevention of anaphylactic transfusion reactions caused by antibodies to IgA. *J. Lab. Clin. Med.* 85:838, 1975.
181. Vyas G.N., Levin A.S., Fudenberg H.H.: Intrauterine isoimmunization caused by maternal IgA crossing the placenta. *Nature* 225:275, 1970.
182. Bachman R.: Studies on the serum IgA level: III. The frequency of IgA globulinemia. *Scand. J. Clin. Lab. Invest.* 17:316, 1965.
183. Schmidt A.P., Taswell F., Gleich G.J.: Anaphylactic transfusion reactions associated with anti-IgA antibody. *N. Engl. J. Med.* 280:188, 1969.
184. Ropars L., Gerbal A., Poncey C., et al.: Accident transfusionnel de type anaphylactique en rapport avec un anticorps anti-IgA. *Rev. Fr. Transfus.* 14:401, 1971.
185. Vyas G.N., Perkins H.A.: Anti-IgA in blood donors, letter. *Transfusion* 16:289, 1976.
186. Vyas G.N., Perkins H.A., Fudenberg H.H.: Anaphylactoid transfusion reactions associated with anti-IgA. *Lancet* 2:312, 1968.
187. Rivat L., Rivat C., Parent P., et al.: Accident sourvenu après injection de gammaglobulines anti-Rh dû à la présence d'anticorps anti-gamma-A. *Presse Med.* 78:2072, 1970.
188. Grumet F.C., Yankee R.A.: Non-red cell reactions, in *New Approaches to Transfusion Reactions*. Washington, D.C., American Association of Blood Banks, 1974, p. 43.
189. Vos G.H., Downing H.J., Vos D.: The incidence of antibodies to leukocytes and gammaglobulin IgG and IgA in a population of multitransfused Southern African Negroes. *Transfusion* 13:437, 1973.
190. Mollison P.L.: *Blood Transfusion in Clinical Medicine*, ed. 7. Oxford, England, Blackwell Scientific Publications, 1983, p. 741.
191. Lieberman R., Humphrey W.: Association of H-2 types with genetic control of immune responsiveness to IgA allotypes in mice. *Proc. Natl. Acad. Sci. USA* 68:2510, 1971.
192. Koistinen J., Leikola J.: Weak anti-IgA antibodies with limited specificity and non-hemolytic transfusion reactions. *Vox Sang.* 32:77, 1977.
193. Widman F.K. (ed.): *Technical Manual*, ed. 8. Washington, D.C., American Association of Blood Banks, 1981, p. 43.
194. Leikola J., Fudenberg H.H., Vyas G.N., et al.: Isoantibodies to IgM: Serologic and immunochemical investigations. *J. Immunol.* 106:1147, 1971.
195. Wells J.V., Bleumers J.F., Fudenberg H.H.: Immunobiology of human anti-IgM iso-antibodies: I. Clinical and serological studies. *Clin. Immunol. Immunopathol.* I:257, 1973.
196. Ropars C., Whylie S., Cartron J., et al.: Anticorps chez les polytransfusés dirigés contre certains immunoglobulins IgM. *Nouv. Rev. Fr. Hematol.* 13:459, 1973.
197. Mollison P.L.: *Blood Transfusion in Clinical Medicine*, ed. 6. Oxford, England, Blackwell Scientific Publications, 1979, p. 615.
198. Berg T.L.O., Johansson S.G.O.: IgE concentration in children with atopic diseases. *Int. Arch. Allergy Appl. Immunol.* 36:219, 1969.
199. Frick O.L.: Immediate hypersensitivity, in Fudenberg H.H., et al. (eds.): *Basic and Clinical Immunology*. Los Altos, Calif., Lange Medical Publications, 1978, pp. 246–266.
200. Cartron J.P., Ropars C., Salmon C., et al.: Teneurs en IgE des sérums des malades polytransfusés. *Rev. Fr. Transfus.* 16:385, 1973.
201. Maunsell K.: Urticarial reactions and desensitization in allergic recipients after serum transfusions. *Br. Med. J.* 2:236, 1944.
202. Ramirez M.A.: Horse asthma following blood transfusion: Report of a case. *JAMA* 73:984, 1919.
203. Hirschfeld J.: The Ag system: Present concepts and immunogenetic models, in Peeters H. (ed.): *Protides of the Biologic Fluids*. Oxford, England, Pergamon Press, 1972, pp. 156–160.
204. Levene C., Blumberg B.S., Vierucci A., et al.: Incidence of antibodies against beta-lipoproteins (Ag system) and the factors influencing isoimmunization in transfused patients in the USA and Italy. *Lancet* 2:582, 1967.
205. Vierucci A., Blumberg B.S., Dettori M., et al.: Isoantibodies to inherited types of beta-lipoproteins (Ag) and immunoglobulins (Gm and Inv). *J. Pediatr.* 72:776, 1968.
206. Huestis D.W., Bove J.R., Busch S.: *Practical Blood Transfusion*, ed. 3. Boston, Little, Brown & Co., 1981, pp. 260–261.
207. Boyan C.P., Howland W.S.: Cardiac arrest and temperature of bank blood. *JAMA* 183:58, 1963.
208. Boyan C.P.: Cold or warmed blood for massive transfusions. *Ann. Surg.* 160:282, 1964.
209. Dybkjaer E., Elkjaer P.: The use of heated blood in massive blood replacement. *Acta Anesthesiol. Scand.* 8:271, 1964.
210. Sheldon G.F.: Hemotherapy in a trauma center, in Barns A. Jr. (ed.): *Hemotherapy in Trauma and Surgery: A Technical Workshop*. Washington, D.C., American Association of Blood Banks, 1979, pp. 17–28.
211. Dalili H., Adriani J.: Effects of various blood warmers on the components of bank blood. *Anesth. Analg.* 53:125, 1974.
212. DeGowin E.L., Hardin R.L., Swanson L.W.: Studies on preserved human blood: IV. Transfusion of cold blood into man. *JAMA* 114:859, 1940.
213. Sharpey-Schafer E.P., Wallace J.: Circulatory overloading following rapid intravenous injections. *Lancet* 2:304, 1942.
214. Mollison P.L.: The survival of transfused erythrocytes, with special references to cases of acquired haemolytic anaemia. *Clin. Sci.* 6:137, 1947.
215. Mollison P.L.: *Blood Transfusion in Clinical Medicine*, ed. 7. Oxford, England, Blackwell Scientific Publications, 1983, p. 127.

216. Sharpey-Schafer E.P.: Transfusion and the anaemic heart. *Lancet* 2:296, 1945.
217. Schwartz S.I.: Hemostasis, surgical bleeding and transfusion, in Schwartz S.I., et al. (eds.): *Principles of Surgery*, ed. 3. New York, McGraw-Hill Book Co., 1979, pp. 99–132.
218. Salant W., Wise L.E.: The action of sodium citrate and its decomposition in the body. *J. Biol. Chem.* 28:27, 1916.
219. Collins J.A.: Massive transfusion: What is current and important? in Nusbacher J. (ed.): *Massive Transfusion: A Symposium*. Washington, D.C., American Association of Blood Banks, 1978, pp. 1–16.
220. Smith N.T., Corbascio A.N.: The interaction of potassium and calcium on the isolated guinea pig atrium. *Fed. Proc.* 23:326, 1964.
221. Bunker J.P., Stetson J.B., Coe R.C., et al.: Citric acid intoxication. *JAMA* 157:1361, 1955.
222. Adams W.E., Thornton T.F., Allen J.G., et al.: Danger and prevention of citrate intoxication in massive transfusions of whole blood. *Ann. Surg.* 120:656, 1944.
223. Nakasone N., Watkins E. Jr., Janeway C.A., et al.: Experimental studies of circulatory derangement following the massive transfusion of citrated blood: Comparison of blood treated with ACD solution and blood decalcified by ion exchange resin. *J. Lab. Clin. Med.* 43:184, 1954.
224. Wexler I.B., Pincus J.B., Matelson S., et al.: The fate of citrate in erythroblastic infants treated with exchange transfusion. *J. Clin. Invest.* 28:474, 1949.
225. Furman R.A.: ECG changes occurring during the course of replacement transfusions. *J. Pediatr.* 38:45, 1951.
226. Wolf P.L., McCarthy L.J., Hafleigh B.: Extreme hypercalcemia following blood transfusion combined with intravenous calcium. *Vox Sang.* 19:544, 1970.
227. Howland W.S.: Calcium, potassium and pH changes during massive transfusion, in Nusbacher J. (ed.): *Massive Transfusion: A Symposium*. Washington, D.C., American Association of Blood Banks, 1978, pp. 17–24.
228. Nahas G.G., Manger W.M., Wittelman A., et al.: Étude experimentale de l'acidose transfusionelle. *Nouv. Rev. Fr. Hématol.* 2:182, 1962.
229. Howland W.S., Schweizer O., Boyan C.P.: The effect of buffering on the mortality of massive blood replacement. *Surg. Gynecol. Obstet.* 121:777, 1965.
230. Simon G.E., Bove J.R.: The potassium load from blood transfusion. *Postgrad. Med.* 49:61, 1971.
231. Miller G., McCoord A.B., Joos H.A., et al.: Studies of serum electrolyte changes during exchange transfusion. *Pediatrics* 13:412, 1954.
232. Moore F.D. (1955), quoted by Mollison P.L.: *Blood Transfusion in Clinical Medicine*, ed. 7. Oxford, England, Blackwell Scientific Publications, 1983, pp. 752–754.
233. Taylor W.C., Gillis C.N., Nash C.W., et al.: Experimental observations on cardiac arrhythmia during exchange transfusion in rabbits. *J. Pediatr.* 58:470, 1961.
234. Spear P.W., Sass M., Cincotti J.J.: Ammonia levels in transfused blood. *J. Lab. Clin. Med.* 48:702, 1956.
235. Mollison P.L.: *Blood Transfusion in Clinical Medicine*, ed. 7. Oxford, England, Blackwell Scientific Publications, 1983, pp. 754–755.
236. Durant T.M., Oppenheimer M.J., Lynch P.R., et al.: Body position in relation to venous air embolism: A roentgenologic study. *Am. J. Med. Sci.* 227:509, 1954.
237. Swank R.L.: Alteration of blood on storage: Measurement of adhesiveness of "aging" platelets and leucocytes and their removal by filtration. *N. Engl. J. Med.* 265:728, 1961.
238. McNamara J.J., Burran E.L., Larson E., et al.: Effect of debris in stored blood on pulmonary microvasculature. *Ann. Thorac. Surg.* 14:133, 1972.
239. Reul G.J. Jr., Beall A.C., Greenberg S.D.: Protection of the pulmonary microvasculature by fine screen blood filtration. *Chest* 66:4, 1974.
240. Tobey R.E., Kopriva C.J., Homer L.D., et al.: Pulmonary gas exchange following hemorrhagic shock and massive transfusion in the babboon. *Ann. Surg.* 179:316, 1974.
241. Brendenburg C.E., in *International Forum: Does a Relationship Exist Between Massive Blood Transfusions and the Adult Respiratory Distress Syndrome? Vox Sang.* 32:311, 1977.
242. Geelhoed G.W., Bennett S.H.: "Shock lung" resulting from perfusion of canine lungs with stored bank blood. *Am. Surg.* 41:67, 1975.
243. Collins J.A.: Massive transfusion: What is current and important? in *Massive Transfusion 1978*. Washington, D.C., American Association of Blood Banks, 1978, p. 2.
244. Solis R.T., Walker B.D., in *International Forum: Does a Relationship Exist Between Massive Blood Transfusions and the Adult Respiratory Distress Syndrome? Vox Sang.* 32:319, 1977.
245. Widman F.K. (ed.): *Technical Manual of the American Association of Blood Banks*, ed. 8. Washington, D.C., American Association of Blood Banks, 1981, p. 281.
246. Marshall B.E., Wurzel H.A., Ellison N., et al.: Microaggregate formation in stored blood: III. Comparison of Bentley, Fenwall, Pall and Swank micropore filtration. *Circ. Shock* 2:249, 1975.
247. Snyder E.L., Bookbinder M.: Role of microaggregate blood filtration in clinical medicine. *Transfusion* 23:460, 1983.
248. Kaplan H.S.: Personal communication, 1978.
249. Wenz B., Gurtlinger K.F., O'Toole A.M., Dugan E.P.: Preparation of granulocyte-poor red blood cells by microaggregate filtration. *Vox Sang.* 39:282, 1980.
250. Hill J.D., Osborn J.J., Swank R.L., et al.: Experience using a new Dacron wool filter during extracorporeal circulation. *Arch. Surg.* 101:649, 1970.
251. Schwartz C.J., et al.: Pathologic sequelae and com-

plications of ventriculotomy. *Arch. Pathol.* 89:56, 1970.
252. Swank R.L., Porter G.A.: Disappearance of microemboli transfused into patients during cardiopulmonary bypass. *Transfusion* 3:192, 1963.
253. Peck C.C., Odom D.G., Friedman H.I., et al.: Di-2-ethylhexyl phthalate (DEHP) and mono-2-ethylhexyl phthalate (MEHP): Accumulation in whole blood and red cell concentrates. *Transfusion* 19:137, 1979.
254. Kaarrianen L., Paloheimo J., Klemola E., et al.: Cytomegalovirus-mononucleosis: Isolation of the virus and demonstration of subclinical infections after fresh blood transfusion in connection with open heart surgery. *Ann. Med. Exp. Fenn.* 44:297, 1966.
255. Spurling C.: Transmissible disease and blood transfusion, in Dawson R.B. (ed.): *New Approaches to Transfusion Reactions: A Technical Workshop.* Washington, D.C., American Association of Blood Banks, 1974, pp. 53–62.
256. Wheeler E.O., Turner J.D., Seannel J.G.: Fever, splenomegaly and atypical lymphocytes: A syndrome observed after cardiac surgery utilizing a pump oxygenator. *N. Engl. J. Med.* 266:454, 1962.
257. Perham T.G.M., Caul E.O., Conway P.J., et al.: Cytomegalovirus infection in blood donors: A prospective study. *Br. J. Haematol.* 20:307, 1971.
258. Suwansirikul S., Rao N., Dowling J.N., et al.: Primary and secondary cytomegalovirus infection. *Arch. Intern. Med.* 137:1026, 1977.
259. Conrad M.: Diseases transmissible by blood transfusion: Viral hepatitis and other infectious disorders. *Semin. Hematol.* 18:122–146, 1981.
260. Turner A.R., MacDonald R.N., Cooper B.A.: Transmission of infectious mononucleosis by transfusion of pre-illness plasma. *Ann. Intern. Med.* 77:751, 1972.
261. Duhl J., et al.: Demonstration of herpes group virus in cultures of peripheral leukocytes from patients with infectious mononucleosis. *J. Virol.* 2:663, 1968.
262. Gerber P., Walsh J.H., Rosenblum E.N., et al.: Association of the EB-virus infection with the postperfusion syndrome. *Lancet* 1:593, 1969.
263. McMonigal K., Horwitz C.A., Henle W., et al.: Post-perfusion syndrome due to Epstein-Barr virus: Report of two cases and review of the literature. *Transfusion* 23:331, 1983.
264. Philip R.N., et al.: The potential for transmission of arbovirus by blood transfusion: With particular reference to Colorado tick fever, in Greenwalt J.J., Jamieson G.A. (eds.): *Transmissible Disease and Blood Transfusion.* New York, Grune & Stratton, 1974, pp. 175–195.
265. Braude A.E., Sandford J.P., Bartlett J.E., et al.: Effects and clinical significance of bacterial contaminants in transfused blood. *J. Lab. Clin. Med.* 39:902, 1952.
266. Gibson T., Norris W.: Skin fragments removed by injection needles. *Lancet* 2:983, 1958.

267. Braude A.E.: Transfusion reactions from contaminated blood: Their recognition and treatment. *N. Engl. J. Med.* 258:1289, 1958.
268. Braude A.E., Carey F.J., Semienski J.: Studies of bacterial transfusion reactions from refrigerated blood: The properties of cold-growing bacteria. *J. Clin. Invest.* 34:311, 1955.
269. Petz L.D., Swisher, S.N.: *Clinical Practice of Blood Transfusion.* New York, Churchill Livingstone, 1981 p. 794.
270. Mollison P.L.: The investigation of haemolytic transfusion reactions. *Br. Med. J.* 529:559, 1943.
271. Habibi B., Kleinknecht D., Vachon F., et al.: Le choc transfusionnel par contamination bactérienne du sang conservé: Analyse de 25 observations. *Rev. Fr. Transfus.* 16:41, 1973.
272. Stenhouse M.A., Milner L.V.: *Yersinia enuerocolica:* A hazard in blood transfusion. *Transfusion* 22:396, 1982.
273. Shubin H., Weil M.H.: Bacterial shock. *JAMA* 235:421, 1976.
274. Rhame F.S., Root R.K., MacLowry J.D., et al.: Salmonella septicemia from platelet transfusions: Study from an outbreak traced to a hematogenous carrier of *Salmonella cholerae-suis. Ann. Intern. Med.* 78:633, 1973.
275. Wood E.E.: Brucellosis as a hazard of blood transfusion. *Br. Med. J.* 1:27, 1955.
276. Seger R., Joller P., Kenney A., et al.: Potential hazards of blood transfusion in clostridia-associated necrotizing enterocolitis. *Lancet* 1:48, 1979.
277. Pavitch M.M., Farmer T.W., Davis B.: Use of blood donors with positive serologic tests for syphilis: With a note on the disappearance of passively transferred reagin. *J. Clin. Invest.* 28:18, 1949.
278. Kalmer A.J.: A note on the survival of *Treponema pallidum* in preserved citrated human blood and plasma. *Am. J. Syphilis* 26:156, 1942.
279. Mollison P.L.: *Blood Transfusion in Clinical Medicine,* ed. 7. Oxford, England, Blackwell Scientific Publications, 1983, p. 776.
280. Turner T.B., Diseker T.K.: Duration of infectivity of *Treponema pallidum* in citrated blood stored under conditions obtained in blood banks. *Bull. Johns Hopkins Hosp.* 68:269, 1941.
281. Buchholtz D.H., Young U.M., Friedman N.R. et al.: Bacterial proliferation in platelets stored at room temperature. *N. Engl. J. Med.* 285:429, 1971.
282. Chambers R.W., Foley H.T., Schmidt P.J.: Transmission of syphilis by fresh blood components. *Transfusion* 9:32, 1969.
283. Centers for Disease Control: Syphilis: Recommended treatment schedules, 1976. *Ann. Intern. Med.* 85:94, 1976.
284. Hoeprich P.D.: *Infectious Diseases,* ed. 2. New York, Harper & Row, 1977, pp. 823–35, 1067–1071.
285. Whillet T.D.: The occurrence and importance of pyrogens. *J. Pharmacol.* 6:304, 1955.
286. Dover A.S., Schultz M.G.: Transfusion induced malaria. *Transfusion* 11:353, 1971.

287. Bruce-Chwatt L.J.: Transfusion malaria. *Bull. WHO* 50:337, 1974.
288. Bruce-Chwatt L.J.: Blood transfusion and tropical disease. *Trop. Dis. Bull.* 69:825, 1972.
289. Conrad M.E., quoted by Spurling C.: Transmissible disease and blood transfusion, in Dawson R.B. (ed.): *New Approaches to Transfusion Reactions: A Technical Workshop.* Washington, D.C., American Association of Blood Banks, 1974, p. 58.
290. Oberman H.L. (ed.): *Standards for Blood Banks and Transfusion Services,* ed. 10. Washington, D.C., American Association of Blood Banks, 1981, p. 6.
291. Miller L.H.: Transfusion malaria, in Greenwalt T.J., Jamieson G.A. (eds.): *Transmissible Disease and Blood Transfusion.* New York, Grune & Stratton, 1975.
292. Jacoby G.A., Hunt J.V., Kosinski K.S., et al.: Treatment of transfusion transmitted babesioses by exchange transfusion. *N. Engl. J. Med.* 303:1098, 1980.
293. Rohwedder R.W.: Chagas infection in blood donors and the possibilities of its transmission by means of transfusion. *Bol. Chil. Parasitol.* 24:88, 1969.
294. Chaffee E.F., Fife E.H., Kent J.F.: Diagnosis of *Trypanosoma cruzi* infection by complement fixation. *Am. J. Trop. Med. Hyg.* 5:763, 1956.
295. Knierim F., Rubinstein P.: The detection of Chagas' disease: A rapid hemagglutination test for special use in blood banks and epidemiological studies. *Vox Sang.* 18:280, 1970.
296. Gutteridge W.E.: Chemotherapy of Chagas' disease: The present situation. *Trop. Dis. Bull.* 73:699, 1976.
297. Vilaseca J.A., Cerisola J.A. Olarte J.A. et al.: The use of crystal violet in the prevention of the transmission of Chagas-Mazza disease (South American trypanosomiasis). *Vox Sang.* 11:711, 1966.
298. Andre R., Brumpt L., Dreyfus B., et al.: Cutaneous leishmaniasis, cutaneous glandular leishmaniasis and transfusional kala-azar. *Trop. Dis. Bull.* 55:379, 1958.
299. Wolfe M.S.: Parasites, other than malaria, transmissible by blood transfusion, in Greenwalt T.J., Jamieson G.A. (eds.): *Transmissible Disease and Blood Transfusion.* New York, Grune & Stratton, 1975.
300. Knott J.: The periodicity of microfilariae: IV. Transfusion of microfilariae into a clean host. *Trans. R. Soc. Trop. Med. Hyg.* 29:59, 1935.
301. Bird G.W.G., Menon K.K.: Survival of *Microfilaria bancrofti* in stored blood. *Lancet* 1:721, 1961.
302. Hawking F.: The transference of *Microfilariae bancrofti* into natural and unnatural hosts. *Ann. Trop. Med. Parasitol.* 34:121, 1940.
303. Siegel S.E., Lunde M.N., Gelderman A.H. et al.: Transmission of toxoplasmosis by leukocyte transfusion. *Blood* 37:388, 1971.
304. Roth J.A., Siegel S.E., Levine A.S. et al.: Fatal recurrent toxoplasmosis in a patient initially infected via a leukocyte transfusion. *Am. J. Clin. Pathol.* 56:601, 1971.
305. Fletcher S.: Indirect fluorescent antibody technique in the serology of *Toxoplasma gondii. J. Clin. Pathol.* 18:193, 1965.
306. Krick J.A., Remington J.S.: Toxoplasmosis in the adult: An overview. *N. Engl. J. Med.* 298:550, 1978.
307. Oberman H.L. (ed.): *Standards for Blood Banks and Transfusion Services,* ed. 10. Washington, D.C., American Association of Blood Banks, 1981, p. 33.
308. Widman F.K. (ed.): *Technical Manual,* ed. 8. Washington, D.C., American Association of Blood Banks, 1981, p. 282.
309. Wilson H.: Aqueous dextrose solutions: A hazard in transfusions. *Am. J. Clin. Pathol.* 20:667, 1950.
310. Vere D.W., Syckes C.H., Armitage P.: Venous thrombosis during dextrose infusion. *Lancet* 2:627, 1960.
311. Weisz-Carrington P.: Experience at NYU Medical Center during 1979, personal observation.
312. Ryden S.E., Oberman H.A.: Compatibility of common intravenous solutions with CPD blood. *Transfusion* 15:250, 1975.
313. Kark R.M.: Two cases of aplastic anaemia: One with secondary haemochromatosis following 290 transfusions in nine years, the other with secondary carcinoma of the stomach. *Guy's Hosp. Rep.* 87:343, 1937.
314. Cartwright G.E.: Hemochromatosis, in Thorn E.W., et al. (eds.): *Harrison's Principles of Internal Medicine,* ed. 8. New York, McGraw-Hill Book Co., 1977, p. 652.
315. Bothwell T., Finch C.A.: *Iron Metabolism.* New York, Churchill Livingstone, 1962, p. 410.
316. Pippard M.J., Callender, S.T., Weatherall D.J.: Intensive iron-chelation therapy with deferoxamine in iron loading anaemias. *Clin. Sci. Mol. Med.* 54:99, 1978.
317. Propper R.D., Cooper B., Rufo R.R., et al.: Continuous subcutaneous administration of deferoxamine in patients with iron overload. *N. Engl. J. Med.* 297:418, 1977.
318. Medical Research Council: Thrombophlebitis following intravenous infusions: Trial of plastic and red rubber giving sets. Report of a subcommittee. *Lancet* 1:595, 1957.
319. Druskin M.S., Siegel P.D.: Bacterial contamination of indwelling intravenous polyethylene catheters. *JAMA* 185:966, 1963.
320. Carter J.F.B.: Reduction in thrombophlebitis by limiting duration of intravenous infusion. *Lancet* 2:20, 1951.
321. Widman F.K. (ed.): *Technical Manual,* ed. 8. Washington, D.C., American Association of Blood Banks, 1981, p. 319.

12

Hepatitis

VIRAL HEPATITIS can be transmitted by transfusion and so is of concern to blood bankers. At least four distinct types of viral hepatitis have been recognized: type A, caused by hepatitis virus A (HAV); viral hepatitis type B (HBV), caused by hepatitis virus B; δ hepatitis; and a fourth which may in fact be more than one disease, designated non-A, non-B (NANB) hepatitis. HBV and NANB hepatitis are more often transmitted by transfusion than is HAV.

VIRAL HEPATITIS TYPE A

HAV, previously called MS-1 hepatitis, has a comparatively short incubation period of 25–30 days.[1] It is usually transmitted by the fecal-oral route, but may occasionally be transmitted parenterally.[2] The HAV virus, otherwise known as the Feinstone particle, is very resistant to heat denaturation, withstanding heating for 30 minutes at 56° C. It is roughly cubic and about 27 nm in diameter, making it a relatively small virus.[3] The capsid has at least four polypeptide determinants termed Vp1–Vp4. This capsid encases a single-stranded RNA core composed of 8,100 bases which at one end possess a Vpg protein thought to function as an anchor to host ribosomes.[4] The viral RNA decodes in a positive polarity, as does messenger RNA. Transmission of the disease has been extensively studied in the marmoset monkey model.[5] Filtrates from infected material allowing passage of 27-nm particles were capable of reproducing HAV hepatitis in these animals. There is no carrier state for HAV in humans, so the continued presence of the disease requires actively infected hosts.

HAV appears to be cyclic, is more frequent in children than in adults, is more frequently seen in areas of poor hygiene (such as some mental institutions), and has a low fatality rate.[6] Antibodies appear 8 days after infection. The titer rises dramatically, sometimes reaching 1:1,280, and decreases during convalescence.[7] The serum glutamic oxaloacetic transaminase (SGOT) and serum glutamic pyruvic transaminase (SGPT) levels rise after the 30-day incubation period (Fig 12–1)[8] and remain elevated 5–10 days. The pathologic changes in the hepatocyte are indistinguishable in HAV, HBV, and NANB.[9] Viral hepatitis A particles are detected by electron microscopy shortly after the onset of the disease. Usually HAV will not develop into either fulminant or chronic viral hepatitis. Liberal bed rest and a diet with balanced electrolytes or intravenous fluid if oral intake is not tolerated have been recommended as the management of choice in controlled studies of patients with hepatitis.[10]

VIRAL HEPATITIS TYPE B

HBV (MS-2 hepatitis) was first described by Lurman after an epidemic of hepatitis in shipyard workers vaccinated with a smallpox vaccine obtained from human lymph.[11]

The transmission of the disease in humans via the MS-2 hepatitis virus was proved by studies in hu-

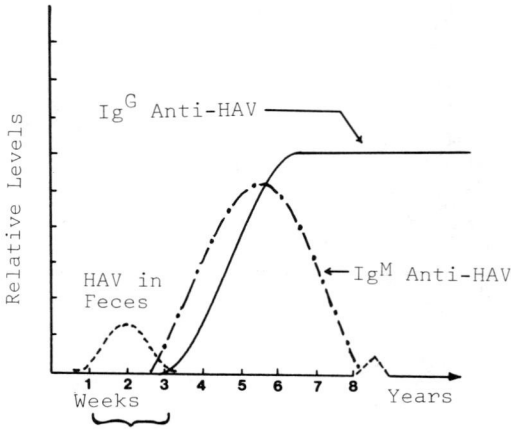

FIG 12–1.—Disease course in viral hepatitis A infections.

mans in 1945,[12] but the hepatitis B virus was discovered as a precipitable agent in 1961.[13] Further studies revealed that the virus was present in multiply transfused patients[14] and its presence correlated with the hepatitis disease state.[15] These findings were later confirmed by other investigators.[16] The virus was successfully transmitted to chimpanzees in 1972.[17]

The Australia antigen, originally described in 1961 and correlated with hepatitis by Blumberg and co-workers,[13–15] has proved to represent part of the capsid of the hepatitis B virus and therefore it is now termed hepatitis B surface antigen (HB_sAg).[18] The entire virus, however, as seen by electron microscopy, was described by Dane and collaborators[8] and has since been termed the Dane particle. The virus particle is a double-shelled sphere measuring 42 nm in diameter. The outer coat is the HB_sAg. Other antigenic molecules compose the Dane particle.[19] The DNA core and DNA polymerases (Fig 12–2) also compose the Dane particle. The core antigen is termed HB_cAg. These particles have been defined by immune electron microscopy.

From recent studies on duck hepatitis virus B, it has been determined that the hepatitis B virus is similar to a retrovirus in that it is originally an RNA virus which by reverse transcription forms two circular strands of DNA from a single strand of RNA. Apparently there is also a genomic analogy between retroviruses and the hepatitis B virus. This observation is important, because retroviruses are known to be oncogenic and HBV has recently been implicated in the pathogenesis of hepatoma.[20]

The capsid of the hepatitis B virus exists in several sizes and in tubular or spherical shapes. The tubular shapes may be over 200 nm long, whereas the more frequent spherical forms are about 20 nm in diameter and are composed of mostly HB_sAg. Particles are about 42 nm in diameter. The complete Dane particle constitutes the 27-nm core and its inner capsid (HB_cAg) and the outer capsid (HB_sAg) (see Fig 12–2).[21] The capsid is composed of a common antigenic subdeterminant, the *a* de-

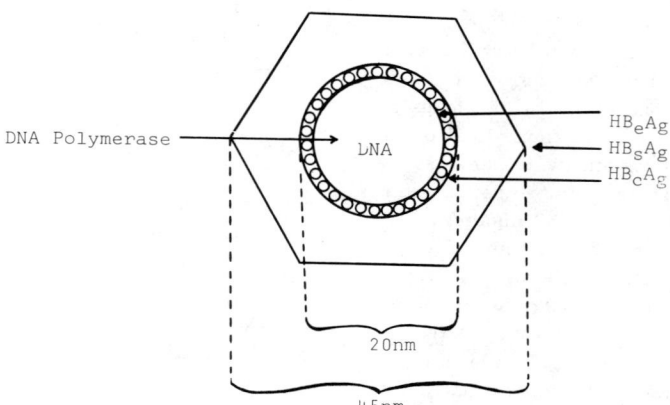

FIG 12–2.—The hepatitis B viral particle. Originally described as the Dane particle, it is composed of a central core containing the viral DNA and DNA polymerase. A protein thought to be surrounding the core is termed the hepatitis B_e antigen (HB_eAg). Another protein surrounding the core is the hepatitis B_c antigen (HB_cAg). The outermost protein capsid is termed hepatitis B surface antigen (HB_sAg). The core diameter measures approximately 20 nm, while the outside diameter of the particle is approximately 45 nm.

terminant. This determinant has at least three antigenic subdeterminants, as demonstrated by monoclonal antibody studies.[22] Other subdeterminants d, y, w, and v are also part of the capsid. The d determinant is dependent on the structural integrity of its 122-lysine residue. This observation may be useful for possible future synthetic production of antigen for vaccines.[22]

The four major combined determinants are adw, adr, ayw, and ayr. Other possible combinations exist but are less frequent.[23] The d and y determinants are mutually exclusive, and so are w and v. These combinations occur with varying frequency in different geographic locations and have been used to study the epidemiology of this disease.[24] These antigens have no prognostic significance on the outcome of the disease.[25] The HB_sAg variants all share the a antigen, and for this reason reinfection is not frequent. The protein component of HB_sAg is a 25,000-dalton chain and a 30,000-dalton chain with almost identical amino acid sequences.[26]

Thus, the HBV viral particle is composed of a capsid hepatitis B surface antigen (HB_sAg); an inner nucleocapsid with distinct antigenic specificity, the HB core antigen (HB_cAg); and a double-stranded circular DNA genome of about 2 million daltons, a segment of which is single-stranded.[27]

The virus particle also contains a DNA-dependent DNA polymerase and a protein kinase. The HB_eAg is a soluble antigen recognized in HBV particles. It probably consists of HB_cAg polypeptides that are not assembled into the HBV core.[27]

Genome Structure of HBV

The HBV DNA is a circular molecule approximately 3,200 nucleotides long,[28] composed of a double-stranded region and a single-stranded region (Fig 12–3). Thus, a long strand (L) and a short strand (S) compose the viral DNA. There is a remarkable difference in the coding capacity of L and S strands. The L strand contains four large potentially coding regions whereas the S strand contains short, poorly conserved open regions. This finding suggests that L strands code for viral proteins but S strands do not.[29]

The four open regions of the L strand are designated S, C, P, and X. Region S can be subdivided into S and pre-S. Gene S codes for a protein PI which is part of the viral envelope.[30] Very few, if any, intervening noncoding sequences are present in this gene. This can be demonstrated by inserting

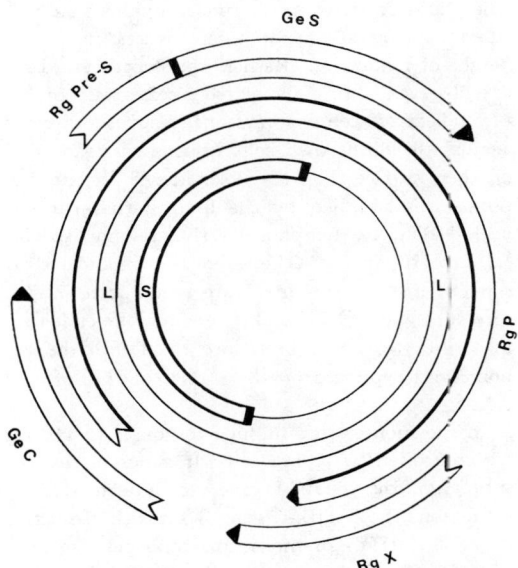

FIG 12–3.—Model of HBV genome. *L*, long strand; *S*, short strand; *Rg*, region; *Ge*, gene (see text).

gene S DNA sequences into *E. coli*, after which the *E. coli* can synthesize HB_sAg.[31] Gene C codes for P 19, which is the major polypeptide of the viral core.[32] Region P, which encompasses 75% of the genome, codes for a large 90,000-dalton protein, probably DNA polymerase.[29]

Region X codes for a short (154 amino acid) polypeptide whose function is not known. Region P overlaps region S. This means that one DNA sequence, as occurs in other viruses, can code for two proteins.[33] It is possible that the single strand has bearing in integrating the viral DNA into the human genome. This viral DNA integration may be significant in the development of hepatocellular carcinoma. This has been suggested by the finding that certain hepatocellular carcinoma cell lines are capable of producing HB_sAg.[34] It has also been possible to induce HB_sAg synthesis by cloning gene S in a recombinant plasmid and inserting this sequence into the DNA of a mammalian cell line such as mouse L cells.[35]

Pathogenesis

The virus penetrates cells, but the cellular damage observed in hepatocytes probably does not represent an immediate cytopathic effect. This is supported by the lack of cytopathic change observed when hepatocytes from infected individuals are cultured in vitro at a time when viruses are at the height of replication. Rather, the hepatocyte damage observed during the active disease state probably reflects a cellular immune response directed against the host's own cells bearing viral antigens on their surface (Fig 12–4). Evidence for this hypothesis is supplied by the finding that patients with HBV have lymphocytes that respond specifically to HB_sAg.[36, 37] The response is modulated by different mechanisms involving lymphocyte inhibitory substances.[38] These antigens may be coded for in viruses that have been integrated into the genome and expressed on the surface of the infected cells.[39]

In the mouse, the immune responses to HB_sAg are controlled by at least two Ir genes in the I-A subregion, the Ir-Hb_s-1 gene, and one in the I-C subregion, the Ir-HB_s-2 gene.[40] Growth of murine hepatitis (MHV) in mouse macrophages has been documented. Resistance to replication in these murine cells is controlled by recessive gene on chromosome 7.[41]

Liver damage is not proportional to antigenemia or to the level of anti-HB_s antibodies. Therefore, it now appears that the cellular immune response of the individual[42] determines the severity of the infection. Thus, fulminant hepatitis may be produced by a heightened cellular immune response,[43] whereas chronic hepatitis develops from a deranged cellular immune response. In summary, this evidence supports the view that liver damage in HBV is not due to a direct viral cytopathic effect but to an interaction between the virus-infected hepatocytes and the immune system.[44] In addition, it appears that cellular rather than humoral elements of the immune system are responsible for the damage, as suggested by the finding of lymphoid cell populations in tissue sections.[45] However, the exact mechanism of injury remains unknown.[46]

The Dudley Hypothesis

Dudley and collaborators[47] have proposed that the extent of the liver damage is in direct proportion to the viral particle load of the infection. Thus, fulminant hepatitis would result after a massive infective dose of viral particles. Cytolytic T cells would recognize only hepatocytes infected by the virus. On the other extreme of the spectrum, a hepatitis carrier would be an individual whose T cells would ignore hepatocytes infected by the virus.[47] Chronic hepatitis would be present in patients who have a partially impaired T cell response. Certain workers have shown enhanced killing by NK-type cells from patients with chronic HBV of liver cells in culture; however, these authors also showed that the cytotoxic effect was nonspecific for HB antigens, or even for liver cells. This was demonstrated by the cytotoxic effect of these cells on Raji cells, which are lymphoblastoid cells devoid of hepatocyte-specific tissue antigens,[48] and on the Mahlaru cell line, which is derived from a hepatoma and lacks HB_sAg antigens. Other authors failed to demonstrate either enhanced or specific cytotoxicity in patients with chronic HBV infections.[49] It has been shown, however, that certain HBV-infected patients with chronic active hepatitis may have very low T4:T8 ratios, and carriers very often have a reversal of normal T4:T8 ratios.[46]

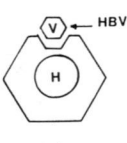

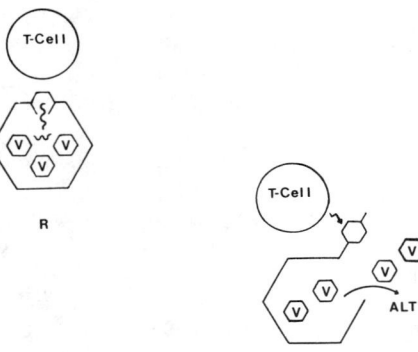

FIG 12–4.—Pathogenesis of hepatitis B. *I*, infection; *R*, replication; *L*, lysis; *V*, virion.

Pathology of HBV

The liver changes seen in HBV can be cytotoxic, inflammatory (hyperplastic and exudative), or regenerative. Damage is more prominent in the centrilobular areas.[9] If the disease becomes chronic it may assume one of two forms, chronic active hepatitis or chronic persistent hepatitis.[50]

In chronic active hepatitis there is progression of the hepatocellular dysfunction; eventually postnecrotic cirrhosis develops. Lymphocytes and plasma cells accumulate in the portal tracts and necrotic hepatocytes trapped in fibrous tissue are seen scattered throughout the lobules. Destruction of the limiting plate is also a feature of chronic active hepatitis. This type of necrosis is termed "piecemeal" necrosis. Clinically there may be episodic jaundice and malaise. Chronic persistent hepatitis B is characterized by a continued inflammatory reaction in the portal triads for months or years, but the destruction is much milder and the outcome usually more benign than in chronic active hepatitis.

T cells and B cells from HBV-vaccinated donors can be shown to respond in vitro to challenge by HB_sAg.[51] Also of interest is the finding that antibodies to HBV can be induced by infusion of anti-idiotypic antibodies in mice. This finding may prove to be useful for the induction of anti-HB_sAg using idiotypes as a primer in lieu of a vaccine.[52]

Clinical Presentation

Most cases of HBV infection are probably subclinical.[53] The symptoms may vary from an insidious presentation, with malaise, arthralgia, and urticaria, to the overt syndrome of anorexia, malaise, and severe icterus which may appear days to weeks after the prodromal stage. In 1% of cases, fulminant hepatitis, a very serious disease, complicated by hepatic failure, develops.[54] Clinical viral hepatitis can be divided into three stages: incubation, the acute phase, and convalescence (Table 12–1).

Incubation.—This period comprises the time of exposure to the onset of symptoms. In subclinical infections HB_sAg antigenemia is used as time of onset.[55] The incubation period for different types of hepatitis is given in Table 12–2. Incubation periods may differ in length because of the size of the inoculum or the route of exposure.[56]

In HBV, the larger the number of viral particles,[56] the shorter the incubation period; furthermore, if the inoculum enters via the oral route, the incubation period is twice as long than if infection occurred via the parenteral route.[57] The route of administration, by contrast, does not appear to affect the incubation time for hepatitis A.[57]

The Acute Phase.—The acute phase is manifested by overt symptoms and signs (see Table 12–2). Most patients with viral hepatitis do not develop icterus. About 25% of patients with NANB hepatitis will become jaundiced.[58] Jaundice is frequently heralded by several days by the appearance of bilirubinuria. When jaundice is eventually manifest, it is usually accompanied by fever, which develops as the jaundice intensifies. Itching and acholic stools appear at the peak of jaundice. About 10% of patients with HBV present with a serum sickness type of syndrome.[59] Soluble immune complexes composed of viral antigens and host antibodies circulate and deposit on tissues as a type III reaction (see Chap. 4).[60]

Nonspecific Laboratory Findings

Atypical lymphocytes and leukopenia may be seen in the preicteric phase. During the prodrome

TABLE 12–1.—CLINICAL CHARACTERISTICS OF VIRAL HEPATITIS B

PHASE	LABORATORY FINDINGS	SYMPTOMS	SIGNS	FREQUENCY AND DURATION
Incubation	Minimal	None	None	3 mo.
Acute	ALT > 1,000 units	Flu	Hepatomegaly	10%–15%, 1 mo.
	AST > 1,000	Fever	Splenomegaly	10%–15%
	Bilirubin > 6%	Anorexia	Icterus	25%
		Nausea		
		Fatigue		
		Serum sickness		10%
Convalescence	ALT < 500 units	Fatigue	None	1–4 mo.
	Bilirubin < 2%			

TABLE 12–2.—MEAN INCUBATION PERIODS FOR
DIFFERENT TYPES OF HEPATITIS

TYPE OF HEPATITIS	INCUBATION (DAYS)	RANGE (DAYS)
A	28–30	15–50
NANB	50	15–180
B	90	15–180

of HBV infection, a serum sickness syndrome may be seen in up to 20% of cases, due to deposition of HB_sAg/anti-HB_s complexes.[61] A fall of plasma C3 and C4 levels[62] may be seen in these cases. Hepatocellular damage is reflected by elevated serum transaminase levels. Elevated transaminase levels are usually detected 8–12 weeks after the onset of infection.

Both alanine aminotransferase (ALT, previously SGPT) and aspartate aminotransferase (AST, previously SGOT) are markedly elevated (100-fold). The creatinine phosphokinase (CPK) level is usually normal. Both ALT and AST levels become abnormal in the late incubation period and are always elevated in the icteric phase of viral hepatitis. In the cholangiolitic variety the serum alkaline phosphatase level may be elevated. Proteinuria and bilirubinuria frequently precede the icteric phase. Acholic stools may be present. Urobilinogenuria may likewise be detected. A broad elevation of serum γ-globulin may be observed.[63] Anicteric hepatitis is not uncommon and may herald chronic hepatitis.[64]

A markedly prolonged prothrombin time not correctable by vitamin K is of poor prognosis and may indicate impending fulminant hepatitis.[4]

Detection of Markers in HBV Hepatitis

One of the hallmarks of HBV laboratory testing is to detect HBV markers. Immunodiffusion and counterimmunoelectrophoresis were used in the past to detect HB_sAg, and were called first- and second-generation tests.[65] The only tests accepted by the FDA today are the so-called third-generation tests, which include radioimmunoassay (RIA) or an enzyme immunoassay, and a reverse passive hemagglutination test (RPHA) or a latex agglutination test, which have a third-generation-type sensitivity.[65, 66]

The RIA test is based on an antigen-antibody "sandwich" principle.[67] Plastic beads are coated with guinea pig antiserum specific for HB_sAg. Patient serum is incubated with the plastic beads and washed. If HB_sAg is present, it will remain attached to the antiserum on the bead.[68] A second antiserum raised in another species with HB_sAg specificity and radiolabeled with ^{125}I is used in a second incubation. The bead is then washed for the second time and counted in a gamma counter (Fig 12–5) to assess the amount of antibody bound to the patient's HB_sAg trapped by the bead. False positive results may result because the test is overly sensitive. A similar test has been designed to detect HB_cAg and many other markers, screening for chronic carriers, as well as for other selected cases (Table 12–3).

The RIA for hepatitis testing is about 1,000 times more sensitive and detects about 15% more positive samples than first-generation tests (e.g., radial immunodiffusion). RIA can detect as few as 1×10^9 particles, whereas first-generation tests detect above 1×10^{13} particles.[69] RIA can also be used to obtain objective numerical values, and the test may be performed on a semiautomated instrument. The results of the gamma counter evaluation in counts per minute are calculated as follows:

Arbitrary cutoff
$$= F \times \frac{\text{Sum of negative controls } (\Sigma NC)}{\text{No. of samples } (n)}$$

$$\text{Ratio of unknown to } \overline{X}NC = \frac{U}{\Sigma NC/n}$$

where $\overline{X}$ = statistical mean, NC = negative controls, U = unknown, and F = a constant factor.

Counts (per millicurie) of radioactivity putatively shown by anti-HB_sAg are considered positive when they are above background radioactivity. For a value to be considered positive, the ratio above (cpm to cpm) must be greater than 2:1.

The negative cutoff value is calculated by first multiplying the mean cpm of the negative controls (usually seven tubes) by 2 and adding the cpm of the background tube.[70] Positive control values are usually 5 times the mean of the negative control.[71] For more details on RIA techniques the reader is referred to work by Linke and Henry.[72]

Some common pitfalls in RIA testing are variability in sensitivity, improperly collected or contaminated samples, and inappropriate incubation times. Inadequate washing, carryover, and radioactive contamination from equipment may also produce spurious results. Positive samples should be retested by RIA or with a manual test such as the RPHA for confirmation. If samples are negative,

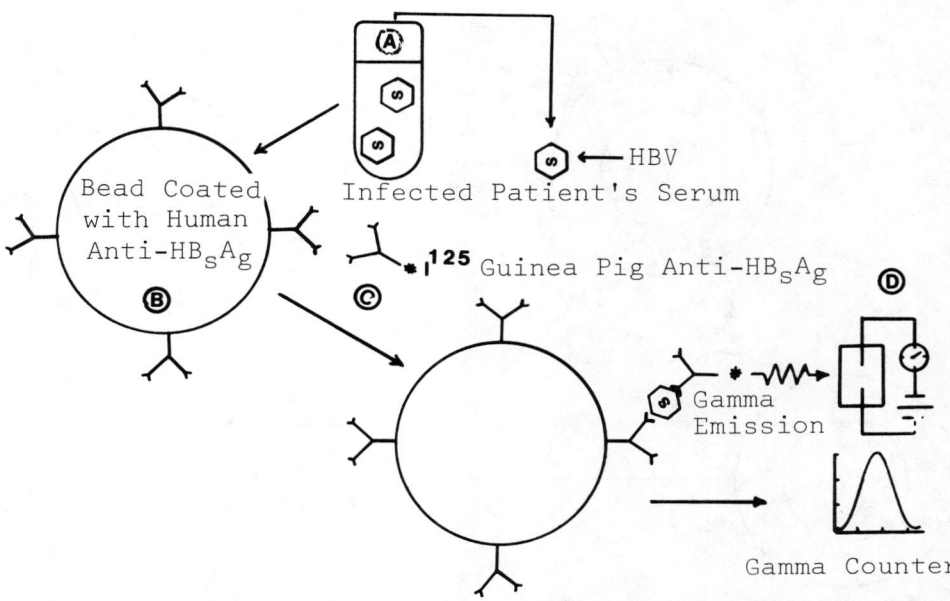

FIG 12–5.—Detection of hepatitis B surface antigen (HB$_s$Ag) by radioimmunoassay. Patient sample *(A)* is incubated with bead coated with anti-HB$_s$Ag *(B)*. Subsequently the bead is incubated with ^{125}I-labeled guinea pig anti-HB$_s$Ag *(C)*. The bead is then washed to eliminate unbound ^{125}I-labeled antibody and counted in a gamma counter *(D)*.

the test is repeated and inhibition of antibody reactivity is attempted using anti-HB$_s$Ag.

Extended turnaround time, high cost of equipment, and radioactive waste disposal problems are some of the drawbacks of RIA hepatitis testing.

RPHA has a third-generation-type sensitivity in hepatitis testing.[73] Tanned RBCs or latex particles are coated with specific antibody (Fig 12–6). If a patient's serum contains HB$_s$Ag, these coated cells will agglutinate on incubation with the infected serum.

RPHA is inexpensive and results are obtained within 2 hours, compared to the 24 hours required for RIA. In addition, no radioactive waste is produced. However, the RPHA method is slightly less sensitive than RIA and test results are interpreted

TABLE 12–3.—SEROLOGIC MARKERS IN HEPATITIS B

ANTIGENS*					ANTIBODIES*				
						anti-HB$_c$			
HB$_s$Ag†	HB$_c$	HB$_e$	DNAP	HBV-DNA	Anti-HB$_s$	IgG	IgM	Anti-HB$_e$‡	INTERPRETATION
+	+	±	+	+	−	−	−	−	Preicteric
+	+	+	+	+	−	±	+	±	Acute (2–6 mo.)
+	+	+	+	+	−	+	−	−	Chronic hepatitis (> 12 mo)
±	+	+	+	+	−	+ +	−	+	Carrier state
−	−	−	−	−	+	+	+	+	Early recovery
−	−	−	−	−	+	+	−	+	Recovery long-term over 1 year§
−	−	−	−	−	+	−	−	−	Immunized HB$_s$Ag

*Last 2–5 months in patients who recover.
†HB$_s$Ag may be positive 2–5 months after exposure.
‡Anti-HB$_e$ appears years after infection in chronic hepatitis and in the carrier state.
§Markers decrease progressively after years.

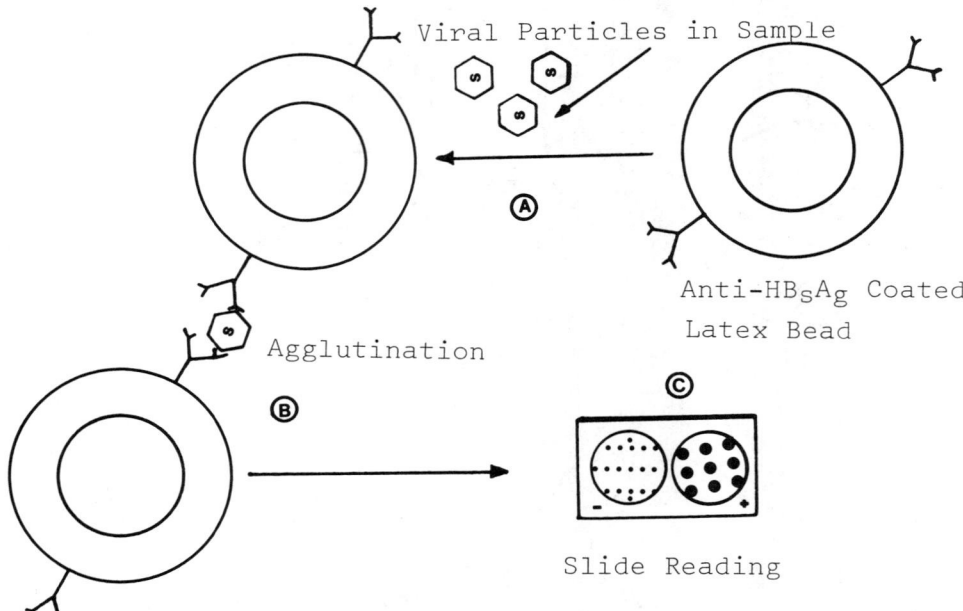

FIG 12–6.—Latex agglutination test for HB_sAg. The patient sample with viral particles (A) is incubated with latex beads coated with anti-HB_sAg antibody. Agglutination will occur if the antibody is present (right circle in C). If no antigen is present, no agglutination will occur (left circle in C).

subjectively rather than by automated reading.

An enzyme-linked immunosorbent assay (ELISA) (Fig 12–7) has been developed that is comparable in sensitivity to RIA, does not produce radioactive waste, and is therefore one of the preferred methods for hepatitis marker detection today.

Anti-HB_s antibodies can also be screened for by RIA techniques. Their detection is helpful in epidemiologic studies, revealing previous infection, or to screen high-risk personnel (e.g., in hemodialysis units).[74] HBV disease progression has been studied by detecting DNA polymerase.[75] Detection of yet another antigen, the HB_e antigen, reveals the degree of infectivity.[76] Furthermore, it has been shown that DNA polymerase and HB_eAg levels correlate in terms of stage of infection.[77] HB_eAg is a viral gene product distinct from HB_cAg and Hb_sAg and may bind to plasma proteins.[78] It is thought that the actual location of the HB_eAg is surrounding the virus core. Hb_eAg can be used to forecast the development of chronic HBV infection. HB_eAg appears early in the disease and should disappear on development of anti-HB_e antibodies, heralding recovery. This usually occurs within 10 weeks of HB_s antigenemia.[25] If HB_eAg does not disappear in 10 weeks, a chronic carrier state can be expected.[79] Furthermore, chronic active hepatitis may develop in patients with persistence of HB_e antigenemia.[80]

The δ Agent

A new agent, the δ agent, has been described.[81] The δ agent is a 35-nm RNA virus which requires HBV for replication and utilizes HB_sAg as a capsid.[4] Thus, the particle has an outer capsid of HB_sAg, a middle coat of δ antigen, and an inner RNA core. The δ agent can present clinically as acute hepatitis concurrently with B hepatitis, as acute δ hepatitis in a chronic HBV carrier, or as chronic δ hepatitis in a chronic HBV carrier. The diagnosis is not routinely made because tests for detecting the δ antigen are not universally commercially available.

However, this diagnosis should be suspected in a case of acute hepatitis developing in a chronic carrier; IgM anti-HB_c testing can disclose these cases,[82] for it may not be elevated in δ hepatitis.[83] Epidemiologically, δ hepatitis is frequently seen in the Middle East and in Mediterranean Europeans with chronic hepatitis, whereas in the U.S.[84] this type of infection is usually seen in high-risk groups

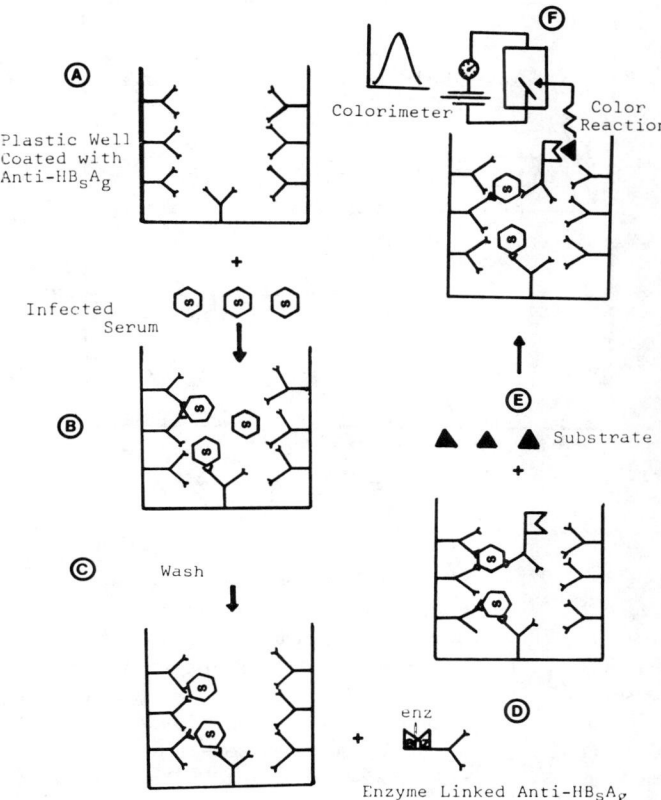

FIG 12–7.—Enzyme immunoassay for the detection of HB$_s$Ag. Plastic well is coated with anti-HB$_s$Ag (A). Infected serum is added to the well (B). Unbound viral particles are washed (C). Chromogeric enzyme-linked anti-HB$_s$Ag is added (D). Essential antibody is washed. Chromogenic substrate is added (black triangles, E). Each resulting color reaction is measured by a colorimeter.

such as hemophiliacs and drug addicts. IV drug abusers may be the reservoir for the δ agent in Western Europe and the U.S.

Laboratory Profiles in the Diagnosis of Hepatitis B

The first laboratory evidence of infection is the detection of HB$_s$Ag in serum about 30 days after exposure (Fig 12–8). Several days after the detection of HB$_s$Ag, HB$_e$Ag and DNA polymerase become apparent. These latter antigens usually disappear by the time jaundice is noted. Abnormal AST (SGOT) and ALT (SGPT) values appear 2 weeks to 2 months after HB$_s$Ag becomes detectable. Serum bilirubin values become elevated 2 weeks after the serum transaminase levels begin to rise. Shortly after the appearance of jaundice, anti-HB$_c$ antibodies become detectable. Anti-HB$_s$Ag antibodies appear weeks or months after the onset of jaundice.

If chronic active hepatitis develops, HB$_s$Ag titers and AST levels remain elevated for longer than 6 months. No antibodies against HB$_s$Ag (anti-HB$_s$) are produced, and titers of HB$_e$Ag, DNA polymerase, and antibodies against HB$_c$Ag remain elevated. Antibodies against HB$_e$Ag and HB$_c$Ag usually remain elevated in the carrier state. Antibodies against HB$_s$Ag do not develop in the majority of these cases (see Table 12–3).[85]

Epidemiology of HBV

About 5%–10% of people infected with HBV become carriers. This carrier state is more frequent in male individuals under the age of 30 and results in about 120 million human carriers in the world population.[86] The carrier state is more prevalent in warm climates and affects noncaucasians of low economic status more frequently.[53] Even though the disease is usually transmitted parenterally, oral transmission and sexual transmission have also been demonstrated and are considered important modes of disease spread.[87] About 70% of male homosexuals have evidence of current or past infection with HBV.[88]

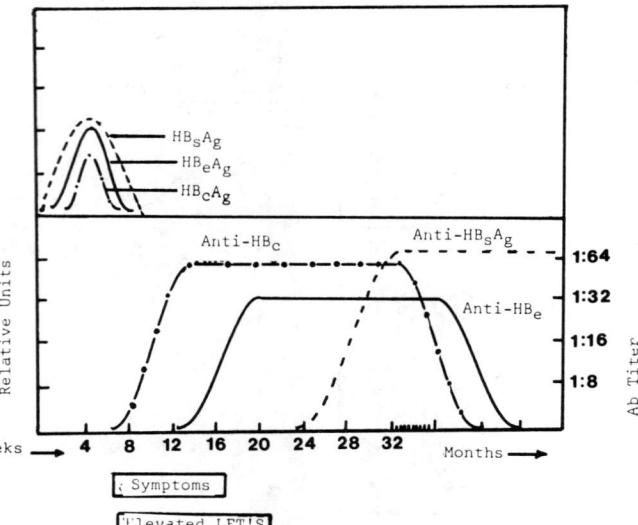

FIG 12–8.—The course of HBV infection. *Top,* antigens s, e, and c; *bottom,* the resulting antibodies. Note that antibodies against HB$_c$ and HB$_e$ decline after the 32d week, but antibodies against HB$_s$ remain elevated for months to years. At *bottom,* the *upper rectangle* depicts the length of duration of the symptoms in weeks; the *lower rectangle* depicts the duration (in weeks) of liver function test results.

Parenteral, oral, and vector transmissions are termed "horizontal" transmissions; transplacental transmission is considered "vertical" transmission. Transplacental transmission is common in immigrants of Asian origin.[89] Transplacental transmission to infants results in a greater number of carriers.[53] Transmission of hepatitis via mosquitoes and bedbugs is less likely, but the virus has been demonstrated in these parasites.[90] Table 12–4 lists the risk groups.

Complications of Hepatitis B

Fulminant Hepatitis

The most dreaded complication of viral hepatitis is fulminant hepatitis. It has a mortality rate of 75%–95%.[91] It may occur in up to 1% of cases of hepatitis B and up to 0.5% of cases of hepatitis A;[92] however, the incidence of fulminant hepatitis is probably much lower. In one series, no cases of fulminant hepatitis occurred in a group of 156 patients.[93] A markedly prolonged prothrombin time may herald this complication.

Hepatic encephalopathy, hepatic failure, and DIC are frequently found in fulminant hepatitis. Supportive measures are the only available treatment. Steroids do not seem to help these patients.[94] Of the few patients that recover from fulminant hepatitis, some do so without residual liver damage.[95]

Relapsing Hepatitis

In this modality, the patient has several episodes of recrudescence rather than resolution into convalescence. These episodes occur over a period of months.[96] Although it appears that these relapses are more frequent in NANB hepatitis,[92] it is quite possible that the disease represents various infections with different agents (i.e., HBV, NANB) such as would occur in high-risk groups such as homosexuals or drug addicts.[97]

Chronic Hepatitis

The criterion to determine if a patient has developed chronic hepatitis is if the patient's liver enzyme levels have not returned to normal after 6 months.[92] Some 5%–10% of patients with HBV[98] and 10%–30% with NANB[99] develop this complication.

There are two types of chronic hepatitis: chronic persistent hepatitis and chronic active hepatitis.

In chronic persistent hepatitis, the hepatitis process is not resolved, yet the hepatocytes are not con-

TABLE 12–4.—Groups at High Risk for HBV Infection

Intravenous drug addicts
Male homosexuals (70% show evidence of exposure)
Hemophiliacs (receiving factor concentrate)
Dialysis nursing personnel
Surgeons
Clinical laboratory personnel
Pathologists
Dentists

tinuously destroyed the way they would be in chronic active hepatitis. Nevertheless, in chronic persistent hepatitis, a lymphocytic infiltrate is seen in the portal triads, but it does not extend to the limiting plate.[100]

This inflammatory process generally resolves, though some cases proceed to chronic active hepatitis.[101] Chronic active hepatitis, in contrast to chronic persistent hepatitis, is characterized by a progressive destruction of hepatocytes, in many cases in the form of piecemeal necrosis. Eventually, cirrhosis develops in many of these cases, and patients die within 3½ years of diagnosis, although recovery may be seen in rare cases.[102]

Recently an inverted T4:T8 ratio has been reported in chronic active hepatitis cases where piecemeal necrosis was observed. This correlates with the current belief that the tissue destruction in chronic active hepatitis is an uncontrolled T-cytotoxic-mediated phenomenon.[103] This finding contrasts with an increased or normal ratio found in primary biliary cirrhosis and non-HBV chronic active hepatitis.[104] No significant numbers of monocytes are observed in these portal infiltrates.

Chronic Immune Complex Disease

Chronic immune complex disease may develop as a complication of hepatitis.[105] The immune complex disease is produced by complexes capable of binding complement via the classical or alternative pathway. The immune complexes in cases where the moieties are recognized are formed of either HB_sAg/anti-HB_sAg or HB_eAg/anti-HB_e.[106] Only a minor fraction of hepatitis carriers develop chronic immune complex disease. Immune complex disease can be manifested as immune vasculitis, glomerulonephritis, or mixed cryoglobulinemia. Necrotizing vasculitis occurs in about 1% of HB_sAg carriers. About 30% of patients with necrotizing vasculitis develop persistent HB_s antigenemia.[107] The disease is similar to other immune-mediated vasculitides. Nodular deposits composed of HB_sAg, immunoglobulin, and complement are present in the elastica of arteries.[108]

Glomerulonephritis can also develop as a consequence of the formation of immune complexes.[109] In Europe and Japan up to 40% of HB_sAg carriers may develop glomerulonephritis.[110] Deposits of immune complexes formed of HB_sAg/anti-HB_sAg or HB_eAg/anti-HB_eAg plus complement form in the subepithelial connective tissue of the glomerulus. These may give rise to membranous glomerulonephritis with the nephrotic syndrome or less commonly to membranoproliferative glomerulonephritis.[106] Some cases resolve spontaneously on disappearance of the HB_s antigenemia.[106] Finally, mixed cryoglobulinemia may be associated with immune complex disease appearing as a consequence of chronic hepatitis.[111] In this disorder, cryoglobulins composed of IgM and IgG, hence the term mixed cryoglobulins, appear in the patient's circulation. Clinically these patients develop arthralgias, weakness, and thrombocytopenia. The association of this disorder and chronic immune complex disease due to hepatitis has not been conclusively proved.[106]

Autoantibodies in HBV Infections

There are three types of chronic hepatitis (Table 12–5):[112]

1. Autoimmune type, or lupoid hepatitis exhibiting autoantibody markers.
2. HBV type showing HB_sAg positivity.
3. Cryptogenic, where neither autoantibodies nor HBV markers are seen.

Autoantibodies to cytoskeletal components are detected by incubating patient serum with cultured fibroblasts, after acetone fixation of the monolayers,[108] and staining by immunofluorescence for actin cables (AC). This type of staining shows parallel fluorescent cytoplasmic lines.

Autoantibodies to liver membrane antigen (LMAg) are detected on monkey liver cells and incubated with patient serum. Radiolabeled protein A is used to detect bound IgG.[112]

Viral Hepatitis and Hepatoma

Hepatoma has recently been considered a complication of viral hepatitis,[113] especially in countries where HBV is endemic, such as some regions of Asia and Africa,[106] where 50%–70% of patients with hepatoma are HB_sAg-positive. Nevertheless,

TABLE 12–5.—Characteristics of HBV and Autoimmune Chronic Active Hepatitis*

	HBV	AUTOIMMUNE
Age (yr)	30–50	Bimodal
Female/male ratio	1:3	5:1
Autoantibodies	±	ANA 3+
	±	(Actin) SMA 3+
	−	LMAg +
Phenotypic markers	HLA-B35	HLA-B8
	−	GMa+x+
Response to steroids	±	Good

*Modified from Gregory et al.[94] by permission.

cocarcinogens such as aflatoxin may be necessary for the development of hepatoma in these cases.

Primary hepatocarcinoma (PHC) is rare in the United States, comprising 1% of all carcinomas. However, it may be the leading carcinoma in the world,[114] accounting for up to 20% of all carcinomas in countries such as China. As we mentioned above, the presence of aflatoxin and HBV in the populations affected by this cancer may prove to have an etiologic correlation.[115] In an epidemiologic study of a Chinese population, the risk of PHC was shown to be dramatically higher in HB_sAg carriers than in noncarriers. In this study, all but one case of PHC was associated with a positive HB_sAg.[116] Aflatoxins may be the cocarcinogens in this disease, and HBV the inducing factor or at least a high-risk factor.[116] HBV has likewise been implicated in the etiology of hepatoma in patients with alcoholic liver disease.[117]

Guidelines for Treatment of Patients With HBV

Since no specific antiviral therapy is available for patients with HBV, treatment continues to be based on the principles set forth by Chalmers et al.[118] In controlled studies, these investigators determined that bed rest is beneficial but not mandatory. For persons who go on to develop chronic hepatitis with high levels of SGOT (AST), the requirement for bed rest will have to be less restricted lest it interfere with customary work and activities. Chalmers et al. suggest an ad libitum diet, remarking that the therapeutic value of high-protein and high-carbohydrate diets with low fat intake is controversial. The use of steroids is not recommended in the treatment of acute viral hepatitis.[119] Human immune globulin, useful in prevention of HBV hepatitis, has been of no use in the treatment of this disease.[120]

In more severe cases, such as fulminant hepatitis, the treatment is supportive, with intravenous fluids and limited protein intake (15–20 gm/day). Neomycin sulfate (8 gm orally q6h) is given to limit bacterial protein breakdown.[121] The prognosis is bad, and mortality varies from 60% to 90%. Steroids have not been shown to be of great value in fulminant hepatitis.[122] From experiments on mice, the use of charcoal in solid-phase filters to eliminate low molecular weight toxins is advocated in patients in hepatic coma.[123] It should be understood that this and many other therapeutic procedures such as exchange transfusion are experimental and do not constitute routine therapy for these patients.

The use of steroids has proved to be of benefit in selected patients with chronic active hepatitis.[124] Nevertheless, in studies by Summerskill et al., it was the HB_sAg-negative patients that benefited most from the immunosuppressive therapy.[124] Recent studies have shown that corticosteroids improve chronic active hepatitis secondary to autoimmune disorders, rather than that caused by HBV.[125]

Prophylaxis of HBV Hepatitis

Active immunization has been recently introduced in the prophylaxis of HBV hepatitis.[126] The vaccine, as it has been used in recent studies, stems from the pioneer work of Krugman et al.,[127] who used heat-inactivated serum from patients with HBV hepatitis. In these studies the MS-2 sera, now known to be HB_sAg positive, were capable of immunizing recipients but were no longer infective. Thus, the DNA replication of viral particles was abrogated but the antigenic determinants of the capsid were preserved.

A more purified vaccine was developed by formalin-inactivation of HB_sAg obtained from plasma of chronic carriers.[128] Trials of this vaccine were conducted in a population of male homosexuals, who are known to have a high prevalence of HBV. A large sample (1,083 volunteers) was vaccinated either with the vaccine or a placebo.[125] Of the vaccinated volunteers, 96% developed antibodies after a booster dose. A 92.3% decrease in the incidence of the disease was observed in the vaccinated population, demonstrating the highly effective nature of this vaccine. The fact that antibody levels were significant after 2 weeks of immunization shows the vaccine is effective after exposure to the virus. Few side effects from the vaccine have been reported. Since the vaccine is produced from human carriers, the possibility that induction of anti-HLA antibodies from hepatocellular debris was raised;[129] however this potential complication has not been documented.[130] Studies of groups of individuals at risk, such as homosexual males and health professionals, show that vaccination programs to prevent HBV would be cost-effective; in one study, accidental exposure to hepatitis by needle punctures in health professionals resulted in hospital expenses ranging from $1,000 to $7,000.[131] Conversely, vaccination of the general population would probably not be cost-effective.[132] It has been suggested that patients undergoing renal transplantation should be immunized with the vaccine, for the complication of hepatitis in patients receiving these transplants is detrimental to the survival of the graft.[133] The vaccine is fully approved by the FDA.[134]

Passive Immunization in Hepatitis

γ-Globulin fractions from serum pools, termed immune human serum globulin (ISG), have been shown to be effective in preventing or modifying HAV infections.[135] Prevention of HBV infections with initial ISG lots, however, was not successful,[136] due to low anti-HB$_s$ titers. More recently, however, ISG lots have been shown to contain variable titers of anti-HB$_s$ content in immunoglobulin fractions. Serum from selected donors has been collected to produce what is termed hepatitis B immunoglobulin (HBIG).[137] HBIG is about 30 times more expensive than ISG and is not recommended for routine prophylaxis of populations at risk. Instead, the U.S. Public Health Service Advisory Committee on Immunization Practices has come forth with specific recommendations on the subject. There are specific recommendations for the use of HBIG where contact with HBV is very likely, such as after puncture with an infected needle or after mucosal contact, as may occur in accidental contact with infected material (e.g., by mouth pipetting). The recommended dose in this case is 0.05–0.07 ml/kg of HBIG given intramuscularly within 7 days of exposure. A second dose in the same amount is given 25–30 days after the first injection.[138] In an extensive study it was shown that only 2% of exposed individuals protected with HBIG developed HBV, compared with 7% of those who received ISG. However, an additional 2% of individuals receiving HBIG developed a delayed type of hepatitis 6–9 months after exposure.[139] This did not occur in the group treated with ISG. The delay in appearance of symptoms suggests that HBIG modifies the incubation period of hepatitis, possibly by suppressing the passive-active immunity response.[139] Furthermore, in a study on staff members of a dialysis unit, who are at high risk of contracting hepatitis, ISG prophylaxis before exposure was as effective as HBIG.[140] It is useful to know if the suspected serum is positive for both HB$_s$Ag and HB$_c$Ag, because the latter antigen is frequently seen in actively infectious cases.[141, 142]

Perinatal Transmission

About 90% of infants born to mothers who are HB$_s$Ag positive become infected at birth. Although few of these infants develop acute disease, up to 90% become chronic carriers, and 25% of carriers eventually develop cirrhosis or hepatoma.[143]

A dose of 0.5 ml of HBIG is given IM to the infant within 12 hours after birth. Three 0.5-ml doses of vaccine should follow this initial dose of HBIG at 7 days, 30 days, and 6 months.[144] After 12 months of this regimen, the baby's serum is tested for anti-HB$_s$ and HB$_s$Ag. If HB$_s$Ag is present, failure of immunization has taken place.

Combined Prophylaxis for Acute Exposure to HB$_s$Ag-Containing Blood or Other Sample

Patients who have an accidental needle puncture with infected blood should be protected with 0.06 ml/kg (5 ml) (for adults) of HBIG IM within 24 hrs of exposure and should receive 20 μg (1 ml) of vaccine at a different injection site within 7 days of exposure. If HBIG is not available, ISG should be given. Sexual partners of patients with HB$_s$Ag-positive serum should receive HBIG (5 ml) IM within 14 days of exposure and vaccine at a different injection site.[144]

The anti-HBV vaccine is probably the best method of protecting high-risk populations. It is recommended that individuals who are at high risk and who are not vaccinated, be protected with ISG in a single 5-ml dose.[145]

There are about 1 million carriers of HBV in the U.S. and about 200 million worldwide. It is expected that widespread active immunization of high-risk groups will decrease these numbers dramatically in the future.[146]

NANB HEPATITIS

After a variety of precautionary measures such as the use of volunteer donor blood and the careful screening of donors, an 85% drop in the incidence of posttransfusion hepatitis (PTH) has been observed in the last two decades. However, 10% of prospectively followed patients continued to present with PTH despite the above-mentioned measures.[147] Thus, transfused patients in whom transfused units were negative for all markers of HBV and HAV must have been infected by a different agent if all other agents such as CMV and EBV viruses could be excluded. A reluctance to call this disease hepatitis C stems from the suspicion that such cases might be caused by more than one agent; therefore the disease is called NANB hepatitis. The transmission of NANB hepatitis was shown experimentally by inoculation of chimpanzees with suspect plasma.[148] Also in chimpanzees, a carrier-state for NANB has been documented.[149] As many as 63%–93% of PTH cases have been caused by NANB.[150] Some differences between HBV and NANB are shown in Table 12–6.[151]

Two types of NANB have been distinguished by electron microscopy of liver biopsy specimens. In this study, spherical particles measuring 20–27 nm in diameter were detected in hepatocyte nuclei of infected chimpanzees. These structures appeared in animals infected with 10^6 particles/ml and were termed strain H.

A second, tubular structure was observed in the endoplasmic reticulum of hepatocytes.[152] These structures were seen in animals inoculated with 10^2 viral particles, which caused a mild hepatitis and were termed strain F. The cellular structures seen after infections with these strains probably reflect cytopathic changes of cell structure, and are not viral particles. In recent studies, strain H has also produced cytoplasmic tubular inclusions, but strain F has not to date produced intranuclear inclusions.[153] This suggests that the H strain may represent two different agents, whereas the F strain may represent only one. Structures morphologically distinct from those described above have subsequently been described.[154] Nevertheless, certain structures previously thought to be HBV particles have been found in unrelated liver diseases and in normal hepatocytes.[155]

Cross-inoculation studies with the two strains (H and F) tend to support the hypothesis that NANB hepatitis is caused by two different agents.

Eighty-nine percent of posttransfusion hepatitis cases in the United States are caused by the agent or agents of NANB hepatitis.[156] Since the disease occurs in two forms with different incubation periods, the concept of two etiologic agents is further supported.[157] DNA hybridization studies have suggested the possibility that NANB hepatitis could be caused, covertly, by HBV.[158] Nevertheless, these results are thought by some to be controversial.[159] Studies in chimpanzees inoculated with plasma from patients with NANB hepatitis also suggest the existence of at least two distinct NANB agents.[160] The magnitude of posttransfusion hepatitis caused by NANB hepatitis is indicated by the 5%–18% incidence of NANB hepatitis in patients receiving 5 units or less of blood or blood products.[161] The transmission of this disease via transfusion of blood and blood products has been conclusively documented by experiments in chimpanzees,[162] the animal model for posttransfusion hepatitis. In biopsies, hexagonal 32-nm virus-like hepatitis negative for HB_sAg and HAV antigens have also been described.[163] Hepatocyte intranuclear virus-like particles have also been seen.[164] There is also evidence that a specific hepatitis C (HC) antigen (not to be confused with HBc) exists in certain NANB hepatitis sera.[165] In spite of this evidence, different investigators are skeptical that the available data pinpoint conclusively the characteristics of the NANB virus.[166] The mean incubation period of NANB hepatitis is about 60 days but may range from 7 to 12 weeks. SGOT elevation is usually prolonged, and in this respect the disease is similar to HBV hepatitis. The disease appears to be somewhat milder than HBV hepatitis[167] but may occasionally progress to chronic liver disease.[168, 169] A chronic carrier state was documented by injecting plasma from chronic NANB hepatitis patients into chimpanzees, which subsequently developed the disease.[170]

Laboratory diagnosis of NANB hepatitis is by exclusion, demonstrating that transaminase elevations and high bilirubin levels are not associated with HAV, HBV, cytomegalovirus, infectious mononucleosis, or any other identifiable etiologic agent. Transaminase elevation is first evident about 60 days after exposure, and 1 week later jaundice usually ensues.[171] It has recently been shown that carriers of NANB hepatitis can be detected by high levels of alanine amino transferase (ALT), especially in those blood donors with ALT levels above 60 IU. It was thus shown that NANB carriers can be detected by screening for high ALT levels.[172] It should be noted that ALT levels in volunteer blood donors vary significantly with different geographical areas and populations, depending on differences in age, sex, and alcohol intake.[173] To assess the economic impact on widespread ALT testing

TABLE 12–6.—CLINICAL CHARACTERISTICS OF VIRAL HEPATITIS

CHARACTERISTICS	VIRAL AGENT		
	HA	HB	NANB
Food-borne	+	+	
Transfusion	+	+ +	+ + +
Vertical	−	+	?
Drug addicts	20%	60%	20%
Male homosexuals	35%	60%	5%
Incubation (days)	15–45	40–180	15–150
Fulminant	5%	60%	35%
Chronic	−	5%–10%	6%–60%
Mortality	0.1%	1%–3%	1%–2%

of donors, more prospective studies are needed.[174]

Another parameter that has been explored as a possible means of identifying potential carriers of NANB virus is the carcinoembryonic antigen (CEA) levels, which seem to be elevated in carriers.[175] However, CEA testing is rather nonspecific, as CEA levels are elevated in 11% of asymptomatic adults and in normal smokers.[176]

CONCEPTS OF HEPATITIS DIRECTLY RELATED TO BLOOD BANKING

Until recently it was felt that hepatitis A was transmitted mostly via an oral-fecal route and HBV was transmitted mostly through transfusion. Since the development of tests allowing the detection of HB_sAg and HAV, it has been shown that both types may be transmitted by transfusion and that at least a third type of hepatitis, NANB hepatitis, exists. NANB hepatitis occurs mostly as posttransfusion hepatitis, although in countries other than the United States, water-borne viruses of the NANB type may be more prevalent.[177] The significance of posttransfusion hepatitis in blood banking is suggested by the fact that 1%–6% of multiply transfused patients of the pre-HB_sAg screening era developed hepatitis as a consequence of transfusion.[178] This incidence did not change dramatically after HB_sAg screening of donors was instituted.[179] The studies mentioned above and those conducted by Okochi and Murakami[180] proved conclusively that the presence of HB_sAg in blood was consistent with the development of hepatitis; however, NANB remained as the main agent (86% of cases) responsible for posttransfusion hepatitis.[181] There is no definitive screening or diagnostic test for NANB hepatitis; therefore, the strategy of using less specific methods, such as serum ALA level determination, has been adopted by some to eliminate potential carriers of NANB hepatitis as donors. Essentially all types of blood units are capable of transmitting hepatitis, including frozen-thawed units.[182] Plasma, cryoprecipitate, and platelets are likewise potentially capable of transmitting hepatitis to recipients. The use of pooled plasma fractions such as fibrinogen has therefore been banned from clinical practice because a high rate of infection develops in recipients of materials obtained from multiple donor pools.[183] Factor VIII and factor IX concentrates have also been implicated in transmitting hepatitis to recipients[184] in as many as 30%–60% of cases.[185] Human albumin is not usually capable of transmitting hepatitis, because in the manufacturing process it is heated to 60° C and then fractionated by chromatography.[186] Occasionally, plasma protein fraction (PPF), which is also heated to 60° C, has been reported to transmit hepatitis; however, this seems to occur when PPF is obtained from pools heavily contaminated with hepatitis virus.[187] It must also be remembered that the minimal dose of virus infective to man is 1×10^6 particles, or 10^{-12} pg. The more sensitive techniques, however, detect only 1×10^9 particles, or 10^{-9} pg/ml of plasma.[188] It is therefore mandatory that blood banks perform screening with the more sensitive third-generation tests; this is an FDA requirement[189] and an AABB standard.[190] The single most important factor in decreasing the incidence of posttransfusion hepatitis, however, has been the careful selection of donors, eliminating those who have a history of jaundice, drug addiction, or other sociopathy.[191] Elimination of commercial blood donors (which increases the risk by 10 times) from the donor pool has also helped remarkably in the decrease of posttransfusion hepatitis, as it has been shown that commercial blood donors have a 10 times greater risk of transmitting hepatitis.[192,193] A donor who has given blood that is subsequently implicated in two cases of hepatitis should be eliminated permanently from the donor pool if the unit was one of several received by the recipient.[70]

Because careful donor selection is still the best preventive measure to reduce transmission of hepatitis, prospective studies are probably more valuable than retrospective studies of cases of clinically apparent hepatitis. This is because subclinical cases are probably missed more frequently in retrospective studies. Up to 60% of cases of posttransfusion hepatitis are seen in recipients of blood from donors with subclinical hepatitis. Nevertheless, prospective studies are more difficult to perform than retrospective studies.

To provide adequate follow-up, hospitals can arrange to get from treating physicians, information regarding the recipients of blood transfusions. All cases of hepatitis must be reported to the patient's private physician, to the infection control committee, and to the health authorities.

Quality Control in Blood Banking Hepatitis Testing

The laboratory area for hepatitis testing should be segregated from all other test areas, and personnel working in this area must not handle blood or blood components for patient care. All waste must be disposed of in sealed, leakproof containers clearly marked with biohazard labels.

Samples from patients with hepatitis are labeled "contaminated" during all phases of testing. When the tests are finished, all potentially contaminated material is disposed of in biohazard, sealed containers.

It is possible that in the future, high-risk personnel such as blood bank technologists may be required to have immunization with an HB vaccine.

Strategy for Donor Recall

When a patient develops hepatitis after multiple transfusions, a rational approach must be adopted, as outlined below, before a massive search for infected donors is launched.[194]

1. Make sure that nonviral causes for jaundice such as anesthetics, thyroid agents, and coumadin therapy are ruled out.

2. If more than 10 units are involved, it will be difficult to eliminate donors from the pool unless a donor has a positive HB_sAg test or a donor develops hepatitis after donation. One should remember that over 80% of cases of posttransfusion hepatitis are caused by NANB hepatitis, for which there is no specific test.

3. In small hospital-based blood banks, the use of a more in-depth evaluation, including assessment of HB_sAg and anti-HB_sAg levels, may be of value in determining the type of hepatitis present and which donor should be eliminated from the pool.[195]

REFERENCES

1. Jawetz E., Melnick J.L., Adelberg E.A.: *Review of Medical Microbiology*, ed. 11. Los Altos, Calif., Lange Medical Publications, 1974, p. 381.
2. Hollinger B.F., Kahn N.C., Oefinger P.E., et al.: Posttransfusion hepatitis type A. *JAMA* 250:2313, 1983.
3. Feinstone S.M., Kapikian A.Z., Purceli R.H.: Hepatitis A: Detection by immune electron microscopy of a virus-like antigen associated with acute illness. *Science* 182:1026, 1973.
4. Hoofnagle J.H.: Symposium: Type A and Type B Hepatitis. *Lab. Med.* 14:705, 1983.
5. Reinhart F., Holmes A.W., Capps R.B., et al.: Studies on the transmission of human viral hepatitis to marmoset monkeys: I. Transmission of disease, serial passage and description of liver lesions. *J. Exp. Med.* 125:673, 1967.
6. Mosely J.W.: The epidemiology of viral hepatitis: An overview. *Am. J. Med. Sci.* 270:253, 1975.
7. Hilleman M.R., Provost P.J., Miller W.J., et al.: Development and utilization of complement fixation and immune adherence tests for human hepatitis A virus and antibody. *Am. J. Med. Sci.* 270:93, 1975.
8. Krugman S.: Viral hepatitis: Overview and historical perspectives. *Yale J. Biol. Med.* 49:199, 1976.
9. Peters R.L.: Viral hepatitis: A pathologic spectrum. *Am. J. Med. Sci.* 270:17, 1975.
10. Carbone J.V., Bandborg L.L., Silverman S.: Alimentary tract and liver, in Krupp M.A., Chatton M.J. (eds.): *Current Medical Diagnosis and Treatment*. Los Altos, Calif., Lange Medical Publications, 1982, p. 387.
11. Lurman A.: Eine Icterusepidemie. *Klin. Wochenschr.* 22:20, 1885.
12. Paul J.R., et al.: Transmission experiments in serum jaundice and infectious hepatitis. *JAMA* 128:911, 1945.
13. Allison A.C., Blumberg B.S.: An immunoprecipitin reaction distinguishing human serum protein types. *Lancet* 1:634, 1961.
14. Blumberg B.S., Alter H.J., Visnich S.: A "new" antigen in leukemia sera. *JAMA* 191:541, 1965.
15. Blumberg B.S., Gersltey B.J.S., Hungerford D.A.: A serum antigen (Australia antigen) in Down's syndrome, leukemia and hepatitis. *Ann. Intern. Med.* 66:924, 1967.
16. Prince A.M.: An antigen detected in the blood during the incubation period of serum hepatitis. *Proc. Natl. Acad. Sci. USA* 60:814, 1968.
17. Maynard J.E., et al.: Experimental infection of chimpanzees with the virus of hepatitis B. *Nature* 237:514, 1972.
18. Committee on Viral Hepatitis of the National Academy of Sciences: WHO Technical Report Series No. 602. Geneva, Switzerland, World Health Organization, 1977.
19. Almeida J., Rubenstein D., Stott E.J.: New antigen antibody systems in Australia-antigen positive hepatitis. *Lancet* 2:1225, 1971.
20. Marx J.L.: Is hepatitis B virus a retrovirus in disguise? *Science* 217:1021, 1982.
21. Almeida J.D., Waterson A.P.: Hepatitis B antigen: An incomplete history. *Am. J. Med. Sci.* 270:105, 1975.
22. Peterson D.L., Paul D.A., Lam J.: Antigenic structure of hepatitis B surface antigen: Identification of the "d" subtype determinant by chemical modification and use of monoclonal antibodies. *J. Immunol.* 132:920, 1984.
23. LeBouvier J., Williams A.: Serotypes of hepatitis B antigen (HBsAg): The problem of "new" determinants as exemplified by "t." *Am. J. Med. Sci.* 270:165, 1975.
24. Courouce A.M., Holland P.V., Muller J.Y., et al. (eds.): *HBs Antigen Subtypes: Proceedings of the Inter-*

national Workshop on HBs Antigen Subtypes. Paris, 1975.
25. Polesky H.F., Hanson M.: Hepatitis B-serologic markers, in Keating L.J. (ed.): *Hepatitis.* Washington, D.C., American Association of Blood Banks, 1981, p. 15.
26. Peterson D.L.: Isolation and characterization of the major protein and glycoprotein of hepatitis B surface antigen. *J. Biol. Chem.* 256:6975, 1981.
27. Purcell R.H.: The hepatitis viruses: An overview and historical perspective, in Szmuness W., et al. (eds.): *Viral Hepatitis: 1981 International Symposium.* Philadelphia, Franklin Institute Press, 1982, p. 3.
28. Tiollais P., Charnay P., Vyas B.N.: Biology of hepatitis B virus. *Science* 213:406, 1981.
29. Tiollais P., Pourcel C., Brechot C., Charnay P., et al.: Structure and expression of the hepatitis B virus genome, in Szmuness W., et al. (eds.): *Viral Hepatitis: 1981 International Symposium.* Philadelphia, Franklin Institute Press, 1982, p. 81.
30. Robinson W.S., Marion P., et al.: The Hepadna virus group: Hepatitis B and related viruses, in Szmuness W., et al. (eds.): *Viral Hepatitis: 1981 International Symposium.* Philadelphia, Franklin Institute Press, 1982, p. 57.
31. Mercereau-Puijalon O., Kourilsky P.: Introns in the chicken ovalbumin gene prevent ovalbumin synthesis in *E. coli* K12. *Nature* 279:647, 1979.
32. Pasek M., Goto T., Gilbert W., et al.: Hepatitis B virus genes and their expression in E. coli. *Nature* 282:575, 1979.
33. Fiers W., Contreras R., Haegeman G., et al.: Complete nucleotide sequence of SV40 DNA. *Nature* 273:113, 1979.
34. Aden D.P., Fogel A., Plotkin S., et al.: Controlled synthesis of HBsAg in a differentiated human liver carcinoma-derived cell line. *Nature* 282:615, 1979.
35. Dubois M.F., Pourcel C., Rousset S. et al.: Excretion of hepatitis B surface antigen particles from mouse cells transformed with cloned viral DNA. *Proc. Natl. Acad. Sci. USA* 77:4549, 1980.
36. Wands J.R., Mann E., Alpert E., et al.: The pathogenesis of arthritis associated with acute hepatitis-B surface antigen-positive hepatitis: Complement activation and characterization of circulating immune complexes. *J. Clin. Invest.* 55:930, 1975.
37. Lee W.M., Reed W.D., Mitchell C.G., et al.: Cell-mediated immunity to hepatitis B surface antigen in blood donors with persistent antigenemia. *Gut* 16:416, 1975.
38. Tomasi T.B., Dattwyler R.J., Murgita R.A., et al.: Immunosuppression by alpha fetoprotein. *Trans. Assoc. Am. Physicians* 88:293, 1975.
39. Hirschman S.Z.: Integrator enzyme hypothesis for replication of hepatitis-B virus. *Lancet* 2:436, 1975.
40. Milich D.R., Leroux-Roels G.G., Louie R.E., et al.: Genetic regulation of the immune response to hepatitis B surface antigen (HBsAg): IV. Distinct H-2-linked Ir genes control antibody responses to different HBsAg determinants on the same molecule and map to the I-A and I-C subregions. *J. Exp. Med.* 159:41, 1984.

41. Smith M.S., Click R.E., Plagemann P.G.W.: Control of mouse hepatitis virus replication in macrophages by a recessive gene on chromosome 7. *J. Immunol.* 133:428, 1984.
42. Edington T.S., Chisiari F.V.: Immunological aspects of hepatitis B virus infection. *Am. J. Med. Sci.* 270:213, 1975.
43. Chisiari F.V., Routenberg J.A., Anderson D.S., et al.: Cellular immune reactivity in HBV-induced liver disease, in Vyas G.N., et al. (eds.): *Viral Hepatitis.* Philadelphia, Franklin Institute Press, 1978, p. 245.
44. Wands J.R., Perrotto J.L., Alpert E., et al.: Cell mediated immunity in acute and chronic hepatitis. *J. Clin. Invest.* 55:921, 1975.
45. Fargion S., Sangalli G., Ronchi G., et al.: Evaluation of T and B lymphocytes in liver infiltrates of patients with chronic active hepatitis. *J. Clin. Pathol.* 32:344, 1979.
46. Dienstag J.L., Bhan A.K., Klingenstein J., et al.: Immunopathogenesis of liver disease associated with hepatitis B, in Szmuness W., et al.: *Viral Hepatitis: 1981 International Symposium.* Philadelphia, Franklin Institute Press, 1982, p. 221.
47. Dudley F.J., Fox R.A., Sherlock S.: Cellular immunity and hepatitis-associated Australia antigen liver disease. *Lancet* 1:723, 1972.
48. Dienstag J.L.: Enhanced in vitro cell-mediated cytotoxicity in chronic hepatitis B virus infection: Absence of specificity for virus-expressed antigen on target cell membranes. *J. Immunol.* 125 2272, 1980.
49. Chisiari F.V., Bieber M.S., Joseph C.A., et al.: Functional properties of lymphocyte subpopulations in hepatitis B virus infection: II. Cytotoxic effector cell killing of targets that naturally express hepatitis B surface antigen and liver specific lipoprotein. *J. Immunol.* 126:45, 1981.
50. Popper H., Schaffner F.: The vocabulary of chronic hepatitis. *N. Engl. J. Med.* 284:1154, 1971.
51. Celis E., Kung P.C., Chang T.W.: Hepatitis B virus-reactive human T lymphocyte clones: Antigen specificity and helper function for antibody specificity. *J. Immunol.* 132:1511, 1984.
52. Kennedy R.C., Melnick J.L., Dreesman G.R.: Antibody to hepatitis B virus induced by injecting antibodies to the idiotype. *Science* 223:930, 1984.
53. Szmuness W., Harley E.J., Ikram H., et al.: Sociodemographic aspects of the epidemiology of hepatitis B, in Vyas G.N., et al. (eds.): *Viral Hepatitis.* Philadelphia, Franklin Institute Press, 1978, p. 297.
54. Redeker A.G.: Advances in clinical aspects of acute and chronic liver disease of viral origin, in Vyas G.N., et al. (eds.): *Viral Hepatitis.* Philadelphia, Franklin Institute Press, 1978, p. 425.
55. Aach R.D.: Clinical manifestations of viral hepatitis, in Keating L.J., Silvergleid A.J.: *Hepatitis.* Washington, D.C., American Association of Blood Banks, 1981, p. 1.
56. Parker, L.F., Murry R.: Relationship of virus dose to incubation time of clinical hepatitis and time of

appearance of hepatitis-associated antigen. *Am. J. Med. Sci.* 263:27, 1972.
57. Krugman S., Giles J.P.: Viral hepatitis: New light on old disease. *JAMA* 212:1019, 1970.
58. Aach R.D., Lander J.J., Sherman L.A., et al.: Transfusion-transmitted viruses: Interim analysis of hepatitis among transfused and non-transfused patients, in Vyas G.N., et al. (eds.): *Viral Hepatitis*. Philadelphia, Franklin Institute Press, 1978, p. 383.
59. Gocke D.J.: Immune complex phenomena associated with hepatitis, in Vyas G.N., et al. (eds.): *Viral Hepatitis*. Philadelphia, Franklin Institute Press, 1978, p. 277.
60. Shusterman N., London W.T.: Editorial retrospective: Hepatitis B and immune complex disease. *N. Engl. J. Med.* 310:43, 1984.
61. Dienstag J.L., Rhodes A.R., Bhan A.K., et al.: Urticaria associated with acute viral hepatitis type B: Studies of pathogenesis. *Ann. Intern. Med.* 89:34, 1978.
62. Alpert E., Isselbacher K.J., Schur P.H.: The pathogenesis of arthritis associated with viral hepatitis: Complement component studies. *N. Engl. J. Med.* 285:185, 1971.
63. Aach R.D., Kahn R.A.: Post-transfusion hepatitis: Current perspectives. *Ann. Intern. Med.* 92:539, 1980.
64. Cooper W.C., Gershon R.K., Sun S.C., et al.: Anicteric viral hepatitis: A clinical pathological follow-up study in Taiwan. *N. Engl. J. Med.* 274:585, 1966.
65. Vandervelde E.M., Goffin C., Megson B., et al.: Users' guide to some new tests for hepatitis B antigen. *Lancet* 2:1066, 1974.
66. Test for hepatitis B surface antigen. *Fed. Reg.* 40:29710, 1975.
67. Ling C.M., Overby L.R.: Prevalence of hepatitis B virus antigen as revealed by direct radioimmune assay with 125 I-antibody. *J. Immunol.* 109:834, 1972.
68. Alter H.J., Holland P.V., Purcell R.H., et al.: The AUSRIA test: Critical evaluation of sensitivity and specificity. *Blood* 42:947, 1973.
69. Gerety R.J., Tabor E., Hoofnagle J.H., et al.: Tests for HBV-associated antigens and antibodies, in Vyas G.N., et al. (eds.): *Viral Hepatitis*. Philadelphia, Franklin Institute Press, 1978, p. 121.
70. Polesky H.F., Hanson M.R.: *Transfusion Associated Hepatitis*. Chicago, American Society of Clinical Pathologists, Check Sample Immunohematology No. 1-107, 1979, p. 5.
71. Miller W.V. (ed.): *Technical Manual of the American Association of Blood Banks*, ed. 5. Washington D.C., American Association of Blood Banks, 1977, p. 259.
72. Linke G.E., Henry B.J.: Clinical pathology: Laboratory medicine, purpose and practice, in Henry B.J. (eds.): *Clinical Diagnosis and Management by Laboratory Methods*. Philadelphia, W.B. Saunders Co., 1984, p. 42.
73. Juji T., Yokochi T.: Hemagglutination technique with erythrocytes coated with specific antibody for detection of Australia antigen. *Jpn. J. Exp. Med.* 39:615, 1969.
74. Szmuness W., Prince A.M., Etling G.F., et al.: Development and distribution of hemagglutinating antibody against the hepatitis B antigen in institutionalized populations. *J. Infect. Dis.* 126:498, 1972.
75. Robinson W.S., Lutwick L.I.: The virus of hepatitis type B. *N. Engl. J. Med.* 295:1168, 1976.
76. Sherlock S.: Predicting the progression of acute type B hepatitis to chronicity. *Lancet* 2:354, 1976.
77. Magnius L.D., Espinar K.J.: New specificities in Australia antigen positive sera distinct from LeBouvier determinants. *J. Immunol.* 109:1017, 1972.
78. Davis D.B., Dulbecco R., Eisen H.N., et al. (eds.): *Microbiology*. New York, Harper & Row, 1980, p. 1221.
79. Norkrans G., Frosner G., Iwarson S.: Determination of HBeAg by radioimmunoassay: Prognostic implications in hepatitis B. *Scand. J. Gastroenterol.* 14:289, 1979.
80. Skinkoj P.: Viral hepatitis in Danish clinical chemistry laboratories 1968-1978: Incidence rates, aetiology and risk factors. *Scand. J. Clin. Lab. Invest.* 40:23, 1980.
81. Rizzetto M., Purcell R.H., Gerin J.L.: Epidemiology of HBV-associated delta agent: Geographical distribution of anti-delta and prevalence in polytransfused HBsAg carriers. *Lancet* 1:1215, 1980.
82. Perillo R.P., Chan K.H., Overby L.R., et al.: Anti-hepatitis B core immunoglobulin M in the serologic evaluation of hepatitis B virus infection and simultaneous infection with type B, delta agent, and non-A, non-B viruses. *Gastroenterology* 85:163, 1983.
83. Angarano G., Monno L., Santantonio T.A., et al.: New principle for the simultaneous detection of total and immunoglobulin M antibodies applied to the measurement of antibody to hepatitis B core antigen. *J. Clin. Microbiol.* 19:905, 1984.
84. Rizzetto, M., Morello C., Mannucci P.M., et al.: Delta infection and liver disease in hemophilic carriers of hepatitis B surface antigen. *J. Infect. Dis.* 145:18, 1982.
85. Koff R.S.: Management of the hepatitis B surface carrier, in *Hepatitis: A Technical Workshop*. Washington, D.C., American Association of Blood Banks, 1981, p. 35.
86. Szmuness W.: Recent advances in the study of the epidemiology of hepatitis B. *Am. J. Pathol.* 81:629, 1975.
87. Krugman S., Giles J.P., Hammon J.: Infectious hepatitis: Evidence for two distinctive clinical epidemiological and immunological types of infection. *JAMA* 200:365, 1967.
88. Murphy B.L., Schreeder M.T., Maynard J.E., et al.: Serological testing for hepatitis B in male homosexuals: Special emphasis on hepatitis Be antigen

and antibody by radioimmune assay. *J. Clin. Microbiol.* 11:301, 1980.
89. Beasley R.P., Trepo C., Stevens C.E., et al.: The e antigen and vertical transmission of hepatitis B antigen. *Am. J. Epidemiol.* 105:95, 1977.
90. Krugman S., Gocke D.J.: *Viral Hepatitis*, vol. XV, in Smith L.H. (ed.): *Major Problems in Internal Medicine*. Philadelphia, W.B. Saunders Co., 1978, p. 27.
91. Blitzer B.L.: Fulminant hepatic failure: A rare but often lethal syndrome. *Postgrad. Med.* 68:153, 1980.
92. Aach R.D.: *Clinical Manifestations of Viral Hepatitis*. Washington, D.C., American Association of Blood Banks, 1900.
93. Aach R.D., Szmuness W., Mosley J.W., et al.: Serum alanine amino transferase of donors in relation to the risk of non-A, non-B hepatitis in recipients: The transfusion-transmitted viruses study. *N. Engl. J. Med.* 304:989, 1981.
94. Gregory P.B., Knauer C.M., Kempson R.L., et al.: Steroid therapy in severe viral hepatitis: A double-blend, randomized trial of methylprednisolone versus placebo. *N. Engl. J. Med.* 294:681, 1976.
95. Karvountzis G.G., Redeker A.G., Peters R.L.: Long-term follow-up of patients surviving fulminant hepatitis. *Gastroenterology* 67:870, 1974.
96. Shirachi R., Shiraishi H., Tateda A., et al.: Hepatitis "C" antigen in non-A, non-B posttransfusion hepatitis. *Lancet* 2:853, 1978.
97. Schreeder M.T., Thompson S.E., Hadler S.C., et al.: Hepatitis B in homosexual men: Prevalence of infection and factors related to transmission. *J. Infect. Dis.* 146:7, 1982.
98. Nielsen J.O., Dietrichson O., Elling P., et al.: Incidence and meaning of persistence of Australia antigen in patients with acute viral hepatitis: Development of chronic hepatitis. *N. Engl. J. Med.* 265:1157, 1971.
99. Knodell R.G., Conrad M.E., Ishak K.G.: Development of chronic liver disease after acute non-A, non-B posttransfusion hepatitis: Role of γ-globulin prophylaxis in its prevention. *Gastroenterology* 72:902, 1977.
100. Scheuer P.J.: Acute and chronic hepatitis revisited: Review by an international group. *Lancet* 2:914, 1977.
101. Chadwick R.G., Galizzi J. Jr., Heathcote J., et al.: Chronic persistent hepatitis: Hepatitis B virus markers and histological follow-up. *Gut* 20:372, 1979.
102. Berman M., Alter H.J., Ishak K.G., et al.: The chronic sequelae of non-A, non-B hepatitis. *Ann. Intern. Med.* 91:1, 1979.
103. Thomas H.C., Brown D., Routheir D., et al.: Inducer and suppressor T-cells in hepatitis B virus induced liver disease. *Hepatology* 2:202, 1982.
104. Alexander G., Williams R.: Characterization of the mononuclear cell infiltrate in piecemeal necrosis (editorial). *Lab. Invest.* 50:247, 1984.
105. London W.T.: Hepatitis B virus and antigen-antibody complex diseases. *N. Engl. J. Med.* 296 1528, 1977.
106. Koff R.S.: Management of the hepatitis B surface antigen carrier, in Keating L.J., Silvergleid A.J. (eds.): *Hepatitis: A Technical Workshop*. Washington, D.C., American Association of Blood Banks, 1981, p. 33.
107. Drueke T., Barbanel C., Jungers P., et al.: Hepatitis B antigen-associated periarteritis nodosa in patients undergoing long-term hemodialysis. *Am. J. Med.* 68:86, 1980.
108. Sergent J.S., Lockshin M.D., Christian C.L., et al.: Vasculitis with hepatitis B antigenemia: Long-term observations in nine patients. *Medicine* 55:1, 1976.
109. Nagy J., Bajtai G., Brasch H., et al.: The role of hepatitis B antigen in the pathogenesis of glomerulonephritis. *Clin. Nephrol.* 12:109, 1979.
110. Takeoshi Y., Tanaka M., Shida N., et al.: Strong association between membranous nephropathy and hepatitis B antigenemia in Japanese children. *Lancet* 2:1065, 1978.
111. Leno Y., Gorevic P.D., Kassab H.J., et al.: Association between hepatitis B virus and essential mixed cryoglobulinemia. *N. Engl. J. Med.* 296:1501, 1977.
112. Mackay I.R., Kronborg I.J., Tait B.D., et al.: Autoantibodies to cytoskeletal proteins and liver membrane in chronic active hepatitis, in Szmuness W., et al. (eds.): *Viral Hepatitis: 1981 International Symposium*. Philadelphia, Franklin Institute Press, 1982, p. 243.
113. Tan A.Y.O., Law C.W., Lee Y.S.: Hepatitis B antigen in the liver cells in cirrhosis and hepatocellular carcinoma. *Pathology* 9:57, 1977.
114. Waterhouse J., Muir C., Correa P., Powell V.: Cancer Incidence in Five Continents, vol. III. Lyon, France, International Agency for Research on Cancer, WHO, 1976.
115. Kew M.C.: In Vyas G.N., et al. (eds.): *Viral Hepatitis*. Philadelphia, Franklin Institute Press, 1978, p. 439.
116. Beasley R.P., Lin C.C., Huang L.Y., et al.: Risk of hepatocellular carcinoma in hepatitis B virus infections: A prospective study in Taiwan, in Szmuness W., et al. (eds.). *Viral Hepatitis: 1981 International Symposium*. Philadelphia, Franklin Institute Press, 1982, p. 261.
117. Brechot C., Nalpas B., Courouce A.M., et al.: Evidence that hepatitis B virus has a role in liver-cell carcinoma in alcoholic liver disease. *N. Engl. J. Med.* 306:1384, 1982.
118. Chalmers T.C.: Treatment of acute infectious hepatitis: Controlled studies of the effects of diet, rest and physical reconditioning on the acute course of the disease and on the incidence of relapses and residual abnormalities. *J. Clin. Invest.* 34:1163, 1955.
119. Gregory P.B., Knauer C.M., Kempson R.L., et al.: Steroid therapy in severe viral hepatitis: A double-blind randomized trial of methylprednisolone versus placebo. *N. Engl. J. Med.* 294:681, 1976.

120. Evans A.S., Nelson R.S., Sprinz H., et al.: Adrenal hormone therapy in viral hepatitis: IV. The effect of gamma globulin and oral cortisone in the acute disease. *Am. J. Med.* 19:783, 1955.
121. Auslander M.O., Gitnick G.L.: Vigorous medical management of acute fulminant hepatitis. *Arch. Intern. Med.* 137:599, 1977.
122. Redeker A.G., Schweitzer I.L., Yamahiro H.S.: Randomization of corticosteroid therapy in fulminant hepatitis. *N. Engl. J. Med.* 294:728, 1976.
123. Guzzard B.G.: Charcoal haemoperfusion in the treatment of hepatitis failure. *Lancet* 1:1301, 1974.
124. Summerskill W.H., Korman M.G., Ammon H.V., Baggenstoss A.H.: Prednisone for chronic liver disease: Titration, standard dose and combination with azathioprine compared. *Gut* 16:305, 1974.
125. Nouri-Aria K.T., Hegarty J.E., Alexander G.J., et al.: Effect of corticosteroids on suppressor-cell activity in "autoimmune" and viral chronic active hepatitis. *N. Engl. J. Med.* 307:1301, 1982.
126. Szmuness W., Stevens C.E., Harley E.J., et al.: Hepatitis B vaccine: demonstration of efficacy in a controlled clinical trial in a high risk population in the United States. *N. Engl. J. Med.* 303:833, 1980.
127. Krugman S., Giles J.P., Hammond J.: Hepatitis virus: Effect of heat on the infectivity and antigenicity of the MS-1 and MS-2 strains. *J. Infect. Dis.* 122:432, 1970.
128. Hilleman M.R., Bertland A.U., Buynak E.B., et al.: Clinical and laboratory studies of HBsAg vaccine, in Vyas G., et al. (eds.): *Viral Hepatitis*. Philadelphia, Franklin Institute Press, 1978, p. 491.
129. Zuckerman A.J.: Hepatitis vaccine: A note of caution. *Nature* 255:104, 1975.
130. Dienstag J.L.: Toward the control of hepatitis B. *N. Engl. J. Med.* 303:874, 1980.
131. Dandoy S., Kirkman-Liff B., Krakowsky F.: Multiple exposure of hospital employees to hepatitis B. *Arch. Intern. Med.* 144:720, 1984.
132. Mulley A.G., Silverstein M.D., Dienstag J.L.: Indicators for use of hepatitis B vaccine, based on cost-effectiveness analysis. *N. Engl. J. Med.* 307:644, 1982.
133. Strom T.B.: Retrospective hepatitis B, transfusions, and renal transplantation: Five years later (editorial). *N. Engl. J. Med.* 307:1141, 1982.
134. Maugh T.H.: FDA approves hepatitis B vaccine. *Science* 214:1113, 1982.
135. Stokes J. Jr., Neeje J.R.: Prevention and attenuation of infectious hepatitis by gamma globulin: Preliminary note. *JAMA* 127:144, 1945.
136. Grady G.F., Rodman M., Larsen L.H.: Hepatitis B antibody in conventional gamma-globulin. *J. Infect. Dis.* 132:474, 1975.
137. Maynard J.E.: Passive immunization against hepatitis B: A review of recent studies and comment on current aspects of control. *Am. J. Epidemiol.* 107:77, 1978.
138. Centers for Disease Control: Recommendations of the Public Health Service Advisory Committee on Immunization: Immune globulins for protection against viral hepatitis. *MMWR* 26(52):441, 1977.
139. Grady G.F., Lee V.A.: Hepatitis B immune globulin: Prevention of hepatitis from accidental exposure among medical personnel. *N. Engl. J. Med.* 293:1067, 1975.
140. Iwarson S., Ahlmen J., Eriksson E., et al.: Hepatitis B immune globulin in prevention of hepatitis B among hospital staff members. *J. Infect. Dis.* 135:473, 1977.
141. Mushahwar I.K., Overby L.R., Frosner G., et al.: Prevalence of hepatitis B antigen and its antibody as detected by radioimmunoassays. *J. Med. Virol.* 2:77, 1978.
142. Alter H.J., Seeff L.B., Kaplan P.M., et al.: Type B hepatitis: The infectivity of blood positive for e antigen and DNA polymerase after needle stick exposure. *N. Engl. J. Med.* 295:909, 1976.
143. Beasley R.P., Hwang L.Y., Lee G.C., et al.: Prevention of perinatally transmitted hepatitis B virus infections with hepatitis B immunoglobulin and hepatitis B vaccine. *Lancet* 2:1099, 1983.
144. Centers for Disease Control: Post exposure prophylaxis of hepatitis B: Recommendation of the Immunization Advisory Committee (ACIP), U.S. Dept. of Health and Human Services. *MMWR* 33:285, 1984.
145. Centers for Disease Control: *MMWR* 25(suppl.):17, 1976.
146. Goldsmith M.F.: Crossing "threshold" of hepatitis B control awaits greater vaccine use. *JAMA* 251:2765, 1984.
147. Alter H.J., Holland P.V., Purcell R.H., et al.: Posttransfusion hepatitis after exclusion of commercial and hepatitis B antigen positive donors. *Ann. Intern. Med.* 77:691, 1972.
148. Alter H.J., Purcell R.H., Holland P.V., et al.: Transmissible agent in non-A, non-B hepatitis. *Lancet* 1:459, 1978.
149. Tabor E., Seeff L.B., Gerety R.J.: Chronic non-A, non-B hepatitis carrier state: Transmissible agent documented in one patient over a six-year period. *Lancet* 2:140, 1980.
150. Alter H.J., Purcell R.H., Feinstone S.M., et al.: Non-A/non-B hepatitis: A review and interim report of an ongoing prospective study, in Vyas G.N., et al. (eds.): *Viral Hepatitis*. Philadelphia, Franklin Institute Press, 1978, p. 359.
151. Ishida N.: Non-A, Non-B hepatitis: An overview, in Szmuness W., et al. (eds.): *Viral Hepatitis: 1981 International Symposium*. Philadelphia, Franklin Institute Press, 1982, p. 275.
152. Shimizu Y.K., Feinstone S.M., Purcell R.H., et al.: Non-A, non-B hepatitis: Ultrastructural evidence for two agents in experimentally infected chimpanzees. *Science* 205:197, 1979.
153. Feinstone S.M., Alter H.J., Dienes H.P., et al.: Studies on non-A, non-B hepatitis in chimpanzees and marmosets, in Szmuness W., et al.: *Viral Hep-*

154. Hantz O., Vitvitski L., Trepo C.: Non-A, non-B hepatitis: Identification of hepatitis-B-like virus particles in serum and liver. *J. Med. Virol.* 5:73, 1980.
155. DeVos R., DeWolf-Peeters C., Vanstapel M.J., et al.: Non-A, non-B hepatitis-like nuclear particles in nonparenchymal cells of the liver. *J. Infect. Dis.* 149:453, 1984.
156. Alter H.J., Holland P.V., Morrow A.G., et al.: Clinical and serological analysis of transfusion-associated hepatitis. *Lancet* 2:838, 1975.
157. Mosley J.W., Redeker A.G., Feinstone S.M., et al.: Multiple hepatitis viruses in multiple attacks of acute viral hepatitis. *N. Engl. J. Med.* 296:75, 1977.
158. Figus A., Blum H.E., DeVirgilis A., et al.: Hepatitis B viral DNA in liver tissues from patients with non-A, non-B hepatitis. *Hepatology* 2:282, 1982.
159. Feinstone S.M., Hoofnagle J.H.: Non-A, maybe-B hepatitis. *N. Engl. J. Med.* 311:185, 1984.
160. Tabor E., Snoy P., Jackson D.R., et al.: Additional evidence for more than one agent of human non-A, non-B hepatitis: Transmission and passage studies in chimpanzees. *Transfusion* 24:224, 1984.
161. Aach R.D., Lander J.J., Sherman L.A., et al.: Transfusion transmitted viruses: Interim analysis of hepatitis among transfused and non-transfused patients, in Vyas G.N., et al. (eds.): *Viral Hepatitis.* Philadelphia, Franklin Institute Press, 1978, p. 383.
162. Tabor E., Peterson D.A., April M., et al.: Transmission of human non-A, non-B hepatitis to chimpanzees following failure to transmit BG agent hepatitis. *J. Med. Virol.* 5:103, 1980.
163. Mori Y., Ogata S., Ata S., et al.: Virus-like particles associated with non-A, non-B hepatitis. *Lancet* 2:317, 1980.
164. Grimand J.A., Peyrols S., Vitvitski L., et al.: Hepatic intranuclear particles in patients with non-A, non-B hepatitis. *N. Engl. J. Med.* 303(14):819, 1980.
165. Gitnick G.: Non-A, non-B hepatitis: Etiology and clinical course. *Lab. Med.* 14:721, 1983.
166. Maugh T.H.: Where is the hepatitis C virus? *Science* 210:999, 1980.
167. Purcell R.H.: Viral hepatitis, in *Current Chemotherapy.* Washington, D.C., International Society of Chemotherapy, American Society for Microbiology, 1978, p. 12.
168. Berman M., Alter H.J., Ishak K.G., et al.: The chronic sequelae of non-A, non-B hepatitis. *Ann. Intern. Med.* 91:1, 1979.
169. Robinson W.S.: The enigma of non A, non B hepatitis. *J. Infect. Dis.* 145:387, 1982.
170. Francis D.P., Maynard J.E.: The transmission and outcome of hepatitis A, B, and non-A, non-B: A review. *Epidemiol. Rev.* 1:17, 1979.
171. Krugman S., Gocke D.J.: *Viral Hepatitis.* Vol. 15 in *Major Problems in Internal Medicine.* Philadelphia, W.B. Saunders Co., 1978, p. 44.
172. Aach R.D., Szmuness W., Mosley J.W., et al.: Serum alanine aminotransferase of donors in relation to the risk of non-A, non-B hepatitis in recipients: The transfusion-transmitted viruses study. *N. Engl. J. Med.* 304:989, 1981.
173. Sherman K.E., Dodd R.Y.: Alanine aminotransferase levels among volunteer blood donors: Geographic variation and risk factors. *J. Infect. Dis.* 145:383, 1982.
174. Hornbrook M.C., Dodd R.Y., Jacobs P., et al.: Reducing the incidence of non-A, non-B posttransfusion hepatitis by testing donor blood for alanine aminotransferase: Economic considerations. *N. Engl. J. Med.* 307:1315, 1982.
175. Molnar I.G., Gitnick G.L.: Carcinoembrionic antigen (CEA): A sensitive test for hepatitis. *Gastroenterology* 73:1235, 1977.
176. Fuks A., Banjo C., Shuster J., et al.: Carcinoembrionic antigen (CEA): Molecular biology and clinical significance. *Biochim. Biophys. Acta* 417:123, 1975.
177. Khuroo M.S., Saleem M., Teli M.R., et al.: Failure to detect chronic liver disease after epidemic non-A, non-B hepatitis. *Lancet* 2:98, 1980.
178. Allen J.G., Sayman W.A.: Serum hepatitis from transfusions of blood. *JAMA* 180:1079, 1962.
179. Walker R.H., in Mollison P.L.: *Blood Transfusion in Clinical Medicine,* ed. 6. Oxford, England, Blackwell Scientific Publications, 1979, p. 617.
180. Okochi K., Murakami S.: Observations on Australia antigen in Japanese. *Vox Sang.* 15:374, 1968.
181. Prince A.M., Grady G.F., Hazzi C., et al.: Long-incubation posttransfusion hepatitis without serological evidence of exposure to hepatitis B virus. *Lancet* 2:241, 1974.
182. Alter H.J., Tabor E., Meryman H.T., et al.: Transmission of hepatitis B virus infection by transfusion of frozen-deglycerolized red blood cells. *N. Engl. J. Med.* 298:637, 1978.
183. Redeker A.G., Hopkins C.E., Jackson B., et al.: A controlled study of the safety of pooled plasma stored in the liquid state at 30 to 32 C for six months. *Transfusion* 8:60, 1968.
184. Snyder E.L. (ed.): *Blood Transfusion Therapy: A Physician's Handbook,* ed. 3. Washington, D.C., American Association of Blood Banks, 1983, pp. 4,5.
185. Oken M.M., Hootkin L., DeJager R.L.: Hepatitis after Konyne administration. *Dig. Dis.* 17:271, 1972.
186. Hoofnagle J.H., Barker L.F., Thiel J., et al.: Hepatitis B virus and hepatitis B surface antigen in human albumin products. *Transfusion* 16:141, 1976.
187. Soulier J.P., Blatix C., Courouce A.M., et al.: Prevention of virus B hepatitis (S H hepatitis). *Am. J. Dis. Child.* 123:429, 1972.
188. Polesky H.F.: Posttransfusion hepatitis: A review and prospectus. *Hum. Pathol.* 2:441, 1971.
189. Test for hepatitis B surface antigen. *Fed. Reg.* 40:29710, 1975.

190. Oberman H.L. (ed.).: *Standards for Blood Banks and Transfusion Services,* ed. 9. Washington, D.C., American Association of Blood Banks, 1978, p. 12.
191. Krugman S., Gocke D.J.: *Viral Hepatitis,* vol. XV, in Smith L.H. (ed.): *Major Problems in Internal Medicine.* Philadelphia, W.B. Saunders Co., 1978, p. 88.
192. Walsh J.H., Purcell R.H., Morrow A.G., et al.: Posttransfusion hepatitis after open-heart operations. *JAMA* 211:261, 1970.
193. Alter H.J., Holland P.V., Purcell R.H., et al.: Posttransfusion hepatitis after exclusion of commercial and hepatitis-B antigen-positive donors. *Ann. Intern. Med.* 77:691, 1972.
194. Schmidt P.J.: Don't jump to conclusions about posttransfusion hepatitis. *Diagn. Med.* Nov./Dec., 1980.
195. Soloway H.B.: Diagnostic decision-making: Interpreting hepatitis profiles. *Diagn. Med.* Jan./Feb., 1980.

13

Acquired Immunodeficiency Syndrome

A RELATIVELY NEW disease termed acquired immunodeficiency syndrome (AIDS) was initially described in 1981.[1,2] It is characterized by a secondary immunodeficiency affecting predominantly T cells and frequently complicated by opportunistic infections and/or tumors such as Kaposi's sarcoma. In many respects the disease is epidemiologically quite similar to HBV hepatitis.

Characteristically, AIDS is a disease wherein previously healthy, often young patients present with nonspecific signs and symptoms (e.g., malaise, fever of unknown origin, marked weight loss, diarrhea, and generalized lymphadenopathy) (Table 13–1), who subsequently develop severe infections with organisms known to be opportunistic (e.g., *Pneumocystis carinii*) or who develop neoplasms such as Kaposi's sarcoma (a disease, until recently, rare [0.05/100,000 per annum], usually present in elderly patients of Mediterranean origin).[4] The full-blown AIDS syndrome is very severe, as reflected by its mortality, which varies from 70% to 100% (Tables 13–2 and 13–3).[5–7]

EPIDEMIOLOGY

In a 1983 review of about 2,000 cases occurring in a span of 2 years, 90% of the cases were in young individuals (ages 20–40). Seventy-one percent were in homosexual males, 7% were in heterosexual females (many of whom were either IV drug abusers or were sexual partners of patients with AIDS), and the remainder were in heterosexual males.[8] IV drug abusers account for about 17% of the cases; in these patients, a history of needle sharing was often found. Eleven percent of the cases were in migrants of Haitian origin. In another study, 1% of AIDS cases were in hemophiliacs requiring factor VIII concentrate therapy.[9]

ANALYSIS OF RISK FACTORS

Homosexual Males

An increased acceptance of homosexuality, accompanied by a greater number of sexually active "functional" homosexual individuals, has occurred in the past 15 years in the United States. In one study, 10% of sexually active homosexuals were "monogamous," whereas 20% were not. Actively "functional" homosexuals accounted for about 15%. These sexual life-style changes are thought to be partially responsible for the current AIDS epidemic among homosexual men.[10] In one study, anal intercourse and multiple sexual partners were demonstrated to be high-risk factors.[11] Trauma to the rectal mucosa has been shown to increase the risk of HBV infection in homosexuals.[12] This finding correlates with the finding of a greater incidence of immune system suppression in recipients of the ejaculate during anal intercourse.[13] Although the cause of immunosuppression in this study was thought to be antisperm antibodies, such antibodies are probably a contributory factor rather than a cause of AIDS. It is now thought that human T

TABLE 13–1.—Frequent Signs and Symptoms of AIDS*

CLINICAL FINDING	% OF CASES
Fever, constant or spiking	100
Candidiasis, oral	100
Weight loss, 10%–30%	90
Chest findings (bilateral pulmonary infiltrates)	65
Malaise	65
Lymphadenopathy	50
Diarrhea, chronic, usually watery	35

*Data obtained from Small et al.[3]

TABLE 13–3.—Mortality From AIDS According to Disease Groups*

DISEASE GROUP	% MORTALITY
KS only	21
PCP only	46
KS and PCP	48

*Data obtained from Jaffe et al.[19] KS, Kaposi's sarcoma; PCC, *Pneumocystis* pneumonia.

lymphocyte virus III (HTLV-III) is a major cause of AIDS. Anti-HTLV-III seropositivity increased from 1% in 1978 to 65% in 1984.[14] The homosexual population in the United States is calculated at 8 million individuals.[11] At least 25% of this population are at risk if the multiple sexual contact risk indicator is used (Table 13–4).

Residence in a Large Metropolitan Area and Sexual Promiscuity

Most of the cases cluster in the larger metropolitan areas such as New York City, Los Angeles, and San Francisco (Table 13–5).[6] In the population of homosexual males with AIDS, there seems to be a preponderance of the disease in persons with multiple sexual partners.[15] This appears to be also true for a group of female patients who develop AIDS and have a history of sexual promiscuity.[16] It is thought that promiscuity is a risk factor of infection rather than a de facto risk factor, as shown in a study of Danish homosexuals: of 78 homosexuals studied, 33% had T4/T8 ratios of less than 1.0. Promiscuity in this group was not a risk factor in itself, but promiscuity plus evidence of travel to the United States represented a 7.7-fold risk factor.[17] These findings support the hypothesis of an infectious agent as the cause of AIDS.

Intravenous Drug Abuse

Nonhomosexual males with AIDS have been identified mostly in another risk group, namely IV drug abusers,[9] especially those with a history of needle sharing. In a recent study of New York City prison inmates, 14 heterosexual inmates developed AIDS. All had a history of IV drug abuse prior to imprisonment.[18] This study helped assess true incubation periods for AIDS related to IV drug abuse, setting it at a mean of 22 ± 9.6 months. Interestingly, the incidence of Kaposi's sarcoma in homosexual men with AIDS is about 45%, whereas it is less than 5% in heterosexual men with AIDS.[19]

Intimate (Sexual and Nonsexual) Contact With Patients With AIDS

Female sexual partners of patients with AIDS or AIDS prodrome have also been reported to develop the syndrome,[20] and their children appear to be at risk, as has been shown by reports of infants born to patients with AIDS or AIDS prodrome who developed AIDS.[16] In one study, 16 mothers of 22 infants with AIDS or AIDS-related complex (ARC) were followed up for 30 months. Fifteen had abnormal T4/T8 ratios but were otherwise well on initial study. AIDS developed in five of the mothers, and AIDS-related complex in seven. Of 12 pregnancies

TABLE 13–2.—AIDS Outcome in NYC (1981–1984)*

OUTCOME	NO. (%)
Total no. of cases studied	1,319
Lost to follow-up	254 (19)
Died during initial hospitalization	136 (14)
Died since first reported	731 (69)
Alive since first reported	331 (30)
Spent > 30% of time hospitalized	484 (59)
Spent > 50% of time hospitalized	332 (40)
Ambulatory	(77)
Continued working	(14)
Received home care	(3)
Developed PCP + other infection	(57)
Developed PCP alone	(32)
Developed KS + PCP or other infection	(35)
Developed KS alone	(22)
Developed KS + PCP	(5)
Median survival with KS alone: 125 wk	
Median survival with KS + infection: 65 wk	
Median survival with PCP + other infection: 48 wk	

*Figures obtained from Evatt et al.[26]

TABLE 13-4.—AIDS RISK FACTORS

RISK FACTOR	COMMENT
Male homosexuality	Most cases (> 70%) are in male homosexuals.
Sexual promiscuity	Would increase the chance of contact with causative agent (virtually certain to be infectious) as well as complicating infections (e.g., CMV). Also true for female prostitutes.
Anal intercourse	Recipients of ejaculate at higher risk. As for hepatitis, rectal mucosal laceration increases the chances of infection.
High-density populations	Metropolitan areas, with increased risk of contact.
Frequent intimate contact	Spouses of patients with AIDS developing AIDS; children of patients with AIDS developing AIDS.
IV drug abusers	Explains presence of AIDS in many heterosexual cases. Direct introduction of agent into bloodstream. More frequent in persons sharing needles.
Hemophiliacs	Those receiving factor VIII concentrates obtained from pools, which would increase likelihood of transmission.
Blood transfusion recipients	Especially those exposed to multiple transfusions (e.g., open heart surgery).
Health professionals	Needle stick from AIDS patient? (Very rare)
Haitians	Probably due to presence of HTLV in Caribbean basin; or belonging to other risk groups mentioned above.
HLA-DR5 and HLA-Bw35	Increased risk for Kaposi's sarcoma.

in 11 mothers subsequent to the initial pregnancy prompting the study, four infants developed AIDS. This study shows that AIDS can be transmitted to infants who have not received blood transfusions and that mothers may harbor the disease and transmit it to infants of subsequent pregnancies.[21]

Spouses of seven men with AIDS or AIDS-related complex were studied for the presence of anti-HTLV-III antibody titers. Five were positive for HTLV-III exposure, and three had evidence of AIDS-related complex. Eleven of their children were studied; only one 17-month-old child was HTLV-III seropositive. This study showed that sexual contact is an effective means for transmission of HTLV-III, but close household contact (e.g., children) is not an effective means of HTLV-III transmission.[22]

Patients Receiving Blood, Blood Components, or Blood Products

Hemophiliacs receiving factor VIII concentrates have been reported to develop AIDS in several recent publications.[23, 24] Hemophiliacs treated with cryoprecipitate are at a lower risk of developing the disease.[25]

More than 85% of 21 hemophilia A patients who received factor VIII concentrate in 1981–1984 revealed seroconversion to HTLV-III/LAV p25 and p41 proteins. These findings reveal simultaneous seroconversion with the outbreak of the AIDS epidemic in 1981.[26]

In a study of 41 spouses of hemophiliacs with reversed T4/T8 ratios, no cases of AIDS were found.[27] Rarely, AIDS is found in the spouses of hemophiliacs with AIDS.[28] Occasionally, multiply

TABLE 13-5.—INCIDENCE OF AIDS: CDC 1983 CENSUS*

AREA OF THE WORLD	NO. OF CASES
United States	2,374
New York	(41%)
San Francisco	(12%)
Miami	(4.5%)
Los Angeles	(7%)
Other	(33%)
Western Europe	44
Haiti	36
Canada	5
Africa	2
South America	2
Mexico	2
Asia	1
Australia	1

*Modified from Drotman and Curran.[160]

transfused patients may develop AIDS.[29] The finding that AIDS can develop in patients who received blood or blood products from donors who had AIDS prodrome or overt cases of AIDS strongly suggests horizontal transmission, transplacental infection as evidenced in AIDs-affected children born to mothers with AIDs suggests vertical transmission. Transfusion-associated AIDS cases now account for 1% of all cases of AIDS.

Haitians

Although Haitians may be considered to be a high-risk group, it has recently been shown that the epidemiology of AIDS in the Haitian population may be similar to that of the U.S. population; that is, many Haitians with AIDS may come from high-risk groups (i.e., male homosexuals, IV drug abusers, and sexually promiscuous individuals).[30] In addition, a recent study shows that Haitians who have emigrated to the United States and who do not belong to other high-risk groups do not show an altered immune system.[31] The data appear to be biased against Haitians because of the unreliability of the clinical history regarding homosexual activity in Haitians with AIDS, because homosexuality is considered a social stigma in that country.[32] It must also be noted that Haiti is an important vacation resort used by homosexual groups.[33]

Another factor against considering Haitians a high-risk group per se is the lack of significant levels of anti-HTLV-III in these patients,[34] although the possibility that a different virus, such as the African swine fever virus (ASFV), which appears to be more prevalent in Haiti, cannot at this point be excluded as a different agent of AIDS.[35]

INCIDENCE AND ETIOLOGY OF AIDS

The search for the specific agent or agents causing AIDS has been a difficult one for a number of reasons. Multiple close exposures to patients with the disease appear to be necessary, such as would occur in sexual intercourse; therefore, the infectivity of the agent is probably low. However, at least 70 new cases every month were reported in 1983.[36] As of March 1985, 8,697 cases have been reported to the CDC, revealing yearly doubling numbers; if the current trend is not modified, 40,000 cases are forecast by the end of 1986.[37] The incubation period seems to be very long (i.e., 1–2 years) before the full-blown disease is apparent.

Although a number of viruses have been suspected as etiologic agents, such as CMV, EBV, herpes viruses,[6] and ASFV,[35] more recent studies point to the human T cell leukemia-lymphoma virus as the direct etiologic agent for this disease.[38] The basis to consider HTLV as the most likely agent stems from the studies of Gallo et al.[38,39] and Essex et al.[40] In these studies, HTLV was isolated from tissues of patients suffering from the disease. Proviral HTLV DNA[39] as well as antibodies to HTLV[40] were described in patients with AIDS and in patients with AIDS-related complex. It must be cautioned, however, that other viruses may also be the cause of this disease, and more data are necessary before these other possibilities can be excluded.

The HTLV Viruses

Of the three known varieties of HTLV (HTLV-I, II, and III), HTLV-III is the causative agent of AIDS. HTLV viruses belong to the family of retroviridae or retroviruses. These viruses are exclusively composed of RNA but are capable of inducing synthesis of proviral double-stranded DNA via reverse transcription.[41] Retroviridae can be (1) spuma viridae (nononcogenic, nontransforming), (2) lentiviridae, or slow viruses, or (3) oncoviridae, or oncogenic viruses. RNA retroviruses are comprised of virions of about 100 nm in diameter, composed of the following:

1. "env" (envelope) proteins derived from infected cell membrane proteins.
2. "gag" proteins (shell).
3. Core, composed of 1x RNA molecule with a 5' cap and a poly A tail at the 3' end. A tRNA "primer" molecule is linked to the genomic viral RNA.
4. Onc sequences may be present in some retroviruses, but no oncogenes have, to date, been found in HTLV. Morphologically, these viruses can be type A (intracellular, noninfectious); type B (excentric core, often carcinogenic); type C (central core, often oncogenic); or type D (intracellular or extracellular). Since HTLV are C-type oncoviruses, a short description of C-type viruses is germaine. C-type viruses can be exogenous or endogenous. HTLV is presumably of the exogenous type. HTLV viruses can be HTLV-I, II, or III. These viruses have been associated with mycosis fungoides (MF), Sézary syndrome, T cell leukemia,[41] and AIDS.

Replication of RNA Tumor Viruses[41]

Replication of RNA retroviruses can be summarized as follows: (1) viral attachment to cellular peplomer glycoprotein, followed by (2) RNA replication. RNA replication takes place in the following manner:

1. Minus DNA strand copy, via reverse transcriptase induced by the tRNA primer.
2. First DNA segment is a "strong stop" segment; by a "molecular jump" it is transferred from the 5' end of one chain of RNA dimer to the 3' end of the other strand of the RNA dimer binding to the R or repeat sequence.
3. Synthesis of the "strong stop" or plus DNA segment.
4. The end product is a 2x DNA provirus with one long terminal repeat (LTR) (Fig 13–1) at each end synthesized by duplication of a segment of the viral RNA.[42] LTRs have relatively constant base sequences and pose an advantage to retroviruses in that during insertion, some base sequences are known to be lost; but they are thought to be expendable sequences due to their homogeneity.[41] LTRs are important to proviral DNA in that (1) They play a crucial role in insertion to host genomic DNA. (2) They contain TATA sequences, termed "TATA boxes," which are important to binding of reverse transcriptase. (3) They contain the signal for poly-A activation and the 5' cap addition. (4) They contain minus DNA (U5) initiation sequences as well as plus DNA (U3) initiation sequences.

Between two LTR regions lie the translational sequences of DNA provirus, as shown in the leukosis retrovirus.

1. Gag and pol gene sequences translate via 35S mRNA into gag-pol polyprotein (MW-180) which on cleavage liberates Pr130, removal of a p15 segment results in the formation of the β subunit of reverse transcriptase. p15 itself is a viral protease. In addition, the removal of the carboxy terminal portion of the β subunit forms the α subunit and a p32 endonuclease.

It should be noted that sequence similarities exist in various retroviruses as shown for region I-III of HBV and the center of the polymerase of cauliflower mosaic virus (CaMV), and region V, which has homology in RSV and HTLV viruses.[43]

2. p63^{env} results from translation of env genes into 25S mRNA, which give rise by cleavage in the endoplasmic reticulum to pr92^{env}, generating viral envelope glycoproteins.

3. Host-derived oncogenes code for 22S mRNA. Many oncogenes have cell-promoting properties, as shown in the SRC-Rous sarcoma oncogene, which codes for products with tyrosine phosphorilase properties which induce intracellular influx of calcium stimulating host protein kinase C.[44] Although no onc genes have been identified in HTLV, a newly defined region, the X region, may have transforming capabilities on infected cells. Both HTLV-I and HTLV-II contain genes gag, pol, env, and the X region, in that sequence. The X region is a 3' terminal segment which codes for a 40-kilodalton protein, a transforming protein.[45]

This protein, termed p42 antigen, is coded for in LOR, a conserved portion of the X region flanked by env genes and LTR. It is possible that p42 is responsible for the transforming properties of HTLV-I.[46]

Mutagenic and Cytopathic Effects of Retroviruses

Proviruses have two properties that suggest mutagenic activity: (1) Since they can insert at several sites in the genome they may, by doing so, inactivate a gene. (2) These viruses also possess regulatory sequences capable of affecting the behavior of host genes and gene products.[41] These viruses have been associated with leukemias and lymphomas.[47] In ad-

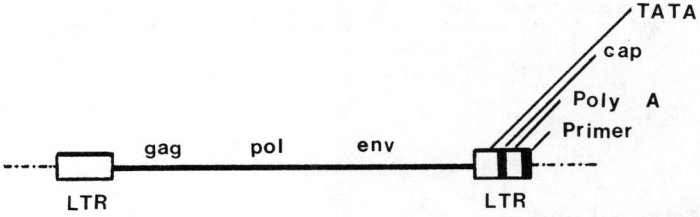

FIG 13–1.—Diagram of a retroviral genome. Note that the genome segment is flanked by two long terminal repeat sequences *(LTR)*. Each *LTR* contains *TATA* sequences, a signal for Poly A activation, a 5' cap, and DNA primer sequences. Genes coded by the genome are thought to occur in sequence: *gag* genes that code for shell proteins, *pol* genes that code for polymerase proteins, and *env* genes that code for envelope proteins.

dition, retroviruses are capable of producing a variety of diseases in animals, characteristically after prolonged incubation periods. It is now known that stretches of viral homology which derive from highly conserved stretches in the host and are host species–specific are capable of cell growth induction. These stretches are termed onc genes, or oncogenes, and can be identified in so-called acute leukemia viruses. These sequences can likewise be activated by chronic leukemia viruses. Nevertheless, of interest to HTLV retroviruses, frequently found oncogenes such as ras^N, ras^H, ras^K, v-sis, v-src, and v-fes have not, to date, been identified in this virus family. In spite of the lack of evidence for an oncogene in HTLV, T cells infected in culture with HTLV-I are capable of dividing and retaining their T helper cell characteristics in vitro, without the addition to the culture of accessory cells.[48]

DNA from an AIDS patient with Kaposi's sarcoma, transfected into NIH 3T3 cells in culture, caused transformation of the 3T3 cells. These cells injected into nude mice were able to produce widely metastatic Kaposi sarcoma–like tumors.[49] HTLV-III has special characteristics of concern to an explanation for the etiology of AIDS: it is tropic for T4 helper cells; it is a cytopathic virus and may be a transforming virus. Cytopathic effects of HTLV-III can be prevented in vitro by the addition to the culture of Suramin. Apparently, Suramin somehow blocks the entrance of the virus into the cells.[50]

Pathogenic role of HTLV Viruses

Although the precise mechanism by which HTLV induces pathology in the cell is not known in detail, it has been demonstrated that HTLV-I is capable of inducing T cell leukemia,[51] and HTLV-II is associated with the induction of lymphoid neoplasms.[52]

Both HTLV-I and HTLV-II have considerable homology at LTR, gag, pol, and env base stretches. A high degree of homology between HTLV-I but especially of HTLV-II and HTLV-III is suspected. This may cause difficulty in defining the presence of HTLV-III and the other two HTLV viruses.[53] Strong evidence that HTLV-III is the prime candidate for the initiating viral agent in AIDS is the demonstration that serum from patients with AIDS and AIDS-related complex recognizes sequences of HTLV-III, as demonstrated by the Western blotting gel chromatography technique (Fig 13–2).[54] The phenotypic gene products of HTLV-I, II, and III also bear homology. For instance, newly expressed proteins of viral origin, p65, p55, p41, p39, p32, and p24, have been identified by Southern blotting by reacting AIDS serum against HTLV-III isolates obtained from immortalized T cell clones (Table 13–6).[55] It appears that the p65 env band represents a viral envelope glycoprotein.[55] In addition, HTLV-III viral products have been isolated from serum samples of 18 of 21 patients with pre-AIDS, 26 of 72 adult and juvenile AIDS patients, and none of 115 controls.[56] About 88% of serum samples of patients with AIDS and 79% of serum samples from homosexual males revealed antibodies against HTLV-III, compared to 1% of serum samples from heterosexual males.[57] It appears that HTLV-III and the "lymphadenopathy virus" (LAV), first described by Montagnier, et al.[58] are the same virus.[59]

In a recent study using ELISA and Western blot

TABLE 13–6.—Comparison of HTLV Proteins From Infected Permissive T Cell Clones*

HTLV-I		HTLV-II		HTLV-III	
Precursor	Mature	Precursor	Mature	Precursor	Mature
Viral Isolates					
$p54^{gag}$	$p24^{wk}$	p55?	p24	$p55^{gag?}$	p24/23(st)
		p48			p48?
Cell Culture					
	p42	p42			p39
		p41?			p41(st)
		p39?			p24
	$wrp65^{env}$	$wrp65^{env}$			$rp65^{env}$
	p61	p61			p61

*Data from references 38–46. Rabbit antiserum against HTLV-III viruses shows greater reactivity with HTLV-II isolates, suggesting similarity between II and III (e.g., crossreactive p. 55).

Abbreviations: wr, weak reactivity; r, reactive; st, structural protein; gag, gag gene product; env, envelope.

analysis, 10 patients with AIDS and 10 patients with AIDS-related complex were all antibody positive for HTLV-III, as were 37 of 103 IV drug abusers, 4 of 40 healthy homosexuals, and 7 of 83 patients with various types of hepatitis, but none of 83 blood donors. Anti-p24 was detected in HTLV-III seropositive pre-AIDS patients and high-risk individuals but was very low in AIDS patients, whereas anti-p41 was only present in patients with AIDS and pre-AIDS but was absent in 10% of seropositive individuals. Thus anti-p24 may well become the screen for pre-AIDS, whereas anti-p41 may be useful for the diagnostic workup of patients with AIDS and AIDS-related complex.[60]

Transmission of HTLV-III has been demonstrated experimentally by transfusing plasma from patients with AIDS or AIDS-related complex to chimpanzees, which subsequently developed anti-HTLV antibodies as well as inverted T4/T8 ratios and lymphadenopathy.[61] Conversely, a type D retrovirus has recently been isolated that arises spontaneously in monkeys and causes the simian AIDS syndrome (SAIDS).[62]

Other Viruses Associated With AIDS

Although it is possible for other viruses to be the etiologic agents of AIDS, these are most probably opportunistic invaders rather than direct causes for the T cell defect. The following must be considered:

1. Epidemiologically, AIDS appears to be a new disease.
2. The viruses proposed have been identified for a long time (e.g., CMV, EBV), making them the primary etiologic agents of a "new" disease unlikely.
3. However, most studies have not analyzed the appearance of either HTLV, CMV, or EBV simultaneously.
4. Truly prospective studies have not been performed.
5. HTLV appears to have special tropism for T4 (helper) cells, with subsequent cytopathic effect on helper T cells.

Since these issues have not been fully elucidated, the data regarding other viruses must be considered here.

In one study, 11 of 30 healthy homosexual men secreted CMV in urine and semen. Eight of 11 CMV "shedders" had IgM anti-CMV antibodies and antibodies against T cell subsets. Only one of 19 "nonshedders" had positive IgM anti-CMV antibodies. No correlation between T4/T8 ratios was noted between CMV "shedders" and "nonshedders" in this study.[63]

Of 419 homosexuals studied, only 7% were seronegative for CMV, and of 644 sexually active homosexuals, only 2% were seronegative for CMV.[64] In a study of 89 sexually active male homosexuals with a history of sodomy, 96% had antibodies to CMV, whereas 94% had antibodies against EBV. Twelve percent of these patients had low T4/T8 ratios, 18% had increased T8, and 3% had T4 cell deficiency.[65]

In another study, 29 of 161 homosexual men (18%) excreted CMV in the urine, compared to 3 of 77 men (4%). In these 29 patients, T4/T8 ratios were depressed (1.13 ± 0.09).[66]

In addition, a separate study showed that multiple CMV infections may presumably cause or complicate a state of immunodeficiency in male homosexual hosts.[67]

Other possible contributory factors in determining the outcome of AIDS may be the effect of cyclosporin immunosuppression on T cells. This substance is found in many strains of fungi frequently found in homosexuals.[68] Nevertheless, the report of cyclosporin in plasma of patients with AIDS has been contested, and today it is believed not to be present in most cases.[69]

PATHOGENESIS AND PATHOLOGY

Viruses such as HTLV are known to inhibit or delete T cell function. T helper cells are essential to an adequate immune response through their cell-cell interaction with effector cells (i.e., cytotoxic lymphocytes or B cells) (see Chap. 4). It is in this way that the immune deficiencies in patients with AIDS have been explained to the present.[70]

The Immunologic Lesion in AIDS: A Working Hypothesis

It has been shown that a direct tropism of HTLV-III or other retroviruses for T4 helper cells exists, with a subsequent specific deletion of T helper cells. It is also possible that a second virus such as EBV then induces a hyperactive B lymphocyte population with inadequate responsiveness to mitogen stimulation.[71] This finding correlates with the frequent finding of a nonspecific increase in most γ-globulins.[72] Enhanced B cell reactivity may be responsible for some of the autoimmune phenomena observed in patients with AIDS, where antibodies to both platelets and cell nuclei have been observed.[73] Furthermore, patients with AIDS and pre-AIDS have antilymphocyte antibody in 61% of cases; some of these antibodies may be reactive against T4 or T8 subsets.[74] However, enhanced B cell responses may be seen in AIDS patients, though the actual qualitative B cell responses are disrupted, as shown in a study in which 18 patients with AIDS were immunized with PPS pneumococcal polysaccharide and keyhole-limpet hemocyanin (KLH). These patients had abnormally low responses to both B cell and T cell antigens.[75] In addition, CMV, also prevalent in these cases, has specific tropism for endothelial cells and may well be responsible for neoplastic proliferation of endothelial cells, with development of Kaposi's sarcoma, which in itself may develop unchecked by the immune system due to a lack of normal T cell function.[76] In addition, acquisition of EBV by AIDS patients may well be followed by the development of lymphomas, which in cases of AIDS have been thought to be associated with EBV.[77] Interestingly, both Kaposi's sarcoma and B cell lymphomas occur more frequently in other immunosuppressed patients, such as transplant recipients.[73]

AIDS associated with opportunistic infections (AIDS-OI) is in many respects different from AIDS associated with Kaposi's sarcoma (AIDS-KS). For instance, in AIDS-OI there is an absolute decrease of T helper cells, whereas in AIDS-KS there is an absolute increase in suppressor cells.[70]

Natural killer (NK) cell activity is markedly depressed, probably secondary to the vigorous suppressor T cell presence in cases of AIDS or pre-AIDS lymphadenopathy.[78] The production of γ-interferon (γ-IFN) by pre-AIDS NK cells may be a reflection of initial viral infection.[79] NK cells have been shown to produce γ-IFN on viral stimulation.[80] α-IFN however, has been noted to be decreased in AIDS patients who are known to produce 100 IU or less.[81] γ-IFN may likewise be decreased in advanced cases. This was shown by assessing production of γ-IFN: 10 of 11 patients with AIDS did not generate effective lymphokine responses on mitogen stimulation; 11 of 16 patients produced abnormal levels. None of 14 patients studied produced lymphokines after stimulation with specific microbial antigens.[82] Nevertheless, γ-IFN production may be induced by incubating AIDS patient cells with T cell growth factors.[83] Another group reported decrements of γ-IFN in 16 "healthy" homosexual men.[84] A profound decrement in the ability to respond to B cell and T cell mitogens has likewise been observed in AIDS-OI and AIDS-KS patients. This decrement was for both phytohemoagglutinin (PHA) as well as for concanavalin A (ConA).[84] Other less specific markers of immunity such as β_2-microglobulin are likewise abnormal. β_2-microglobulin was found to be elevated in 24 patients with AIDS and in 2 of 40 asymptomatic male homosexuals who later developed AIDS.[56]

Other Abnormalities of the Immune System

Though macrophage functions do not appear to be altered in patients with AIDS, as assessed by ingestion of IgG-coated RBCs (personal observation), the killing capability of macrophages in AIDS is impaired, as shown in infections with *Mycobacterium avium-intracellulare*.[6] In addition, epidermal antigen presenting cells such as Langerhans cells have decreased Ia antigens and decreased ATPase activity.[85]

Thymosin α_1 levels are reported to be abnormally high in patients with AIDS and pre-AIDS, compared to elevations in only 2% of the normal population.[86] Finally, other less specific changes, such as defective polymorphonuclear functions, have also been reported in homosexuals with persistent lymphadenopathy.[87]

HISTOPATHOLOGY OF TISSUES FROM AIDS PATIENTS

Aside from the pathology induced by infections and tumors present in these patients, there appear to be consistent pathologic findings in the lymph nodes of patients with AIDS or AIDS prodrome who do not have opportunistic infections. These findings in lymph nodes are: markedly enlarged, irregular germinal centers containing abundant nuclear debris, focal necrosis with neutrophils, and focal areas of hemorrhage. In contrast, patients who are infected with opportunistic organisms have mostly atrophic germinal centers, fibrosis, and proliferation of blood vessels in the germinal centers.[88] A persistent lymphadenopathy as the only symptom has also been observed in some patients from high-risk groups (e.g., homosexual males, IV drug abusers, or Haitians). This type of disease is the so-called prodrome of AIDS, also termed AIDS-related complex. In these cases, an atypical follicular hyperplasia with multinucleated lymphoid cells but with preservation of lymph sinusoids has been observed. A peppering of neutrophils and plasma cells is likewise noted.[89] Lymph node planimetry in many of these cases reveals decreased T4/T8 ratios.[90] In many of these cases, cell suspensions of lymph nodes quantitated by flow cytometry showed decreased T4/T8 ratios; however, the values were not entirely correlative with peripheral blood T4/T8 values.[91] In bone marrow biopsies, there appears to be a distinctive AIDS pattern, where hematopoietic cells (often immature) separate the fat cells individually.[92] In children with AIDS, the thymus gland may appear depleted of Hassal's corpuscles as well as of lymphocytes.[93]

The physiopathology of diarrhea in patients with AIDS may be related to a Whipple's disease–like syndrome.[94] Interestingly, patients with AIDS who have presented with life-threatening infections with *Mycobacterium avium-intracellulare* showed unusual small bowel lesions with foamy macrophages resembling those found in Whipple's disease.[95] These foamy macrophages were seen infiltrating the intestinal mucosa as well as the regional lymph nodes. The authors of this study suggest that the diarrhea so often found as one of the symptoms of AIDS may be due to this Whipple-like syndrome. Furthermore, an immunodeficiency state is also found in Whipple's disease,[96] making a correlation of physiopathology, albeit not of direct etiology, between these two diseases quite plausible. It should be added here that disseminated infections with *M. avium-intracellulare* is not uncommon in populations at risk for AIDS.[97] For autopsy findings in AIDS see Table 13–7.

Ultrastructural Changes

At the electron microscopic level, the major finding in lymphocytes of patients with AIDS is the tubuloreticular structure, which consists of a 20- to 30-nm tubular structure within the cysterns of the smooth endoplasmic reticulum.[98] Other structures are the vesicular rosette, also described in lymphocytes of patients with AIDS,[99] and a rod-shaped structure.[100] It has been suggested that these rosettes are possibly infective particles, or degenerative changes of lympholysis.[98] Rosette-type structures have also been described in poorly fixed material and may not be a specific finding for AIDS.[101] Rather, test tube–like structures have been reported in lymph nodes from homosexuals and drug addicts examined by electron microscopy.[101, 102] These structures are similar to those described in lymphocytes of patients with the Japanese variety of the T cell virus-associated adult T cell leukemia.[103] Furthermore, other authors have found rosette-like structures in cells obtained from amniocentesis and cultured, which eventually showed other degenerative changes.[104]

TABLE 13–7.—AUTOPSY FINDINGS IN PATIENTS WITH AIDS*

FINDING	NO. (%) OF PTS.
Total cases	36
Multiple OI	35
Respiratory tract	(64%)
Meninges	(11%)
Organism:	
C. albicans	(81%)
CMV	25 (69%)
PCP	23
Kaposi's sarcoma	18 (50%)
Metastatic	10 (28%)
Confined to skin	8 (22%)
Lymphoma	4 (11%)

*Data from Welch et al.[161] OI, opportunistic infections; CMV, cytomegalovirus; PCP, *Pneumocystis carinii* pneumonia.

CLINICAL PRESENTATION OF PATIENTS WITH AIDS

AIDS usually manifests in one or a combination of three clinical patterns, as described below.

Type I

Patients with type I disease have fever of unknown origin (constant or episodic and spiking to up to 39° C), diarrhea (usually associated with malabsorption, and evidence of a histopathologic process with lymphocytic infiltration in the lamina propria of the small intestine and colon[105]), weight loss (20%–30% of body weight), malaise, lymphadenopathy for weeks or months, often complicated by oral candidiasis, and no history of steroid or antibiotic therapy. This is termed AIDS prodrome.[106, 107]

Type II

The above signs and symptoms plus a severe infection (e.g., abscess formation, pneumonia) with an opportunistic infectious agent such as *Pneumocystis carinii*, disseminated tuberculosis, or atypical mycobacterial infection in the absence of a known cause for diminished resistance to these diseases constitutes the full-blown syndrome of AIDS (see Table 13–1). Other diseases presenting without a clear-cut explanation for the presence of immunosuppression that have likewise been outlined by the CDC as possibly constituting part of the AIDS syndrome are:

1. Pneumonia, meningitis, encephalitis, or esophagitis caused by viruses such as CMV or herpes simplex; bacteria such as atypical mycobacteria, *Nocardia, Aspergillus, Zygomycosis;* or parasitic diseases such as amebiasis, strongiloidiasis, or toxoplasmosis.

2. Unusually severe mucocutaneous herpes simplex of more than a month's duration.

3. Chronic enterocolitis longer than a month, due to cryptosporidiosis with or without accompanying interstitial pneumonia.[108]

4. Disseminated or CNS infections with histoplasmosis, cryptococcosis, or coccidiomycosis.

5. Other unusual diseases such as progressive leukoencephalopathy and lymphoma limited to the brain[109] in young, previously healthy individuals belonging to high-risk groups for AIDS.[110]

Disseminated infections with *Listeria monocytogenes* or with *Nocardia asteroides,* which are often seen in immunosuppressed patients, are not often seen in patients with AIDS.[110]

Type III

The patient presents with an insidious set of symptoms and develops Kaposi's sarcoma of the invasive type with lymph node and intestinal involvement.[5] Less frequently, advanced AIDS patients may develop Hodgkin's[111] or non-Hodgkin's lymphomas[112] or other tumors, frequently in the oral cavity or the anus. Other complications such as autoimmune thrombocytopenic purpura have also been described in these patients.[113] Persistent generalized lymphadenopathy alone in individuals of AIDS high-risk groups has also been described[114] and is often punctuated by oral candidiasis, which may be a harbinger of full-blown AIDS in up to 50% of cases of AIDS;[115] esophageal candidiasis should also be searched for.[116] Dermatomal herpes is likewise seen in this so-called AIDS-related complex.

OTHER COMPLICATIONS FOUND IN AIDS

About 50% of patients with AIDS have proteinuria, and about 10% develop nephrosis. Acute renal insufficiency developed in 14 of 75 patients in one study.[117] In another group, 11 of 92 patients developed the nephrotic syndrome. Six of the 11 patients did not have a history of IV drug abuse; hence nephrosis was probably directly associated with AIDS.[118] It is possible that some of the nephrotic lesions are secondary to immune complexes found in certain cases of AIDS.[119]

LABORATORY FINDINGS

The main laboratory test that supports the diagnosis of AIDS is a recently introduced ELISA screen for HTLV-III; however confirmatory test by a Western blot electrophoresis must be performed in positive cases. Other tests to help in the diagnosis of AIDS are at best nonspecific. Nevertheless, the diagnosis can be achieved by combining the clinical history, findings on physical examination, and results of other laboratory tests such as T4/T8 ratios. T helper (inducer) and T suppressor (cytotoxic) cells are assessed by monoclonal antibodies against T4 (Leu-3) and T8 (Leu-2) antigens, respectively. These antigens are usually assessed by immunofluorescence, and their assay is an important test in the assessment of the disease. Normally, a 2:1 ratio exists between T4 (helper) and T8 (suppressor) cells. In bona fide AIDS cases, this ratio is frequently inverted (e.g., 0.01 to 0.30). Nevertheless, AIDS-related complex should be suspected if T4/T8 ratios fall to .75 to 1.1.[15, 120] Lymphocyte stimulation tests reveal 10%–50% of normal values.[121]

One should remember that these test results are frequently altered in patients who are immunosuppressed for other reasons, such as those receiving steroid therapy or immunosuppressive therapy, as is used in tissue transplantation, or chemotherapy. Severely infected patients and/or severely debilitated patients with other systemic diseases may also have altered T4/T8 ratios. Furthermore, T4/T8 testing has not been fully standardized for general laboratory use, and results should be interpreted cautiously.[122] Serum protein electrophoresis may be normal or may reveal a polyclonal gammapathy.[6] Since many patients in the high-risk AIDS group are also at high risk of developing hepatitis, it has been suggested that screening for antibodies to hepatitis B core antigen (HB_c) be used to supplement the screening of populations at risk of developing AIDS. Anti-HB_c antibodies are present in 90% of the AIDS population.[123]

Another parameter is the β_2-microglobulin level in plasma, which is usually elevated twofold in patients with AIDS.[110] Other tests have been suggested to screen for AIDS patients; however, these are exclusively investigational and not available in most clinical laboratories. These tests include α_1-thymosin levels (which appear to be increased twofold in patients with AIDS and AIDS prodrome)[124] and acid-labile α-interferon, which is also elevated in patients with AIDS.[125] A higher incidence of patients with AIDS-KS carrying the HLA-DR5 phenotype has been found, compared to the general population. HLA-Bw44, HLA-A29, and HLA-Cw4 were also associated with AIDS-KS.[126] Some hematologic and immunologic changes seen in AIDS and AIDS-related complex are summarized in Table 13-8.[127]

Other Laboratory Studies

Since patients with AIDS often present with opportunistic infections, microbiologic studies to identify these organisms must be performed. The list of opportunistic organisms is as extensive as that described for other immunodeficient patients. In a study of 53 patients the five most common infections were CMV (31 patients), *Candida* (29), *P. carinii* (26), *M. avium-intracellulare* (15),[128] and *Cryptococcus neoformans* (8).[6] Organisms such as *Klebsiella*, *Mycobacterium tuberculosis*, and other atypical mycobacteria have likewise been cultured in these cases. *Toxoplasma gondii*[129] (common in CNS lesions of AIDS patients), *Entamoeba histolytica*, *Pneumocystis carinii*, CMV, EBV, and disseminated herpes simplex infections have often been found in blood cultures, bone marrow cultures and cell cultures of these patients.[6, 110] If chronic, watery diarrhea is present, stool sucrose flotation may be helpful in diagnosing cryptosporidia.[110] *Entamoeba histolytica*, *Giardia lamblia*, *Shigella*, and *Salmonella* should likewise be searched for.[110]

Some infections are characteristically frequent, as has been mentioned above. *Pneumocystis carinii* is one of them. Fifty-five percent of the cases of AIDS reported to the CDC had evidence of *P. carinii* pneumonia. Over 95% of the deaths of AIDS followed with autopsy showed evidence of *P. carinii*. This type of pneumonia is fulminant. Dyspnea is characteristic, but cough may be absent. Chest x-ray films show bilateral pulmonary infiltrates. The diagnosis is achieved by pulmonary brushings or transbronchial biopsy. Another protozoan infection common in AIDS is toxoplasmosis. Toxoplasmosis serology in patients with AIDS is usually negative. *M. avium-intracellulare*, an organism infrequently isolated in other cases, has been documented in 40 cases of AIDS. The disease has resisted most conventional antimycobacterials. *Cryptococcus neoformans* is a fungal infection often seen in patients with AIDS who present with CNS symptoms. Some patients respond to antifungal therapy, but this therapy is quite toxic. Oral candidiasis has very often been documented in patients with both AIDS and AIDS-related complex. A dreaded complication of candidiasis in these patients is candidial esophagitis. Viral infections with *Herpes simplex* in AIDS patients present as extensive genital and perirectal ulcerations,[130] but esophagitis and tracheobronchitis have likewise been reported. The diagnosis is often made by finding multinucleated giant cells on scrapings from lesions. Disseminated CMV is very frequently found in AIDS patients. Seropositivity is present in over 90% of healthy homosexuals. In patients with AIDS, CMV infections are disseminated and present clinically as diffuse pneumonia, ulcerative gastroenteritis, encephalitis, and hepatitis.

TABLE 13-8.—HEMATOLOGY/IMMUNOLOGY WORKUP IN AIDS*

GROUP†	NO. OF CASES	ANEMIA	LEUKOPENIA	T4/T8 RATIO < 1	THROMBOCYTOPENIA	CUTANEOUS ANERGY	DECREASED		
							IgG	IgA	IgM
I	11	91	45	89	36	88	56	67	22
II	39	17	23	69	23	62	21	8	29
III	32	...	9	4	15	37	10	13	37
IV	57	...	4	52	...	18	...	5	24
V	39	...	...	18	12	23	...	9	11

*Data from Kalish et al.[127] unless otherwise indicated, numbers in table are percentages of totals.
†Group I: AIDS; group II: homosexuals or bisexuals with two or more of the following: lymphadenopathy, fever, weight loss, mucosal herpes, candidiasis; group III: only one feature of group II; group IV: asymptomatic homosexuals; group V: control healthy heterosexuals.

TREATMENT OF PATIENTS WITH AIDS

The treatment of patients with AIDS is, to date, supportive. Some patients with *P. carinii* pneumonia are treated successfully with Pentamidine, a drug provided by the CDC.[131] Trimethoprim-sulfamethoxazole has also been used and appears to be less toxic,[110] although frequent reactions are seen with this drug.[6] Infections by other organisms are treated according to the specific infectious agent. Often the dosages must be increased in order to overcome the infections, due to the patient's immunologic status. Deterioration after improvement or lack of response to therapy may warrant bronchial lavage or biopsy to obtain a definitive diagnosis of the causative agent. Treatment for some of the opportunistic infections may be successful (e.g., *P. carinii* pneumonia, which is slowly responsive to pentamidine in AIDS; cryptococcal meningitis, occasionally responsive to flucytosine; mucocutaneous *Candida,* responsive to ketoconazole or amphotericin; and herpes, which may respond to acyclovir).[6] However, disseminated infections with *M. intracellulare,* disseminated CMV, or disseminated cryptosporidiosis are usually resistant to therapy.[6]

Experimentally, some treatments have been attempted to improve or try to reconstitute the immune system. Interleukin-2 (IL-2) has been proposed as a possible therapeutic agent to circumvent the T helper block. A phase 1 clinical trial has been started using IL-2 preparations,[132] although the results on this study have not been published at the time of writing this manuscript. Response does not appear to be significant,[133] although cells for AIDS patients, which have TAC+ (IL-2) receptors, respond in vitro to isoprinosine, an IL-2 stimulator drug.[133] Likewise, leukocyte-A interferon (IFLrA) has also been used experimentally, with encouraging results. Of 12 AIDS patients with Kaposi's sarcoma, five had objective responses, with improved T4/T8 ratios and a decrease in tumor load.[134] Transient remissions (up to 12 months, in one case) can be achieved rarely with combined chemotherapy in Kaposi's associated to AIDS.[6]

A transient improvement of immune responses was obtained with adoptive transfer of peripheral blood lymphocytes coupled with bone marrow transplantation in one patient; however, this patient subsequently died.[135]

PREVENTION

The epidemiology of AIDS and the results of screening tests undertaken with the HTLV ELISA screen prove, a viral infectious agent. These findings imply horizontal as well as vertical transmission, and therefore infectious disease guidelines must be observed. The lack of information on the actual infectivity of the agent or agents producing AIDS is the main cause of concern and anxiety in dealing with patients at the clinical level and with samples at the laboratory level. Intimate contact between carrier and recipient appears to be a condition for transmission of AIDS. Furthermore, actual exchange of body fluids such as would occur during sexual intercourse, sharing of infected needles in drug abusers, and blood or blood product transfusion seems to be the most frequent scenario in the transmission of this disease. Thus, casual contact with patients with AIDS is very probably not a reason for concern. Furthermore, the relatively low infectivity of AIDS has been recently assessed in a study in which none of 85 hospital employees (including several individuals who experienced needle-punctures while trying to obtain samples from AIDS patients, endoscopists, pathologists, and laboratory technologists) developed HTLV-III antibodies by ELISA or Western blotting techniques as evidence of infection with HTLV-III.[136]

The incubation period varies from 6–8 months up to 2 years, underscoring the difficulty in exercising retrospective preventive measures. In spite of the above-stated facts, the concern for transmission of AIDS is warranted, especially in hospitals and other health care facilities. The CDC has, therefore, made the following recommendations for health care personnel:[137]

1. Avoid contact of potentially infective material with broken skin. Wear gloves and gowns when potential for soiling with infective material exists.

2. Hands should be washed immediately after handling potentially contaminated material.

3. Label specimens from AIDS patients prominently with labels such as "AIDS precautions." Clean potentially contaminated surfaces with a 1:10 dilution of 5.25% sodium hypochlorite (household bleach).

4. Disposable supplies used in specimen collection or otherwise potentially contaminated must be incinerated.

5. Dispose of needles in containers designed for

disposal. Do not attempt to replace needles in sheaths, as this is a common cause of accidental needle stick.

6. Reusable instruments are first decontaminated with hypochlorite, then autoclaved.

7. Private rooms for patients too ill to care for themselves are recommended.

8. These guidelines are likewise recommended to morticians[138] and dentists.[139]

Special Recommendations for Laboratories:

1. Conduct tests in class I or II laminar flow cabinets when the potential for aerosol production is present (e.g., vigorous shaking, centrifugation, etc.).

2. Use mechanical pipetting during laboratory tests.

3. Use gloves and gowns when working with AIDS samples.

4. Avoid accidental needle punctures, as outlined above.

5. Decontaminate animal cages and incinerate bedding, animal carcasses, and excreta.

AIDS IN REFERENCE TO BLOOD BANKING

The American Association of Blood Banks and the American Red Cross have made the following recommendations regarding AIDS:[140]

1. Continue to caution physicians regarding the risks of blood transfusions.

2. Autologous transfusion should be encouraged.

3. Blood banks should be cautioned as to a possible increase in the requests for cryoprecipitate, brought on by reports that hemophiliacs treated with cryoprecipitate have less chance of developing T cell abnormalities than those treated with factor VIII concentrates.

4. Donor screening should probe possible AIDS symptoms (e.g., night sweats, diarrhea, weight loss, lymphadenopathy, etc.).

5. Recruiters should not target their recruiting efforts to high-risk groups for AIDS.

6. It is not appropriate at this time to institute directed donations.

Routine laboratory tests to screen for HTLV are currently available, and used in blood banks. Positive units are not used for transfusion. Positive samples are corroborated by the Western blot technique, and the results reported to the patient's physician (see Fig 13–2). In addition to posttransfusional AIDS, a major concern to blood banks is the hazard of AIDS transmission to hemophiliacs requiring factor VIII concentrates. It has been fully documented that hemophiliacs receiving factor VIII concentrate are at a higher risk of developing AIDS and AIDS-related complex T lymphocyte abnormalities than are patients treated with cryoprecipitate.[141] Bona fide cases of AIDS have usually been reported in hemophiliacs receiving large amounts of

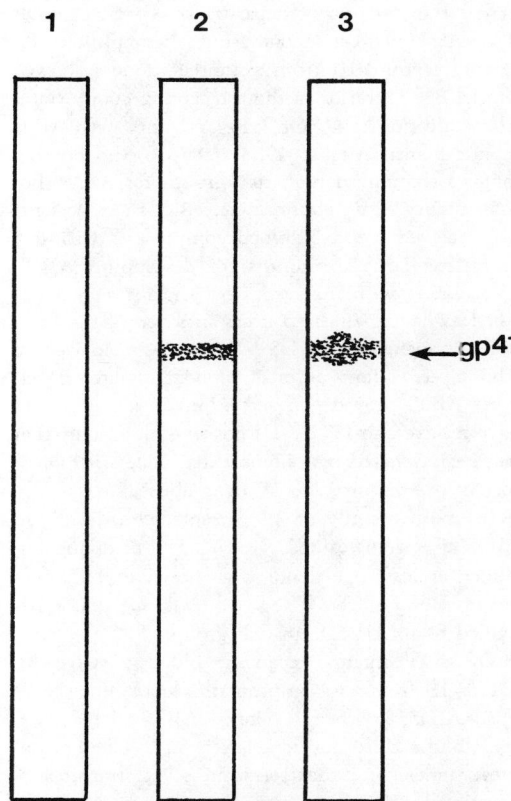

FIG 13–2.—Diagram of a Western blot test. Purified disrupted virus is run on a polyacrilamide gel strip. The protein bands are transferred electrophoretically to a nitrocellulose gel and immobilized. This nitrocellulose gel is then incubated with the patient's serum. After washing, the strips are incubated with peroxidase labeled antihuman Ig antibodies, washed again, and developed with a peroxidase substrate to visualize the bands. *1* = negative control; *2* = positive control; *3* = patient sample showing compatible *gp41* of control # 2.

factor VIII concentrates.[142] Seventeen cases of hemophiliac patients with AIDS were reported from 1981 to 1983. Two of these patients belonged to other high-risk groups for AIDS. Of the remaining 15 not belonging to other risk groups, 10 died, which underscores the seriousness of the disease in these patients.[143] Patients with hemophilia B receiving factor IX concentrates appeared to be at a lesser risk of developing AIDS than patients receiving factor VIII.[144] It should be noted here that donors of plasma for the production of factor VIII concentrate are, in the vast majority of cases, paid donors, a group that, compared to volunteer donors, has historically had a much higher incidence in the transmission of hepatitis B as well as other diseases. However, in one study, hemophiliacs receiving factor VIII from volunteer donors showed similar T4/T8 ratios as those receiving concentrates from paid donors.[145] Of 2,157 patients with AIDS reported until August 1983, 64 (3%) did not belong to recognized high-risk groups for AIDS (homosexuality, drug abuse, etc.); 18 of these patients had received blood or blood components within 5 years (median, 27 months) of developing AIDS. Five donors with inverted T4/T8 ratios were identified as having donated units in seven of the cases of posttransfusional AIDS.[146] A 60-year-old woman who received four units of blood and later developed AIDS proved, on screening of the units, to have received an HTLV-III-positive blood unit that had been donated by a homosexual male with a history of promiscuity and IV drug abuse.[147]

In another study of 12 patients who developed AIDS after transfusions, 9 of 12 sets of donors included at least one donor with positive HTLV exposure. In 6 of the 9 sets, at least one donor belonged to an AIDS high-risk group.[148]

Of three infants receiving blood positive for HTLV-III from an asymptomatic donor, one developed AIDS, another developed AIDS-related complex, and a third developed AIHA.[149] These examples underscore the seriousness of transfusion-associated AIDS.

The general consensus at present is that the screening of plasma donors for AIDS will have to rely mainly on the donor's HTLV-III seropositivity as well as the clinical history of belonging to a high-risk group. Screening for HTLV-III may be accompanied by several logistic, economical, sociological and psychological problems:

1. It redefines the role of blood collecting facilities, (e.g., testing, notifying, counseling donors).

2. It may attract persons at high risk for AIDS who wish to get free testing for AIDS.

3. The problem of handling the expected 1% HTLV-seropositive healthy donors, half of whom will be falsely positive, will entail expensive confirmatory testing and counseling.

4. If a donor whose plasma is in a pool for factor VIII production eventually develops AIDS, it may not be feasible to recall the factor VIII lots,[143] for this practice could jeopardize national supplies of factor VIII concentrate.

5. Legal liability of a blood bank is possible from transmission of AIDS via blood or blood products[150] and will increase if blood has not been tested for HTLV-III if other blood banks are routinely testing their units.

The risk of developing AIDS after blood transfusion appears to be less than that following transfusion with factor VIII concentrates,[151] but AIDS in multiple transfusion cases has been frequently documented.[29,152]

AIDS IN REFERENCE TO HEPATITIS B VACCINE

It is unlikely that the hepatitis B vaccine transmits AIDS, if the disease is indeed caused by an infective agent such as a viral particle. The vaccine is derived from plasma from individuals with HB_sAg. It is inactivated in three steps: treatment with pepsin at pH 2, inactivation with 8M urea, and treatment with Formalin. These steps are known to inactivate all forms of viruses infective to man.[153]

Two cases of AIDS have been described in recipients of the vaccine or vaccine placebo during the hepatitis B vaccine trials. One AIDS patient receiving the vaccine developed AIDS 4 years after receiving the vaccine; the other received a placebo.[153] During the vaccine trial, 442 medical staff members, 660 patients in dialysis units, 549 sexually active homosexuals, and 227 placebo recipients in the original trial received the vaccine. The only case of AIDS reported in all these recipients was the one mentioned above, and it occurred in a patient from a high-risk group, developing 2 years after the mean incubation period for AIDS.[153]

The finding of AIDS in recipients of the vaccine who also belong to a group at high risk for AIDS should not be surprising because high-risk groups for hepatitis B and AIDS generally overlap.[154] In a recent report, serum from 212 HBV vaccine participants was tested for anti-HTLV-III antibodies by ELISA and by Western blotting techniques. Of this group, 35.4% were seropositive. Seven of the 212 had been seroconverted to HTLV-III before the vaccine was given. However, seroconversion to HTLV-III antigens was not statistically different in vaccinated versus placebo groups ($P > 0.50$). It was decided, on the basis of these data, that the HBV vaccine produced in the United States does not induce anti-HTLV antibodies, does not protect against HTLV infection, and does not transmit HTLV virus.[155] In addition, in another report, 200 health care personnel not at risk of acquiring AIDS and who received the HBV vaccine did not produce anti-HTLV-III antibodies more than a year after vaccination.[156] Furthermore, T4/T8 ratios were not altered in recipients of the vaccine nor in AIDS risk groups more than 3 years after vaccination.[157]

All things considered, the benefits far outweigh the unlikely and, to date, undocumented risk to HBV recipients of developing AIDS as a consequence of the vaccine. The vaccine prevents most of the new 200,000 cases of hepatitis B appearing yearly. Of these cases, 10,000 patients will require hospitalization, 10,000–20,000 patients will develop chronic hepatitis, and 1,000 patients will die of fulminant hepatitis,[158] a calculated 25 patients per 100,000 of the general population.[159]

FUTURE DEVELOPMENTS

Much has been clarified in terms of AIDS since the disease was first described. However, the key issues in this disease have not been resolved. Although the most likely etiologic agent (HTLV-III) has been isolated and a specific test to diagnose the disease is available, an effective preventive treatment such as a vaccine remains to be developed, and implementation of a curative treatment for this ominous disease is not yet available at the time of writing this manuscript. The outlook for patients with full-blown AIDS is not encouraging; usually patients die of an opportunistic infection or of disseminated Kaposi's sarcoma or other tumors 2–4 years after the initial diagnosis of AIDS.[26] One cannot expect to find a cure for the disease until a way is found to reverse the immunologic defect in these patients.

REFERENCES

1. *Pneumocystis* pneumonia—Los Angeles. *MMWR* 30:250, 1981.
2. Kaposi's sarcoma and *Pneumocystis* pneumonia among homosexual men—New York City and California. *MMWR* 30:305, 1981.
3. Small C.B., Klein R.S., Friedland G.H., et al.: Community-acquired opportunistic infections and defective cellular immunity in heterosexual drug abusers and homosexual men. *Am. J. Med.* 74:433, 1983.
4. Mansell P.W.A.: Acquired immune deficiency syndrome, leading to opportunistic infections, Kaposi's sarcoma, and other malignancies. *CRC Crit. Rev. Clin. Lab. Sci.* 20:191, 1984.
5. Rivin B.E., Monroe J.M., Hubschman B.P., et al.: AIDS outcome: A first follow-up (letter). *N. Engl. J. Med.* 311:857, 1984.
6. Fauci A.S., Macher A.M., Longo D.L., et al.: Acquired immunodeficiency syndrome: Epidemiologic, clinical, immunologic, and therapeutic considerations. *Ann Intern. Med.* 100:92, 1984.
7. Fauci A.S.: The acquired immunodeficiency syndrome: The ever-broadening clinical spectrum. *JAMA* 249:2375, 1983.
8. Leads from the MMWR. Update: Acquired immunodeficiency syndrome (AIDS)—USA. *JAMA* 250:1016, 1983.
9. Curran J.W.: AIDS—Two years later. *N. Engl. J. Med.* 309:609, 1983.
10. William D.C.: The changing life-styles of homosexual men in the last 15 years, in Freidman-Kien A., Laubenstein L.J. (eds.): *AIDS: The Epidemic of Kaposi's Sarcoma and Opportunistic Infections.* New York, Masson Publishing U.S.A., Inc., 1984, p. 258.
11. Epidemiologic aspects of the current outbreak of Kaposi's sarcoma and opportunistic infections. *N. Engl. J. Med.* 306:248, 1982.
12. Schreeder M.T., Thompson S.E., Hadler S.C., et al.: Hepatitis B in homosexual men: Prevalence of infection and factors related to transmission. *J. Infect. Dis.* 146:7, 1982.
13. Mavligit G.M., Talpaz M., Hsia F.T., et al.: Chronic immune stimulation by sperm alloantigens. *JAMA* 251:237, 1984.
14. Antibodies to a retrovirus etiologically associated with acquired immunodeficiency syndrome (AIDS) in populations with increased incidences of the syndrome. *MMWR* 33:377, 1984.
15. Kornfeld H., Vande Stone R.A., Lange M., et al.:

T lymphocyte subpopulations in homosexual men. *N. Engl. J. Med.* 307:729, 1982.
16. Rubinstein A., Sicklick M., Gupta A., et al.: Acquired immunodeficiency with reversed T4/T8 ratios in infants born to promiscuous and drug-addicted mothers. *JAMA* 249:2358, 1983.
17. Biggar R.J., Melbye M., Ebbesen P., et al.: Low T-lymphocyte ratios in homosexual men: Epidemiologic evidence for a transmissible agent. *JAMA* 251:1441, 1984.
18. Hanrahan J.P., Wormser G.P., Reilly A.A.: Prolonged incubation period of AIDS in intravenous drug abusers: Epidemiological evidence in prison inmates. *J. Infect. Dis.* 150:263, 1984.
19. Jaffe H.W., Bregman D.J., Selik R.M.: Acquired immune deficiency syndrome in the United States: The first 1,000 cases. *J. Infect. Dis.* 148:339, 1983.
20. Harris C., Butkus Small C., Klein R.S., et al.: Immunodeficiency in female sexual partners of men with the acquired immunodeficiency syndrome. *N. Engl. J. Med.* 308:1181, 1983.
21. Scott G.B., Fischl M.A., Klimas N., et al.: Mothers of infants with the acquired immunodeficiency syndrome: Evidence for both symptomatic and asymptomatic carriers. *JAMA* 253:363, 1985.
22. Redfield R.R., Markham P.D., Salahuddin S.Z., et al.: Frequent transmission of HTLV-III among spouses of patients with AIDS related complex and AIDS. *JAMA* 253:1571, 1985.
23. *Pneumocystis carinii* pneumonia among persons with hemophilia A. *MMWR* 31:365, 1982.
24. Weintraub P., Ammann A.J., Abrams D.I., et al.: Altered T-cell immunity in hemophiliacs receiving frequent factor VIII concentrate. *Blood* 60: (suppl. 1):224a, 1982.
25. Menitove J.E., Aster R.H., Casper J.T.: T-lymphocyte subpopulations in patients with classic hemophilia treated with cryoprecipitate and lyophilized concentrates. *N. Engl. J. Med.* 308:83, 1983.
26. Evatt B.L., Gomperts E.D., McDougal J.S., et al.: Coincidental appearance of LAV/HTLV-III antibodies in hemophiliacs and the onset of the AIDS epidemic. *N. Engl. J. Med.* 312:483, 1985.
27. Kreiss J.K., Kasper C.K., Fahey J.L., et al.: Nontransmission of T-cell subset abnormalities from hemophiliacs to their spouses. *JAMA* 251:1450, 1984.
28. Pitchenik A.E., Shafron R.D., Glasser R.M., et al.: The acquired immunodeficiency syndrome in the wife of a hemophiliac. *Ann. Intern. Med.* 100:62, 1984.
29. Possible transfusion-associated acquired immunodeficiency syndrome (AIDS)—California. *MMWR* 31:652, 1982.
30. Marmor M., Friedman-Kien A.E., Laubenstein L., et al.: Risk factors for Kaposi's sarcoma in homosexual men. *Lancet* 1:1083, 1982.
31. Nicholas P., Masci J., deCatalogne J., et al.: Immunocompetence in Haitians living in New York (letter). *N. Engl. J. Med.* 309:1187, 1983.
32. Pape J.W., Liautand B., Thomas F., et al.: Characteristics of the acquired immunodeficiency syndrome (AIDS) in Haiti. *N. Engl. J. Med.* 309:945, 1983.
33. Medgyesy S.L.: Physician criticizes coverage of AIDS. *American Medical News,* Sept. 9, 1983, p. 6.
34. Landesman S.H., Ginzburg H.M., Weiss S.H.: The AIDS epidemic. *N. Engl. J. Med.* 312:521, 1985.
35. Burnet J.B., Bouvet E., Leibowitch M.: Acquired immunodeficiency syndrome in France. *Lancet* 1:700, 1983.
36. Acquired immunodeficiency syndrome (editorial). *Lancet* 1:162, 1983.
37. Hardy A.M., Allen J.R., Morgan W.M., et al.: The incidence rate of acquired immunodeficiency in selected populations. *JAMA* 253:215, 1985.
38. Gallo R.C., Sarin P.S., Gelmann E.P., et al.: Isolation of human T-cell leukemia virus in acquired immune deficiency syndrome. *Science* 220:865, 1983.
39. Gellman E.P., Popovic M., Blayney D., et al.: Proviral DNA of a retrovirus, human T-cell leukemia virus, in two patients with AIDS. *Science* 220:862, 1983.
40. Essex M., McLane M.F., Lee T.H., et al.: Antibodies to human T-cell leukemia virus membrane antigens (HTLV-MA) in hemophiliacs. *Science* 221:1061, 1983.
41. Varmus H.E.: Form and function of retroviral proviruses. *Science* 216:812, 1982.
42. Hsu T.W., Subran J.L., Mark G.E., et al.: Analysis of unintegrated avian RNA tumor virus double stranded DNA intermediates. *J. Virol.* 28:810, 1978.
43. Patarca R., Haseltine W.A.: Sequence similarity among retroviruses: Erratum. *Nature* 309:728, 1984.
44. Macara I.G., Marinetti G.V., Balduzzi P.C.: Transforming protein of avian sarcoma virus UR2 is associated with phosphatidylinositol kinase activity: Possible role in tumorigenesis. *Proc. Natl. Acad. Sci. USA* 81:2728, 1984.
45. Slamon D.J., Shimotohno K., Cline M.J., et al.: Identification of the putative transforming protein of human T-cell leukemia viruses HTLV-I and HTLV-II. *Science* 226:61, 1984.
46. Lee T.H., Coligan J.E., Sodroski J.G., et al.: Antigens encoded by the 3′-terminal region of human T-cell leukemia virus: Evidence for a functional gene. *Science* 226:57, 1984.
47. Gallo R.C., Wong-Staal F.: Human T-cell leukemia-lymphoma virus (HTLV) and human virion onc-homologies, in O'Connor T.E., Rauscher F.J. Jr. (eds.): *Oncogenes and Retroviruses: Evaluation of Basic Finding and Clinical Potential.* New York, Alan R. Liss, Inc., 1983, pp. 223–243.
48. Mitsuya H., Guo H.-G., Cossman J., et al.: Functional properties of antigen-specific T-cells infected by human T-cell leukemia-lymphoma virus (HTLV-I) *Science* 225:1484, 1984.
49. Lo S.-C., Liotta L.A.: Vascular tumors produced by

NIH/3t3 cells transfected with human AIDS Kaposi's sarcoma DNA. *Am. J. Pathol.* 118:7, 1985.
50. Mitsuya H., Popovic M., Yarchoan R., et al.: Suramin protection of T cells in vitro against infectivity and cytopathic effect of HTLV-III. *Science* 226:172, 1984.
51. Longo D.L., Gelman E.P., Cossman J., et al.: Isolation of HTLV-transformed B-lymphocyte clone from a patient with HTLV-associated adult T-cell leukemia. *Nature* 310:505, 1984.
52. Wachsman W., Shimotohno K., Clark S.C., et al.: Expression of the 3' terminal region of human T-cell leukemia viruses. *Science* 226:177, 1984.
53. Shaw G.M., Gonda M.A., Flickinger G.H., et al.: Genomes of evolutionarily divergent members of the human T-cell leukemia virus family (HTLV-I and HTLV-II) are highly conserved, especially in pX. *Proc. Natl. Acad. Sci. USA* 81:4544, 1984.
54. Schüpbach J., Popovic M., Gilden R., et al.: Serological analysis of a subgroup of human T-lymphotropic retroviruses (HTLV-III) associated with AIDS. *Science* 224:503, 1984.
55. Schüpbach J., Sarngadharan M.G., Gallo R.C.: Antigens on HTLV-infected cells recognized by leukemia and AIDS sera are related to HTLV glycoprotein. *Science* 224:607, 1984.
56. Gallo G., Salahuddin S.Z., Popovic M., et al.: Frequent detection and isolation of cytopathic retroviruses (HTLV-III) from patients with AIDS and at risk of AIDS. *Science* 224:500, 1984.
57. Sarngadharan M.G., Popovic M., Bruch L., et al.: Antibodies reactive with human T-lymphotropic retroviruses (HTLV-III) in the serum of patients with AIDS. *Science* 224:506, 1984.
58. Montagnier L., Chermann J.C., Barre-Sinoussi F., et al.: A new human T lymphotropic retrovirus: Characterization and possible role in lymphadenopathy and acquired immunodeficiency syndrome, in Gallo R.C., Essex M., Gross L. (eds.): *Human T-Cell Leukemia Virus.* Cold Spring Harbor Laboratory, Cold Spring Harbor, N.Y., 1984, p. 363.
59. Evatt B.L., Gomperts E.D., McDougal J.S., et al.: Coincidental appearance of LAV/HTLV-III antibodies in hemophiliacs and the onset of the AIDS epidemic. *N. Engl. J. Med.* 312:483, 1985.
60. Schupbach J., Haller O., Vogt M., et al.: Antibodies to HTLV-III in Swiss patients with AIDS and pre-AIDS and in groups at risk for AIDS. *N. Engl. J. Med.* 312:265, 1985.
61. Alter H.J., Eichberg J.W., Masur H., et al.: Transmission of HTLV-III infection from human plasma to chimpanzees: An animal model for AIDS. *Science* 226:549, 1984.
62. Marx P.A., Maul D.H., Osborn K.G., et al.: Simian AIDS: Isolation of a type D retrovirus and transmission of the disease. *Science* 223:1083, 1984.
63. Lange M., Klein E.B., Kornfield H., et al.: Cytomegalovirus isolation from healthy homosexual men. *JAMA* 252:1908, 1984.
64. Dylewsky J.S., Rasmussen L., Mills J., et al.: Large scale serological screen of cytomegalovirus antibodies in homosexual males by enzyme linked immunosorbent assay. *J. Clin. Microbiol.* 19:200, 1984.
65. Detels R., Visscher B., Fahey J.L., et al.: The relation of cytomegalovirus and Epstein-Barr virus antibodies to T-cell subsets in homosexually active men. *JAMA* 251:1719, 1984.
66. Greenberg S.B., Linder S., Baxter B., et al.: Lymphocyte subsets and urinary excretion of cytomegalovirus among homosexual men attending a clinic for sexually transmitted disease. *J. Infect. Dis.* 150:330, 1984.
67. Spector S.A., Hirata K.K., Neuman T.R.: Multiple infections by cytomegalovirus in patients with acquired immunodeficiency syndrome: Documentation by Southern-blot hybridization. *J. Infect. Dis.* 150:952, 1984.
68. Sell K.W., Folks T., Kwon-Chung K.J., et al.: Cyclosporin immunosuppression as the possible cause of AIDS. *N. Engl. J. Med.* 309:1065, 1983.
69. Schran H.F., Hassell A.E., Winter D.L., et al.: Cyclosporin-like substance not detected in patients with AIDS (letter). *N. Engl. J. Med.* 310:1324, 1984.
70. Mildvan D., Mathur U., Enlow R.W.: Opportunistic infections and immune deficiency in homosexual men. *Ann. Intern. Med.* 96:700, 1982.
71. Lane H.C., Masur H., Edgar L., et al.: Abnormalities of B-cell activation and immunoregulation in patients with the acquired immunodeficiency syndrome. *N. Engl. J. Med.* 309:453, 1983.
72. Zolla-Pazner S., William D., El-Sadr W., et al.: Quantitation of β_2-microglobulin and other immune characteristics in a prospective study of men at risk for acquired immune deficiency syndrome. *JAMA* 251:2951, 1984.
73. Millard P.R.: AIDS: Histopathological aspects. *J. Pathol.* 143:223, 1984.
74. Williams R.C. Jr., Masur H., Spira T.S.: Lymphocyte-reactive antibodies in acquired immune deficiency syndrome. *J. Clin. Immunol.* 4:118, 1984.
75. Ammann A.J., Schiffman G., Abrams D., et al.: β-cell immunodeficiency in acquired immune deficiency syndrome. *JAMA* 251:1447, 1984.
76. Levine A.S.: Viruses, immune dysregulation, and oncogenesis: Inferences regarding the cause and evolution of AIDS, in Friedman-Keen A.E., Laubenstein L.J. (eds.): *AIDS: The Epidemic of Kaposi's Sarcoma and Opportunistic Infections.* New York, Masson Publishing, USA, Inc., 1984, p. 7.
77. Ziegler J.L., Miner R.C., Rosenbaum E.R., et al.: Outbreak of Burkitt's-like lymphoma in homosexual men. *Lancet* 2:631, 1982.
78. Cunningham-Rundles S.: Analysis of altered immune function in acquired immunodeficiency syndrome, in Ma P., Armstrong D. (eds.): *The Acquired Immune Deficiency Syndrome and Infections of Homosexual Men.* New York, Yorke Medical Books, 1984, p. 331.
79. Cunningham-Rundles S., Safai B., Metroka C.: Lymphocyte effector function in vitro in the ac-

quired immune deficiency syndrome, in Friedman-Kien A., Laubenstein L.J. (eds.): *AIDS: The Epidemic of Kaposi's Sarcoma and Opportunistic Infections.* New York, Masson Publishing USA, Inc., 1984, p. 153.
80. Djeu J.Y., Stocks N., Aooni K., et al.: Positive self regulation of cytotoxicity in human natural killer cells by production of interferon upon exposure to influenza and herpes virus. *J. Exp. Med.* 156:1222, 1982.
81. Lopez C., Fitzgerald P.A., Siegal F.P.: Immunologic alterations in acquired immune deficiency syndrome, in Ma P., Armstrong D. (eds.): *The Acquired Immune Deficiency Syndrome and Infections of Homosexual Men.* New York, Yorke Medical Books, 1984, p. 342.
82. Murray H.W., Rubin B.Y., Masur H., et al.: Impaired production of lymphokines and immune (gamma) interferon in the acquired immunodeficiency syndrome. *N. Engl. J. Med.* 310:883, 1984.
83. Moore J.L., Poiesz B., Tomar R.H., et al.: Gamma interferon and AIDS (letter). *N. Engl. J. Med.* 312:443, 1985.
84. Buimovici-Klein E., Lange M., Ramey W.G., et al.: Cell mediated immune responses in AIDS (letter). *N. Engl. J. Med* 310:328, 1984.
85. Belsito D.V., Sanchez M.R., Baer R.L., et al.: Reduced Langerhans cell Ia antigen and ATPase activity in patients with the acquired immunodeficiency syndrome. *N. Engl. J. Med.* 310:1279, 1984.
86. Reuben J.M., Hersh E.M., Marsell P.W., et al.: Immunological characterization of homosexual males. *Cancer Res.* 43:897, 1983.
87. Valone F.H., Payan D.G., Abrams D.I., et al.: Defective polymorphonuclear leukocyte chemotaxis in homosexual men with persistent lymph node syndrome. *J. Infect. Dis.* 150:267, 1984.
88. Ioachim H.L.: Lymphadenopathies in homosexual men: Relationships with the acquired immunodeficiency syndrome. *JAMA* 250:1307, 1983.
89. Domingo J., Chin N.W.: Lymphadenopathy in a heterogeneous population at risk for the acquired immunodeficiency syndrome (AIDS): A morphologic study. *Am. J. Clin. Pathol.* 80:649, 1983.
90. Raphael M., Pouletty P., Cavaille-Coll M., et al.: Lymphadenopathy in patients at risk for acquired immunodeficiency syndrome: Histopathology and histochemistry. *Arch Pathol. Lab. Med.* 109:128, 1985.
91. Chan W.C., Brynes R.K., Spira T.J., et al.: Lymphocyte subsets in lymph nodes of homosexual men with generalized unexplained lymphadenopathy: Correlation with morphology and blood changes. *Arch. Pathol. Lab. Med.* 109:133, 1985.
92. Geller S.A., Muller R., Greenberg M.L., et al.: Acquired immunodeficiency syndrome: Distinctive features of bone marrow biopsies. *Arch. Pathol. Lab. Med.* 109:138, 1985.
93. Joshi V.V., Oleske J.M.: Pathologic appraisal of the thymus gland in acquired immunodeficiency syndrome in children. *Arch. Pathol. Lab. Med.* 109:142, 1985.
94. Autran B., Gorin I., Leibowitch M., et al.: AIDS in a Haitian woman with cardiac Kaposi's sarcoma and Whipple's disease (letter). *Lancet* 1:767, 1983.
95. Strom R.L., Gruninger R.P.: AIDS with *Mycobacterium avium-intracellulare* lesions resembling those of Whipple's disease. *N. Engl. J. Med.* 309:1323, 1983.
96. Dobbins W.O. III: Is there an immune deficit in Whipple's disease? *Dig. Dis. Sci.* 26:247, 1981.
97. Greene J.B., Sidhu G., Lewin S.: *Mycobacterium avium-intracellulare:* A cause of disseminated life-threatening infection in homosexuals and drug abusers. *Ann. Intern. Med.* 97:539, 1982.
98. Zucker-Franklin D.: "Looking" for the cause of AIDS. *N. Engl. J. Med.* 308:837, 1983.
99. Ewing E.P. Jr., Spira T.J., Chandler F.W., et al.: Unusual cytoplasmic body in lymphoid cells of homosexual men with unexplained lymphadenopathy: A preliminary report. *N. Engl. J. Med.* 308:819, 1983.
100. Burrage T., Andiwan W., Katz B.Z., et al.: Virus-like rods in a lymphoid line from an infant with AIDS. *N. Engl. J. Med.* 310:1460, 1984.
101. Sidhu G.S.: Ultrastructure of AIDS lymph nodes (letter). *N. Engl. J. Med.* 309:1188, 1983.
102. Sidhu G., Stahl R.E., El-Sadr W., et al.: Ultrastructural markers of AIDS. *Lancet* 1:990, 1983.
103. Shamoto M., Murakami S., Zenke T.: Adult T-cell leukemia in Japan: An ultrastructural study. *Cancer* 47:1804, 1981.
104. Miller S.E., Rogers F.J.: Ultrastructure of AIDS lymph nodes (letter). *N. Engl. J. Med.* 309:1188, 1983.
105. Kotler D.P., Gaetz H.P., Lange M., et al.: Enteropathy associated with the acquired immunodeficiency syndrome. *Ann. Intern. Med.* 101:421, 1984.
106. Persistent generalized lymphadenopathy among homosexual males. *MMWR* 31:249, 1982.
107. Stahl R.E., Friedman-Kien A., Dubin R., et al.: Immunologic abnormalities in homosexual men: Relationship to Kaposi's sarcoma. *Am. J. Med.* 73:171, 1982.
108. Ma P., Villanueva T.G., Kaufman D., et al.: Respiratory cryptosporidiosis in the acquired immune deficiency syndrome: Use of modified cold Kinyoun and Hemacolor stains for rapid diagnoses. *JAMA* 252:1298, 1984.
109. Fernandez R., Mouraclian J.A., Metroka C., et al.: Malignant lymphoma with central nervous system involvement in six homosexual men with acquired immunodeficiency syndrome (abstract). *Lab. Invest.* 48:25A, 1983.
110. Macher A.M., Masur H., Lane H.C., et al.: *AIDS: Diagnosis and Management,* monograph. Baltimore, Burroughs Wellcome Co., 1983.
111. Schoeppel S.L., Hoppe R.T., Dorfman R.F., et al.: Hodgkin's disease in homosexual men with generalized lymphadenopathy. *Ann. Intern. Med.* 102:68, 1985.
112. Ziegler J.L., Beckstead J.A., Volberding P.A., et al.: Non-Hodgkin's lymphoma in 90 homosexual men: Relation to generalized lymphadenopathy and

113. Morris L., Distenfeld M.L., Amorosi E., et al.: Autoimmune thrombocytopenic purpura in homosexual men. *Ann. Intern. Med.* 96:714, 1982.
114. Persistent, generalized lymphadenopathy among homosexual males. *MMWR* 31:249, 1982.
115. Klein R.S., Harris C.A., Small C.B., et al.: Oral candidiasis in high-risk patients as the initial manifestation of the acquired immunodeficiency syndrome. *N. Engl. J. Med.* 311:354, 1984.
116. Joy M.: Oral candidiasis and AIDS (letter). *N. Engl. J. Med.* 311:1379, 1984.
117. Pardo V., Aldana M., Colton R.M., et al.: Glomerular lesions in the acquired immunodeficiency syndrome. *Ann. Intern. Med.* 101:429, 1984.
118. Rao T.K.S., Filippone E.J., Nicastri A.D., et al.: Associated focal and segmental glomerulosclerosis in the acquired immunodeficiency syndrome. *N. Engl. J. Med.* 310:669, 1984.
119. Gupta S., Licorish K.: Circulating immune complexes in AIDS (letter). *N. Engl. J. Med.* 310:1530, 1984.
120. Fahey J.L., Detels R., Gottlieb M., et al.: Immune cell augmentation (with altered T-subset ratio) is common in healthy homosexual men. *N. Engl. J. Med.* 308:842, 1983.
121. Pitchemik A.E.: Acquired immune deficiency syndrome in low risk patients. *JAMA* 250:1310, 1983.
122. Greenberg F.: Screening for acquired immune deficiency syndrome (letter). *N. Engl. J. Med.* 307:1521, 1982.
123. Spira T., quoted by Marx J.L.: Health officials seek ways to halt AIDS. *Science* 219:271, 1983.
124. Hersh E.M., Reuben J.M., Rios A., et al.: Elevated thymosin alpha-1 levels associated with evidence of immune dysregulation in male homosexuals with a history of infectious diseases or Kaposi's sarcoma. *N. Engl. J. Med.* 308:45, 1983.
125. Eyster M.E., Goedert J.J., Poon M.C., et al.: Acid-labile alpha interferon: A possible preclinical marker for the acquired immunodeficiency syndrome in hemophilia. *N. Engl. J. Med.* 309:584, 1983.
126. Prince H.E., Schroff R.W., Ayoub G., et al.: HLA studies in acquired immune deficiency syndrome patients with Kaposi's sarcoma. *J. Clin. Immunol.* 4:242, 1984.
127. Kalish S.B., Ostrow D.G., Goldsmith C.C.S., et al.: The spectrum of immunologic abnormalities and clinical findings in homosexually active men. *J. Infect. Dis.* 149:148, 1984.
128. Zakowski P., Fligiel S., Berlin G.W., et al.: Disseminated *Mycobacterium avium-intracellulare* infection in homosexual men dying of acquired immunodeficiency. *JAMA* 248:2980, 1982.
129. Luft B.J., Conley F., Remington J.S.: Outbreak of central nervous system toxoplasmosis in Western Europe and North America. *Lancet* 1:781, 1983.
130. Seigal F.P., Lopez C., Hammer G.S., et al.: Severe acquired immunodeficiency in male homosexuals manifested by chronic perianal ulcerative herpes simplex lesions. *N. Engl. J. Med.* 305:1439, 1981.
131. Gottlieb M.S., Schroff R., Schanker H.M., et al.: *Pneumocystis carinii* pneumonia and mucosal candidiasis in previously healthy homosexual men: Evidence of a new acquired cellular immunodeficiency. *N. Engl. J. Med.* 305:1425, 1981.
132. Marwick C.: Interleukin-2 trial will try to spark flagging immunity of AIDS patients. *JAMA* 250:1125, 1983.
133. Tsang K., Fudenberg H.H., Galbraith G.M.P.: In vitro augmentation of interleukin-2 production and lymphocytes with TAC antigen marker in patients with AIDS (letter). *N. Engl. J. Med.* 310:987, 1984.
134. Krown S.E., Real F.X., Cunningham-Rundles S., et al.: Preliminary observations on the effect of recombinant leukocyte A interferon in homosexual men with Kaposi's sarcoma. *N. Engl. J. Med.* 308:1071, 1983.
135. Lane H.C., Masur H., Longo D.L., et al.: Partial immune reconstitution in a patient with the acquired immunodeficiency syndrome. *N. Engl. J. Med.* 311:1099, 1984.
136. Hirsch M.S., Wormer G.P., Schooley R., et al.: Risk of nosocomial infection with human T-cell lymphotropic virus III (HTLV-III). *N. Engl. J. Med.* 312:1, 1985.
137. Acquired immune deficiency syndrome (AIDS): Precautions for clinical and laboratory staffs. *MMWR* 31:577, 1982.
138. Guidelines on infection control: Guidelines for hospital environmental control (continued). *Infect. Cont.* 3:52, 1982.
139. Cooley R.L., Lubow R.M.: AIDS: An occupational hazard? *J. Am. Dent. Assoc.* 107:28, 1983.
140. Joint statement on acquired immunodeficiency syndrome (AIDS) related to transfusion (editorial). *Transfusion* 23:87, 1983.
141. Lederman M.M., Ratnoff O.D., Scillian J.J., et al.: Impaired cell-mediated immunity in patients with classic hemophilia. *N. Engl. J. Med.* 308:79, 1983.
142. *Pneumocystis carinii* pneumonia among persons with hemophilia A. *MMWR* 31:365, 1982.
143. Marwick C.: "Contaminated" plasma: No automatic recall. *JAMA* 250:1126, 1983.
144. Hager T.: What is the role of factor VIII therapy in inducing helper suppressor ratios? *JAMA* 249:3277, 1983.
145. Cable R.G., Hoyer L., Marchesi S., et al.: Influence of plasma source on T-lymphocyte subpopulations in hemophiliacs using factor VIII concentrate. *N. Engl. J. Med.* 309:1057, 1983.
146. Curran J.W., Lawrence D.N, Jaffe H., et al.: Acquired immunodeficiency syndrome (AIDS) associated with transfusions. *N. Engl. J. Med.* 310:69, 1984.
147. Groopman J.E., Salahuddin S.Z., Sarngadharan M.G., et al.: Virologic studies in a case of transfusion-associated AIDS. *N. Engl. J. Med.* 311:1419, 1984.

148. Jaffe H.W., Francis D.P., McLane M.F., et al.: Transfusion associated AIDS: Serologic evidence of human T-cell leukemia virus infection of donors. *Science* 223:1309, 1984.
149. Wykoff R.F., Pearl E.R., Saulsbury F.T.: Immunologic dysfunction in infants infected through transfusion with HTLV-III. *N. Engl. J. Med.* 312:265, 1985.
150. Landfield R.: Some thoughts about AIDS, blood products, and products liability laws. *Plasma Q.* 4:69, 1983.
151. Check W.A.: Preventing AIDS transmission: Should blood donors be screened? *JAMA* 249:567, 1983.
152. Jett J.R.: Acquired immunodeficiency syndrome associated with blood product transfusions. *Ann. Intern. Med.* 99:621, 1983.
153. Stevens C.E.: No increased incidence of AIDS in recipients of hepatitis B vaccine. *N. Engl. J. Med.* 308:1163, 1983.
154. Macek C.: AIDS transmission: What about the hepatitis B vaccine? *JAMA* 249:685, 1983.
155. Stevens C.E., Taylor P.E., Rubinstein P., et al.: Safety of the hepatitis B vaccine (letter). *N. Engl. J. Med.* 312:375, 1985.
156. Dienstag J.L.: Safety of the hepatitis B vaccine (letter). *N. Engl. J. Med.* 312:376, 1985.
157. Jacobson I.R., Dienstag J.L., Zachoval R., et al.: Lack of effect of hepatitis B vaccine on T-cell phenotypes. *N. Engl. J. Med.* 311:1030, 1984.
158. Gerety R.J., Tabor E.: Newly licensed hepatitis B vaccine: Known safety and unknown risks. *JAMA* 249:746, 1983.
159. Sacks H.S., Rose D.N., Chalmers T.C.: Should the risk of acquired immunodeficiency syndrome deter hepatitis B vaccination? *JAMA* 252:3375, 1984.
160. Drotman P.D., Curran J.W.: AIDS: An epidemiologic overview, in Friedman-Kien A., Laubenstein L.J. (eds.): *AIDS: The Epidemic of Kaposi's Sarcoma and Opportunistic Infections*. New York, Masson Publishing U.S.A., Inc., 1984, p. 279.
161. Welch K., Finkbeiner W., Alpers C.E., et al.: Autopsy findings in the acquired immunodeficiency syndrome. *JAMA* 252:1152, 1984.

14

Concepts of Medical Genetics Useful in Immunohematology

To understand how some cell membrane markers, and more specifically, red blood cell (RBC) antigens are inherited, it is useful to review some basic concepts in genetics. This chapter provides a short and simplified approach to a subject of ever-growing complexity. It also contains material pertinent to chapter 15, which discusses paternity testing.

BASIC CONCEPTS IN GENETICS

The combination of genetic information that takes place in the formation of a new being with the union of two gametes, the ovum and the spermatozoid, permits hereditary transmission from one generation to the next. Twenty-three pairs of chromosomes from each parent are normally contributed to a new individual. Twenty-two of these chromosome pairs are similar in males and females and called autosomes. In one pair, chromosomes differ in shape in males (XY) and are similar in females (XX); these are the sex chromosomes or heterochromosomes.

Each chromosome (Fig 14–1) consists of a short "p" arm, a centromere, and a long "q" arm. Chromosomes can be subdivided in regions and subregions defined by chromosome banding techniques.[1]

Chromosome Identification

Lymphocytes that are first stimulated to divide, arrested in mitosis with Colcemid, and stained by a simple staining technique can be analyzed for their chromosome content, and their chromosomes divided into seven groups. These groups have been determined by observing differences in the relative size of the chromosome arms and the position of the centromere. Thus, seven groups have been identified with this method: A (1, 2, 3); B (4, 5). C (6 to 12 and sex chromosome X); D (13, 14, 15); E (16, 17, 18); F (19, 20); and G (21, 22, and sex chromosome Y).[2] However, by this simple staining method, the identification of each individual chromosome is not possible. To identify each chromosome, it is necessary to apply a relatively more modern technique called chromosome banding. This can be achieved by Giemsa staining (G banding),[3] or by quinacrine banding (Q banding).[4] With these techniques, a much more accurate analysis and grouping of chromosomes has been made possible. Furthermore, reverse banding (R banding), which is another fluorescent method,[5] helps corroborate accurate interpretation of Q banding, and C banding, another transmitted light method, helps further define chromosomes and chromosome abnormalities.[6]

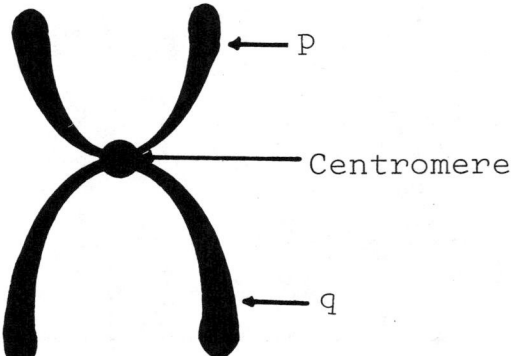

FIG 14–1.—An autosomic chromosome. The short arms are labeled *p* and the long arms are labeled *q*.

Nomenclature of Banded Chromosomes

An international convention held in Paris in 1971 proposed a nomenclature that is used as the protocol for banding classification.[7] Using this nomenclature, the chromosome number, the arm, the region, and the band number are given together without punctuation. For instance, 6p23 defines chromosome 6, arm p, region 2, band 3. If subbands are defined, a period separates the band from the subband. Using the example given above, in 6p23.2, the .2 on the right refers to subband number 2.

Clinically, a method which defines the type of abnormal chromosomic material present is utilized. The chromosome number is given first, followed by the sex chromosomes present, then one or more of the following symbols may be used to define abnormalities: r (ring chromosome), t (translocation), del (deletion), dup (duplication), ins (insertion). (Other symbols are used as well.[1]) For instance, 46 XX, t(2;6) (9^{34}; p12) denotes a female with a reciprocal translocation (t) between chromosomes 2 and 6 (2;6) and with break points in region 3, band 4, of the long arm (q) of chromosome 2 and in region 1, band 2, of the short arm of chromosome 6.

Uses of Chromosomal Studies

The medical uses of chromosomal analysis are multiple. Hereditary disorders have been better defined since banding techniques were introduced. Trisomy is one of the more frequently identified disorders and is usually caused by nondisjunction during mitosis. Trisomy 21, trisomy 13, trisomy 9, and trisomy 8 are examples of this disorder. They can all be detected by chromosome analysis techniques. The "cat-cry" syndrome has been very frequently associated with del 5p; del 18q has likewise been associated with multiple organ defects and mental retardation. The Turner syndrome, classically a monosomy of chromosome X, can be identified as a mosaic by chromosome analysis, as can other sex chromosome defects such as the Klinefelter syndrome (XXY) or, less frequently, mosaics of this pattern.

More recently, patients with myeloproliferative disorders can be found to have chromosomal abnormalities. For instance t(9,22) frequently occurs in chronic myelogenous leukemia and acute lymphocytic leukemia, whereas t(8,21) is frequently seen in acute myelogenous leukemia. Burkitt's lymphoma frequently exhibits t(8,14), and retinoblastoma shows 13q14 translocations.[8] The list of chromosomal abnormalities continues to grow. Details of other chromosomal abnormalities related to hematologic disease are given in chapter 2.

Identification of blood group mapping on chromosomes is also the result of chromosomal analysis. Possible assignment of Jk to chromosome 7 was due to abnormally inherited Jk in a del (7)q case.[9]

Chromosomes contain genetic material expressed in units called genes. Genes are, in essence, sections of DNA strands about which factors affecting phenotypic expression are clustered. Genes are paired in chromosomes (Fig 14–2). If two genes exist in two or more forms and occupy the same locus they are called *alleles* (see Fig 14–2,A). An individual is *homozygous* for a certain trait when the coding genes are alike at one locus, and *heterozygous* for that trait when two genes at a certain locus are not alike (see Fig 14–2,B). If a gene product is expressed only in homozygous individuals, the trait is called *recessive*.

Codominant genes are genes which are always expressed when present, even in the heterozygous state. In sex-linked inheritance, a male receiving an X chromosome bearing the trait from an affected mother is called hemizygous.

Prior to mitosis, each chromosome synthesizes a duplicate copy of itself. When division takes place, each chromosome separates sagitally in half. Thus the two daughter cells have the same 23 chromosome pairs as the mother cell. However, when gamete division takes place, a reduction division, or meiosis, occurs. In brief, during meiosis, cells divide twice while chromosomes divide only once (Fig 14–3). The result is that each chromosome pair separates and the new individual receives only one chromosome from each parental pair. Thus, each

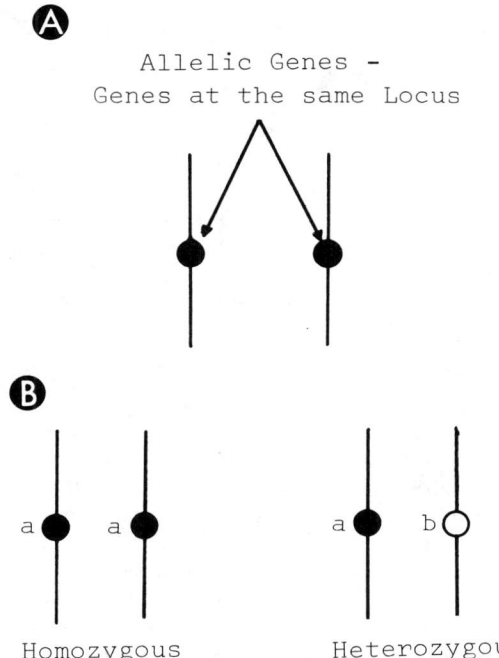

FIG 14–2.—**A**, location of allelic genes on chromosomes. These genes occupy reciprocal locations on each of the two sides of the chromosome. **B**, homozygous genes are identical allelic genes (at the same locus). Heterozygous genes are different allelic genes (at the same locus).

gamete contains only 23 chromosomes instead of 46 chromosomes.

During meiosis there is an assortment of genes within each pair of chromosomes so that each germ cell receives a different combination of maternal and paternal chromosomes. This produces an enormous diversity in the possible genotype combinations of the progeny. For each of the 23 pairs of chromosomes there are 2^{23} combinations that could occur in a gamete. Therefore, the likelihood that one set of parents will produce two identical offspring (precluding identical twins) is 1 in 8 million. Genetic recombination also adds to diversity. Recombination occurs during meiosis. When homologous chromosomes pair, bridging occurs at corresponding regions of the homologous chromosome; the chromosome breaks and rejoins at these so-called chromata. The result is a "crossover" of information between two identical chromosomes, resulting in a recombination of genes. Crossing-over (Fig 14–4) during meiosis occurs relatively frequently in humans. The farther apart two genes are on a chromosome, the greater is the likelihood of crossing-over. Thus, genes that are close together are said to be linked, because they will "travel" together during recombination. The study of phenotypes resulting from linkage helps in mapping genes on chromosomes. Mapping is done by calculating the frequency of crossover between two different genes. Linked or closely positioned genes form groups of genes called haplotypes (e.g., HLA, MNS, Rh systems). Genes in the same chromosome that may or may not be in immediate proximity to each other are called syntenic genes.

Genes may be "expressed" with differing degrees of *penetrance*. The degree of penetrance is modified by both genotype and environment. If an abnormal gene cannot be detected phenotypically, it is said to be nonpenetrant.

THE MOLECULAR BASIS OF GENETIC INFORMATION

The genetic code is located in the chromosomal DNA, which, by virtue of combination possibilities, functions as the code template. The DNA molecule is shaped like a spiral staircase folded in plectonemic coils, which in turn are folded into supercoils. The steps of the staircase are composed of complementary pairs of pyrimidine and purine bases in the form of nucleotides. The two pyrimidine bases are adenine and guanine; the two purine bases are cytosine and thymine.[10] The handrails of the staircase are composed of phosphate and a pentose linked together by hydrogen bonds. The com-

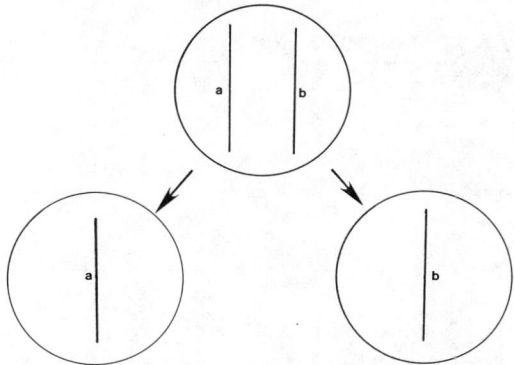

FIG 14–3.—The reduction of chromosomal material during meiosis. Genes located on the *a* side of the chromosome will go to one gamete and genes located on the *b* side will go to a different gamete. A net reduction of 50% of the chromosomal material is observed in the second division.

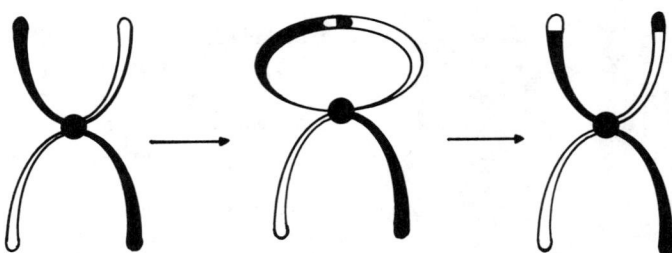

FIG 14–4.—Chromosomal crossing-over. Note that information located at the tip of the p arms is exchanged. Closely linked genes so exchanged will travel from one arm to the other arm of the chromosomes during crossing-over.

bination of phosphate, pentose and a base is termed a nucleotide. The nucleotides are connected by 3′,5′-phosphodiester bonds. The 5′ terminal is conventionally placed at the left, whereas the 3′-OH terminal is to the right of the sequence, so sequences are read from left to right. Bases approximate each other at the midpoint of each step in distances ranging from 0.29 nm to 0.30 nm, forming hydrogen bonds.

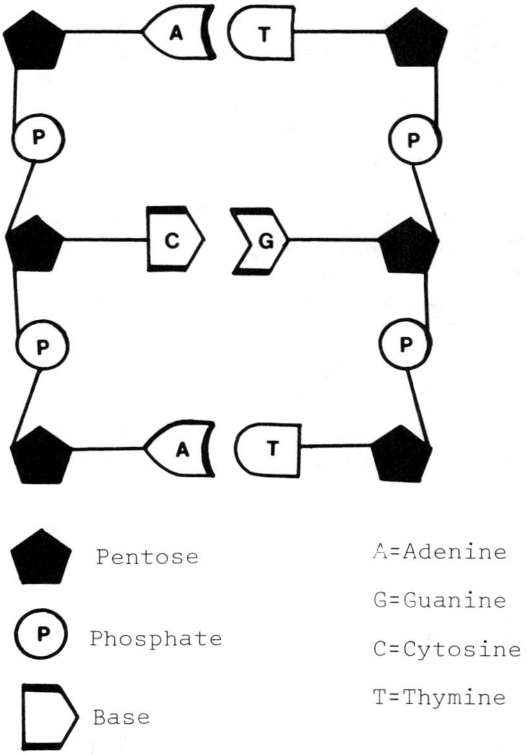

Adenine always pairs with thymine and cytosine always pairs with guanine (Fig 14–5). A typical gene consists of a DNA strand of about 500–1000 bases. The main genetic unit is the codon, which is composed of three consecutive bases. Each codon codes for one amino acid on translation at the ribosomal level. The array of bases will be such that upon decoding at the ribosomal RNA, the arrays result in messages translated as protein amino acid sequences.

Apparently only one strand codes for the amino acid sequences, the other functioning as a complementary strand during DNA replication.

Replication constitutes the biosynthesis of new DNA during cell division. This DNA replication occurs in a complementary sequence at each of the DNA strands and takes place when these strands separate (Fig 14–6).[11] The process is catalyzed by DNA polymerase. DNA polymerase will add nucleotides sequentially only when there is a template DNA strand. Addition of nucleotides by DNA polymerase begins at the 3′-hydroxyl primer. Biosynthesis of nucleotide segments, as mentioned above, grow in a 5′ to 3′ direction. DNA polymerase will add about 1,000 nucleotides per minute per mole of enzyme.[12]

Replication occurs in short fragments, termed Okasaki fragments,[13] and appears to be initiated by a DNA-dependent RNA polymerase which produces a short RNA segment, as shown by rifampicin block, which affects RNA polymerase, inducing paralysis of the DNA replication process.

FIG 14–5.—Diagram of the DNA structure. Note that nucleotides are linked to each other by a chain of pentose and phosphate molecules. Bases are indicated by capital letters (see code). The shape of the bases depicts "key lock" compatibility of the molecules.

Transcription of the DNA Code

Messages are transmitted from the nucleus of the cell to the cytoplasm via messenger RNA (mRNA), which is a single-stranded nucleoprotein.[14] RNA

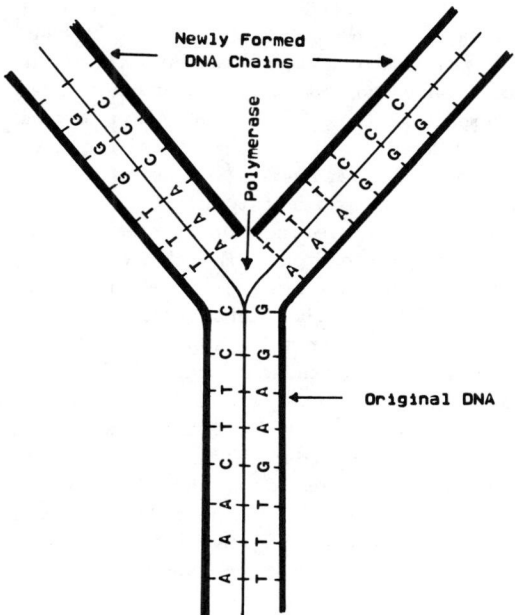

FIG 14–6.—DNA replication. Nucleotides are placed on newly formed DNA chains by DNA polymerase junction sites.

also differs from DNA in that it is composed of uracil bases instead of thymine. RNA is formed in alignment with one of the DNA strands by a process called transcription. At least three types of RNA are recognized: mRNA, 5%–10% of the total; transfer RNA (tRNA), 10% of the total; and ribosomal RNA (rRNA), 75%–80% of the total. RNA is *transcribed* from the DNA template, which unfolds and separates at the transcription site serving as a template for mRNA formation. Transcription takes place under the influence of DNA-dependent RNA polymerase, a 500-kilodalton molecular complex. Initiation of transcription is via a sigma factor which does not have enzymatic activity, but recognizes start code sequences on DNA. As mRNA is formed, DNA strands recouple behind it, causing the mRNA strand to peel off. The message is terminated by the rho(p) factor, a 60-kilodalton protein, which causes detachment of the newly synthesized mRNA. Three RNA polymerases are recognized, I, II, and III. RNA polymerase I is involved in rRNA synthesis in the nucleoplasm; RNA polymerase II is involved in mRNA synthesis in the nucleotides; and RNA polymerase III is involved in the synthesis of tRNA and the 5S rRNA portion. Transcription is thought to take place mainly in the cell's nucleolus. Messenger RNA proceeds to unhook from the transcriptional site migrating to the cytoplasm. In the cytoplasm mRNA attaches to ribosomes or groups of ribosomes (polysomes). Ribosomes and 80S subcellular structures are composed of two subunits, a 50S subunit and a 30S subunit. Each subunit contains rRNA and 34 other proteins.

Protein Synthesis

In a way similar to mRNA transcription, protein synthesis can be considered in three stages: initiation, elongation, and termination. The initiation process involves aggregation of the 30S subunits of ribosomes with tRNA, GTP, and initiation factors IF-1, IF-2, and IF-3, plus the mRNA strand.

Each tRNA recognizes a triple-base codon which codes for an amino acid, thus aligning amino acids into chains that eventually polymerize into polypeptides, or proteins, via a polymerase.

In all prokaryotic cells, the first amino acid at the amino terminal portion of all proteins is N-formyl methionine (f-Met). Transfer-RNA combines with f-Met during initiation of synthesis and binds only to the 30S ribosomal subunit, whereas nonformylated methionine binds to the 50S subunit.

Ribosomes have two binding sites, the A or (aminoacyl-tRNA) site and the P (or peptide) site. The A site is the recognition or decoding site, where tRNA will meet complementarity for mRNA via its anticodon end. The codon end "holds" an amino acid to be added to the nascent polypeptide. In the 50S ribosomal unit, catalysis of peptide bonds takes place in the amino acid–binding site of tRNA. Thus, the process of elongation is started and continued until the message on mRNA is read. Not all DNA base sequences have translational meaning which would result in the synthesis of peptide chains. Intervening sequences that do not appear to translate into amino acid sequences are thought to function as stop codes.[15]

Ultimately the ribosome reaches the end of the message or cystron. A terminating codon, usually UAA, UAG, or UGA bases, flags the end of the mRNA translation. When these sequences enter the A site, instead of a new aminoacyl tRNA, an R1 or R2 terminating protein enters the site and causes detachment of the newly formed protein. During transcription, nascent mRNA does not always have meaningful sequences. This has been shown to be the case, for immunoglobulins, as reviewed in chapter 4. The nonmeaningful stretches or introns between genes occur in so-called immature mRNA, which purportedly, via maturases, is spliced and rejoined, at each step of RNA maturation, eliminating intervening introns and approximating meaningful sequences.[16] This process appears to occur in many eukaryotic genes and is also significant when attempting recombinant DNA technology with eukaryotic genes.

Gene Regulation

Genes appear to be organized according to the model set forth by Jacob and Monod,[17] which is based on findings of bacterial genetic regulation. According to this model, the phenotypic product is coded for by a structural gene located between an initiator sequence which induces the synthesis of RNA and a termination sequence which ends the translation. One or more of these structured genes may tie in sequence and are controlled by an operator gene capable of switching the gene "on" or "off." The complex of one or more structural genes and its operator gene is termed an operon and its components are usually close to each other, in sequence.

A regulator gene, which may be located at a distant site from the operon, produces a small protein or peptide, which combines with the operon, blocking the synthesis of mRNA by the operon.[17] An inducer substance is capable of combining with the repressor blocking its action. Alternatively, corepressors may reactivate a repressor, with a resulting block of RNA synthesis.

Recombinant DNA

Recombinant DNA technology holds great promise in the development of genetic engineering. Recombinant DNA implies selecting or preparing a small segment of DNA with a desired gene coding. This genetic material is then inserted into bacteria that, after replication, will produce the genetic product. The genetic product can then be harvested (e.g., synthetic factor VIII).

With present-day technology, it is possible to insert DNA carriers into bacteria; in addition, it is also possible to splice and join specific segments of DNA to bacterial DNA, allowing these codes to be integrated into the bacterial genome with resulting recombinant DNA (rDNA). On replication, these bacteria synthesize the phenotypic products of the adoptive encoded genes. Various methods can be used; involving plasmids, bacteriophage λ, cosmids, or bacteriophage M13.[18] Plasmids are extrachromosomal genetic elements, are normally found in a variety of bacteria, and constitute closed, circular double-stranded DNA. These circular DNA segments may confer phenotypes to their bacterial hosts such as resistance to antibiotics, enterotoxin synthesis, and other functions that otherwise would not be present in the host bacteria. Copies of most plasmids are restricted and coupled to the cell host's metabolism. Relaxed plasmids, on the other hand, can produce several copies and are useful for recombinant technology. The number of plasmids can be increased if the bacterial host's protein synthesis is stopped (e.g., using chloramphenicol).[19] Cloning in plasmid DNA can be achieved by cleaving the circular DNA with restriction endonuclease and joined in vitro to foreign DNA. The resulting recombinant plasmids are used to transform a suitable bacterial host. If antibiotic resistance plasmids are used in the insertional process, only bacteria containing this plasmid will grow in the presence of the antibiotic.

Another method of DNA insertion to bacteria is by using the bacteriophage λ.[20] The λ-phage can be used during lysogeny when it is possible to integrate recombinant DNA between the J and N genes, which are unnecessary for the lysogenic process. Selective segments of λ-phage DNA can be prepared for foreign DNA targeting by using restriction endonucleases (which are enzymes capable of cleaving DNA at palindromic message sites), inserting the message and ligating it using DNA-ligase. This process can be attained while retaining phage infectivity.[21] Eco RI is a very useful endonuclease, because it causes DNA nicks at sites which become sticky. However, λ-phage has a limited capacity of about 23 kilobases. To circumvent this shortcoming, cosmids have been developed. Cosmids consist of (1) a drug resistance marker and a plasmid origin of replication; (2) one or more cloning restriction sites; and (3) a fragment of DNA containing the cohesive (COS) end of a λ-phage. Cosmids are usually small, so the eukaryotic DNA message (usually 45 KB or smaller) can be accommodated in a λ-phage package.[22]

When recombination is attempted with eukaryotic genes, introns are usually attached to meaningful DNA sequences. Introns cannot be excised by bacteria, for these organisms do not appear to possess the enzymes necessary to excise these sequences from the meaningful DNA sequences, with the result that the message cannot be read.[23] To circumvent this problem the message is obtained from mature RNA; this RNA does not contain introns, and with the aid of enzymes termed reverse transcriptases, which use the polyadenine terminus present in most mRNA,[24] the RNA message is converted into a DNA copy, or cDNA.[25] This cDNA must then be joined to plasmids acceptable to bacterial insertion.

Mutant bacteria lacking DNA are capable of cleaving the "foreign" sequences and are selected as recipients of the transferred DNA. To isolate a desired mRNA message, a probe is needed. These probes can be synthetically produced if the sequence of the polypeptide is known by preparing a complementary oligonucleotide chain. The probe is then radiolabeled and used to screen a genomic library, which consists of short DNA segments (24 KB) obtained by endonuclease cleavage. The radioactive probe is hybridized with the library and then searched for by Southern blotting (after Dr. E. M. Southern),[26] which involves separating DNA fragments on gel electrophoresis and then running perpendicular fluid currents to make the DNA bands migrate into nitrocellulose gels; the bands can then be separated and eluted for cloning. A similar method, termed Northern blotting, has been developed for RNA.[27]

Gene cloning has far-reaching possibilities in terms of basic immunohematology research (e.g., cloning genes for blood groups) to further understand the biology of blood group antigens, as well as therapeutic applications (e.g., cloning the genes of factor VIII) which would solve many problems in the therapy of hemophiliacs, including the prevention of AIDS in these patients. Evidently this technology will be the forerunner of immunohematology research for several decades to come.

MENDELIAN GENETICS

Monohybrid Cross

It was through the study of the monohybrid cross that Gregor Mendel discovered the basic laws governing inheritance; his findings were published in 1866.[28] In experiments using garden peas, Mendel demonstrated that in the first generation, F_1, pairing of two individuals (P_1) with homozygous traits AA (dominant) and aa (recessive) results in a heterozygous progeny Aa, which exhibits the dominant phenotype Aa. However, in the second generation, F_2, the segregation of phenotype is 25% AA homozygotes, 50% Aa heterozygotes, and 25% aa homozygotes.[28]

The phenotype is the observable expression of the genotype or genetic code. In this type of segregation, 75% of offspring would exhibit the dominant phenotype (25% AA, 50% Aa), and 25% would exhibit the recessive aa phenotype, which is only expressed in the homozygous aa genotype.

Dihybrid Cross

In this trial cross, two sets of different genes are studied. The F_1 generation is $1:1:1:1$. In the F_2 generation genes segregate in a ratio of $9:3:3:1$ and can be diagnostically predicted by the Punnet's checkerboard diagram (Fig 14–7).[29]

Probability

Probability is the mathematical study of events occurring by chance. Since the segregation of genes during meiosis is random, it follows the laws of probability. The expected probability of a certain genetic combination may or may not be seen in the second generation, but the probability that it may occur exists. Therefore, observed ratios vary in small numbers above or below the expected ratios of a given event.

Law of Coincidental Happenings

The law of coincidental happenings may be described this way: *the chance of any number of events happening together is equal to the product of the chances of each happening separately*.[30] For example, the chance of a coin toss resulting in heads is the same as the chance of a coin toss resulting in tails. So, from the principle of coincident happenings, if we toss two coins, the chance of two heads turning up is $½ \times ½ = ¼$. There is a one-in-four chance that both coins will turn up heads or tails. If six coins are tossed, the chance of six heads turning up is $½ \times ½ \times ½ \times ½ \times ½ \times ½ = ¹⁄₆₄$.

Law of Effect of Previous Events

Events that occur independently of each other do not influence the probability of those same events occurring again. However, if the events are not entirely independent, they may influence the probability of an event occurring. For instance, if in a

	GW	Gw	gW	gw
GW	GG WW	GG Ww	Gg WW	Gg Ww
Gw	GG wW	GG ww	Gg wW	Gg ww
gW	gG WW	gG Ww	gg WW	gg Ww
gw	gG wW	gG ww	gg wW	gg ww

9:3:3:1 Ratio

FIG 14–7.—Possible permutations in dihybrid cross generations.

deck of cards there are four aces and one is drawn at random, this will influence the probability of the other three being drawn by decreasing the chances of their appearance.

Chances may be calculated by expanding the binomial $(a + b)^n$, where a = the chance of one event occurring, b = the chance of another event occurring, and n = the total number of events occurring. For example, for two events, $(a + b)^2 = a^2 + 2ab + b^2$, and for four events, $(a + b)^4 = a^4 + 4a^3b + 6a^2b^2 + 4ab^3 + b^4$. Using this binomial, we can predict the simultaneous tossing of four coins 16 times. The probability of heads or tails combinations will be:

1 out of 16 times all coins will be heads;
4 out of 16 times, 3 will be heads, 1 will be tails;
6 out of 16 times, 2 will be heads, 2 will be tails;
4 out of 16 times, 3 will be tails, 1 will be heads;
1 out of 16 times all 4 will be tails.

This produces a gaussian distribution of the event sample plot similar to many other biologic sample plots. To calculate the likelihood that a particular event will occur out of a combination of events, the binomial method is used. The exponents of the first variable decrease by 1 in the sequence of the polynomial, as follows:

$$(a + b)^4 = a^4 + 4a^3b + 6a^2b^2 + 4ab^3 + b^4$$

Conversely, the exponents of the second variable increase by 1. To calculate the value of the coefficients, these steps are observed:[31] the first coefficient is 1, the second coefficient is the value of the first exponent, and the third coefficient is the product of the first two exponents divided by the number of the coefficients' ordinal numeric value:$(4 \times 3)/2 = 6$. Therefore, $a^4 + 4a^3b + 6a^2b^2 + 4ab^3 + b^4$.

Statistical Equations to Analyze the Validity of Results

A simple method for calculating the validity of the results of a statistical study is to calculate the standard error (SE). This is done by using the following formulas:[32]

$$SE = \sqrt{\frac{p \times q}{n}}$$

or, if the sample is large:

$$SE = \sqrt{\frac{p \times q}{n - 1}}$$

where p = the expected number of the first group with phenotype a, q = the expected number of the second group with phenotype b, and n = number of variables.

We can take as an example a population phenotyped for the MN blood group system. Assume that 150 people type M and 50 people type N, for a total population sample of 200. By using the formula for deriving SE, given above:

$$SE = \sqrt{\frac{150 \times 50}{200}} = 6.1$$

To convert the value to percentage of probability, we do the following:

$$\frac{\delta}{SE} = \frac{6}{6.1} = .98 \text{ (not significant)}$$

where δ = difference from the expected percentage.

When the SE value is 2 or higher, the result is considered statistically significant. The standard deviation (SD) of the values can be calculated as follows:

$$SD = \sqrt{\frac{\Sigma(\delta^1 - \delta^2)^2}{n}}$$

Concepts of Medical Genetics Useful in Immunohematology

or, if the sample is large:

$$SD = \sqrt{\frac{\Sigma\,(\delta^1 - \delta^2)^2}{n-1}}$$

Gene Linkage

The discovery of gene linkage was made by Sutton in 1903.[33] Linkage is said to occur with the simultaneous appearance of two different genes occurring in a ratio higher than that expected by chance alone.

It can be demonstrated by calculating the frequency with which these two separate genes are found together during crossing-over (Fig 14–8).

Two genes lying close to each other have a low incidence of crossing-over. If genes on a single chromosome are separated by a large distance, the probability of crossover is high. Since the frequency of crossing-over is proportional to the distance between genes, the genes on a particular chromosome can be mapped, once the crossover incidence is known. If the number of recombinants in a test cross is high, it indicates a high crossover rate, and therefore the genes are probably far apart on the chromosome. However, if the number of recombinants is low, the genes probably travel together and are therefore linked. One percent of the crossover frequency is 1 unit of length, otherwise known as a centimorgan. Double crossover may take place in certain cases and results in restoration of the original position of genes on the chromosome. Linked genes on the same side of the chromosome are said to be in the *cis* position:

A   a
B   b

Nonallelic genes located in different chromosomes are said to be in the *trans* position:

A   a
b   B

The Hardy-Weinberg Principle

The Hardy-Weinberg principle[34] has many applications in the determination of homozygous frequencies based on heterozygous frequencies. Initially, one must know the frequency of occurrence of homozygous recessive individuals in the general population by using the binomial,

$$(a + b)^2 = a^2 + 2ab + b^2$$

where a = the frequency of the dominant allele and b = the frequency of the recessive allele.

If b = the frequency of the recessive trait and b^2 = the total population with the recessive trait, then $b^2 = b$, or the frequency of the recessive trait.

A second equation gives us the frequency of the dominant allele:

$$a = 1 - b \quad \text{or} \quad 1 - \sqrt{b^2}$$

If b^2 = 1/16th of a certain population, then

$$\sqrt{1/16} = 1/4\,a = 1 - 1/4 = 3/4$$

Therefore, homozygotes = $\dfrac{(3)^2}{(4)^2} = \dfrac{9}{16}$

If we solved the problem with decimals, it would be:

rr (or b^2) = .0625 or 1/16
r = .0625 = .25
R = 1.0 − .25 = .75 or 3/4
Rr = 2 × .75 × .25 = .3750
RR = (.75)² = .5625

Therefore, heterozygotes will be $2ab$, or 2 × 3/4 × 1/4 = 6/16.

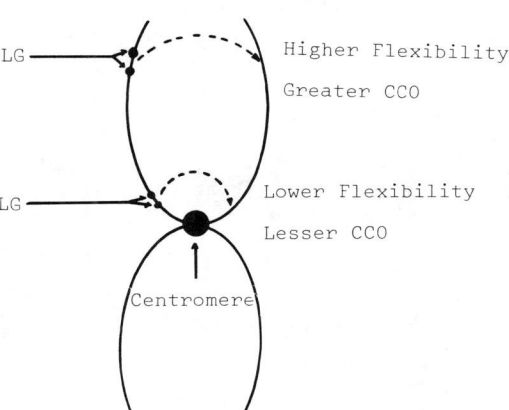

FIG 14–8.—Figure depicting the chance of linked genes *(LG)* crossing over to the opposite arm of a chromosome. Linked genes will travel together in such circumstances. Genes located in the distal portion of the arms of the chromosome have a greater chance of crossing over *(CCO)*.

Morton's Formula for Linkage

This analysis poses the question of linkage when odds are computed on the basis of random assortment. Morton's formula for linkage[33] states that the relative probability of linkage is as follows:

$$\frac{\text{Probability of linkage on the basis of 10 recombinations}}{\text{Probability of random assortment} (> .50)}$$

The Lod score represents the logarithm of relative odds or reciprocals. The greater the Lod score, the greater the probability that the genes are linked.

Gene Mutations

For the most part, genes are extremely stable units. However, mutations do occur. Mutations play an important part in evolution and in inheritable disease. Most mutations are harmful, but selection due to environmental factors tends to abolish such defects.

Mutations can occur in gametes and be transmitted to the progeny, or they may be somatic, affecting the cells in the developed organism. Several clinical and physical agents, such as x-rays and some carcinogens, can cause mutations on the genome of cells.

Pedigree Charts

Pedigree charts represent graphically the patterns of inheritance. Certain symbols are used by convention (Fig 14–9). The proband is the individual who prompted the study by the appearance of a determined phenotypic marker. The proband is usually indicated on the pedigree chart by an arrow.

Each generation is indicated by a Roman numeral. Each subject within a generation is indicated by an Arabic numeral to the left of the symbol on the pedigree chart. In small pedigrees the Arabic numerals may be omitted.[35] The sibship (family of brothers and sisters) is indicated by a coupling bar which unites the persons born to the same parents (see Fig 14–9). The marriage coupling bar unites husband and wife. A double coupling bar indicates that husband and wife are blood relatives.

Squares designate males and circles designate females. Affected persons are designated by filled-in squares or circles. Heterozygotes are designated by half-squares or half-circles. Carriers are indicated by a central dot in the square or circle.

Calculation of Probability by Fisher's Method

This method is useful to determine whether the probability of an event occurring is statistically significant.[36] The symbols used in Table 14–1 are defined as follows:

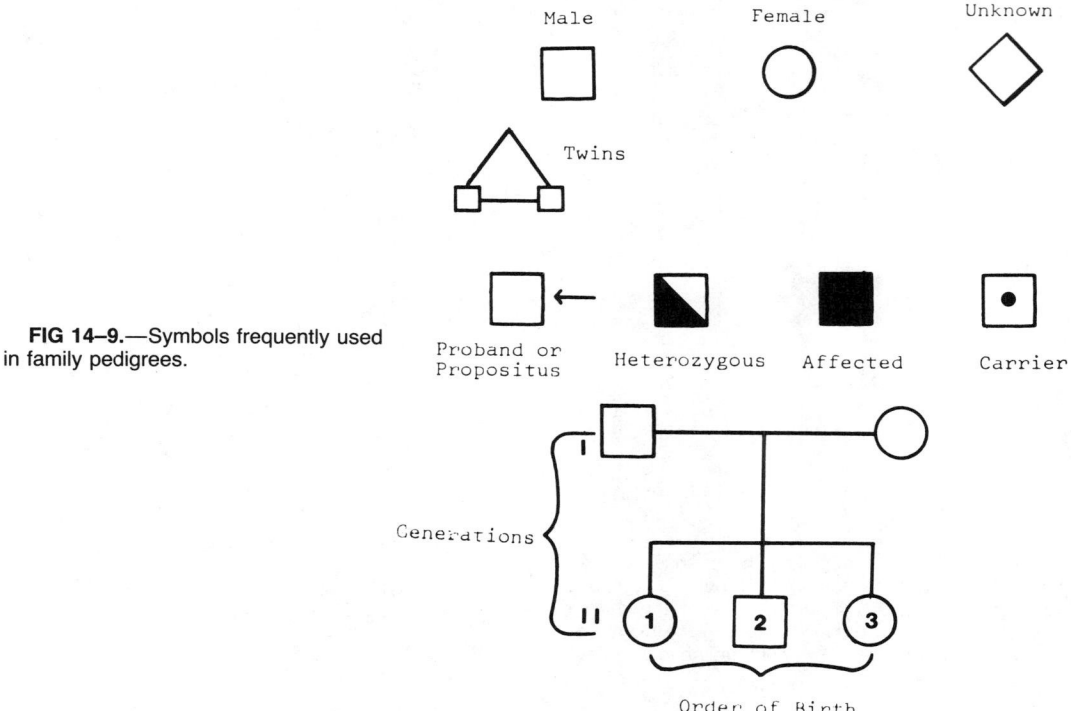

FIG 14–9.—Symbols frequently used in family pedigrees.

TABLE 14–1.—CALCULATION OF PROBABILITY BY THE FISHER METHOD

REACTION	CONDITION PRESENT	CONDITION ABSENT	TOTALS
+	A	B	A + B
−	C	D	C + D
TOTALS	A + C	B + D	N

A, positive finding, the condition searched for is present.

B, positive finding, the condition searched for is absent.

C, negative finding, the condition searched for is present.

D, negative finding, the condition searched for is absent.

N, total number of reactions observed.

P, probability.

The formula is applied in factorials (!):

$$P = \frac{(A+B)!\,(C+D)!\,(A+C)!\,(B+D)!}{(N!)\,(A!)\,(B!)\,(C!)\,(D!)}$$

A factorial is the product of all of the whole integers from 1 to the integer listed (e.g., $5! = 5 \times 4 \times 3 \times 2 \times 1$).

REFERENCES

1. Yunis J.J., Chandder M.E.: Cytogenetics, in Henry B.J. (ed.): *Clinical Diagnosis and Management by Laboratory Methods*, ed. 16. Philadelphia, W.B. Saunders Co., 1979, p. 801.
2. Patau K.: The identification of individual chromosomes especially in man. *Am. J. Hum. Genet.* 12:250, 1960.
3. Wang H.C., Federoff S.: Banding in human chromosomes treated with trypsin. *Nature* 235:52, 1972.
4. Casperson T., Zech L., Johansson C., et al.: Identification of human chromosomes by DNA-binding fluorescent agents. *Chromosoma* 30:215, 1970.
5. Dutrillaux B., LeJeune J.: Sur une nouvelle technique d'analyse du caryotype humain. *CR Acad. Sci. (D) (Paris)* 272:2638, 1971.
6. Arrighi F.E., Hsu T.C.: Staining constitutive heterochromatin and Giemsa crossbands of mammalian chromosomes, in Yunis J.J. (ed.): *Human Chromosome Methodology*, ed. 2. New York, Academic Press, 1974, p. 1.
7. Paris Conference: Standardization in human genetics. *Birth Defects* 3(7), 1971.
8. Rowley J.D.: The role of cytogenetics in hematology. *Blood* 48:1, 1976.
9. Shokeir M.H.K., Ying K.L., Pabello P.: Deletion of the long arm of chromosome no. 7: Tentative assignment of the Kidd (Jk) locus. *Clin. Genet.* 4:360, 1973.
10. Watson J.D., Crick F.H.C.: Molecular structure of nucleic acids. *Nature* 171:737, 1953.
11. Elgin S.C.R., Weintraub H.: Chromosomal proteins and chromatin structure. *Annu. Rev. Biochem.* 44:725, 1975.
12. Orten J.M., Neuhaus O.: *Human Biochemistry*, ed. 10. St. Louis, C.V. Mosby Co., 1982, p. 164.
13. Lehman I.R., Uyamura D.G.: DNA polymerase I: Essential replication enzyme. *Science* 193:963, 1976.
14. Brawerman G.: Eukaryotic messenger RNA. *Annu. Rev. Biochem.* 43:621, 1974.
15. Rich A., Raj Bhandary U.L.: Transfer RNA: Molecular structure, sequence and properties. *Annu. Rev. Biochem.* 45:805, 1976.
16. Chambon P.: Split genes. *Sci. Am.* 244:60, 1981.
17. Jacob F., Monod J.: Genetic regulatory mechanisms in the synthesis of proteins. *J. Mol. Biol.*, 3:318, 1961.
18. Maniatis T., Fritsch E.F., Sambrook J.: *Molecular Cloning: A Laboratory Manual*. Cold Spring Harbor, N.Y., 1982, pp. 1–55.
19. Clewell D.B.: Nature of Col E1 plasmid replication in *Escherichia coli* in the presence of chloramphenicol. *J. Bacteriol.* 110:667, 1972.
20. Hendrix R.W., Roberts J.W., Stahl F.W., Weisberg R.A.: *Lambda II*. Cold Spring Harbor Laboratory. Cold Spring Harbor, N.Y., 1983.
21. Williams B.G., Blattner F.R.: Bacteriophage λ vectors for DNA cloning, in Setlow J.K., Hollaender A. (eds.): *Genetic Engineering*. New York, Plenum Press, 1980, vol. 2, p. 201.
22. Hohn B., Collins J.: A small cosmid for efficient cloning of large DNA fragments. *Gene* 11:291, 1980.
23. Stroup M.: Genetic manipulation and control of disease, in Garraty G. (ed.): *Blood Group Antigens and Disease*. Arlington, Va., American Association of Blood Banks, 1983, pp. 85–123.
24. Watson J.D., Tooze J., Kurtz D.: *Recombinant DNA: A Short Course*. New York, Scientific American Books, 1983, pp. 72–90.
25. Temin H.M.: RNA-directed DNA synthesis. *Sci. Am.* 226:25, 1972.
26. Southern F.M.: Detection of specific sequences among DNA fragments separated by gel electrophoresis. *J. Mol. Biol.* 98:503, 1975.
27. Almine J.C., Kemp D.J., Stark G.R.: Method for detection of specific RNAs in agarose gels by transfer to diazobenzyl oxymethyl-paper and hybridization with DNA probes. *Proc. Natl. Acad. Sci. USA* 74:5350, 1977.
28. Altenburg E.: *Genetics*. New York, Henry Holt & Co., 1957, p. 25.
29. Strickberger M.W.: *Genetics*. New York, Macmillan Publishing Co., 1968, p. 109.
30. Gardner E.J.: *Principles of Genetics*. New York, John Wiley & Sons, 1968, p. 47.
31. Winchester A.M.: *Heredity: An Introduction to Genetics*, ed. 2. New York, Barnes & Noble, 1966, p. 74.

32. Bradford-Hill A.: *A Short Textbook of Medical Statistics*. Kent, England, Hodder & Stoughton, 1977, p. 287.
33. Winchester A.M.: *Heredity: An Introduction to Genetics*, ed. 2. New York, Barnes & Noble, 1966, p. 141.
34. Winchester A.M.: *Heredity: An Introduction to Genetics*, ed. 2. New York, Barnes & Noble, 1966, p. 230.
35. Frazer-Roberts J.A., Pembrey M.E.: *An Introduction to Medical Genetics*, ed. 7. Oxford, England, Oxford Medical Publications, 1978, p. 14.
36. Widman F.K. (ed.): *Technical Manual*, ed. 8. Washington, D.C., American Association of Blood Banks, 1981, p. 420.

Paternity Testing and Forensic Immunohematology

EVER SINCE the U.S. Congress passed Public Law 93-647 in 1975,[1] ruling the right of a child to have a father and relieving the public of the economic burden of supporting illegitimate children, the demand for paternity testing has increased. Laboratory tests for paternity should be undertaken only by the specialized laboratory, because the complexities involved in performing the tests are usually beyond the realm of routine blood banking, and the legal responsibility of correctly interpreting them requires specialized experience. One of the more crucial aspects of paternity testing is the proper identification of the probands in the presence of witnesses. The guidelines summarized below are derived from those reached by concensus of the American Medical Association (AMA) and the American Bar Association (ABA).[2]

IDENTIFICATION, TESTING, AND REPORTING

The name of the institution and its location are identified on the record, which becomes a legal document. Witnesses must show a signed identification document bearing a photograph (such as a passport or license). Age, sex, race, and address and telephone number of the individuals tested are entered into the record, which is signed by them and by the witnesses. Fingerprints of the alleged parents as well as the child's footprint, if the child is less than 1 year old, also become part of the record.

Blood samples and saliva samples are obtained in duplicate and identified by the proband's name and social security number. Sample containers should be signed and dated by the technologist taking the sample. All tests are run in duplicate, with positive and negative controls. All tests are performed with licensed reagents where possible. Tests are performed by expert senior technologists versed in paternity testing. Results are recorded as they are read and reactions are graded. Records of electrophoretic patterns are secured once they have been developed. A physician in charge of the laboratory supervises, interprets, and reports the results.

Family Studies

To study gene distribution it is sometimes necessary to study family distribution. Family distribution can be graphically represented by pedigree charts (Fig 15-1). The proband or individual under study is indicated by an arrow. Each generation is assigned a roman numeral.

Types of Markers Used

The markers used in paternity testing should (1) follow mendelian laws and (2) be polymorphic, to allow variation in the population without exhibit-

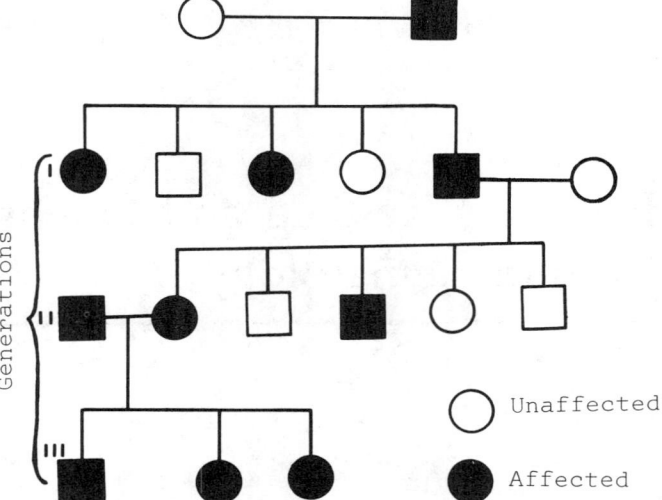

FIG 15–1.—A family pedigree representing a non-sex-linked trait.

ing extreme polymorphism, which would not be useful. Nevertheless, some rare alleles, such as Mg in the MNS system, are useful in paternity testing.

The following rules apply to paternity testing:[3]

1. The child cannot exhibit a genetic marker not found in the parents. (A direct exclusion is determined if this type of extraneous marker is observed.)

2. The child must inherit one of each of the genes in a marital pair. (A direct exclusion is present if this phenomenon is not observed.)

3. A child cannot be homozygous for a trait unless both parents carry the marker. (An indirect exclusion is established in this case.)

4. A child must inherit one of the genes from a homozygote pair. (An indirect exclusion is established if this is not the case).

Blood groups or other markers used in paternity actions must show unequivocal patterns of inheritance, must show a relatively high frequency of each of the alleles, and must not be affected by age or environmental factors. In addition, reliable, reproducible techniques for detecting the phenotype must be available. Blood groups used in paternity usually have distinct predictable patterns of inheritance, and most are codominant.[4] A first-order exclusion can only very rarely be justified on the basis of suppressor genes. Mutation is very rarely accepted as an argument for the presence of an unexpected antigen because mutations are rare events. Chimerism may be a source of confusion and should be considered in rare cases. It should be noted that only exclusions, not incontroversial proof of paternity, can be obtained by paternity testing. Certain blood group antigens comply with the conditions described above and are therefore useful in paternity testing.

Red Blood Cell (RBC) Antigens

The ABO System in Paternity Testing

Because of its known genetic inheritance patterns, relative polymorphism, and well-established techniques for detection, the ABO system is always tested for in paternity cases. It is also the blood type most judges involved in paternity actions are acquainted with.

In many cases ABO testing can provide direct exclusion, such as, for example; if the mother is group A, the child is AB, and the alleged father is O. ABH substances can be found in secretions, so this system is also used in various types of criminology studies.

However, paternity exclusion testing is never limited to the ABO system. Although rare, there are some pitfalls which should be considered in ABO testing. Newborns and infants may have weakly expressed antigens. Certain patients with intestinal infections or intestinal inflammation may have acquired group substances (e.g., acquired B antigen).[5] Bombay-group individuals are very rare but should be readily detectable. Chimeras may give rise to ABO typing abnormalities (for more details, see Chap. 5).

AB antigens in the *cis* position on a chromosome may be a source of confusion, but these cases are exceptionally rare.[6] Subgroups of A may be a more frequent source of discrepancy, but laboratory methods are readily available to clarify these cases.

Rh System in Paternity Testing

The Rh system is also useful because it is widespread and polymorphic. By itself, it can exclude as many as 25% of cases in paternity testing.[3] At least 35 different antigenic determinants have been described for alleles and combinations of alleles in the Rh system. Again, only the phenotype can be tested for, the genotype remaining mostly unknown unless the family of the proband can be fully phenotyped. The Rh null phenotype is a possible source of misleading results, but it is so rare that its significance in paternity testing is mostly of academic interest. Deletions in the Rh system are similarly rare and should not be of concern in most cases. As was described earlier in the chapter on Rh antigens, weakened forms of the Rh antigen exist and are more frequent than deletions or other rare Rh antigenic determinants. These weakened forms should be considered when interpreting Rh phenotypes in paternity studies. Most Rh antigens are codominant and are therefore expressed in the heterozygote state. In the Rh system antisera exist that are specific for combination of antigens (e.g., anti-ce or f), which help determine the position of the genes on either side of the genome (e.g., CDe/ce versus CDe/cE) (see Chap. 5).

Other RBC Antigens

The MNS system is also very useful in paternity testing, having a 30% exclusion probability. Care must be taken, however, with rare alleles such as M^g or M^x, which may give apparently mistaken results. The Duffy system is also useful, providing about an 18% probability when Fy^a and Fy^b are included. The Kidd system gives an 18% exclusion probability. The Kell system by itself excludes only about 5% of alleged parents. Lutheran, Lewis, and P systems are not routinely used in paternity testing because their exclusion probabilities are inconstant. Care must be exercised with antigens that show a dosage effect. In general, the cumulative exclusion percentage for the RBC antigens listed above is about 60%–65%.

The HLA System in Paternity Testing

The HLA system is the single most useful system to exclude paternity. It provides a 60%–82% cumulative chance of exclusion, using readily available antisera. However, the test is not available in many blood banks. HLA-A has 18 known alleles, B has 23, C has 6, and D has 11; the DR antigen has 7 defined alleles. The use of HLA-A and B antigens is the most practical approach because the methods are simpler and reagents can be obtained commercially. The possible combinations of the HLA-A and HLA-B alleles amount to 210 haplotypes, more than 22,000 genotypes, and more than 12,000 phenotypes. Blood samples should be collected in heparin and studied while they are fresh. The A and B HLA loci are the ones most commonly tested for. This is done by cytotoxicity, using antisera obtained commercially. Values are compared with national standards provided by the National Institutes of Health.

Because of linkage disequilibrium, the gene frequencies in any given individual are not calculated independently but as a haplotype. Recombination between genes occurs in about 0.8% of meiotic divisions, a fact which is taken into account in probability calculations. A diagram of an HLA paternity exclusion test is shown in Figure 15–2.

Only direct exclusions are accepted using the HLA system, because of cross-reactivity of antisera, possible crossover, and lack of good statistical data for different ethnic groups.

RBC Enzyme Phenotyping in Paternity Testing

RBC enzymes were introduced into paternity testing relatively recently. These proteins can be detected by electrophoresis, and the equipment is usually accessible to blood bank laboratories.

Furthermore, some of these proteins are expressed widely in the population in a desirable degree. Both the polymorphism and codominance of phenotypic expression of these enzymes make these markers useful in paternity testing.

The polymorphism of RBC enzymes allows definition between populations and at times helps differentiate one individual from another. RBC enzymes supplement blood groups in paternity studies and in blood studies in criminology. Protein sequences are coded for by nuclear DNA and transmitted to the cytoplasm via mRNA. Some of these proteins, including those to be discussed in this section, exhibit enzyme activity. Because they are coded for directly by DNA, their hereditary patterns can be traced. These proteins change little, if at all, and their phenotypic products are readily identifiable.[7]

The enzymes used for paternity, forensic, or an-

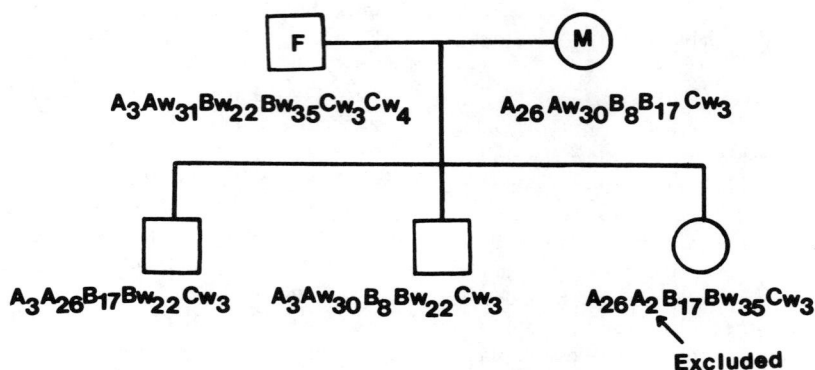

FIG 15–2.—Paternity exclusion by HLA testing. The progeny has HLA genes compatible with the mother's phenotype (HLA26, B17, and Cw3). However, the HLA2 gene is not found in either parent. The alleged father was therefore excluded.

thropologic studies are those that have a useful degree of polymorphic expression, are (usually) codominant, and have clear-cut, predictable genetic segregation patterns.

Proteins, which are composed of sequences of amino acids, have an amino terminal and a carboxyl terminal. As such, they behave as zwitterions or dipolar ions. This characteristic determines the dissociation constant and makes them travel on an electrically charged gel matrix as positively or negatively charged molecules, the degree of charge depending on the pH of the solution in which they are suspended. The matrix is usually a protein with a gel consistency. Test proteins are inoculated and given an electrical charge (electrophoresis). The differential charge allows separation of proteins. It is this difference in migration patterns that allows distinction of the various phenotypes. The type of matrix, running time, strength of the current, and concentration of the buffer are factors that may influence the rate of migration as well.

The staining procedure involves either (1) application of specific substrate, which reacts with the enzyme, or (2) direct dye chromophore, such as Coomassie blue stain. In the first case, enzymes are reacted specifically by one of the following methods: (a) chromogenic substrate, (b) fluorogenic substrates, or (c) electron transfer dyes. These substrates are applied to the gel by agar overlay or by segments of filter paper saturated with the substrate.

Sample Collection

Blood samples are usually collected in acid-citrate-dextrose solution. Hemolysates from the washed RBCs can be obtained by freezing and thawing or by sonication. Stroma-free hemolysates can also be obtained by addition of digitonin. Many of these RBC enzymes can be run on hydrolyzed starch as well. Texts by Giblett,[7] Dykes et al.,[8] and Shanfield et al.[9] can be consulted for collection methods for the more frequently used enzymes in paternity testing.

The samples are run by inoculating the gel at the cathodal end. Four different enzymes can be studied on one slab. Brinkman's method is a good method for staining.[10]

Some Characteristics of Frequently Used Enzyme Phenotypes (Table 15–1)

Erythrocyte Acid Phosphatase.—This enzyme participates in the hydrolysis of monophosphate esters. It is present in high amounts in semen, on erythrocytes, and in saliva[11] and can therefore be used in forensic determinations. Three allelic markers are common: pa, pb, and pc. Other less common alleles are p^r and p^d.

Phosphoglucomutase.—PGM converts glucose-1-phosphate to glucose-6-phosphate. At least three genetic loci are identified: PGM_1, PGM_2, and PGM_3. PGM_1 is commonly used in forensic medicine because of its ease of identification as well as its stability. Common phenotypes of PGM are PGM_1-1, PGM_1-2-1, and PGM_1-2. Many rare phenotypes have been defined.[12] PGMs appears to be linked to HLA and MNS.[13]

Glucose-6-Phosphate Dehydrogenase (G6PD).—G6PD converts gluconate-6-phosphate

TABLE 15–1.—Some Enzymes Used in Paternity Testing*

ENZYME IN CAUCASIANS	LOCI	SUBUNITS	COMMON PHENOTYPES	FREQUENCY (%)
Acid phosphatase	EAP^a	RBC	AA	11.5
	EAP^b	β	AB	42
	EAP^c	α	BB	34.5
			BC	7
Phosphogluconate mutase	PGM_1	"a"	1–1, 2–1, 2–2	63, 32, 5
	PGM_2	"e"		
	PGM_3	"h"		
Glucose-6-phosphate dehydrogenase	$G6PD^A$		A-A	95.8
	$G6PD^B$		A-B	4
			B-B	0.05
Glutamate pyruvate transaminase	GPT_1		1–1	26.4
	GPT_2		2–1	47.8
	GPT_3		2–2	25.1
Esterase D	EsD_1		1–1	80
	EsD_2		2–1	18
	EsD_3		2	1.5
			3–1	<0.05
Adenosine	ADA_1		1–1	88
	ADA_2		2–1	11.5
			2–2	0.5
Glyoxalase I	GLO_1		1–1	17
	GLO_2		2–1	50
			2–2	32
Adenylate kinase	AK_1		1–1	92.5
	AK_2		2–1	7.45
			2–2	0.05

*Most of these enzymes are present in a variety of other tissues aside of RBCs. PGM_3 is not present on RBCs.

to ribulose-5-phosphate in the pentose cycle. This enzyme is quite polymorphic and hence useful in population studies. The main alleles are PGD^A and PGD^B.

Glutamine Pyruvate Transaminase (GPT).—GPT transfers amino acids to ketoacids in the urea cycle. GPT_1, GPT_2, and GPT_3 have been described. Three phenotypes are common GPT_1, GPT_{2-1} and GPT_2.[14] Several isotypes have been described. They are detected by starch electrophoresis and developed with formazan.

Esterase D (EsD).—Three common alleles are known for EsD—EsD^1, EsD^2, and, rarely, EsD^3. It is a good enzyme to investigate forensic cases because of its good phenotypic population distribution.

Adenosine Deaminase (ADA).—Adenosine deaminase is an aminohydrolase that catalyzes the deamination of adenosine to inosine in the purine metabolism. ADA has two common alleles: ADA_1 and ADA_2. Rarely ADA_{3-7} are observed.

Glyoxalase I (GLO).—GLO is quite polymorphic[15] and is likewise useful in paternity testing.

Adenylate Kinase (AK).—AK catalyzes conversion of ADP into ATP and AMP. Two frequent alleles are known AK_1 and AK_2. It can be identified by starch electrophoresis.

Erythrocyte acid phosphatase (EACP), alanine amino transferase (ALT or GPT), glyoxalase (GLO), and phosphoglucomutase (PGM) offer a 13%–18% chance of exclusion when used individually. Esterase D (EsD), adenylate kinase (AK), adenosine deaminase (ADA), and glucose-6-phosphate dehydrogenase (G6PD) offer an additional 1%–8% exclusion. The cumulative chance of exclusion by using the eight enzymes combined may be 66.3% in whites and 55.6% in blacks. Most of the enzymes listed have two common different alleles, except ACD, which has three alleles. These alleles migrate differently in the electrophoretic matrix and are distinguished either as type 1/type 2 or as type A/type B, depending on the enzyme. Therefore, genotypes are expressed as 1–1, 1–2 or AA, AB.[16] When the samples are run on a gel, AK, G6PD, and ADA are run in one half of the gel and the remainder of the gel is used for acid phosphatase. PGM and EsD can also be used. A frequently found allele combination for ADA is ADA (1,2); for EsD, EsD (1,2) is the most frequent combination. G6PD is sex-linked and usually used in paternity exclusion for female children.

Enzyme results should not be interpreted by inexperienced personnel because amorphs and alleles with low activity do exist. About 37.3% of alleged fathers can be excluded by just using enzymes, but the figure may be greater, depending on the ethnic group studied.[3]

Other Proteins[17]

Proteins in plasma are often polymorphic enough to be of use in paternity testing. The plasma proteins most suitable for testing are those found in serum. Polyacrylamide gels are suitable as a matrix for separation of these proteins. Controls of each protein are run in parallel and stained with amido black, Coomassie blue, or other protein stains.

Some useful proteins in paternity testing are the following: Gc-globulin, or group-specific component, has two common alleles, Gc^1 and Gc^2. The probability of exclusion varies from 15% in the white population to 8% in the black population. Ceruloplasmin is also useful: Cp^A and Cp^B are the common alleles. The probability of exclusion varies from 0.5% in the white population to 5% in the black population. Haptoglobin is frequently used in paternity exclusion (Fig 15–3). Hp^1 and Hp^2 are the two common alleles. The probability of exclusion is 18% in the white population and 15% in the black population. The Gm γ-globulin heavy chain marker as well as Inv and Km from light chains are also polymorphic and can be used in exclusions. However, deletions, crossing-over, failure to appear at an early age, and changes during certain diseases make these proteins somewhat less reliable than the more stable markers such as the ABO system. The addition of RBC enzymes and plasma proteins to RBC antigen testing gives a cumulative chance of exclusion of about 93.3%.

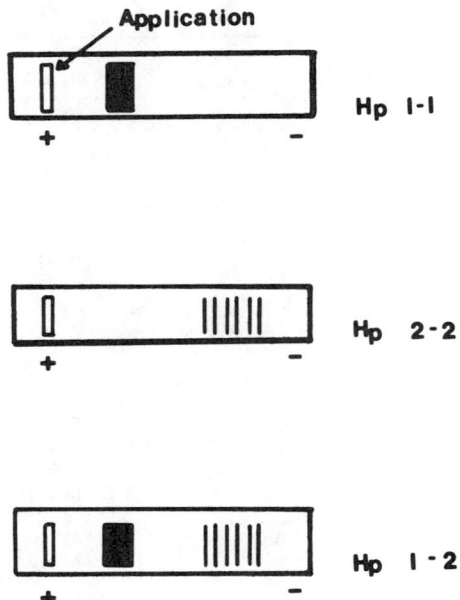

FIG 15–3.—Electrophoretic patterns of haptoglobin phenotypes. Phenotype 1–1 has one single solid band. Phenotype 2–2 has several faint bands. Phenotype 1–2 exhibits one heavy band close to the positive charge and several finer bands close to the negative charge.

How Valid is Paternity Testing?

The person being tried in a paternity case has the right to know how accurate was the test or combination of tests used to determine his case. To assess the validity of the combination of tests used, single gene frequencies as well as the probability of gametes containing certain genes are used. These values are found in most standard textbooks on paternity testing.[18–20] This section briefly reviews some of the formulas used in determining the validity of a test or group of tests in paternity exclusion.

Approach to Paternity Test Results[18]

1. List the phenotypes of the alleged father *(AF)*, the mother *(M)*, and the child *(C)*, and compare them with random man *(RM)* in the population.

2. How frequently would each phenotype of the trio *(AF, M, C)* occur at random?

3. Compute the probability of exclusion by adding the individual exclusion frequencies. This is done by using the phenotype frequency of *AF* and calculating the genotype frequencies of the mother, which are compatible with the phenotype of the child.

Hardy-Weinberg Law

As reviewed in Chapter 14, gene frequencies are obtained from the general population by the Hardy-Weinberg Law,[21] which states that the ratio between homozygous individuals and heterozygous individuals remains constant from generation to generation. The formula for this probability equilibrium is:

$$p^2 + 2pq + q^2$$

which results from the sum of all possible permutations of genetic marker p and its allele q. Thus the genotypes of a and b can be combined as: aa × aa, aa × ab, aa × bb, ab × aa, ab × ab, ab × bb, bb × ab, and bb × bb. This expression is summarized as follows: if $a = p$ and $b = q$ to generalize for any gene marker, and $2pq$ represents the heterozygote, by factoring we get $pp(pp + 2pq + qq) + 2pq(pp + 2pq + qq) + qq(pp + 2pq + qq)$, or $p^2 = 2pq + p^2$, which is the Hardy-Weinberg formula.

Together, $p + q = 1$ accounts for all the population. We can then infer the following: if p is the trait, then p^2 represents the homozygous distribution of p in a population. Similarly, if q is the other allele, then q^2 represents the homozygous distribution of q in a population, and $2pq$ will represent the heterozygous population. Hence,

$$\sqrt{p^2} = p$$
$$1 - p = \% \text{ of } q$$
$$\sqrt{q^2} = q$$
$$1 - q = \% \text{ of } p$$

Let AF represent the alleged father, M the mother, and C the child. Suppose one marker (e.g., Kell) is used, and AF is Kell negative, M is Kell negative, and C is Kell positive. Then:

$$AF = kk = q^2$$
$$M = kk = q^2$$
$$C = p$$

where p = gene frequence of RBC marker P (in this case Kell antigen) and q = gene frequency of marker Q (in this case k).

By multiplying,

$$q^2 \times q^2 \times p = pq^4$$

which is the combined set of frequencies.

pq^4 is the probability of exclusion for P and q^2 is the chance that AF or M is homozygous (negative for p; in this case, negative for K or Kell antigen). $q^2 \times q^2 = q^4$ represents the chance that AF and M are homozygous and negative for p. If pq^4 is the probability of exclusion for P, the p^4q is the probability of exclusion for Q.

When two alleles are tested for in combination, rather than one only, a greater probability of exclusion is obtained. Two criteria are used, one for each antigen. The formula for two antisera is:[22]

$$pq^4 + p^4q + 2p^2q^2 = pq(p^3 + q^3 + 2pq)$$

Simplifying, this expression becomes:

$$pq(1 - pq)$$

An example is given below with only M and N RBC antigen phenotypes given as markers in a caucasian paternity exclusion case.

Gene frequency of M in whites: $p = 0.5536$ (from tables).

Gene frequency of N in whites: $q = 0.4464$ (from tables).

From the Hardy-Weinberg formula, the chance of exclusion with anti-M antiserum will be pq^4, or $0.5536 \times (0.4464)^4 = 0.0219$, or a 2% chance of exclusion. The chance of exclusion with anti-N antiserum is p^4q, or $(0.5536)^4 \times 0.4464 = 0.0419$, or a 4% chance of exclusion. Using the two antisera, $0.5536 \times 0.4464(1 - 0.5536 \times 0.4464) = 0.1860$, or 19%. This means that using both antisera there is a 19% chance of exclusion if only the MN system is used.

Cumulative Probability of Exclusion—More Than One System

Let CPE be the cumulative probability of exclusion[22] and PE be the probability of exclusion. Then PE_1 (system 1; e.g., ABO) = 0.185 (from tables) and PE_2 (system 2; e.g., MNS) = 0.316 (from tables).

When the two systems are combined (ABO + MNS), $PE_1 + PE_2 - (PE_1 \times PE_2) = 0.190 + 0.316 - (0.190 \times 0.316) = 0.45$ or 45% CPE. Thus, the cumulative probability of exclusion using ABO and MN blood groups is 45%.

Generalizing for more than two systems, the formula would be:[23]

Two systems:

$$PE_1 + PE_2 - (PE_1 \times PE_2) = 1 - (1 - PE_1)(1 - PE_2)$$

More than two systems:

$$1 - (1 - PE_1)(1 - PE_2)(1 - PE_3) \ldots (1 - PE_n)$$

The probability of exclusion does not give us sufficient information to do a relative comparison with a given population. It, therefore, becomes necessary to compare the frequencies of each of the genes found in the group under study, namely, M, C, and AF, with the frequencies of each gene in the random population. For this comparison to be of use in determining the validity of a test, the paternity index or the plausibility of paternity should be calculated.

Paternity Index and Plausibility of Paternity

First, list all the possibilities of the mother's genotypes compatible with the offspring, then list all the genotype possibilities of the alleged father which could be compatible with the phenotype of the offspring. Let X equal the combined probability that AF contributed the gene and Y equal the combined probability that RM contributed the gene.

The plausibility of paternity is calculated with the Essen-Moller formula:

$$W = X/(X + Y) = \frac{X}{Y} \frac{(X+Y)}{Y} = \frac{X}{Y} / \frac{X}{Y} + 1 = \frac{PI}{PI + 1}$$

Conversely,

$$PI = X/Y$$

Generalizing:

$$1/[(1 + Y_1/X_1)(Y_2/X_2)(Y_3/X_3)(Y_nX_n)]$$

where X = chance of paternity of AF, Y = chance of paternity of RM, and W = plausibility of paternity.

Example:
Alleged father AF types as ABO group A_1.
The mother M types as A_2.
Possible genotypes of C: A_2A_2 or A_2O
Possible genotypes of M: A_2A_2 or A_2O
Possible genotypes of AF: A_2A_2, A_1A_1, or A_1O
The obligatory gene OG is either A_2 or O.

First possibility:
If M transmitted an A_2 gene with the frequency 0.525 (from tables), then AF transmitted A_2 (.525) or O (.475). The probability will then be the product $A_2 \times O$ or $(.525)(.475) = 0.231$, or a 23% probability that this combination may have happened.

Second possibility:
If M transmitted a group O gene (0.475) then the alleged father AF must have contributed an A_2 gene (.04) (from table), which is less likely, because AF is phenotyping as A_1, and A_1/A_2 is a rare combination, found in only 4% of the population. Therefore, the probability is $(.475)(.04) = 0.019$.

Let X = total probability that AF is the father. X is obtained by adding the first and second possibilities. Therefore, $0.231 + .019 = .250$. If a random man RM were considered in the case given above, then we would restate the two possibilities as follows: if M transmits A_2 (.525), then RM must contribute A_2 (.525) or O (.7304), in which case the probability would be $(.525)(.7304) = .3834$. If M contributed the O gene (.475), then RM must have contributed the A_2 gene of C. This possibility is remote (.07); thus $(.475)(.07) = .0332$.

Let Y equal all the possibilities that RM is the father. The likelihood is the sum of the first and second possibilities:

$$Y = 0.3834 + 0.0332 = .4166$$

Several phenotypes must be tested for this study to be of value. This procedure is repeated for each phenotype determined and the product of multiplying each X value obtained, then obtain the product of each of the Y values for each system analyzed. The products are termed composite X values and composite Y values. Let's assume that the following values were obtained as composites of AF, or $X = .28$, as compared to composite Y, $RM = .014$. Then:

$$\frac{X}{X + Y} = \frac{.28}{.28 + .014} = 0.95$$

This means there is a 95% chance that AF cannot be excluded. In other words, it is almost certain that AF is the father.

Legal Aspects of Paternity Testing

Close to 2 million illegitimate children were born in the United States in the past 5 years, accounting for more than 10% of all births. A significant number of these children will be dependent on subsidy from the state. The legal protection for an illegitimate child, in terms of custody or inheritance, may also be jeopardized if paternity is unclear. However, today a child is considered legitimate by common law in any alliance that can be compared to a formal marriage. For these reasons, Congress passed PL 93-647, which articulates the concept that every child is entitled to a legal father and therefore economic support, as stated in the introduction to this chapter.[1] This law, if enforced, will shift the burden of financial care from society to the parents of the children.

Laboratory testing of genetic markers that can clarify the paternity status of individuals involved in these cases has become crucial. Children born out of wedlock have a legal right to a paternal name, as well as to inheritance rights in many states, provided paternity can be proved in a court of law. This ruling relies heavily on paternity testing. However, there is still a substantial inequality in legislation against illegitimate children.

Welfare laws are not always clear whether the benefits cover illegitimate as well as legitimate children, leaving the decision up to the lawyer or judge. Thus, in many cases paternity must be proved before children can benefit from these provisions. The courts ruling for child support by the father rely on paternity testing when the paternity of the child is in question, as is the case when the mother was sexually involved with two men at the time of conception.

In a recent survey, about 10% of judges did not use laboratory tests as evidence in paternity cases, and only 7.6% used it in all their cases.[24] This probably is due to the inability of many laboratories to provide incontrovertible evidence to the courts. The AMA and ABA have therefore developed guidelines to ensure quality in paternity testing by laboratories. As a result, paternity testing has tended to become centralized in highly qualified laboratories such as blood banks in larger hospitals or blood centers.

Depending on each state's laws, exclusion by blood typing may or may not be accepted as conclusive. If paternity cannot be excluded but the probability calculations permit reasonable conclusions, these conclusions are accepted by some courts of law. However, in many states such a decision may be overridden. Substantial evidence must be provided by the laboratory that no errors occurred during the collection and testing of the specimens.

Paternity testing reports should provide clear explanations of the tests performed, documentation of the validity of these tests, and documentation of double testing conducted independently by two technicians. The forms should include certification by the director of the laboratory that the tests were performed in compliance with the AMA and ABA regulations on paternity. Conclusions reached on the plausibility of paternity should be clearly spelled out.

USE OF RBC ANTIGEN TESTING, RBC ENZYMES, AND PLASMA PROTEINS IN CRIMINOLOGY

In cases of murder, accidental death, or identification of a deceased person, RBC antigen testing, enzyme testing, and protein phenotypic identification may be of help in the crime laboratory. As in paternity testing, these tests must not be undertaken or interpreted by the novice. The consequences of interpretation may result in the imprisonment or release of an individual accused of a crime. It is, therefore, obvious that these tests are to be conducted by experts and that they should be performed with the utmost care and responsibility.

If a murderer gets the blood of his victim on his clothing and the police laboratory workup reports the putative evidence sample as probably belonging to the deceased, this represents helpful evidence to clarify the circumstances of the crime and may be used as such by a court of justice.

Although it is not yet possible to identify an individual exclusively by RBC phenotyping, exclusionary data based on statistical analysis of the frequency can be helpful in solving a case. Since the amount of RBC material available to the crime laboratory is usually very small, testing methods are somewhat different from paternity cases. Often micromethods are used, in which very small amounts of RBC substances or proteins from plasma can be detected. Samples from all the individuals that may have been involved in a case are grouped and sent to the crime laboratory with full identification of each suspect. Eliminating suspects who could not have shed blood and thus could not have contributed to the stains can save the crime laboratory a substantial amount of time. Blood phenotyping should be entered in the criminal record of a suspect, along with the fingerprints.

RBC Antigens

In fluid blood, the main method of RBC antigen identification is by agglutination, so long as the RBCs are intact. However, if the cells are disrupted, the absorption inhibition micromethod is employed. In this method, aliquots with different dilutions of antisera are added to extracts of stains. A reduction in the titer of the antiserum indicates the presence of the antigen.

A more sensitive method employs the teasing out of fabric fibers from the blood-stained cloth. This method is termed the Howard Martin technique.[25] These blood-stained fibers are incubated in high-titer antiserum specific for a suspected group. After a period of absorption, the fibers are washed to rid them of excess antiserum. Indicator cells with antigen specific for the antiserum are added.

If the suspected antigen is present on the strands the indicator cells will attach to the fibers. Conversely, if the antigen is absent, indicator cells will not adhere to strands. This procedure is useful for ABO typing but not for Rh or MNS typing.

If many stains are to be tried, the blood-stained fiber strands are attached to a sheet of cellulose acetate soaked in acetone. In this way, several samples can be processed at the same time.

The ABO system is always tested for and has certain advantages. The antigenic determinants are quite resistant to denaturation and withstand both drying and temperature changes. The samples are tested with anti-A, anti-B, and anti-A,B. Anti-H testing with *Ulex europaeus* is also used. A_1, B, and O cells are used as indicator cells. Some false results may be caused by denaturation by heating or chemical denaturation, as well as by bacterial contamination of samples.

Absorption elution, as described in chapter 6, has been useful in identifying ABO, Rh, and MN groups, in suspected blood stains.

In the future, radioimmunoassay and fluorescence-labeled antibodies may be used for identification and detection purposes. However, false positive results plague current technology in these areas.

ABO grouping of muscle, skin, and other tissues can also be undertaken with the absorption inhibition studies. The MN system is also tested for, but variability in antisera to detect it give confusing results. Rh antigens can be detected most suitably by the absorption elution method. Antisera against D, C, c, E, e, and C^w are commonly used in detection of Rh antigens. However, the Rh system is more susceptible to denaturation by drying and chemical denaturation than other systems. In modern criminology laboratories, an autoanalyzer similar to that used in large blood centers may be used to handle several samples. Results with this instrument are usually reliable and reproducible.

Study of Secretions in the Crime Laboratory[25]

The study of secretions is especially informative in the segment of the population exhibiting the secretor gene (Se) (approximately 80%). The secretion of A, B, and H substances and Lewis substances is detected by either agglutination inhibition with test antisera and cells or absorption inhibition and absorption elution methods.

This type of testing is not always clear-cut, and results should be analyzed very critically. Prozoning in the inhibition reaction is common and should be considered in the interpretation of results. All samples are tested against doubling dilutions of antiserum for correct interpretation. Dried samples of serum or saliva can be tested by redissolving substances from the sample materials.

RBC Enzymes and Plasma Proteins in Criminology[25]

These phenotypic markers can be used for the same purposes as RBC antigen studies in criminology. Some advantages to using RBC and plasma proteins are (1) they withstand a certain degree of drying and denaturation, (2) they are good phenotypic markers to identify individual samples, and (3) testing is performed with relatively simple equipment. The genetic inheritance is straightforward in most RBC enzyme systems and results are very often clear-cut, to the degree of representing evidenciary material. The enzymes and proteins studied are the same as those studied in paternity cases.

Some pitfalls to RBC enzyme and plasma protein testing include weak representation of the phenotype (e.g., in children), drying of the sample with subsequent degradation of proteins, phenotypic variants, and denaturation of proteins by other physical or chemical agents with appearance of accessory bands on the gels.

REFERENCES

1. Public Law 93–647. 93rd U.S. Congress, Jan. 4, 1975. Hr17045, Title IV-D of the SSA as amended.
2. Abbott J.P.: Joint AMA-ABA guidelines: Present states of serologic testing in problems of disputed parentage. *Family Law Q.* 10:247, 1976.
3. Lee C.L., Henry J.B.: Laboratory evaluation of dis-

puted paternity, in Henry J.B. (ed.): *Clinical Diagnosis and Management by Laboratory Methods*. Philadelphia, W.B. Saunders Co., 1979, p. 1507.
4. Holland P.V.: Transmission patterns, in Wilson J.K. (ed.): *Genetics for Blood Bankers*. Washington, D.C., American Association of Blood Banks, 1980, pp. 19–30.
5. Cameron C., Graham F., Dunsford I., et al.: Acquisition of a B-like antigen by red blood cells. *Br. Med. J.* 2:29, 1959.
6. Seyfried H., Waleska I., Werblinska B.: Unusual inheritance of ABO group in a family with B antigens. *Vox Sang.* 9:268, 1964.
7. Giblett E.R.: *Genetic Markers in Human Blood*. Oxford, England, Blackwell Scientific Publications, 1969, pp. 424–554.
8. Dykes D.D., Polesky H.F.: Application of tests for serum proteins and red cell enzymes in determination of parentage, in Silver H. (ed.): *Paternity Testing: A Seminar*. Washington, D.C., American Association of Blood Banks, 1978, p. 44.
9. Schanfield M.S., Polesky H.F., Sebring, E.S.: *Paternity Testing*. Chicago, Ill., American Society of Clinical Pathologists, 1975, p. 45.
10. Brinkman B., Thomas G.: Simultaneous three-isoenzyme polymorphisms: 6-phosphogluconate dehydrogenase (6-PGD), adenosine deaminase (ADA), adenyl kinase (AK). *Vox Sang.* 21:90, 1971.
11. Tan S.G., Ashton G.L.: Saliva acid phosphatases: Genetic studies. *Hum. Hered.* 26:81, 1976.
12. Dykes D.D., Polesky H.F.: Review of isoelectric focusing for Gc, PGM_1, Tf and Pi. *Clin. Lab. Sci.* 20:115, 1984.
13. Bissbort S., Kompf J., Bethge R., et al.: Population genetics of human red cell phosphoglucomutase isoenzyme PGM_3. *Humangenetik* 27:57, 1975.
14. Sonneborn H.H.: *Human Erythrocyte Iso-enzyme Polymorphism: Theory and Methods*. Frankfurt, Germany, Biotest Serum Institut, 1978, pp. 1–32.
15. Kompf J., Bisbort S., Gussmann S., et al.: Polymorphism of red cell glyoxalase I (E.C. 4.4.1.5): A new genetic marker in man. *Humangenetik* 27:141, 1975.
16. Harris H.: *The Principles of Human Biochemical Genetics*, ed. 2. Amsterdam, Elsevier North-Holland, 1975, pp. 30–90.
17. Dykes D.D., Polesky H.F.: The usefulness of serum protein and erythrocyte enzyme polymorphisms in paternity testing. *Am. J. Clin. Pathol.* 55:982, 1976.
18. Walker R.H.: Probability in the analysis of paternity test results, in Silver H. (ed.): *Paternity Testing: A Seminar*. Washington, D.C., American Association of Blood Banks, 1978, p. 69.
19. Boyd W.C.: Tables and nomogram for calculating chances for excluding paternity. *Am. J. Hum. Genet.* 6:426, 1954.
20. Hummel V.K.: *Biostatistical Opinion of Parentage Based Upon the Results of Blood Group Tests*. Stuttgart, Gustav Fisher Verlag, 1971.
21. Winchester A.M.: *Heredity: An Introduction to Genetics*, ed. 2. New York, Barnes & Noble, 1966, p. 230.
22. Weiner A.S., Lederer M., Polayes S.H.: Studies in isohemagglutination: IV. On the chances of proving nonpaternity with special reference to blood groups. *J. Immunol.* 19:259, 1930.
23. Sussman L.M.: *Paternity Testing by Blood Grouping*, ed. 2. Springfield, Ill., Charles C Thomas, Publisher, 1976.
24. Krause H.D.: Paternity testing: Legal considerations, in Silver H. (ed.): *Paternity Testing: A Seminar*. Washington, D.C., American Association of Blood Banks, 1978, p. 145.
25. Culliford B.J.: Polymorphic enzyme systems, in *The Examination and Typing of Blood Stains in the Crime Laboratory*. Washington, D.C., U.S. Dept. of Justice, Law Enforcement Assistance Administration, National Institute of Law Enforcement and Criminal Justice, 1971, pp. 106–207.

Perinatal Blood Banking

PEDIATRIC IMMUNOHEMATOLOGY, due to its special characteristics, can be considered a subspecialty of the general field of immunohematology. Its study can be divided into three areas: (1) prenatal immunohematology, (2) perinatal immunohematology, and (3) pediatric immunohematology.

PRENATAL IMMUNOHEMATOLOGY

Hemolytic Disease of the Newborn

Prenatal immunohematology has developed mainly as a result of preventing and treating hemolytic disease of the newborn (HDN). The description of serologic studies of a case of HDN by Levine and Stetson led to the understanding of the serologic basis of HDN, as well as to the discovery of the Rh system.[1]

Just how an antibody produced by the maternal immune system is capable of destroying the red blood cells (RBCs) of the conceptus, causing very serious disease and often death of the fetus in utero, or very high perinatal morbidity, has been the object of intense research for several decades. It has been known for some time that most of the IgG circulating in the fetus is of maternal origin, whereas IgM in the fetus is of fetal origin.[2]

The assumption was made that the presence of maternal IgG in the fetal circulation and the absence of maternal IgM was due to the smaller size of IgG in comparison to IgM. Immunoglobulin transport across the placental barrier, however, has proved to be more complex and not merely determined by the size of the molecules. It has been demonstrated, for instance, that Fc fragments of IgG, but not of IgM, can cross the placenta, whereas F(ab) fragments of neither IgG nor IgM are capable of crossing the placental barrier.[3] In addition, Fc transport across the placenta requires intact C_H2 and C_H3 domains.[4]

Transplacental IgG crossing appears to be an active transport phenomenon[5] rather than a simple diffusion phenomenon and appears to be mediated by a receptor for IgG in the trophoblast.[3,5] The receptor must be highly specific, for not only does it discriminate between IgG and IgM, but it favors the transport of certain subclasses of IgG. For instance, the rate of transport of IgG subclasses occurs in the following order: IgG1 > IgG4 > IgG3 > IgG2.[6,7]

This transport does not parallel the serum concentrations of these subclasses,[4] nor does it parallel the binding affinity of the IgG subclasses to the placental receptor.[8] It is possible that the sequence of disulfide bonds (IgG1 = 2, IgG2 = 3, IgG3 = 4, IgG4 = 1[9]) has a bearing on receptor selectivity. Unfortunately, Rh antibodies are usually of the IgG1 and IgG3 subclasses and readily cross the placenta.[10] A subclass restriction to IgG1 and IgG3 appears to hold for RBC antibodies of the IgG class.[11] Exceptions to this rule do exist; for example, in one series eight cases of strong IgG2 anti-D and three cases of IgG4 anti-D were observed.[12] Antibodies to bacterial polysaccharides are usually of the IgG2 subclass[11] and antibodies to factor VIII are consistently of the IgG4 subclass but may have a simultaneous component of IgG1 or IgG3.[13] IgG3 and IgG1 readily bind C1q (IgG3 > IgG1 > IgG2 > IgG4 at approximate ratios of 41:7:1:0)[14] and promote phagocytosis, IgG3 proving to be the most active, followed by IgG1. IgG2 and IgG4 do not appear to promote phagocytosis.[15] The binding affinity of IgG subclasses to FcR on monocytic phagocytes appears to depend on the integrity of the amino acid sequence between amino acids 407 and 416 in the C_H3 domain.[16]

Furthermore, RBCs coated with IgG3 are more effectively removed by splenic macrophages than those coated with IgG1,[17] and cells coated with IgG2 or IgG4 may survive normally.[18] These observations correlate with the finding that splenic macrophages possess receptors for IgG1 and IgG3 but not for IgG2 and IgG4.[19] This phenomenon becomes relevant when it is remembered that RBCs coated with antibody of the IgG1 and IgG3 subclasses are preferentially removed by the spleen. Two factors are clearly important in the development of HDN: the development of antigenic determinants on the fetal RBCs sufficient to induce an antibody response, and the potential for the antigen of inducing an IgG3 or IgG1 response in the mother.

Antigens of the Rh, Kell, Duffy, Kidd, and MNS systems are well developed at birth. ABH, P, and Lutheran antigen systems are less well developed, while Lewis, I, and Kell antigen systems are poorly developed.[20] Several of these antigens (e.g., Rh, Kell, Duffy) induce mostly IgG responses and are therefore likely to appear as the causative antibody of HDN, whereas other antigens, eliciting mostly IgM responses, will not be seen as causative of HDN (e.g., Lewis, I, and P [excluding a-Tj[a], which is usually IgG]).

The severity of HDN correlates linearly with levels of antibodies of subclass IgG1, but correlation with IgG3 antibodies is not so clear.[21] When HDN is caused by antibodies to antigens other than those of the Rh system, the disease is less severe, with few exceptions.[22]

When maternal antibodies cross the placental barrier, gaining access to the fetal circulation, and coat fetal RBCs, the potential for the development of HDN exists. When HDN develops, the life of fetal RBCs is shortened.[23] Many antibodies are capable of producing HDN, but the more important ones are those directed against the ABO and the Rh systems, for they account for 98% of all cases. The remaining 2% are attributed to non-ABO, non-Rh antigenic systems. ABO HDN affects between 7 and 53.4 per 1,000 births in certain populations, a distribution which may depend on socioeconomic factors rather than genetic factors.[24] The incidence of HDN secondary to Rh immunization before the advent of preventive treatment was similar to ABO, namely, about 7 per 1,000 births, 60% of which required therapy.[25] About 12% of the immunized mothers had stillbirths.[26] Since the introduction of Rh immune globulin (RhIG) prophylaxis, the incidence decreased from 40.5 cases per 10,000 births to 14.3 per 10,000 births in a span of 10 years (1970–1979).[27]

Pathophysiology of HDN and Erythroblastosis Fetalis

The pathophysiology of HDN and erythroblastosis fetalis (EF) centers on the effect of maternal antibodies directed against fetal RBCs that cross the placenta, coat fetal RBCs, and promote their destruction. An increase in anti-D titer from 1:16 to 1:32 is significant and may mean active EF.[28] This titer increment applies to other antibodies as well (e.g., Kell and Kidd system antibodies). Antibody titers below 1:16 within 10 days of delivery usually have a good prognosis.

Antibodies crossing the placenta coat the fetal RBCs (Fig 16–1) and are trapped by fetal splenic macrophages and destroyed completely or pitted, producing spherocytes. Thus, the main pathology of EF is anemia of varying degrees. The anemia stimulates extramedullary hemopoiesis, which can be detected in the fetal liver, kidneys, lymph nodes, lungs, and spleen.[29] Bone marrow studies reveal erythroid hyperplasia as a reflection of compensatory mechanisms for the continued extravascular hemolysis occurring in the spleen. In severe cases, hepatosplenomegaly is present due to a combination of increased destruction of RBCs in the spleen in addition to the extramedullary hemopoiesis.

Eventually anasarca and ascites due to heart failure secondary to anemic hypoxia, and hypoalbuminemia due to hepatic damage, develop. Anasarca and ascites are aggravated by the increased venous return resulting from hepatosplenomegaly and by the increased portal venous pressure secondary to extramedullary hemopoiesis[30] and a drop in plasma protein (which may be as low as 2 gm/100 ml)[29] brought on by hepatic dysfunction and failure. This syndrome, when severe, is called hydrops fetalis.

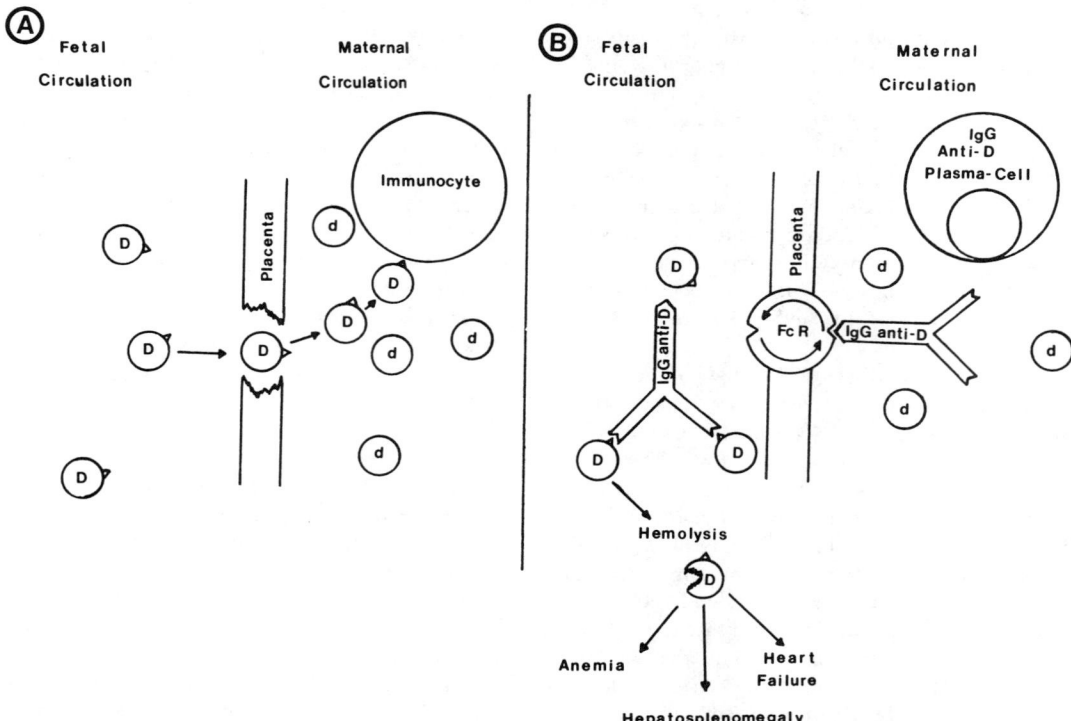

FIG 16–1.—A, fetomaternal hemorrhage. D-positive cells cross into the maternal circulation; the maternal circulation has immunocytes which recognize D-positive cells as foreign. D cells represent maternal Rh-negative cells in the circulation. **B,** an IgG anti-D maternal plasma cell is shown synthesizing IgG anti-D. Cells in the placenta contain Fc receptors *(Fc-R)* specific for IgG that function as transport molecules, allowing IgG anti-D to cross selectively into the fetal circulation. This antibody coats Rh_o (D)–positive cells, destroying them. The main clinical signs then ensue: hepatosplenomegaly, anemia, and heart failure.

The hemolytic process produces an increase in the indirect bilirubin levels. Indirect bilirubin is water soluble, lipophilic, and causes CNS toxicity. However, because the maternal liver handles toxic materials in the fetal plasma via the placenta, bilirubin does not represent the same degree of threat to the fetus as after delivery, when the maternal circulation no longer clears the fetal bilirubin.[31] Despite placental clearance of bilirubin, levels in severely affected fetuses may be as high as 8–10 mg/dl of plasma. A significant portion is direct bilirubin due to fetal liver damage. In severe cases of hydrops fetalis, the placenta is affected as well. The cotyledons are large and edematous. Round or polygonal epithelioid lipid-laden Hofbauer cells may be seen.[29]

Clinical Aspects of Rh Immunization

Two factors influence the development of Rh immunization: the volume of RBCs to which the host is exposed, and an individualized immune response of the host on exposure to the antigen.[32] In one series of 28 Rh-negative volunteers, 24 developed anti-D antibodies within 6 months of being immunized with 200 ml of Rh_o (D)–positive blood. A second immunization raised the number of immunized individuals to 26.[33] Another study revealed that these immune responses are dose dependent; for instance, when 1 ml is used to immunize, about 5 of 12 individuals can be expected to respond in the first immunization and about 9 of 12 in the second.[34] As little as 0.03 ml of RBCs is capable of immunizing an Rh-negative recipient, as was demonstrated by a study in which 6 of 8 individuals formed anti-D antibodies after repeated injections with very small amounts of RBCs.[35] The overall risk of an Rh-negative woman carrying an Rh-positive fetus in the general population is about 1 in 10 pregnancies.[36] Of these patients, about 4% will be immunized 6 months after the first delivery.[37]

After the second pregnancy, the incidence of immunized mothers increases to 17%.[38] About 2% of Rh-negative women at risk are sensitized to Rh_o (D) during pregnancy.[39] ABO incompatibility offers protection against immunization by Rh_o (D) mothers with Rh-positive pregnancies, as follows: group A incompatibility offers 90% protection, group B incompatibility offers 55% protection.[40] Sensitization occurs in 7%–8% of ABO-compatible pregnancies, but only in 2% of ABO-incompatible pregnancies.[41]

Different Factors Affecting the Severity of HDN

Titer of the antibody in the maternal and fetal circulation.[42] As mentioned above, titers greater than 1:16 (e.g., 1:32) are usually significant in relation to the severity of HDN; however, these values do not fully predict the outcome of the disease.[42]

Nature of the immunoglobulin class, subclass, and rate of placental transfer. IgG1 is transported across the placenta earlier and exceeds maternal and fetal levels earlier than other subclasses in Rh immunization, whereas IgG3 may never reach maternal levels.[42] These findings suggest that measuring IgG1 anti-Rh_o (D) levels in maternal samples is more significant than measuring total IgG in terms of predictive value. Sufficient numbers of antibody molecules must be bound to the fetal RBCs for phagocytosis to occur.[21] The antibody binding constant must be high for adequate RBC destruction to occur. "Monogamous" bivalency likewise appears to be crucial in antibody binding equilibrium and for more effective phagocytosis, as has been shown for IgG, which is the prototype of "monogamous" bivalent antibody.[43]

Antigenic representation on fetal tissues. It is suggested that the low reactivity of cord cells with anti-A and B, as well as P1, P, and Pk, is the result of the paucity of binding sites for double binding by monogamous bivalent antibodies.[44] However, this cannot be the only cause, for M, N, and S are similarly distributed yet can cause HDN. Representation of various RBC antigens in the fetus were discussed earlier.

Capacity of fetal RES for RBC lysis.

Ability of the fetal liver to metabolize bilirubin. This ability is impaired due to fetal immaturity and due to erythroblastosis, which, per se, is capable of damaging the liver in severe cases.

Erythropoiesis as a response to anemia by hemopoietic tissues of the fetus.

Intrauterine Therapy for HDN

Assessment of patients for intrauterine therapy of HDN includes the following parameters:[45] (1) obstetric history; (2) medical complications (eclampsia, diabetes); (3) estimate of fetal maturity (ultrasound and L/S ratios); (4) assessment of immunologic response (maternal antibody titer and IgG subclass); and (5) analysis of amniotic fluid.

Obstetric History and Medical Complications.—A previous history of pregnancy, miscarriage, or abortion is very important for the prognosis of HDN. A previous history of an affected infant is useful in determining the outcome of HDN as well. During the first pregnancy anti-Rh antibodies are usually low and a rise is usually detected in the 35th week of gestation.[46] In the first affected infant, the rate of stillbirths is about 6%, whereas in the second and following pregnancies, the rate of stillbirths rises to about 29%.[47]

Accompanying medical complications such as eclampsia worsen the prognosis in HDN.

Estimate of Fetal Maturity.—Ultrasound can successfully be used to determine gestational age. It is usually performed before 14 weeks to determine fetal age, then repeated at 31 weeks to assess head diameters and again at 36 weeks to assess cephalic, thoracic, and abdominal dimensions.[45] Hydramnios, ascites, hepatosplenomegaly, and other signs of edema are searched for at this stage.

The fetal maturity is assessed from amniotic fluid measurements of lecithin/sphingomyelin (L/S) ratios.[48] L/S ratios less than 1 indicate immature lungs, which may result in severe respiratory distress syndrome at birth. L/S ratios above 2 usually indicate mature lungs and may indicate good infant thriving.[44]

Assessment of the Maternal Immunologic Response.—Antibody titers are a useful parameter. If they are below 1:16, the prognosis is usually good.[45] Significant elevations are titers greater than 1:16.[30] However, in many cases when titers are above 1:32, levels remain elevated but plateau; nevertheless, progression of EF continues.[45] Thus, maternal serum titers are not always useful to assess progression of EF. Two tube dilutions are considered significant elevations. Titers are usually assessed monthly the first 6 months, biweekly the last trimester, and a week before the estimated date of delivery.[45]

Analysis of Amniotic Fluid.—Increments in antibody titers above 1:16 are an indication for amniocentesis. The procedure is not free of hazards; in one study, fetal loss was 2.6% compared to 1.1% in a control group.[49] Potential complications include pneumothorax, splenic laceration, umbilical artery laceration, placental laceration with or without subsequent maternal immunization, and spontaneous abortion.[50]

The purpose of the procedure is to obtain a spectrophotometric scan of the amniotic fluid, which reflects quite accurately the severity of hemolysis in the fetus. However, L/S ratios and chromosome analysis, as well as other special tests, can be performed on the amniotic fluid sample in addition to the bilirubin scan.

Amniocentesis can be performed as early as the 24th week of gestation and may have to be repeated thereafter. The detailed technique has been described by Werch[51] (Fig 16–2).

The fetal contour must first be delineated by ultrasonography prior to amniocentesis. A location for entering the amniotic sac is then selected; this is usually in the maternal lower abdomen, suprapubic, and contralateral to the presenting fetal parts. Following preparation of the skin, a 3-inch, 20-gauge needle is inserted into the amniotic sac, with every effort made to avoid placental laceration, which can result in dangerous hemorrhage and primary immunization or immunologic booster.[52] In all cases of amniocentesis to assess Rh-induced EF or where other potential for Rh immunization exists, RhIG must be given prior to the procedure; one dose is usually sufficient in uncomplicated cases.[53]

Amniotic Fluid Spectrophotometry

Amniotic fluid spectrophotometry is the routine method for assessing the severity of EF. Significant hemolysis usually starts at about the 16th week of gestation. Fetal hemoglobin (Hb F) is catabolized to indirect bilirubin. A portion of indirect bilirubin will be converted to direct bilirubin by the fetal hepatic glucuronyl transferase system.[49] Protein-bound bilirubin then gains access to the amniotic fluid by a mechanism which is not fully understood.[54] Bilirubin remains at fairly constant levels in spite of rapid amniotic fluid turnover and is therefore of great use as an index of fetal hemolysis.[55]

The sample obtained by amniocentesis should be collected in a sterile amber glass tube. Usually a 5-ml sample is sufficient for the spectrophotometric study, but 10 ml may be indicated if other studies are performed (e.g., L/S ratios, cell cultures, chromosome analysis). All separation procedures such as filtering and centrifugation must be performed in the dark to avoid light-induced bilirubin breakdown, which may result in spurious bilirubin values.[50] The spectrophotometry studies are performed with a narrow bandwidth recording spectrophotometer using distilled water as a blank. Readings are performed at 365 nm, 450 nm, and 550 nm. Spectrophotometric studies can predict the severity of EF and were first used for this purpose by Liley.[56]

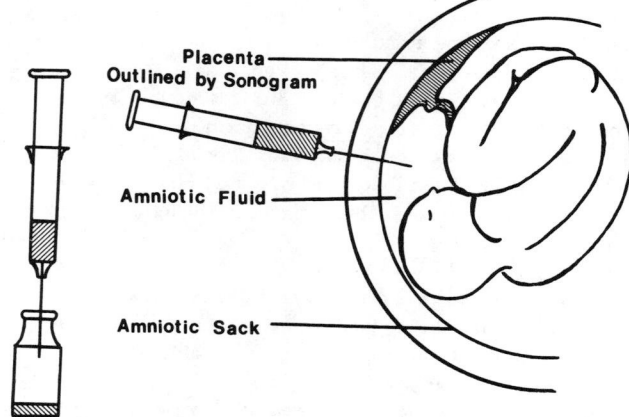

FIG 16–2.—Amniocentesis. The placenta is outlined by sonography before amniocentesis to prevent accidental puncture. The amniotic fluid removed is protected from direct exposure to white light by placing the sample in an amber bottle. The site of amniocentesis in practice is at a suprapubic location, as defined in the text.

The net optical density at 450 nm represents the bilirubin peak and is measured from the baseline, as shown in Figure 16–3. Liley stipulated that the net optical density at 450 nm should decrease as pregnancy progresses, probably because of a dilutional effect of increased amniotic fluid later in gestation. Therefore, relatively severe disease is present if the optical density at 450 nm is smaller than in previous weeks. Because this decrement is logarithmic, values for different stages of gestation can be plotted on log or semilog graphs. Conclusions are drawn based on plotted values. Liley based his prediction of severity of EF on the graph points for the 450-nm readings and described three zones (Fig 16–4). The upper zone, with high optical density readings, correlated with severely ill infants and neonatal deaths. The middle zone represented moderately affected infants, and the lower zone (small net optical density) represented mildly affected or unaffected infants. Liley subsequently divided the middle zone in zones *a* and *b* to predict poor prognosis (upper half of the middle zone) and good prognosis (lower half of the middle zone).[57] Trends may vary upward or downward during gestation. Guidelines for management can be given based on Liley graphs (see Fig 16–4).

The decision to perform an intrauterine transfusion may have to be based on values obtained before 32 weeks' gestation. The decision to induce labor and perform an exchange transfusion is based on data obtained after the 32d week of gestation. The therapeutic plan thus is based on the results of Liley chart plotting.

Other authors consider the developmental status of the fetus and the degree of fetal jeopardy, rather than the degree of EF alone,[51] before deciding on intrauterine transfusion.[51] One drawback to exhaustive time studies of fetal condition is that repeated amniocentesis is necessary.

In spite of the fairly accurate assessment of EF severity by Liley charts, some pitfalls to amniotic fluid scanning must be recognized. For instance, if blood contaminates the amniotic fluid due to rupture of a small vessel during amniocentesis, a peak will be present at 400 nm (Fig 16–5). Meconium, conversely, will give a broad curve on the scan (Fig 16–6). Peaks of bilirubin may be obscured by these extraneous substances, and certain procedures such as chloroform extraction may have to be performed on the sample (see Fig 16–6).[50]

Intrauterine Transfusion

The decision to transfuse in utero must be carefully weighed against the hazards of the procedure. Fetuses of 26 to 32 weeks' gestational age are too immature to survive outside the uterus and may be too ill to wait for induction and early delivery. The decision is made on the basis of high amniotic fluid bilirubin values and determination of L/S ratios.[58] If, for instance, spectroscopy of amniotic fluid reveals high values (e.g., 0.41Δ optical density at 450 nm) with an L/S ratio below 1, an intrauterine

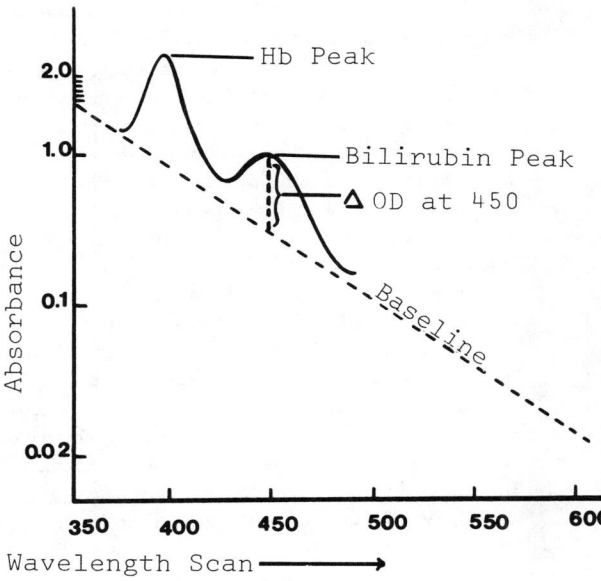

FIG 16–3.—Spectrophotometric scan of an amniotic fluid sample. The *x* axis represents sequential variations in the wavelength scan. The *y* axis depicts absorbance. The baseline is represented by the *dotted line*. The significant distance measured, representing the bilirubin peak, is the peak present at 450 nm. The significant distance is optical density and is measured from the baseline to the apex of the peak, not from the *x* axis to the apex of the peak.

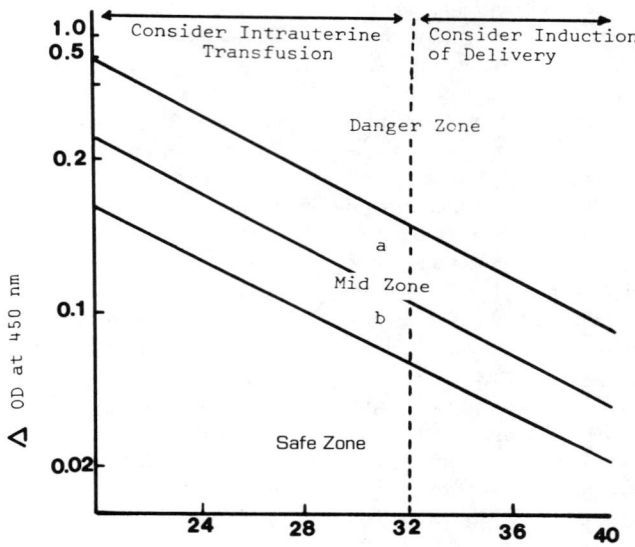

FIG 16–4.—A modified Liley graph. The top zone is considered the danger zone. The middle zone is separated into two subzones, a and b. The safe zone is at the bottom. The decision to give an intrauterine transfusion must be made before 32 weeks of gestation if the values fall within the danger zone. The decision to induce delivery is made after 32 weeks, when extrauterine survival is more favorable. Mid-zone a and mid-zone b are "gray areas" and the decision to transfuse intrauterinely or to induce delivery must be made in borderline cases of hemolytic disease of the newborn when other parameters of fetal viability are available.

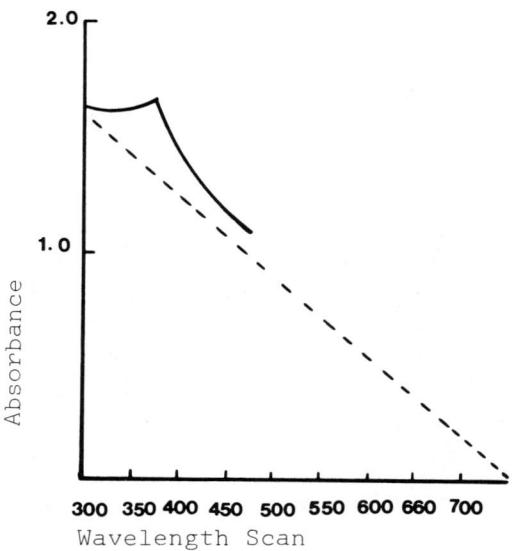

FIG 16–5.—Spectrophotometric scan of amniotic fluid that is stained with a small amount of meconium.

transfusion may be the only way to save the fetus.

Intrauterine transfusion was first done by Liley,[59] who used the fetal intraperitoneal route as the preferred site because of its accessibility.[60] Approximately 50% of cells transfused appear in the circulation 4 days after intraperitoneal transfusion (Fig 16–7).[61] In the method reported by Liley, approximately 20 cc of contrast medium (60% meglumine iothalamate in aqueous solution[45]) is injected into the amniotic cavity. The radiopaque material dissolves in the amniotic fluid, which is swallowed by a viable fetus. If the contrast medium is not present in the fetal stomach by 24 hours, the fetus is considered in severe jeopardy.[45]

The swallowed radiopaque material helps the transfusionist visualize the intestinal tract of the fetus and allows positioning of a 16-gauge Touhy needle for intraperitoneal transfusion. A metal grid placed on the mother's abdomen is used for orientation during fluoroscopy. In early intrauterine transfusions (i.e., 28 weeks) the volume of blood transfused is 40–50 cc; fetuses transfused later, around 30–32 weeks' gestation, will tolerate approximately 100–120 ml of transfused cells.[28]

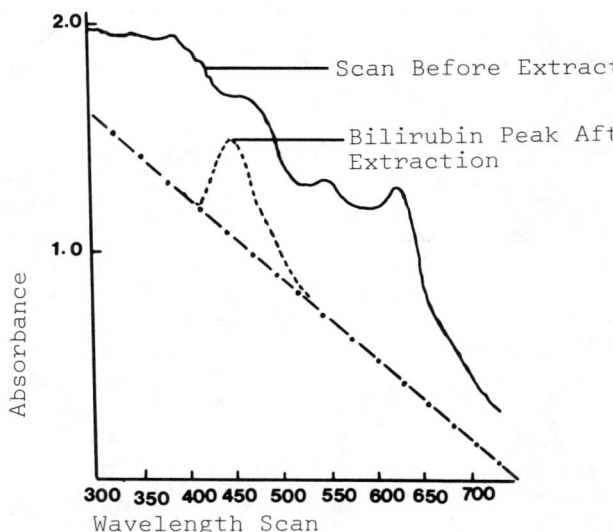

FIG 16–6.—Spectrophotometric scan of an amniotic fluid sample that has been heavily contaminated with blood. The sample is subjected to chloroform extraction. The extracted material will now reveal a bilirubin peak *(dotted line peak).*

It must be stressed that intrauterine transfusion carries a high morbidity and mortality and must not be performed by the inexperienced. Although experienced operators report fetal death rate from intrauterine transfusions at 10%–30%,[28] others put the figure at 40% 7 days post transfusion,[62] or 50% overall fetal mortality after intrauterine transfusion.[63] These figures should be considered very carefully before intrauterine transfusion is performed. Furthermore, in an extensive retrospective study undertaken by Robertson et al.,[64] 40% of infants from mothers with a previous stillbirth due to EF survived, compared to 52% of infants who had received intrauterine transfusions. However, the long-term survival rate did not significantly differ between the two groups. If intrauterine transfusion is to be performed at all, it should be done in specialized centers, and only when failure to transfuse may cause high fetal morbidity or death.

The component of choice is a frozen-thawed Rh-negative unit that has been packed sufficiently (i.e., hematocrit of 75%–80%) to deliver the product with the most concentrated oxygen-carrying capacity. Frozen-thawed cells are chosen because most of the WBCs have been eliminated, thus reducing the hazard of lymphocyte engraftment.[28] However, the complication of graft-versus-host disease (GVHD) is perhaps somewhat overestimated. This conclusion stems from the finding that attempts to engraft splenic cells in the fifth month of pregnancy were

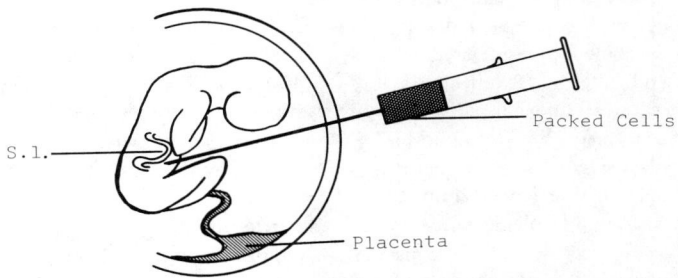

FIG 16–7.—Intrauterine transfusion. Highly packed cells are given through a syringe. The needle is passed through the amniotic sac and into the fetal peritoneal cavity, where the packed cells are injected. The small intestine of the fetus is visualized by injecting radiopaque material into the amniotic fluid a few days before intrauterine transfusion. The fetus swallows the amniotic fluid, thus allowing the small intestine to be visualized. This helps in the adequate identification of fetal abdominal parts. Sonography is used to guide needle placement to avoid rupturing the placenta.

unsuccessful.[65] Nevertheless, since GVHD has occasionally been reported after intrauterine transfusions,[66] the precaution of transfusing frozen-thawed cells seems warranted. These units should be irradiated with 2,000 rad before transfusion, for even frozen-thawed units may contain viable, engraftable lymphocytes.[67]

If intrauterine transfusion is performed through catheters, care must be taken not to use catheters that are too narrow, for they tend to produce hemolysis.[68]

Prophylaxis of Rh Immunization

The most important aspect of Rh immunization today is its prophylaxis, since for the most part it is a fully preventable disease. The mechanisms of how RhIG prevents immunization are not entirely clear. A simple explanation is that antibody injected into the host might coat Rh-positive RBCs and immune clearance might take place before immunization could occur.[69] However, immune clearance cannot be documented as the sole mechanism of immune suppression experimentally. Immune suppression to rabbit hemoglobin was undertaken, without immune clearance prior to treatment with specific antibody.[70] Another possibility is that antibody may act by competitive inhibition by covering Rh immunogenic sites. However, F(ab) or F(ab')$_2$ fragments of the suppressive antibody did not produce suppression in vivo at the usual doses.[71] Furthermore, if RhIG at a dose of 25 µg (which is sufficient to protect against immunization with 1 ml of Rh-positive blood) were distributed after the injection, in about two times the volume of plasma in the body, only 5% of the antigen and 1% of the antibody would bind to each other at equilibrium.[72] It is more likely that immune suppression by antibody, with subsequent development of tolerance, is in some way associated with idiotypic recognition and block of T cell clones.[69] This would, in essence, create a feedback mechanism, which has been termed the "immunostat" mechanism, with regulation similar to a thermostat, switching on and off particular immunocytes.[73, 74] It appears that rapid splenic sequestration of immune complexes is necessary for adequate Rh immune suppression, as shown in one case where suppression by RhIG failed due to prior splenectomy.[72] Interestingly, one antibody (anti-K) given together with Rh$_o$ (D)-positive, Kell-positive cells will induce suppression against both antigens in an Rh-negative, Kell-negative individual.[75] For details on immune suppression by RhIG and the development of its use in humans, see chapter 5. A discussion of some practical aspects on the use of RhIG is given below.

Evaluation of a Fetomaternal Bleed

In order to calculate the dose of RhIG to be given to an Rh-negative mother for immune suppression, the extent of the fetomaternal bleed at delivery must be calculated. Since Rh$_o$ (D) is the most immunogenic of the Rh antigens,[76] it is sometimes recommended that D-positive cells be counted in a maternal sample. This can be done by experimental techniques such as enzyme-linked antiglobulin[77] and by fluorescence.[78] A simple and routinely used method for calculating the amount of fetomaternal bleeding is by assessing the number of fetal cells in the maternal circulation by using the Kleihauer-Betke method, modified by Clayton et al.[79] This is an acid elution test based on the principle that HbF is more resistant than maternal hemoglobin to denaturation by a decrement in pH.

Most maternal cells appear as ghosts or as bleached RBCs in the blood film, compared to the more deeply staining fetal RBCs. At least 2,000 cells in the smear, maternal and fetal cells included, are counted and the percentage of fetal cells is calculated. This percentage is then multiplied by 50 to determine the ratio in an assumed total maternal blood volume of 5,000 ml, the average blood volume of a 70-kg adult.

The following formula is used: Percentage of fetal cells from a total of 2,000 cells counted in maternal sample × 50 = volume of fetal blood that entered the maternal circulation. For example, assume 20 of 2,000 cells in a smear were fetal. As 20 = 1% of 2,000, 1% × 50 = 50 ml. So 50 ml of fetal blood has entered the maternal circulation. As detailed in chapter 4, the dosage of RhIG is 1 unit (300 µg)/30 ml of whole blood. In the above example of a fetomaternal bleed, 50 ml/30 = 1.6 vials, 1.2 × 2 (twice the amount as recommended recently by the AABB) will result in administration of 3–4 vials.[80]

Before RhIG is given, a small portion of the immunoglobulin may be reacted with the maternal sample. This is termed RhIG crossmatch. This procedure is no longer followed in most hospitals and is no longer required by the AABB. In certain cases it could be used to detect possible missed D^u mothers or large fetomaternal bleeds. A positive reaction is manifested as agglutination of fetal Rh-positive cells against a maternal Rh-negative RBC background.

Antepartum RhIG Prophylaxis

In a study of 210 Rh-negative mothers with no previous sign of immunization prior to pregnancy, five mothers showed evidence of immunization at delivery, revealing they had become Rh immunized during pregnancy.[41] In another study by the same authors, 62 (1.8%) of 3,533 Rh-negative women given RhIG after delivery or abortion proved to have become immunized during the pregnancy. Five of the 62 women were immunized by the conceptus before 28 weeks of gestation.[41] These findings suggested that RhIG given prophylactically before 28 weeks' gestation and then repeated would prevent most of these "RhIG failures." This idea proved to be correct in a clinical trial in which 1,357 mothers were given RhIG antenatally: only one mother became Rh immunized in spite of RhIG protection (0.07% of cases).

This type of program has been criticized because of the additional cost it would be expected to add to health care. However, a Canadian study has revealed this concern to be unfounded.[41]

Artificial Reduction of Circulatory Anti-D

Intensive plasma exchange of the mother in the antenatal period may induce significant decrements of anti-D antibody titers.[81] In one series of 12 mothers, 9 gave birth to live infants following antenatal plasma exchange. Of the 12, 5 had had stillbirths in earlier untreated pregnancies.[81] Though complications have not been very frequent following plasma exchange to reduce anti-D titers during pregnancy, three cases of pulmonary edema were reported in a total of 663 procedures, one case being fatal, and two patients had sepsis following plasmapheresis.[81] In one series in which small volumes were removed (i.e., 250 ml/week), the levels of antibody paradoxically decreased to 20% of the original levels.[82] More data are necessary before definitive protocols can be suggested. Though results using these techniques appear encouraging, a prospective, controlled clinical trial is mandatory before plasma exchange can be accepted as the procedure of choice for pregnant Rh-immunized mothers. Immune adsorption columns and immune suppression with promethazine have been used successfully in selected cases, but again, the data are scant and the procedures considered experimental.[81]

ABH Hemolytic Disease of the Newborn

ABH hemolytic disease of the newborn is the more frequent cause of HDN today, occurring twice as often as other causes of HDN.[83] As was mentioned at the beginning of this chapter, the incidence ranges from 7 to 53.4 per 1,000 births.[24] Afro-Americans, Hispanics, and American Indians have a higher rate of ABH HDN.[84] In one study of 8,007 infants, 418 infants had a positive direct antiglobulin test, in 390 cases due to ABO incompatibility between mother and infant, and in 19 cases due to anti-Rh antibodies.[85]

ABO hemolytic disease of the newborn is almost always confined to group O mothers with a group A, B, or AB conceptus.[86] However, it sometimes occurs in A or B mothers with an ABO-incompatible conceptus, though very rarely (0.8% in A or B mothers; 37.9% in group O mothers).[83] The reason for this distribution appears to be that group O mothers produce monospecific and cross-reactive anti-A and anti-B antibodies of the IgG class.[87] Most of the eluted antibodies from neonates with ABO HDN are nevertheless monospecific anti-A or anti-B.[85] The likelihood of group A or group B infants developing ABO HDN is reported to be higher in group A caucasian babies, in whom the ratio is 3.7:1.[88] The disease appears to be equal in distribution between A and B infants when the population is predominantly black and Hispanic.[85] Although in one study, baby girls were more affected than boys,[89] in another series no sex difference was noted.[85] Up to 38% of ABH-incompatible pregnancies may have a positive DAT,[83] but only 6%–10% of these infants require treatment for HDN.[4] ABO-incompatible babies from group O mothers should have cord bilirubin tested and screened for spherocytes.[4] Eluates from cord cells may be performed but have not proved useful in determining the clinical course of ABH HDN.[83] For the most part, HDN caused by ABH incompatibility is much less severe than that caused by Rh immunization,[86] probably due to absorption of the antibodies by non-RBC cells and fluids containing ABH substances.[90]

Antigens Other than ABH or Rh Causing HDN

Antigens other than the Rh_o (D) or ABH can cause HDN, but less frequently, and usually the disease is less severe.[91] Some of the more frequent ones are outlined in Table 16–1.

MANAGEMENT OF EXTRAUTERINE PROBLEMS CAUSED BY EF

A laboratory evaluation of cord blood should be immediately undertaken to evaluate the primary problem in the early neonatal period (first 48 hours), namely, the anemia caused by intrauterine destruction of RBCs.

The newborn normally has higher hemoglobin values (17 gm/dl) than the older infant.[92] Values below 15 gm/dl may indicate anemia, and values of 8–10 gm/dl indicate severe anemia. Similarly, hematocrits of less than 30% represent severe anemia and are considered pediatric emergencies warranting correction by transfusion.[93] These infants should receive a complete hematologic workup by a pediatric hematologist.

Reticulocyte counts should be interpreted cautiously, for newborns usually have increased reticulocyte counts, sometimes as high as 6%–7%.[94] A hemorrhagic tendency secondary to thrombocytopenia and capillary endothelial damage is usually present.

Physiopathology of Hyperbilirubinemia in HDN

As was mentioned above, unconjugated bilirubin in utero for the most part is cleared by the placenta and metabolized by the maternal liver to bilirubin diglucuronide and excreted. On delivery, however, the infant's hepatic Y-transport and glucuronyltransferase mechanisms for bilirubin conjugation are not fully developed. Therefore, the newborn is unable to conjugate the large amounts of unconjugated bilirubin produced by the immune hemolytic process. Untreated, HDN will soon produce a saturation of the albumin transport and binding capacity (1 gm of albumin will normally bind 17 mg of bilirubin).[95] This allows unconjugated bilirubin, which is lipid soluble, to traverse neuron membranes, interfering with neuronal metabolism. The areas most often affected by this phenomenon are the cerebellar tonsils, the hippocampal gyrus, the midbrain, and the medullary nuclei. This pathologic entity is termed kernicterus.[96] A critical factor in deciding to exchange transfuse a newborn is the bilirubin level. When kernicterus is a possibility,[93] it is best to be conservative and place the threshold of danger somewhat below the originally stipulated 20 mg/dl of indirect bilirubin.[94] This recommendation is based on the observation that kernicterus may develop at levels considerably lower than the standard cutoff point of 20 mg/dl (i.e., 6–10 mg/dl).[97] In general, an increment of more than 0.5 mg/dl/hour indicates severe disease.[98] A quick rise in the indirect bilirubin level is much more significant than a slow rise over several days. A useful rule of thumb is to decrease the cutoff value of 20 mg/dl by 1 mg for one of each of the clinical factors that will influence the prognosis of the newborn negatively. For instance, if an APGAR value is two points less than optimal, the cutoff point is 18 mg/dl of indirect bilirubin. Any other factor such as low birth weight or a diabetic mother will lower the cutoff point considerably.

Other factors include prematurity, anemia, hypoxia, acidosis, hypoglycemia, infection, and high nonesterified fatty acids.[99] As was mentioned above, most of the indirect bilirubin in the newborn infant is bound to albumin. Sulfasoxasole, which competes

TABLE 16–1.—Some Antigens Other Than $Rh_O(D)$ or ABH Causing HDN*

ANTIGENS	SEVERITY	FREQUENCY	STUDY
ABH	Usually mild		Hardy and Napier[22]
E	Moderate to severe	55/99	Kornstad[91]
c	Most severe, after Rh_o (D)	23/99	Kornstad[91]
E + c	Moderate to severe	5/99	Kornstad[91]
C^w	Moderate to severe	13/99	Kornstad[91]
Fy	Severe	1/35 non-D	Hardy and Napier[22]
K^u	Severe	1/35 non-D	Hardy and Napier[22]

*Although many other RBC antigens may cause HDN, they do so less frequently, and immunization is usually secondary to transfusion rather than pregnancy.

with bilirubin for its binding site, will allow kernicterus to develop at lower levels of serum bilirubin (18 mg/dl) than in non-sulfasoxasole-treated neonates;[100] this proves the importance of bound to nonbound albumin/bilirubin ratios. Free to bound ratios equal to or greater than 6.4 are an indication for exchange. Conversely, if the reserve albumin is equal to or less than 1.25 gm/dl, exchange is indicated.[101] One of the best single indicators for assessing the severity of HDN is the cord hemoglobin level. Infants with hemoglobin levels of 12 gm/dl or lower have significantly more severe hemolysis than those with levels of 14 gm/dl, as compared with bilirubin levels, which vary more widely.[102]

Exchange Transfusion in the Neonate

Exchange transfusion in the neonate is not a risk-free procedure, so care must be exercised while performing it. In experienced hands, mortality is about 1%.[103] Once the conceptus is separated from the placental bilirubin clearance mechanism and the maternal liver no longer metabolizes the fetal bilirubin, the newborn must handle the toxic effects of indirect bilirubin. In most cases, neonates are doubly compromised: by anemia, which increases susceptibility to the toxic effects of indirect bilirubin, and by the increased levels of nonconjugated bilirubin.

Exchange transfusion of a neonate has three main advantages: it corrects the anemia, it eliminates plasma bilirubin, and it eliminates infant RBCs that carry antigens incompatible with the passively acquired circulating maternal IgG.

Pre-exchange Plan

Blood selected for transfusion should be relatively fresh. Units up to 5 days old are acceptable, acid-citrate-dextrose (ACD) or citrate-phosphate-dextrose (CPD) units are useful for this procedure, for older units contain unacceptable levels of potassium.[104] Furthermore, the content of citrate in a unit has an additive effect on potassium toxicity.[105]

Heparinized units are inadequate because of the short expiration time (48 hours) and because they have not proved to be more advantageous than citrated units despite the claims of a more physiologic pH.[106] Furthermore, heparin inhibits the ability of albumin to bind to bilirubin.[107] The use of CPD adenine units for exchange transfusion has been controversial due to the potential of renal damage secondary to 2,8-dioxyadenine crystal formation in renal tubules.[108] However, one study did not demonstrate such an occurrence with ACD-adenine units,[109] and another study with CPD-adenine units did not reveal a significant risk.[108]

Frozen-thawed units reconstituted with fresh frozen plasma (FFP) have been used successfully in exchange transfusions of infants. Advantages are the preservation of 2,3-DPG and a reduction in potassium, granulocytes, and platelets.[110] A disadvantage is the increasing risk of hepatitis or AIDS due to the use of added extraneous plasma.

If clotting factors are needed, as revealed by coagulation profiles, FFP may have to be given. The following basic rules must be observed in neonatal exchange transfusion:

1. The blood selected for the exchange must be compatible with the maternal serum.

2. In the absence of such a sample, the infant's serum and the eluate must be compatible with the unit selected.

3. All infants with Rh HDN are given Rh-negative blood.

4. All Rh-negative infants are transfused with Rh-negative blood.

5. All infants with ABO HDN should receive group O blood. These units may be resuspended in AB plasma.[110]

Some aspects of laboratory testing must be kept in mind. For instance, infants with Rh HDN may type as Rh negative because of excessive binding of anti-Rh antibodies to the RBCs. The Coombs reaction in these cases is strongly positive. The eluate is always tested against a cell panel in these cases to define the specificity of the coating antibody.

In ABO HDN, the Coombs test is weak in most instances, possibly because the low levels of antibody coating fall in the lower limits of Coombs test sensitivity; these can be enhanced using albumin solutions.[111] An eluate is always tested in these instances for anti-A or anti-B activity. Regardless of the reason for a high indirect bilirubin level, dangerously high levels of unconjugated bilirubin must be decreased, and the usual treatment in severe cases is exchange transfusion.

Infants previously transfused in utero may have cord samples with group O, Rh-negative RBCs or a mixed field of group O and the baby's ABO and Rh type. In addition, the serum may contain IgG anti-D antibodies.[112]

The first exchange transfusion for the treatment of HDN was performed by Wallerstein in 1945.[113] However, the procedure did not become an established therapeutic modality until later because of the high morbidity and mortality of early exchange transfusions. Disposable sets for exchange transfusion have decreased infant morbidity due to a reduced rate of infection following the exchange. Small volumes of blood are removed and replaced through a plastic catheter passed into the umbilical vein. The catheter is connected to a three-way stopcock syringe (Fig 16–8). This intermittent method is preferred to a continuous infusion/extraction method because it is more efficient.[114] The volume removed and exchanged can be calculated by the following formula:[115]

$$R = \left(\frac{V - S}{V}\right)^n$$

where R = residual volume in the infant's circulation, V = infant's blood volume calculated on the basis of weight (10% of weight in kilograms), S = volume removed by the syringe at any single volume withdrawn, and n = number of syringe volumes replaced.

Another useful formula calculates the remaining concentration of the toxic substance after each volume exchanged:

$$Xn = X_o \left(1 - \frac{b}{v}\right)^n$$

where Xn is the remaining concentration of substance X after n units of blood have been exchanged, X_o is the initial concentration of substance X, b is the volume of a unit of blood, v is the recipient's blood volume, and n is the number of volumes exchanged.

A double-volume exchange (approximately 1 unit of whole blood) removes about 90% of the infant's cells.[116] This amount (1 unit) is usually the maximum volume recommended in most cases.

The amount of bilirubin removed varies, depending on the stage after birth at which exchange transfusion is performed. A rebound phenomenon may be seen because bilirubin accumulates extravascularly. This sudden increment in bilirubin after an exchange transfusion is usually seen when the ex-

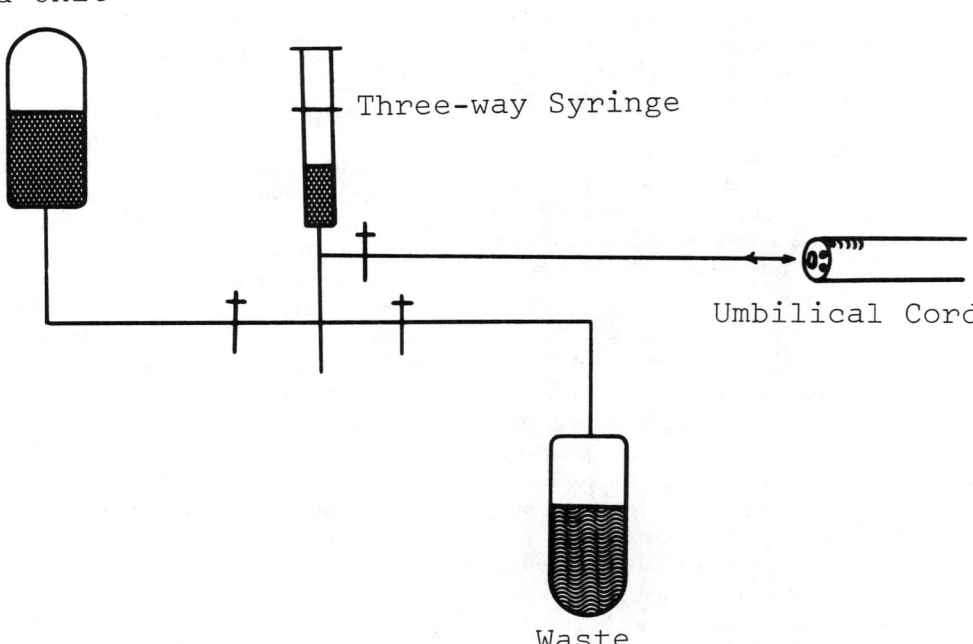

FIG 16–8.—Components of an exchange transfusion set. A unit of blood hangs in the inverted position with the portals of exit facing downward. By gravity, the blood penetrates the tubing system and comes to the three-way syringe. The transfusion takes place through the umbilical cord vein. Small volumes are transfused sequentially, with small volume removal of the baby's blood through the cannulated umbilical vein. The blood removed from the baby is transferred to the satellite bag labeled "waste."

change is performed rapidly.[117] It is therefore suggested that exchange transfusions be performed slowly, to permit the extravascular space bilirubin and the intravascular space bilirubin to reach equilibrium. If the umbilical vein has become inaccessible, as frequently occurs in multiple exchanges and in older infants, the saphenous vein and the radial artery may be used as an alternative transfusion route.[118]

Complications of Exchange Transfusions

In experienced hands, mortality from exchange transfusion should be less than 1%,[119] but in training centers mortality from exchange transfusions may be as high as 4.7%.[120] Most deaths occur within 6 hours of the exchange and are due to high pressure and volume variations. Necrotizing enterocolitis appears to be the most common complication of exchange tranfusion, probably secondary to ischemia due to mesenteric artery thrombosis.[95]

Erythropoiesis has been known to be suppressed in infants that have had exchange transfusions, to the point that the infant's RBCs may temporarily disappear from the circulation.[121] Platelets may decrease significantly in number and may reach low levels (30% of normal) after an exchange transfusion.[122]

Infections still pose a threat to these newborns. The most dreaded infections are osteomyelitis of the hip (more frequently seen in infants catheterized via the umbilical artery) and osteomyelitis of the shoulder joints and elbow (more frequently seen when the umbilical vein is used).[123] Cytomegalovirus infection occurs in up to 30% of infants that have had exchange transfusion.[124] Posttransfusion hepatitis may also be a complication,[125] and malaria has been reported.[126] AIDS is also a potential complication of exchange transfusion. Other less frequent but dreaded complications include air embolism,[127] umbilical vein perforation,[128] small bowel perforation (secondary to a mesenteric vessel embolism or thrombosis),[129] and paralysis of lower extremities due to ischemia of the lumbar spinal cord.[130] Metabolic disturbances have also been described, including acidosis[131] and potassium toxicity,[132] when older blood units were used in the exchange.[131] An increase in plasma free fatty acids may be observed when heparinized units are used.[133] Using cold blood units to exchange transfuse an infant is dangerous and may result in cardiac arrhythmias.[133]

Though mortality from exchange transfusion in experienced hands is reported to be as high as 0.7% of cases, many of these infants are already compromised by underlying disease, a fact which eventually determines the final survival rates.

Other Methods for Decreasing Bilirubin Levels

Severe hyperbilirubinemia in the newborn is treated mainly with exchange transfusion. Once the exchange has taken place and levels of bilirubin begin to decrease gradually, they can be controlled by noninvasive methods. Phototherapy to decrease bilirubin levels is one such method. It was first introduced into pediatric practice by Cremer et al.[134] Daylight or blue spectrum–emitting light of 450–460 nm wavelengths degrades bilirubin both in vivo and in vitro.[135]

Neurotoxic, indirect bilirubin is converted in the presence of light into harmless water-soluble dipyrroles which are readily eliminated by the body. This process probably occurs in the superficial capillaries of the skin and the outer 2 mm of the skin.[136] White fluorescent light has been used most effectively in phototherapy.

The infant is placed under a transparent plastic shield to avoid unwanted ultraviolet light, and the light source is placed 40–45 cm away from the infant.[136] Phototherapy can reduce serum bilirubin levels by 2 mg/10 L every 24 hours, providing an excellent adjunct therapy to exchange transfusion.[92] Phototherapy is usually employed in full-term infants with serum bilirubin levels of 10–12 mg/dl and in premature infants with serum bilirubin levels of 10 mg/dl. However, phototherapy is not acceptable as the sole mode of therapy in severe cases of HDN (e.g., 20 mg/dl).[136] The infant's eyes are shielded with dark glasses to avoid light-induced retinitis. Potential complications of phototherapy include diarrhea secondary to phototherapy-induced lactose deficiency, "bronze baby" syndrome, and dehydration.

Certain drugs such as phenobarbital enhance the development of the glucuronidase system in the newborn necessary for the metabolism and degradation of bilirubin.[137] Some experience has accumulated on the positive effects of barbiturates in infants with HDN.[138] However, because these substances are capable of inducing activation of other enzyme systems, may cause CNS depression, and can potentially cause habituation, they are rarely used to treat HDN.[139]

SPECIAL ASPECTS OF TRANSFUSION IN PEDIATRIC PRACTICE

Development of Hemopoiesis and Maturation of Hemoglobin

Pediatric hematology as a subspecialty of hematology is practiced using laboratory values which reflect the somewhat different physiology of neonates. Some of these pediatric hematology aspects are reviewed in more detail in chapter 2. Blood cells originate in the yolk sac about the 19th day of gestation.[140] Mesenchymal cells from the yolk sac progressively develop into blood vessels and hemocytoblasts.[141] However, erythropoiesis also takes place in the liver (from 5 weeks to 6 months, when erythroid precursors prevail).[142] Erythroid cells appear in the marrow between the 10th and 11th gestational week.[141] Granulopoiesis starts at about 7 weeks, and lymphocytes appear about the 9th week of gestation.[143] The earliest fetal hemoglobins contain a ζ chain (similar to α) and ϵ chains (similar to γ chains) termed Gower hemoglobin.[144] Later Hb F ($\alpha 2$, $\gamma 2$) predominates[145] until the 34th week, when adult hemoglobin (Hb A) synthesis increases and Hb F synthesis decreases. However, Hb F at term may range from 53% to 95% of the total hemoglobin.[146] HB F then progressively decreases by 3%/week after birth to reach negligible levels (less than 2%–3%) by 6 months of extrauterine life. This decrement in Hb F is a maturation process unaffected by oxygen tension or environment at birth.[147] This difference in distribution of Hb F during intrauterine life has significant physiologic implications. Hb F has a greater affinity for oxygen than does Hb A, causing a shift to the left in oxygen affinity curves. The shift of the P50 during oxygen saturation is in part due to a difference in binding of 2,3-DPG to the globin chains of Hb F at a serine residue rather than a histidine residue of Hb A.[148] Another factor is the pH shift at the placenta, which favors formation of 70% oxygen saturation as oxygen leaves the placenta.[149] Premature infants have a decreased offloading capacity, which is a disadvantage under hypoxic stress.[150]

Hematologic Parameters in the Neonate

Hemoglobin levels in the neonate are higher than in adults. The mean hemoglobin level in the neonate is 16.8 gm/dl,[151] probably reflecting perinatal hypoxia. Thus, a hemoglobin value of 14 gm/dl in a newborn is a sign of anemia. Hemoglobin levels, however, drop in the first 5–8 weeks of extrauterine life to about 11 gm/dl.[152] In the premature infant, hemoglobin levels drop at a faster rate and at a lower level than in term infants, to as low as 9.4 gm/dl after 2 months.[153] Reticulocytes are high at birth but fall to less than 1% 1 week after birth.[154]

Hemoglobin values in the newborn are about 3 gm/dl higher in capillary samples than in venous samples.[151] To stress this finding, in one study of 41 infants almost twice the number of anemias were diagnosed from venous rather than from capillary blood samples.[155] The mode of delivery is likewise important, for a significant and rapid placental transfusion may take place at birth (up to 125 ml of blood is contained at birth in the placenta).[156] This phenomenon will make cord hemoglobin and hematocrit values vary widely. At birth, the mean corpuscular volume (MCV) is about 106.4 in the full-term infant, whereas premature or low birth weight infants have MCVs of about 115, revealing a degree of macrocytosis.[157] In addition, these cells have a shorter life span—16.6 days in the premature infant and about 23.3 days in term infants[158] (normal adult, 26–35 days).[159]

The blood volume in term infants is about 85 ml/kg.[160] Prematures have a greater blood volume (89–105 ml/kg), mostly due to higher plasma volume.[161] Nevertheless, the infant is less well equipped to compensate for acute hypovolemia than is the adult, as shown by acute distress after losses of as little as 10% of the blood volume.[159] Neutrophil counts increase in prematures and term infants during the first 24 hours after birth.[162] Occasional early blast forms may be seen in a peripheral smear.[162] Platelet counts are similar in prematures, term newborns, and adults.[163]

PEDIATRIC DISEASES NEEDING BLOOD BANKING CONSULTATION

Anemia of the Newborn

As in the adult, anemia in the newborn can be caused by increased destruction (e.g., hemorrhage, hemolysis) or decreased production (e.g., aplasia, cytopenias). Hemorrhage can be due to obstetric accident, occult hemorrhage, or traumatic internal hemorrhage.[159]

Acute blood losses in the newborn may be attributed to twin-to-twin transfusion, fetomaternal transfusion,[164] early clamping of the umbilical cord, cesarean intervention, or emergency resuscitation of the neonate.[156] These neonates may then go on to develop respiratory distress syndrome (RDS) due to hypoxia and prematurity.[156] However, whether RDS is a cause of or an accompanying effect of a low RBC mass is controversial.[165] Nevertheless, a higher RBC mass in these infants often increases viscosity, with a decrease in tissue perfusion.[166] These premature infants may develop acute RDS in the presence of normal hemoglobin;[167] thus, the decision to transfuse may depend solely on p50 values[168] and clinical judgment. An important cause of chronic anemia of the newborn is iatrogenic; blood sampling for laboratory workups of sick neonates. These neonates have been known to lose an average of 12.4 ml of blood in neonatal intensive care units,[164] which is over 10% of the blood volume of prematures (100–200 ml) and about 5% of the blood volume of term infants (200–350 ml).[167] These findings warrant restriction of testing to tests which are essential.

BLOOD TRANSFUSION IN THE NEONATAL PERIOD

Although few guidelines have been established for correcting anemia in neonates, the work of Kevy is quite helpful.[169] Kevy recommends that if hemoglobin levels are below 5 gm/dl, the volume of packed cells given should be about 4.5 ml/kg of body weight, depending on the needs and the hemodynamic state of the child. In prematures and in neonates in whom overload is anticipated, the volume should be decreased to 2.25 ml/kg.[169] Providing frozen-thawed units is indicated in these cases. In this way aliquots from a single donor can be thawed out as needed.[170] This strategy is preferred to the use of blood from "walking donors," which poses the threat of casual blood banking procedures and catastrophic cases of hepatitis or AIDS.[171] For most pediatric transfusion purposes, 5-day-old or fresher CPD and CPDA units are adequate. Microaggregate filters can be used to decrease WBC contamination. In order not to waste valuable components, hospitals with a significant pediatric population draw units into an integral multiple-bag system with smaller volumes destined for these purposes. These "smaller" units have the same expiration date as units routinely collected in a closed system.

Exchange Transfusion for Diseases Not Directly Associated With HDN

Exchange transfusion can be used as a therapeutic modality for diseases other than HDN. The more common indication is disseminated intravascular coagulation (DIC) secondary to septicemia or other causes.[172] Other bleeding abnormalities of the newborn, such as vitamin K deficiency, have also been treated successfully by exchange transfusion.[173] In addition, sepsis appears to improve in newborns treated by exchange transfusion of fresh (up to 5-day-old) blood. Reasons for this improvement have been the observation of an improved opsonic activity,[174] improved neutrophil function,[175] and removal of toxins.[176] Exchange transfusion may be used in the treatment of RDS. The rationale for exchange transfusion in these infants is to eliminate as much Hb F as possible, and by transferring relatively fresh adult-type blood (less than 5 days old), to improve 2,3-DPG levels and oxygen offloading. In addition, acidosis in premature infants worsens their oxygenation problem.[177] Other uses include removing toxic drugs from the infant's circulation[178] and reducing ammonia levels in infants with liver failure.[179]

Common Complications of Transfusion in the Neonate

Perhaps the most common complication of administering blood perinatally is transfusion-associated infection with cytomegalovirus (CMV). When symptomatic, neonatal posttransfusional CMV infection may be quite severe and characterized by respiratory difficulty, hepatosplenomegaly, gray pallor, and atypical lymphocytes in the peripheral smear.[180] Characteristically, the infection has a worse prognosis in premature infants than in term infants.[180] This fact is emphasized by a report in which 14 of 43 term infants who received CMV-seropositive blood became seropositive, but none of the infants developed the syndrome outlined above.[181] Conversely, 16 of 51 premature infants receiving multiple transfusions became seropositive for CMV. Of the 16, 14 developed the CMV syndrome, and 3 died of it.[180] Infants born to CMV-seropositive mothers transfused with seropositive blood fare better than those born to CMV-seronegative mothers.[182] These findings strongly suggest the need for screening blood units for seropositivity and eliminating them from transfusion pools to be used for prematures and other newborns.[182] The transmission of other blood-borne infections such as hepatitis and AIDS is reviewed in chapters 12 and 13, respectively. Intravascular hemolysis is a potential complication in neonates who have circulating T-activated RBCs induced by clostridial necrotizing enterocolitis and who have been transfused with plasma containing components harboring anti-T antibody.[183]

A noninfectious complication from multiple transfusion in the neonate is iron overload in the multiply transfused neonate. This iron overload may increase the risk of infections due to block of the bacteriostatic effect of lactoferrin and transferrin due to iron binding at active sites.[184]

Citrate toxicity is another complication of blood transfusion to neonates. Citrate toxicity is manifested as hypocalcemia, either due to the direct chelating effect of citrate on Ca^{++} or due to conversion of citrate to bicarbonate in the liver and other tissues and mobilization of calcium by parathormone.[185] Neonates present this toxicity on saturation of the homeostatic mechanisms that eliminate citrate, and they do so more readily due to their relative hepatic and renal immaturity, as well as their relative hypoparathyroidism.[185] If hypocalcemia develops as a result of citrate toxicity, 0.5–1 cc of 10% calcium gluconate per kg of body weight can be given to correct the hypocalcemia.[185] Neonates are also more vulnerable than adults to hypoglycemia and hypothermia induced by transfusion of blood and components.[185] Retrolental fibroplasia developing in premature neonates, presumably as a result of the higher oxygen-carrying capacity of adult blood, may be a tragic complication of transfusion.[186] However, this complication may be mostly a disease associated with neonatal prematurity, rather than a direct effect of transfusion.

Although theoretically GVHD may develop in neonates due to immaturity of their immune system, most infants who have developed this complication were exchange-transfused neonates who had received intrauterine transfusions.[187]

OTHER DISEASES OF THE NEWBORN REQUIRING COMPONENTS

Thrombocytopenia in the newborn may be due to maternal autoimmune thrombocytopenia or to alloimmunization, usually secondary to previous pregnancies. Maternal autoimmune thrombocytopenia, with the production of mostly IgG1 antiplatelet antibodies,[188] may also be associated with other autoimmune disease (e.g., SLE).[189] Alloimmune thrombocytopenia occurs at an incidence of about one case in 10,000 births.[190] The antibody, an IgG antibody,[191] is usually directed against P1A1, an antigen present on a major platelet membrane protein (glycoprotein IIIa).[192] If a history of maternal autoimmune thrombocytopenia or maternal platelet alloimmunization with previously affected children exists, delivery by cesarean section must be considered to prevent delivery-induced intracranial hemorrhage in the newborn.[193] A platelet count from a fetal scalp vein sample can be obtained by amniotomy prior to delivery. If the count is below 100,000 platelets/mm^3, a cesarean delivery is mandatory.[194]

P1A1 antigens are present in 98% of random donor platelets. Therefore, platelets from random donors are not indicated, for they are quickly destroyed by maternal antibodies circulating in the newborn infant.[195] Washed maternal platelets are therefore the component of choice in alloimmune thrombocytopenia, but not in autoimmune thrombocytopenia.[195] Maternal platelets should be given, ideally after the exchange transfusion to reduce the circulating antibody load.[189] Maternal platelets are obtained by plateletpheresis, and the platelets are washed in saline and resuspended in AB plasma before transfusion.[196] Platelet plasma volume must be concentrated to 15 or 20 ml prior to infusion by centrifugation in alloimmune neonatal thrombocytopenia, and units given when the neonate's platelet count drops below 50,000/mm^3.[185] Another cause of immune mediated thrombocytopenia is seen in non-DIC associated severe bacterial and viral infections.[197]

Infections such as toxoplasmosis, rubella, CMV, and herpes simplex are all capable of producing neonatal thrombocytopenia.[185] Maternal ingestion of hydralazine and tolbutamide may produce transient neonatal thrombocytopenia and neutropenia.[185] Ingestion of aspirin by the mother 5 days prior to delivery has occasionally been the cause of neonatal bleeding.[198]

Alloimmune Neonatal Neutropenia

This disease occurs due to maternal immunization against several neutrophil antigens prior exposure to these antigens via previous pregnancies or due to autoimmune neutropenia. The main antigens involved in alloimmune immunization are

NA1 and NB1, which are each responsible for about 40%–50% of cases.[199] Autoimmune neutropenia has been observed against NA1 and ND1. Most cases which have been studied for IgG subclass have been IgG1.[200]

Clotting Deficiencies in the Neonate

Coagulopathies affect about 3% of infants in active neonatology intensive care units.[185] Routine screening tests when a coagulopathy is suspected in these newborns are APTT, PT, and TT. These tests and their interpretation are discussed in more detail in chapter 3. An abnormal APTT usually points to intrinsic factor abnormalities.

The major diseases producing factor deficiencies in the newborn are hemophilia A (factor VIII deficiency), von Willebrand's disease (factor VIII vW deficiency), and hemophilia B (factor IX deficiency). The vast majority of these diseases occur in male neonates. Bleeding in these cases is usually less severe than in profound thrombocytopenia and usually develops a few days after birth, when circumcision is performed.[201] Even after circumcision, less than half of the severely affected hemophiliacs will have external bleeding.

If the above-mentioned factors (III, VIII vW, and IX) are not too decreased, and if volume handling by the infant's circulation is not compromised, one may use FFP as therapy for the hemophilias. Nevertheless, it must be remembered that the suggested dose of 20–30 ml/kg will only increase the patient's clotting factor activity by 20%–30%.[202] One unit of factor VIII per kilogram of body weight (which is the activity found in 1 ml of plasma) will raise the plasma level of factor VIII by 2%.[108] However, if a patient with hemophilia A has a compromised circulatory system, then cryoprecipitate, which contains mostly factor VIII, VIII vW, and fibrinogen, must be used. When calculating the dose of cryoprecipitate for these patients it should be remembered that a unit of cryoprecipitate contains an average of 80 units per bag. For prematures or volume-compromised neonates, the volumes of FFP may have to be decreased to 10 cc/kg. These doses are given every 6–8 hours over 2 days.[185]

If large amounts of factor VIII are needed to correct values in hemophilia A, factor VIII concentrates may be used. These products are usually used preoperatively to correct hemostasis. Nevertheless, use of factor VIII concentrates entails a high risk of hepatitis. In the neonatal period, 30–50 units/kg are recommended.[182] Factor VIII concentrates are not used in von Willebrand's disease.

Hemophilia B (factor IX deficiency) is usually corrected in neonates with FFP alone.

One unit of factor IX per kilogram of body weight will raise the patient's factor IX level 1.5%. Factor IX concentrates available contain factors II, VII, IX, and X (prothrombin complex). However, these concentrates carry the danger of causing thrombotic phenomena, and the risk of hepatitis is higher than with concentrates of factor VIII.[202] The risk of AIDS when factor VIII or factor IX concentrates are used is discussed in chapter 13. When factor VIII or factor IX concentrates are used preoperatively, the goal is to achieve 100% levels, especially when major surgery is contemplated. Levels above 60% should be maintained 4 days postoperatively.[202]

Probably the most common acquired coagulopathy of the neonate is "hemorrhagic disease of the newborn" associated with vitamin K deficiency. This problem has been circumvented by routine administration of vitamin K1. The vitamin can be given IV in a dose of 1–2 mg. If, however, the need for vitamin K–dependent factors (II, VII, IX, and X) is emergent, these can be supplemented by giving FFP at doses of 10 cc/kg of body weight.[185]

Another cause of bleeding in the neonatal period is DIC. DIC usually accompanies other serious diseases, such as HDN, which in themselves may affect clotting factor levels. This condition may occur as a complication of abruptio placentae or amniotic fluid embolism. Both the PT and PTT are prolonged.[203] The differential diagnosis and treatment of this condition are discussed in chapter 3.

Other diseases of children that concern the blood bank, such as leukemia, thalassemia, sickle cell disease, and autoimmune hemolysis, are discussed in chapter 2.

REFERENCES

1. Levine P., Stetson R.: An unusual case of intragroup agglutination. *JAMA* 113:126, 1939.
2. Brambell F.W.R.: The transmission of immunity from mother to young and the catabolism of immunoglobulins. *Lancet* 2:1087, 1966.
3. Brambell F.W.R.: The relative transmission of the fraction of papain by hydrolyzed homologous gammaglobulin from the uterine cavity to the fetal circulation in the rabbit. *Proc. R. Soc. Biol.* 151:478, 1960.

4. Schanfield M.: Antibody-mediated perinatal diseases. *Clin. Lab. Med.* 1:239, 1981.
5. Kohler P.F., Farr R.S.: Elevation of cord over maternal IgG immunoglobulin: Evidence for an active placental IgG transport. *Nature* 210:1070, 1966.
6. Morell A., Skvaril F., van Loghem E., et al.: Human IgG subclasses in maternal and fetal serum. *Vox Sang.* 21:481, 1971.
7. Schur P.H., Alpert E., Alper C.: Gamma G subgroups in human fetal cord and maternal sera. *Clin. Immunol. Immunopathol.* 2:62, 1973.
8. McNabb T., Koh T.Y., Dorrington K.J., et al.: Structure and function of immunoglobulin domains: V. Binding of immunoglobulin G and fragments to placental membrane preparations. *J. Immunol.* 117:882, 1976.
9. Frangione B., Milstein C.: Variations in the disulfide bridges of immunoglobulin G: Interchain disulfide bridges of γ3 myeloma proteins. *J. Mol. Biol.* 33:983, 1968.
10. Devey M.E., Voak D.: A critical study of the IgG subclasses of Rh anti-D antibodies formed in pregnancy and in immunized volunteers. *Immunology* 27:1073, 1974.
11. Schanfield M.S.: Immunoglobulins: Genetic markers, in Fudenberg H.H., Sites D.P., Caldwell J.L., et al. (eds.): *Basic and Clinical Immunology*. Los Altos, Calif., Lange Medical Publishers, 1980, p. 79.
12. Engelfriet C.P., quoted by Mollison P.L., in *Blood Tranfusion in Clinical Medicine*, ed. 7. Oxford, England, Blackwell Scientific Publications, 1983, p. 350.
13. Hulting M.B., London F.S., Shapiro S.S., et al.: Heterogeneity of factor VIII antibodies: Further immunochemical and biological studies. *Blood* 49:807, 1977.
14. Augener W., Grey H.M., Cooper N.R.: The reaction of monomeric and aggregated immunoglobulins with C1. *Immunochemistry* 8:1011, 1971.
15. Spiegelberg A.L.: Biological activities of immunoglobulins of different classes and subclasses. *Adv. Immunol.* 19:259, 1974.
16. Cicimarra F., Rosen F.S., Merler E.: Localization of the IgG effector site for monocyte receptors. *Proc. Natl. Acad. Sci. USA* 72:2081, 1975.
17. Engelfriet C.P., von dem Borne A.E.G., Beckers D., et al.: Autoimmune haemolytic anemia: Serological and immunochemical characteristics of the autoantibodies, in *Mechanisms of Cell Destruction. Ser. Haematol.* 7:328, 1974.
18. Von Dem Borne A.E.G., Beckers D., van der Muellen F.W., et al.: IgG4 autoantibodies against erythrocytes, without increased haemolysis: A case report. *Br. J. Haematol.* 37:137, 1977.
19. Abramson N., Lo Buglio A.F., Jandl J.H., et al.: The interaction between human monocytes and red cells: Specificity for IgG subclasses and IgG fragments. *J. Exp. Med.* 132:1207, 1970.
20. Kline W.E.: Chemistry of blood group antigens and antibodies in hemolytic disease of the newborn, in Bell C.A. (ed.): *A Seminar on Perinatal Blood Banking*. Washington, D.C., American Association of Blood Banks, 1978, p. 21.
21. Schanfield M.S., Schoeppner S.L., Stevens S.O.: New approaches to detecting clinically significant antibodies in the laboratory, in Sandler S.G., Nusbacher J., Schanfield M.S. (eds.): *Immunobiology of the Erythrocyte*. New York, Alan R. Liss, 1980, p. 305.
22. Hardy J., Napier J.A.F.: Red cell antibodies detected in antenatal tests on rhesus positive women in South Wales, 1948–1978. *Br. J. Obstet. Gynaecol.* 88:91, 1981.
23. Mollison P.L.: *Blood Transfusion in Clinical Medicine*, ed. 7. Oxford, England, Blackwell Scientific Publications, 1983, p. 675.
24. Peevy K.J., Wiseman H.S.: ABO hemolytic disease of the newborn: Evaluation of management and identification of racial and antigenic factors. *Pediatrics* 61:475, 1978.
25. Walker W.: The changing pattern of haemolytic disease of the newborn (1948–1959). *Vox Sang.* 3:225, 1958.
26. Wykowsky P.K., Flint J.W., Goldberg M.F., et al.: Rh hemolytic disease, in *Epidemiologic Surveillance in the United States, 1968 to 1975. JAMA* 242:1376, 1979.
27. Current Trends: Rh hemolytic disease—Connecticut, United States, 1970–1979. *MMWR* 30:13, 1981.
28. Werch A.: Prenatal evaluation of hemolytic disease of the fetus, in Bell C.A. (ed.): *A Seminar on Perinatal Blood Banking*. Washington, D.C., American Association of Blood Banks, 1978, p. 56.
29. Robbins S.L., Cotran R.S.: *Pathologic Basis of Disease*. Philadelphia, W.B. Saunders Co., 1979, pp. 578–580.
30. Driscoll S.G.: Hydrops fetalis. *N. Engl. J. Med.* 275:1432, 1966.
31. Gorman J.G.: *The Role of the Laboratory in Hemolytic Disease of the Newborn*. Philadelphia, Lea & Febiger, 1965, p. 64.
32. Mollison P.L.: Some aspects of Rh hemolytic disease and its prevention, in Garraty G. (ed.): *Hemolytic Disease of the Newborn*. Arlington, Va., American Association of Blood Banks, 1984, pp. 1–32.
33. Urbaniak S.J., Robertson A.E.: A successful program of immunizing Rh-negative male volunteers for anti-D production using frozen/thawed blood. *Transfusion* 21:64, 1981.
34. Samson D., Mollison P.L.: Effect on primary Rh immunization of delayed administration of anti-Rh. *Immunology* 28:349, 1975.
35. Jacobowicz R., Williams L., Silberman F.: Immunization of Rh negative volunteers by repeated injections of very small amounts of Rh positive blood. *Vox Sang.* 23:376, 1972.
36. Mollison P.L.: *Blood Transfusion in Clinical Medicine*, ed. 7. Oxford, England, Blackwell Scientific Publications, 1983, p. 377.
37. Eklund J., Nevanlinna H.R.: Rh prevention: A report and analysis of a national programme. *J. Med. Genet.* 10:1, 1973.

38. Mollison P.L.: *Blood Transfusion in Clinical Medicine,* ed. 7. Oxford, England, Blackwell Scientific Publications, 1983, pp. 379, 380.
39. Blajchman M., Zipursky A., Bartsch F.R., et al.: McMaster conference on prevention of Rh immunization. *Vox Sang.* 36:50, 1979.
40. Murray S., Knox E.G., Walker W.: Rhesus haemolytic disease of the newborn and the ABO groups. *Vox Sang.* 10:6, 1965.
41. Bowman J.M.: Controversies in Rh prophylaxis, in Garraty D. (ed.): *Hemolytic Disease of the Newborn.* Arlington, Va., American Association of Blood Banks, 1984, p. 67.
42. Hughes-Jones N.C., Irona M., Ellis J., et al.: Anti-D concentration in mother and child in haemolytic disease of the newborn. *Vox Sang.* 21:135, 1971.
43. Schanfield M.S., Marguelies M.: Interrelación entre las subclases de IgG y el desarrollo clínico de la enfermedad hemolítica neonatal. *Rev. Argent. Transfusión* 3:383, 1979.
44. Romans D.G., Tilley C.A., Dorrington K.J.: Monogamous bivalency of IgG antibodies: I. Deficiency of branched ABHI-active oligosaccharide chains on red cells of infants causes the weak antiglobulin reaction in hemolytic disease of the newborn due to ABO incompatibility. *J. Immunol.* 124:2807, 1980.
45. Freda V.J.: *The Antepartum Management of Rh Disease in Hemolytic Disease of the Newborn.* Arlington, Va., American Association of Blood Banks, 1984, p. 33.
46. Bowman J.M., Chown B., Lewis M., et al.: Rh-immunization during pregnancy: Antenatal prophylaxis. *Can. Med. Assoc. J.,* 118:623, 1978.
47. Mollison P.L.: *Blood Transfusion in Clinical Medicine,* ed. 7. Oxford, England, Blackwell Scientific Publications, 1983, p. 680.
48. Freda V.J., Robertson J.G.: Antepartum management: Amniocentesis and experience with hysterotomy and surgery in utero. *Jewish Mem. Hosp. Bull. (NYC)* 10:47, 1965.
49. The risk of amniocentesis (editorial). *Lancet* 2:1287, 1978.
50. Wenk R.E., Rosenbaum J., Statland B.E.: Assessment of fetal condition and amniotic fluid analysis, in Henry B.J. (ed.): *Clinical Diagnosis and Management by Laboratory Methods,* ed. 17. Philadelphia, W.B. Saunders Co., 1984, p. 502.
51. Werch A.: Amniocentesis: Indications, technique and complications. *South. Med. J.* 69:824, 1976.
52. Peddle L.J.: Increase of antibody titer following amniocentesis. *J. Obstet. Gynecol.* 100:567, 1968.
53. Mollison P.L.: *Blood Transfusion in Clinical Medicine,* ed. 7. Oxford, England, Blackwell Scientific Publications, 1983, p. 398.
54. Broderson R., Jacobsen J., Hertz H., et al.: Bilirubin conjugation in the human fetus. *Scand. J. Clin. Lab. Invest.* 20:41, 1967.
55. Walker A.H.C.: Liquor amnii studies in the prediction of haemolytic disease of the newborn. *Br. Med. J.* 2:376, 1957.
56. Liley A.V.: Liquor amnii analysis in the management of the pregnancy complicated by rhesus sensitization. *Am. J. Obstet. Gynecol.* 82:1359, 1961.
57. Liley A.W.: Errors in the assessment of hemolytic disease from amniotic fluid. *Am. J. Obstet. Gynecol.* 93:485, 1963.
58. Gluck L., Kulovich M.V.: Lecithin sphingomyelin ratios in amniotic fluid in normal and abnormal pregnancy. *Am. J. Obstet. Gynecol.* 115:539, 1973.
59. Liley A.W.: Intrauterine transfusion of foetus in haemolytic disease. *Br. Med. J.* 2:1107, 1963.
60. Pritchard J.A., Weisman R. Jr.: The absorption of labelled erythrocytes from the peritoneal cavity of humans. *J. Lab. Clin. Med.* 49:756, 1957.
61. Mollison P.L.: *Blood Transfusion in Clinical Medicine,* ed. 7. Oxford, England, Blackwell Scientific Publications, 1983, pp. 122–123.
62. Palmer A., Gordon R.R.: A critical review of intrauterine fetal transfusion. *Br. J. Obstet. Gynaecol.* 83:688, 1976.
63. Queenan J.T.: Intrauterine transfusion: A cooperative study. *Am. J. Obstet. Gynecol.* 104:397, 1969.
64. Robertson E.G., Brown A., Ellis M.I., et al.: Intrauterine transfusion in the management of severe rhesus isoimmunization. *Br. J. Obstet. Gynaecol.* 83:694, 1976.
65. McClure-Brocone J., cited by Mollison P.L : *Blood Transfusion in Clinical Medicine,* ed. 6. Oxford, England, Blackwell Scientific Publications, 1979, p. 694.
66. Parkman R., Mosier D., Umansky I., et al : Graft versus host disease after intrauterine transfusions for hemolytic disease of the newborn. *N. Engl. J. Med.* 290:359, 1974.
67. Kevy S.V., Jacobson M., Button L.: Clinical uses of frozen-thawed erythrocytes in pediatrics, in *Clinical Uses of Frozen-Thawed Red Blood Cells.* New York, Alan R. Liss, 1976, p. 89.
68. Bowman J.M., Pollock J.M.: Haemolysis of donor red cells at fetal transfusion due to catheter trauma. *Lancet* 2:1190, 1980.
69. Pollack W.: Mechanisms of Rh immune suppression by Rh immune globulin, in Garraty G. (ed.): *Hemolytic Disease of the Newborn.* Arlington, Va., American Association of Blood Banks, 1984, p. 53.
70. Pollack W., Ascari W.Q., Crispen J.R., et al.: Studies on Rh prophylaxis: II. Rh immune prophylaxis after transfusion with Rh-positive blood. *Transfusion* 11:340, 1971.
71. Chan P.L., Sinclair N.R.: Regulation of the immune response: VI. Inability of (Fab')$_2$ antibody to terminate established immune responses and its ability to interfere with IgG antibody-mediated immune suppression. *Immunology* 24:289, 1973.
72. Mollison P.L.: *Blood Transfusion in Clinical Medicine,* ed. 7. Oxford, England, Blackwell Scientific Publications, 1983, pp. 243–244.
73. Pollack W., Gorman J.G.: Rh immune suppression: An immunostat hypothesis, in *Rh Antibody Mediated Immunosuppression.* Raritan, N.J., Ortho Diagnostics, 1976, p.115.

74. Siskind G.W.: The role of circulating antibody in the control of antibody synthesis: Mechanism for the suppressive effect of passive antibody on active antibody synthesis. *Transfusion* 8:127, 1968.
75. Woodrow J.C., Clarke C.A., Donohue W.T.A., et al.: Mechanism of Rh prophylaxis: An experimental study on specificity of immunosuppression. *Br. Med. J.* 2:57, 1975.
76. Huestis D.W., Bove J.R., Busch S.: *Practical Blood Transfusion*, ed. 2. Boston, Little, Brown & Co., 1976, p. 278.
77. Ness P.M.: The assessment of fetal maternal hemorrhage by an enzyme-linked antiglobulin test for Rh immune globulin recipients. *Am. J. Obstet. Gynecol.* 143:788, 1982.
78. Medearis A.L., Hensleigh P.A., Parks D.R., et al.: Detection of fetal erythrocytes in maternal blood postpartum with the fluorescence-activated cell sorter. *Am. J. Obstet. Gynecol.* 148:290, 1984.
79. Clayton E.M. Jr., Foster E.B., Clayton E.P.: New stain for fetal erythrocytes in peripheral blood smears. *Obstet. Gynecol.* 35:642, 1970.
80. Widman F.K. (ed.): *Technical Manual*. Washington, D.C., American Association of Blood Banks, 1981, p. 259.
81. Rock G.: Amelioration of Rh disease, in Garraty G. (ed.): *Hemolytic Disease of the Newborn*. Arlington, Va., American Association of Blood Banks, 1984, p. 119.
82. Rubinstein P.: Repeated small volume plasmapheresis in the management of hemolytic disease of the newborn, in Frigoletto F.D., Jewett J.F., Konungres A.A., et al. (eds.): *Rh Hemolytic Disease: New Strategy for Eradication*. Cambridge, Mass., Harvard University Press, 1982.
83. Dufour D.R., Monoghan W.P.: ABO hemolytic disease of the newborn: A retrospective analysis of 254 cases. *Am. J. Clin. Pathol.* 73:369, 1980.
84. Kirkman H.N.: Further evidence for a racial difference in frequency of ABO hemolytic disease. *J. Pediatr.* 90:717, 1977.
85. Chan-Shu S-Y.A., Blair O.: ABO hemolytic disease of the newborn. *Am. J. Clin. Pathol.* 71:677, 1979.
86. Rosenfield R.E., Ohno G.: A.B. hemolytic disease of the newborn. *Rev. Hematol.* 10:231, 1955.
87. Voak D.: The serologic specificity of the sensitizing antibodies in ABO heterospecific pregnancy of the group-O mother. *Vox Sang.* 14:271, 1968.
88. Mollison P.L.: *Blood Transfusion in Clinical Medicine*, ed. 7. Oxford, England, Blackwell Scientific Publications, 1983, p. 690.
89. Grundbacher F.J.: ABO incompatibility and hemolytic disease of the newborn. *S. Afr. Med. J.* 44:221, 1970.
90. Moulds J.J.: Immunosuppression by passive antibody, in Bell C.A. (ed.): *A Seminar on Perinatal Blood Banking*. Washington, D.C., American Association of Blood Banks, 1978, p. 81.
91. Kornstad L., quoted by Mollison P.L.: *Blood Transfusion in Clinical Medicine*, ed. 7. Oxford, England, Blackwell Scientific Publications, 1983, p. 677.
92. Oski F.A., Naiman J.L.: *Hematologic Problems in the Newborn*, ed. 2. Philadelphia, W.B. Saunders Co., vol. 4, 1972.
93. Michaels-Hills R., Cabrera-Meza G.: Utilization of blood components in neonatal medicine, in Bell C.A. (ed.): *A Seminar on Perinatal Blood Banking*. Washington, D.C., American Association of Blood Banks, 1978, p. 119.
94. Allen F.H. Jr., et al.: Erythroblastosis fetalis: VI. Prevention of kernicterus. *Am. J. Dis. Child.* 80:77a, 1980.
95. Bowman J.M.: Neonatal management, in Quenan J.T. (ed.): *Modern Management of the Rh Problem*, ed. 2. Hagerstown, Md., Harper & Row, 1977, p. 208.
96. Bowman J.M.: Alloimmune hemolytic disease of the newborn, in Williams W., Beutler E., Erslev A.J., et al. (eds.): *Hematology*, ed. 3. New York, McGraw-Hill Book Co., 1983, p. 653.
97. Gartner L.M., Snyder R.N., Chabon R.S., et al.: Kernicterus: High incidence in premature infants with low serum bilirubin concentrations. *Pediatrics* 45:906, 1970.
98. Huestis D.W., Bove J.R., Busch S.: *Practical Blood Transfusion*, ed. 2. Boston, Little, Brown & Co., 1981, pp. 396–397.
99. Michaels-Hill R., Cabrera-Meza G.: Utilization of blood components in neonatal medicine, in Bell C.A. (ed.): *A Seminar on Perinatal Blood Banking*. Washington, D.C., American Association of Blood Banks, 1978, p. 115.
100. Silverman W.A., Anderson D.N., Black W.A., et al.: A difference in mortality rate and incidence of kernicterus among premature infants allotted to two prophylactic antibacterial regimens. *Pediatrics* 18:614, 1956.
101. Sacher R.A., Lenes B.: Exchange transfusion. *Clin. Lab. Med.* 1:265, 1981.
102. Mollison P.L.: *Blood Transfusion in Clinical Medicine*, ed. 7. Oxford, England, Blackwell Scientific Publications, 1983, p. 684.
103. Boggs T.R., Westphal M.C.: Mortality of exchange transfusion. *Pediatrics* 26:745, 1960.
104. Michael J.M., Dorner I., Bruns D., et al.: Potassium load in CPD-preserved whole blood and two types of packed red cells. *Transfusion* 15:144, 1975.
105. Taylor W.C., Gillis C.N., Nash C.W., et al.: Experimental observations on cardiac arrhythmia during exchange transfusion in rabbits. *J. Pediatr.* 58:470, 1961.
106. Abelson N.M.: *Topics in Blood Banking*. Philadelphia, Lea & Febiger, 1974, p. 142.
107. Widman K.F. (ed.): *Technical Manual*, ed. 8. Washington, D.C., American Association of Blood Banks, 1981, p. 54.
108. Kreuger A.: Adenine metabolism during and after exchange transfusion in newborn infants with CPD-adenine blood. *Transfusion* 16:249, 1976.
109. Kreuger A.: Exchange transfusion with ACD-adenine blood: A follow-up study. *Transfusion* 13:69, 1973.

110. Grajwer L.A., Pildes R., Zarif M., et al.: Exchange transfusion in the neonate: A controlled study using frozen-stored erythrocytes resuspended in plasma. *Am. J. Clin. Pathol.* 66:117, 1976.
111. Hsu T.C.S., Rosenfield R.E., Rubinstein P.: Instrumented PVP-augmented antiglobulin tests: III. IgG-coated cells in ABO incompatible babies, depressed hemoglobin levels in type A babies of type O mothers. *Vox Sang.* 26:326, 1974.
112. Wallace J.: Hemolytic disease of the newborn, in *Blood Transfusion for Clinicians.* Edinburgh, Churchill Livingstone, 1977, p. 177.
113. Wallerstein H.: Treatment of severe erythroblastosis by simultaneous removal and replacement of blood of newborn infant. *Science* 103:583, 1946.
114. Mollison P.L.: *Blood Transfusion in Clinical Medicine,* ed. 7. Oxford, England, Blackwell Scientific Publications, 1983, p. 699.
115. Allen F.H. Jr., Diamond L.K.: *Erythroblastosis Fetalis.* Boston, Little, Brown & Co., 1957, pp. 52–83.
116. Huestis D.W., Bove J.R., Busch S.: *Practical Blood Transfusion,* ed. 3. Boston, Little, Brown & Co., 1981, p. 399.
117. Brown A.K., Zuelzer W.W., Robinson A.R.: Studies in hyperbilirubinemia: 2. Clearance of bilirubin from plasma and extravascular space in newborn infants during exchange transfusion. *Am. J. Dis. Child.* 93:274, 1957.
118. Srinivasan G., Shaukar H., Yeh T.F., et al.: A critical care problem in neonates: Exchange transfusions through peripheral artery. *Crit. Care Med.* 8:338, 1980.
119. Dorand R.D., Cook L.N., Andrews B.F.: Umbilical vessel catheterization: The low incidence of complications in a series of 200 newborn infants. *Clin. Pediatr.* 16:569, 1977.
120. Weldon V.V., Odell G.B.: Mortality risk of exchange transfusion. *Pediatrics* 41:797, 1968.
121. Mollison P.L.: The survival of transfused red cells in haemolytic disease of the newborn. *Arch. Dis. Child.* 18:161, 1943.
122. Desforges J.F., O'Connel L.G.: Hematologic observations of erythroblastosis fetalis. *Blood* 10:802, 1955.
123. Michels-Hill R., Cabrera-Meza G.: Utilization of blood components in neonatal medicine, in Bell C.A. (ed.): *A Seminar on Perinatal Blood Banking.* Washington, D.C., American Association of Blood Banks, 1978, p. 120.
124. Tobin J. O'H., MacDonald H.: Cytomegalovirus infection and exchange transfusion. *Br. Med. J.* 4:404, 1975.
125. Paxson C.L., Morriss F.H., Adock E.W.: Neonatal exchange transfusion with blood containing hepatitis B antigen. *J. Pediatr.* 88:357, 1976.
126. Mallin W.S., Alter A.A., Ritz N.D., et al.: Posttransfusion malaria in a newborn. *Postgrad. Med.* 54:219, 1973.
127. Van Loghem J.J., vanBolhuis J.H., Soeters J.M., Veeneklaas G.M.H.: Treatment of 160 cases of erythroblastosis foetalis with exchange transfusion. *Br. Med. J.* 2:49, 1949.
128. Sundal A., Kass A.: Morbus hemolyticus neonatorum. *Acta Pediatr.* 43:579, 1954.
129. Hilgartner M.W., Lanzkowsky P., Lipsitz P.: Perforation of small and large intestine following exchange transfusion. *Am. J. Dis. Child.* 120:79, 1970.
130. Michels-Hill R., Cabrera-Meza G.: Utilization of blood components in neonatal medicine, in Bell C.A. (ed.): A Seminar on Perinatal Blood Banking. Washington, D.C., American Association of Blood Banks, 1978, p. 122.
131. Povey M.J.C.: pH changes during exchange transfusion. *Lancet* 2:339, 1964.
132. Mollison P.L.: *Blood Tranfusion in Clinical Medicine,* ed. 7. Oxford, England, Blackwell Scientific Publications, 1983, p. 752.
133. Schiff D., Aranda J.V., Chan G. et al.: Metabolic effects of exchange transfusions: I. Effect of citrated and heparinized blood on glucose, nonsterified fatty acids, 2-4 hydroxybenzeneazo-benzoic acid binding, and insulin. *J. Pediatr.* 78:603, 1971.
134. Cremer R.J., Perryman P.W., Richards D.F.: Influence of light on the hyperbilirubinemia of infants. *Lancet* 1:094, 1958.
135. Seligman J.W.: Recent and changing concepts of hyperbilirubinemia and its management in the newborn. *Pediatr. Clin. North Am.* 24:509, 1977
136. Michels-Hills R., Cabrera-Meza G.: Utilization of blood components in neonatal medicine, in Bell C.A. (ed.): *A Seminar on Perinatal Blood Banking.* Washington, D.C., American Association of Blood Banks, 1978, p. 126.
137. Trolle D.: Decrease of total serum bilirubin concentration in newborn infants after phenobarbitone treatment. *Lancet* 2:705, 1968.
138. McMullin G.P., Hayes M.F., Arora S.C.: Fhenobarbitone in rhesus haemolytic disease: A controlled trial. *Lancet* 2:949, 1970.
139. Bowman J.M.: Rh-isoimmunization 1977. *Med. Can.* 32:17, 1977.
140. Gilmour J.R.: Normal hemopoiesis in intrauterine and neonatal life. *J. Pathol.* 52:25, 1942.
141. Oski F.A., Naiman J.L.: *Hematologic Problems in the Newborn,* ed 3. Philadelphia, W.B. Saunders Co., 1982, p. 1.
142. Fakuda T.: Fetal hematopoiesis: II. Electron microscopic studies on human hepatic hematopoiesis. *Virchows Arch. Cell Pathol.* 16:249, 1974.
143. Gupta S., Pahwa R., O'Reilly R., et al.: Ontogeny of lymphocyte subpopulation in human fetal liver. *Proc. Natl. Acad. Sci. USA* 73:919, 1976.
144. Gale R.E., Clegg J.B., Huehns E.R.: Human embryonic haemoglobins Gower 1 and Gower 2. *Nature* 280:162, 1979.
145. Pataryas H.A., Stomatoyannopoulos G.: Hemoglobins in human fetuses: Evidence of adult hemoglobin production after the 11th gestational week. *Blood* 39:688, 1972.
146. Kazazian H.H., Woodhead A.P.: Hemoglobin A

synthesis in the developing fetus. *N. Engl. J. Med.* 289:58, 1973.
147. Bard H.: Postnatal fetal and adult hemoglobin synthesis in early preterm newborn infants. *J. Clin. Invest.* 52:1789, 1973.
148. Cooper H.A., Hoagland H.C.: Fetal hemoglobin. *Mayo Clin. Proc.* 47:402, 1972.
149. Delivoria-Papadoupolos M., Roncevic N.P., Oski F.A.: Postnatal changes in oxygen transport of term, premature and sick infants: The role of adult hemoglobin and red cell 2,3-diphosphoglycerate. *Pediatr. Res.* 5:235, 1971.
150. Bertles J.H.: Human fetal hemoglobin: Significance in disease. *Ann. NY Acad. Sci.* 241:638, 1974.
151. Linderkamp O., Versmold H.T., Messow-Zahn K., et al.: The effect of intrapartum and intrauterine asphyxia on placental transfusion in premature and full-term infants. *Eur. J. Pediatr.* 127:91, 1978.
152. Saarinen U.M., Siimes M.A.: Developmental changes in red blood cell counts and indices of infants after exclusion of iron deficiency by laboratory criteria and continuous iron supplementation. *J. Pediatr.* 92:412, 1978.
153. Lundstrom U., Siimes M.A.: Red blood cell values in low-birth weight infants: Ages at which values become equivalent to those of term infants. *J. Pediatr.* 96:1040, 1980.
154. Seip M.: The reticulocyte level and the erythrocyte production judged from reticulocyte studies in newborn infants during the first week of life. *Acta Pediatr. Scand.* 44:355, 1955.
155. Moe P.J.: Umbilical cord blood and capillary blood in the evaluation of anemia in erythroblastosis fetalis. *Acta Pediatr. Scand.* 56:391, 1967.
156. Yao A.C., Lind J., Tisala R., et al.: Placental transfusion in the premature infant with observation on clinical course and outcome. *Acta Pediatr. Scand.* 58:561, 1969.
157. Stockman J.A., Oski F.A.: Erythrocytes of the human neonate. *Curr. Top. Hematol.* 1:193, 1978.
158. Pearson H.A.: Life span of the fetal red blood cell. *J. Pediatr.* 70:166, 1967.
159. Luban N.L.C.: Physiology of normal and premature infants, in Luban N.L.C., Keating L.J. (eds.): *Hemotherapy of the Infant and Premature.* Arlington, Va., American Association of Blood Banks, 1983, pp. 1–20.
160. Mollison P.L.: *Blood Transfusion in Clinical Medicine,* ed. 7. Oxford, England, Blackwell Scientific Publications, 1983, p. 88.
161. Sisson T.R., Knutson S., Kendall N.: The blood volume of infants: IV. Infants born by cesarean section. *Am. J. Obstet. Gynecol.* 117:351, 1973.
162. Xanthou M.: Leucocyte blood picture in healthy full term and premature babies during the neonatal period. *Arch. Dis. Child.:* 45:242, 1970.
163. Sell E.J., Corrigan J.J.: Platelet counts, fibrinogen concentrations and factor V and factor VIII levels in healthy infants according to gestational age. *J. Pediatr.* 82:1028, 1973.
164. Wallas C.H.: Considerations and indications for the use of red blood cell products, in Luban N.L.C., Keating L.J. (eds.): *Hemotherapy of the Infant and Premature.* Arlington, Va., American Association of Blood Banks, 1983, pp. 21–36.
165. Robinson R.O., Emerson P.M., Howes D., et al.: Red cell mass and blood volume in low birth weight infants. *J. Perinat. Med.* 6:213, 1978.
166. Hakanson D.O., Oh, W.: Hyperviscosity in the small for gestational age infant. *Biol. Neonate* 37:109, 1980.
167. Wardrop C.A., Holland B.M., Veale K.E.A., et al.: Nonphysiological anaemia of prematurity. *Arch. Dis. Child.* 53:855, 1978.
168. Jones J.G., Holland B.M., Veale K.E.A., et al.: "Available oxygen": A realistic expression of the ability of the blood to supply oxygen to tissues. *Scand. J. Haematol.* 22:77, 1979.
169. Kevy S.V.: Pediatric transfusion therapy, in Dawson R.B. (ed.): *Transfusion Therapy: A Technical Workshop.* Washington, D.C., American Association of Blood Banks, 1974, pp. 55–76.
170. Valeri C.R., Valeri D.A., Gray A., et al.: Cryopreserved red blood cells for pediatric transfusion: Frozen storage of small aliquots in polyvinyl chloride (PVC) plastic bags. *Transfusion* 21:527, 1981.
171. Kakaiya R.M., Morrison F.S., Halbrook J.C., et al.: Problems with walking donor programs. *Transfusion* 19:577, 1979.
172. Sacher R.A., Jacobson R.J., Davitt M.K., et al.: Blood component utilization in neonatal intensive care (abstract), *Proceedings of 1st International Congress of Pediatric Laboratory Medicine.* Jerusalem, 1980, p. 194.
173. Glader B.E., Buchanan G.R.: Care of the critically ill child: The bleeding neonate. *Pediatrics* 58:548, 1976.
174. Stoerner J.W., Pickering C.K., Adock E.W., et al.: Polymorphonuclear leukocyte function in newborn infants. *J. Pediatr.* 93:862, 1978.
175. DeCurtis M., Vetiano G., Romano G., et al.: Improvement of phagocytosis and nitroblue tetrazolium reduction after exchange transfusion in two preterm infants with severe septicemia. *Pediatrics* 70:829, 1982.
176. Ishikawa A., Hafter R., Graeff H.: The effect of heparinized blood exchange transfusion on endotoxin induced disseminated intravascular coagulation. *J. Pediatr. Med.* 7:250, 1979.
177. Delivoria-Pappadoupolos M., Morrow G. III, Oski F.A.: Exchange transfusion in the newborn infant with fresh and old blood: The role of storage on 2,3-diphosphoglycerate hemoglobin oxygen affinity, and oxygen release. *Pediatrics* 79:898, 1971.
178. Kessler D.L. Jr., Smith A.L., Woodrum D.E.: Chloramphenicol toxicity in a neonate treated with exchange transfusions. *Pediatrics* 96:140, 1980.
179. Donn S.M., Swartz R.D., Thoene J.G.: Comparison of exchange transfusion, peritoneal dialysis and hemodialysis for the treatment of hyperammonemia in an anuric newborn infant. *J. Pediatr.* 95:67, 1979.

180. Ballard R.A., Drew W.L., Hufnagle K.G., et al.: Acquired cytomegalovirus infection in preterm infants. *Am. J.Dis. Child.* 133:482, 1979.
181. Kumar A., Nankervis G.A., Cooper A.R., et al.: Acquisition of cytomegalovirus infection in infants following exchange transfusion: A prospective study. *Transfusion* 20:327, 1980.
182. Yeager A.S., Grumet F.C., Hafleigh E.B., et al.: Prevention of transfusion-acquired cytomegalovirus infections in newborn infants. *J. Pediatr.* 98:281, 1981.
183. Seger R., Yoller P., Kenny A., et al.: Potential hazards of blood transfusion in clostridia-associated necrotizing enterocolitis. *Lancet* 1:48, 1979.
184. Bullen J.J., Rogers H.J., Leigh L.: Iron binding proteins in milk and resistance to *Escherichia coli* infection in infants. *Br. Med. J.* 1:69, 1972.
185. Kevy S.V., Fosburg M., Wolfe L.: The use of platelets, plasma and plasma derivatives in the newborn, in Luban N.L.C., Keating L.J. (eds.): *Hemotherapy of the Infant and Premature.* Arlington, Va., American Association of Blood Banks, 1983.
186. Adamkin D.H., Schott R.J., Cook L.N., et al.: Nonhyperoxic retrolental fibroplasia. *Pediatrics* 60:828, 1977.
187. Parkman R., Mosier D., Umansky I., et el.: Graft versus host disease after intrauterine and exchange transfusion for hemolytic disease of the newborn. *N. Engl. J. Med.* 290:359, 1974.
188. Rosse W.F., Adams J.P., Yount W.J.: Subclasses of IgG antibodies in immune thrombocytopenic purpura (ITP). *Br. J. Haematol.* 46:109, 1980.
189. Noto T.A., Steib M.D.: Use of exchange transfusions in neonatology. *Lab. Med.* 12:609, 1981.
190. Shulman N.R., Marder V.J., Hiller M.C., et al.: Platelet and leukocyte isoantigens and their antibodies: Serologic, physiologic and clinical studies. *Prog. Hematol.* 4:22, 1964.
191. von Dem Borne A.E.G.Kr., van Leeuwen E.F., von Riesz L.E., et al.: Neonatal alloimmune thrombocytopenia: Detection and characterization of the responsible antibodies by the platelet immunofluorescence test. *Blood* 57:649, 1981.
192. Kuniki T.J., Aster R.H.: Isolation and immunologic characterization of the human platelet alloantigen, Pl^{A1}. *Mol. Immunol.* 16:353, 1979.
193. Sitarz A.L., Driscoll J.M., Wolff J.A.: Management of isoimmune neonatal thrombocytopenia. *Am. J. Obstet. Gynecol.* 124:39, 1976.
194. Scott J.R., Cruikshank D.P., Kochenour N.K., et al.: Fetal platelet counts in the obstetric management of immunologic thrombocytopenic purpura. *Am. J. Obstet. Gynecol.* 136:495, 1980.
195. McIntosh S., O'Brien R.T., Schwartz A.D., Pearson H.A.: Neonatal isoimmune purpura response to platelet infusions. *J. Pediatr.* 82:1020, 1973.
196. Wolfe L., Epstein M., Kevy S.: Blood transfusion for the neonatal patient. *Hum. Pathol.* 14:256, 1983.
197. Tate D.Y.: Immune thrombocytopenia in severe neonatal infections. *J. Pediatr.* 98:449, 1981.
198. Stuart M.J., Gross S. J.: The effect of prenatal acetylsalicylic ingestion on maternal and neonatal hemostasis. *Pediatr. Res.* 12:475, 1978.
199. Lalezari P., Radel E.: Neutrophil-specific antigens: Immunology and clinical significance. *Semin. Hematol.* 11:281, 1974.
200. Veheught F.W.A., von dem Borne A.E.G., V. Noord-Bokhorst J.C., et al.: Serological, immunochemical and immunocytological properties of granulocyte antibodies. *Vox Sang.* 35:294, 1978.
201. Baehner R.L., Strauss H.S.: Hemophilia in the first year of life. *N. Engl. J. Med.* 275:524, 1966.
202. Hilgartner M.W.: The management of hemophilia, in Mallory D. McG. (ed.): *Hemophilia: A Technical Workshop.* Washington, D.C., American Association of Blood Banks, 1978, p. 17.
203. Michels-Hill R., Cabrera-Meza G.: Utilization of blood components in neonatal medicine, in Bell C.A. (ed.): *A Seminar on Perinatal Blood Banking.* Washington, D.C., American Association of Blood Banks, 1978, p. 124.

17

Quality Control and Legal Aspects of Immunohematology

THE DIFFERENCE BETWEEN quality control exercised as a bureaucratic procedure and quality control exercised for the sake of preserving excellence lies in the attitude one adopts toward it. The term quality control as used in industry[1] is different from the term (and concept) as used in the laboratory, for the main goal of a good laboratory is the delivery of good patient care rather than the achievement of monetary reward. This attitude is expressed both in good will on the part of personnel and in good science in the application of laboratory technology to medical practice. Scientifically, the term quality control denotes the study of physical and chemical phenomena in a rational, well-organized manner. Unknown data (patient data) are compared with known standards (controls) to determine the presence of an abnormality caused by disease, genetic polymorphism, or individual variation.

This chapter approaches the subject of quality control from two points of view: overall quality control in the laboratory, and specific blood bank quality control techniques. Most tests performed in the blood bank produce binary discrete variates; that is, tests yield either positive or negative results. However, quantitative assessments are also used, and reactions are graded subjectively in terms of strength of reaction. It is anticipated that in the future, blood bank test results will be truly quantitative, as testing will be done with instruments that provide a numerical value rather than a semi-quantitative evaluation. In fact, some larger blood centers possess instruments capable of measuring hemagglutination in a quantitative manner.

For numerical data, a statistical analysis must be done to assess machine and operator performance and to determine standards for accuracy and precision.

Precision denotes the capacity to obtain reproducible readings under the same conditions, but such measurements have no validity if they are not compared within the framework of a standardized system. If control values fall within the range of expected, standard values the test is said to be accurate. The two concepts of precision and accuracy are graphically expressed in Figure 17–1. To obtain accuracy, it is necessary to know the concentration of numerical values of the normal value whenever feasible. However, all laboratory procedures are subject to bias as well as analytical inaccuracies.

To establish standards, pools of normal samples are obtained from a specific population. A crucial facet of a quality control program is the careful selection and preparation of standards. When the standards are compared, there are acceptable degrees of variability. The expected values and the reported values should cluster around a mean.

Values may be charted on a Levey-Jenings chart (Fig 17–2).[2] These charts reflect trends in the quality of laboratory procedures and may help detect

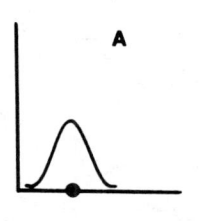
Accurate and Precise

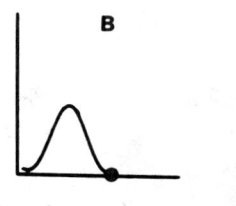
Precise but Inaccurate

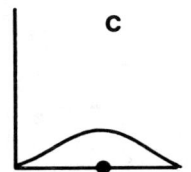
Accurate but Imprecise

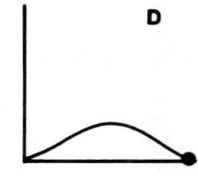
Imprecise and Inaccurate

FIG 17–1.—Types of quality control profiles. *A*, the expected value *(black dot)* is placed at the center of a gaussian curve. This represents accurate and precise results. *B*, the expected value is skewed to either side of the gaussian curve. These results are precise but inaccurate. *C*, the distribution of the gaussian curve is expanded; however, the expected value is at the center of the curve. These results are accurate but imprecise. *D*, the distribution of the gaussian curve is expanded and the expected value is skewed off-center. These results are both imprecise and inaccurate.

problems related to machine function or operation. Usually, values clustered around the mean should fall within ± 1 SD of the mean. Steady upward or downward trends may reflect a shift in standardization of equipment; a zigzag, up-and-down trend may indicate poor precision on the part of the operator.

QUALITY CONTROL IN THE BLOOD BANK

Even though testing in a blood bank is at best semiquantitative and is often subjectively evaluated, the chances of error probably mean more here in terms of patient welfare than in any other laboratory. The blood bank is the only laboratory that delivers a product *and* a test result rather than a test result only, such as, for instance, a clinical chemistry laboratory would provide. It is therefore mandatory to approach a "zero defect status" to ensure the delivery of a safe product. A physician treating a patient in the ward has no way of telling what type of blood is in a blood unit just by looking at it, and relies totally on the accurate testing performed in the immunohematology laboratory. The safety of a product delivered by the blood bank is largely determined by accuracy on the part of the technical and clerical staff, adequate machine function, and appropriate choice of reagents.

Personnel

Well qualified and trained personnel are important to quality blood banking. It is a good practice to conduct in-house training and retraining of staff as part of the quality control process. This is especially indicated for laboratory personnel who have reduced access to continuing medical education, such as those working the midnight shifts. These persons can be rotated sequentially to day shifts for retraining and continuing medical education. Accreditation in blood bank technology by major accrediting associations is highly recommended. The clerical workers in a blood bank are perhaps the most crucial factor in the accurate delivery of a safe product, especially those individuals involved in the chain of events that leads to the direct delivery of a unit. It is therefore mandatory that these individuals have a good understanding of the principles of blood transfusion and be acutely aware of the disastrous consequences that a mistake may have on the welfare of a patient. In a recent survey, 33 of 37 fatalities caused by errors in the chain of events leading to transfusion were attributed to clerical mistakes.[3]

Quality Control of Blood Bank Equipment

Fortunately, the equipment in the blood bank is usually simple and not prone to excessive malfunction. The following section reviews the quality assessment of equipment according to whether it is temperature-dependent equipment or non-temperature-dependent equipment. Only cursory mention is made of how these instruments are checked; interested readers are referred to special texts on the subject.

Temperature-dependent Equipment

Refrigerators.—Refrigerators in the blood bank are used for two purposes: storage of blood and blood products and storage of reagents. Different refrigerators should be used for these two different functions when feasible. Blood bank refrigerators are manufactured commercially to meet the specifications of the Bureau of Biologics, Food and Drug Administration (FDA), which inspects and accredits blood banks. These standards require that these refrigerators maintain the blood, plasma, or reagents within specified temperatures. The American Association of Blood Banks (AABB), which accredits blood banks on a voluntary basis, reviews the requirements in its standards manual.[4] Blood and blood component refrigerators should contain only these products. The storage temperature for blood units should be within 1° to 6°C throughout the refrigerator. All areas within the refrigerator should be clearly labeled to enable quick identification of the different products stored and should be equipped with visual alarms to warn the technologist if out-of-control temperatures are reached. These alarms must be tested periodically (every 2–4 months) and the results recorded in a quality control book.

The sensors of the alarm systems must be immersed in 10% glycerol in water.[5] These sensors are periodically tested to be sure the alarm sounds at low and high temperatures. The high temperature can be assessed by holding the sensor in one hand or immersing it in warm water and observing the needle on the recorder or the digital temperature display. The low temperature can be checked by immersing the sensors in a slush of crushed ice and water and observing the recorder. These tests are best performed by two persons.

A mercury thermometer immersed in 10% glycerol should be left at all times in the higher portion

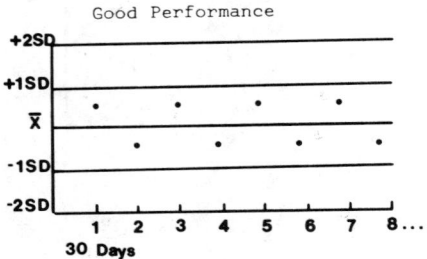
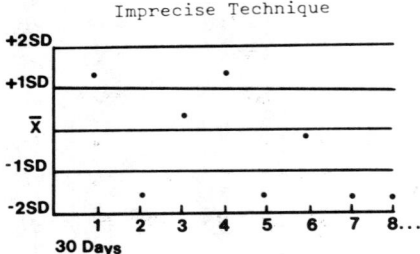
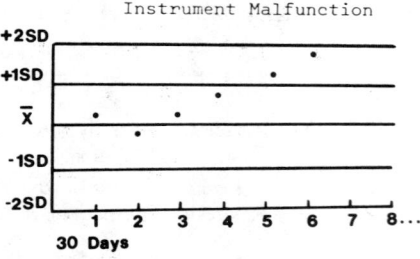

FIG 17–2.—A monthly cumulative quality control. *Top,* good performance results. The values are distributed in close proximity to the average ($\bar{x}$). *Middle,* random distribution of results, denoting imprecise technique. *Bottom,* results are distributed close to the average line ($\bar{x}$) in the first days of the month. Thereafter there is an upward trend, indicating instrument malfunction.

of the refrigerator and another one in the lower portion. Records of the charted temperature from the recorder should be signed and dated by the person performing the quality control check of the refrigerators. The manual reading from mercury thermometers is also recorded in the quality control book. These records are usually kept for at least 5 years. Ordinary household-type refrigerators can be used for storing reagents. These are kept at 1°–8° C.

Freezers.—Deep freezers for blood banks are commercially available and used for storage of plasma and cryoprecipitate. Although one usually checks the temperature by checking the recording chart, it is a good practice to check the sensors occasionally. However, these are less accessible than the sensors in a blood component refrigerator. Plasma and cryoprecipitate are kept at $-18°C$, although $-30°C$ is better for preservation of plasma and cryoprecipitate.[6] There should be an audible temperature alarm system that rings at a site other than the blood bank, such as the telephone room, where other personnel are advised of the problem. A visual alarm is recommended as well.

Labels on blood products and on storage shelves are advisable. Temperature records are kept for at least 5 years. Both refrigerators and freezers should be kept clean and used only for the designated purpose (i.e., blood components or reagents, respectively).

The electrical supply for these machines should be connected to an emergency electrical supply system and clear instructions as to where to relocate the components in case of electrical malfunction must be stated in the laboratory manual and on the storage machines.

Water Baths, Dry Baths, and View Boxes.—Thermometers are immersed in the water of water baths to a marked line in order to assess the required temperatures. Temperatures are recorded daily and logged in the quality control book. Water in the water baths for thawing plasma is changed frequently to minimize contamination. This water must be changed immediately if a bag breaks while in the water. It is recommended that plasma units be thawed in a second bag to avoid spills of plasma into the water bath.

Dry baths are metal blocks kept at the required temperature. They are monitored by means of a manual thermometer inserted in a tube with a fluid level.

Although tube testing is recommended for testing in the blood bank, some laboratories still use view boxes for various tests. Temperatures in view boxes are unreliable and it is difficult to maintain proper temperature quality control over the boxes. All thermometers should be calibrated as suggested by Swindles.[7]

Non-Temperature-Dependent Equipment

Centrifuges.—Centrifuges are used for two main purposes in a blood bank: for the preparation of components and for laboratory testing. Centrifuges for the preparation of components must be kept meticulously clean and must be routinely calibrated. Although most user manuals provide charts to calculate centrifugal force, the following formula can be used:

$$RCF \times G = .00001118 \times (rpm)^2 \times r \times 1.0$$

where RCF = relative centrifugal force, G = gravity, rpm = revolutions/minute, and r = radius in centimeters.

The rpm of the centrifuge is determined with a tachometer. The most popular model is the strobe light tachometer.

Centrifuges used for hemagglutination testing are checked as follows: A nonhemolytic antiserum giving a 1+ reaction (e.g., anti-A, typing serum) is used. Appropriate red blood cells (RBCs) at 5% suspension and a negative control should be used. The manufacturer's instructions for use of all reagents should be followed. After samples are centrifuged they are checked for supernatant clarity, delineation of cell button, difficulty of resuspension of cells, and strength of agglutination.

Hematocrit centrifuges are similarly checked for speed and performance. All readings are entered in the quality control book. Variations in voltage may produce variation in centrifugal rotation speed.

SUPPLIES

Disposable Supplies

Most laboratories use disposable serologic tubes, pipets, and droppers. This ensures a degree of safety and cleanliness that is not as easily achieved with reusable glassware. It is therefore suggested that disposable materials be used whenever possible. Nevertheless, disposable tubes and other supplies should be routinely checked for foreign particles and defects. It is a useful learning exercise to perform quality control checks on volumetric supplies in the laboratory. For detailed methods, the reader is referred to the work of Linke et al.[8]

Reagents

The minimum requirements for reagents are specified in the Code of Federal Regulations and should be consulted for quality control programs. The first rule for using reagents is to read and follow the supplier's instructions. Slight alterations in procedure may result in serious errors. A uniform method of performing every test is one element of good laboratory technique. Attention to detail will also contribute to good, clear-cut results. These principles are essential to maintaining high quality control of reagents.

Antisera

Several aspects of an antiserum are measured in a quality control program. Antisera are used as reagents to detect antigenic determinants because of their specificity. This specificity must be unique in order to provide accuracy in typing RBCs or demonstrating antigenic determinants in other systems. Antisera must also be potent. A potent antiserum is assessed by its titer (i.e., how many serial twofold dilutions it withstands before producing a negative agglutination test), and by its avidity, which is a measure of the speed and strength of the reaction. Avidity is influenced by antigenic representation on the cell, by the concentration of cells in the suspension, by the medium in which the antiserum is suspended, and by the temperature at which the reactants are incubated.

The titer is quality controlled by incubating serial twofold dilutions of serum. In the blood bank, lectins are also assessed for specificity and titer of reactivity. These values are recorded in a log book, along with the expiration dates of each vial. To preserve the agglutination strength of the sera, vials should be stored only for a limited period of time, as indicated by the expiration date, and at recommended temperatures, lest their reactivity become suboptimal for safe testing.

The antiglobulin serum used in the routine Coombs test should be capable of detecting human γ-globulins and C3 and C4 components of complement. The minimum requirements for blood bank reagents are specified in the Code of Federal Regulations,[9-11] as are the titer values suggested for reagents routinely used in blood grouping and Rh typing. These requirements are also reviewed by Hedlund Hoppe.[12] Readers are advised to consult these references for specific information on required reactivity of reagents. The following section briefly reviews some required characteristics of reagents frequently used in the blood bank.

ABO Antisera

ABO antisera obtained from donors immunized with Witebsky substances will produce high-titer typing reagents.[13] These sera must be controlled for avidity. Usually this is done by mixing a drop of a 40% solution of type A or B cells with 1 drop of specific typing serum. The time between mixture of the drops and the first evidence of agglutination is measured. By 2 minutes after mixing the cell button must be 1 sq mm or larger.[14]

The titer of a typing antiserum is assessed by preparing serial twofold dilutions of the antiserum. A drop of the dilution and a drop of a 2% cell suspension are incubated and timed for the appearance of a 1+ hemagglutination reaction. The end point is the highest dilution giving this degree of reaction. Specificities of ABO blood grouping sera are checked against control sera. To exclude possible unwanted specificities, the antisera are checked against group O cells to demonstrate negative reactivity. All antisera should be stored below 8°C. Rare sera can be stored frozen.

Rh Antisera

Antisera for Rh typing are obtained from donors who have anti-Rh antibodies in their sera. The most important of the Rh typing antisera, and the most widely used in routine blood banking, is anti-Rho(D). On avidity testing, agglutination should begin at 60 seconds and formation of 1-sq mm clumps at 2 minutes after a drop of reagent is mixed with a drop of 40% RBC suspension in saline on a slide. The agglutination titer should be at least 1:32, as detected by testing serial dilutions of the antiserum with a drop of 2% suspension of Rh-positive cells. Serial dilutions of incomplete antibodies are performed with albumin.

Other Antisera

The FDA requires that sera other than the ABO and Rh typing sera be specific and capable of detecting the antigen in heterozygous individuals. Control tests for the quality assessment of these sera should be performed. In control tests, heterozygous cells are tested and negative controls are used to dispel any other specificity. Most reagents are obtained from individuals who lack an antigen and have produced an antibody against it. However, some reagents, such as anti-M, are produced in other species, such as rabbits. Monoclonal antibodies are becoming available for detection of various antigens.

Antiglobulin Antiserum

Coombs antisera with anti-human globulin specificity are usually produced in rabbits. The avidity and titer are tested with precoated cells. Since the cells must be manipulated, it is necessary to determine titers both of the coating antiserum and of the antiglobulin reagent. Usually anti-D-coated Rh-positive cells are used to test the antiglobulin antiserum.[15] Anti-D antisera must show at least 1+ reaction at 1:64 dilutions. These aliquots are then incubated with serial dilutions of the antiglobulin reagent. Each of the highest dilutions of anti-D coating the cells and of antiglobulin must give a 1+ reaction, and the first three dilutions of antiglobulin reagent should not vary in strength. All dilutions are made with albumin. These tests are called block titrations, because dilutions of the two antisera are compared against each other.

The next step is to check the non-γ activity of the antiserum. The reactivity of most good Coombs sera is purported to also contain antibodies that react against β-globulins (i.e., complement components and immunoglobulins other than IgG). This test is done by coating cells with C3 or C4 complement components with an anti-Lewis antibody or an anti-I antibody, respectively.[16]

Other Reagents

Many problems can arise from the use of the more mundane reagents such as saline or albumin. Therefore, these reagents should be routinely checked for contamination or impurities. Although these materials may be prepared in the blood bank, this is rarely done; instead, commercially available products that are readily available, save time for the staff, and are subjected to strict factory quality control.

Several proteolytic enzymes, such as papain, ficin, and bromelin, are used in the blood bank. These reagents may be difficult to quality control because of the variation in reactivity among different lots. However, positive and negative controls should be used whenever possible in tests using enzymes, and close attention should be paid to the required pH at which these substances act. Some guidelines are given in AABB as well as other publications.[17, 18]

Reagent RBCs

Reagent RBCs are usually obtained commercially. They should be washed before use because some patient sera contain antibodies against some of the reagents used in the preservation of these cells[19] and may cause misinterpretation of results. All reagent cells are checked daily for hemolysis, and notes on expiration times should be readily available so that out-of-date cells can be discarded.

The specificity and reactivity of the typing cells for the ABO system are routinely checked. Panel cells may be tested routinely for reactivity with a cold antibody (e.g., of the Lewis system) and a warm antibody (e.g., anti-D).

QUALITY CONTROL OF BLOOD COMPONENT PREPARATION

Institutions that regularly draw blood from donors must exercise quality control over the blood products. All of the various steps, from the screening of the donor to the preparation of the individual components, must be checked in a quality control program. Records of donors must be kept scrupulously in order to facilitate rapid retrieval of information. Such records should include information on past donations, date of last donation, adverse reactions to donation, etc.

It is best to have accredited nurses working in blood bank donation or outpatient transfusion and apheresis areas, for many of the problems encountered are of a clinical nature. A physician responsible for the blood bank should be available at all times in case of donor reactions or in case there are questions on the acceptability of potential donors. All medications used in emergencies in the blood bank should be within date, and the expiration times should be checked routinely. The preparation of phlebotomy sites should be inspected routinely by the head nurse or the blood bank director to insure the donor room personnel are exercising good technique. Venipuncture techniques should also be reviewed (see Chap. 8).

Weighing devices to assess the amount of blood drawn should be checked periodically and values recorded in the quality control log. Unit identification procedures, labels, and records should be checked frequently to ensure that all steps are being adhered to. Since most components are obtained by centrifugation, quality control of the blood component centrifuge is mandatory. A log book is kept to record correct speeds and utilization of the centrifuge. The scale used to weigh blood units and centrifuge buckets should be checked periodically for accuracy with weights of known values.

Units of blood collected as whole blood for separation into components accommodate 450 ml ± 10%, in addition to the weight of the bags and the anticoagulant. These units are centrifuged at room temperature to obtain packed cells, fresh frozen plasma (FFP), granulocytes, and platelets. Packed cells have a hematocrit of about 70%–80%,[20] which should be periodically checked. Packed cells expire in 21–35 days, depending on the anticoagulant, and are obtained by centrifugation, usually in multiple bags. They should be stored at 1°–6°C in a blood bank refrigerator.

When leukocyte-poor RBCs are prepared, the goal is to keep the number of cells below 1.0×10^9. A sample is taken from a portion of the quality control unit after thorough mixing. A 1:500 dilution is prepared from the sample portion.

To calculate the blood volume in a bag, the weight of the empty bag is subtracted from the weight of the full bag and the result is divided by 1.09, which gives the number of milliliters of blood in the unit.

Total unit WBC count = volume of blood in unit (ml) $\times$ WBC/mm^3 $\times$ 1,000

$$\% \text{ WBC removed} = \frac{\text{WBCs in Buffy coat-poor unit}}{\text{Total WBCs in pre-Buffy-coat unit}} \times 100$$

The full procedure is described in the AABB technical manual.[21]

Frozen-Thawed Blood

The use of frozen-thawed cells in blood banking is commonplace and has definite indications, as discussed in chapter 8. However, careful quality control is necessary to provide a sterile product with minimal debris as well as optimal RBC survival. Units selected for freezing are subjected to the same screening as ordinary units. However, units selected for freezing must not be over 5 days old, to preserve adequate 2,3-DPG and adenosine triphosphate levels.[22] Incubators for glycerolization should be checked for accuracy. Freezing is usually performed at high glycerol (40%) concentrations in the United States.[23] These units are stored in −85°C freezers. The recording chart of these freezers is to be checked routinely and a log kept on daily inspection of charts. The low-glycerol method, which is less popular in the United States, uses 14% glycerol and freezing in liquid nitrogen at gas phase temperatures below −120° C.[24]

Most of the glycerol should be removed on thawing. It is suggested that less than 1% glycerol be present in the supernate.[25] Although glycerol may be measured enzymatically,[26] this is not the most practical way for blood banks to perform quality control checks on frozen cells. A better method is to measure the osmolarity of the supernate.[27] The osmolarity should not be above 420 mOsm; if it reaches 450 mOsm, hemolysis may occur.[28]

Another parameter that can be used to determine the adequacy of the deglycerolizing method is the free hemoglobin level in the supernate. A level below 200 mg/dl is considered adequate.[29] RBC recovery from a frozen-thawed unit should be in the range of 90%. Deglycerolized cells expire in 24 hours because washing is performed in an open system.

Fresh Frozen Plasma

FFP is generally used to correct deficiencies in coagulation factors. Freezing should take place within 2 hours to avoid significant losses of factor VIII activity. FFP must be maintained frozen at −30°C. The clotting activity of the product may be measured by assessing the prothrombin time (PT) and the partial thromboplastin time (PTT) of the product and comparing them with normal values. PT and PTT measurement is recommended in patients receiving plasma as a check on the biologic activity of the product.

Cryoprecipitate

Cryoprecipitate has a relatively low volume per unit (3–5 ml). On average, each unit should contain 100 units of AHF activity. One unit of AHF is the AHF activity in 1 ml of normal plasma. To assay factor VIII activity, a sample of factor VIII deficient plasma is incubated with a test sample of cryoprecipitate and tested for correction of the PTT.[30] However, since this test is not routinely performed in the blood bank, it is advisable to have the coagulation laboratory perform it. In vivo correction of the PTT as well as correction of factor VIII activity are measures of factor VIII activity in cryoprecipitate units. The factor VIII activity in a unit of cryoprecipitate is calculated as follows:

Units of factor VIII/bag
$$= \frac{\text{Plasma volume (ml)} \times (\text{postinfusion} - \text{preinfusion factor VIII levels})}{\text{No. of bags infused} \times 100}.$$

At least four bags should be quality controlled every month, both by in vivo and in vitro methods, in facilities manufacturing this product. In vitro assays are done on dilutions of 20%, 10%, 5%, and 2.5%, and a graph is constructed to assess each concentration against clotting times in seconds.[31]

Platelets

Platelets are labile products and their survival is short. It is therefore necessary to perform all the testing required to ensure a safe product (i.e., typing, grouping, and hepatitis testing) as soon as possible, lest the survival time of this high-demand component be further reduced. The FDA[32] and the AABB standards[33] require counts of 5.5×10^{10} platelets in at least 75% of the concentrates after 72 hours. At least 4 units each month should be checked to ascertain whether these requirements are being met. A good unit usually contains 0.5×10^{11} platelets.[34]

Since units of platelets are obtained by centrifugation, a quality control check must be done on the centrifuge as usual.

If platelets are obtained by automated plateletpheresis, maintenance logs and quality control records of platelet products must be kept for these instruments as well.

Platelet counts can be achieved by manual chamber counting, using phase microscopy, or by counting in an electronic chamber counter.

A count on a fresh EDTA sample from the donor is performed as well as on a portion of the well-mixed platelet concentrate.

The ratio of these values will give the percentage yield. The number of platelets in the concentrate is calculated as follows:

Number of platelets/unit = platelet count/mm^3 $\times$ 1,000 $\times$ volume

Another portion is used for determining pH, which must be above 6.

A good quality control program of platelets also includes determination of platelet count increments in the patient receiving these products at 1 hour and 24 hours after infusion as well as correction of the bleeding time.

The hematocrit of the unit should also be measured so that units with excess RBC contamination can be discarded (i.e., hematocrit > 0.4 ml of blood/unit).[35] This point is particularly important when Rh-positive platelets are given to Rh-negative patients. If this occurs, Rh immunoglobulin (RhIG) is given to prevent immunization.[36]

It is recommended that platelets be stored at 22°C on a rotator (quality controlled by means of a temperature chart) and that they be suspended in a 50-ml residual plasma volume.[37] Another recommendation is that platelet pools be given as group and type specific because of the presence of RBCs and because potentially large amounts of ABO incompatible plasma may have to be transfused.

Granulocyte Concentrates

Granulocyte concentrates should contain 1×10^{10} cells. Since these units contain substantial amounts of RBCs, they should be type specific and compatible, and a crossmatch should be performed on the product. The same rules apply to granulocytes obtained by cytapheresis. The expiration time for both components is 24 hours.

RPR AND VDRL TESTING OF DONOR SAMPLES

In many donor facilities, the blood bank laboratory is still responsible for performing nontreponemal testing, including the VDRL and RPR tests, as a screen for syphilis. Adherence to the instructions supplied by the manufacturers is mandatory. A quality control record book for testing of reagents with both positive and negative controls is suggested.[38] Control of rotation speeds should also be documented.[39] Positive tests are reconfirmed by fluorescent treponemal antibody testing. Hepatitis screen testing can be performed with a latex agglutination test and confirmed by a radioimmunoassay or ELISA. Both methods are third-generation tests[40] as required by the FDA. A quality control check on these tests is performed as suggested by the supplier and documented in a log. The area for RPR and hepatitis testing is to be kept meticulously clean and isolated from areas where units for transfusion are handled. Good asepsis must be observed. After testing, all specimens and materials must be placed in special containers labeled "biohazard" and disposed of by incineration. Confirmed cases of syphilis and hepatitis are to be reported to the patient's physician and to the FDA. The AABB no longer requires screening of donors for syphilis. Testing of units for HTLV-III is now required (see Chap. 8).

QUALITY CONTROL OF FORMS AND RECORD-KEEPING

Donor records are kept for at least 5 years. These records must include the donor's name, age, date of birth, sex, and other pertinent identifying information. A medical history revealing potentially harmful diseases, drug therapy, and physical examination findings are noted in the record, as are laboratory values of hemoglobin, Hct, CBC, pulse, blood pressure, height, and weight. An identification number is assigned to each donor. This number accompanies the unit throughout laboratory testing and transfusion. All records on laboratory instruments are kept for 5 years. For more details consult chapter 8 on components.

Labels used on all items must comply with FDA standards. Sample drawing procedures as well as patient sample identification must also meet FDA standards. A laboratory manual with frequent updating by the blood bank director must be available at all times in the blood bank. A similar manual stating donor room procedures must be available in the donor room. A transfusion reaction record book must be kept, reviewed by the blood bank director, and must meet FDA standards. All lethal transfusion reactions must be reported to the FDA. Transfusion request forms, compatibility, other laboratory test records, and shipping plus transportation records must all be kept for 5 years. These standards and requirements are listed in an FDA publication.[41]

INVENTORY CONTROL

Inventory control should also be part of a quality control program in the blood bank. A guideline for ordering blood for elective surgical procedures should be available.[42] The percentage of expired blood products should be reviewed. Crossmatch to transfusion ratios must be reviewed to determine utilization. A transfusion committee should be convened to review transfusion practices, and the meetings should be documented as part of the quality control program in a hospital blood bank.

LEGAL ASPECTS OF BLOOD BANKING

In the last few decades the medical profession has increasingly become the target of legal actions. Among medical professionals, the pathologist has been relatively spared by the lawsuit epidemic. However, lawyers are discovering that suing the laboratory is both possible and profitable; as a result, there has been an increase in lawsuits brought against the blood bank in recent years.[43] The laboratory most exposed to liability, owing to the nature of its products, is the blood bank.

To understand some of the legal problems affecting blood banking, it is first necessary to review some terms frequently used by the judiciary profession in relation to medicolegal problems.

Tort: any wrongful act, damage, or injury done willfully, negligently, or in circumstances involving strict liability, but not involving breach of contract, for which a legal suit can be brought.[44]

Proximate cause: an event without which the injury would not have occurred.

Negligence: failure to observe adequate care. In medicine, this may be a wide variety of improperly applied precautions or deviations from standard procedure which will be considered as potential liability when brought to court.

Absolute liability: liability without negligence. This relieves the plaintif from the burden of proving negligence.

Assault and battery: construed as performing a procedure such as a blood transfusion, taking a donation, or performing plasmapheresis without the full consent of the party.

Res ipsa loquitur: "the thing speaks for itself;" substitutes for evidenciary proof. The typical case in blood banking is a case of negligence in which a unit of the wrong ABO blood type is given to a patient, resulting in an incompatible transfusion reaction.[45]

Respondeat superior: the doctrine that holds that "the captain of the ship" (the laboratory director) is ultimately responsible for what occurs in the laboratory. This means that the director is legally liable for negligence that occurs in the laboratory, regardless of who actually committed the mistake or negligent practice.[46]

Charitable immunity: presently not a defensible position in most states, although in the past, charitable institutions were largely immune to legal suits.[47]

A more detailed explanation of some of these concepts are presented below.

Negligence

Negligence is the most common basis for liability in medical malpractice.[48] One can object strenuously to legal suits brought against a profession that helps fellow human beings recover their health or alleviates the pain of disease. However, ill individuals who do not receive optimal medical treatment have a right to justice. There is little excuse for poor medical judgment, and society provides a mechanism for citizens to defend themselves against potential medical malpractice. In the blood bank, negligence typically occurs when a patient receives the wrong type of blood because of clerical or technical mistakes. Although in most cases the person responsible for the mistake is held directly responsible, in some cases the doctrine of *respondeat superior* is applied and the blood bank director is held responsible for the mistake. For negligence to be defensible, the following elements must be present: (1) duty, (2) breach of duty, (3) proximate cause, and (4) actual harm.

In a tort of negligence, the injured party must prove that the proximate cause of injuries was dereliction of duty by the defendant.[45] Such dereliction is judged in comparison with accepted medical behavior and current practices of the profession. Any case in which standards were not met may be subject to greater liability than if all the accepted rules were met. Lawyers usually consider FDA and AABB standards for blood banks and transfusion services in these cases. An expert witness is usually present to document veracity of claims. In hemolytic reactions, proof of negligence is usually needed. In a few cases, such as a straightforward case of blood group incompatibility, the doctrine of *res ipsa loquitur* may be introduced by the claimant's attorneys. *Res ipsa loquitur* will hold when the following conditions are met:[43]

1. The accident could not have occurred in the absence of negligence.
2. Preventing the accident from happening was under the exclusive control of the defendant.
3. No voluntary part was played by the injured party in causing the accident.
4. Knowledge of the causes of the accident was more accessible to the defendant than to the injured party.

In cases of emergency, the physician may decide to change standard procedure. However, liability will be determined according to the severity of the emergency, and no excuse for lack of judgment is defensible, no matter how severe the emergency.

Clerical errors are usually more clear-cut than laboratory errors, because courts consider that reading a label with the patient's name is a matter of routine skill and judgment, whereas laboratory testing is not, as was shown in a court action involving a patient in a Mississippi hospital.[49]

Strict or Warrant Liability

This is a "no fault" liability where, despite lack of negligence on anyone's part, courts decide for the plaintiff because a so-called contract of warranty has not been kept, and medication that was supposed to be guaranteed pure transmitted an infection (e.g., hepatitis). It is therefore mandatory (in the blood bank's interest) to use labels bearing disclaimers of full warranty to prevent this type of lawsuit. Furthermore, the AABB has rallied to declare this type of lawsuit invalid, based on the premise that the law provides this type of protection mostly for commercial products, while blood and blood components are considered a medical service and not a sale of goods. At least 43 states do not honor "implied warranty" regarding transfusion of blood or blood components.[50] An example of this type of case is *Perlmutter v. Beth David Hospital*, New York.[51] Because of the implied liability concept, blood provided by noncommercial means must be clearly stated. Furthermore, if charges are made to the patient (such as a processing fee), these must be very clearly defined if one is to avoid prosecution under the above-mentioned terms. Most cases of the implied warranty type have arisen out of the transmission of hepatitis. In these cases the prosecution has pressed suit even when hospitals or blood centers adequately screened blood donors for hepatitis. In the case of *DeBatista v. Argonaut Insurance Co.*,[52] for instance, the Louisiana Supreme Court held a blood bank liable on a "no fault" basis despite adherence to good hepatitis screening. Since the State of Louisiana does not consider blood a commercial commodity, it was surprising that the courts fined against the blood bank; however, it does reflect the tendency of sympathy by the courts toward the plaintiff who has contracted disease from transfusion.[53]

If units are *not* adequately tested, the case becomes a tort of negligence, violating the federal or state Pure Food and Drugs Act (see FDA Regulations, *Federal Food, Drug and Cosmetics Act,* 21 U.S. Congress, Section 351).

Assault and Battery

Giving a blood transfusion, performing plasmapheresis, or drawing a blood sample without proper consent may constitute a case of assault and battery. Evidence must be available that a donor or a recipient has given appropriate "informed consent." Children, demented persons, and unconscious individuals may be transfused only after the proper consent form has been secured from the legal guardian. Drawing blood from underage donors or donors not mentally fit may constitute a legal liability unless the appropriate legal mentor is present to give written consent. In emergencies these laws may be overruled, but legal consultation should be obtained from the legal advisor of the hospital or blood center. This is especially true for cases involving patients whose religious faith does not permit the transfusion of blood (such as Jehovah's Witnesses[54]). In certain cases where transfusion of blood is life-saving, patients of the Jehovah's Witness faith have been transfused without consent of legal guardians; however, a court order was secured before transfusion in these cases.[55]

These legal proceedings are undertaken under the State's statute of *parens patriae*,[56] whereby the State undertakes custody of a child's care under the legal argument of child negligence. In adults, however, matters are very different, and *parens patriae* cannot be exercized unless there is evidence that the person cannot reason at the time the decision to transfuse was undertaken. Expert legal advice is usually necessary in these cases before proceeding with the transfusion.

Charitable Immunity

Charitable immunity has been subjected to critical evaluation in different states of the United States, to the extent that 38 states no longer have a charitable immunity clause. The doctrine states that a charitable institution is exempt to a large extent from liability stemming from torts that would affect other organizations not holding charitable philosophies. The doctrine is extremely variable.[43] A few states, including Arkansas, Maine, and Virginia, still grant complete immunity to hospitals.[57]

The blood bank director and other top managers must be fully acquainted with the laws governing the state they operate in, concerning transfusions, donations, and laboratory procedures. They should also know specific laws of states they may be getting blood from or shipping blood to. This will protect the institution as well as these individuals against potential liability.

Statute of Limitations

Injured parties who choose to sue must file suit within a specified time following the injury. These times vary from state to state but are often 13 years. In cases of negligence, this statute is usually determined from the date the injured party became aware of the misdeed.[50]

LEGAL MATTERS AFFECTING BLOOD BANK MANAGEMENT

Taxes

Because blood banks may be located in a hospital or may be independent institutions, they are often considered for administrative purposes as part of a corporation or as an independent corporation. Nonprofit organizations are essentially tax exempt.[58] Tax-exempt blood banks grossing over $5,000 a year must file information returns. State taxes must be cleared by the blood bank through the Attorney General.

Licensing

The FDA requires by law that blood banks be registered. Furthermore, blood banks that ship blood or blood products across state lines must be licensed by the FDA. Registration forms may be obtained from:

    Bureau of Biologics
    Food and Drug Administration
    5600 Fishers Lane
    Rockville, MD 20857
    Tel. 301-496-1911

Actual licensing is granted by the Centers for Disease Control, Atlanta.

For state licensing it is suggested that the blood bank administration investigate the local state requirements for registration and licensing.

SUGGESTIONS REGARDING LEGAL ACTIONS AGAINST THE BLOOD BANK

Preventative Measures

All possible precautions must be taken to keep the quality, precision, and accuracy of the blood bank operations at their highest level of excellence. Legal actions may affect any blood bank, but liability can be reduced if rules and regulations promoting safe, high-quality blood banking are strictly followed. Above all, FDA regulations must be met and exceeded. It is advisable that blood banks undergo voluntary inspection by organizations such as the AABB and the CAP to ensure that a high quality of work, installations, equipment, and procedures is maintained. Detailed records must be kept scrupulously and made available for consultation. Donor procedures must be up to date and must follow accepted standards, and all precautions must be taken to ensure the health of donors during and immediately after donation. The same quality and precautions must be applied to therapeutic apheresis procedures. All accidents or abnormal reactions relating to transfusions, donations, or apheresis must be carefully documented in the event they become the basis for a court action.

The content of printed labels and disclaimers must be reviewed by the legal representative of the institution.

Technical training, licensing (which is compulsory in certain states), expertise, and coverage must be adequate to ensure the best possible testing and transfusion practices. Coverage must be available for night and weekend shifts, when staffing may be less optimal than at other times. Adequate medical coverage must be available wherever patients are being transfused or apheresed or normal donors are being drawn.

Detailed consent forms must be available containing printed explanations of procedures; each point of a procedure should be verbally reviewed before any patient or donor undergoes a procedure. Experimental therapeutic procedures are to be avoided unless special consent forms are obtained and only after careful legal consideration has been given to the potential hazards of such practices.

Suits Filed Against the Blood Bank

Any event which may conceivably result in a lawsuit should immediately be brought to the attention of the attorneys representing the hospital or the transfusion service, as well as the insurance carrier for the institution. A great degree of tact and discretion in treating patients and donors is preferable to a lawsuit. This must be stressed to the laboratory personnel so that wrong information is not generated or transmitted to outsiders. All records pertinent to matters under litigation must be sequestered and kept by the legal representative of the hospital blood bank or the blood center lawyer. Summons or letters from lawyers representing the plaintiff must be routed to the legal representative of the blood bank.

BLOOD BANKING ORGANIZATIONS

The adequate availability of blood and blood components has created a need for organization of community efforts to better obtain and distribute blood and blood components. This type of institution is different in many ways from hospital-based blood banks, which are essentially laboratories geared to test patient samples and provide blood directly to patients.

Regulation of Community Blood Banks

Community blood banks have arisen from the need to have a more centralized organization where blood can be collected, stored, and distributed to hospitals needing blood products. Community blood banks are usually nonprofit organizations that take the onus of self-sufficiency away from the hospital blood banks. Today's busy surgical centers can rarely be truly self-sufficient in terms of blood supply.

Two major organizations regulate the activities of most community blood centers, these are the American National Red Cross (ANRC) and the AABB. The Council of Community Blood Centers (CCBC) is a third organization that regulates some community blood centers not belonging to the ANRC or the AABB. The ANRC considers blood donation a community responsibility, whereas the AABB considers blood donation an individual responsibility of replacement for usage. The two organizations promote voluntary blood donation and do not accept commercial blood donation.

The ANRC supplies about 50% of the blood and blood components used in the United States. Through its network of community blood centers it functions under a single license. Many of the activities of each blood center are regulated by the ANRC central office in Washington. The ANRC has an active plasma fractionation program as well as a research program.

The AABB includes over 100 community blood banks and counts over 2,000 institutions among its members. Through its publications, *Standards for Blood Banks and Transfusion Services*, the *Technical Manual*, *Blood Component Therapy: A Physician's Handbook*, as well as many specialized publications that appear every year, this organization provides guidance for high standards and quality blood banking. The AABB also provides an inspection and accreditation program that certifies blood banks which voluntarily submit to such programs.

Role of the College of American Pathologists (CAP) and Other Organizations

The CAP has a voluntary quality control program in which problem samples are regularly sent to blood banks to determine precision, accuracy, and performance compared to other participating members. Results on such problem samples determine CAP accreditation. Biannual inspection of all laboratories, including the blood bank, is conducted by the CAP.

The AMA has a committee on blood banking that has joined forces with the ANRC and the AABB to plan for a national blood policy.

Role of the Federal Government

The U.S. Department of Health, Education and Welfare has recently increased its efforts to participate more aggressively in creating a nationwide blood program. This effort has arisen in conjunction with increasing attempts to create some form of national health insurance. The FDA has also attempted to institute inspection and accreditation programs but has decided to accept AABB and CAP inspection and accreditation results as a valid accreditation system.

The federal government requested the AMA, ANRC, AABB, and CCBC to form a nationwide resource study group, now known as the American Blood Commission, to regulate collection, distribution, and costs of blood and blood components.[59]

ANTITRUST LAWS REGARDING BLOOD BANKING

Various federal and state laws prohibit restraints on free competition. One such law is the Sherman Act of the Federal Trade Commission. These laws can affect nonprofit organizations. For example, an agreement between two blood banks to avoid trading with a third blood bank would constitute a violation of the Sherman Act. Sometimes these agreements are made justifiably, to avoid purchasing products of questionable quality. However, it is best to consult the blood bank attorney regarding antitrust laws.

REFERENCES

1. Shewhart W.A.: *Economic Control of Quality of Manufactured Products.* New York, Van Nostrand Co., 1931.
2. Levey S., Jennings E.R.: The use of control charts in the clinical laboratory. *Am. J. Clin. Pathol.* 20:1959, 1950.
3. Honig C.L., Bove J.R.: Transfusion-associated fatalities: Review of Bureau of Biologics reports 1976–1978. *Transfusion* 20:653, 1980.
4. Oberman H.L. (ed.): *Standards for Blood Banks and Transfusion Services,* ed. 11. Washington, D.C., American Association of Blood Banks, 1984, p. 15.
5. Widman F.K. (ed.): *Technical Manual of the American Association of Blood Banks,* ed. 8. Washington, D.C., American Association of Blood Banks, 1981, pp. 52–55.
6. Austal H.B., Grove-Rasmussen M., Shaw R.S.: Optimal conditions for storage of fresh frozen plasma. *Transfusion* 1:87, 1961.
7. Swindles J.F.: *Calibration of Liquid in Glass Thermometers.* Washington, D.C., National Bureau of Standards, Monograph 90, 1965, p. 23.
8. Linke E.G., Henry B.J.: Clinical pathology/laboratory medicine: Purposes and practice, in Henry B.J. (ed.): *Clinical Diagnosis and Management by Laboratory Methods,* ed. 17. Philadelphia, W.B. Saunders Co., 1984, p. 16.
9. Potency test without reference preparations. Code of Federal Regulations 21, part 600.24. Washington, D.C., U.S. Government Printing Office, 1981, pp. 151–152.
10. Potency test without reference preparations. Code of Federal Regulations 21, part 660.25. Washington, D.C., U.S. Government Printing Office, 1981, pp. 152–153.
11. Avidity testing. Code of Federal Regulations 21, part 660.27. Washington, D.C., U.S. Government Printing Office, 1981, p. 155.
12. Hedlund Hoppe P.A.: Performance criteria for blood grouping sera, in Myhre E.A. (ed.): *A Seminar on Performance Evaluation.* Washington, D.C., American Association of Blood Banks, 1976, p. 1.
13. Witebsky E., Klendsho N.C., McNeil C.: Potent typing sera produced by treatment of donors with isolated group specific substances. *Proc. Soc. Exp. Biol. Med.* 55:167, 1944.
14. Widman F.K. (ed.): *Technical Manual of the American Association of Blood Banks,* ed. 8. Washington, D.C., American Association of Blood Banks, 1981, p. 356.
15. Widman F.K. (ed.): *Technical Manual of the American Association of Blood Banks,* ed. 8. Washington, D.C., American Association of Blood Banks, 1981, p. 357.
16. Widman F.K. (ed.): *Technical Manual of the American Association of Blood Banks,* ed. 8. Washington, D.C.,

American Association of Blood Banks, 1981, pp. 395–396.
17. Widman F.K. (ed.): *Technical Manual of the American Association of Blood Banks*, ed. 8. Washington, D.C., American Association of Blood Banks, 1981, pp. 388–389.
18. Issitt P.D., Issitt C.H.: *Applied Blood Group Serology*, ed. 2. Oxnard, California, Spectra Biologicals, 1975, pp. 24–27.
19. Beattie K.M., Ferguson S.J., Burmie K.L., et al.: Cloramphenicol antibody causing interference in antibody detection and identification tests. *Transfusion* 16:174, 1976.
20. Chaplin H. Jr.: Packed red blood cells. *N. Engl. J. Med.* 281:364, 1969.
21. Miller W.V. (ed.): *Technical Manual of the American Association of Blood Banks*, ed. 7. Washington, D.C., American Association of Blood Banks, 1977, p. 292.
22. Oberman H.L. (ed.): *Standards for Blood Banks and Transfusion Services*, ed. 10. Washington, D.C., American Association of Blood Banks, 1981, p. 9.
23. Valeri C.R.: *Blood Banking and the Uses of Frozen Blood Products*. Cleveland, Ohio, CRC Press, 1976, p. 56.
24. Oberman H.L. (ed.): *Standards for Blood Banks and Transfusion Services*, ed. 10. Washington, D.C., American Association of Blood Banks, 1981, p. 16.
25. Valeri C.R.: Principles of cryobiology: High glycerol and storage at -80 C and low glycerol and storage at -150 C, in Guy R.L. (ed.): *Red Cell Freezing: A Technical Workshop*. Washington, D.C., American Association of Blood Banks, 1973, pp. 1–30.
26. Bucolo G., David H.: Quantitative determination of serum triglycerides by the use of enzymes. *Clin. Chem.* 19:476, 1973.
27. Roberts S.C., Franks M.L., Griep J.A.: A quality assurance program for deglycerolized red cells (human), abstracted. *Transfusion* 16:519, 1976.
28. Davey R.: Discussion I, in Griep J.A. (ed.): *Clinical Uses of Frozen-Thawed Red Blood Cells*. New York, Alan R. Liss, 1976, p. 53.
29. Miller W.V. (ed.): *Technical Manual of the American Association of Blood Banks*, ed. 7. Washington, D.C., American Association of Blood Banks, 1977, p. 292.
30. Myhre B. (ed.): *Quality Control: A Practical Workshop*. Washington, D.C., American Association of Blood Banks, 1970, p. 92.
31. Myhre B. (ed.): *Quality Control: A Practical Workshop*. Washington, D.C., American Association of Blood Banks, 1970, p. 94.
32. Food and drugs. Code of Federal Regulations, Title 21, parts 640.20–640.26. Washington, D.C., U.S. Government Printing Office.
33. Oberman H.L. (ed.): *Standards for Blood Banks and Transfusion Services*, ed. 10. Washington, D.C., American Association of Blood Banks, 1981, p. 12.
34. Cavins J.A.: Clinical effectiveness of platelet concentrates prepared with or without acidification of the plasma. *Transfusion* 8:289, 1968.
35. Walker R.H.: Preparation of blood components, in Myhre B. (ed.): *Quality Control in the Blood Bank*. Chicago, American Society of Clinical Pathologists, 1973, p. 82.
36. Mollison P.L.: *Blood Transfusion in Clinical Medicine*, ed. 7. Oxford, England, Blackwell Scientific Publications, 1983, p. 168.
37. Widman F.K. (ed.): *Technical Manual of the American Association of Blood Banks*, ed. 8. Washington, D.C., American Association of Blood Banks, 1981, pp. 48–49.
38. Pusch A.L.: Serodiagnostic tests, in Henry B.J. (ed.): *Clinical Diagnosis and Management by Laboratory Methods*, ed. 16. Philadelphia, W.B. Saunders Co., 1979, p. 1886.
39. Myhre B. (ed.): *Quality Control: A Practical Workshop*. Washington, D.C., American Association of Blood Banks, 1970, p. 24.
40. Ray G.C., Hicks M.H.: Laboratory diagnosis of virus, *Rickettsia* and *Chlamydia*, in Henry B.J. (ed.): *Clinical Diagnosis and Management by Laboratory Methods*, ed. 16. Philadelphia, W.B. Saunders Co., 1979, p. 1867.
41. Food and drugs. Code of Federal Regulations, title 21, parts 600–1299. Washington, D.C., U.S. Government Printing Office.
42. Boral L.I., Henry J.B.: The type and screen: A safe alternative and supplement in selected surgical procedures. *Transfusion* 17:163, 1977.
43. Randall C.H. Jr.: *Medico-Legal Problems in Blood Transfusion*, rev. ed. Washington, D.C., American Association of Blood Banks, 1969.
44. Dean Prosser: *Prosser on Torts*, ed. 2, 1955, p 788, quoted in Randall C.H. Jr. (ed.) *Medico-Legal Problems in Blood Transfusion*. Washington, D.C., American Association of Blood Banks, 1969, p. 14.
45. Holder A.R.: Mismatched blood. *JAMA* 228:1606, 1974.
46. Greenwalt T.J., et al. (ed.): *General Principles of Blood Transfusion*, rev. ed. Chicago, American Medical Association, 1977, p. 89.
47. Kammerer R.C. (ed.).: *Administrative Procedure and Practices: A Guide for Blood Banks and Transfusion Services*, ed. 2. Washington, D.C., American Association of Blood Banks, 1974, pp. 91–112.
48. Willett D.E.: Transfusion service liability, in Mayer K. (ed.): *Guidelines to Transfusion Practices*. Washington, D.C., American Association of Blood Banks, 1980, pp. 167–175.
49. *Mississippi Baptist Hospital v. Holmes*, 214 Miss 906, 55, So, 2d, 142 (1952) affd. 56, So, 2d, 709 (1952).
50. Huestis D.W., Bove J.R., Busch S.: *Practical Blood Transfusion*, ed. 2. Boston, Little, Brown & Co., 1976, pp. 369–382.
51. *Perlmutter v. Beth David Hospital*, 308 NY 100, 123 NE 2d 792 (1954).
52. 403 So. 2d 26 (La. 1981), cert. denied 103 S. ct. 82(1982).
53. Clark G.A.: *Medicolegal Aspects of Blood Collection and Transfusion*. Arlington, Va., American Association of Blood Banks, 1983, p. 25.
54. Blood transfusions: Jehovah's Witnesses (editorial). *JAMA* 263:660, 1957.

55. *People ex Rel. Wallace v. Labrenz,* 411, Ill. 618, 104, N.E., 2d 269 (1952).
56. Clark G.A.: *Medicolegal Aspects of Blood Collection and Transfusion* Arlington, Va., American Association of Blood Banks, 1983, p. 3.
57. Clark G.A.: *Medicolegal Aspects of Blood Collection and Transfusion* Arlington, Va., American Association of Blood Banks, 1983, p. 46.
58. Internal Revenue Code Regarding Federal Income Tax 501 (c) (3), ruling 66–323.
59. National blood policy: Departmental response to private sector implementation plan. *Fed. Register* 39:32702–32711, 1974.

18

Transfusion Practices

THIS CHAPTER describes some systems for regulating blood processing and blood transfusion which ensure that good transfusion practices are observed. These can be divided into external regulatory bodies and internal regulatory bodies. Thereafter, transfusion practices for special conditions not fully described elsewhere are reviewed.

EXTERNAL REGULATORY BODIES

As we reviewed in the previous chapter, all blood banks are subject to regulations imposed by the Bureau of Biologics of the Food and Drug Administration (FDA). These regulations, which are mandatory for certification and operation of a blood bank, are designed to ensure that the minimum standards applicable to blood banks are being adhered to. In some states, state regulatory agencies have their own regulatory programs. Most blood banks and transfusion services, however, voluntarily attempt to meet quality standards set by specialized external institutions, as well as their own internal system of quality standards. As mentioned before, the American Association of Blood Banks (AABB) is one such private institution that promulgates quality control standards and conducts inspections regularly. The College of American Pathologists (CAP) is another nongovernmental institution that has a regulatory program to ensure quality control and to upgrade standards of blood banks.

INTERNAL REGULATORY BODIES

Internal regulatory bodies include the transfusion committee of a hospital transfusion service and the medical director and technical supervisors of the blood bank.[1]

The Transfusion Committee

The AABB recommends that every hospital form a transfusion committee to ensure that the highest quality product and best care are delivered to the patient. This committee preferably includes membership from the major areas of hospital staff. For instance, the medical service should be represented by a hematology staff person as well as an oncology staff person. The surgical service should be represented by a physician from thoracic surgery, and so on. Nursing services should also be represented. A member of the hospital administration must participate and the director of the blood bank should either chair the committee or at least be a member of the committee. The committee reviews and establishes policies of transfusion practices pertinent to the hospital. It also provides a mechanism for transmitting these policies to the hospital staff. The transfusion committee thus serves as an internal review committee on hospital policies and practices regarding blood transfusion. The committee should meet at least quarterly and the minutes should be recorded. The minutes must be informative and

459

The Medical Director

In no other laboratory is the presence of a medical doctor more important than in the blood bank. It is in the transfusion service that complications due to faulty laboratory results or improper handling of blood products have most impact on patient care. Therefore, the FDA as well as voluntary regulatory agencies such as the CAP and the AABB mandate that the blood bank be directed by an M.D.

The functions of a blood bank director include clinical consultation, administration, technical consultation, and education and training.[1]

The blood bank director provides direct medical consultation in cases of donor reaction, transfusion reaction, coagulopathy, calling for blood or blood components, platelet therapy, and therapeutic plateletpheresis or plasmapheresis, as well as many other clinical conditions for which the blood bank is consulted. Failure to have a specialized physician direct treatment in these situations will compromise the patient and jeopardize the legality of transfusion practices in a blood center, a transfusion service, or on services where patients are treated with blood or blood products. Because of experience in dealing with laboratories and personnel, the blood bank director is also the person best able to guide and administer the operations of the blood bank. Budget allocation, equipment acquisition, and licensing standards regulation are but a few of these activities.

The medical director must be a physician who, because of training in the field and clinical knowledge of the pathology, physiopathology, and treatment of diseases treated with blood and components, is best able to guide the technical staff toward the solution of complicated cases. The development of new techniques and the establishment of new policies, protocols, and regulations in the blood bank are also the domain of the medical director. A good supervisor in this setting is crucial to ensuring that the technical staff understand the procedures.

Education and training of residents in immunohematology and training of supervisors and technical staff at different levels are important aspects of the blood bank director's responsibilities.

GOOD PRACTICES IN THE USE OF BLOOD AND BLOOD COMPONENTS

Blood is a scarce commodity. Its use must be closely supervised. The misuse of blood (a vital fluid donated by individuals, mostly for altruistic reasons) is inconsiderate and wasteful. Furthermore, blood transfusion carries definite risks. In spite of these risks, clinicians continue to expose patients unnecessarily to transfusion.[2] Often the question must be asked: Is it really necessary to transfuse a particular patient? The answer, unfortunately, is not always straightforward. Many patients will tolerate relatively low hematocrit levels without too many complications.

This question does not arise in cases of massive bleeding when there is no doubt as to the necessity of immediate replacement of volume as well as oxygen-carrying capacity, but in the transfusion of a chronically anemic patient with a single unit of blood. It should be stressed here that the transfusion of 1 unit of blood will raise the hematocrit only 3% in a 70-kg adult.[3] Before long-term transfusion of a patient is recommended, a full study of the cause of anemia is mandatory. For instance, if a chronically anemic patient needs blood, the use of packed cells is more logical than whole blood. Whole blood will expose the patient to an unnecessary volume of plasma as well as toxic substances (potassium, ammonium, and cellular debris), as well as potentially immunogenic material (WBCs and platelets). However, the use of whole blood is indicated in cases of hypovolemia. Transfusing plasma from another unit by reconstituted packed cells with fresh frozen plasma (FFP) may unnecessarily increase the risk of hepatitis.[4]

Once initial screening tests in hematology have been performed, and if a clue to the cause of the anemia is not discernible, it is a good idea to investigate the survival time of transfused cells with a chromium survival study. These RBC survival studies often provide the clinician with a clue to the source of anemia. A large number of single-unit transfusions is indicative of poor transfusion practices. Single-unit transfusions should not exceed 10% of all transfusions.[5] This does not mean that if 1 unit is indicated, 2 are justified.

The relatively high use of whole blood instead of components is evidence of a poorly educated medical staff. The rationale for using specific components for therapy is that in most cases, patients lack specific components of blood.[6] Furthermore, the use of components allows more than one patient to profit from 1 unit of blood,[1] thus making the utilization of this resource more intelligent and practical. Using stored whole blood to correct a blood volume problem in which there is a complicating coagulopathy is also a poor transfusion practice, for coagulation factors are not optimal in units of blood that have been stored for relatively short periods of time.

The term "fresh blood" is to be banned from the transfusion vernacular, for it is not only impractical to supply, but indications for its use are unclear,[7] and the practice of drawing blood from "walking" donors is hazardous to the patient and legally unsound for the blood bank. The mystique of using freshly drawn blood for its "magical" properties is not based on a scientific approach to transfusion therapy.

THE TRANSFUSION OF BLOOD

When Does One Transfuse?

Blood replacement is mandatory in acute blood loss; however, the main aspect of blood replacement (at least in the first 1,000 cc of bleeding) is the replacement of volume, which can be achieved with crystalloid.[8] Blood loss of up to 25% of the blood volume can be sustained as long as volume is replaced with crystalloid.[9] This has been shown in major surgery such as open heart surgery[10] as well as in combat trauma.[11] Patients who are chronically anemic may tolerate hemoglobin concentrations of as low as 8–10 gm/100 ml.[12] Furthermore, patients with severe chronic anemia may develop cardiac failure from overload,[12] and hemopoiesis may be suppressed by RBC plethora after transfusion.[13] Therefore, it is advisable to treat anemic patients when they are symptomatic, rather than panicking, if the hemoglobin value remains above 10 gm/100 ml. Transfusing an anemic patient and immunizing him or her against a variety of RBC antigens may rob the individual of the benefit of a life-saving transfusion when the person really needs it.

Packed cells should be used when possible, for a greater oxygen-carrying capacity is available in a smaller volume. Furthermore, when a unit of whole blood is centrifuged into components, the granulocytes may be removed, rendering it leukocyte poor. This kind of unit has less chance of producing febrile reactions than a unit of cells containing WBCs. If a patient has frequent febrile reactions to WBCs, Buffy coat–poor cells must be supplied. Buffy coat–poor cells can be made more granulocyte free by adding microaggregate filtration to the process of eliminating WBCs. If the patient continues to react to granulocytes, the patient can be premedicated with Tylenol, or, as a last resort, transfused with frozen-thawed cells. A similar stepwise treatment can be undertaken for preventing urticarial reactions to plasma. By packing units, plasma is eliminated. A note should be entered in the patient's chart to alert the physician to avoid, if possible, the use of components containing plasma in these patients. Premedication with Benadryl can prevent the reaction. If patients continue to exhibit urticarial reactions or have a history of more severe reactions, frozen-thawed cells should be used.

Patients who are IgA deficient, have had severe anaphylactic reactions, and need transfusions should always be transfused with IgA-deficient plasma or blood. The next best alternative is to transfuse them with frozen-thawed blood. A clearly marked note in the hospital chart or medical record should state that such patients are not to be transfused with blood or blood components (including γ-globulin) that might contain IgA, for this may cause death.

All patients that react severely to transfused blood and blood products must be studied extensively. A history of the transfusion must be obtained. The possibility of incompatible fluid infusion in cases where hemoglobinuria has been reported or documented must be ruled out as well as in cases where no RBC incompatibility has been found. Hematuria must not be confused with bona fide hemoglobinuria in the differential diagnosis. This finding is more frequent in catheterized patients, especially if they are on anticoagulants or have a coagulopathy (e.g., hemophiliacs, leukemics, or patients with thrombocytopenia of other types). Diagnostic evidence of hemoglobinuria or hematuria must always be sought by the blood bank physician, and a note should be entered in the chart of the patient, explaining the finding.

The misuse of frozen RBCs is extremely costly and wasteful. Clear indications for the use of frozen-thawed cells have been given in chapter 8. These include intrauterine transfusion, transfusion of patients with paroxysmal nocturnal hemoglobinuria, transfusion of patients with a history of severe febrile or urticarial reactions, transfusion of patients with aplastic anemia, and transfusion of immunosuppressed patients. Frozen-thawed cells may have to be irradiated before transfusion into patients with severe immunodeficiency to prevent graft-versus-host disease. Furthermore, once the decision to use frozen-thawed units is made, the blood bank staff must inform the attending physician when such units are ready for use. This will prevent outdating these units, which can only be kept for 24 hours. The same is true for units that have been Buffy coated after they have been collected as whole blood. Units that have been filtered, washed or manipulated in any way also have a 24-hour expiration time and must be transfused quickly. In large blood banks it may be necessary to assign to a specific person the task of reminding the attending physicians that the units are ready for use. If high wastage of these types of units is detected in the quarterly analysis of blood use statistics, the causes must be investigated and the transfusion committee must establish guidelines to prevent such events from occurring.

Issuing Blood

Before the blood is released from the blood bank, the technologist must compare the ABO, Rh type, and the unit number on the component labels with the information on the compatibility slip and blood requisition form. This is best done by two people and the release form cosigned by two individuals. The technologists must ascertain that the component is the one requested. The name of the individual releasing the component and the name of the person to whom it is released must be recorded in a laboratory log.[7] Careful attention to this procedure will prevent most catastrophic mistakes. It is worth reiterating here that clerical mistakes are the cause of at least 90% of fatal transfusion reactions,[14] and it is in the issuing transaction that many of these mistakes occur.

Hanging a Unit

Usually two individuals—two physicians, a physician and a nurse, or two nurses—should be involved in hanging a unit. Before the unit is hung, these persons verify the name and hospital identification number on the requisition form and on the caution tag on the unit. Verbal identification is advised if the patient is conscious. Under no circumstances is blood to be transfused if recipient identification is lacking (i.e., bracelet I.D.). The only exception to this rule is emergency transfusion of uncrossmatched blood to a patient in the emergency room, in which case the transfusionists check the ABO and Rh type of the recipient. These must be compatible. In large hospitals it is best to have a transfusion team. These individuals are trained in the technology of venipuncture and are knowledgeable in immunohematology principles.

Venipuncture

Blood products are infused intravenously in a great majority of cases. A vein of sufficient diameter to accommodate a 19-gauge or larger needle is selected.[7] Large-bore needles are used when fast infusion rate is required. Exceptions to the use of large-sized needles are pediatric transfusions, where a 23-gauge needle may be used. Butterfly needles and sets with a "flashback" feature that allow the transfusionist to know if a vein has been entered are recommended.[15] In an adult patient, large veins are most accessible in the antecubital fossa. Veins in the forearm or hand are possible alternatives, but venipuncture in these sites is more painful. The administration set is vented before transfusion.

In multiple trauma patients, two access ports are recommended, one above and one below the diaphragm. For this purpose a pediatric feeding catheter, No. 8–10 French, can be used.[16] These catheters are checked daily and the site is disinfected with antibacterial ointments. Indwelling catheters must be removed as soon as possible.

Although blood is transfused intravenously in the great majority of cases, the intraperitoneal route[17] has been used to transfuse infants when cardiac overload must be avoided at all costs, and the intrasternal route has been used in burn patients when other ports were inaccessible.[18] The intrasternal route is infrequently used because venipuncture here may be extremely painful and hazardous.

Rate of Transfusion

One must calculate the rate of transfusion, especially in patients who cannot tolerate rapid volume changes, such as patients with cardiac or renal insufficiency. The rate of transfusion can be calculated as follows: a unit of whole blood (500 ml) will be transfused in about 3 hours if the drop rate in the drop chamber is adjusted to 40 drops a minute, in 2 hours if the drop rate is 60 drops a minute, and in 30 minutes if the drop rate is 200 drops a minute.[19] Transfusions should be completed in less than 4 hours to avoid bacterial proliferation.[20] If transfusions are to be given very slowly, the unit should be split into pedipacks and the unused portion refrigerated in a blood bank refrigerator. Under no circumstances is blood to be stored in a refrigerator not designed for blood storage. For this reason, it is probably a good policy not to release more than 1 unit of blood at a time for any single patient, unless the need for massive transfusion is anticipated. Conservative release of transfusion units avoids the potential hazard of transfusing wrong units to other patients in the ward.

Increased rates of infusion are recommended only in emergencies and can be achieved manually or with a pressure cuff. Packed cells usually run quite slowly, (it takes 10 minutes to infuse a unit of packed cells using a completely open line). However, if 50 ml of saline is infused in the unit from a sterile saline bag for IV use through the unit line, the unit will run in 4 minutes (personal experience).

Filters

The FDA mandates in-line filters for every transfusion.[15] The standard filter has a 170-μ pore size. The filter sets have a stylet cannula at one end to enter the component bag. Care must be taken not to touch any of the sterile end points of the cannula. In multiple transfusions, filters must be changed every 8 hours to avoid contamination. Filters screening particles 20 μ or larger in diameter are recommended in massive transfusion (5 units or more),[21] in open heart surgery cases when pulmonary capillary filtration is bypassed, or in multiply transfused patients, to minimize granulocyte contamination. All filters must be properly primed and vented. Multiple transfusions using the same filter set will result in an increased screening filtration rate. Using infusion sets with in-line microfilters results in a more economical practice. Infusion sets with a Y set permit priming with saline or increasing packed cell rheology and flow rates, as suggested above. However, users tend to use these Y sets for infusion of incompatible fluids into the unit.[15]

All blood transfusions should be constantly monitored by a nurse. The starting time and the finishing time must be recorded. The patient should be observed for reactions for at least 30 minutes after the transfusion.

Transfusion Practices in Platelet Therapy

Platelet therapy should be preplanned whenever possible, owing to the paucity of these units in most institutions. Units must not be pooled until the blood bank staff is assured these will be used. The expiration time of pooled platelets is 24 hours. ABO types are pooled according to type. ABO-compatible platelets should be given when possible. The next best alternative is to use ABO-incompatible platelets from which excess plasma has been removed by centrifuging and expressing the plasma out of the pooled units with a donor room bag clamp. If this is done, platelets must be resuspended by gentle rotation on a platelet rotator for at least 1 hour, or until aggregates are minimal. Platelet manipulation of this sort may decrease the viable platelet population in the pool.

Rh type for platelets must be respected in recipients not immunized to the D antigen. This rule is mandatory in Rh-negative women of child-bearing age. If platelets are given to these individuals and Rh immunization is a possibility, Rh immunoglobulin (RhIG) administration is mandatory as a preventative measure. Pooled platelets are to be kept in platelet incubators under gentle rotation until used. Issued platelets may not be accepted back into the blood bank. Platelets may have to be washed by a special protocol if plasma is to be avoided (e.g., in patients with anti-IgA antibodies). It is not a good practice to give platelets to patients who have massive bleeding of a mechanical cause until bleeding is controlled, because of a washout phenomenon. In adults, pools usually consist of 5 units of platelets. The dosage for pediatric transfusions is discussed in chapters 8 and 16. Issuing platelets without first obtaining a platelet count is a poor practice. If the platelet count is normal and platelets are still requested from the blood bank, the blood bank physician must ask to see a platelet function study. The bleeding time is an excellent test to assess in vivo platelet function.[22] All these recommendations may be waived in emergencies when it is believed that platelets will contribute to hemostasis. Platelets are not released from the blood bank until hepatitis and HTLV-III testing has been performed.

Platelets from plateletpheresis machines have an expiration time of 24 hours. In such cases, hepatitis testing is usually performed the day before the procedure. These platelet units are also kept at room temperature under gentle rotation. Treating physicians who request HLA-matched platelets must be informed of the procedure for obtaining such units so that patients and donors can be HLA tested in optimal time. Patients must be tested before they become leukopenic, after which HLA testing is more difficult. Possible donors must be identified in advance, not when the patient is bleeding from thrombocytopenia or profoundly leukopenic. Transfusion with HLA-matched platelets is usually started when patients have become unresponsive to random donor platelets. In patients chronically transfused with this component, platelet counts must be determined 1 hour and 24 hours after transfusion. Platelets are usually given through a regular 170-μ infusion set, followed by a saline flushing rinse to ensure complete infusion of platelets possibly trapped in the residual space. Platelets can be given through microaggregate filters if infusion through the filter is followed by a saline rinse.[23] Platelets given to febrile patients have a shortened survival time.[24] Similarly, patients with hepatosplenomegaly will not have a good platelet increment after transfusion.[25] It is a good idea to remember these facts before deciding that a patient is unresponsive to random donor platelet units.

Platelets given to immunosuppressed individuals may have to be irradiated to avoid graft-versus-host disease, since these units are contaminated with viable lymphocytes.[26] Exposing the components to 2,000 rad is sufficient to render lymphocytes nonmitotic. Arrangements to irradiate the units must be made with the nuclear medicine department of the hospital if the machine for irradiating components is not available in the blood bank.

Transfusion of Granulocytes

Good granulocyte transfusion practice entails, above all, careful assessment of patients in whom this component is believed needed. Criteria for such assessment are given in chapter 8.

Granulocytes from random donors are transfused in pools of 2 or 3 units. In this way those unit pools causing fever can be discarded. Granulocytes must always be ABO compatible and must be crossmatched with a patient sample, because these units are heavily contaminated with RBCs. Treatment should continue uninterrupted for at least 5 days. Eight to fifteen units are given each day. A trial with three antibiotics for 48 hours is usually attempted before deciding to use granulocytes. Granulocytes are routinely irradiated before use, in a similar protocol as that for platelets. The expiration time for granulocytes is 24 hours, and the treating physician must be informed of this fact before granulocyte transfusion is selected. Physicians ordering granulocytes must be advised not to expect peripheral count increments after transfusion, but rather a clinical improvement of the infection under treatment. This component *must not* be infused through a microaggregate filter. Fever is frequently encountered after infusing granulocytes; however, patients requiring granulocytes are often febrile due to infection or underlying disease. Patients are usually premedicated with Tylenol before transfusion.

Transfusion of Plasma

Plasma may be given through 170-μ filters or through microaggregate filters. Often cryoprecipitate aggregates are found in plasma and are a good indication that the component should be given through a microaggregate filter set. Plasma transfusion has few indications, and therefore its use in hospitals should be monitored.

Patients undergoing open heart surgery routinely require 2 or more units of plasma during the postperfusion recovery phase. Patients receiving massive transfusion may also require plasma after 6–8 units of blood have been given. Elective use of plasma is justified only in patients who are actively bleeding and have a prolonged prothrombin time (PT) and partial thromboplastin time (PTT). Patients with disseminated intravascular coagulation (DIC) or liver failure may require FFP before PT and PTT studies can be done.

Giving plasma to reconstitute packed cells is justified only when there is a clear need for procoagulant (e.g., DIC, washout in massive transfusion, or factor XIII deficiency). Giving plasma or FFP instead of whole blood when whole blood is needed for volume is not a good transfusion practice because it increases the risk of hepatitis and is economically unsound.[4] FFP must not be used as a volume expander; other expanders such as crystalloid and dextran solutions will achieve volume expansion without the potential hazards that FFP carries (e.g., hepatitis, AIDS, immune reactions). FFP should be ABO compatible[27] but is given without testing for compatibility and within 24 hours after thawing if it has been refrigerated at 4°–6° C in the interim.[28]

Cryoprecipitate

Cryoprecipitate is usually used as a source of factor VIII or fibrinogen. Its use in DIC is justified, as well as in other causes of hypofibrinogenemia (e.g., hepatic failure). It is the component of choice in the therapy of von Willebrand's disease. It can be used within 6 hours after thawing[28] and should be ABO compatible, especially in patients with a small blood volume (e.g., pediatric patients).[27] Cryoprecipitate may be given in pools of 5–10 units, and saline may be used to facilitate resuspension and infusion of the component. Elective use of cryoprecipitate is warranted only in cases of renal calculi extraction or if a coagulopathy such as hemophilia A, von Willebrand's disease, or hypofibrinogenemia has been documented.

Plasma Fractions

Several plasma fractions are utilized in a hospital setting, although not all are handled by the blood bank. In some institutions, for example, they may be dispensed by the pharmacy. However, in most hospitals it is the blood bank that handles these products.

Factor VIII Concentrates

Factor VIII concentrates are used in the home treatment of hemophilia A and to prepare hemophiliacs for surgery. Since factor VIII concentrates are prepared from pools, transfusion of the product carries a relatively high risk of hepatitis and AIDS. Nevertheless, it is the only product that will increase the plasma factor VIII concentration to hemostatic levels. Factor VIII concentrates *must not* be used to correct bleeding in patients with von Willebrand's disease because they do not contain optimal levels of vW factor VIII.[29] As stated earlier, von Willebrand's disease is treated with cryoprecipitate. Chronic hemophiliacs are at risk not only of developing hepatitis and AIDS but also of developing antibodies against factor VIII. About 10%–15% of patients with hemophilia A will develop antibodies.[30] These antibodies are of the IgG4 subclass and do not bind complement[31] but do produce a refractory state to factor VIII concentrate. These patients are difficult to treat. The following alternatives may be tried to override the inhibitors:[30]

1. Total bed rest with immobilization. This option is not the most popular.
2. Large doses of factor VIII to neutralize antifactor VIII antibodies.
3. Nonactivated factor IX for active bleeding. For life-threatening hemorrhage, use activated factor IX preparations to override the factor VIII deficiency.
4. Animal factor VIII preparations are presently experimental and should be used as a last resort.

Hepatitis in Hemophiliacs.—Most patients with hemophilia A who have been treated with concentrates will develop antibodies against hepatitis B; 2%–4% will develop a positive HB_sAg. Most patients will have transient transaminase elevation, but only 30% will develop chronic transaminase elevation.[32]

Factor IX Concentrates

The prothrombin complex contains factors IX, II, VII, and X and is used mainly in the treatment of hemophilia B, but deficiencies of factors II, VII, and X are also treated with these concentrates.

Complications such as thrombosis may be seen in patients taking high doses of factor IX concentrates because some activated factor IX is present in these preparations.

Inhibiting antibodies may also develop in patients with hemophilia B treated with factor IX concentrate.

Other Complications From Procoagulant Concentrates

A rare complication from procoagulant concentrate therapy (both factor VIII and factor IX concentrate) is hemolysis from isoantibodies in the concentrates against ABH antigens.[33] AIDS in hemophiliacs is reviewed in chapter 13.

γ-Globulin Preparations

Most centers dispense γ-globulin preparations through the pharmacy. However, some blood banks may be involved in issuing units of γ-globulin, or the blood bank physician may be requested to give information on the use of γ-globulin.

Immune serum globulin (ISG) is a 10%–16% concentrate of γ-globulin obtained by the Cohn fractionation procedure. It is mainly used for prophylaxis of contacts of persons with hepatitis A, but it may be used as replacement therapy for patients with agammaglobulinemia or hypogammaglobulinemia and as prophylaxis for measles.[34] Travelers to areas where hepatitis A is endemic may benefit from prophylaxis with γ-globulin. This drug must not be used in patients with antibodies to IgA, because it may result in a severe anaphylactic reaction due to IgA contamination.

Hepatitis is not thought to be transmitted in these preparations,[35] although passive-active immunization against herpes virus type B has been documented after intramuscular injection of ISG.[36] Immunoglobulin preparations licensed in the United States for IM use must not be used intravenously.[35] If they are given intravenously, microaggregates may trigger thromboembolic phenomena. IV preparations of ISG are currently available in this country. For more details on γ-globulin (ISG), see chapter 8.

Special hyperimmune γ-globulin preparations against hepatitis (HBIG) and Rh (RhIG) exist. These are usually readily available in blood banks or the pharmacy. Guidelines for use are given in chapter 8.

Other types of hyperimmune γ-globulin that are less frequently used are zoster immune globulin, vaccinia immune globulin, rabies immune globulin, and tetanus immune globulin. These are available from the Immunological Activity Branch of the Centers for Disease Control, Atlanta. The telephone numbers are 404-633-3311, 8 A.M. to 4:30 P.M. weekdays, or 404-633-2176 for emergencies. These telephone numbers must be checked periodically for possible number changes.

Albumin (Crystalloid Versus Colloid)

The extensive use of albumin is attested to by the fact that most hospitals spend more on albumin than on antibiotics.[37] This increased use of albumin has arisen from the knowledge that pooled plasma transmits hepatitis. Albumin characteristically does not transmit hepatitis because of the Cohn fractionation process. This feature of albumin has made it one of the more popular colloids used for volume replacement in surgical patients. Plasma protein fraction, which is a less pure albumin preparation, has fallen into disfavor due to kallikrein-induced vasoactive reactions. Despite the popularity of albumin, this product is not necessarily more advantageous for volume expansion than plain crystalloid replacement.[38] The controversy of volume replacement with colloid versus crystalloid does not arise from clinical experience but from misconceptions about the physiology of fluid replacement.

Albumin usually produces increased intravascular volume but decreased diuresis.[39] Crystalloid replacement advocates suggest that triple the amount of crystalloid per volume of plasma lost should be replaced to offset the loss of oncotic pressure.[40] In the long run, diuresis is much better after crystalloid solution infusion than after colloid infusion. Furthermore, the respiratory function is much better after crystalloid for massive replacement than after colloid, which tends to produce edematous lungs.[41] Massive volume replacement with crystalloid alone has been achieved most successfully in Vietnam casualties[38] and in elderly patients.[42]

Despite these general guidelines, fluid therapy must be individualized. Burn patients have traditionally been treated with crystalloid for the first 24 hours to expand the constricted extracellular volume, followed by intravenous replacement with albumin.[43] However, it is not recommended that albumin use be continued as nutritional support for these patients. Albumin is not a high-quality protein in terms of amino acid content and is not a substitute for adequate nutrition. Amino acids should be replaced orally as soon as possible.

Although albumin has been used extensively in burn patients and in patients with hepatic failure, hypoalbuminemia, and even malnutrition, its use in the treatment of these conditions is controversial.[38] Two other points in the controversy are (1) on a volume-per-volume basis, albumin is 100 times more expensive than crystalloid,[38] and (2) the continued misuse of albumin promotes the exploitation of undernourished and underprivileged commercial donors in the United States and abroad.[44]

In summary, crystalloid solutions should be used instead of albumin whenever possible, including the treatment of burn patients. Using albumin for nutritional purposes is not a good transfusion practice, nor is the use of packed cells and albumin for massive replacement of blood a good practice. These patients are best given whole blood and, if procoagulants are needed, FFP is given separately or as FFP-reconstituted whole blood.

SPECIAL PROBLEMS IN TRANSFUSION PRACTICE

The blood bank physician is often confronted with multifaceted problems that require consultation with the treating physician. Some of these problems are reviewed below.

Emergency Transfusion Therapy

Emergency transfusion therapy must be addressed individually because of its important clinical implications.

The life of a patient may depend on how fluid replacement is handled in the first hour, often termed the "golden hour" in emergency centers. This section reviews a few concepts of emergency room care in general, followed by the role of the blood bank in such a setting.

An advance communications system is extremely important to convey an estimated time of arrival and to notify the blood bank immediately if the need for large amounts of blood is anticipated. A specialized team of physicians and nurses must be available in the emergency room. These individuals should have thoroughly assimilated their roles in the team. A prestocked cart containing emergency supplies and equipment should be ready in each emergency unit area. Thoracotomy kits, vein cutdown equipment, and the like should be on these carts and ready for immediate use.[45] Operating room staff must be ready to set up in a matter of minutes. Staff are prepared in teams with each individual focusing on one aspect of patient treatment, and rigid protocols should be followed. A consensus on therapy in the emergency room is essential. Disordered activity introduces chaos into an already pressing situation and results in loss of valuable time. For victims in shock or suffering from major trauma, emergency treatment is started before diagnostic procedures are begun.

The first steps in treating an emergency patient are:

1. Establish an airway and give oxygen.
2. Stop blood or fluid loss.
3. Replace fluid loss.
4. Treat with vasopressors.
5. If only one line is available, stabilize the patient with fluids before attempting restoration of central venous pressure.

Restoration of Volume

The following decisions must be made immediately:[45]

1. Selection of an infusion site.
2. Selection of type of fluid replacement.
3. Treatment methods in case of possible complications from infusions.

Site of Infusion.—Choose the easiest, most accessible site. If a percutaneous subclavian line cannot be placed, perform a medial cubital vein cutdown. Attempt to put a line into each extremity.

Type of Fluid Replacement.—Depending on the cause of the trauma, crystalloid or crystalloid and colloid may be selected (if crystalloid is used, give 3 times the amount of plasma lost). Acute hemorrhage should be treated with packed cells and crystalloid after the first 1,000 cc of blood lost. Uncrossmatched O-negative packed cells are used if there is no time to type and crossmatch, after the first 1,000 cc of crystalloid is given. However, a sample is sent to the blood bank so that work can begin on a rapid type and crossmatch as soon as the patient arrives in the emergency room. If group O Rh-negative cells are not available, use O-positive packed cells. In the meantime, AB plasma can be thawed immediately to be ready for posttransfusion needs, since it takes approximately 10–15 minutes to thaw. Two units of plasma are given for every 10 units of blood.[45] The decision to give uncrossmatched blood must be made to salvage patients in acute severe hemorrhagic shock (requiring 10 or more units). Hesitation or delays at this point may result in death of the patient.[45] After 20 units of blood are given, 5–6 units of platelets must be given.[45]

Massive Transfusion

Pathophysiology of Hypovolemic Shock

With loss of blood volume, the cardiac output decreases, as well as the stroke volume and stroke work, thereby decreasing oxygen transport. In response to these decrements, the heart rate, the peripheral resistance, and oxygen extraction increase.[46] When these compensatory mechanisms fail, cellular hypoxia will result, leading to metabolic acidosis. Eventually irreversible shock may develop and the patient will die, in spite of increased intravascular pressure.

It is thought that the mechanisms contributing to the irreversibility of shock are (1) vascular vasoconstriction, (2) microemboli resulting from sludging in small capillaries, and (3) acidosis. These pathologic changes further promote tissue damage and hypoxia. To avoid the onset of irreversible shock, the patient must be treated immediately with fluids that restore volume as well as oxygen-carrying capacity. As much as 1,000 ml of fluid may be lost without a concomitant fall in blood pressure, due to the physiologic compensatory mechanisms of the body.[47] This comes about through the action of baroreceptors triggered by hypovolemia. Triggering of baroreceptors induces release of epinephrine from the adrenal gland and norepinephrine from postganglionic sympathetic nerve endings.[48] A vasoconstriction and redistribution of flow from the periphery to the heart, brain, and adrenals are produced.[49] However, if hypovolemia persists unchecked, cellular hypoxia will produce a fall in pH because of increased release of lactic acid due to cellular anaerobic glycolysis. This fall in pH may induce precapillary arteriolar dilation[50] with persistent postcapillary venule constriction, resulting in stagnation and "vicious cycle" hypoxia.

Fluid is also preserved physiologically via a decrease in glomerular filtration rate brought on by the renin-angiotensin mechanism triggered by hypovolemima.[51] Antidiuretic hormone release also inhibits diuresis and contributes to fluid retention[52] in cases of hemorrhagic shock. To maintain adequate volume, adequate perfusion, and sufficient oxygen-carrying capacity, severely traumatized patients often undergo what is called massive transfusion.

In hypovolemic shock, complications from "too little blood, too late" are much more severe than problems caused by the net negative effect of massive blood transfusion.[53] Massive transfusion is defined as the replacement of 90% of the total blood volume within 3 hours.[54]

Three major problems may arise in the massively transfused patient: bleeding diathesis, potentially toxic levels of substances present in stored blood, and overload.

Bleeding Diathesis Secondary to Massive Transfusion

About 30% of patients develop a bleeding diathesis after massive transfusion. The major bleeding problem arising from massive transfusion of stored blood is dilutional thrombocytopenia,[55] which occurs in about 63% of patients that develop a diathesis. The remaining 27% bleed because of the development of DIC. The notion that massive transfusion may produce depletion of factor VIII and factor V, based on the observation that these factors decrease during storage of blood, is more theoretical than real. In practice, factor VIII is rapidly synthesized by the liver in the successfully resuscitated trauma patient,[54] and the factor V level may drop to 15% of normal before it becomes clinically significant.[12] It is therefore unlikely that any bleeding tendency in the massively transfused patient results from depletion of these factors. Nevertheless, certain authors recommend infusion of 2 units of FFP after transfusion of 10 units of blood.[45] Platelets can be given in a dose of 5 units for every 10 units of blood transfused to avoid dilutional thrombocytopenia.

Toxic or Injurious Substances Transfused During Massive Transfusion

Some of the potentially toxic substances that accumulate in the plasma of stored units have proved to be not as significant as initially thought.[56] Potassium levels may be as high as 14 mEq/L in stored blood after 1 week. However, patients undergoing massive transfusion usually have increased potassium elimination via the kidneys, owing to increased diuresis,[54] and hyperkalemia is not usually a frequent problem unless patients are transfused at very rapid rates (100–150 ml/minute). Potassium intoxication is indicated by the appearance of peaked T waves on the ECG. Hypocalcemia due to the chelating effect of citrate may be present after massive transfusion, because there is a decrease in ionized calcium. Prolonged QT intervals may appear on the ECG but are not always significant.[57] Calcium supplementation has been recommended for massive transfusion-induced hypokalemia because of the narrow margin of safety with low calcium levels. However, indiscriminate calcium supplementation (i.e., without monitoring) is a poor transfusion practice and may be deleterious to the patient.[56] Calcium salts must never be infused via a blood transfusion line, as clots may form and DIC may result.

Citrate toxicity in general will not appear in otherwise intact adults receiving 1 unit of blood every 5 minutes. The combination of high potassium and low calcium levels is an undesirable complication that may result from massive transfusion.[58] Potentiation of both is possible during massive transfusion, thus, the toxicity of hypocalcemia or hypokalemia is higher when both conditions are present together. Careful monitoring of the patient's potassium and ionized calcium levels is necessary for adequate replacement. Laboratory testing may not be immediately available in emergencies, in which case an ECG may be of some value in assessing hypokalemia or hypocalcemia.

Stored blood that has been refrigerated for several days (26–35 days) may have markedly decreased levels of 2,3-DPG. This decrement results in a decrease of the oxygen-releasing function of hemoglobin and eventually in poor oxygen delivery to the tissues. Transfused cells recover normal 2,3-DPG levels in 12–24 hours.[59] This lag is usually not significant in elective transfusion but must be considered in the massively transfused patient. It is therefore advisable to give relatively fresh blood (less than 1 week old) to patients undergoing massive transfusion; however, older units should be given first, since they are almost immediately lost. Transfusion of untested and potentially infected blood from walk-in donors is a poor practice and has legal implications.

The formation of microaggregates has been thought to be significant in the massively transfused patient. The true importance of this cell debris in the pathology of massive transfusion is not fully documented and today is believed not to be very significant.[60] Furthermore, interposing a microaggregate filter in the transfusion line may reduce the infusion rate, and multiple unit transfusion through the same filter may increase the screen filtration pressure; either of these practices compromises the speed of replacement blood transfusion.

The release of kinins in the trauma patient should be considered. Leukocytes present in blood may conceivably trigger the kinin-kallikrein system, thus activating the kininogen-kinin system. Depletion of the proteins in this system may reduce perfusion and oxygen levels and deplete glucose at the cellular level. Infusion of FFP and washed cells has been recommended.[61] However, neither the significance of depletion of kininogen nor the use of various recommended therapies has been assessed in controlled clinical trials.

Rapid transfusion of cold blood may produce cardiac standstill, so blood warmers must be available in emergency room bays. Volume overload is another potential complication of massive blood transfusion. It can be avoided by monitoring the central venous pressure with an intravenous catheter. Subclavian vein catheters are routinely used in such emergencies to monitor fluid balance.

Therapeutic Strategies in the Hypovolemic Patient

The following procedures are followed in the emergency room for hypovolemic patients, in coordination with the blood bank:

1. Start replacement with crystalloid. Loss of up to 1,000 cc of blood or plasma can be corrected with crystalloid alone.

2. Send a blood sample for typing and crossmatching to the blood bank, immediately.

3. Get O-negative packed cells, uncrossmatched, ready for use should lack of time preclude completion of tests. O-positive packed blood cells may be given if O-negative units are not available.

4. Typing usually takes 5–10 minutes and a rapid modified crossmatch may take 15 minutes; this blood is used next, if less than 4 group units have been given. Otherwise continue the transfusion with crossmatched group O packed cells.[52]

5. Thawing AB plasma is a good practice, if use of 10–20 units is anticipated in a short period of time (it takes approximately 15 minutes to thaw a unit, and starting the thawing process as soon as possible saves time).

6. Get units of platelets pooled after the first 10 units of blood are given.

BLOOD BANK READINESS PLAN

Blood banks dealing with transfusion emergencies must have emergency protocols to avoid chaos, confusion, and poor time response. The blood bank staff must be ready to respond. The only way to achieve this is through training. In large trauma centers, it is better to have a specialized team in the blood bank to deal with emergencies. This team should be well practiced in emergency procedures and expert in the blood bank technology pertinent to emergencies.

Releasing uncrossmatched blood is unappealing to most people who work or have worked in a blood bank. However, if blood is not given immediately during an acute massive hemorrhage emergency (2–3 units in 5–10 minutes), time will be wasted and the patient may die. Insisting on the completion of a crossmatch in a massively bleeding patient only reveals inexperience in handling this type of emergency.

The following protocol can be adopted by blood banks that anticipate massive bleeding emergencies.

Phase 1: Requisition and Sample Identification

A patient blood sample is necessary for typing and crossmatching, although in urgent circumstances it may not be available immediately. However, if a sample is brought to the blood bank, it must be properly identified. In a massive casualty situation, identification may have to be done by assigning a special and individual number to each patient sample. A label bearing the same number is affixed to the wrists of patients who lack personal identification and are unconscious.

The emergency request form *must* be secured from the treating physician. This form should contain the following items:[63]

1. Patient's name, if available, or an identification number if the name is not available.

2. Number of units requested by the physician.

3. Patient's blood type if available; if not, label "group O packed cells."

4. Units are labeled "uncrossmatched." When crossmatched units become available, the uncrossmatched units are returned to the blood bank. The identification of units as "uncrossmatched" will alert physicians to the possibility of a reaction.

5. Number and group and type of units issued; identification number of each unit issued.

6. Units issued this way are usually given as packed cells. This should be stated on the release form.

7. Statement from the physician as to why the units must be released uncrossmatched.

8. The physician's signature. The form then becomes a legal document to protect the blood bank.

9. The technician's signature. The technician also witnesses the issuing process.

10. The date and time of release of a unit from the blood bank. Releasing a unit without filling in this form must be a very rare event and only with permission by the blood bank physician or designated person.

Phase 2: The Test

One technologist ideally should handle one emergency sample. Confusion is a main problem leading to release of the wrong unit; overworking a technologist is an invitation to disaster.

One set of tubes is prepared for typing and grouping immediately (timetable: 5 minutes).

The crossmatch is set in duplicate:

1. An immediate spin is done using saline technique (timetable: 5–10 minutes, if no incubation at 37° C is performed).

2. In an abbreviated crossmatch, an immediate spin is done, plus 10 minutes at 37° C in albumin. Cells are then washed and prepared for Coombs testing (timetable: 15 minutes).

A screen is performed (timetable: 45 minutes).

All testing must be taken to completion regardless of the outcome of the emergency. If the patient dies the tests may be abbreviated but must be completed for legal purposes.[63]

Phase 3: Release Triage

Blood release after infusion of uncrossmatched units is given in the following priority:[63]

1. Uncrossmatched type- and group-specific units are given if available and if no more than 4 units of uncrossmatched group O blood have been given to the patient. If more than 4 units of group O blood have been given, continue giving group O blood until bleeding subsides and sequential isoantibody titers in the patient's plasma do not show reaction with the patient's type-specific cells. Type A packed cells are usually available and should be given to group AB patients in whom large transfusion needs are anticipated.

2. Crossmatched units "on the spin" are available next and should immediately be substituted for units that were released uncrossmatched.

3. Units that have been crossmatched with a modified crossmatch technique become available next and should be substituted for all previously released units.

4. Units completely screened and crossmatched are available last. These units are substituted for any previous units incompletely tested to that moment.

All units are released with a form bearing full patient identification and unit identification plus a description of the stage of testing completed until release time. Forms are dated, timed, and signed both by the person responsible for transfusing the unit and by the technologist releasing the units.

Patients who have a screen test completed may receive all subsequent units after a modified crossmatch. Since this emergency crossmatch system has been introduced in a large hospital setting, a negligible number of transfusion incidents have occurred.[64]

In a very acute case, more than one technician works on the sample if the staff are available. One person does the typing and the other does the crossmatch.

In any massive hemorrhage case with anticipated needs of 10–20 units of blood, 1 or 2 units of AB plasma may be thawed as soon as the patient's arrival time is known. For FFP and platelet replacement, every attempt to determine the PT, PTT, and platelet count should be made before giving these components, thus providing a rational approach to platelet therapy. Standardized replacement with components of any sort is excusable only in extreme emergencies. As soon as coagulation laboratory results and other laboratory results become available, they must be used in selecting further replacement therapy.

Blood Component Replacement in DIC

Blood bank physicians are often consulted in the management of DIC. DIC may be seen in various conditions that cause tissue damage with release of thromboplastin, including tumor necrosis, obstetric complications, trauma, extensive surgery, and so forth. Other substances and conditions can also activate the clotting cascade, including the immune complexes (such as in hemolytic reactions), endothelial injury, and gram-negative septicemia. Gram-negative endotoxins may trigger DIC via thromboplastin release from granulocytes.[65] However, of all these causes, infection and neoplasia are the most common.[66] When blood clots, there is consumption of fibrinogen and factors V and VIII, as well as factor II and antithrombin III. Platelets are trapped in the clot fibrin mesh. The same changes occur in DIC, along with other changes occasioned by the in vivo setting, such as concurrent fibrinolysis via plasmin activation.

Diagnosis of DIC

The most useful tests are (1) the PT, which is usually prolonged, (2) fibrinogen, which is usually low (< 100 mg/100 ml), (3) fibrin split products, which are increased, (4) platelet count (decreased), and (5) the presence of schistocytes in the peripheral smear.

Therapy for DIC[67]

There is no standard treatment for DIC. Each patient is treated individually. The following plan of action is suggested:

1. Eliminate the cause of DIC and treat shock and/or acidosis.
2. Replace volume with FFP, which will also provide factors V, VIII, and XIII.
3. Give cryoprecipitate to supply fibrinogen and factor VIII.
4. Give platelets as needed on the basis of a platelet count.
5. Give heparin as needed in selected cases. Heparin is not indicated when massive bleeding from DIC is present. If the decision to give heparin is made, an initial bolus of 5,000–10,000 units is given, followed by 1,000 units/hour by continuous infusion.
6. Give packed cells if massive bleeding is present.

TRANSFUSION PRACTICES IN OPEN HEART SURGERY REPLACEMENT THERAPY

A major user of blood and blood components in a tertiary care hospital is the thoracic surgery department, especially the subdivision of cardiovascular surgery. In a comprehensive surgery department, it was found that the average number of blood units used in nearly 40,000 cases of open heart surgery was 8.[68] However, this study was conducted in 1973, and the quality of surgery as well as the equipment has since improved considerably.[69] Some authors report many less units used per case (averaging 2 units per open heart operation).[70]

Cardiopulmonary Bypass System (CPB)

The cardiopulmonary bypass machine (Fig 18–1) has revolutionized open heart surgery. This machine has three main components, as described below.[71]

1. Oxygenator.—Anticoagulated venous blood is routed by gravity from the vena cava into the oxygenator. The oxygenator functions as a respiratory system for the patient on bypass. It bubbles oxygen with small amounts of CO_2 through venous blood, oxygenating it. A debubbling system is incorporated into the system to prevent air embolism; this portion of the oxygenator is called the debubbling chamber. The blood temperature is maintained at 37° C by a water bath. Oxygenation and pH are checked and corrected via a pH and oxygen monitoring system.

2. Main Oxygenator Pump.—As the oxygenated blood leaves the oxygenator, it enters a flexible plastic tubing system, which is compressed rhythmically by a peristaltic roller pump. This makes the blood progress into the arterial system of the patient.

3. Suction System and Accessory Pump.—A suction system which uses an accessory peristaltic roller pump removes blood from the cardiotomy site into a reservoir with a microaggregate filter that eliminates debris and allows blood salvage. The blood is then circulated by gravity from the reservoir through the oxygenator and returned to the patient via the main oxygenator pump (see Fig 18–1).

Other types of oxygenators, called membrane oxygenators, are recommended for prolonged pump runs.[72] The surgeon may decide not to reinfuse the blood remaining in the reservoir (as much as 1 L) to avoid circulatory overload. In this case the blood is sent to the blood bank, following a protocol similar to that for autotransfusion: the bag is carefully

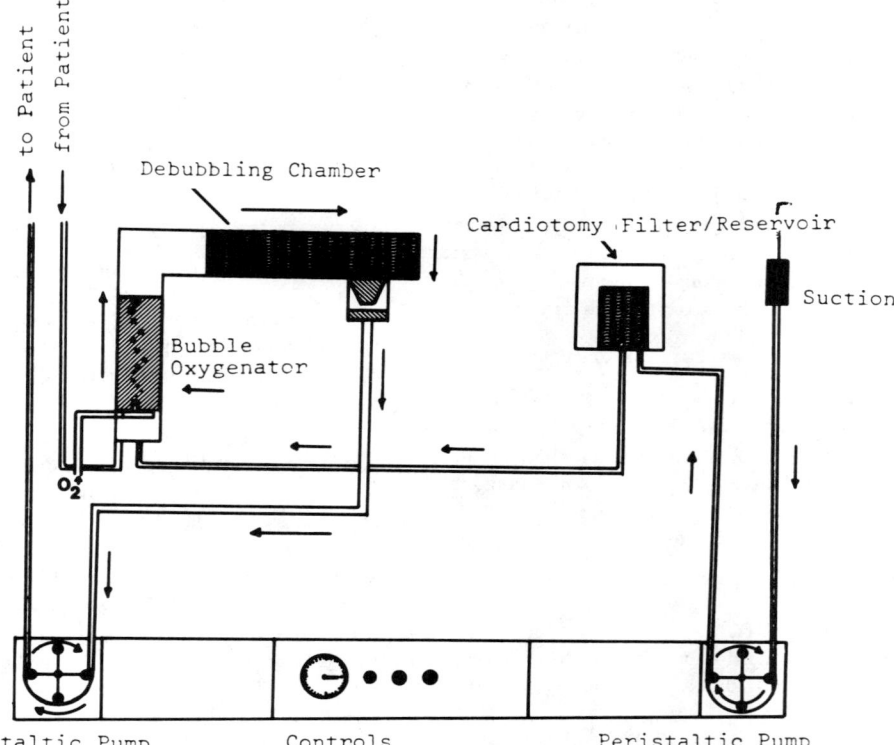

FIG 18–1.—Cardiopulmonary bypass oxygenator pump with five components. The first component is a pump that promotes circulation from the vena cava of the patient *(top left)*. The blood is pumped into the second component, the bubble oxygenator chamber *(left)*, then through a fine metal mesh which functions as a debubbling chamber (third component). The pump then returns the blood to the patient *(top left)*. *Large arrows* represent the flow of blood through the system. The fourth component is a second peristaltic pump, which promotes suction *(right side of figure)* from the cardiotomy area. This blood is then pumped into a cardiotomy filter reservoir, the fifth component of the system, and circulated through the bubble oxygenator *(left)*. The controls shown at *bottom* regulate variables such as rate of flow and rate of oxygenation.

labeled with the patient's name and hospital identification number to avoid transfusion incompatibility. The blood may then be washed, either mechanically or manually with saline, to eliminate hemoglobin and some cellular debris.

Evaluation of Fluid Therapy and Component Replacement in CPB

Very often patients undergoing CPB have blood volume imbalance.[73] Monitoring prebypass fluid needs is probably best undertaken by a pulmonary capillary wedge pressure (PCWP) monitor with a Swan-Ganz catheter. Pressure must be maintained at 8–10 mm Hg.[69] Most institutions use crystalloid to maintain PCWP during induction.

Increased bleeding after CPB may occur due to a coagulopathy if a patient has been bleeding at a rate of 200 ml/hour for 3 or more hours.[74] Causes for this excessive bleeding after open heart surgery are multiple and range from surgical technique to true depletion of clotting factors and platelets. Experience in terms of numbers of open heart operations performed often determines which institutions have high or low usage of blood per case. For example, institutions where fewer than 75 CPB operations per year are performed use an average of 10–11 units per case, while institutions where more than 175 CPB operations are performed use an average of 7 units per case.

The following factors decrease the amount of blood used per case:[70]

1. Hemodilution using a crystalloid prime rather

than whole blood prime for the oxygenator.[75] This procedure is not recommended in patients with left ventricular failure, in whom hematocrit values of 40 or more are recommended.[76]

2. Autotransfusion of blood shed during the procedure.

3. Accepting a hematocrit in the high teens as patients come off bypass, and accepting a hematocrit in the mid-20s in the immediate postbypass period.

Derangement of Hemostasis in Patients Undergoing Open Heart Surgery

Mechanical bleeding not due to coagulopathy but to poor surgical technique is a major cause of bleeding. Once this cause can be ruled out, a coagulopathy or thrombocytopenia should be searched for. A coagulopathy may be present in up to 20% of cases.[77] The main coagulopathies associated with CPB are DIC, depletion, and fibrinolysis. However, the major cause of bleeding is the consequence of complete neutralization of heparin, heparin rebound, and thrombocytopenia.

In about 25% of all CPB cases, increased fibrinolytic activity can be documented.[78] Occasionally fibrinolysis and hypofibrinogenemia are the cause of severe postbypass hemorrhage, which responds to cryoprecipitate therapy.[79] About 2% of patients may have overt DIC. This complication usually occurs in patients with low cardiac output and has a 50% mortality.[80] There are two main reasons why DIC is not a frequent complication of CPB. One is the widespread use of hemodilution when clotting factors are decreased in the plasma secondary to the use of a crystalloid prime, and the other is the use of heparin to anticoagulate CPB patients.[81] Reinfusion of unwashed RBCs from cardiotomy suction promotes a higher incidence of coagulopathy, probably due to release of tissue thromboplastin at this site.[69] Therefore, reservoir blood washing as well as better surgical technique with less reservoir volume reinfusion results in fewer complications.

Heparin in CPB

Heparin is used to prevent blood from clotting in the oxygenator and to prevent the development of DIC.

In the first case, if blood must be used to prime the pump, heparin is added to citrate-phosphate-dextrose (CPD) units and recalcified with 0.8 ml of 10% calcium gluconate per 100 ml of CPD blood.[81] In the second case, the patient is heparinized systemically (200–300 units of heparin per kilogram of body weight).[82] Once the operation is completed and the patient can be taken off bypass, heparin neutralization with protamine is necessary to avoid hemorrhage. The usual dose is 1.5–2.5 mg of protamine per 1 mg of heparin given during the procedure.[83] Paradoxically, protamine has a mild anticoagulant effect even after neutralizing heparin, but this does not seem to result in increased bleeding.[84] The bleeding observed after heparin reversal is thought to be due to circulating nonneutralized heparin in the postbypass patient. Furthermore, the tissue distribution of heparin[85] apparently responsible for heparin rebound warrants increasing doses of protamine to neutralize this effect.[86]

Laboratory Control of Heparin

Although the thrombin time is a quite sensitive test to monitor heparin activity, the activated PTT is the laboratory test of choice to follow up CPB cases.[87] Monitoring with these tests does not help predict whether a patient will bleed or not, or how severe the bleeding will be.[88] A rapid test for anticoagulation that can be performed in the operating room is the Hemochron System (International Technidyne Corp., Metuchen, N.J.), which is essentially an activated clotting time (ACT).[89] This test is routinely performed in most centers to monitor heparin effect. The principle of the test is activation of factor XII by diatomaceous sand and glass beads. The tube is then put into the Hemochron reader, which automatically provides the clotting time values. The normal ACT range by this method for preoperative patients is 201–317 seconds.[90]

Thrombocytopenia and Platelet Disorders Resulting From CPB

Most patients undergoing CPB surgery develop some degree of thrombocytopenia, which may last up to 8 days.[91,92] However, a postbypass platelet count does not necessarily reveal the degree of platelet damage and malfunction.[93] A template bleeding time is essential to get a clear picture of true platelet function in vivo. The platelet depletions and abnormalities developing during bypass are multifactorial.

Platelets may decrease as a direct heparin effect,[94] by sequestration in the liver,[95] or by platelet deposition on foreign surfaces.[96] Platelet levels usually decrease sharply at the beginning of bypass to as low as 26% of prebypass levels[97] and then stabilize to about 70% of prebypass levels[95] if the pump run is not too long (i.e., 2 hours).

Replacement Therapy in Open Heart Surgery

The hematocrit (Hct) which a patient will have upon starting bypass can be calculated as follows:[69]

$$\text{New Hct} = \frac{\text{TBV} \times \text{Hct} \times 0.91 \times 100}{\text{TBV} + \text{AV}}$$

where TBV is the total blood volume (which is equal to body weight $\times$ blood volume in ml/kg), 0.91 is the correction value for central hematocrit, and AV is the volume added during perfusion.

If 1,000 ml of prime is added to the volume of a 70-kg individual with a blood volume of 50 ml/kg (normal = 70 ml/kg) and an initial hematocrit of 42%, the predicted hematocrit is figured as follows:

$$\frac{70 \times 50 \times .42 \times 0.91 \times 100}{70 \times 50 + 1,000} = 29.72\%$$

The new hematocrit will be about 30%. Incrementing the hematocrit before CPB requires evaluating whether the patient can tolerate low hematocrit levels. Experience has shown that correcting the plasma clotting factors, hematocrit, and oncotic pressure is not warranted in most patients in the prebypass period unless the hematocrit drops below 25%.[69] However, if blood is used, packed RBCs rather than whole blood should be used in the oxygenator. Residual pump fluid after bypass can be washed by centrifugation to recover most of the RBCs, which can be reinfused after bypass. Approximately 44% of patients undergoing bypass may not have to be transfused if adequate technique is used.

The use of whole blood is not warranted during bypass.[69] This has been proved with the use of hemodilution techniques in CPB, where hemodilution is considered a beneficial practice.[98]

Use of FFP has traditionally been relegated to the postbypass period after the heparin effect has been reversed with protamine, for FFP has no function as long as heparin is circulating in the patient. The rationale for using FFP has stemmed from the assumption that since the patient has been infused with banked blood, replacement with FFP is warranted. However, most studies have not been controlled with PT, PTT, and thrombin time values. For rational component therapy, these coagulation tests should be done before using FFP. If the patient is actively bleeding, a mechanical cause can be ruled out, and if a template bleeding time is normal, use of FFP can be attempted to curtail bleeding. However, FFP should be used scientifically, not as an automatic response to a bleeding patient.

The use of cryoprecipitate is usually warranted when dangerously low levels of fibrinogen are present. This can be assessed only by measuring fibrinogen, which should be done before the patient is exposed unnecessarily to several units of cryoprecipitate.

Platelets should be administered only after the patient has been weaned from CPB. It is useless to infuse platelets earlier, as they will only be damaged in the oxygenator. As with plasma, use of platelets after bypass should not be automatic. A platelet count and a template bleeding time should be determined if the patient is to be treated rationally. The only reason for transfusing platelets without first performing these tests is life-threatening hemorrhage, which, by the way, is almost always mechanical in origin in CPB.

In vivo hemostatic platelet function is normal in about 90% of patients in the postbypass period.[99] The decision to reoperate is based on the absence of coagulation or platelet abnormalities that could explain continuous excessive bleeding through the drainage tubes (75 ml/hour or more).[69]

A protamine titration and activated PTT studies are useful in the diagnosis. If coagulation profiles and platelet function studies are abnormal, FFP and platelets may be warranted. Additional protamine may correct the bleeding tendency. If fibrinogen is low, less than 100 mg/100 ml, then cryoprecipitate is indicated. Reexploration must not be postponed if all these studies appear normal and the patient continues to lose blood.

Hemolysis

Hemolysis is another complication of CPB. It may be produced mechanically by the pump[96] or when blood makes contact with the pericardium or the pleural surface.[100]

BLOOD COMPONENTS IN PATIENTS WITH CANCER

Patients with a variety of neoplasms (including leukemia) frequently develop anemia, leukopenia, and thrombocytopenia, either as a direct result of disease or as a side effect of the therapy. Since patients on certain chemotherapy protocols almost invariably develop these complications, phenotyping and HLA typing of these individuals and their families should be done at an early stage.

RBC Transfusions

RBCs are usually given as packed cells in cancer patients unless a massive transfusion must be given. Granulocyte-poor units should be given whenever possible. This delays the development of unpleasant febrile transfusion reactions. The use of microaggregate filters eliminates unwanted WBCs, and combining this method with centrifugation may abrogate most WBC febrile reactions. In-line integrated filter sets are more economical. Premedicating cancer patients with Tylenol may also prevent febrile transfusion reactions. Although these preventative measures may add to the unit cost of the blood, they pay off in the long run by making these very ill patients more comfortable and by decreasing the time spent on laboratory workups. The advantage of early RBC phenotyping is obvious, as these patients often have multiple transfusions at a later stage in therapy, making crossmatching more difficult. Frozen-thawed blood is used in patients who have severe reactions to granulocytes or who require special units, to avoid certain RBC antigens they have become sensitized to.

Platelet Transfusions

Before platelet transfusions became available, thrombocytopenia was a major cause of death in patients with neoplastic diseases. Today patients can be supported for long periods of time by using platelet units. There is an increased likelihood of spontaneous bleeding in patients with neoplastic disease when platelet counts reach 20,000/μl,[101] and 26% of patients will develop major bleeding when the count reaches 10,000/μl.[102] Giving approximately 5 or 10 units to patients with counts of 25,000 prophylactically to avoid bleeding seems to have comparable results, with the obvious advantage of requiring lower doses.[102]

A major problem that can develop with platelet therapy is the appearance of a refractory state, in which patients no longer respond with increments in their peripheral count. Although the appearance of the refractory stage is variable, it may develop as early as 1 week or 10 days after the initiation of therapy. Therefore, if the patient is not bleeding, it is a good practice to allow the platelet count to drop to approximately 20,000. Thereafter therapy can be started with random donor platelets. Many physicians have heard about HLA-matched platelets and like the novelty of the term, but it is not a good practice to initiate transfusions with HLA-matched platelets without using random donor platelets first, and then proving that this type of platelet preparation does not produce hemostasis. This will save HLA platelets for the patient in later stages of disease, when random units are no longer effective. Platelets from both related and nonrelated HLA-matched donors may prove effective.[103] However, patients matched for HLA antigens may not respond to HLA-matched platelets due to the development of platelet-specific antibodies.[104] If HLA-matched donors cannot be recruited, siblings should always be tried as donors before parents.[105] These units are usually obtained by automated plateletpheresis. This procedure is very time-consuming, uncomfortable, and potentially dangerous to the donor—all factors that must be considered before subjecting donors to this ordeal. It is a good practice to give donors a full information package before starting a therapy for a recipient. Relatives will usually cooperate, but if HLA-matched nonrelated donors can be found every effort should be made to relieve the burden on the relatives if they must donate more than once a week but not to discourage them from donation. These components have a 24-hour expiration time. Therefore, hepatitis and HTLV-III testing of the donor is usually performed beforehand and repeated at least every 4 months, along with a review of cumulative laboratory data for donor suitability.[106] A consent form must always be signed.[107] Once the plateletpheresis procedure is completed, the platelets must be made available to the patient as soon as possible to avoid expiration of the component. These units are stirred under gentle rotation in a room-temperature, 22° C incubator. The possibility of using frozen deglycerolized platelets[108] or platelets stored in DMSO[109] in the frozen state has been studied. However, up to 70% attrition of viable platelets may occur, so the procedure remains experimental.

Platelet therapy is best assessed by combining the platelet count with a template bleeding time. The latter test is very useful, because in some cases, even though platelet counts may not increase in the periphery, the units will improve hemostasis.

Complications of Platelet Transfusion Therapy.—Patients who receive platelets on a chronic basis develop complications other than the

refractory state. These complications are frequently in the form of febrile and urticarial reactions, pulmonary infiltrates, or reactions to infused IgA in the suspending plasma. However, patients with neoplastic disease have special problems. They are frequently immunosuppressed and therefore are especially prone to infections (a problem now seen more frequently due to storage of platelets at room temperature).[110] Graft-versus-host disease (GVHD) due to infusion of viable lymphocytes in units of platelets is a dreaded complication which can be prevented by irradiating the units.[111] To prevent febrile reactions in patients who do not respond to premedication with Tylenol, a method for eliminating granulocytes from platelet units by slow centrifugation at 800 G has been developed and should be employed.[112] To avoid GVHD, platelet units must be irradiated with 2,000 rad before transfusion.[113] These units must be labeled "irradiated." Irradiation of units should be available on a 24-hour basis. Urticarial reactions and other plasma-related reactions can be minimized by using washed platelets.[114]

Transfusion of Granulocytes to Leukopenic Patients

After thrombocytopenia, probably the most ominous complication seen in patients treated with chemotherapy is the development of infection due to leukopenia.[115] This complication has been recently treated with granulocyte transfusions. Granulocyte transfusions are effective if given continuously for at least 5 days. A dose-related response is noted, and therefore 8–15 units of granulocytes are administered daily. A culture should show evidence of infection. Fever is not always a good indicator of the presence of infection, because many leukopenic patients have fever for other reasons (e.g., tissue necrosis). All components potentially containing viable WBCs and which are given to immunosuppressed individuals must be irradiated to prevent GVHD; 2,000–3,000 rad is an optimal dose.

As stated above, granulocytes have a 24-hour expiration time. If they are obtained from random donors, they should be given as pools of 2 or 3 units. Granulocytes are never infused through a microaggregate filter. If possible, granulocytes should be HLA matched, unless the patient is awaiting a bone marrow transplant, in which case it might be advisable to curtail transfusions, if possible.

Granulocyte units are always crossmatched with the patient's serum to avoid RBC reactions caused by RBC contamination of these units. The two best methods for obtaining granulocytes are the continuous-flow centrifugation method and the discontinuous-flow centrifugation method. Both of these are made easier by premedication with steroids and hydroxyethyl starch (for details, see Chap. 8).

Filtration leukapheresis is no longer employed to obtain granulocytes, for it yields mostly nonfunctional WBCs.

Other Complications in Patients with Neoplasms

Patients with neoplasms often develop acute or chronic DIC. This complication is very serious. Supportive therapy with FFP and cryoprecipitate as well as platelets may be necessary. The use of heparin may be considered for selected patients.

OTHER DISEASES IN WHICH SPECIAL TRANSFUSION PRACTICES ARE RECOMMENDED

There are other diseases which often require direct consultation between the treating physician and the blood bank physician. A few selected diseases requiring special transfusion techniques are reviewed below.

Autoimmune Hemolytic Anemia

One of the most agonizing problems in blood banking is when to transfuse a patient with warm autoimmune hemolytic anemia. These patients are virtually "uncrossmatchable." The clinician must decide if the development of hemolysis is acute and rapidly progressive or stable and tolerated. It has been shown that patients with warm autoimmune hemolytic anemia tolerate low levels of hemoglobin relatively well if bed rest is employed.[116] Furthermore, these patients may respond to steroids quite quickly after therapy is instituted.[117] Hemoglobin levels maintained at 8–11 gm/100 ml are considered optimal in these patients.[118] However, severe anemia with hemoglobin levels of 4 gm/100 ml or a hematocrit of 12% usually results in angina and/or neurologic symptoms.[118] These patients must be treated with transfusions in the form of packed cells.[118]

Blood for these patients must be phenotyped using special techniques, such as warm autoabsorption[119] and differential absorption techniques.[118] The Rh of the patient is always respected in these cases.[118] The workup of patients with warm autoimmune hemolytic anemia is very difficult and best undertaken by laboratories in large hospitals and reference centers.

Once alloantibodies have been ruled out (if this is possible), the next step is to select a compatible unit. Many blood bankers eventually release the least incompatible unit. However, in vivo compatibility testing is probably the test that best indicates how long a unit will survive in the circulation.[120] If the least incompatible units have a shortened survival time, they should still be transfused to relieve the patient's symptoms.[119] Transfusing patients who have hemoglobin values above 10 gm/100 ml and who are not severely symptomatic (do not have angina or neurologic symptoms) is a poor practice and may ruin the patient's chance for treatment when severe symptoms appear. Relief of symptoms is achieved in some patients by infusion of as little as 100 ml of blood, which can be given twice daily,[121] and the hemoglobin level may not have to be raised above 8 gm/100 ml.[121]

Transfusion of Patients with Cold Autoimmune Hemolysis.—Compatibility testing for these patients is performed using the warm technique at 37° C.[118] Cold autoabsorption may be necessary, but this technique is time-consuming if blood is needed urgently.[119] Other methods to study alloantibodies in these patients are mercaptoethanol IgM inactivation[122] and the dithiothreitol method.[123] These patients may have to be transfused in a warmed room (37° C) and the blood transfused through a blood warmer.[118] Steroids[124] and splenectomy[125, 126] are less effective in cold than in warm autoimmune hemolytic anemia and are not routinely used. Plasma exchange has been attempted.[127] These patients must avoid cold temperatures, to the extent of changing their residence (see Chap. 10).[118]

Components in Renal and Bone Marrow Transplantation

It has been reported that patients undergoing cadaver kidney transplant and who have received more than 10 blood transfusions have a better successful transplant rate than those who never receive transfusion.[128] In one series patients who did not develop cytotoxins after 10 blood transfusions had a greater success rate than those who did develop cytotoxins. The conclusion of these rather surprising findings is that patients who tolerate the graft better have developed immune unresponsiveness.[129] This finding has been documented experimentally in rhesus monkeys matched at the A and B loci of their histocompatibility antigen system. One group was pretransfused and another was not. Immunosuppressive therapy was given to the two study groups but not to a control group. The pretransfused group showed a fourfold increase in mean survival time. Immunosuppressive therapy did not alter survival.[130]

In contrast, patients awaiting bone marrow transplantation must not be transfused. Transfusion in these patients reduces the chance of a good transplant outcome,[131] probably by sensitization to minor histocompatibility antigens.[132] Bone marrow grafting is done with marrow from donors who are ABO and HLA compatible. Large volumes of bone marrow are required (250–900 cc). Complications include graft rejection (30% in patients with aplastic anemia[133]) and GVHD (in about 70% of bone marrow recipients).[134, 135]

Experimental Stem Cell Transplant.—It is possible now to obtain stem cells capable of repopulating the bone marrow via cytapheresis of peripheral blood. This method may replace the way in which bone marrow grafts are currently performed.

PLATELETPHERESIS AND CYTAPHERESIS PRACTICES

Chapters 8 and 9 examined this topic in detail. The following section reviews basic apheresis practices and topics not covered elsewhere.

All requests for apheresis must be cleared by the blood bank physician. This is especially important in therapeutic plasmapheresis.

The following criteria must be met:[136]
1. Valid reasons for performing the procedure.
2. Choice of appropriate technique.
3. Adequate equipment and knowledgeable staff.
4. Monitoring of parameters to be changed by the apheresis procedure.
5. A signed consent form bearing an explanation of the procedure.

Therapeutic plasmapheresis is accepted for the following diseases: (1) Multiple myeloma and macroglobulinemia. These diseases can be treated by plasmapheresis when hyperviscosity is present secondary to disease (i.e., when viscosity is above 3 when compared to water at 37° C[137] or when hemostatic complications due to paraproteins are present).[136] Plasmapheresis in these diseases is only supportive. (2) Cryoglobulinemia[138] plasmapheresis is performed to remove immune complexes (IC), which results in temporary improvement. (3) Thrombotic thrombocytopenic purpura. Plasmapheresis is probably beneficial because it removes IC and because of infusion of special factors in FFP used as replacement,[139] though some authors consider the use of plasmapheresis in TTP still controversial. (4) In Goodpasture's disease, plasmapheresis removes causative antibodies.[140]

Use of plasmapheresis is to date investigational in primary biliary cirrhosis, thyrotoxicosis, myasthenia gravis, amyotrophic lateral sclerosis, factor VIII inhibitors, idiopathic thrombocytopenic purpura, hemolytic disease of the newborn, pemphigus, systemic lupus erythematosus, rheumatoid arthritis, and polyarteritis. Therefore, its use is not accepted practice and requires controlled research protocols.

Therapeutic phlebotomy is an accepted practice in polycythemia vera[141] and in hemochromatosis.[142]

Therapeutic Leukapheresis

This procedure is acceptable to remove large numbers of WBCs to prevent leukostasis, such as might occur in acute myelogenous leukemia.[143] Therapeutic leukapheresis in other hematologic disorders such as chronic lymphocytic leukemia must be considered experimental.[144]

REFERENCES

1. Mayer K.: *Guidelines to Transfusion Practices.* Washington, D.C., American Association of Blood Banks, 1980, pp. 1–9.
2. Dietrich E.B.: Evaluation of blood transfusion. *Transfusion* 5:82, 1965.
3. Borucki D.T. (ed.): *Blood Component Therapy: A Physicians Handbook,* ed. 3. Washington, D.C., American Association of Blood Banks, 1981, p. 5.
4. Schmidt P.J.: Red cells for transfusion. *N. Engl. J. Med.* 299:1411, 1978.
5. Masouredis S.P.: Preservation and clinical use of erythrocytes and whole blood, in Williams W.J., et al. (eds.): *Hematology,* ed. 2. New York, McGraw-Hill Book Co., 1977, chap. 166.
6. Greenwalt T.J.: *General Principles of Blood Transfusion.* Chicago, Ill., American Medical Association, 1978.
7. Widman F.K. (ed.): *Technical Manual of the American Association of Blood Banks,* ed. 8. Washington, D.C., American Association of Blood Banks, 1981, pp. 263–288.
8. Rigor B., Bosomworth P., Rush B.F. Jr.: Replacement of operative blood loss of more than 1 liter with Hartman's solution. *JAMA* 203:111, 1968.
9. Gardner R.J.: Blood loss after fractures of the hip. *JAMA* 208:1005, 1969.
10. Gollub S., Bailey C.P.: Management of major surgical blood loss without transfusion. *JAMA* 198:1171, 1966.
11. Mendelson J.A.: The selection of plasma volume expanders for mass casualty planning. *J. Trauma* 14:987, 1974.
12. Caggiano V.: Red blood cell transfusions, in Silver H. (ed.): *Blood, Blood Components and Derivatives in Transfusion Therapy: A Technical Workshop.* Washington, D.C., American Association of Blood Banks, 1980, pp. 1–28.
13. Mollison P.L.: *Blood Transfusion in Clinical Medicine,* ed. 7. Oxford, England, Blackwell Scientific Publications, 1983, pp. 118–119.
14. Honig C.L., Bove J.R.: Transfusion-associated fatalities: Review of Bureau of Biologics reports 1976–1978. *Transfusion* 20:653, 1980.
15. Solis R.T., Wurzel H.A.: Equipment, devices and instruments associated with transfusion therapy, in Mayer K. (ed.): *Guidelines to Transfusion Practices.* Washington, D.C., American Association of Blood Banks, 1980, pp. 15–23.
16. Gill W.: Volume resuscitation in critical major trauma, in Guy R.L. (ed.): *Transfusion Therapy: A Technical Workshop.* Washington, D.C., American Association of Blood Banks, 1974, p. 77.
17. Scopes J.W.: Intraperitoneal transfusion of blood in newborn babies. *Lancet* 1:1027, 1963.
18. Tocantins L.M., O'Neill J.F.: Infusion of blood and other fluids into the general circulation via the bone marrow: Technique and results. *Surg. Gynecol. Obstet.* 73:281, 1941.
19. Mollison P.L.: *Blood Transfusion in Clinical Medicine,* ed. 7. Oxford, England, Blackwell Scientific Publications, 1983, p. 127.
20. Braude A.I., Carey F.J., Siemenski J.: Studies of bacterial transfusion reactions from refrigerated blood: The properties of cold growing bacteria. *J. Clin. Invest.* 34:311, 1955.
21. Solis R.T., Walker B.D., in *International Forum: Does a Relationship Exist Between Massive Blood Transfusions and the Adult Respiratory Distress Syndrome? Vox Sang.* 32:319, 1977.
22. Harker L., Slichter S.: The bleeding time as a

screening test for evaluation of platelet function. *N. Engl. J. Med.* 287:155, 1972.
23. Snyder E.L., Grum P., Cooper-Smith M., et al.: Transfusion of platelets through microaggregate filters. *Anesthesiology* 51(suppl.): S205, 1979.
24. Grumet F.C., Yankee R.A.: Long term platelet support of patients with aplastic anemia. *Ann. Intern. Med.* 73:1, 1970.
25. Harker L.A.: The role of platelet thrombokinetics. *J. Lab. Clin. Med.* 77:247, 1971.
26. Cohen D., Weinstein H., Mihm M., et al.: Non fatal graft-versus host disease occurring after transfusion with leukocytes and platelets obtained from normal donors. *Blood* 53:1053, 1979.
27. Schmidt P. (ed.): *Standards for Blood Banks and Transfusion Services,* ed. 11. Arlington, Va., American Association of Blood Banks, 1984, p. 26, 27.
28. Schmidt P. (ed.): *Standards for Blood Banks and Transfusion Services,* ed. 11. Arlington, Va., American Association of Blood Banks, 1984, p. 30, 31.
29. Blatt P.M., Brinkhouse K.M., Culp H.R., et al.: Antihemophilic factor concentrate therapy in von Willebrand's disease. *JAMA* 236:2770, 1976.
30. Cederbaum A.I.: The appropriate use of plasma and plasma components in clinical medicine, in Silver H. (ed.): *Blood, Blood Components and Derivatives in Transfusion Therapy: A Technical Workshop.* Washington, D.C., American Association of Blood Banks, 1980, pp. 105–131.
31. Andersen B.R., Terry W.D.: Gamma G4-globulin antibody causing inhibition of clotting factor VIII. *Nature* 217:174, 1968.
32. Cederbaum A.I., Blatt P.M., Levine P.H.: Abnormal serum transaminase levels in patients with hemophilia, quoted by Cederbaum A.I.: The appropriate use of plasma and plasma components in clinical medicine, in Silver H. (ed.): *Blood, Blood Components and Derivatives in Transfusion Therapy: A Technical Workshop.* Washington, D.C., American Association of Blood Banks, 1980, p. 119.
33. Orringer E.P., Koury M.H., Blatt P.M., et al.: Hemolysis caused by factor VIII concentrates. *Arch. Intern. Med.* 136:1018, 1976.
34. Solis T.R., Smith D., Barker L.F.: Transfusion of plasma and plasma derivatives, including albumin, in Mayer K. (ed.): *Guidelines to Transfusion Practices.* Washington, D.C., American Association of Blood Banks, 1980, pp. 101–108.
35. Borucki D.T. (ed.): *Blood Component Therapy: A Physician's Handbook,* ed. 3. Washington, D.C., American Association of Blood Banks, 1981, pp. 34–36.
36. Hoofnagle J.H., Seeff L.B., Bales Z.B., et al.: Passive-active immunity from hepatitis B immunoglobulin. *Ann. Intern. Med.* 91:813, 1979.
37. Silver H.: Normal serum albumin and plasma protein fraction, in Silver H. (ed.): *Blood, Blood Components and Derivatives in Transfusion Therapy: A Technical Workshop.* Washington, D.C., American Association of Blood Banks, 1980, pp. 89–95.
38. Mayer K.: Crystalloids versus colloid, in Silver H. (ed.): *Blood, Blood Components and Derivatives in Transfusion Therapy: A Technical Workshop.* Washington, D.C., American Association of Blood Banks, 1980. p. 97.
39. Lucas C.E., Ledgerwood A.M., Higgins R.F.: Impaired salt and water excretion after albumin resuscitation for hypovolemic shock. *Surgery* 86:544, 1979.
40. Cervera A.L., Moss G.: Crystalloid distribution following hemorrhage and hemodilution: Mathematical model and prediction of optimum volumes for equilibration at normovolemia. *J. Trauma* 14:506, 1974.
41. Weaver D.W., Ledgerwood A.M., Lucas C.E., et al.: Pulmonary effects of albumin resuscitation for severe hypovolemic shock. *Arch. Surg.* 113:387, 1978.
42. Virgilio R.W., Rice C.L., Smith D.E., et al.: Crystalloid vs. colloid resuscitation: Is one better? *Surgery* 85:129, 1979.
43. Tullis J.L.: Albumin: 1. Background and use. 2. Guidelines for clinical use. *JAMA* 237:355, 1977.
44. International Forum: *Can a National All Voluntary Blood Transfusion Service by Adequate Blood Component Therapy Cover Actual Future Needs of Albumin? Vox Sang.* 31:225, 1976.
45. Gill W., Champion H.R.: Volume resuscitation in critical major trauma, in Guy R.L. (ed.): *Transfusion Therapy: A Technical Workshop,* Washington, D.C., American Association of Blood Banks, 1974, pp. 77–105.
46. Shoemaker W.C.: Pathophysiologic basis for therapy of shock and trauma syndromes. *Semin. Drug Treat.* 3:211, 1973.
47. Shenkin H.S.: On the diagnosis of hemorrhage in man: A study on volunteers bled large amounts. *Am. J. Med. Sci.* 208:421, 1944.
48. Sohmer P.R.: The pathophysiology of hemorrhagic shock, in Barns A. Jr. (ed.): *Hemotherapy in Trauma and Surgery: A Technical Workshop.* Washington, D.C., American Association of Blood Banks, 1979, p. 1.
49. Zinner M.J., Gurll N.J., Reynolds D.G.: The effect of hemorrhagic shock and resuscitation on regional blood flow in cynomulgus monkeys. *Circ. Shock* 4:291, 1977.
50. Lillehi R.C., Dietzman R.C.: Circulatory collapse and shock, in Schwartz S.I., et al (eds.): *Principles of Surgery,* ed. 2. New York, McGraw-Hill Book Co., 1974, p. 133.
51. Peart W.S.: Renin-angiotensin system. *N. Engl. J. Med.* 292:302, 1975.
52. Weinstein H., Berne R.M., Sachs H.S.: Vasopressin in blood: Effect of hemorrhage. *Endocrinology* 66:712, 1960.
53. Collins J.A.: Massive blood transfusion. *Clin. Haematol.* 5:201, 1976.
54. Sheldon G.F.: Hemotherapy in a trauma center, in Barns A. Jr. (ed.): *Hemotherapy in Trauma and Sur-*

gery: A Technical Workshop. Washington, D.C., American Association of Blood Banks, 1979, p. 17.
55. Counts R.B., Haisch C., Simon T.L., et al.: Hemostasis in massively transfused trauma patients. Ann. Surg. 190:91, 1979.
56. Howland W.S.: Calcium, potassium and pH changes during massive transfusion, in Nusbacher J. (eds.): Massive Transfusions: A Symposium. Washington, D.C., American Association of Blood Banks, 1978, p. 17.
57. Howland W.S., Schweizer O., Carlon G.C., et al.: The cardiovascular effects of low levels of ionized calcium during massive transfusion. Surg. Gynecol. Obstet. 145:581, 1977.
58. Smith N.T., Corbascio A.N.: The interaction of potassium and calcium on the isolated guinea pig atrium. Fed. Proc. 23:326, 1964.
59. Sheldon G.F.: Massive transfusion: A metabolic and hemodynamic lesion. Surg. Forum 24:17, 1973.
60. Collins J.A.: Massive transfusion: What is current and important, in Nusbacher J. (ed.): Massive Transfusion 1978. Washington, D.C., American Association of Blood Banks, 1978, p. 2.
61. McConn R.: Massive transfusion and its effect on hemodynamic function in the recipient, in Barns A. Jr. (ed.): Massive Transfusion 1978: A Symposium. Washington, D.C., American Association of Blood Banks, 1978, p. 25.
62. Barnes A. Jr. (ed.): The Blood Bank in Hemotherapy for Trauma and Surgery: A Technical Workshop. Washington, D.C., American Association of Blood Banks, 1979, p. 77.
63. Schmidt P. (ed.): Standards for Blood Banks and Transfusion Services, ed. 11. Washington, D.C., American Association of Blood Banks, 1984, pp. 29, 30.
64. Mayer K.: A different view of transfusion safety: Type and screen, transfusion of Coombs incompatible cells, fatal transfusion-induced graft-versus-host disease, in Polesky H.F., Walker R.H., (eds.): Safety in Transfusion Practices. Skokie, Ill., College of American Pathologists, 1982.
65. Rapaport S.I.: Defibrination syndromes, in Williams W.J., et al. (eds.): Hematology, ed. 2. New York, McGraw-Hill Book Co., 1977, chap. 161.
66. Colman R.W., Robboy S.J., Minna J.D.: Disseminated intravascular coagulation: A reappraisal. Annu. Rev. Med. 30:359, 1979.
67. Gaston L.W.: Component use in the treatment of disseminated intravascular coagulation, in Silver H. (ed.): Blood, Blood Components and Derivatives in Transfusion Therapy: A Technical Workshop. Washington, D.C., American Association of Blood Banks, 1980, p. 211.
68. Roche J.K., Stengle J.M.: Open heart surgery and the demand for blood. JAMA 225:1516, 1973.
69. Fleming A.W., Garcia C.S.: Use of blood components in cardiac surgery, in Silver H. (ed.): Blood, Blood Components and Derivatives in Transfusion Therapy: A Technical Workshop. Washington, D.C., American Association of Blood Banks, 1980, p. 173.
70. Tector A.J., Gabriel R.P., Matericka W.E., et al.: Reduction of blood usage in open heart surgery. Chest 70:454, 1976.
71. Milam J.D., Austin S.F.: Red cell salvage in open heart surgery, in Barns A. Jr. (ed.): Hemotherapy in Trauma and Surgery: A Technical Workshop. Washington, D.C., American Association of Blood Banks, 1979, pp. 67–75.
72. Heiden D., Mielke C.H. Jr., Rodvien R., et al.: Platelets, hemostasis and thromboembolism during treatment of acute respiratory insufficiency with extracorporeal membrane oxygenation. J. Thorac. Cardiovasc. Surg. 70:644, 1975.
73. Cohn L.H., Klovekorn P., Moore F.D., et al.: Intrinsic plasma volume deficits in patients with coronary artery disease. Arch. Surg. 108:57, 1974.
74. Pike O.M., Marquiss J.E., Weiner R.S., et al.: A study of platelet counts during cardiopulmonary bypass. Transfusion 12:119, 1972.
75. Cooley D.A., Beall A.C. Jr., Gronden P.: Open heart operations with disposable oxygenators: 5% dextrose prime and normothermia. Surgery 52:713, 1962.
76. Johnson W.D., Flemma R.J., Manley J.C., et al.: The physiologic parameters of ventricular function as affected by direct coronary surgery. J. Thorac. Cardiovasc. Surg. 60:483, 1970.
77. Marengo-Rowe A.J., Lambert C.J., Leveson J.E., et al.: The evaluation of hemorrhage in cardiac patients who have undergone extracorporeal circulation. Transfusion 19:426, 1979.
78. Kevy S.V., Glickman R.M., Bernhard W.F., et al.: The pathogenesis and the control of the hemorrhagic defect in open heart surgery. Surg. Gynecol. Obstet. 123:313, 1966.
79. Phillips L.L., Malm J.R., Deterline R.A.: Coagulation defects following extracorporeal circulation. Ann. Surg. 157:317, 1963.
80. Boyd A.D., Engelman R.M., Beaudet R.L., et al.: Disseminated intravascular coagulation following extracorporeal circulation. J. Thorac. Cardiovasc. Surg. 64:685, 1972.
81. Solis R.T.: Extracorporeal circulation, in Mayer K. (ed.): Guidelines to Transfusion Practices. Washington, D.C., American Association of Blood Banks, 1980, p. 83.
82. Bull B.S., Korpman R.A., Huse W.M., et al.: Heparin therapy during extracorporeal circulation: I. Problems inherent in existing heparin protocols. J. Thorac. Cardiovasc. Surg. 69:674, 1975.
83. Douglas A.S., McNicol G.P., Bain W.H., et al.: The haemostatic defect following extracorporeal circulation. Br. J. Surg. 53:455, 1963.
84. Ellison N., Ominsky A.J., Wollman H.: Is protamine a clinically important anticoagulant? Anesthesiology 35:621, 1971.
85. Gollub S.: Heparin rebound in open heart surgery. Surg. Gynecol. Obstet. 124:337, 1967.

86. Ellison N., Beatty C.P., Blake D.R., et al.: Heparin rebound. *J. Thorac. Cardiovasc. Surg.* 67:723, 1974.
87. Spector I., Corn M.: Control of heparin therapy with activated partial thromboplastin times. *JAMA* 201:75, 1967.
88. Bauer G.: Clinical experience of a surgeon in the use of heparin. *Am. J. Cardiol.* 14:29, 1964.
89. Hill J.D., Dontigny L., DeLeval M., et al.: A simple method for heparin management during prolonged extracorporeal circulation. *Ann. Thorac. Surg.* 17:129, 1974.
90. Schriever H.G., Epstein S.E., Mintz M.D.: Statistical correlation and heparin sensitivity of activated partial thromboplastin time, whole blood coagulation time, and automated coagulation time. *Am. J. Clin. Pathol.* 60:323, 1973.
91. Schmidt P.J., Peden J.C. Jr., Brecher G., et al.: Thrombocytopenia and bleeding tendency after extracorporeal circulation. *N. Engl. J. Med.* 265:1181, 1961.
92. de Leval M.R., Hill J.D., Mielke C.H. Jr., et al.: Blood platelets and extracorporeal circulation. *J. Thorac. Cardiovasc. Surg.* 69:144, 1975.
93. Hardin S.A., Shakoor M.A., Grindon A.J.: Platelet support for cardiopulmonary bypass surgery. *J. Thorac. Cardiovasc. Surg.* 70:350, 1975.
94. Gollub S., Ulin A.W.: Heparin-induced thrombocytopenia in man. *J. Lab. Clin. Med.* 59:430, 1962.
95. de Leval M., Hill J.D., Mielke H., et al.: Platelet kinetics during extracorporeal circulation. *Trans. Am. Soc. Artif. Intern. Organs* 18:355, 1972.
96. Andersen M.N., Kuchiba K.: Blood trauma produced by pump oxygenators. *J. Thorac. Cardiovasc. Surg.* 57:238, 1969.
97. de Jong J.C., ten Duis H.J., Smit Sibinga C.T., et al.: Hematologic aspects of cardiotomy suction in cardiac operations. *J. Thorac. Cardiovasc. Surg.* 79:227, 1980.
98. Messmer K.: Hemodilution. *Surg. Clin. North Am.* 55:659, 1975.
99. Umlas J.: In vivo platelet function following cardiopulmonary bypass. *Transfusion* 15:596, 1975.
100. Morris K.N., Kinross F.M., Stirling G.R.: Hemolysis of blood in the pericardium: The major source of plasma hemoglobin during total body perfusion. *J. Thorac. Cardiovasc. Surg.* 49:250, 1965.
101. Gaydos L.A., Freireich E.J., Mantel N.: The quantitative relation between platelet count and hemorrhage in patients with acute leukemia. *N. Engl. J. Med.* 266:905, 1962.
102. Roy A.J., Jaffen N., Djerassi I.: Prophylactic platelet transfusions in children with acute leukemia: A dose response study. *Transfusion* 13:283, 1973.
103. Yankee R.A., Grumet F.C., Rogentine G.N.: Platelet transfusion therapy: The selection of compatible platelet donors for refractory patients by lymphocyte HLA typing. *N. Engl. J. Med.* 281:1208, 1969.
104. Bucher U., Weck A de, Spengler H., et al.: Platelet transfusion: Shortened survival of HL-A-identical platelets and failure of in vitro detection of antiplatelet antibodies after multiple transfusions. *Vox Sang.* 25:187, 1973.
105. Schiffer C.A., McCredie K.B.: Cell component therapy for patients with cancer, in Guy R.L. (ed.): *Transfusion Therapy: A Technical Workshop*. Washington, D.C., American Association of Blood Banks, 1974, p. 29.
106. Widman F.K. (ed.): *Technical Manual of the American Association of Blood Banks and Transfusion Services,* ed. 10. Washington, D.C., American Association of Blood Banks, 1981, pp. 24–25.
107. Schmidt P. (ed.): *Standards for Blood Banks and Transfusion Services,* ed. 10. Washington, D.C., American Association of Blood Banks, 1984, p. 21, 22.
108. Cohen P., Gardner F.H.: Platelet preservation: IV. Preservation of human platelet concentrates by controlled slow freezing in a glycerol medium. *N. Engl. J. Med.* 274:1400, 1966.
109. Djerassi I., Farber S., Roy A., et al.: Preparation and in vivo circulation of human platelets preserved with combined dimethyl sulfoxide and dextrose. *Transfusion* 6:572, 1966.
110. Buchholz D.H., Young V.M., Friedman N.R., et al.: Bacterial proliferation in platelet products stored at room temperature: Transfusion-induced *Enterobacter* sepsis. *N. Engl. J. Med.* 285:429, 1971.
111. Hong R., Gatti R.A., Good R.A.: Hazards and potential benefits of blood transfusion in immunological deficiency. *Lancet* 2:388, 1968.
112. Herzig F.G.: Correction of poor platelet transfusion responses from donors matched for HL-A antigens. *Clin. Res.* 22:393, 1974.
113. Crosson J.T.: Platelet Transfusions, in Mayer K. (ed.): *Guidelines to Transfusion Practices*. Washington, D.C., American Association of Blood Banks, 1980, pp. 87–93.
114. Silvergleid A.J., Hafleigh E.B., Harabin M.A.: Clinical value of washed-platelet concentrates in patients with nonhemolytic transfusion reactions. *Transfusion* 17:33, 1976.
115. Levine A.S., Schimpff S.C., Graw R.G. Jr., et al.: Hematologic malignancies and other marrow failure states: Progress in the management of complicating infections. *Semin. Hematol.* 11:141, 1974.
116. Pirofsky B.: Immune haemolytic disease: The autoimmune haemolytic anaemias. *Clin. Haematol.* 4:167, 1975.
117. Pirofsky B.: Clinical aspects of autoimmune hemolytic anemia. *Semin. Hematol.* 13:251, 1976.
118. Petz L.D., Garraty G.: *Acquired Immune Hemolytic Anemias*. New York, Churchill Livingstone, 1980, pp. 358–391.
119. Petz L.D., Garraty G.: Laboratory correlations in immune hemolytic anemias, in Vyas G.N., et al. (eds.): *Laboratory Diagnosis of Immunologic Disorders*. New York, Grune & Stratton, 1975, p. 139.

120. Mayer K., Bettigole R.E., Harris J.P., et al.: Test in vivo to determine donor compatibility. *Transfusion* 8:28, 1968.
121. Rosenfield R.E., Jagathambal K.: Transfusion therapy for autoimmune hemolytic anemia. *Semin. Hematol.* 13:311, 1976.
122. Deutsch H.F., Morton J.I.: Dissociation of human serum macroglobulins. *Science* 125:600, 1957.
123. Pirofsky B., Rosner E.R.: DTT test: A new method to differentiate IgM and IgG erythrocyte antibodies. *Vox Sang.* 27:480, 1974.
124. Dacie J.V., Worlledge S.M.: Autoimmune hemolytic anemias. *Prog. Hematol.* 6:82, 1969.
125. Swisher S.N., Burk E.R.: Cryptopathic hemolytic syndromes, in Williams W.J., et al. (eds.): *Hematology*. New York, McGraw-Hill Book Co., 1977, p. 598.
126. Schubothe H.: The cold hemagglutinin disease. *Semin. Hematol.* 3:27, 1966.
127. Taft E.G., Propp R.P., Sullivan S.A.: Plasma exchanges for cold agglutinin hemolytic anemia. *Transfusion* 17:173, 1977.
128. Opelz G., Sengar D.P., Mickey M.R., et al.: Effect of blood transfusions on subsequent kidney transplants. *Transplant. Proc.* 5:253, 1973.
129. Opelz G., Terasaki P.I.: Poor kidney-transplant survival in recipients with frozen-blood transfusions or no transfusions. *Lancet* 2:696, 1974.
130. van Es A.A., et al.: Blood-transfusions induce prolonged kidney allograft survival in rhesus monkeys. *Lancet* 1:506, 1977.
131. Storb R., Epstein R.B., Rudolph R.H., et al.: The effect of prior transfusion on marrow grafts between histocompatible canine siblings. *J. Immunol.* 105:627, 1970.
132. Storb R., Thomas E.D., Buckner C.D., et al.: Allogeneic marrow grafting for treatment of aplastic anemia. *Blood* 43:157, 1974.
133. Storb R.: Aplastic anemia treated by allogeneic marrow transplantation, in Perkins H.A. (ed.): *Human Bone Marrow Transplantation: Symposium*. Washington, D.C., American Association of Blood Banks, 1976, p. 35.
134. Thomas E.D., Storb R., Clift R.A., et al.: Bone marrow transplantation. *N. Engl. J. Med.* 292:832, 1975.
135. Goldman J.M., Catovsky D., Hows J., et al.: Cryopreserved peripheral blood cells functioning as autografts in patients with chronic granulocytic leukaemia in transformation. *Br. Med. J.* 1:1310, 1979.
136. Reich L.M.: Therapeutic phlebotomy or removal of selected blood components (leukapheresis, plateletpheresis or exchange plasmapheresis), in Mayer K. (ed.): *Guidelines to Transfusion Practices*. Washington, D.C., American Association of Blood Banks, 1980, pp. 155–165.
137. Russell J.A., Toy J.L., Powels R.L.: Plasma exchange in malignant paraproteinemia. *Exp. Hematol.* 5:105, 1977.
138. Lockwood C.M.: Plasma exchange in cryoglobulinemia, quoted by Reich L.M., in Mayer K. (ed.): *Guidelines to Transfusion Practices*. Washington, D.C., American Association of Blood Banks, 1980, p. 155.
139. Bukowski R.M., King J.W., Hewlett J.S.: Plasmapheresis in the treatment of thrombotic thrombocytopenic purpura. *Blood* 50:413, 1977.
140. Lockwood C.M.: The treatment of Goodpasture's syndrome and glomerulonephritis. *Plasma Ther.* 1:19, 1979.
141. Dameshek W.: The case for phlebotomy in polycythemia vera: A panel discussion. *Blood* 32:488, 1968.
142. Williams R., Smith P.M., Spicer E.J., et al.: Venisection therapy in idiopathic hemochromatosis. *Q. J. Med.* 149:1, 1969.
143. Oliver R.T.D., Lister T.A., Russel J.: Leucopheresis in the management of patients with acute leukemia, in Goldman J.M., Lowenthal R.M. (eds.): *Leucocytes: Separation, Collection and Transfusion*. New York, Academic Press, Inc., 1975, p. 471.
144. Curtis J.E., Hersh E.M., Freireich E.J.: Leukapheresis therapy of chronic lymphocytic leukemia. *Blood* 39:163, 1972.

Index

A

ABH (*see* Blood groups, ABH)
ABO
  (*See also* Blood groups, ABO)
  incompatibility, and DIC, 89
  substances, chemical analysis of, 3
  transfusion reactions
    ABO hemolytic, 122
    ABO-incompatible, 88
Abortion: spontaneous, and anti-Tj^a antibodies, 159
Acanthocytes, 14
Acanthocytosis: in McLeod syndrome, 15
Acetaminophen: and platelet survival, 251
Acetylation, 76
Acetyl cholinesterase, 15
  platelet production and, 73
Acid
  -base equilibrium, 7
  hydrolases, 18
  load in banked blood, 339–340
  mucopolysaccharide, 18
  phosphatase, 18
    isoenzyme, 3, 38
Acidosis: diabetic, 16
Acquired immunodeficiency syndrome (*see* AIDS)
Acriflavin: natural, 152
Actin, 14, 20
  platelet, 74, 75
Actinomycin: effect on marrow, 42
Actomyosin, 74
  platelet aggregation in, 75
Addiction: drug, and blood donation, 237

Adenine: in RBC rejuvenation, 263
Adenosine
  deaminase, in paternity testing, 413
  diphosphate, 72
  monophosphate, 72
    cyclic, 22
Adenylate kinase: in paternity testing, 413–414
Adolescence: diffuse lymphoma during, 48
ADP, 72
  aspirin, 76
  in platelet aggregation, 74, 76, 77
  in platelet release type 1, 75
  receptor, platelets possessing, 75
Adrenalin, 28
Adriamycin: in acute myelogenous leukemia, 36
Adsorption: of plasma proteins, 316
African trypanosomiasis: transfusion transmitting, 344
Agammaglobulinemia
  acquired primary, 130
  X-linked Bruton type, in infant, 130
Age populations: hematologic values by, 6
Aged
  ABO system of, 153
  hematologic values in, 6
  hemoglobin in, 6
  marrow in, 6
  susceptibility to infection, 6
  T cells in, 6
Agglomeration method, 244

Agglutination, 2, 111, 215
  antibodies and, 110
    monoclonal, 113
  inhibition
    techniques for blood group A substances, 150
    test, RBC, 90
  isoantigen by anti-A and anti-B, 204
  latex agglutination test for hepatitis B surface antigen, 362
Agglutinin
  cold (*see* Cold agglutinin disease)
  IgM cold, 49
  peanut, 184
Aggregometer curves: of platelets, 77
Aggregometric studies, 76
Agnogenic myeloid metaplasia, 43
Agote, L., 1
Agranulocytosis
  etiology, 25
  genetic, in infant, 25, 26
  neutropenia in, 27
AIDS, 73, 130–131, 377–396
  autopsy findings in, 385
  blood banking and, 389–390
  blood components and, 379–380
  blood donation and, 237
  blood products and, 379–380
  clinical presentation, 385–386
  complications, 386
  drug abuse and, intravenous, 378
  epidemiology, 130, 377
  etiology, 380–383
  future developments, 391

483

AIDS (cont.)
  Haitians and, 380
  hematology workup in, 387
  hemophilia A and, 85
  hemophilia B and, 85
  hepatitis B vaccine and, 390–391
  histopathology of tissues from patients, 384–385
  homosexual males, 377–378
  immunologic lesion in, working hypothesis of, 383–384
  immunology workup in, 387
  impairment of macrophage killing capability in, 384
  incidence, 379, 380–383
  intimate contact with patients with AIDS, 378–379
  laboratory findings, 386–387
  lymphocytes in, ultrastructural changes, 385
  mortality, 378
  outcome in New York City, 378
  pathogenesis, 383–384
  pathology, 383–384
  prevention, 388–389
  risk factors, analysis of, 377–380
  sexual promiscuity in large metropolitan area and, 378
  signs, 378
  special recommendations for laboratories, 389
  symptoms, 378
  transmission, vertical, 380
  treatment, 388
  type I, 385
  type II, 385–386
  type III, 386
Air embolism (see Embolism, air)
Albumin
  anaphylaxis after, 260
  crystalloid vs. colloid, 466
  discussion of, 259–260
  practices with, 466
  vasoactive reactions to, 260
  zeta potential and, 205
Alcoholism, 75
Alder-Reiley anomaly, 23
Aldomet: causing immune hemolysis, 315–316
Aleutian disease virus, 50
Alkaline phosphatase, 30
  leukocyte, 32
  test, leukocyte, 28
Alkylating agents
  effect on marrow, 42
  in myeloma, plasma cell, 50
Alkylators, 41
Allelic gene: on chromosome, 399

Allergy
  basophils and, 22
  blood donation and, 238
  eosinophilia and, 21
Alloimmune neutropenia: in newborn, 436–437
Alloimmunization: assessment, 227
Allotypes, 16, 105–106
  heavy chain, 106
  Inv, 105
  transfusion reactions to, 105
Alpha$_2$-antiplasmin, 84
Alpha$_1$-antitrypsin, 83
Alpha-globulin inhibitor, 83
Alpha granules, 74, 90
  type 2 platelet release in, 75
Alpha$_2$-macroglobulin inhibitor, 83
Alpha-methyldopa: in immune hemolysis, 316
Amebiasis, 21
Aminco continuous flow centrifugation rotor: cross section of, 284
Amino acid
  groups, different, bonds produced by, 111
  sequences of heavy chains of immunoglobulin, 104
  terminal, of MNSs antigens, 161
Aminopyrine, 25
Ammonium load: and transfusion, 340
Amniocentesis: in hemolytic disease of newborn, 424
Amniotic fluid
  analysis in hemolytic disease of newborn, 424
  embolism, and DIC, 89
  spectrophotometry, 424–425, 426
  in meconium stain, 427
AMP, 72
Ampicillin, 25
Amyloidosis: in gammopathy, 131
Analgesics: and neutropenia, 25
Anaphylactic reactions, 21, 132
  to anti-immunoglobulin A antibodies, prevention of, 338
  epinephrine in, 132
  management, 132
Anaphylatoxin
  C5a as, 118
  1, 121
  2, 122
Anaphylaxis
  after albumin, 260
  anti-immunoglobulin A antibodies causing, 337
  in immunoglobulin A deficiency after cryoprecipitate, 337

  after platelet transfusion, 253
Androgens: in aplastic anemia, 9
Anemia
  α-hypochromic, 9
  aplastic, 8–9, 75
    causes, idiopathic, 9
    chronic, 9
    complicating paroxysmal nocturnal hemoglobinuria, 15
    endocrine diseases causing, 9
    infection causing, 9
    leukemia and, 30
    lymphocytopenia in, 29
    marrow transplant in, 265
    pancytopenia in, 28
    in preleukemia, 29
    transfusions in, 9
    treatment, 9
  blood donation in, 238
  causes of, main, 8
  of cold agglutinin disease
    pathophysiology, 310–311
    therapy of, 312
  enzyme defects causing, 17
  Fanconi's, in leukemia, 30
  in gammopathy, 131
  glucose metabolism defects causing, 14
  in hemoglobinuria, paroxysmal nocturnal, 15
  hemolytic
    autoimmune (see below)
    drug-induced, 123
    in G6PD deficiency, 16
    in lymphadenopathy, immunoblastic, 49
    in myeloid metaplasia, agnogenic, 43
    nonspherocytic, hereditary, 16
  hemolytic, autoimmune, 38, 123, 158, 303–313
    cold, 310–313
    Coombs test in, 2–4
    drug-induced, pathogenesis, 313
    in Hodgkin's disease, 45
    in SLE, 213
    tabular data on, 304
    transfusion in, 476–477
  hemolytic, autoimmune, warm-type, 44, 303–310
    clinical aspects, 306–307
    compatibility testing in, in vivo, drawbacks of, 308
    drug therapy of, 309
    immunohematology workup in, 308–309
    laboratory aspects, 306–307
    laboratory workup in, 308–309

monocyte in vitro assay in, 308
pathophysiology, 303–304
prognosis, 310
red blood cell survival studies in, 307–308
steroids in, 309
transfusion in, 309–310
hypochromic, 9
hemoglobin in, heme defect, 10
hemoglobin in, porphyrin defect, 10
iron deficiency, 9–10
iron store decrease causing, 9
in leukemia, chronic lymphocytic, 38
megaloblastic, 10
neutropenia of, 26
unresponsive to vitamin B12, 10–11
in myeloid metaplasia, agnogenic, 43
of newborn, 434–435
nonsideroblastic, in preleukemia, 29
packed red blood cells and, 241
pernicious
ABH antigens and, 154
gastric carcinoma and, 10
pancytopenia in, 28
polymorphonuclear cells in, segmented, 18
pyridoxine-responsive, 9
red blood cell
abnormal production causing, 8–10
decrease causing, 8–10
destruction increase, 11–17
maturation defect in, 10–11
membrane defects, 14
metabolism defects causing, 16–17
sickle cell, 7, 12
laboratory testing in, 12
transfusions in, 12
treatment, 12
sideroblastic, 30
ABO antigen weakening in, 154
refractory, and preleukemia, 29
in spherocytosis, hereditary, 14
of thalassemia, 14
Angioedema
complement genetic deficiency causing, 120
hereditary, 123, 135
Angiotensin II, 72
Anomalies
Alder-Reiley, 23

chromosome (see Chromosome, abnormalities)
May-Hegglin, 23, 77
Pelger-Huët, 30
Anthracycline
effect on marrow, 42
in leukemia, acute myelogenous, 37
Antibiotics
effect on marrow, 42
in neutropenia, 25
committed stem cell, 26
semisynthetic, 27
vitamin K and, 87
Antibody(ies)
absorption, 207
techniques, 207–208
against reagent substances, 204
agglutination and, 110
anticomplement hybridoma, 112
anti-D, 207
-antigen (see Antigen, -antibody)
anti-H, in Bombay phenotype, 154
anti-I, 208
after infectious mononucleosis, 209
antiidiotypic, 106
anti-immunoglobulin A (see Anti-immunoglobulin A antibodies)
anti-immunoglobulin G, 336
anti-Lewis, in kidney transplant rejection, 156
anti-M, 112
anti-N, 112
anti-NB1, 26
antireceptor, 133
anti-Rh₀(D), 173
bivalent, 109
cold, antigens that elicit, 146–163
combining site, 103–104
complementarity of antibody and antigen, 111
detection, 204–205
diversity of, 3
generation of, 106
genetics of, 107
elution, 208–209
ferritin-labeled, 145
genetic markers on, 105–107
to high-incidence antigens, transfusion with, 182
in hypersensitivity, 133
hypervariable regions, 103
identification, 205–206
IgG antineutrophil maternal, 26
after immunization by transfusion, 38
to immunoglobulins, 338

interaction with antigens, 110–111
J segment, 106
laboratory techniques for, special, 206–211
to lipoproteins, 338
molecule, structure of, 3
monoclonal (see Monoclonal antibodies)
neutralization, 209
oligoclonal, in cold agglutinin disease, 158
platelet, 77, 251
polyclonal, 111
production, 126–127
red blood cell, 214–215
complement binding by, 123
Rh antigen-antibody testing, laboratory aspects of, 171–172
Rh, in pregnancy, 172–173
valence, 109
V regions, 106
warm, 214–215
panel showing two, 212
warm-reacting, 163–181
Anticoagulants, 240
Anticomplement hybridoma antibodies, 112
Anticonvulsants: and neutropenia, 25
Anti-D
antibody, 207
circulatory, artificial reduction of, 429
Antieosinophil antiserum, 21
Antigen(s), 108–113
ABH (see Blood groups, ABH, antigens)
administration route, 109
ALL, 39
-antibody
lattice formation, 110
reactions, 2
reactions, Heidelberger's curve of, 110
reactions, kinetics of, 109
reactions, laboratory methods for detecting, 113
specificity of, 145
testing, 201–202
Australia, 356
Berrens, 183
blood group (see Blood group, antigens)
carcinoembryonic, in colorectal carcinoma, 154
complementarity of antibody and antigen, 111
cross-reacting, 132
cryptantigen, 160, 184

Antigen(s) *(cont.)*
D
  CE deletion with enhancement of, 169
  enhanced forms of, 169–170
determinants, 109
dose of, 109
Duffy
  Plamodium parasites infecting RBCs, 175
  production of, suggested pathway for, 176
  statistical frequencies of, 177
En^a, 182
excess causing immunoparalysis, 132
Forssman-like, 158
Fy, 177
Gerbich system, 182
hemolytic disease of newborn and, 429–430
hepatitis B surface (*see* Hepatitis, B, surface antigen)
high-frequency, 181–182
  clinical significance, 183
high-incidence, transfusion with antibodies to, 182
histocompatibility, 3, 218
HLA (*see under* HLA)
in hypersensitivity, 133
"i," 29
  in leukemia, chronic lymphocytic, 38
Ia, in acute lymphocytic leukemia, 40
Ii, clinical aspects of, 157–158
immunogenicity of, 128
interaction with antibodies, 110–111
Kell, 24, 179, 202
  chronic granulomatous disease and McLeod syndrome, 181
  complex, genetic pathway for, 180
  statistical frequencies of, 177
Kx, 24
Landsteiner-Wiener, 170
Langeris, 182
leukemia-associated, 36
Lewis, 155
  clinical aspects of, 156
of low incidence, 182–183
M, contrasted with N antigens, 160
MNSs (*see* MNSs antigens)
as multivalent, 108, 109
N, contrasted with M antigens, 160
neutrophil
  NA, 26
  NB, 26

red blood cell (*see* Red blood cell, antigens)
Rh (*see* Rh antigens)
Rogers, 122
Sid, 182
Swann, 183
T cell-independent, 126
Vel system, 181
Antigenicity, 108
Antiglobulin antiserum: in quality control, 448–449
Antiglobulin test (*see* Coombs test)
Anti-H antibody: in Bombay phenotype, 154
Antihemophilia A factor: characteristics of, 79
Antihemophilia B factor: characteristics of, 79
Antihemophilic factor, 246
Antihistamines
  mastocytosis and, malignant, 43
  neutropenia and, 25
  platelet function after, 77
Anti-I antibodies, 208
  after infectious mononucleosis, 209
Antiidiotypic antibodies, 106
Anti-immunoglobulin A antibodies
  anaphylactic reactions due to, prevention, 338
  anaphylaxis due to, 337–338
Anti-immunoglobulin G antibodies, 336
Anti-inflammatories: and neutropenia, 25
Anti-Lewis antibodies: in kidney transplant rejection, 156
Anti-M antibodies, 112
Antimalarials: and neutropenia, 25
Antimetabolites
  anemia and, megaloblastic, 10
  effect on marrow, 42
Anti-N antibodies, 112
α_2-Antiplasmin, 84
Antipurines: in chronic myelogenous leukemia, 33
Antipyrimidines: in chronic myelogenous leukemia, 33
Antireceptor antibodies, 133
Anti-Rh$_o$(D) antibodies, 173
Antisera
  cross-reactivity to HLA antigens, 219
  quality control and, 448
    ABO, 448
    Rh, 448
Antithrombins, 83
  I, 83
  control mechanisms of coagulation and, 83
  III, 83

deficiency, 87
in DIC, 90
-heparin, 82
inactivation, 72
-thrombin III complexes, 72
II, 83
Antitrust laws: regarding blood banking, 456
α_1-Antitrypsin, 83
Apheresis, 281–302
  blood volume change calculation, 284
  bowl, massive clotting in, 287
  control, 293–294
  donor, 281–288
    centrifugation, continuous flow, 283
    centrifugation, continuous flow, Aminco, 284
    centrifugation system, discontinuous flow, 281–282
    donation frequency, 285–286
    donor management, 286
    donor medical history, 284
    donor reactions, 286–288
    donor reactions, mild, 287
    donor reactions, severe, 287–288
    donor selection, 283–284
    effects of apheresis on donor, 285–286
    reactions to infused materials, 284–285
    recruitment, 293
  facilities for, 293
  Haemonetics system for, 282
  personnel for, 293
  plasmapheresis (*see* Plasmapheresis)
  preapheresis laboratory testing, 285
  products, uses and storage procedures, 288
  program, management techniques, 293–294
  therapeutic, 288–293
    death during, 256
Aplasia
  in leukemia, acute myelogenous, 36
  megakaryocytic, isolated, 77
  pure RBC, 9
  thrombocytopenia and, 77
Aplastic (*see* Anemia, aplastic)
Ara-C: effect on marrow, 42
Arginil groups, 80
Arginine: C-terminal, 122
Arthritis (*see* Rheumatoid arthritis)
Arthropathy: complicating hemophilia A, 85

Index

Arthropodes, 21
Ascorbic acid, 72
ASD acetate, 35
Ashby method, 215
Asparaginase, 41
Aspergillus, 24
Aspirin, 25
  blood donation and, 237
  platelet function and, 76
  platelets after, 248
  -treated donors, 76
Assault and battery, 452, 453–454
Asthma, 21
  blood donation and, 238
Ataxia telangiectasia, 29
Atomic bomb: and leukemia, 31
ATP, 72, 74
  after aspirin, 76
  in platelet release type 1, 75
Auer rods, 30, 32
  in leukemia, acute myelogenous, 35
Australia antigen, 356
Autoantibody
  cold, weak, panel showing, 211
  in hepatitis B, 365
Autoimmune
  anemia (*see* Anemia, hemolytic, autoimmune)
  disease, 72, 303
    basophils and, 22
    DIC and, 89
    HLA in, 230
    purpura and, idiopathic thrombocytopenic, 78
  hepatitis, characteristics, 365
  neutropenia, 25, 26
Autoimmunity, 131–132
  HLA-B8 antigen and, 131
  as loss of immunologic tolerance, 131
Autologous (*see* Transfusion, autologous)
Autosomic chromosome, 398
Autotransfuser: Bentley ATS-100, 296
Autotransfusion, 281–302
5-Azacytidine: in acute myelogenous leukemia, 36
Azathioprine: in idiopathic thrombocytopenic purpura, 78
6-Azauridine: in chronic myelogenous leukemia, 33

B

Babesiosis, 343
Bacterial disease: transmitted by transfusion, 341–342
Band forms, 18

Banking (*see* Blood, banking)
Basophil(s), 22–23
  circulating, increase in, diseases associated with, 22
  comparison with mast cells, 22
  degranulation of, 22
Basophilia, 22
  in leukemia, 31, 33
Basophilopenia, 22
Baths: water and dry, and quality control, 447
B cells, 123, 125
  in AIDS, 131
  antigens and, 109
  becoming plasma cells, 125
  binding Fc fragments, 125
  deficit in Wiskott-Aldrich syndrome, 130
  development into plasma cells, 127
  disorders with neutropenia, 25–26
  functions in Hodgkin's disease, 44
  germinal centers and, 124
  hapten-specific response mediated by, 127
  in humoral immunity, 124
  immature, 104
  immunity and, humoral, 102
  immunogenes in lymph node hyperplasia, 43
  immunoglobulin found on, 125
  immunologic tolerance and, 129
  in leukemia, hairy cell, 42
  in lymphoma
    diffuse, 48
    follicular, 48
    nodular, 48
  in macroglobulinemia, Waldenström's, 131
  macrophage presenting antigen to, model, 224
  markers
    in leukemia, acute lymphocytic, 40
    in lymphoma, non-Hodgkin's, 46
  memory cell stage of, 50
  monoclonal antibodies and, 111
  primitive, 49
  RNA transcript and, 50
  stimulation, 126
  surface, 127
  type I pre-B, 49
Benacerraf, 3
  two-receptor theory of, 128
Bence Jones protein: in gammopathy, 131
Bentley ATS-100 autotransfuser, 296

Benzene
  leukemia due to, 31
    acute lymphocytic, 40
  as leukemogenic, 30
  pancytopenia due to, 28
  toxicity, 8
Berbich system, 182
Bernard-Soulier syndrome, 76, 81
  treatment, 76
Bernstein, 3
Berrens antigen, 183
Bilirubin: decreasing, 433
Biopsy
  liver, in non-Hodgkin's lymphoma, 48
  marrow
    in anemia, aplastic, 9
    in lymphoma, non-Hodgkin's, 48
Blankets: warming, 214
Blast counts: in acute lymphocytic leukemia, 40
Blast crisis, 33
  discussion of, 32
  in leukemia, 31
Bleeding
  (*See also* Hemorrhage)
  diathesis after massive transfusion, 468
  time, 76
Bleomycin: and cell cycle, 41
Blindness: color, 16
Blood
  bank
    complement in, significance of, 123
    laboratory testing in Waldenström's macroglobulinemia, 50
    legal actions against (*see* Legal actions, against blood bank)
    medical director for, 460
    readiness plan, 469–471
    serology in hemoglobinuria, cold paroxysmal, 313
    studies, in cold agglutinin disease, 311–312
    support, for marrow transplant, 265–266
    testing, in disseminated intravascular coagulation, 88
  banked, acid load in, 339–340
  banker, concepts from chemotherapy useful to, 41–42
  banking
    AIDS and, 389–390
    antitrust laws regarding, 456
    community, regulation of, 455–456

Blood *(cont.)*
    consultation, diseases in children needing, 434–435
    hepatitis and, concepts in, 369–370
    hepatitis testing, quality control in, 369–370
    laboratory aspects, 201–217
    legal aspects of, 452–454
    management, legal matters affecting, 454
    organizations, 455–456
    organizations, role of College of American Pathologists in, 456
    perinatal, 420–443
    quality control in *(see* Quality control, in blood banking)
    role of Federal Government in, 456
  cells
    red *(see* Red blood cells)
    white *(see* White blood cells)
  coagulation *(see* Coagulation)
  cold, transfusion of, 338–339
  compatibility, 145
  component(s), 236–280
    AIDS and, 379–380
    in cancer, 474–476
    after marrow transplant, 477
    in newborn diseases, 436–437
    obtained from whole blood by centrifugation, 242
    practices for, good, 460–461
    preparation, 240–245
    preparation, quality control in, 449–451
    replacement in cardiopulmonary bypass, evaluation, 472–473
    replacement in disseminated intravascular coagulation, 470–471
    storage of, 240–245
    units, reactions to toxic substances in, 339
    uses of, 240–245
  dissociation curve, 241
  donor *(see* Donor)
  dyscrasias, platelet transfusion in, 249
  flow, and control mechanisms of coagulation, 83
  freezing, 333
  fresh frozen plasma, quality control in, 450
  frozen-thawed, 243–244
    quality control in, 450
  group *(see below)*
  heating, 333
  incompatibility, 215
  issuing, 462
  practices, good, 460–461
  product, and AIDS, 379–380
  samples in paternity testing, 409
  substitutes, 262–263
  thawing, 244
  as a tissue, normal aspects, 5
  volume
    changes, calculation for apheresis, 284
    total, in newborn, 6
    total, in prematurity, 6
  warmers, 214
  whole
    indications for, 240–241
    preparation, 240–241
    storage, 240–241
Blood group(s)
  A, 148
    substances, agglutination inhibition techniques for, 150
    synthesis, 148
  ABH
    antigens, 29
    antigens, disease and, 154
    antigens and transplantation, 154
    substances, biochemistry of, 146–147
    substances, genes involved in synthesis of, 152
    substances, monoclonal antibodies to, 152–154
    substances in secretions, 147–148
  ABO
    (See also ABO)
    antisera, quality control, 448
    groups that are compatible, 153
    inheritance in, codominant, 3, 146
    laboratory determination of, 146
    synthesis from group I substance, 157
    system, 146–154
    system, aspects of clinical significance, 153–154
    system, chromosome 9 and, 151
    system, discovery of, 2
    system, genetics of, 151–152
    system, groups in, 148–152
    system, in laboratory, 152
    system, in paternity testing, 410–411
    system, permutations in, possible, 147
    system, serologic aspects of, 150–151
    typing, discrepancies in, 152–153
  antigens, 145–200
    eliciting cold antibodies, 146–163
    weakening of, 154
  B, 150
    synthesis of, 148
  Duffy system, 175–177
    biochemistry, 175
    clinical aspects, 177
    gene frequencies, 176
    genetics of, 175–176
    laboratory studies, 176–178
    in paternity exclusion tests, 176
  H substance
    Bombay group lacking, 151–152
    in subgroups of A, relative proportion of, 149
    sugar sequence of, 155
  I
    molecule, 156
    substances, content in adult and fetal cells, 156
    substances, synthesis of ABO groups from, 157
    subtypes of, 157
    system, biochemistry of, 156–157
    system, serology of, 157
  Ii, 156–158
    antigens, clinical aspects of, 157–158
    substances, content in adult and fetal cells, 156
    system, genetics of, 157
  Kell system, 178–181
    antigenic, biochemistry of, 178–179
    genetics of, 179–180
    at laboratory level, 180–181
  Kidd system, 177–178
    biochemistry, 177
    clinical aspects, 178
    genetics, 177–178
    laboratory studies, 178
  Lewis system *(see* Lewis system)
  Lutheran system, 162–163
    biochemistry of, 162–163
    clinical aspects, 163
    genetics of, 162–163
    serology of, 163
    Swann antigen and, 183
  MNSs system, 159–162

biochemistry of, 159–161
clinical aspects of, 162
genetics of, 161
serology of, 161–162
in paternity testing, 410
P system, 158–159
  biochemistry, 158
  clinical aspects of, 159
  serology of, 158–159
  substances, biosynthesis of, 158
  substances, possible gene action for synthesis of, 159
subgroup A_1, 148
subgroup A_2, 148–149
subgroup A_3, 149–150
subgroups of A, serologic characterization, 149
subgroups of B, 150
substances on cell membranes, 147
theories of Landsteiner, 2
Xg system, 181
Bloom's syndrome: converting to leukemia, 30
Blundell, James, 1
Bohr effect, 7
Bombay group: lacking H substance, 151–152
Bombay phenotype, 147, 148
  anti-H antibody in, 154
  I antigens in, 156
Bombay-type transfusion recipients, 147
Bone
  infarction and sickle cell anemia, 12
  marrow (see Marrow)
Bordet, 2
Bordetella pertussis, 29
Boyle, Sir Robert, 1
Bradykinin, 81
Brucellosis, 29
  blood donation and, 237
Budd-Chiari syndrome: complicating hemoglobinuria, 15
Buffy coat, 243
Burkitt's lymphoma (see Lymphoma, Burkitt's)
Burns: crystalloid in, 260
Bursa of Fabricius, 45–46
Busulfan
  effect on marrow, 42
  in leukemia, chronic myelogenous, 33
  in myeloid metaplasia, agnogenic, 43
Bypass (see Cardiopulmonary bypass)

C

Cad polyagglutination, 185
Calcium
  characteristics of, 79
  factor X activation and, 82
  ions, 74
  in platelet aggregation, 74
  in platelet release type 1, 75
Cancer
  blood components in, 474–476
  DIC and, 89, 476
  eosinophilia and, 21
  platelet transfusion in, 249, 475
  red blood cell transfusion in, 475
  thrombocytosis in, 79
Candida, 44
Caprilate, 214
Carbenicillin: platelet function after, 77
Carbohydrate
  glycolysis, 74
  moiety, NANA, 160
γ-Carboxyglutamic acid, 80
Carboxylase: hepatic, 87
Carcinoembryonic antigen: in colorectal carcinoma, 154
Carcinogens: initiating preleukemia, 29
Carcinoma
  basophils and, 22
  blood donation and, 238
  colon, and ABO discrepancy, 153
  colorectal, carcinoembryonic antigen in, 154
  lymphocytopenia in, 29
  ovaries, 37
    leukemia in, 34
  pancytopenia due to, 28
  stomach
    ABH antigens and, 154
    anemia and, pernicious, 10
    HLA and, 228
  thrombocytosis in, 79
Carcinomatosis: and ABO discrepancy, 153
Cardiopulmonary bypass, 27, 78, 471–474
  accessory pump for, 471–472
  blood component replacement in, 472–473
  complement during, 123
  DIC and, 89
  fluid therapy in, evaluation, 472–473
  hemolysis after, 474
  hemostasis alterations in, 90
  heparin in, 473
  oxygenator for, 471
    with five components, 472
    main oxygenator pump, 471
  platelet disorders after, 473–474
  suction system for, 471–472
  thrombocytopenia after, 252, 473–474
Cardiopulmonary pump, 77
Cardiopulmonary resuscitation: in blood donor reactions, 239
Carmustine
  effect on marrow, 42
  in myeloma, 37
  in myeloma, plasma cell, 50
Cataract: congenital, 158
Catecholamines, 74
Catepsins, 75, 83
Cation permeability disorders, 14
CCNU, 41
Cell(s)
  B (see B cells)
  blood (see Blood, cells)
  colony-forming unit, 8
  complement receptors in, 120–121
  cycle, effect of chemotherapy on, 41
  effect of surface-bound immunoglobulin on, 108
  endothelial (see Endothelium, cells)
  frozen deglycerolized, physiology, 244
  hypotetraploid, 44
  killer, 125
  Kupffer, 121
  mast (see Mast cells)
  membranes, blood group substances on, 147
  mononuclear, Fc receptors on, 108
  plasma (see Plasma, cell)
  polymorphonuclear, segmented, 18
  progenitor, disorders, 26
  Reed-Sternberg, 44, 45
  Rhesus monkey, 3
  sickle cell (see Sickle cell)
  stem (see Stem cells)
  T (see T cells)
  tumor, kinetics, 40–41
Cellular immunity, 123–129
Celsus, 1
Centimorgans, 222
Central nervous system: lymphoma, 47
Centrifugation
  in apheresis, donor (see Apheresis, donor, centrifugation)

Centrifugation *(cont.)*
  differential, 113
  in granulocyte preparation, 254
Centrifuges: quality control in blood banking, 447
Cephalothin, 25
Cestodes, 21
CFU, 18
  -C, 8, 33
  cells, 8
  -E, 8
  -EOS, 17
  -M, 19, 73
  -M1, 73
  -M2, 73
  for monocytes, 30
  -N, 19
  for neutrophils, 30
  -NM, 17, 19
  -S, 8, 18, 19
    deficiency (in mice), 18
Chagas' disease: transmitted by transfusion, 344
Charcot-Leyden crystal protein, 21
Charitable immunity, 452, 454
Chédiak-Higashi syndrome, 23–24
  neutrophil granules in, 23
Chemicals: causing acute lymphocytic leukemia, 40
Chemotherapy
  antimetabolite, 27
  combination, 41
  concepts from, useful to blood banker, 41–42
  effect on cell cycle, 41
  effect on marrow, 42
  in Hodgkin's disease, 45
  of leukemia, 41
    chronic lymphocytic, 38
    chronic myelogenous, 33–34
    leukemic transformation after, 30
  lymphocytopenia after, 29
  of lymphoma, diffuse, 49
  nadir of, 41
    prolonged, 41
  poor response to platelets after, 251
Children
  diseases needing blood banking consultation, 434–435
  granulomatous disease *(see* Granulomatous disease, chronic, in children)
  lymphoma, diffuse, 48
  transfusion for, special aspects of, 434
Chills: after apheresis, 287
Chimerism: in paternity testing, 410

Chlorambucil
  effect on marrow, 42
  in leukemia, 30
    chronic lymphocytic, 38
    chronic myelogenous, 33
  in lymphoma, diffuse, 49
  in myeloma, plasma cell, 50
  in polycythemia vera, 43
  in Waldenström's macroglobulinemia, 50, 131
Chloramphenicol, 27
  toxicity, 8
Chloroacetate esterase, 32
Chlorothiazide, 25
Chlorpromazine, 27
  in immune hemolysis, 317
Cholelithiasis: and sickle cell anemia, 12
Christmas disease, 85
Christmas factor: characteristics of, 79
Chromatography: affinity, 113
Chromogenic enzyme-linked assay, 204
Chromosome(s)
  abnormalities
    in Hodgkin's disease, 44
    in leukemia, acute lymphocytic, 40
    in leukemia, acute myelogenous, 35–36
    in lymphoma, non-Hodgkin's, 48
  polycythemia vera and, 43
  alterations in preleukemia, 30
  autosomic, 398
  banded, nomenclature of, 398
  crossing-over, 400
  8, 35
  15, 35
  14q+ in non-Hodgkin's lymphoma, 48
  gene, allelic, 399
  identification, 397
  material reduction during meiosis, 399
  9, and ABO system, 151
  Philadelphia, 30, 31, 34
    in leukemia prognosis, acute lymphocytic, 40
  7, 35
  17, 35
    H2 histocompatibility complex on, 225
  6
    deletion in lymphocytic leukemia, 40
    HLA genes on short arm of, 223

  studies, uses of, 398–399
  t(8;21), 35
  translocation, 30
    8;21, 35
    in leukemia, acute lymphocytic, 40
    in lymphoma, non-Hodgkin's, 48
  12, trisomy in chronic lymphocytic leukemia, 37
  21 deletions and thrombocytopenia, 30
  X, 35
    factor VIII in, 81
    G6PD synthesis and, 16
  Y, 35
Chymotrypsin, 160
Cimetidine, 25
  thrombocytopenia due to, 78
Circulation: extracorporeal, 123
Cisplatin: effect on marrow, 42
Citrate toxicity, 339
Clone amplification, 106
Clotting
  activation of, 88–89
  activity, tissue factor, 72
  cascade, activation in DIC, 88
  deficiencies, in newborn, 437
  disorders, major acquired, laboratory findings, 87
  factor
    (See also Factor)
    abnormalities causing abnormal platelet aggregation, 76
    biochemistry, 79–81
    characteristics of, 79
    inhibitors, acquired, 87–88
    monoclonal antibodies in analysis of, 113
    produced by endothelial cells, 72
    restoration with fresh frozen plasma, 246
  rouleaux formation and, 213
CNS lymphoma, 47
Coagulation, 78–91
  abnormalities, 84–90
    laboratory evaluation, 84
  cascade, 82
  chemoattractants and, 19
  control mechanisms of, 83–84
    local, 83
  diffuse intravascular, major causes, 89
  disorders, congenital, 84–87
  disseminated intravascular, 75, 88–90
    acute, 88–89

blood component replacement
    in, 470–471
  in cancer, 476
  chronic, 89
  complement activation
    triggering, 88
  diagnosis, 471
  diagnosis, laboratory, 89–90
  platelet destruction and, 78,
    249
  therapy, 90, 471
  inhibitors, 83
    humoral, 83
  pathway, factor XIII in, 81
  physiology of, 81–83
Coagulopathy
  acquired, 87–90
  disseminated intravascular
    in leukemia, chronic
      myelogenous, 35
    in leukemia, promyelocytic,
      36
    treatment, 36
  liver disease, 87
  of vitamin K deficiency, 87
Cobalophilin, 18
Cold
  agglutinin, 38
  agglutinin disease, 157,
    130–132
    anemia in, pathophysiology,
      310–311
    blood bank studies in,
      311–312
    clinical findings, 311
    laboratory findings, 311
    monoclonal antibodies in, 158
    oligoclonal antibodies in, 158
    pathogenesis, 310
    therapy of, 312
  autoantibody, weak, panel
    showing, 211
  autoimmune hemolytic anemia,
    310–313
  hemoglobinuria (see
    Hemoglobinuria, cold)
Colitis: ulcerative, 21
Collagen
  abnormal, 72
  bands in Hodgkin's disease, 45
  biosynthesis, 72
  degenerative changes, 72
  factor XI activated by, 88
  factor XII and, 81
  factor XII and intrinsic system,
    82
  fibers, 72
    AB_2, 71
    type IV, 71
    type V, 71

  in platelet aggregation, 74, 76
  platelets adhering to, 74
  subendothelial types, 72
Collagenase, 18
Collapse curve: of Mollison, 215
College of American Pathologists:
  role in blood banking, 456
Colonic carcinoma
  ABO discrepancy and, 153
  carcinoembryonic antigen in,
    134
Colony-forming unit (see CFU)
Colony-stimulating activity, 8
  I, 8
  II, 8
  III, 8
  IV, 8
Colony-stimulating factors, 19
Color blindness, 16
Complement, 113–123
  abnormalities, 122
  activation, 114–116
    alternative pathway, 116,
      118–120
    alternative pathway,
      amplification, 119–120
    alternative pathway,
      enhancing, 118
    alternative pathway, initiation
      of, 118–119
    alternative pathway, proteins
      involved in, 119
    chemotactic effect of, 121
    classical activation interacting
      with alternative activation,
      119
    classical pathway, 116–117
    properdin pathway, 118
    triggering DIC, 88
    unit, 115
    vasoactive effect of, 121
  in anaphylatoxin production,
    114
  binding, 116
    immunoglobulin, 104
    by RBC antibodies, 123
  in blood bank, significance of,
    123
  C5, 73
  C5a, 19, 27
  C4a, 19
  characteristics, 113–114
    by components and pathways,
      115
  chemoattractants, 19
  components
    biosynthesis of, 116–118
    plasmin degrading, 84
    soluble, 121–122
  C1-inactivator, 83

  C1 and recognition unit, 117
  C1q
    deficiency and X-linked
      hypogammaglobulinemia,
      134
    IgM binding of, 116
    receptor, and trypsin, 120
  control of, 120
  CR1 electrophoretic mobility,
    120
  C7 deficiency, and Raynaud's
    phenomenon, 135
  C3 cleavage products, 117
  C3a, 19
  C3b, 21
  C3c, 73
  C3d, 73
  deficiencies, 134–135
  in disease, 122–123
  factors, 19
  genetics of, evolutionary,
    122
  in hemoglobinuria, paroxysmal
    nocturnal, 15
  immunoglobulin and, 116
  lytic functions, 114
  -mediated intravascular
    hemolysis, 163
  membrane attack unit, 115,
    117–118
    lytic activity of, 118
  neutrophils with Fc receptors
    for, 20
  nomenclature, 113–114
  in phagocytosis, 121
  proteins, 122
  receptors, 23, 121
    on cells, 120–121
    on macrophages, 304–306
  recognition unit, 115
  sensitization of cells during
    opsonization, 114
  transmembrane channels, 118
Components (see Blood,
  components)
Concanavalin, 127
  A, 19
Coombs panels, 204
Coombs reagents, 112, 203
Coombs test, 38, 202–204
  direct, 202
  in hemolytic anemia,
    autoimmune, 303
  indirect, 202
  in lymphoma, diffuse, 49
  pitfalls, 203–204
  uses of, 204
Copper sulfate, 238
Copperhead venom: and
  fibrinopeptide B, 80

Corticosteroids, 21
    white blood cell count and, 255
Costs: of therapeutic plasmapheresis, 292
Coumadin, 214
CPK-MM isoenzymes, 24
Crime laboratory: study of secretionsin, 418
Criminology, 417–418
    proteins in, 418
    red blood cell antigens in, 417–418
    red blood cell enzymes in, 418
Crohn's disease: plasmapheresis in, 291
Crossing-over phenomenon, 222
Crossmatch, 211–214
    incompatibilities, 213
    major, 212
    minor, 211–212
    pitfalls, common, 212–214
Cryoglobulinemia: complicating Waldenström's macroglobulinemia, 131
Cryoprecipitate, 76, 246–248
    complications, 247–248
    in DIC, 90
    dosage, 247
    factor VIII and AIDS, 379
    in hemophilia A, 85
    practices for, good, 465
    preparation, 246–247
    quality control and, 450
    uses, clinical, 247
    in von Willebrand's disease, 86
Cryoprotecting agents, 243
Cryptantigen: T, 160, 184
Crystalloid: in burns, 260
CSA (*see* Colony-stimulating activity)
Cyanocobalamine, 10
Cyanomethemoglobin method, 7
Cyclo-oxygenase, 76
Cyclophosphamide, 41
    effect on marrow, 42
    in leukemia
        chronic lymphocytic, 38
        chronic myelogenous, 33
    in lymphoma
        Burkitt's, 48
        diffuse, 49
    in myeloma, 37
        plasma cell, 50
    in polycythemia vera, 43
Cysticercosis, 21
Cytapheresis, 256
    hydroxyethyl starch for, 284
    practices in, 477–478
    therapeutic, 292–293
Cytarabine
    cell cycle and, 41
    in leukemia, acute myelogenous, 37
Cytochalasin B, 134
Cytomegalovirus infection, 237
Cytosine arabinoside
    in leukemia, acute myelogenous, 36
    megakaryocytes after, 77
Cytosol: of platelets, 248
Cytotoxic drugs, 34
Cytotoxicity, 224

D

D antigen (*see* Antigen, D)
Daunomycin: in acute myelogenous leukemia, 36
Dausset, 3
DDAVP: in von-Willebrand's disease, 86
1-Deamino-8-D-arginine vasopressin: in von Willebrand's disease, 86
Decarbazine: effect on marrow, 42
Deglycerolization, 244
Deglycerolized
    cells, frozen, physiology of, 244
    RBC transfusion, 245
    RBCs, frozen, 244–245
Delta agent: in hepatitis B, 362–363
Denys, Jean, 1
Deoxynucleotydil transferase: terminal, 31
Dermatitis herpetiformis, 21
    blood donation in, 238
Dexamethasone: and granulocytes, 255
Dextran(s), 261
    in hemoglobinuria, paroxysmal nocturnal, 15
    platelet function after, 77
    in rouleaux formation prevention, 261
Diabetes mellitus
    acidosis of, 16
    type I in DR3 and DR4 phenotypes, 230
Dialysis tubing: formalin treatment of, 162
Diamond-Blackfan syndrome, 9
Diathesis: bleeding after massive transfusion, 468
Dibromannitol: in chronic myelogenous leukemia, 33
DIC (*see* Coagulation, disseminated intravascular)
DiGeorge syndrome, 29, 129
Digestive tract inflammation: and basophils, 22
Digitonin method, 308
Di Guglielmo's syndrome, 35
Dilantin: in immune hemolysis, 317
Diphenylhydantoin, 25
Disgammaglobulinemia, 25
Disproteinemia, 75
Diuretics: and neutropenia, 25
Dizziness: after aphresis, 287
DNA
    code, transcription of, 400–401
    EBV, in Burkitt's lymphoma, 47
    hybridization, 3
    recombinant, 402–403
    replication, 401
    structure, diagram of, 400
    synthesis, 41
        mercaptopurine inhibiting, 40
        methotrexate inhibiting, 40
        vitamin B12 and, 10
Dohle body(ies), 23
    -bearing granulocytes, 77
Donath-Landsteiner phenomenon: and P system, 158
Donation, 238–240
    adverse reactions to, 239–240
    donor care after, 239
    granulocyte, complications from, 256–257
Donor
    adverse reactions of, treatment, 239–240
    apheresis (*see* Apheresis, donor)
    care after donation, 239
    with leukemia, myelogenous, leukocytes from, 255
    leukocyte, of granulocytes, 254–255
    medical history, 236–238
    paid, 236
    physical examination, 238
    selection, 236–238
    single, and HLA-matched platelets, 250–251
    temperature of, 238
    voluntary, 236
Down's syndrome, 28
    converting to leukemia, 30
    Philadelphia chromosome contrasted with, 30
Doxorubicin, 41
    effect on marrow, 42
Dreyer-Bennet hypothesis, 107
Drug(s)
    abuse, IV, and AIDS, 378
    addiction, and blood donation, 237
    in anemia, hemolytic, autoimmune, warm-type, 309

haptenic, conjugation with red
 blood cells, 313–315
hemolysis due to (*see* Hemolysis,
 immune, drugs causing)
for leukemia, chronic
 myelogenous, 33
neutropenia due to, 27
platelet defects due to, 75,
 76–78
platelet production inhibited by,
 77
thrombocytosis due to, 79
Dudley hypothesis: in hepatitis,
 358
Duffy antigens (*see* Antigens,
 Duffy)
Dyscrasias: blood, platelet
 transfusion in, 249
Dyserythropoiesis: inherited, 185
Dysgenesis: reticular, 25

E

EBV (*see* Epstein-Barr virus)
Edelman, 3
Ehlers-Danlos syndrome, 72
Ehrlich, 2, 3
Elastin, 71
Elderly (*see* Aged)
Electron microscopy
 freeze-etching, 145
 immunoferritin, 146
 in platelet release type 1, 75
Electrophoresis, 113
 of complement, 115
 CR1 mobility, 120
 of haptoglobin phenotypes, 414
 hemoglobin, 12
 in leukemia, chronic
  lymphocytic, 38
 SDS-agarose, 86
 zone, 113, 114
Electrostatic forces: in bonding,
 111
Elliptocytosis: hereditary, 14
Elongation factor, 11
Elution: of antibodies, 208–209
Embden-Meyerhof pathway, 7, 15
Embolism
 air
  after blood donation, 240
  after transfusion, 340
  amniotic fluid, and DIC, 89
Emergency (*see* Transfusion,
 emergency)
En[a] antigens, 182
En[a]-negative phenotype, 182
Endocrine disease
 anemia due to, aplastic, 9
 basophils and, 22
Endonucleases, 107

Endothelium
 cells, 71
 activating factor XII, 72
 clotting activity and, tissue
  factor, 72
 clotting factors produced by,
  72
 neutrophils adhering to, 20
 synthesizing factor VIII, 81
 in thrombin removal, 83
 in von Willebrand's disease
  defect, 85
 derangement causing abnormal
  hemostasis, 72–73
 integrity in hemostasis, 72
 vascular, 75
Endotoxemia: and thrombosis, 89
Endotoxins, 88, 119
 platelet release induced by, 88
Enteritis: regional, 21
Entropy, 109
Enzyme
 chromogenic enzyme-linked
  assay, 204
 defects causing anemia, 17
 immunoassay for hepatitis B
  surface antigen, 363
 leukocyte, 122
 phenotypes (*see* Paternity testing,
  red blood cell enzyme
  phenotypes)
 red blood cell
  in criminology, 418
  membrane, 14
  testing, 17
Eosinopenia, 21
 infection causing, 21
Eosinophil(s), 20–22
 cationic protein, 21
 functions, 20–21
 granules in, 21
 in Hodgkin's disease, 45
 kinetics, 20
 in leukemia, 31
 receptors for Fc portion of IgE,
  21
 -releasing factor, 20
 role in host defenses, 21
 survival of, 20
Eosinophilia, 21–22
 causes, major, 21
Eosinophilopoietic factor: tumor-
  derived, 21
Epinephrine
 in anaphylactic reactions,
  132
 eosinopenia due to, 21
 in platelet aggregation, 74, 76
Epithelium: of intestine,
 synthesizing complement,
 116

Epitopes, 219
 "private," 219
 "public," 219
Epstein-Barr virus, 31
 in Burkitt's lymphoma, 40
 in Hodgkin's disease etiology,
  44
 in lymphoma etiology, non-
  Hodgkin's, 47
Equations: to analyze validity of
 results, 404–405
Equipment for blood banking
 quality control, 446–447
  non-temperature-dependent,
   447
  temperature-dependent,
   446–447
Erythroblastic hyperplasia, 33
Erythroblastic multinuclearity
 hereditary, 158
Erythroblastosis fetalis, 75
 extrauterine problems,
  management, 430–435
 pathophysiology, 421–422
Erythrocytapheresis: in sickle cell
 disease, 292
Erythrocyte (*see* Red blood cells)
Erythroid precursors, 73
Erythroleukemia, 15, 35, 36
Erythropoiesis: and thrombopoiesis,
 78
Erythropoietin, 8, 78
 CFU-M and, 73
Escherichia coli, 27
 in leukemia, acute myelogenous,
  37
Essen-Molar formula, 416
Esterase
 activity of factor VII, 80
 D, in paternity testing, 413
Estrogen, 77
 effect, 78
Ethanol, 77
Ether elution method, 308
Etiocholanolone: and white blood
 cell count, 255
Eukaryotic initiating factor, 11
Exchange transfusion (*see*
 Transfusion, exchange)
Exercise
 increasing granulocyte count, 19
 neutrophilia after, 28
Extracorporeal circulation, 123
Extrinsic system, 82–83

F

Fab fragment: of immunoglobulin
 monomer, 103
Factor(s)
 (*See also* Clotting, factors)

Factor(s) *(cont.)*
  antihemophilia A, characteristics of, 79
  antihemophilia B, characteristics of, 79
  antihemophilic, 246
  B, 114, 115
    genetics of, 122
  Christmas, characteristics of, 79
  consumption, evidence of, 90
  D, 114, 115
  VIII, 76, 77, 79
    activation, 81
    C, 76
    concentrates, 257–258
    concentrates, complications from, 258
    concentrates, practices for, 465
    concentrates, replacement therapy with, 257–258
    C portion of, 85
    cryoprecipitate and, 246
    deficiency, 84
    discussion of, 80–81
    inhibitors, 87, 88
    in platelet aggregation, 74
    in platelet release type 1, 75
    protein C and, 72
    replacement therapy, hepatitis after, 258
    R:R CO, 76
    in transfusion, massive, 246
    von Willebrand portion of, 72
  XI, 81, 82
    collagen activating, 88
    deficiency, in people with European Jewish ancestry, 86
  XIa, 80, 82
  Fitzgerald, characteristics of, 79
  V, 72, 80
    activation of, 80
    activation, protein C in, 80
    deficiency, 86
    inhibitors, 88
  Va, 82
  Fletcher, 82
    characteristics of, 79
  H, 121
  Hageman
    characteristics of, 79
    deficiency, 86
  labile, characteristics of, 79
  in newborn, 6
  IX, 80
    activity assays, 85
    concentrates, 258–259
    concentrates, clinical uses of, 258–259
  concentrates, complications of therapy, 259
  concentrates, practices for, 465
  deficiency, 84, 85, 87
  excess, 85
  IXa, 82
  non-vitamin K-dependent, 80–81
  I, 79–80
  Ia, 80
  plasmin degrading, 84
  VII, 80, 82
    deficiency, 86
    deficiency, treatment, 86
  Stuart-Prower, characteristics of, 79
  X, 80, 82
  Xa
    antithrombin III inhibiting, 83
    factor VIII activity and, 82
  XIII, 74, 81
    deficiency, 86
    deficiency, therapy, 86
  XIIIa, 81
  III, 81
    deficiency, diagnosis, 86
    tissue, 81
  XII, 81
    activation, 81, 82
    deficiencies, 86
    endothelial cells activating, 72
  XIIa, 20, 82
    factor VII activity and, 82
  II, 80
  vitamin K-dependent, 80
  von Willebrand, 81
    characteristics, 79
Family
  pedigree representing a non-sex-linked trait, 410
  studies in paternity testing, 409
Fanconi's anemia: in leukemia, 30
Fatty acids: factor XII and intrinsic system, 82
Favism: in G6PD deficiency, 16
Fc binding capacity: distortion of, 108
Fc-dependent characteristics: of immunoglobulin, 116
Fc fragment, 103
  B cells binding, 125
Fc on macrophages, 304–306
Fc portion
  of immunoglobulin, 125
  of molecule, 116
Fc receptors, 23
  binding of, 108
  expression on platelets, 78
  of macrophages, 108
  on mononuclear cells, 108
  platelet surface, 78
Ferritin, 9
  -apoferritin cycle, 9
  granules, 74
  -labeled antibodies, 145
Fetal hemoglobin, 7
  hereditary persistence, 13–14
Fetomaternal hemorrhage *(see* Hemorrhage, fetomaternal)
Fetus
  liver, primitive B cells in, 49
  maturity estimate in hemolytic disease of newborn, 423
Fever: platelet survival in, 251
Fibrin
  control mechanisms of coagulation and, 83
  degradation
    fragment E, 84
    fragment X, 84
    fragment Y, 84
    product detection, 84
    products, 89
    steps of, 84
  fibrinogen conversion to, 78, 84
  macrophages and, 83
  microthrombosis, 89
  monomers, 89
  split products, 84
  -stabilizing factor, 79
    characteristics of, 79
Fibrinogen, 79–80, 84
  characteristics of, 79
  conversion to fibrin, 78, 84
  deficiency, 259
    congenital, 86
  depletion, 87
  discussion of, 259
  inhibitors, 88
  lyophilized, in cryoprecipitate, 247
  molecule, thrombin in, 78
  monomers, free, 78
  in platelet aggregation, 74
  in platelet release type 1, 75
  in platelets, 74
  thrombin and, 82
Fibrinolysis, 83–84
  endothelial cells in, 72
  evidence of, 90
Fibrinolytic system, 83
  anticoagulant properties of, 83
Fibrinopeptide
  A, 79
    in coagulation, 80
    thrombin and, 82
  B, 20, 80
    thrombin and, 82

thrombin and, 87
Fibroblasts, 72
Fibronectin, 71, 240
Fibrosis: in Hodgkin's disease, 45
Filariasis: transfusion transmitting, 344
Filters: for transfusion, 463
Fisher method: for calculation of probability, 406–407
Fisher-Race nomenclature: for Rh system, 164
Fitzgerald factor: characteristics of, 79
Fletcher factor, 82
  characteristics of, 79
Fluid therapy: in cardiopulmonary bypass, evaluation, 472–473
Fluorescent spot test, 17
5-Fluorouracil, 41
  effect on marrow, 42
Fluosol-DA, 263
FMLP, 20
Folate
  in anemia, megaloblastic, 10
  deficiency, 10
Folic acid: in myelogenous leukemia, 35
Forbol ester TPA test, 39
Forensic immunohematology, 409–419
Formalin treatment: of dialysis tubing, 162
Forms: quality control of, 451–452
Formula: of Morton for linkage, 405–406
Forssman-like antigen, 158
Fractions, 236–280
  plasma, 257–263
Fractures: and DIC, 89
Franklin's disease, 50
Freeze-etching electron microscopy, 145
Freezers: in blood banking, quality control, 446–447
Freezing: of blood, 333
Fresh frozen plasma (see Plasma, fresh frozen)
Frozen
  deglycerolized cells, physiology of, 244
  deglycerolized RBCs, 244–245
  marrow, 263
  plasma (see Plasma, fresh frozen)
  storage, processing units for, 244
  -thawed blood, 243–244
Fucosyltransferase, 154
  presence or absence in epithelium, 155
Fy antigens, 177

G

Galactosyl residues: in platelet adhesion, 74
Gamma-carboxyglutamic acid, 80
Gamma-globulin preparations: practices for, 465–466
Gammopathy, 131
  benign monoclonal, 131
  melphalan in, 131
Gangrene: and ABO discrepancy, 153
Gastric (see Stomach)
Gastrointestinal
  disease, 21
  disorders, blood donation in, 238
  infection, acquired group antigens in, 154
  symptoms in non-Hodgkin's lymphoma, 48
Gaucher-like cells, 32
Gaucher's disease, 77
Gelatin, 261–262
  rouleaux formation after, 262
Gelatin tests, 90
Gene(s)
  in ABH substance synthesis, 152
  ABO, 151
  action for synthesis of P substances, 159
  allelic, location on chromosome, 399
  arrangement according to Fisher-Race theory, 164
  associated with immune system, assignment of, 222
  β, 11
  D, 107
  δ, 11
  duplication, tandem, 122
  ϵ, 11
  V, 107
  frequencies, and Duffy system, 176
  γ, 11
  in genome, complement of, 107
  globin, 11
  in G6PD synthesis, 16
  HLA, on short arm of chromosome 6, 223
  Ir, 224
  light chain, 107
  linkage, 405
    disequilibrium and HLA system, 222–223
    Morton's formula for, 405–406
    megagene characteristics of HLA locus, 221–222
  mutations, 406
  pathway for Kell antigenic complex, 180
  regulation, 402
  responsible for immunoglobulin isotype expression, 125
  Rh (see Rh gene)
  shuffling, 107
  splicing, 3
  suppressor, in paternity testing, 410
Generation time: for cells, 18
Genetic
  deficiency, complement, causing angioedema, 120
  factors in acute lymphocytic leukemia, 40
  information, molecular basis of, 399–403
  markers on antibodies, 105–107
Genetics, 397–408
  of ABO system, 151–152
  of antibody diversity, 107
  basic concepts, 397–399
  of complement, evolutionary, 122
  cross
    dihybrid, 403
    dihybrid, possible permutations in, 404
    monohybrid, 403
  of HLA system, 221–223
  of Ii system, 157
  in immunohematology, 397–408
  of Kell system, 179–180
  of Kidd system, 177–178
  of Lutheran system, 162–163
  Mendelian, 403–407
  of MNSs system, 161
Genome
  genes in, complement of, 107
  of hepatitis B virus, model of, 357
  retrovirus, diagram, 381
  structure of hepatitis B virus, 357
Gentamicin: in myelogenous leukemia, 37
Germinal centers: and B cells, 124
Glanzmann's thrombasthenia, 76
Glass: factor VII and intrinsic system, 82
Globin
  gene, 11
  molecule synthesis, 11–12
α-Globulin inhibitor, 83
Glomerulonephritis:
  membranoproliferative, and complement, 122

Glucocorticoids, 19
    eosinopenia due to, 21
    in neutrophilia, 28
Glucose
    G6PD (see G6PD)
    metabolism defects causing anemia, 14
Glutamic acid, 87
Glutamine, 82
    pyruvate transaminase, in paternity testing, 413
Glutaraldehyde: and hemagglutination, 146
Glutathione, 17
Glycerol, 243–244
Glycogen, 74
    synthesis, 74
Glycolysis
    anaerobic, in chronic granulomatous disease of children, 24
    carbohydrate, 74
Glycophorin, 160
    A, 163, 211
Glycoproteins, 116, 128
    class I, 219
    class II, 219
    Ib, 76
    Is, 76
    150,000-dalton, 156
    P substance and, 158
    red cell membrane, and MNSs antigens, 160
    III, 76
    IIIa, 76
    IIb, 76
Glycosidases, 18
Glycosphingolipids, 146
    in P substance, 158
Glyoxalase I: in paternity testing, 413
GMP: effect on marrow, 42
Gompertzian growth: of tumors, 41
Goodpasture's syndrome, 133
    plasmapheresis in, 290
Graft: marrow, in paroxysmal nocturnal hemoglobinuria, 15
Graft-vs.-host disease, 134
    chronic, 134
    in immunodeficiency, 130
    after marrow transplant, 134, 226
    transfusion complicated by, 335
Graft-vs.-host reaction: after marrow transplant, 34
Graham's method, 204
Granulocyte(s), 8, 17, 253–257
    abnormalities
        acquired, 23–24

congenital, 23–24
collections, 19
concentrates, and quality control, 451
count, 19
    exercise increasing, 19
destruction of, mechanisms for, 27
Döhle body-bearing, 77
donation, complications from, 256–257
elimination by centrifugation, 243
endothelium and, 72
functions, 19–20
    in leukemia, 33
HLA-matched, 254
kinetics, 18–19
leukocyte donor, 254–255
mature, 18
morphological changes in, 23
-poor blood units, preparation by centrifugation, 243
precursors, 73
preparation of units, 254
    automated methods, 254
    manual methods, 254
progenitors, 34
after radiotherapy, 77
transfusion (see Transfusion, granulocyte)
yield, increments in, 255
Granulocytic sarcoma, 36
Granulocytopenia
    chemotherapy and, 41
    platelet transfusions and, 227
Granuloma: marrow in, 9
Granulomatous disease, chronic, in children, 24–25
    immunohematology of, 24–25
    maternal systemic lupus erythematosus and, 25
    McLeod syndrome and Kell antigens, 181
Graph: modified Liley, 426
Graves' disease, 133
Gross virus, 230
Growth
    gompertzian, of tumors, 41
    -promoting factor, 74
G6PD
    A, 16
    B, 16
    deficiency
        anemia in, hemolytic, 16
        drugs in, 16
        hemolysis in, 16
        infection in, 16
        Hektoen variant of, 16
        in hemoglobinuria, paroxysmal nocturnal, 15

leukemia and, 31
myeloid metaplasia and, agnogenic, 43
in paternity testing, 412–413
synthesis, genes controlling, 16

H

Haemonetics system: for hemapheresis, 282
Hageman factor
    characteristics of, 79
    deficiency, 86
Hair dyes: causing pancytopenia, 28
Hairy cell leukemia, 37, 42
Haitians: and AIDS, 380
Ham test, 15
Haplotype, 222
Hapten(s), 78, 109
    in drug-induced immune hemolysis, 315
    -specific response mediated by B cells, 127
Haptenic drug: conjugation with red blood cells, 313–315
Haptoglobin phenotype: electrophoretic patterns of, 414
Hardy-Weinberg law: and paternity testing, 415
Hardy-Weinberg principle, 405
HAT medium, 112
Hb
    (See also Hemoglobin)
    A, 14
    A2, 13
    Bart, 13
    C, 12
    F, 13, 14, 29
    H disease, 14, 29
    S, 11
Heart
    failure, and packed red blood cells, 241
    open surgery, 237
        hemostasis derangement during, 473
        replacement therapy in, 474
        replacement therapy in, transfusion practices, 471–474
    surgery, hemostasis in, 90–91
Heating: of blood, 333
Heidelberger's curve: of antibody-antigen reactions, 110
Heinz bodies, 16
Hemagglutination, 102
    inhibition immunoassay, RBC, 84
    reactions, 145

Hemangioma
  cavernous, 78
  giant, and DIC, 89
Hemapheresis: Haemonetics system for, 282
Hemarthroses: complicating hemophilia A, 85
Hematocrit, 5
  in females, 5
  in males, 5
  in newborn, 6
Hematologic disease: converting to leukemia, 30
Hematologic values
  by age populations, 6
  in aged, 6
  in infant, 6
  in newborn, 6
Hematology
  perinatal, 6
  workup in AIDS, 387
Hematopoiesis: ineffective, and pancytopenia, 28
Hematopoietic cells: neoplastic disorders of, 29
Heme defect: causing hypochromic anemia, 10
Hemochromatosis: and transfusion, 345
Hemodialysis, 27
Hemoglobin
  (See also Hb)
  affinity for oxygen, 7
  in aged, 6
  chains during development, composing, 13
  determination
    cyanomethemoglobin method, 7
    specific gravity (see Specific gravity)
  disease, sickle cell, 12
  electrophoresis, 12
  embryonic, 13
  fetal, 7
    hereditary persistence, 13–14
  globulin portion, 7
  Gower 1, 13
  Gower 2, 13
  heme portion, 7
  maturation, in children, 434
  mean corpuscular, 5, 9
    concentration, 5
  mean, in newborn, 6
  molecule, 11
    structure, 11
  in newborn, 6
  in oxygen transport, 7
  Portland, 13
  stroma free, 262
  variants, biochemical functions of, 11–12

Hemoglobinuria
  cold, paroxysmal, 158, 159, 304, 312–313
    blood bank serology, 313
    clinical manifestations, 312
    laboratory findings, 312–313
    management, 313
    pathophysiology, 312
Hemoglobinuria, paroxysmal nocturnal, 15, 332–333
  clinical manifestations, 15
  complement in, 15
  complications, 15
  diagnosis, 15
  in leukemia, 30
  pancytopenia in, 28
  in preleukemia, 29
  stem cell monoclonality in, 15
  treatment, 15
Hemolysis
  anti-P antibodies in, 159
  after cardiopulmonary bypass, 474
  cold autoimmune, transfusion in, 477
  complement-mediated intravascular, 163
  in elliptocytosis, 14
  extravascular, 331
    predominantly, clinical symptoms in, 332
  in G6PD deficiency, 16
  in hemoglobinuria, paroxysmal nocturnal, 15
  immune, 303–324
    Aldomet in, 316–317
    drugs causing, 313–317
    drugs causing, examples of, 315
    drugs causing, laboratory testing in, 317
    drugs causing, mechanisms, 314
    drugs causing, pathogenesis, 316–317
    drugs causing, via suppressor T cell inhibition, 316–317
    immune complex mechanism in, 315–316
    tabular data on, 304
  intravascular
    DIC and, 89
    transfusion reactions leading to, 326
  non-antibody-mediated, 332
  red blood cell alloimmunization causing, 304
  red blood cell deficiencies causing, 333
  red blood cell, physical agents causing, 333

  reticulocytes in, 314
Hemolytic
  anemia (see Anemia, hemolytic)
  β-hemolytic streptococcal infection, 73
  disease of newborn, 3, 420–430
    ABH, 429
    ABO system and, 153
    amniocentesis in, 424
    amniotic fluid analysis in, 424
    amniotic fluid spectrophotometry in, 424–425
    antigens causing, 429–430
    complications, medical, 423
    Coombs test in, 204
    fetal maturity estimate in, 423
    hyperbilirubinemia in, pathophysiology, 430–431
    intrauterine therapy, 425
    maternal immunologic response assessment in, 423–424
    obstetric history in, 423
    pathophysiology, 421–422
    severity, different factors affecting, 423
    transfusion in, intrauterine, 425–428
  process, 306
  reactions, 2
    acute, management scheme for, 330
    immune, intravascular, clinical findings in, 327–328
  transfusion reactions (see Transfusion, reactions, hemolytic)
  uremic syndrome, T activation in, 184
Hemophilia
  A, 16, 84, 85
    classification, 85
    cryoprecipitate in, 247
    management, 85
  B, 84, 85
    incidence, 85
    Leyden, 85
  as sex-linked recessive trait, 85
  complications, 85
  hepatitis in, 465
Hemopoiesis
  development, in children, 434
  extramedullary, 8
  hypoplastic, in preleukemia, 29
  infective, and preleukemia, 29
Hemorrhage
  (See also Bleeding)

Hemorrhage *(cont.)*
  coagulation abnormalities and, 84
  fetomaternal, 422
    evaluation of, 428–429
    Rh immunization and, 173
  in leukemia, acute myelogenous, 36
  after marrow transplant, 227
  during minor surgery in hemophilia A, 85
  producing "washout" effect and thrombocytopenia, 78
  thrombocytosis and, 79
  transfusion, massive, 91
  vitamin K deficiency causing, in newborn, 87
Hemosiderin, 9
Hemostasis, 71–101
  abnormal, due to endothelial derangement, 72–73
  derangement during open heart surgery, 473
  endothelial integrity in, 72
  in heart surgery, 90–91
  platelets in, 73–78
  physiology, 74–75
  soluble phase of, coagulation as (*see* Coagulation)
Henoch-Schönlein purpura, 73, 122
Heparin, 22
  as anticoagulant, 240
  -antithrombin III, 82
  in cardiopulmonary bypass, 473
  coagulation altered by, 90
  cofactor
    I, 83
    II, 83
  in DIC, 90
  laboratory control of, 473
  rebound phenomenon, 90
Hepatitis
  A, 355
    course, 356
  B, 355–367
    acute phase, 359
    autoantibodies in, 365
    chronic, 364–365
    clinical characteristics, 359, 365
    clinical presentation, 359
    complications, 364–366
    course of, 364
    delta agent in, 362–363
    diagnosis, laboratory profiles in, 363
    fulminant, 364
    groups at high risk for, 364
    immunization in, passive, 367
    incubation period, 359
    laboratory findings, nonspecific, 359–360
    markers in, serologic, 361
    pathogenesis, 357–358
    prophylaxis, 366–367
    relapsing, 364
    surface antigen, exposure to, prophylaxis for, 367
    surface antigen, immunoassay for, enzyme, 363
    surface antigen, latex agglutination test for, 362
    surface antigen, radioimmunoassay of, 361
    treatment guidelines, 366
    vaccine, and AIDS, 390–391
    virus epidemiology of, 363–364
    virus, genome, model of, 357
    virus, genome structure of, 357
    virus, markers in, detection of, 360–362
    virus particle, 356
    virus, pathology of, 359
  blood banking, concepts, 369–370
  blood banking testing, quality control, 369–370
  blood donation and, 237
  chronic active, autoimmune, characteristics, 365
  clinical characteristics, 368
  Dudley hypothesis in, 358
  in factor VIII replacement therapy, 258
  in hemophilia, 465
  hepatoma and, 365–366
  immunoglobulins in, 261
  incubation periods for, mean, 360
  NANB, 367–369
  neutropenia of, 26
  non-A, non-B, 367–369
  perinatal transmission, 367
  platelet units and, 249
  after transfusion, 130
    strategy for donor recall, 370
  viral, causing aplastic anemia, 9
Hepatocytes, 79
Hepatoma: and hepatitis, 365–366
Hepatomegaly: in lymphocytic leukemia, 38
Hepatosplenomegaly, 30
  in lymphoma, non-Hodgkin's, 48
Hexose monophosphate shunt, 16
  deficiency, 16
  pathway, 15
Histamine, 22
  degranulation and release of, 122
  IgE and, 105
Histocompatibility
  antigens, 3, 218
  complex(es)
    HLA, and disease, proposed theories, 229
    H2, on chromosome 17 (in mice), 225
    immune response and, 3, 128–129
  major histocompatibility region (in mice), 224
HLA, 112
  -A, 218
    class I, 220
    cross-reactivity of antisera to, 219
    currently accepted, 219
    identification, laboratory, 224–225
    in leukemia, acute lymphocytic, 40
    on platelets, significance of, 227
  -A2, 220
  -B, 218
  -B8 antigen and autoimmunity, 131
  blanks, 219
  -B7, 220
  -B27, 27
  -C, 218
  compatibility in platelet transfusions, 251
  cross-reactive groups in common HLA types, 220
  -D, 218
  in disease, 228
    associations, 231
    examples of associations, 230
    mechanisms of disease susceptibility, 229–230
    selection of samples, 228
    statistical evaluation, 228–229
  -DR, 220, 221
  -DR antigens, 36
  -DS, 221
  factor B and, 122
  genes, on short arm of chromosome 6, 223
  histocompacibility complex and disease, proposed theories, 229
  locus, megagene characteristics of, 221–222
  -matched granulocytes, 254
  -matched platelets, 251
    single donor and, 250–251
  matching
    for granulocyte transfusion, 228

marrow transplant and, 226–227
molecular complex, biochemistry of, 219–221
in paternity testing, 228
phenotype, and categories of disease associations, 230–231
system, 218–235
  genetics of, 221–223
  immunobiology of, 223–224
  linkage disequilibrium, 222–223
  nomenclature, 218–219
  in paternity testing, 411
  testing, for paternity exclusion, 412
  in transplant (*see* Transplantation, kidney, HLA)
-typed platelets, 36
typing
  in paternity testing exclusion, 222
  in platelet transfusion, 227–228
Hodgkin's disease, 21, 44–45
  chromosomal abnormalities, 44
  classification, 44–45
    Ann Arbor, 45
    histologic, 45
    Rye, 44
  fibrosis, diffuse, 45
  immunologic abnormalities, 44
  leukemia and, 30, 34
  lymphocyte depletion, 45
  lymphocyte predominance, 45
  lymphocytopenia in, 29
  mixed cellularity, 45
  morphological abnormalities, 44
  prognosis, 45
  radiotherapy of (*see* Radiotherapy, of Hodgkin's disease)
  sclerosis, nodular, 45
  stage I, 45
  stage II, 45
  stage III, 45
  stage IV, 45
  stages, 45
  survival, 45
  symptoms, 45
  thrombocytosis in, 79
Hog stomach mucosa, 150
Homosexual males
  AIDS and, 377–378
  blood donation and, 237
Horse stomach mucosa, 150
Host defenses: eosinophils in, 21
5-HPETE, 22

H substances (*see* Blood groups, H substances)
HTLV
  proteins from infected permissive T cell clones, 382
  virus, 380–383
    pathogenic role, 382–383
Hübner-Thomsen-Friedenreich phenomenon, 183
Humoral
  immunity (*see* Immunity, humoral)
  inhibitors of coagulation, 83
Hurler's disease, 23
Hustin, A., 1
Hybridization, 107
Hybridoma
  antibodies, anticomplement, 112
  technology, 3
Hydantoin: causing aplastic anemia, 9
Hydration envelope: and RBCs, 111
Hydrochloroquine, 25
Hydrocortisone sodium succinate: in anaphylactic reactions, 133
Hydrogen bonding, 111
Hydrolases, 75
Hydrophobic, 108
  bonding, 111
Hydroxyethyl starch, 261
  for cytapheresis, 284
5-Hydroxyperoxyeicosatetraenoic acid, 22
Hyperbilirubinemia: in hemolytic disease of newborn, pathophysiology, 430–431
Hypergammaglobulinemia: polyclonal, in immunoblastic lymphadenopathy, 49
Hyperimmunoglobulin E syndrome, 24
Hyperkalemia: after transfusion, 340
Hyperplasia
  erythroblastic, 33
  lymph node (*see* Lymph nodes, hyperplasia)
  marrow, and preleukemia, 29
Hyperproteinemia, 213
Hypersensitivity
  delayed, 132–135
  immediate, 132–135
  lymphocytosis and, 29
  mast cells and, 132
  type I reactions, 132–133
  type II reactions, 133
  type III reactions, 133
  type IV reactions, 133–134

Hypersplenism
  pancytopenia in, 28
  platelet destruction and, 78
Hyperuricemia, 35
Hyperventilation: after apheresis, 287
Hyperviscosity
  in gammopathy, 131
  syndrome, plasmapheresis in, 289–290
  in Waldenström's macroglobulinemia, 50
Hypoadrenocorticism, 21
Hypochromia: causes of, 9
Hypochromic (*see* Anemia, hypochromic)
Hypocomplementemia: in rheumatoid arthritis, 122
Hypogammaglobulinemia
  ABO discrepancy and, 153
  in leukemia, lymphocytic
    acute, 40
    chronic, 38
  X-linked, and C1q deficiency, 134
Hypoplasia: of thymus, 129
Hypotetraploid cells, 44
Hypothermia, 214
  in P system, 159
Hypovolemia: after apheresis, 287
Hypovolemic (*see* Shock, hypovolemic)
Hypoxia, 72
  platelet destruction and, 78

I

Icterus: in newborn, 16
Idiotypes, 106
  T cell, 127
Ig (*see* Immunoglobulin)
Ii blood group (*see* Blood groups, Ii)
Immune
  complex(es)
    circulating, diseases with, plasmapheresis in, 290–292
    disease, 133
    disease, chronic, 365
    in leukemia, acute myelogenous, 37
    mechanism, 315–316
    in purpura, Henoch-Schönlein, 73
    RBCs as carriers of, 120
    reduction, and plasma exchange, 286
  deficiency (*see* Immunodeficiency)
  hemolysis (*see* Hemolysis, immune)
  -mediated
    neutropenia, 26

Immune *(cont.)*
    thrombocytopenia, 78
    reaction, hypersensitivity *(see* Hypersensitivity)
    response
        cell-cell interactions in, 127–128
        cell cooperation in, 126–127
        cell cooperation in, theories of, 126
        genes, 224
        histocompatibility complex and, 3
        histocompatibility complex and, major, 128–129
        in leukemia, acute lymphocytic, 38
        lymphocytes and, 23
        pathology, 129–131
        Rh antigens and, 172
    system
        assignment of genes associated with, 222
        deficiencies and Hodgkin's disease, 44
        modulation, 230
Immunity
    cell-mediated, testing, 226
    cellular, 2, 123–129
        T cells in, 124
    charitable, 452, 454
    humoral, 102–113
        B cells in, 124
    humoral theory of, 2
Immunization
    active, against anthrax, 2
    conception of term, 2
    in vitro, 112
    passive, in hepatitis, 367
    Rh *(see* Rh immunization)
    by transfusion, antibodies after, 38
Immunoassay
    hemagglutination inhibition, RBC, 84
    for hepatitis B surface antigen, 363
Immunobiology: of HLA system, 223–224
Immunoblastic lymphadenopathy, 49
Immunocytes, 151
Immunodeficiency
    acquired, 130–131
    acquired immunodeficiency syndrome *(see* AIDS)
    combined, severe, 130
    congenital, 129–130
    converting to leukemia, 30
    diagnosis, 112
    lymphocytopenia due to, 29
    secondary, 130

thrombocytopenia and, 77
Immunodiffusion
    in antigen-antibody reactions, 113
    double technique, 113
Immunoelectrophoresis, 113, 114
    in myeloma, plasma cell, 50
Immunoferritin electron microscopy, 146
Immunofluorescence, 113
Immunogenes: in lymph node hyperplasia, 43
Immunogenicity, 108
    of antigens, 128
    Rh, 172
Immunoglobulin, 102–108
    A, 104–105
        complexes in purpura, 73
        deficiency, anaphylaxis after cryoprecipitate in, 247
        in leukemia, chronic lymphocytic, 38
        nephritis, 122
        reactions to, 337
    in agammaglobulinemia, 130
    antibodies to, 338
    binding to membranes, 107–108
    biologic properties of, 104
    C, 102
    chemical properties of, 104
    class switching, 107
    classes, 104–105
    combining sites, sizes of, 103
    complement and, 116
    complement-binding, 104
    constant region, 102
    D, 105
    deficiency, selective, 130
    E, 105
        eosinophils with receptors for, 20
        Fc portion of, eosinophil receptors for, 21
        reactions due to, 338
        receptors for, 22
    Fc-dependent characteristics of, 116
    Fc portion of, 125
    found on B cells, 125
    G, 104
        antineutrophil maternal antibodies, 26
        binding to platelets, 78
        injected, reactions to, 336
        subclasses, 105
    heavy chains, 102–103
        amino acid sequence of, 104
        domains, 102–103
    in hepatitis, 261
    hinge region, 103
    isotype expression, genes responsible for, 125

light chains, 102
M, 104
    binding Clq, 116
    cold agglutinin, 49
    heavy chain of, 104
    intracytoplasmic, 49
    in Waldenström's macroglobulinemia, 50
monomer Fab fragment, 103
preparations, 260–261
    uses of, 260–261
specific binding, determinant of, 103–104
surface, in B cell leukemia, 39
surface-bound, effect on cells, 108
V, 102
variable region, 102
Immunohematology
    forensic, 409–419
    genetics in *(see* Genetics)
    of granulomatous disease of children, chronic, 24–25
    historical outline, 1–4
    prenatal, 420–430
    quality control in, 444–452
    workup in autoimmune hemolytic anemia, 308–309
Immunologic markers: in acute leukemia, 35
Immunologic phenomena: chemical analysis of, 2
Immunologic tolerance, 129
    autoimmunity as loss of, 131
Immunology, 102–144
    workup in AIDS, 387
Immunoparalysis: due to antigen excess, 132
Immunosuppression
    leukemia after, 30
    in purpura, idiopathic thrombocytopenic, 78
Incompatibility, 215
Indomethacin, 25
    platelet release and, 77
Infant
    agranulocytosis, genetic, 25, 26
    hematologic values in, 6
    leukemia of, acute myelogenous, 34
    X-linked agammaglobulinemia of, Bruton type, 130
Infarction: bone, and sickle cell anemia, 12
Infectious mononucleosis
    anemia due to, aplastic, 9
    anti-i antibodies in, 157–158, 206, 209
    neutropenia of, 26
Inheritance patterns: in paternity testing, 410

Inosine: in RBC rejuvenation, 263
Interleukin, 129
Intestine
  (See also Gastrointestinal)
  infection, and ABO discrepancy, 153
  sterilization syndrome, 87
Intrauterine transfusion: in hemolytic disease of newborn, 425–428
Intravenous injection, 1
Intrinsic factor: in pernicious anemia, 10
Intrinsic pathway
  of factor VIII, 81
  factor XI in, 81
Intrinsic system, 82
Inventory control, 452
Ionizing radiation (see Radiation)
Ir genes, 224
Iron
  in anemia, aplastic, 9
  deficiency
    anemia, 9–10
    hypochromia due to, 9
  serum, decrease, 9
  store decrease causing anemia, 9
  total body, 9
Isoagglutinin
  anti-T, 184
  discussion of term, 2
Isoantibodies, 152
Isoimmune neutropenia: in newborn, 26
Isotransferrin, 9

J

Jaundice: in graft-vs.-host disease, 134
Jenner, 2
Jerne network theory, 106

K

Kabat, 3
Kala-azar
  pancytopenia in, 28
  transfusion transmitting, 344
Kallikrein, 20
  factor VII activity and, 82
  factor XII and, 81
  factor XIIa and, 82
Kaposi's sarcoma, 73
Kawasaki's disease: neutropenia of, 26
Kell antigen (see Antigens, Kell)
Kell system (see Blood groups, Kell system)
Kidd antigens: statistical frequencies of, 177
Kidd system (see Blood groups, Kidd system)
Kidney
  disease
    blood donation and, 238
    chronic, 21
    factor VII and, 80
  failure
    anemia due to, aplastic, 9
    red blood cells and, packed, 241
    thrombocytopenia due to, 77
  transplant (see Transplantation, kidney)
Killer cells, 125
Kinin-generating system: chemoattractants, 19
Kininogen
  characteristics of, 79
  high molecular weight, 82
  kallikrein activating, 81
Klebsiella, 27
  pneumoniae, in acute myelogenous leukemia, 37
Kleihauer-Betke method: to calculate a fetomaternal bleed, 174
Kostmann's disease, 26
Kupffer cells, 121
Kx antigen, 24

L

"Labeling index," 18
Labile factor: characteristics of, 79
Lactic dehydrogenase: in autoimmune hemolytic anemia, 307
Lactoferrin, 18
Lactosyl ceramide: in P system substances synthesis, 158
Laminin, 20
Landsteiner, 2, 3, 109
  blood group theories of, 2
  rule, 146
Landsteiner-Wiener antigen, 170
Langeris antigens, 182
Langmuir plots, 110
LAP: in paroxysmal nocturnal hemoglobinuria, 15
Latex agglutination test, 84, 90
  for hepatitis B surface antigen, 362
Latham bowl
  modified, 249
  principle for donor apheresis, 281
Law(s)
  antitrust, regarding blood banking, 456
  of coincidental happenings, 403
  of effect of previous events, 403–404
  Hardy-Weinberg, in paternity testing, 415
LDH: increase in acute myelogenous leukemia, 35
Le^a substances: sugar sequence of, 155
Le^b substances: sugar sequence of, 155
Lead
  interfering with cation pump, 10
  poisoning, 9
  porphyria after, 10
Lectins, 209–210
  reactivity, 184
Leder, 3
Leg ulcers: in sickle cell anemia, 12
Legal actions, against blood bank, 454–455
  preventive measures, 454–455
  suits filed against blood bank, 455
Legal aspects
  of blood banking, 452–454
  of paternity testing, 416–417
Legal matters: affecting blood bank management, 454
Leukapheresis, 254
  filtration
    complications, 287–288
    neutropenia during, 27
  in leukemia, 32
    chronic myelogenous, 34
  neutrophilia and, 28
  preleukapheresis testing, 253–254
  therapeutic, 478
Leukemia, 29–43
  ABO antigen weakening in, 154
  ABO discrepancy and, 153
  acute, classification, differentiated morphological, 32
  acute, immunologic markers in, 35
  acute lymphocytic, 38–40
    B cell, 39
    Burkitt's-like, 40
    classification, FAB, 39
    common type, 39
    cytochemical characterization, 39
    differentiation from acute myelocytic leukemia, 39
    etiology, 40
    immunologic characterization, 39

Leukemia (cont.)
  morphological
    characterization, 39
    null cell, 39
    prognosis, 40
    T cell, 39
    therapy, 40
    undifferentiated, 39
  acute, marrow transplant in, 265
  acute myeloblastic, and
    agnogenic myeloid
    metaplasia, 43
  acute myelogenous, 34–37
    chromosomal abnormalities in, 35–36
    classification, FAB, 35
    combination therapy of, 36
    correlation of subclassification with clinical outcome, 36
    diagnosis, differential, 36
    differentiation from acute lymphocytic leukemia, 39
    laboratory features, 36
    laboratory findings in, 35
    prognosis, 36, 37
    remission, complete, 37
    treatment, 36–37
    variants, 35
  acute nonlymphocytic, 30
  acute, after preleukemia, 29
  acute promyelocytic, 35
  -associated antigens, 36
  basophilic, 33
  basophils and, 22
  chemotherapy of, 41
  chronic granulocytic, leukostasis, 293
  chronic lymphocytic, 37–38
    B cell, 37, 38
    clinical features, 38
    familial tendency in, 37
    "lymphosarcoma type," 38
    monoclonality of, 38
    prognosis, 38
    staging of, 38
    subtypes, 37
    survival with therapy, 38
    T cell, 37
    therapy, 38
  chronic myelocytic
    diagnosis, differential, 33
    prognosis, 34
  chronic myelogenous, 30–34
    chemotherapy, 33–34
    clinical presentation, 31
    drugs for, 33
    etiologic agents associated with, 31
    laboratory findings, 31–33
    leukocyte donors with, 255
    monoclonality of, 31
    remission, 34
    therapy of, 33
    variants of, 33
  chronic neutrophilic, 31
  complicating paroxysmal nocturnal hemoglobinuria, 15
  conditions leading to, 30
  DIC and, 89
  hairy cell, 37, 42
  I antigen weakening in, 157
  lymphoblastic, 39
  lymphocytic, and lymphocytosis, 29
  marrow transplant in
    complications, 265
    with prior treatment, 264
  mastocytosis and, malignant, 43
  myeloblastic, 36
  myelomonocytic, 15, 32, 36
  oligoblastic, 29
  pancytopenia due to, 28
  prolymphocytic, 37
  promyelocytic, 36
  T cell
    human, 40
    Japanese, 128
  virus, Rauscher murine, 44
Leukemoid reaction, 28
  eosinophilic, 22
  leukoerythroblastic type, 28
Leukoagglutinins, 253
  lung infiltrates due to, 335
Leukocyte (see White blood cells)
Leukocytosis-inducing factor, 19
Leukoerythroblastic phenomenon, 9
Leukoerythroblastic reactions, 33
Leukopenia
  DIC and, 89
  granulocyte transfusion in, 476
  in hemoglobinuria, paroxysmal nocturnal, 15
Leukostasis, 34
  in leukemia, granulocytic, 293
Leukostatic lesions, 32
Leukotrienes, 122
  complement and, 121
  IgE and, 105
Leu-3, 112
Levamisole, 27
Levine, 1
Levodopa: in immune hemolysis, 317
Lewis antigens, 155
  clinical aspects of, 156
Lewis system, 154–156
  biochemistry, 154–155
  serologic aspects of, 155–156
Lewishon, R., 1
Liability
  absolute, 452
  strict, 453
  warrant, 453
Libavius, Andreas, 1
Licensing: and blood bank management, 454
Liley graph: modified, 426
Linkage (see Gene, linkage)
Lipid
  bilayer of red blood cells, 6–7
  composition abnormality, 14–15
  storage diseases, pancytopenia in, 28
Lipoprotein: antibodies to, 338
β-Lipoproteinemia, 15
Lithium carbonate, 27
Liver
  biopsy in non-Hodgkin's lymphoma, 48
  carboxylase, 87
  damage in graft-vs.-host disease, 134
  disease
    blood donation and, 238
    coagulopathy, 87
    platelet defects in, 75
    prothrombin lyophilized concentrates in, 87
  fetal, primitive B cells in, 49
  macrophages, trapping by mechanism of, 308
  platelets and, 73
  procoagulants and, activated, 83
  synthesizing factor VIII, 81
Lomustine, 41
  effect on marrow, 42
Lower, Richard, 1
Lung
  (See also Pulmonary)
  infiltrates due to leukoagglutinins, 335
Lupus erythematosus-like syndrome (in mice), 132
Lupus erythematosus, systemic, 25
  blood donation and, 238
  DIC and, 89
  factor VIII inhibitors and, 88
  granulomatous disease of children and, chronic, 25
  hemolytic anemia in, autoimmune, 213
  lymphocytopenia in, 29
  pancytopenia in, 28
  thrombocytopenia and, 78
Lutheran system (see Blood groups, Lutheran system)
Lymph nodes
  anatomy, functional, 124
  acute, 43
  acute, germinal centers in, 43
  chronic nonspecific 43–44
  in leukemia, chronic

Index

lymphocytic, 38
pathology, 43–50
peripheral, functional anatomy, 124
Lymphadenopathy
  immunoblastic, 49
  in leukemia
    chronic lymphocytic, 38
    myeloblastic, 36
Lymphatic
  afferent, 124
  flow, 124
  organs, 124
  system, 123–126
Lymphoblast, 17
Lymphocyte(s), 17, 22–23
  activation, 127
  in AIDS, ultrastructural changes, 385
  endothelium and, 72
  enumeration, 112
  in Hodgkin's disease, 45
  killer, 121
  -macrophage interactions, 128
  -myeloma cells, 112
  origin of, 8
  after radiotherapy, 77
  subpopulations, 124–126
  suppression, 127
  T cell, 102
B Lymphocytes
  differentiation of, 105
  disorder, 25
  plasma cells and, 23
T Lymphocyte disorder, 25
Lymphocytopenia, 29
  causes, major, 29
Lymphocytosis, 28–29, 157
  causes, major, 29
  -promoting factor, 29
Lymphoma, 44–49
  ABO antigen weakening in, 154
  Burkitt's
    cyclophosphamide in, 48
    Epstein-Barr virus in, 40
    Epstein-Barr virus DNA in, 47
    translocation in, 48
  CNS, 47
  diffuse, 48
    B cells in, 48
    cell marker analysis, 49
    laboratory, 49
    prognosis as poor, 48
    treatment, 49
  follicular, 48
    B cells in, 48
  monoclonal antibodies and, 158
  nodular, 48
    B cells in, 48
  non-Hodgkin's, 37, 44, 45–49

B cell, 47
  B cell markers in, 46
  cell surface monoclonal markers, 49
  cells as large cleaved, 46
  cells as large noncleaved, 47
  cells as small cleaved, 46
  cells as small noncleaved, 46
  chromosomal abnormalities of, 48
  classification, Ann Arbor, 45
  classification, histopathologic, 46–47
  classification of Lukes-Collins, 47
  classification of NCI working formulation study, 47
  classification of Rappaport, 46
  clinical aspects, 48
  correlation of histopathology with stage and prognosis, 48
  etiology, 47–48
  pathogenesis, 47–48
  stage I, 45
  stage II, 45
  stage III, 45
  stage IV, 45
  staging procedures, 48
  T cell, 47
  T cell receptors in, 46
pancytopenia due to, 28
splenomegaly and, 306
Lymphoproliferative disorders, 303
Lymphosarcoma, 37
Lysine, 82
  humoral inhibitors of coagulation and, 83
  in platelet adhesion, 74
  in platelets, 75
Lysis, 118
  membrane, 114
Lysosomes
  in platelet, 74
  as primary granules, 18
Lysozyme, 18
  in leukemia, 32

M

a_2-Macroglobulin inhibitor, 83
Macroglobulinemia: Rouleaux formation in, 213
Macroglobulinemia, Waldenström's, 37, 50, 131
  chlorambucil in, 131
  intravascular paraprotein component of, 50
  melphalan in, 131
  Rouleaux formation in, 50

Macrophages, 121, 125–126
  binding sites, 215
  complement receptors on, 304–306
  Fc on, 304–306
  fibrin and, 83
  impairment of killing capacity in AIDS, 384
  liver, mechanisms of trapping by, 308
  -lymphocyte interactions, 128
  precursors, 73
  presenting antigen to B and T cells, model, 224
  procoagulants and, activated, 83
  splenic, mechanism of trapping by, 308
Magnesium: in platelet release type 1, 75
Majocchi-Schamberg purpura, 72
Malaria: after transfusion, treatment, 343
Malignancy (see Cancer)
Mancini plate, 113, 114
Mannosidosis, 25
M antigens: contrasted with N antigens, 160
Marfan's syndrome, 72
Marrow
  in aged, 6
  aspiration, 226
  autologous, 34
  B cells in, primitive, 49
  biopsy (see Biopsy, marrow)
  culturing, 36
  effect of chemotherapy on, 42
  frozen, 263
  graft in paroxysmal nocturnal hemoglobinuria, 15
  hyperplasia and preleukemia, 29
  in leukemia, 32
  in myeloid metaplasia, agnogenic, 43
  in pancytopenia, 28
  in platelet removal, senescent, 73
  stress, 157
  suppression, 41
  thrombocytopenia and, 77
  transplant (see Transplantation, marrow)
  trapping platelets, 74
Mast cells, 22–23
  comparison with basophils, 22
  degranulation of, 22
  hypersensitivity and, 132
Mastocytosis
  basophils and, 22
  malignant, 42–43
Maternal
  fetomaternal hemorrhage, 422

Maternal (cont.)
   Rh immunization and, 173
   immunologic response assessment in hemolytic disease of newborn, 423–424
May-Hegglin anomaly, 23, 77
MCH, 5
MCHC, 5
McLeod syndrome
   acanthocytosis in, 15
   granulomatous disease of children and, chronic, 24
   Kell antigens and, 181
MCV, 5
Mean corpuscular
   hemoglobin, 5
      concentration, 5
   volume, 5
Measles: and blood donation, 237
Mechlorethamine, 41
   effect on marrow, 42
Meconium stain: for amniotic fluid spectrophotometry, 427
Mefananic acid: in immune hemolysis, 317
Megagene characteristics: of HLA locus, 221–222
Megakaryoblasts, 73
Megakaryocytes, 8, 32
   after cytosine arabinoside, 77
   membranes, 73
   precursors, 73
Megaloblastic (see Anemia, megaloblastic)
Meiosis: chromosomal material reduction during, 399
Melphalan
   effect on marrow, 42
   in gammopathy, 131
   in macroglobulinemia, Waldenström's, 131
   in myeloma, 37
      plasma cell, 50
   platelet function after, 77
   in polycythemia vera, 43
Mendelian genetics, 403–407
Meningococcal infection, 135
Mercaptopurine: inhibiting DNA synthesis, 40
6-Mercaptopurine in leukemia, myelogenous
   acute, 36
   chronic, 33
Metabisulfite test, 12
Metamyelocytes, 18
Metaplasia: agnogenic myeloid, 43
Metchnikoff, Elie, 2
Methicillin: and platelet survival, 251

Methionine, 160
Methotrexate
   cell cycle and, 41
   inhibiting DNA and RNA synthesis, 40
α-Methyldopa: in immune hemolysis, 316
MHC molecules: model of, 221
Microaggregate(s)
   filters, 243
   of leukocytes, 340–341
   of platelets, 340–341
Microcytosis, 9
Microscopy (see Electron microscopy)
Microthrombosis: fibrin, 89
Microtubules, 73
Milstein, 3
Miltenberger complex, 159
Minigene, 103
Mithramycin: effect on marrow, 42
Mitochondria, 74
Mitomycin: effect on marrow, 42
MNSs antigens
   amino acids of, terminal, 161
   red cell membrane glycoproteins and, 160
MNSs system (see Blood groups, MNSs system)
Model
   of hepatitis B virus genome, 357
   Jerne network, 106
   of macrophage presenting antigen to B and T cells, 224
   of MHC molecules, 221
   of Rh molecule, 164
   Rosenfield, for Rh genes, 165
   Singer's bilayer, of biologic membranes, 7
Mollison collapse curve, 215
Monoclonal antibodies, 111–113, 210–211
   to ABH substances, 152–154
   against factor VIII, 85
   against T cell markers, 125
   B cells and, 111
   binding, radiolabeled, logarithmic index of, 113
   in clotting factor analysis, 113
   in cold agglutinin disease, 158
   in factor IX, 85
   to group A, 211
   to group B, 211
   lymphoma and, 158
Monoclonal gammopathy: benign, 131
Monocytes, 17, 22–23, 305
   -free platelet, 252

   in granulomatous disease of children, chronic, 24
   in vitro assay in autoimmune hemolytic anemia, 308
Mononuclear cells: Fc receptors on, 108
Mononucleosis (see Infectious mononucleosis)
Morquio's syndrome, 23
Mortality: in AIDS, 378
Morton's formula: for linkage, 405–406
MTY: effect on marrow, 42
Mucopolysaccharides, 71
Mucosa
   hog stomach, 150
   horse stomach, 150
Multimers, 76
Multiple sclerosis: plasmapheresis in, 291
Muramidase, 10
Mutagenic effects: of retroviruses, 381–382
Mutation(s)
   gene, 406
   in paternity testing, 410
   somatic, 106–107
Myasthenia gravis: plasmapheresis in, 290
c-Myc oncogene, 47, 48
Mycobacterial infections, 25
   basophils and, 22
   disseminated, pancytopenia in, 28
Mycosis fungoides, 42
Myeloblast, 17
Myelocytes, 17
   from promyelocytes, 17–18
   secondary granules, 18
   specific granules, 18
   type A granules, 17
   type B granules, 17
Myelofibrosis
   in leukemia, 30
   marrow in, 9
   myeloid metaplasia and, agnogenic, 43
   pancytopenia due to, 28
   and polycythemia vera, 43
Myeloid metaplasia: agnogenic, 43
Myeloma, 111
   cells, drug-marked, 112
   -lymphocyte cells, 112
   pancytopenia due to, 28
   plasma cell, 50
      diagnosis, laboratory, 50
      etiology, 50
      treatment, 50
   rouleaux formation in, 213
Myeloperoxidase, 18, 19, 32
   granules, 35

Myelophthisis, 9
Myeloproliferative disorders, 43
  platelets in, 252
  thrombocytopenia in, 79
Myelosuppression
  of polycythemia vera, 43
  thrombocytopenia due to, 77
Myosin, 20

N

NADPH, 17
  hexose monophosphate shunt as source of, 16
"Nail-patella" syndrome: and ABO system, 151
NANA carbohydrate moiety, 160
N antigens: contrasted with M antigens, 160
Naphthylacetate esterase, 32
Natural selection, 223
  phenomenon, 222
Nausea: after apheresis, 287
Necrosis: and DIC, 89
Negligence, 452–453
Nematodes, 21
Neocytes, 245
Neonatal (see Newborn)
Neoplastic disorders (see Tumors)
Neostigmine, 73
Nephelometry, 113
Nephritic factor, 122
Nephritis: IgA, 122
Nervous system: central, lymphoma, 47
Network theory: of Jerne, 106
Neuraminidase, 160
Neutropenia
  alloimmune, in newborn, 436–437
  autoimmune, 25, 26
  B cell disorders and, 25–26
  chronic hypoplastic, 25
  classification
    by cell kinetics, 26
    by etiology, 25
  cyclic, 26
    (in gray collie dogs), 26
  drug-induced, 27
  findings in, 27
  hypoplastic, in preleukemia, 29
  immune-mediated, 26
  of infections, 26, 27
  isoimmune, in newborn, 26
  management, 27–28
  organisms isolated in, 27
  presentation, 27
  stem cell
    committed, 26
    noncommitted, 25–26

  stem cell disorders leading to, acquired, 26
  T cell disorders and, 25–26
  therapy, 27
  type I, 26
  type II, 26
  type III, 26
  type IV, 26
  type V, 26
Neutrophil(s), 120
  adhering to endothelial cells, 20
  antigens (see Antigens, neutrophil)
  chemotaxis, 19–20
  degranulation, 19
  disorders, quantitative, 25
  as Fc receptors for immunoglobulin and complement, 20
  granule
    azurophilic, 18
    characteristics of, 18
    specific, 18
  in granulomatous disease of children, chronic, 24
  hypersegmentation, 10
  kinetics, 19
    three compartments, 19
  polymorphonuclear, 18
Neutrophilia, 28
  mechanisms of, 28
Newborn
  ABH antigens in, 148
  anemia of, 434–435
  blood volume in, total, 6
  clotting deficiencies in, 437
  diseases requiring blood components, 436–437
  exchange transfusion for (see Transfusion, exchange, in newborn)
  factors in, 6
  hematocrit, 6
  hematologic parameters in, 434
  hematologic values, 6
  hemoglobin, 6
    mean, 6
  hemolytic disease (see Hemolytic, disease of newborn)
  hemorrhage due to vitamin K deficiency, 87
  icterus, 16
  neutropenia
    alloimmune, 436–437
    isoimmune, 26
  oxygen affinity curve in, 6
  platelet counts in, 6
  prothrombin in, 6
  reticulocyte counts in, 6
  thrombocytopenia, 436

  transfusion for, 435–436
    complications, 435–436
  white blood cells in, 6
Night sweats: in non-Hodgkin's lymphoma, 48
Nitroblue tetrazolium screen: for chronic granulomatous disease of children, 24
Nitrogen mustard, 41
  in Hodgkin's disease, 45
  in leukemia, chronic myelogenous, 33
Nitrosourea, 41
  effect on marrow, 42
Nocturnal (see Hemoglobinuria, paroxysmal nocturnal)
Nucleoli: in myeloblastic leukemia, 36
Nucleotides, 74
Nystatin: in acute myelogenous leukemia, 37

O

Obstetric history: in hemolytic disease of newborn, 423
OKT4, 112
OKT8, 112
Oligoclonal antibodies: in cold agglutinin disease, 158
Oligoclonality, 88
Oncogenes, 47
  c-myc, 47–48
Ontogeny, 106
  of T cells, 127
Opsonization: sensitization of cells during, 114
Oral surgery: and blood donation, 238
Osmotic shock: to red blood cells, 333
Osteopetrosis: causing pancytopenia, 28
Ouchterlony
  plate, 113
  technique, 113
Ovarian carcinoma, 37
  leukemia in, 34
Oxygen
  affinity
    of cord blood, 6
    curve in newborn, 6
  carrier, artificial, 262
  hemoglobin affinity for, 7
  saturation curves, 7
  transport
    during blood storage, 240
    hemoglobin in, 7
Oxygenator for cardiopulmonary bypass, 471

Oxygenator for cardiopulmonary
    bypass (cont.)
  five components of, 472
  main oxygenator pump, 471

P

Pancytopenia, 28
  causes, main, 28
  pathogenesis, 28
  in preleukemia, 29
Paraglobiside: conversion of
    lactosyl ceramide to, 158
Parasitic diseases: transmitted by
    transfusion, 343
Parasitic infections, 21
Parasitoses, 21
Paresthesias: after apheresis, 287
PAS, 36
PAS-positive granules, 35
Pasteur, 2
Paternity exclusion tests: Duffy
    system in, 176
Paternity index, 416
Paternity: plausibility of, 416
Paternity testing, 105, 409–419
  ABO system in, 410–411
  adenosine deaminase in, 413
  adenylate kinase in, 413–414
  blood samples in, 409
  direct exclusion in, 410
  esterase D in, 413
  exclusion
    cumulative probability of,
      415–416
    by HLA testing, 412
    by HLA typing, 222
  family studies, 409
  glucose-6-phosphate
      dehydrogenase in, 412–413
  glutamine pyruvate transaminase
      in, 413
  glyoxalase I in, 413
  Hardy-Weinberg law and, 415
  HLA in, 228
  HLA system in, 411
  identification, 409–417
    of probands, 409
  indirect exclusion in, 410
  legal aspects of, 416–417
  markers used, types, 409–410
  phosphoglucomutase in, 412
  proteins in, 414
  red blood cell acid phosphatase
      in, 412
  red blood cell enzyme
      phenotypes, 411–414
    characteristics of frequently
        used enzyme phenotypes,
        412–414
    sample collection, 412
  reporting, 409–417
  results, approach to, 414–417
  Rh system in, 411
  saliva samples in, 409
  validity of, 414
Pediatric (see Children)
Pedigree
  charts, 406
    symbols used in, 406
  family, representing a non-sex-
      linked trait, 40
Pelger-Huët anomaly, 30
Pelger-Huët cells, 35
Penicillin, 88
  anemia due to, aplastic, 9
Peptic ulcer: and ABH antigens,
    154
Perfluorocarbons, 262–263
Perfluorodecalin, 263
  structure, 262
Perinatal blood banking, 420–443
Perinatal hematology, 6
Perinatal transmission: of hepatitis,
    367
Pernicious (see Anemia, pernicious)
Peroxide ion, 19
Personnel: in blood banking, 445
Pfeiffer, 2
Phagocytosis: complement in, 121
Phenothiazines, 27
Phenotype
  Bombay (see Bombay phenotype)
  En^a-negative, 182
  haptoglobin, electrophoretic
      patterns of, 414
  HLA, and categories of disease
      associations, 230–231
  RBC enzyme (see Paternity
      testing, red blood cell
      enzyme phenotypes)
  Rh null, 168
Phenotyping: multiply transfused
    patient, 210
Phenylbutazone: causing aplastic
    anemia, 9
Phenytoin, 88
Philadelphia chromosome, 30, 31,
    34
  in acute lymphocytic leukemia
      prognosis, 40
Phlebotomy: predeposit, screening
    patients for, 294–295
Phorbol esters, 19
Phosphate: in RBC rejuvenation,
    263
Phosphoglucomutase: in paternity
    testing, 412
Phospholipid
  extrinsic system and, 83
  factors X activation and, 82
  for thrombin, 73

Phosphorus: radioactive, in
    polycythemia vera, 43
Physiogel, 261
Phytohemagglutinin: and T cells,
    125
Pigeon-breeders: and anti-P1
    antibodies, 159
Placenta
  abruptio, and DIC, 89
  immunoglobulin G crossing,
      104
  primitive B cells in, 49
Plasma
  capacity to clot of, 78
  cells, 22–23
    B cells becoming, 125
    in Hodgkin's disease, 45
    myeloma (see Myeloma,
        plasma cell)
  exchange
    continuous, noxious
        substances removed after,
        289
    partial, in rheumatoid
        arthritis, 291
  expanders, 261–262
  fractions, 257–263
    practices for, 465
  fresh frozen, 245–246
    in DIC, 90
    quality control in, 450
    storage, 246
    thawing, 246
    use of, clinical, 246
  hemolyzed, 244
  incompatible, 153
    reactions due to, 332
  platelet-rich, 248
  reactions, prevention, 336–337
  transfusion, practices, 464
Plasmapheresis, 286
  in diseases with circulating
      immune complexes, 290–
      292
  experimental techniques, 292
  for hyperviscosity syndrome
      treatment, 289–290
  marrow transplant rejection and,
      154
  in neutropenia, 26
  in Rh immunization, 174
  therapeutic, 288–289
    applications, 291
    costs of, 292
    hazards of, 292
  in Waldenström's
      macroglobulinemia, 50
Plasmin
  activation, 83
  alpha$_2$-macroglobulin inhibitor
      and, 83

degradation products of fibrin, 89
degrading factors, 84
  factor VII activity and, 82
  factor XII and, 81
  inhibition, 84
  inhibitor, 83
  regulating fibrinolytic system, 83
  substrates, 84
Plasminogen
  activator, 72
  kallikrein activating, 81
  regulating fibrinolytic system, 83
Plasmodium parasites: infecting RBCs bearing Duffy antigens, 175
Platelet(s), 73–78, 248–253
  in adhesion, 73, 74
    defects, 75, 76
  aggregation, 74–75
    abnormal due to clotting factor abnormalities, 76
    defects, 75, 76
    dense bodies during, 74
    factor VIII in, 81
    first-phase, 73
    primary, 74
    secondary, 74
  aggregometer curves, 77
  antibodies, 77, 251
  canalicular system, 76
  contractile phases, 73
  contractility, 248
  counts
    in DIC, 90
    in leukemia, 32
    in leukemia, acute myelogenous, 36
    in newborn, 6
    normal, 73
    before transfusion, 250
  crossmatches, 251
  cycle of adhesion-release-aggregation, 73
  defects
    acquired qualitative, 76–78
    congenital, 75–76
    drugs causing, 76–78
    major, 75
    storage pool, "acquired," 77
  disorders after cardiopulmonary bypass, 473–474
  dosage, calculation of, 250
  factor 4, 74
  factor X activation and, 82
  factor XI and, 82
  function
    impairment, 73
    secretory, 73

giant, 76
in hemostasis, 73–78
HLA antigens on, significance, 227
HLA-matched, 251
  single donor and, 250–251
HLA-typed, 36
microaggregates of, 340–341
monocyte-free, 252
organelle zone, 74
pathology, 75–78
peripheral zone, 73
  amorphous coat, 73
  membrane, 73
  submembrane, 73
physiology during hemostasis, 74–75
-pools, 91
poor response to, 251–252
postoperative, in heart surgery, 90–91
preparation of unit, 248–249
  automated methods, 248–249
  manual method, 248
production
  drugs inhibiting, 77
  kinetics, 73
  lack of causing thrombocytopenia, 77
quality control and, 451
after radiotherapy, 77
receptors on, 72
reduction in number, 73
release
  accelerating DIC, 88
  reaction, 75
  type 1, 75
  type 2, 75
-rich plasma, 248
senescent, marrow in removal of, 73
sol-gel zone, 73, 74
  canalicular system, open, 74
  cytoskeleton, 74
  microcanalicular system, 74
  tubular system, 74
  tubular system, dense, 74
in special clinical situations, 252–253
structure, 73–74
survival, 74, 248
survival time, 73
transfusion (*see* Transfusion, platelet)
turnover, 74
use in clinical practice, 249–250
Plateletpheresis, 286
  practices in, 477–478
  in thrombocytosis, 292
Pneumonia: viral, 158

PNH (*see* Hemoglobinuria, paroxysmal nocturnal)
Podophylotoxin, 41
Poisoning
  lead, 9
    porphyria after, 10
Poisons: snake, 88
Polyagglutinability, 153, 184
Polyagglutination, 78, 183–185
  Cad, 185
  clinical aspects, 185
  at laboratory level, 185
T-Polyagglutination, 183
Polyarteritis: and DIC, 89
Polybrene, 184
Polycythemia vera, 43
  converting to leukemia, 30
  thrombocytosis in, 79
Polyethylene glycol, 111
Polymorphonuclear cell: segmented, 18
Polyolefin containers: for platelet storage, 248
Polyploidy: 2N, 73
Pope Innocent VIII, 1
Porphyria
  erythropoietic, 10
  after lead poisoning, 10
  true, 10
Porphyrin defect: causing hypochromic anemia, 10
Porter, 3
Potassium: and blood storage, 241
Preapheresis laboratory testing, 285
Pre-B lymphocyte markers, 31
Precipitin reaction, 109–110
Prednisone
  in Hodgkin's disease, 45
  in leukemia, chronic lymphocytic, 38
  in myeloma, plasma cell, 50
  in purpura, idiopathic thrombocytopenic, 78
Pregnancy
  blood donation during, 237
  Rh antibodies in, 172–173
Prekallikrein, 20, 81
  activation of, 72
  characteristics of, 79
  factor XII and, 81
  factor XIIa and, 82
Preleukapheresis testing, 253–254
Preleukemia, 25, 26, 29–30
  conditions leading to, 30
  management, 30
  marrow transplant in, 30
  "promoter" phase, 29
  syndrome of, 29
Premature condensation analysis, 36
Prematurity, 6

Prematurity (cont.)
  blood volume in, total, 6
  thrombocytosis in, 79
Prenatal immunohematology, 420–430
Primaquine, 16
Pristane: in plasma cell myeloma, 50
Proaccelerin: characteristics of, 79
Probability, 403
  calculation by method of Fisher, 406–407
Procainamide: in immune hemolysis, 317
Procarbazine
  effect on marrow, 42
  in Hodgkin's disease, 45
Procoagulant(s)
  activity of prekallikrein, 81
  cellular clearance of, 83
  concentrates, complications from, 465–466
Proconvertin: characteristics of, 79
Progenitor cell disorder, 25, 26
Promyelocytes, 17
  myelocytes deriving from, 17–18
  type A azurophilic, nonspecific granules, 17
Pronase, 160
Properdin, 114
  pathway in complement activation, 118
Prostacyclin, 72
Prostaglandins, 72
  E_2
    in platelet release reaction, 75
    synthesis, 76
    eosinopenia due to, 21
  $F_{2\alpha}$
    in platelet release, 75
    synthesis, 76
  I_2, 72
    indomethacin inhibiting, 77
    in platelet release, 75
Protamine sulfate, 90
  gelation test, 90
Protease(s)
  inhibitor, 120
  neutral, 18
Proteins
  acidic, 18
  Bence Jones, in gammopathy, 131
  C, 72, 80
    in factor V deficiency, 86
  Charcot-Leyden crystal, 21
  complement, 122
  in criminology, 418
  derivative test, positive purified, 237
  eosinophil cationic, 21
  factor VIII-related, 81
  HTLV, from infected permissive T cell clones, 382
  involved in alternative pathway of complement activation, 119
  major basic, 21
  in paternity testing, 414
  plasma
    adsorption of, nonspecific, 316
    sensitivity causing transfusion reactions, 335–338
  S, and factor X, 80
  synthesis
    elongation, 401
    initiation, 401
    termination, 401
  thrombin-sensitive, 74
Prothrombin
  characteristics of, 79
  complex (see Factor, IX, concentrates)
  complex concentrates in hemophilia B, 85
  factor II, 80
  in factor VII deficiency, 86
  lyophilized concentrate in liver disease, 87
  in newborn, 6
  time, 84
  -vitamin K complex, 87
Prothrombinase: and factor X, 80
Protozoans, 21
Proximate cause, 452
Prozone, 113
"Prozoning," 110
Pseudomonas aeruginosa, 27
  in leukemia, acute myelogenous, 37
Pseudoneutropenia: acquired, 26–27
Pseudoxanthoma elasticum, 72
Psoriasis, 21
P system (see Blood groups, P system)
Pulmonary
  cardiopulmonary (see Cardiopulmonary)
  thrombosis, and sickle cell anemia, 12
Pump: cardiopulmonary, 77
Puromycin, 118
Purpura, 75
  Henoch-Schönlein, 73, 122
  Majocchi-Schamberg, 72
  nonthrombocytopenic, 72
  infections in, 72
  senile, 72
  stasis causing, chronic, 72
  thrombocytopenic, idiopathic, 78
Pyridoxine-responsive anemia, 9
Pyrogens: causing transfusion reactions, 343
Pyruvate: in RBC rejuvenation, 263

Q

Quality control, 444–452
  antiglobulin antiserum, 448–449
  antisera (see Antisera)
  in baths, water and dry, 447
  in blood banking, 445–447
    of equipment, 446–447
    for equipment, non-temperature-dependent, 447
    for equipment, temperature-dependent, 446–447
    freezers, 446–447
    personnel, 445
    supplies, 447–449
    supplies, disposable, 447
    view boxes, 447
  in blood component preparation, 449–451
  of forms, 451–452
  in immunohematology, 444–452
  inventory, 452
  monthly cumulative, 446
  profiles, types of, 445
  reagents, 447–448
  in record-keeping, 451–452
Quinidine, 25
  purpura and, idiopathic thrombocytopenic, 78

R

Radiation
  actinic, 72
  anemia due to, aplastic, 9
  initiating preleukemia, 29
  leukemia due to, 31
    acute lymphocytic, 40
    chronic myelocytic, 37
  as leukemogenic, 30
  pancytopenia due to, 28
Radiography
  in lymphoma, non-Hodgkin's, 48
  in thalassemia major, 14
Radioimmunoassay
  of antigen-antibody reactions, 113
  of hepatitis B surface antigen, 361
  of monoclonal antibodies, 112

Radiotherapy
  granulocytes after, 77
  in Hodgkin's disease, 45
    inverted Y pattern, 45
    mantle pattern, 45
  of lymph nodes in chronic
    lymphocytic leukemia, 38
  lymphocytes after, 77
  lymphocytopenia after, 29
  of lymphoma, diffuse, 49
  platelets after, 77
  of testes in leukemia, 40
Radius: absent radius syndrome, 77
Random distribution, 222
Rapaport, 3
Rapoport-Luebering shunt, 15
Rash: after cryoprecipitate, 247
Rauscher murine leukemia virus, 44
Raynaud's phenomenon
  complicating
    macroglobulinemia,
    Waldenström's, 131
  C7 deficiency and, 135
  plasmapheresis in, 291
RBC (see Red blood cell)
Reagents
  quality control and, 447–448
  RBCs, and quality control, 449
Recognition unit: and C1, 117
Record-keeping: quality control of, 451–452
Rectum: carcinoma,
  carcinoembryonic antigen in, 154
Red blood cell(s), 6–17
  acid phosphatase in paternity testing, 412
  alloimmunization causing hemolysis, 304
  in anemia (see Anemia, red blood cell)
  antibodies, 214–215
    complement binding by, 123
  antigens
    in criminology, 417–418
    in paternity testing, 410–411
  aplasia, pure, 9
  Bombay group, 145
  conjugation with haptenic drug, 313–315
  count, normal
    in females, 5
    in males, 5
  damage mechanisms in transfusions, 326–327
  deficiency causing hemolysis, 333
  development, 8
  enzyme phenotypes (see Paternity testing, red blood cell

enzyme phenotypes)
  enzymes in criminology, 418
  fragility, increase, 14
  frozen, deglycerolized, 244–245
  hemolysis due to physical agents, 333
  leukocyte-poor, 241–243
  membrane
    components, 14
    damage, and blood storage, 241
    lipid bilayer of, 145
    metabolism defects, 15–16
  morphology, 6–8
  packed, 241
    disadvantage of, 241
  panels, 205–206
    approach to reading, 205–206
    with combination of two antibodies, 210
    typical, 206
  pathology, 8–17
  physiology, 6–8
  prephenotype, 202
  reagents, and quality control, 449
  salvage, intraoperative, 296–297
    automated, 297
    contraindications, 297
    filtration method, 296–297
  sensitization by pharmacologic agents, 204
  shock to, osmotic, 333
  survival studies in autoimmune hemolytic anemia, 307–308
  transfusion (see Transfusion, red blood cell)
Reed-Sternberg cells, 44, 45
Refrigerators: for blood banking, quality control, 446
Renal (see Kidney)
Rendu-Osler-Weber syndrome, 72
Reptilase: in DIC, 90
Res ipsa liquitur, 452
Respiratory
  burst, 19
  disease, and blood donation, 238
  infection, bacterial, 158
  viral syndromes, 158
Respondeat superior, 452
Results: validity of, equations to analyze, 404–405
Resuscitation: cardiopulmonary, in blood donor reactions, 239
Reticulocyte
  count
    in newborn, 6
    normal, 8
    vitamin B12 deficiency and, 10

in hemolysis, 314
Reticulum: sarcoplasmic, 74
Retrovirus
  cytopathic effects, 381–382
  genome, diagram, 381
  mutagenic effects, 381–382
Rh antibodies: in pregnancy, 172–173
Rh antigen(s)
  altered expression of, 168–170
  -antibody testing, laboratory aspects of, 171–172
  chemistry of, 165–167
  D^u, 168–169
  immune response and, 172
  immunogenicity of, 172
Rh antigenic specificities: resulting from probable antigen proximity, 170–171
Rh antisera: and quality control, 448
Rh genes
  amorphic, 168–170
  combinations of, and frequency of combinations, 166
  deletion, 168–170
  inheritance, 165
    suggested mechanism, 167
  null, homozygous, 168
  Rosenfield model for, 165
  suppression, 168–170
Rh immunization
  clinical aspects of, 422–423
  clinical significance of, 172
  fetomaternal bleeding and, 173
  plasmapheresis in, 174
  prevention of, 173–174
  prophylaxis of, 428
  of Rh-negative mothers, 174
Rh molecule: model of, 164
Rh-negative mothers, 111
  Rh immunization of, 174
Rh null phenotype, 168
Rh system, 163–168
  discovery of, 3
  genetics of, 167–168
  nomenclature for, 164–167
    Fisher-Race, 164
    frequently used, 166
    Rosenfield, 165
    Wiener, 164
  in paternity testing, 411
  specificities of, 170–171
$Rh_o(D)$ deletion, 169
$Rh_o(D)$ molecule: inheritance of mosaic structure of, 170
Rhesus monkey cells, 3
Rheumatoid arthritis
  blood donation in, 238
  hypocomplementemia in, 122
  plasma exchange in, partial, 291

Rheumatoid arthritis (cont.)
  thrombocytosis in, 79
RhIG failures, 174
RhIG prophylaxis: antipartum, 429
Ristocetin
  aggregation test, 76
  cofactor, 81
  factor VIII, 81
  -induced aggregation, 86
  in platelet aggregation, 74, 76
RNA
  synthesis, methotrexate
    inhibiting, 40
  transcript, and B cells, 50
  tumor viruses, replication of,
    381
  virus
    in preleukemia, 29
    type C, 47
Rogers antigen, 122
Rosenfield nomenclature: for Rh
  system, 165
Rouleaux formation, 153, 213
  dextran to prevent, 261
  after gelatin, 262
  granulocytes and, 255
RPR testing: of donor samples,
  quality control, 451
Rubella
  ABO antigen weakening and,
    154
  thrombocytopenia and, 77

S

Saliva samples: in paternity testing,
  409
Sarcoid: lymphocytopenia in, 29
Sarcoma
  granulocytic, 36
  Kaposi's, 73
Scabies, 21
Schilling test, 10
Schistocytes, 89
Scleroderma: and
  thrombocytopenia, 89
Sclerosis: nodular and Hodgkin's
  disease, 45
Semustine, 34, 41
  effect on marrow, 42
Sepsis: bacterial, severe, 25
Septicemia: T activation in, 184
Serine esterase, 108
  factor XII and, 81
  heparin-antithrombin III and, 82
Serine protease activity: of factor
  Xa, 80
Serotonin, 22
  after aspirin, 76
  in platelet release, 75
    reaction, 75

type 1, 75
storage, 74
Serum sickness, 21
Sexual promiscuity: in large
  metropolitan area and
  AIDS, 378
Sézary's syndrome, 37, 42, 128
Shock
  DIC and, 89
  hypovolemic
    pathophysiology, 467–468
    therapeutic strategies in, 469
  osmotic, to red blood cells, 333
Shwartzman reaction, 88
  classic, 89
Sickle cell
  anemia (see Anemia, sickle cell)
  crisis, 12
  disease, erythrocytapheresis in,
    292
  hemoglobin disease, 12
  trait, 12
Sickle thalassemia, 12
Sid antigens, 182
Sideroblast(s), 30
Sideroblastic (see Anemia,
  sideroblastic)
Sigmoid curve: in interaction of
  antibodies in antigens, 110
Singer's bilayer model: of biologic
  membranes, 7
Snake bites
  DIC and, 89
  platelet destruction and, 78
Snake poisons, 88
Sodium fluoride, 36
Somatic mutation, 106–107
Somatic recombination, 107
Sorenson ATS system, 296
Specific gravity, 7
  normal
    for men, 7
    for women, 7
Spectrin, 14
  in elliptocytosis, 14
Spectrophotometry, amniotic fluid,
  424–425, 426
  in meconium strain, 427
Spherocytes, 14
Spherocytosis, hereditary, 14
  splenectomy in, 14
Spleen
  macrophages, trapping by,
    mechanism of, 308
  in myeloid metaplasia,
    agnogenic, 43
  platelets and, 73, 78
  trapping platelets, 74
Splenectomy
  in cation permeability disorders,
    14

in leukemia, hairy cell, 42
in purpura, idiopathic
  thrombocytopenic, 78
in spherocytosis, 14
in thrombocytopenia, 77
thrombocytosis after, 79
Splenomegaly
  in leukemia, chronic
    lymphocytic, 38
  lymphoma and, 306
  pancytopenia in, 28
  platelet survival in, 251
Splicing, 11
Staphylococcus
  aureus, 27
  in leukemia, acute
    myelogenous, 37
  clumping test, 90
Statute of limitations, 454
Stem cell(s), 8
  disorders, 25
    acquired committed, 26
    acquired, leading to
      neutropenia, 26
    leukemia and, 36
  eosinophils and, 20
  granulocytes from, 18
  megakaryocytes and, 73
  monoclonality in paroxysmal
    nocturnal hemoglobinuria,
    15
  neutropenia (see Neutropenia,
    stem cell)
  totipotent hematopoietic, 18
  transplant, 477
Steroids, 41
  androgenic, in agnogenic
    myeloid metaplasia, 43
  in anemia, hemolytic,
    autoimmune, warm-type,
    309
  basophilopenia and, 22
  eosinophils after, 20
  lymphocytopenia after, 29
  in neutropenia
    autoimmune, 26
    cyclic, 26
  neutrophils after, 28
  platelets and, 78
Stetson, 3
Stoichiometry, 109
Stomach
  (See also Gastrointestinal)
  carcinoma
    ABH antigens and, 154
    anemia, pernicious, 10
    HLA and, 228
  disease, and blood donation, 238
Stomatocytes, 14
Storage: frozen, processing units
  for, 244

Streptococcal infection: β-hemolytic, 73
Streptomycin, 88
Stress
  marrow, 157
  neutrophilia after, 28
Stuart-Prower factor: characteristics of, 79
Sudan black B, 36
Sugar sequence: of H, Le^a and Le^b, 155
Sulfhydryl groups: free, in platelet adhesion, 74
Sulfisoxazole, 25
Sulfonamides: and neutropenia, 25
Sulfonic acid esters: in chronic myelogenous leukemia, 33
Sun-exposed areas: hematomas of, 72
Swann antigen, 183
Sweats: night, in non-Hodgkin's lymphoma, 48
Syphilis
  blood donation and, 237
  after platelet transfusion, 253
  transfusion transmitting, 342–343

T

Taxes: and blood bank management, 454
T cells, 123, 125, 304–305
  in aged, 6
  in AIDS, 131
  carrier-specific response mediated by, 127
  in cellular immunity, 124
  clones, and HTLV proteins, 382
  deficit in Wiskott-Aldrich syndrome, 130
  disorders with neutropenia, 25–26
  function derangement in Hodgkin's disease, 44
  helper, 42, 127
  helper/inducer, 112
  idiotypes, 127
  immunogens in lymph node hyperplasia, 43
  in immunologic tolerance, 129
  -independent antigens, 126
  leukemia (see Leukemia, T cell)
  in leukemia, chronic lymphocytic, 38
  lymphocytes, 102
  in lymphoma, diffuse, 48
  macrophage presenting antigen to, model, 224
  markers, monoclonal antibodies against, 125
  migrating to thymus, 125
  ontogeny, 127
  phytohemagglutinin and, 125
  receptors in non-Hodgkin's lymphoma, 46
  response and delayed hypersensitivity, 132
  stimulation of, surface, 127
  subdivisions of, 112
  suppression and thrombocytopenia, 78
  suppressor, 40, 48
T cryptantigen, 160, 184
Testes: radiotherapy in leukemia, 40
Tetracycline: causing aplastic anemia, 9
Tetrasaccharides: Thomas-Winkler, 162
Thalassemia, 7, 13–14, 157
  anemia of, 14
  classification of syndromes, 13
  forms of, main, 13
  RBC morphology in, 14
  sickle, 12
α-Thalassemia, 14
β-Thalassemia, 13
  anemia and, aplastic, 9
  in blacks, 13
Thawed: frozen-thawed blood, 243–244
Thawing: blood, 244
Thiazide, 75
  thrombocytopenia due to, 77
Thioguanine: in chronic myelogenous leukemia, 33
Thomas-Winzler tetrasaccharides, 162
Thoracic duct drainage, 29
Thorotrast, 89
Thrombasthenia: Glanzmann's, 76
Thrombin, 72
  alpha$_2$-macroglobulin inhibitor and, 83
  -antithrombin III complexes, 72
  control mechanisms of coagulation and, 83
  extrinsic system and, 83
  factor VII activity and, 82
  factor VIII and, 81
  factor X activation and, 82
  in fibrinogen molecule, 78
  fibrinopeptide and, 87
  fibrinopeptide A and, 79
  inhibitor, 83
  in platelet aggregation, 74
  in platelet release reaction, 75
  prothrombin and, 80
  receptor, 73
  removal, 83
  -sensitive protein, 74
  time test, 90
Thrombocythemia: essential, 75
Thrombocytopenia, 77
  after cardiopulmonary bypass, 252, 473–474
  causes, two basic, 249
  congenital, 77
  dilutional, and fresh frozen plasma, 246
  in gammopathy, 131
  in hemoglobinuria, paroxysmal nocturnal, 15
  hereditary, 75
  immune
    drug-induced, 315
    -mediated, 78
  in leukemia
    acute myelogenous, 36
    chronic lymphocytic, 38
  after marrow transplant, 227
  in myeloid metaplasia, agnogenic, 43
  in newborn, 436
  platelet(s) in, 249, 252
  platelet destruction increase causing, 78
  platelet production lack causing, 77
  after surgery, 252–253
Thrombocytosis, 78
  causes, major, 79
  drugs causing, 79
  plateletpheresis in, 292
Thromboembolism
  in factor VII deficiency, 86
  in liver disease, 87
β-Thromboglobulin: in platelets, 74
Thrombophlebitis: and transfusion, 345
Thromboplastin, 81
  characteristics of, 79
  plasma thromboplastin antecedent, characteristics of, 79
  time, activated partial, 84
Thrombopoietic substance, 78
Thrombopoietin, 73, 78
Thrombosis, 71–101
  endotoxemia and, 89
  microthrombosis, fibrin, 89
  pulmonary, and sickle cell anemia, 12
Thromboxane
  A$_2$, 72
  in platelet aggregation, 75
  synthesis, 76
Thrombus: phospholipids for, 73
Thymidine kinase, 10
Thymoma, 9
Thymopoietin, 127

Thymus
  eosinophils and, 20
  hypoplasia, 129
  in origin of diffuse lymphoma, 48
  T cells migrating to, 125
Thyroguanine: in leukemia, acute myelogenous, 36
Thyrotoxicosis: and lymphocytosis, 29
Tissue factor, 81
Tn-polyagglutinability, 36
Tonegawa, 3
Tort, 452
Toxic substances
  in blood causing reactions, 339
  transfused during massive transfusion, 468–469
Toxicity
  of benzene, 8
  of chloramphenicol, 8
  citrate, 339
Toxoplasma gondii, 29
Toxoplasmosis: transfusion transmitting, 344
TPA test: forbol ester, 39
Transferrin, 9
Transfusion(s), 459–482
  ammonium load and, 340
  in anemia
    aplastic, 9
    hemolytic, autoimmune, 309–310, 476–477
    sickle cell, 12
    with antibodies to high-incidence antigens, 182
  autologous, 238, 294–297
    methods for, current, 295–296
    predeposit, 295
    predeposit, clinical uses, 296
    predeposit, frozen storage, 295–296
    predeposit, liquid storage, 295
  cell survival in patients without detectable antibodies, 332
  Chagas' disease after, 344
  in children, special aspects of, 434
  circulatory overload, 339
  of cold blood, 338–339
  committee, 459–460
  deglycerolized RBC, 245
  embolism after, air, 340
  emergency, 466–467
    infusion site, 467
    type of fluid replacement, 467
    volume restoration, 467
  exchange, in newborn, 431
    complications of, 433
    diseases not associated with hemolytic disease of newborn, 435
    pre-exchange plan, 431–433
    set for, components of, 432
  exchange, in sickle cell anemia, 12
  fatalities, reportable cases in U.S., 345
  filariasis transmitted by, 344
  filters for, 463
  first, 1
  graft-vs.-host disease complicating, 335
  granulocyte
    autologous, 34
    complications, 256
    criteria for, 255–256
    in granulomatous disease of children, chronic, 25
    HLA matching for, 228
    indications, 255–256
    in leukopenia, 476
    in neutropenia, 27
    practices, 464
  hemochromatosis and, 345
  in hemoglobinuria, paroxysmal nocturnal, 15
  in hemolysis, cold autoimmune, 477
  hepatitis after, 130
    strategy for donor recall, 370
  human-to-human, first, 1
  hyperkalemia after, 340
  immunization by, antibodies after, 38
  incompatible, 153
  indications for, 461–462
  infection transmitted by, 341–344
    bacterial, 341–342
    viral, 341
  intrauterine, in hemolytic disease of newborn, 425–428
  IV fluids, incompatible, 344–345
  kala-azar transmitted by, 344
  before kidney transplant, 226
  malaria after, treatment, 343
  massive, 467–469
    bleeding diathesis after, 468
    factor VIII and, 246
    hemorrhage after, 91
    injurious substances transfused during, 468–469
    toxic substances transfused during, 468–469
  multiple, phenotyping, 210
  in newborn, 435–436
    complications, 435–436
  in open heart surgery replacement therapy, practices, 471–474
  parasitic diseases transmitted by, 343
    nonmalarial, 344
  plasma, practices, 464
  platelet, 76, 249
    anaphylaxis after, 253
    in cancer, 475
    clinical response to, 227–228
    complications from, 253, 475–476
    HLA compatibility in, 251
    HLA typing in, 227
    platelet count before, 250
    practices in, 463–464
    reactions to, 335
    syphilis after, 253
  practices, 459–482
    special problems in, 466–469
  rate, 462–463
  reaction(s), 1, 325–354
    ABO hemolytic, 122
    ABO-incompatible, 88
    to allotype antibodies, 105
    delayed, 330–331
    delayed, anti-P1 antibodies in, 159
    delayed, MNSs system in, 162
    febrile, 243, 245
    febrile, management, 334–335
    hemolytic (*see below*)
    leading to intravascular hemolysis, 326
    nonhemolytic, immune mediated, 333–335
    nonhemolytic, non-immune-mediated, 338–341
    protein sensitivity causing, 335–338
    pyrogens causing, 343
    to toxic substances in blood and blood component units, 339
  reactions, hemolytic, 25, 153, 325–333
    causes, 332
    extravascular hemolysis causing, management, 332
    immune, intravascular, prevention, 328–329
    immune, intravascular, treatment, 328–329
    immune, management, algorithm for, 331
    immune mediated, 325–330
    immune mediated, epidemiology, 325–326

immune mediated,
  pathophysiology, 326
immune, prognosis, 330
laboratory findings in, 328
non-ABO, 330
recipients, Bombay-type, 147
red blood cell
  in cancer, 475
  deglycerolized, 245
regulatory bodies
  external, 459
  internal, 459–460
syphilis transmitted by, 342–343
thrombophlebitis and, 345
toxoplasmosis after, 344
trypanosomiasis transmitted by, African, 344
unit for, hanging, 462
Translocation: of V-D-J complex, 125
Transplantation
  ABH antigens and, 154
  kidney
    anti-Lewis antibodies in, 156
    characteristics of, 227
    HLA and, 225–226
    HLA and, follow-up, 226
    HLA and, pretransplantation workup, 225–226
    HLA and, survival for 1 year, 225
    HLA and, transfusion before, 226
    rejection, MNSs system in, 162
  marrow, 154, 264–266
    in anemia, aplastic, 9, 265
    blood bank support for, 265–266
    blood components after, 477
    characteristics of, 227
    definition, 264
    graft-vs.-host disease after, 134, 226
    in granulomatous disease of children, chronic, 25
    HLA matching in, 226–227
    in immunodeficiency, 130
    indications, 265
    in leukemia, acute, 265
    in leukemia, acute lymphocytic, 40
    in leukemia, acute myelogenous, 37
    in leukemia, complications, 265
    in leukemia, with prior treatment, 264
    in neutropenia, committed stem cell, 26

  in preleukemia, 30
  scientific rationale, 264
  rejection and platelet destruction, 78
  stem cell, 477
Trendelenburg position: for blood donor reactions, 239
Trichinosis, 21
Trisomy: of chromosome 12 in chronic lymphocytic leukemia, 37
Trypanosomiasis: African, transfusion transmitting, 344
Trypsin, 160
  in Clq receptor, 120
  factor XI and, 81
  factor XII and, 81
Tuberculosis
  miliary, 77
  anemia in, aplastic, 9
  neutrophilia and, 28
Tumor(s)
  cell kinetics, 40–41
  clonality of, 16
  -derived eosinophilopoietic factor, 21
  growth as gompertzian, 41
  of hematopoietic cells, 29–43
  RNA, viruses, replication, 381
Twitching: after blood donation, 239
Typhus: and blood donation, 237

U

Ulcer
  leg, and sickle cell anemia, 12
  peptic, and ABH antigens, 154
Ulcerative colitis, 21
Ultrastructure: changes in lymphocytes in AIDS, 385
Uremia: platelet defects in, 75, 77
Uremic hemolytic syndrome: T activation in, 184
Uroporphyrins, 10
Urothelium: synthesizing complement, 116
Urticaria pigmentosa: and malignant mastocytosis, 43

V

Vaccination
  blood donation and, 237
  discussion of term, 2
Vaccine: hepatitis B, and AIDS, 390–391
Validity: of results, equations to analyze, 404–405

van der Waals forces, 111
Vancomycin: in acute myelogenous leukemia, 37
Vasoactive reactions: to albumin, 260
Vasopressin
  DDAVP in von Willebrand's disease, 86
  deamino-8-D-arginine, 77
  in platelet aggregation, 74
V-D-J complex: translocation of, 125
VDRL testing: of donor samples, quality control in, 451
Vel antigen system, 181
Velban: effect on marrow, 42
Venipuncture, 462
  for blood donation, 238–240
Venoms: viper, and fibrinopeptide A, 80
Vessels
  endothelium, 75
  walls, structural integrity of, 71–73
Vinblastin-loaded platelets, 78
Vinblastine: in chronic myelogenous leukemia, 33
Vinca alkaloids: effect on marrow, 42
Vincristine
  effect on marrow, 42
  in Hodgkin's disease, 45
  in leukemia, acute lymphocytic, 40
Viper venoms: and fibrinopeptide A, 80
Virus(es)
  Aleutian disease, 50
  cytomegalovirus infection, 237
  Epstein-Barr (see Epstein-Barr virus)
  Gross, 230
  hepatitis (see under Hepatitis)
  HTLV (see HTLV virus)
  infection
    in thymic hypoplasia, 129
    transmitted by transfusion, 341
  leukemia, Rauscher murine, 44
  in lymphoma etiology, non-Hodgkin's, 47
  retrovirus (see Retrovirus)
  RNA (see RNA virus)
Vitamin
  B12
    daily requirements, 10
    deficiency, 10
    deficiency, megaloblastic anemia in, 10
    in leukemia, acute myelogenous, 35

Vitamin *(cont.)*
  megaloblastic anemia unresponsive to, 10–11
  C deficiency, 72
  deficiencies and pancytopenia, 28
  K
    deficiency, coagulopathy of, 87
    -dependent factors, 80
    prothrombin complex, 87
von Willebrand factor, 81
  characteristics of, 79
von Willebrand's disease, 75, 76, 84, 85–86
  classification, 86
  cryoprecipitate in, 247
  diagnosis, differential, 85
  inheritance of, 86
  therapy, 86
  type I, 76
  type II, 76

W

Waldenström's *(see* Macroglobulinemia, Waldenström's)
Warm-reacting antibodies, 163–181
WBC *(see* White blood cells)
Weight loss
  in Hodgkin's disease, 45
  in lymphoma, non-Hodgkin's, 48
Western blot test: diagram of, 389
Whipple's disease, 29
White blood cells, 17–43
  count
    corticosteroids and, 255
    etiocholanolone and, 255
    in DIC, 89
    from donors with myelogenous leukemia, 255
    immature forms, 17–18
  leukocyte donor of granulocytes, 254–255
  leukocyte-poor red blood cells, 241–243
  microaggregates of, 340–341
  morphology, 17–23
  in newborn, 6
  pathology, 17–43
  physiology, 17–23
  reactions against, 333–334
Whole blood *(see* Blood, whole)
Wiener, Alexander, 3
Wiener nomenclature: for Rh system, 164
Wiskott-Aldrich syndrome, 77, 130
Witebsky substances, 150, 152
Wren, Sir Christopher, 1

X

X chromosome *(see* Chromosome, X)
Xg system, 181
X-linked agammaglobulinemia: Bruton type, in infant, 130
X-linked hypogammaglobulinemia: and Clq deficiency and, 134
X-ray *(see* Radiography, Radiotherapy)

Y

Y chromosome, 35

Z

Zeta potential
  albumin and, 205
  of RBCs, 111
  on surface of cells, 202
Zwitterions, 412